D1626177

A Textbook of Epilepsy

For Churchill Livingstone:
Publisher: Michael Parkinson
Project Editor: Dilys Jones
Copy Editor: Leslie Smillie
Production Controller: Lesley W Small
Sales Promotion Executive: Marion Pollock

A Textbook of Epilepsy

Edited by

John Laidlaw FRCP (Edin)
Formerly Consultant Physician to the Epilepsy Centre,
Quarrier's Homes, Bridge of Weir, Scotland; Formerly
Physician-in-charge of the Chalfont Centre for Epilepsy,
Chalfont St Peter, Buckinghamshire, and Honorary
Consultant to the National Hospitals, London, UK

Alan Richens PhD FRCP
Professor of Pharmacology and Therapeutics,
University of Wales College of Medicine, Heath Park,
Cardiff, UK

David Chadwick DM FRCP
Consultant Neurologist, The Walton Centre for Neurology
and Neurosurgery, Liverpool, UK

FOURTH EDITION

CHURCHILL LIVINGSTONE
EDINBURGH LONDON MADRID MELBOURNE NEW YORK AND TOKYO 1993

CHURCHILL LIVINGSTONE
Medical Division of Longman Group UK Limited

Distributed in the United States of America by Churchill
Livingstone Inc., 650 Avenue of the Americas, New York,
N.Y. 10011, and by associated companies, branches and
representatives throughout the world.

First edition 1976
Second edition 1982
Third edition 1988
Fourth edition 1993
  Reprinted 1993

ISBN 0-443-04473-2

British Library of Cataloguing in Publication Data
A catalogue record for this book is available from the British
Library.

Library of Congress Cataloging in Publication Data
A Textbook of epilepsy / edited by John Laidlaw, Alan
Richens, David Chadwick. — 4th ed.
    p.   cm.
  Includes bibliographical references and index.
  1. Epilepsy.   I. Laidlaw, John.   II. Richens, Alan.
III. Chadwick, David.
  [DNLM: 1. Epilepsy.   WL 385 T355]
RC372.T48   1993
616.8'53—dc20
DNLM/DLC
for Library of Congress   92-12309

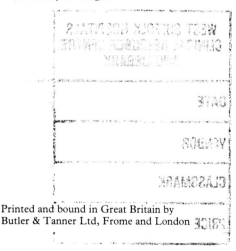

Printed and bound in Great Britain by
Butler & Tanner Ltd, Frome and London

The
publisher's
policy is to use
**paper manufactured
from sustainable forests**

Preface

In this fourth edition the two original editors, John Laidlaw and Alan Richens, have been joined by a new editor, David Chadwick. He replaces Jolyon Oxley, who has moved from a primary clinical role in the field of epilepsy to a key position in postgraduate medical education. Dr Oxley continues as an author of the chapter on social aspects of epilepsy, reflecting his continuing interest and commitment in this area.

Several important new chapters have been commissioned for this edition: status epilepticus (Treiman), neuropharmacology (Richens and Davies), assessment of new drugs (Gram, Schwabe and Jensen), the legal aspects of epilepsy (Treiman), clinical audit (Morrow and Baker) and, finally, coping with epilepsy (Scambler). We believe that these additions make the new edition a more comprehensive account of epilepsy and its management, as well as providing glimpses of new things to come.

New authors have joined us for some of the chapters: Annegers and Hauser have compiled the chapter on genetics, as has Chadwick on seizures in adults, Jeffreys on pathophysiology, Shorvon on epilepsy in developing countries, Schmidt on epilepsy in women, and Duncan on medical services. Also Perucca has joined Richens as a co-author on clinical pharmacology and medical treatment, and Thompson has collaborated with Oxley on the social aspects of epilepsy. These changes have allowed major revisions of many chapters so that the Textbook remains an up-to-date reference source about all aspects of epilepsy.

The first edition was produced in 1976. It is exciting to see so many areas of new knowledge and understanding about epilepsy in this fourth edition compared with the first. This has happened both on the medico-scientific and the socio-medical fronts, and augurs well for the person with epilepsy.

As always, we thank all those people, un-named in the credits, without whom this book would never have been produced.

1992

J.L.
A.R.
D.C.

Contributors

V. Elving Anderson PhD
Professor Emeritus of Genetics, University of
Minnesota, Minneapolis, Minnesota, USA

John F. Annegers PhD
Professor of Epidemiology, Division of
Epidemiology, University of Texas, School of
Public Health, Houston, USA

Gus A. Baker BA MClinPsychol CPsychol AFBPsS
Principal Clinical Neuropsychologist; Senior
Clinical Research Associate, Department of
Neurosciences, University of Liverpool, Walton
Hospital, Liverpool, UK

Tim Betts MB ChB DPM FRCPsych
Senior Lecturer in Psychiatry, University of
Birmingham, Queen Elizabeth Psychiatric
Hospital, Birmingham, UK

Nadir E. Bharucha MD MRCP (UK) FRCP(C)
MNAMS
Assistant Professor, Department of Neurology,
Seth G. S. Medical College and K. E. M.
Hospital; Honorary Consultant Neurologist,
Bombay Hospital and Medical Research Centre;
Chief, Department of Neuroepidemiology,
Medical Research Centre and Bombay Hospital,
Bombay, India

Colin D. Binnie MD MA
Consultant Clinical Neurophysiologist and
Clinical Director of Neurosciences, The
Bethlem Royal and Maudsley Hospitals, London,
UK

David Chadwick DM FRCP
Consultant Neurologist, The Walton Centre for
Neurology and Neurosurgery, Liverpool, UK

John A. Corbett FRCP FRCPsych DPM(Acad) DCH
AKC
Professor of Developmental Psychiatry,
University of Birmingham, Queen Elizabeth
Psychiatric Hospital, Birmingham, UK

John A. Davies PhD CBiol MIBiol
Senior Lecturer, Department of Pharmacology
and Therapeutics, University of Wales College of
Medicine, Cardiff, UK

Carl B. Dodrill PhD
Professor, Departments of Neurological Surgery,
and Psychiatry and Behavioral Sciences,
University of Washington School of Medicine,
Seattle, Washington, USA

John S. Duncan MA DM MRCP
Senior Lecturer in Neurology, Institute of
Neurology; Consultant Neurologist, Chalfont
Centre for Epilepsy and National Hospitals for
Neurology and Neurosurgery, London, UK

Lennart Gram MD DrMedSci
Associate Professor, University Clinic of
Neurology, Hvidovre Hospital, Hvidovre,
Denmark

Yvonne M. Hart MB MRCP
Senior Registrar in Neurology, Atkinson
Morley's Hospital, London, UK

W. Allen Hauser MD
Professor of Neurology and Public Health,
Columbia University, New York, USA; Visiting
Professor, Section of Epidemiology and Medical
Information, Institute of Advanced Biomedical
Technology, National Research Council, Milan,
Italy

John G. R. Jefferys BSc PhD
Wellcome Senior Lecturer, Department of
Physiology and Biophysics, St Mary's Hospital
Medical School, Imperial College, London
University, London, UK

Peder Klosterskov Jensen MD
Director of CNS/Allergy and Asthma Research,
Schering-Plough Corporation Clinical Research,
New Jersey, USA

Brian Kendall FRCP FRCS FRCR FFRRCSI(Hon)
Radiologist, National Hospital for Neurology and
Neurosurgery, London; Neuroradiologist,
Hospital for Sick Children, London, UK

John Laidlaw FRCP(Edin)
Formerly Consultant Physician to the Epilepsy
Centre, Quarrier's Homes, Bridge of Weir,
Scotland; Formerly Physician in charge of the
Chalfont Centre for Epilepsy, Chalfont St Peter,
Buckinghamshire, and Honorary Consultant to
the National Hospitals, London, UK

Mary V. Laidlaw SRN
Formerly Rehabilitation Adviser to the Epilepsy
Centre, Quarriers Homes, Bridge of Weir,
Scotland, and to the Chalfont Centre for Epilepsy,
Chalfont St Peter, Buckinghamshire, UK

Gordon Mathieson MSc FRCP(C)
Professor and Chairman, Discipline of
Pathology, Memorial University of
Newfoundland, St John's, Newfoundland,
Canada

James I. Morrow MB MRCP
Consultant Neurologist, Royal Victoria Hospital,
Belfast, N. Ireland, UK

Jolyon Oxley MA MB BChir FRCP
Secretary, Standing Committee on Postgraduate
Medical Education, London; Chairman,
Employment Commission of the International
Bureau for Epilepsy; Honorary Physician,
National Society for Epilepsy, London, UK

E. Perucca MD PhD
Associate Professor of Clinical Pharmacology,
University of Pavia, Clinical Pharmacology Unit,
Pavia, Italy

C. E. Polkey MD FRCS
Consultant Neurosurgeon, The Bethlem Royal
and Maudsley Hospitals, London, UK

Roger J. Porter MD
Deputy Director, National Institute of
Neurological Disorders and Stroke, National
Institutes of Health, Bethesda, Maryland, USA

Alan Richens PhD FRCP
Professor of Pharmacology and Therapeutics,
University of Wales College of Medicine,
Cardiff, UK

Graham Scambler BSc PhD
Senior Lecturer in Sociology, Academic
Department of Psychiatry, UCL, University of
London, London, UK

Dieter Schmidt MD
Professor and Chairman of the Department of
Neurology, Free University of Berlin, Berlin,
Germany

Stefan Schwabe BS MD
Head of Epilepsy and Research, Ciba-Geigy,
Basel, Switzerland

S. D. Shorvon MA MD FRCP
Senior Lecturer in Neurology, Institute of
Neurology, London; Consultant Neurologist,
National Hospital for Neurology and
Neurosurgery, London; Medical Director,
Chalfont Centre for Epilepsy, UK

Pamela Thompson PhD AFBPsS DipPsych
Head of Psychological Services, Chalfont Centre
for Epilepsy, UK

David M. Treiman MD
Professor of Neurology, UCLA School of
Medicine, Los Angeles, California; Co-Director,
DVA Southwest Regional Epilepsy Center, DVA
Medical Center, West Los Angeles, California,
USA

Sheila J. Wallace MB FRCPE
Consultant Paediatric Neurologist, University
Hospital of Wales, Cardiff, UK

Contents

1. Classification of epileptic seizures and epileptic syndromes

R. J. Porter

INTRODUCTION

The epilepsies are one of the most common of the neurological disorders; only stroke has a higher incidence. If one estimates that 1% of the world's population has epilepsy, then about 50 million persons worldwide suffer from the disorder. Data from the US Presidential Commission (1978) suggest that about 10% of patients have seizures more than once per month; worldwide, therefore, approximately 5 million persons are severely disabled by their epileptic seizures.

Efforts to generate empirical classifications of any disorder are, by their very nature, surrounded by controversy. Each expert views the clinical world in a slightly different way, sees patients who differ slightly from those studied by other experts, and formulates unique understandings of the disorder to be classified. The efforts to classify epileptic seizures and epileptic syndromes afford excellent examples of this problem; each epileptologist's synthesis of the disorder varies from that of his or her colleagues. When an epileptologist is confronted with a construct (classification) created by someone else, this synthesis is challenged and resistance to the classification often occurs. The various classifications of epileptic seizures and epileptic syndromes, however—even if less than fully accepted— provide a framework within which we improve our understanding of what we see and what others see as well as providing a vocabulary for our interactions. This chapter will consider the definitions of seizures and epilepsy; the seizure classification is based on the 1981 Classification of Epileptic Seizures (Appendix A), and the epilepsy classification is based on the 1989 Classification of Epileptic Syndromes (Appendix B). Each

of these has been approved by the International League Against Epilepsy. I have borrowed liberally from these documents and from the data and analyses the Porter (1989) for the construction of this chapter.

SEIZURES, EPILEPSY AND DIAGNOSIS

Definitions

A seizure is a finite event; it has a beginning and an end. It can be defined, as did Hughlings Jackson in 1870, as a 'symptom . . . an occasional, an excessive and a disorderly discharge of nerve tissue.' (Taylor 1931). Epilepsy, on the other hand, is 'a chronic disorder characterized by recurrent seizures . . .' (Gastaut 1973). As epilepsy is a symptom complex and not a disease per se, a discussion of epilepsy requires reference to one of three levels: 1. the aetiology, 2. the seizure type, or 3. the epilepsy syndrome. Appropriate diagnosis follows naturally from appropriate classification (Porter 1990a).

The value of each of these diagnostic levels will be delineated. The *aetiological diagnosis* is fundamentally useful in guiding standard neurological evaluation and intervention, e.g. antibiotics for meningitis or surgery for tumours. The *seizure diagnosis* is most useful in determining the appropriate antiepileptic drug therapy; it also is critical for surgical evaluation. The *epilepsy syndrome diagnosis* is most helpful for determining prognosis and duration of therapy.

Aetiology

It is beyond the scope of this chapter to consider the various aetiologies that may be responsible

Table 1.1 Important causes of seizures in children and adults in order of probable incidence

Infants and children	Adults
No definite cause determined	No definite cause determined
Birth and neonatal injuries	
Vascular insults (other than above)	Vascular lesions
Congenital or metabolic disorders	Head trauma
	Drug or alcohol abuse
Head injuries	Neoplasia
Infection	Infection
Neoplasia	Heredity
Heredity	

(From Porter 1989)

for epilepsy. It is noteworthy, however, that epilepsy can be caused by virtually any major category of serious disease or disorder of humans. It can result from congenital malformations, infections, tumours, vascular diseases, degenerative diseases, or injury. In more than three-quarters of patients with epilepsy, the seizures begin before the age of 18 years (Commission 1978). The reason for this age of onset is not clear, but the increased vulnerability of the young nervous system to seizure development is known clinically and documented experimentally. Any categorization of the causes of epilepsy should, therefore, attempt to distinguish between the causes in children and the causes in adults. Table 1.1 lists, in descending order of probable incidence, the main causes of seizures in children and adults (Porter 1989).

Neurological history and intensive monitoring

Most seizures can be classified by taking an appropriate neurological history from the patient. Only rarely is special monitoring necessary to establish the correct diagnosis. These topics are dealt with in Chapters 5 and 9 and will not be considered further here.

CLASSIFICATION OF SEIZURES—THE FUNDAMENTALS

Introduction

Of the classifications of epileptic seizures, the 1981 Classification of Epileptic Seizures is the most pragmatic for clinical use; it is reproduced

as Appendix A to this chapter. This classification is extraordinarily empirical, ignoring such factors as anatomical substrate, aetiology, and age of onset, in favour of the videotaped clinical event and its accompanying electroencephalogram. There are at least two reasons why such a classification is logical. First, the eliminated factors of anatomical substrate, aetiology, and age of onset are actually the criteria on which a classification of epileptic syndromes must be based (see below). Second, the availability of videotaped seizures, with their accompanying EEGs, has allowed experts to construct a data-oriented classification for most groups of seizures. Although the seizure is admittedly viewed in isolation, it is, apart from the patient's age, the only useful information available on many patients.

Pragmatic application is a function of any classification. The classification of Epileptic seizures assists the physician in determining the seizure diagnosis and may also assist in establishing the aetiological diagnosis in those cases in which aetiology can be ascertained. Such determinations will assist directly in planning appropriate therapy for both the patient's seizures and their underlying cause (Porter 1989).

Epileptic seizures are fundamentally divided into two groups—partial and generalized, as can be noted in the abbreviated form of the classification in Table 1.2. Partial seizures have clinical or electroencephalographic evidence of a localized onset; the word 'partial' is deliberately chosen to avoid the implication that a highly discrete focus exists, as such is often not the case. Arguments against the use of the term 'partial' relate to semantics of the English language rather than to the concept proposed.

Generalized seizures have no evidence of a localized onset. Generalized seizures are, as a group, much more heterogeneous than partial seizures. Our inability to localize the onset of generalized attacks, however, may reflect either a multifocal onset or our current technical incapability of determining the single locus of onset.

Important factors in seizure classification

Consciousness and responsiveness

Among the more controversial aspects of classi-

Table 1.2 1981 International classification of epileptic seizures

---

I. PARTIAL SEIZURES (seizures beginning locally)
    A. Simple partial seizures
       (consciousness not impaired)
       1. With motor symptoms
       2. With somatosensory or special sensory symptoms
       3. With autonomic symptoms
       4. With psychic symptoms
    B. Complex partial seizures (with impairment of consciousness)
       1. Beginning as simple partial seizures and progressing to impairment of consciousness
          a. With no other features
          b. With features as in A.1–4
          c. With automatisms
       2. With impairment of consciousness at onset
          a. With no other features
          b. With features as in A.1–4
          c. With automatisms
    C. Partial seizures secondarily generalized

II. GENERALIZED SEIZURES (bilaterally symmetrical and without local onset)
    A. 1. Absence seizures
       2. Atypical absence seizures
    B. Myoclonic seizures
    C. Clonic seizures
    D. Tonic seizures
    E. Tonic-clonic seizures
    F. Atonic seizures

III. UNCLASSIFIED EPILEPTIC SEIZURES (inadequate or incomplete data)

Abstracted from: Commission on Classification and Terminology of the International League Against Epilepsy. This classification was approved by the International League Against Epilepsy in September 1981.

fying epileptic seizures, especially partial seizures, is the role of alteration in consciousness. Consciousness has been defined as 'the state of awareness of the self and the environment' (Plum & Posner, 1980), an empirical definition subject to much philosophical interpretation. Penfield & Jasper (1954) noted, when confronted with the issue of consciousness in patients with epilepsy: 'Thus, the clinician is brought to a consideration of the consciousness and unconsciousness, in spite of himself and however insecure he may feel, when forced to pass over so much deep water on the thin ice of his own psychological insight.' Clearly the issue of consciousness is unavoidable. We can, for example, establish that consciousness is present by communicating with a conscious subject (Gloor 1986), and fragments of behaviours requiring intact consciousness are common

in epilepsy; careful analysis of these behavioural patterns may be of value in understanding the patient (Porter 1990b), even if we lack a satisfactory overall understanding of consciousness.

Although consciousness is exceedingly difficult to define, a working definition has evolved in which *responsiveness* is the critical factor. If the patients have some decrement in their ability to respond to exogenous stimuli, then responsiveness is considered to be altered. Obviously, the degree of difficulty of the task presented will affect the application of this definition to individual patients. Exceptional patients with discrete lesions may be unresponsive but aware (e.g. those with aphasia); in such patients, whose recall of ictal events is normal, consciousness is considered to be intact. Although responsiveness clearly represents a limited view of consciousness, this definition has the special advantage of being testable (Porter 1989).

Data from a wide variety of clinical events, ranging from metabolic diseases to vascular insults and head trauma allow generalizations about the anatomy of consciousness (Porter, 1990b). In general, consciousness is preserved as long as the brainstem and at least one cerebral hemisphere are functional. Widespread bilateral cerebral dysfunction or failure of the brainstem (at the pons or above) causes a decrement in consciousness that is, to a large degree, proportionate to the size and extent of the insult (Plum & Posner 1980).

There is some dissent, however, regarding the proposed necessity of bilateral hemispheric involvement for alteration of consciousness. Gloor et al (1980) evaluated 69 complex partial seizures and found 'no evidence for bilateral spread' of the discharge in 19 using depth EEG recordings, and concluded that bilateral spread was not required for altered consciousness. This sophisticated study attempted to prove the nonexistence of an electrical discharge in part of the brain by inference from depth electrode recordings. The degree of uncertainty associated with such inferences is unknown, but may be considerable— especially in view of the limitations of depth electrodes in detecting distant generators (Gloor 1984).

Most agree, however, that partial loss of consciousness can occur and that epilepsy is an especially good model for documenting such in-complete alterations. A particularly good example is given by Gloor (1986), who noted that amnesia for an event, such as might occur in a perfectly conscious patient with Korsakoff's syndrome, may have direct implications for patients with epilepsy. Testing for amnesia in a patient who has had an epileptic seizure is common; should amnesia be present, the physician may erroneously conclude that loss of consciousness occurred during the seizure. The elements of consciousness can, at least on theoretical grounds, be dissected into memory, speech, motor impairment, and alert-ness or attention. Unfortunately, it is rarely pos-sible to test all of these functions during or immediately after an epileptic seizure; an evalua-tion of consciousness, therefore, especially in a complex partial seizure, is usually incomplete (Porter 1990b).

Evaluation of consciousness is not only compli-cated by the fragmentary nature of its loss, as noted above, but also by the change in the altera-tion of consciousness over time. During an absence seizure, for example, the patient will, from moment to moment, vary greatly in ability to respond to exogenous stimuli (Browne et al 1974).

Clearly, therefore, responsiveness represents a limited view of consciousness. This working defi-nition, however, has great clinical utility, as the ability of the patient to respond during the seizure can usually be measured. The ability to respond during a seizure is not only some indication of the extent of seizure spread but is also, obviously, a functional test of the patient during an attack.

Seizure progression

Although the concept of seizure progression has long been recognized, the 1981 classification embodied the concept for partial seizures in a way which allows easy classification of this group. If one accepts the tenets that simple partial seizures are associated with preserved responsiveness and that complex partial seizures are associated with altered responsiveness, the concept of seizure progression in partial seizures is quickly limited to three fundamental possibilities: 1. a simple par-tial seizure may occur in isolation, 2. a complex partial seizure may be characterized by alteration of consciousness at onset, and 3. a complex partial seizure may be preceded by a simple partial sei-zure (often then called an 'aura'). An example of the third possibility would be a foul odour which leads directly to altered responsiveness and fumbling of the hands (an automatism) followed by a gradual return to normal consciousness. The foul odour may occur without progression as in the first possibility, or the complex partial seizure may occur without the aura as in the second pos-sibility. Assuming that partial seizures progress in only one direction (as is most often the case), the possibilities including secondary generalization, are summarized in Table 1.3.

That seizures in the 'generalized' category may also progress has been documented by Oller-Daurella (1974), Niedermeyer (1976), Porter & Sato (1982) and by Stefan (1982). The usual progression observed is from an absence or a clonic seizure to a generalized tonic-clonic attack. The concept of progression in generalized seizures was not included in the 1981 classification, an oversight that will require eventual redress (Wolf 1985). A considerable semantic difficulty arises when a seizure in the 'generalized' category progresses secondarily to a generalized tonic-clonic attack; this problem has been addressed by Porter & Sato (1982) who suggest that the gener-alized tonic-clonic seizure is the maximal neuronal expression of an epileptic attack and may, in fact, be the only seizure type worthy of being called 'generalized'.

Table 1.3   Possible progression of partial seizures

Seizure progression	Seizure name
SP	Simple partial seizures
SP→CP	Complex partial seizures (with SP onset)
CP	Complex partial seizures
SP→GTC	Partial seizures secondarily generalized—generalized tonic-clonic seizures
CP→GTC	Partial seizures secondarily generalized—generalized tonic-clonic seizures
SP→CP→GTC	Partial seizures secondarily generalized—generalized tonic-clonic seizures

(From Porter 1989)

PARTIAL SEIZURES

Simple partial seizures

Simple partial seizures are those attacks which show evidence of a localized onset, but during which consciousness (responsiveness) is preserved. The discharge is usually confined to a single hemisphere, and the symptoms are specific to the affected brain region. Four major groups of simple partial seizures need to be considered: 1. simple partial seizures with motor signs, 2. simple partial seizures with sensory symptoms, 3. simple partial seizures with autonomic symptoms or signs, and 4. simple partial seizures with psychic symptoms. Most commonly, patients experience either a motor event, such as clonic jerking of an extremity, or a sensory event, such as a bad odour or taste.

The varieties of simple partial seizures have been well described by Engel (1989). Simple partial seizures with motor signs include clonic motor seizures, tonic motor seizures, asymmetrical dystonic posturing, adversive head turning, and aphasic seizures or speech arrest. Simple partial seizures with sensory symptoms include simple hallucinations or illusions, somatosensory seizures, and ictal visual, auditory, olfactory, gustatory, or vertiginous symptoms. Simple partial seizures with autonomic symptoms include epigastric sensations, pallor, flushing, sweating, piloerection, pupillary dilatation, alterations in heart and respiratory rate, urination, defaecation, and penile erection. Simple partial seizures with psychic symptoms include ictal dysmnesic events, cognitive disturbances, affective symptoms, and complex illusions and hallucinations—including various experiential phenomena, micropsia, macropsia, polyopsia and metamorphopsia.

An aura is nothing more than a simple partial seizure. The word aura (from the Greek, meaning 'breeze') traditionally has been used in epilepsy to refer to the onset of a seizure which the patient is able to describe because consciousness is preserved during the event. The seizure that follows the aura, again from tradition, is usually associated with alteration of consciousness and is usually a complex partial or generalized tonic-clonic seizure. There is nothing fundamentally erroneous about this description, but a broader view is useful. First, the aura often does not progress further; the aura itself is the seizure. It is the reflection of abnormal neuronal discharge as perceived by the patient. Second, since consciousness is preserved during an aura, and since only a portion of the brain is involved, the attack is, by definition, a simple partial seizure. Any partial seizure may progress to another seizure type, and an aura is just one kind of simple partial seizure. A simple partial seizure may precede either a complex partial seizure or a generalized tonic-clonic seizure (Table 1.3). This progression is apparent to those who treat many patients with partial seizures; treatment often decreases the frequency of the secondary attacks but leaves the patient with the simple partial seizures (auras) (Porter 1989).

A special type of simple partial seizure with motor signs is that in which spread occurs to contiguous cortical areas producing a sequential involvement of body parts in an 'epileptic march' (Commission 1981). Hughlings Jackson contributed to the understanding of such seizures and referred to them as 'cortical epilepsy'. Charcot, however, is credited with popularizing the term 'Jacksonian seizure' for the simple partial motor seizure which 'marches' along the cortex and body parts (Kelly 1939).

Although the vast majority of simple partial seizures have only unilateral hemispheric involvement, very rarely a simple partial seizure will involve both hemispheres simultaneously with sparing of consciousness (Weinberger & Lusins, 1973). These seizures apparently occur because of an abnormal bilateral discharge of limited extent. An actual recorded example documented a patient who had twitching of the left face and right arm simultaneously, with normal communication during the attack. One might call such an attack a 'bilateral simple partial seizure' (Porter 1989).

The prognosis of simple partial seizures is exceedingly variable and is mostly dependent on the aetiology (Porter 1989). A small cortical venous malformation that causes contralateral focal motor signs may be surgically correctable with minimal deficit. A gustatory or olfactory simple partial seizure is sometimes a premonitory sign of a glioma (not always, as shown by Howe &

Gibson 1982); the prognosis may be poor. Some patients have continuous simple partial seizures (epilepsia partialis continua), which are often unresponsive to either medical or surgical therapy (Porter 1989).

Simple partial seizures can be quite difficult to record electrographically. In one series, scalp electrodes were effective in recording only 10% of the attacks, whereas subdural electrodes detected almost 90% of the simple partial seizures in the same patient group (Devinsky et al 1989).

The temporary weakness or paralysis (Todd's paralysis) that sometimes follows simple partial seizures is more likely to be caused by active inhibition of neuronal function than by 'neuronal exhaustion'; in this regard one cannot discern ictal from postictal paralysis with any certainty (Efron 1961).

The occurrence of psychic symptoms as the sole manifestation of a simple partial seizure is both uncommon and controversial; most psychic symptoms occur as part of complex—not simple— partial seizures. Video recording, however, has provided evidence that some patients with a seizure involving higher cortical function (e.g. forced thinking) may have preservation of responsiveness during the attack. On the other hand, one must be very cautious in ascribing to epilepsy such psychic phenomena as depersonalization, derealization, jamais vu, and deja vu (Harper & Roth 1962).

Complex partial seizures

Complex partial seizures are those attacks which show evidence of a localized onset and in which consciousness (responsiveness) is altered. In most instances the alteration results from bihemispheric involvement (see above). On occasion, a complex partial seizure will be preceded by an aura (a simple partial seizure); such an ictal event may simply by called a complex partial seizure (see Table 1.3) or more specifically a 'complex partial seizure with simple partial onset'.

The characteristics of complex partial seizures are a function of their origin and their spread. The most fundamental subdivision of these attacks, therefore, is achieved by dividing them into

temporal, frontal, parietal and occipital complex partial seizures. Ironically, one of the most thorough sources for the logic of such categorization is to be found in the latest international classification of epileptic *syndromes* (Commission 1989). The reason that epileptic seizures are so well described in the syndrome classification of partial seizures is that the syndromes related to partial seizures are almost totally based on the seizure characteristics. The fundamentals are reiterated here (Commission 1989); for the fullest description see Appendix B.

Complex partial seizures of *temporal lobe origin* often begin with motor arrest followed by oroalimentary automatisms; other automatisms frequently follow. The attacks last less than one minute and are followed by postictal confusion and gradual recovery. Further subdivision has been accomplished (Appendix B).

Complex partial seizures of *frontal lobe origin* are usually short with prominent motor manifestations and gestural automatisms; they may not have associated postictal confusion. The seizures frequently progress to secondary generalization. Further subdivision has been accomplished (Appendix B).

Complex partial seizures of *parietal lobe origin* and *occipital lobe origin* are uncommon, as most are sensory (simple partial) events. Spread of the discharge to other areas may be required for alteration of responsiveness.

It has been argued that by equating 'complex' with 'altered consciousness' the 1981 seizure classification sacrifices some of the intent of the original 1969 classification. This author agrees with Wolf's assessment of the controversy (Wolf, 1985). He notes that opponents of the current use of the term 'complex' generally belong to one of two groups: 1. those who hold that the term 'complex' should not be redefined but kept in its old meaning and 2. those who, while willing to accept a separation between seizures with impaired and seizures with preserved consciousness, are unwilling to accept 'complex' and 'simple' as appropriate labels for this dichotomy. Since, as Wolf points out, the 1969 classification lacked a precise definition of the term 'complex', it is difficult to know what meaning the first group wishes to retain.

The complex partial seizure has characteristics which have been reviewed in detail using video-tape techniques (Escueta et al 1981, Theodore et al 1983). Automatisms are typical, occurring in 96% of complex partial seizures in one series (Theodore et al 1983); an automatism, or automatic behaviour, has been defined as complicated behaviour which requires integration of higher cortical structures and for which the patient has no recollection. A classification of automatisms is helpful and suggests that many such events are not very specific to either the locus of the seizure onset or even to the seizure type. Although a highly detailed classification of automatisms is available (Penry & Dreifuss 1969), most such events can be categorized into one of three fundamental groups (Porter 1989):

1. *De novo automatisms from internal stimuli* (including 'release' phenomena), for example, chewing, lip smacking, swallowing, scratching, rubbing, picking, fumbling, running and disrobing.

2. *De novo automatisms from external stimuli*, for example, responding to pin prick, drinking from a cup, chewing gum placed in the mouth and pushing in response to restraint.

3. *Perseverative automatisms* (the continuation of any complex act initiated prior to loss of consciousness), for example, chewing food, using fork or spoon, drinking and walking.

Secondarily generalized partial seizures

It is a matter of some debate whether most generalized tonic-clonic (grand mal) seizures are secondary to another seizure type. In the population reviewed by Porter & Sato (1982), most such attacks were preceded by a partial seizure and very few were considered 'primary'; however, this study was based on a referral population and almost certainly does not reflect the large numbers of patients who have infrequent grand mal seizures with no evidence of any other seizure type. On the other hand, many patients do experience a variety of seizure types in conjunction with grand mal attacks; these concomitant attacks often go unrecognized for variable periods of time. The clinical nature of the secondarily generalized seizure itself does not appear to differ from that of the primary attack.

GENERALIZED SEIZURES

Introduction

The generalized seizures are an exceedingly heterogeneous group. Whether seizures in this group truly arise in both hemispheres simultaneously, or whether our ability to pinpoint the locus of onset is merely deficient, is not yet determined. The term 'generalized' has deficiencies as noted earlier in this chapter.

The generalized tonic-clonic (grand mal) seizure

Although the generalized tonic-clonic seizure may progress directly from another seizure as noted above, some such attacks appear to be generalized at onset. The generalized tonic-clonic seizure has certain well defined characteristics, summarized in Tables 1.4 and 1.5. In addition, autonomic changes are observed, including increased heart rate and blood pressure, increased bladder pressure, pupillary mydriasis, and glandular hypersecretion.

The absence seizure

The absence (petit mal) seizure begins in childhood or early adolescence and is characterized by unresponsiveness and a variety of associated

Table 1.4 Tonic phase of generalized tonic-clonic seizures

1. Usually lasts from 10 to 20 seconds

2. Begins with brief *flexion*:
   a. muscles contract
   b. the eyelids open; eyes look up
   c. the arms are elevated, abducted, and externally rotated; elbows are semiflexed
   d. the legs are less involved, but may be flexed

3. The *extension* phase is more prolonged:
   a. involves first the back and neck
   b. a tonic cry may occur—lasts 2–12 seconds
   c. the arms extend
   d. legs are extended, adducted, and externally rotated

4. The *tremor* begins:
   a. the tremor is a repetitive relaxation of the tonic contraction
   b. starts at 8 per second, gradually coarsens to 4 per second
   c. leads to the clonic phase

(From Gastaut & Broughton 1972)

Table 1.5 Clonic phase of generalized tonic-clonic seizures

1. Usually lasts about 30 seconds
2. Begins when the muscular relaxations completely interrupt the tonic contraction
3. Brief, violent flexor spasms of the whole body
4. The tongue is often bitten

(From Gastaut and Broughton 1972)

phenomena (Fig. 1.1). Automatic behaviour is common. As automatism are frequently observed in both absence and complex partial seizures, such behaviour should not be used to distinguish between the two types of attacks. Some features of the absence seizure may be helpful in establishing the diagnosis: the attacks are short, usually less than 10 seconds and rarely longer than 45 seconds; the onset is paroxysmal and without warning; the cessation is likewise sudden and without postictal depression or malaise. Automatisms are more common in longer attacks; clonic motion, usually of the eyelids, is common in shorter seizures (Penry et al 1975). A patient with absence seizures has a good prognosis if normal or above-average intelligence and a normal neurological examination are present (Sato et al 1983).

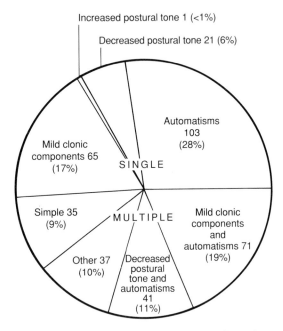

Fig. 1.1 Relative frequency of different types of 374 absence seizures. Reproduced with permission from Penry et al 1975.

Holmes et al (1987) studied 926 videotaped absence seizures and differentiated between typical and atypical absence attacks. Patients with atypical attacks have a much higher likelihood of having developmental delay or retardation, additional seizure types (other than partial seizures), and EEGs with interictal abnormalities. Typical absence seizures are more likely to be characterized by automatisms and eye blinking, whereas atypical absence seizures are typified by more prominent increases or decreases in muscle tone. Atypical absence seizures are significantly longer than typical absence seizures. Abrupt onset and cessation were noted in both types, and neither was useful in distinguishing between the two groups. Automatisms were found in 44% of typical absence seizures but in only 22% of patients with atypical attacks, a statistically significant difference. The investigators concluded that typical and atypical absence attacks are not discreet entities but form a continuum.

The myoclonias

The myoclonias are very heterogeneous; furthermore, clonic motion is a frequently-observed phenomenon which is a part of other seizure types. The terms which are commonly used to describe the phenomena (myoclonus, myoclonic, clonus, clonic) have been discussed (Porter 1989), and a volume has been written about epileptic myoclonus (Charleton 1975); classifications of myoclonus continue to evolve (Gastaut 1968, Marsden et al 1982).

An unambiguous clinical definition of myoclonus is lacking. Myoclonus has been defined as a 'quick movement of muscle'. Unfortunately, common usage varies greatly, and other entities such as tic, chorea, dystonia, fasciculations, and myokymia, for example, may also involve quick movements of muscle but are not considered to be myoclonia (Hallett 1986).

Clonic jerking, when observed in an epileptic attack, is a surprisingly stereotyped movement; it is not a random flailing about. The characteristics of clonic jerking can sometimes be used to distinguish epileptic attacks from pseudoseizures (Porter 1986).

Clonic seizures

Clonic seizures are usually those generalized convulsive seizures which lack a tonic phase and are, in fact, a fragment of a generalized tonic-clonic seizure. In addition, certain patients with epileptic attacks characterized by repetitive myoclonic jerks must be considered to have 'clonic seizures'. These attacks may progress to generalized tonic-clonic seizures (Porter 1986).

Clonic seizures are also seen in isolation from generalized tonic-clonic attacks. When these seizures progress to generalized tonic-clonic attacks, some have labelled them clonic-tonic-clonic seizures. In fact, such an event is just one example of a fundamental seizure type progressing to a generalized tonic-clonic seizure (Porter 1989).

Tonic seizures

Tonic seizures are uncommon, especially in the absence of at least a minimal amount of clonic jerking; they are usually a fragment of a generalized tonic-clonic attack. Such seizures are usually seen either in the Lennox–Gastaut syndrome or, less commonly, in multiple sclerosis. In a series of patients with severe epilepsy of various types studied by Spencer et al (1988), seven of 22 patients had tonic seizures. These attacks were considered to be secondarily generalized by the authors; such observations are consistent with the thesis that such seizures are fragments of generalized tonic-clonic seizures. Of the seven, six also had generalized tonic-clonic seizures.

Atonic seizures

Atonic seizures are those often severely incapacitating attacks in which precipitous loss of tone, usually postural, causes the patient to have a sudden nodding of the head or to fall to the floor. Although less sudden losses of tone have been described, the patients are usually at risk for injury, especially to face and head, and may require protective helmets (Porter 1986). Previous terms for atonic seizures include 'akinetic' and 'astatic'; the reasons for the abandonment of these terms have been reviewed (Porter 1989).

NEONATAL SEIZURES

Although most neonatal seizures can, at least theoretically, be placed into either the partial or generalized categories, these seizures are much more poorly described than seizures in adults, Even the concept of whether a particular event is or is not a seizure is often controversial. Two classifications have been proposed; the earlier is by Volpe (1981) (Table 1.6) and more recent is by Mizrahi & Kellaway (1987) (Table 1.7). The details have been summarized (Porter 1989). The Commission on Classification and Terminology of the International League Against Epilepsy fully recognizes the deficiencies of the current classification of neonatal seizures and is vigorously addressing this issue.

EPILEPTIC SYNDROMES

An epileptic syndrome may be defined as a disorder characterized by a cluster of signs and symptoms customarily occurring together (Commission 1985). As epilepsy is more a group of syndromes than a disease, 'the epilepsies' or 'epileptic syndromes' classify patients and emphasize the heterogeneity of these symptom-

Table 1.6 Neonatal seizure types (order of decreasing frequency)

1. Subtle
2. Generalized tonic
3. Multifocal clonic
4. Focal clonic
5. Myoclonic

(From Volpe 1981)

Table 1.7 Neonatal seizure types

I. Seizures with consistent electrical signature
   1. Focal clonic seizures
   2. Myoclonic seizures
   3. Focal tonic seizures
   4. Apnoea

II. Seizures with inconsistent electrical signature
   1. Motor automatisms
   2. Generalized tonic seizures
   3. Myoclonic seizures

III. Infantile spasms

IV. EEG seizures without clinical seizures

(From Mizrahi and Kellaway 1987)

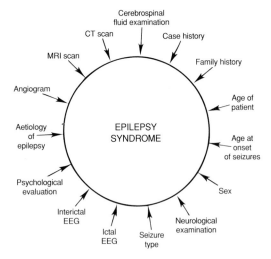

Fig. 1.2 The epileptic syndrome diagnosis is achieved by evaluating all factors relevant to the patient. This view of the syndrome diagnosis is complementary to that of Table 1.8. Reproduced with permission from Porter 1989.

Table 1.8 Data needed to provide a syndrome diagnosis

I. Informaton on *aetiology*
   A. Aetiological diagnosis is either definitively known or definitively unobtainable (idiopathic), *or*
   B. Aetiological diagnosis is suggested by some of the following:
      1. Neurological history, including age of onset and family history
      2. Neurological examination
      3. Electroencephalogram
      4. Radiological (and related) examinations
      5. Other tests, including psychological examinations

II. Information on *seizure type*
   A. Seizure type is definitively known, *or*
   B. Seizure type is suggested by some of the following:
      1. Neurological hisotry, including age of onset
      2. Neurological examination
      3. Direct or indirect (i.e. videotape) observation of a seizure
      4. Electroencephalogram, ictal and interictal
      5. Other tests, as above

(From Porter 1989)

complexes. The classification of the epilepsies depends on the determination of a framework of similarity in patient characteristics—including seizures and many other factors (Porter 1989).

The data required to establish an epilepsy syndrome diagnosis can be viewed in two different ways. First (Fig. 1.2), one can construct a diagram of all the different data which individually contribute to the epilepsy syndrome diagnosis. Alternatively (Table 1.8), one might consider that the aetiological and seizure diagnoses provide all the fundamental data required for establishing a syndrome diagnosis, and that all other data are subsets thereof.

The most important division of the epilepsies is between epilepsy with a recognizable cause (symptomatic) and epilepsy without a recognizable cause (cryptogenic or idiopathic—see Appendix B for distinction between these two). The cryptogenic group of patients has been gradually getting smaller as diagnostic techniques improve. The terms 'primary epilepsy' (meaning that the aetiology is unknown) and 'secondary epilepsy' (meaning that the aetiology is clinically identifiable) have also been used in a similar way to differentiate the epilepsies. From the 1989 Commission, the fundamental outline of the classification of the epilepsies is, therefore:

1. Localization-related (partial) epilepsies

   1.1 Idiopathic (with age related onset)
   1.2 Symptomatic
   1.3 Cryptogenic
2. Generalized epilepsies and syndromes
   2.1 Idiopathic (with age-related onset)
   2.2 Cryptogenic or symptomatic
   2.3 Symptomatic
3. Epilepsies and syndromes undetermined whether partial or generalized
   3.1 With both generalized and focal seizures
   3.2 Without unequivocal generalized or focal features
4. Special syndromes
   4.1 Situation-related seizures.

The next subdivision below partial/generalized and idiopathic/symptomatic, especially for the generalized epilepsies, is the relationship of age to epilepsy onset—one of the most important variables underlying the classification. Where appropriate, the classification progresses from the youngest affected group to the oldest. Relationship to age is most important in the generalized idiopathic epilepsies and least important in the partial symptomatic epilepsies (Porter 1989).

The following is a summary, based on the above outline, of the most important and relevant syndromes as viewed by this author. The data come primarily from Porter (1989) and the 1989 Commission report.

Partial epilepsies, idiopathic

Benign childhood epilepsy with centrotemporal spikes

This syndrome typically occurs between the ages of 3 and 13, and is characterized by brief, simple partial hemifacial motor seizures; these attacks tend to secondarily generalize. A genetic predisposition is frequent; males predominate.

Childhood epilepsy with occipital paroxysms

This syndrome is similar to the one above. Visual symptoms may occur at the onset; some patients have an associated migraine headache.

Primary reading epilepsy

Most seizures are precipitated by reading aloud; the attacks are partial and involve masticatory muscles. The syndrome may be inherited, but is generally benign.

1.2 Partial epilepsies, symptomatic

Chronic progressive epilepsia partialis continua of childhood (Kojewnikow's syndrome)

The syndrome is characterized by Jacksonian march of clonic jerking of a body part as well as myoclonias of the same area. It typically begins with between ages 2 and 10; the course is malignant (Delgado-Escueta & Treiman 1987).

Syndromes characterized by seizures with specific modes of precipitation

This group of syndromes, in which the aetiology of the seizures is known or suspected, is largely characterized by the seizure type, which is very much determined by the locus of onset of the attacks. Included are syndromes characterized by simple and complex partial seizures as well as secondarily generalized seizures. Obviously this group encompasses the most frequent and severe epilepsy problems of adults. The anatomically designated syndromes are:

1. temporal lobe epilepsies
2. frontal lobe epilepsies
3. parietal lobe epilepsies
4. occipital lobe epilepsies

Our understanding of these syndromes is still evolving. Although the medical therapy for all of these syndromes is usually similar, their individual recognition is important when considering surgical therapy for the patient's epilepsy.

1.3 Cryptogenic

Same as above, but of unknown aetiology.

2.1 Generalized epilepsies, idiopathic

Benign neonatal convulsions

These clonic or apnoeic seizures occur in the first few days of life and may be familial or sporadic.

Benign myoclonic epilepsy in infancy

These patients have bursts of myoclonus in the first or second year of life; the EEG shows generalized spike-waves. Treatment is usually effective.

Childhood absence epilepsy

The absence seizure is described above. The syndrome of absence epilepsy includes an onset during childhood, genetic predisposition, and predominance in girls. The EEG is typically 3/second spike-waves. Generalized tonic-clonic seizures may occur. Whether this entity differs from *juvenile absence epilepsy* is debatable; the latter may simply represent a continuum from the former.

Juvenile myoclonic epilepsy

Juvenile myoclonic epilepsy is a common, benign myoclonic syndrome. In general, it is a rewarding disorder to recognize and treat. The onset of sudden, sometimes explosive, uncontrollable myoclonic jerks in a teenager is typical. The jerks will be embarrassing, more frequent in the morning or on arising from sleep, and bothersome at the table when eating. The attacks occasionally progress to generalized tonic-clonic seizures, which may follow directly from an especially severe series of clonic seizures. Mental retardation does not occur. Attacks worsen with anxiety, sudden stimuli, or sleeplessness. The EEG typically shows generalized polyspike and wave abnormalities;

photic stimulation may elicit an attack. The largest study of this disorder is by Janz & Christian (1957), who described 47 patients with juvenile myoclonic epilepsy. The usual age at onset of the disorder was between 10 and 23 years, and all but two patients had occasional generalized tonic-clonic seizures in addition to the myoclonic attacks. In a more recent review, Janz (1985) considered the syndrome in detail and has termed it 'epilepsy with impulsive petit mal' because of its close relationship to absence epilepsy. Some evidence suggests that the genetic abnormality for juvenile myoclonic epilepsy may reside on chromosome number six (Delgado-Escueta et al 1988).

2.2 Generalized epilepsies, cryptogenic or symptomatic

Infantile spasms (West syndrome)

Infantile spasms is an epileptic syndrome encompassing a group of attacks with remarkably diverse aetiologies, in which most patients have the onset of seizures before the age of one year. The recurring attacks, which are brief contractions of the neck, trunk, and extremities, are usually associated with mental retardation and hypsarrhythmia in the EEG. The seizures are usually divided into three different clinical types (Kellaway et al 1979): 1. flexor spasms, 2. extensor spasms, and 3. mixed flexor-extensor spasms. The causes are extremely diverse. Classically, the EEG shows hypsarrhythmia, although it is most typical only in the early stages of the disorder (Hrachovy 1982). The prognosis of patients with infantile spasms is poor. Of the 214 patients followed for at least 3 years by Riikonen (1982), 19.6% had died and only 12% had developed normally. More recent data reported by Glaze et al (1988) are even more pessimistic; only three of 64 patients had 'normal development or mild impairment'. Many patients progress to the Lennox–Gastaut syndrome.

Lennox–Gastaut syndrome

The Lennox–Gastaut syndrome usually begins between the ages of 1 and 6 years, though rarely it may occur as late as 10 years of age or older. It may develop in patients who have had infantile spasms, but more often occurs spontaneously. The aetiologies are diverse. Most patients are mentally retarded. The most devastating seizures are atonic; the head may drop suddenly onto the breakfast table, or the patient may fall precipitously to the floor. The absence seizures are usually brief and atypical (Holmes et al 1987). Either the atonic or absence attacks may be accompanied by myoclonic jerks. The EEG commonly demonstrates continuous spike-and-wave abnormalities, usually at a rate which is less than 3/second, and the complexes are often irregular and asymmetrical; multifocal spikes are also common. As the patient gets older, complex partial and generalized tonic-clonic seizures may become predominant.

Epilepsy with myoclonic-astatic seizures

This subdivision may be a mild form of the Lennox–Gastaut syndrome. Heredity may play a role.

Epilepsy with myoclonic absences

This rare form of absence epilepsy is characterized by severe bilateral jerking and a relatively poor prognosis.

2.3 Generalized epilepsies, symptomatic

Early myoclonic encephalopathy

This poorly defined syndrome has its onset before 3 months; the prognosis is poor.

3.1 Uncertain—either partial or generalized epilepsies

Neonatal seizures

Although listed as a syndrome, this entity is more a collection of seizure types. Individual syndromes may eventually emerge. See previous discussion under 'neonatal seizures.'

Epilepsy with continuous spike-waves during slow wave sleep

Generalized tonic-clonic seizures are typical in

these patients who have a epileptic pattern during slow wave sleep.

Acquired epileptic aphasia (Landau–Kleffner syndrome)

This syndrome in childhood is characterized by an acquired aphasia and multifocal EEG spikes and spike-waves. Epileptic seizures and psychomotor disturbances occur in two-thirds of patients.

4.1 Special epileptic syndromes

Febrile convulsions

Febrile seizures occur in 2–5% of the population (Hauser 1981); the attacks are usually benign. They occur between 3 months and 5 years of age, and are associated with fever, but are not associated with intracranial infection or any other defined cause specifically related to the central nervous system. The risk of subsequent epilepsy to most children who experience febrile seizures is minimal (Annegers et al 1987). There is little evidence that recurrent febrile seizures cause any type of subsequent epilepsy. Patients with uncomplicated febrile seizures, even if several eventually occur, are not usually considered to have epilepsy, the chronic recurrent disorder.

Single seizures

Single seizures are another epilepsy syndrome for which the patient may not require treatment. Some controversy, however, exists regarding the likelihood of recurrence where there has been only a single attack. Hauser et al (1982) and Hauser (1986) suggested that the 3-year recurrence rate may be as low as 27%, whereas Elwes et al (1985) found a recurrence rate of 71%, and Hopkins et al (1988), a rate of 52%. The low rate of the first studies may be due to a higher percentage of treated patients and to a less rapid entry into the study following the first event (Elwes & Reynolds 1988). One consideration which is often uncontrolled in such studies is the heterogeneity of the patients and their epilepsy.

Seizures occurring only in response to an acute metabolic or toxic events

These attacks usually disappear when the abnormality is rectified or the offending agent removed.

SUMMARY

The epilepsies are a heterogeneous symptom complex. Classifications have been designed both for epileptic seizures and for epileptic syndromes. The 1981 Classification of Epileptic Seizures is pragmatic and can be applied to every patient in which epilepsy is in the differential diagnosis. The 1989 Classification of Epileptic Syndromes will, in many patients, provide prognosis and expectation of the duration of therapy. The thorough use of these classifications by the practicing physician, an effort which is highly dependent upon an adequate medical history, will greatly benefit the patient with epilepsy.

APPENDIX A

The material in Appendix A is reprinted with the permission of Raven Press Ltd from Commission on Classification and Terminology of the International League Against Epilepsy 1981.

I. PARTIAL (FOCAL, LOCAL) SEIZURES

Partial seizures are those in which, in general, the first clinical and electroencephalographic changes indicate initial activation of a system of neurons limited to part of one cerebral hemisphere. A partial seizure is classified primarily on the basis of whether or not consciousness is impaired during the attack. When consciousness is not impaired, the seizure is classified as a simple partial seizure. When consciousness is impaired, the seizure is classified as a complex partial seizure. Impairment of consciousness may be the first clinical sign, or simple partial seizures may evolve into complex partial seizures. In patients with impaired consciousness, aberrations of behaviour (automatisms) may occur. A partial seizure may not terminate, but instead progress to a generalized motor seizure. Impaired consciousness is defined as the inability to respond normally to exogenous stimuli by virtue of altered awareness and/or responsiveness (vide infra: Definition of Terms).

There is considerable evidence that simple partial seizures usually have unilateral hemispheric involvement and only rarely have bilateral hemispheric involvement; complex partial seizures, however, frequently have bilateral hemispheric involvement.

Partial seizures can be classified into one of the following three fundamental groups:

A. Simple partial seizures
B. Complex partial seizures
   1. With impairment of consciousness at onset
   2. Simple partial onset followed by impairment of consciousness
C. Partial seizures evolving to generalized tonic-clonic convulsions (GTC)
   1. Simple evolving to GTC
   2. Complex evolving to GTC (including those with simple partial onset)

Clinical seizure type	EEG seizure type	EEG interictal expression
A. *Simple partial seizures* (consciousness not impaired)	Local contralateral discharge starting over the corresponding area of cortical representation (not always recorded on the scalp)	Local contralateral discharge
1. With motor signs		
(a) Focal motor without march		
(b) Focal motor with march (Jacksonian)		
(c) Versive		
(d) Postural		
(e) Phonatory (vocalization or arrest of speech)		
2. With somatosensory or special-sensory symptoms (simple hallucinations, e.g. tingling, light flashes, buzzing)		
(a) Somatosensory		
(b) Visual		
(c) Auditory		
(d) Olfactory		
(e) Gustatory		
(f) Vertiginous		
3. With autonomic symptoms or signs (including epigastric sensation, pallor, sweating, flushing, piloerection and pupillary dilatation)		
4. With psychic symptoms (disturbance of higher cerebral function). These symptoms rarely occur without impairment of consciousness and are much more commonly experienced as complex partial seizures		
(a) Dysphasic		
(b) Dysmnesic (e.g. déjà-vu)		
(c) Cognitive (e.g., dreamy states, distortions of time sense)		
(d) Affective (fear, anger, etc.)		
(e) Illusions (e.g. macropsia)		
(f) Structured hallucinations (e.g. music, scenes)		
B. *Complex partial seizures* (with impairment of consciousness; may sometimes begin with simple symptomatology)	Unilateral or, frequently bilateral discharge, diffuse or focal in temporal or frontotemporal regions	Unilateral or bilateral generally asynchronous focus; usually in the temporal or frontal regions
1. Simple partial onset followed by impairment of consciousness		
(a) With simple partial features (A.1.–A.4.) followed by impaired consciousness		
(b) With automatisms		
2. With impairment of consciousness at onset		
(a) With impairment of consciousness only		
(b) With automatisms		

Clinical seizure type	EEG seizure type	EEG interictal expression
C. *Partial seizures evolving to secondarily generalized seizures* (This may be generalized tonic-clonic, tonic, or clonic) 1. Simple partial seizures (A) evolving to generalized seizures 2. Complex partial seizures (B) evolving to generalized seizures 3. Simple partial seizures (A) evolving to complex partial seizures (B) evolving to generalized seizures	Above discharges become secondarily and rapidly generalized	

II. GENERALIZED SEIZURES (CONVULSIVE OR NONCONVULSIVE)

Generalized seizures are those in which the first clinical changes indicate initial involvement of both hemispheres. Consciousness may be impaired and this impairment may be the initial manifestation. Motor manifestations are bilateral. The ictal electroencephalographic patterns initially are bilateral, and presumably reflect neuronal discharge which is widespread in both hemispheres.

Clinical seizure type	EEG seizure type	EEG interictal expression
A. 1. *Absence seizures*	Usually regular and symmetrical 3 Hz but may be 2–4 Hz spike-and-slow-wave complexes and may have multiple spike-and-slow-wave complexes. Abnormalities are bilateral	Background activity usually normal although paroxysmal activity (such as spikes or spike-and-slow-wave complexes) may occur. This activity is usually regular and symmetrical

(a) Impairment of consciousness only
     (b) With mild clonic components
     (c) With atonic components
     (d) With tonic components
     (e) With automatisms
     (f) With autonomic components
     (b through f may be used aalone or in combination)		

2. *Atypical absence*	EEG more heterogeneous; may include irregular spike-and-slow wave complexes, fast activity or other paroxysmal activity. Abnormalities are bilateral but often irregular and asymmetrical	Background usually abnormal; paroxysmal activity (such as spikes or spike-and-slow-wave complexes) frequently irregular and asymmetrical

May have:
     (a) Changes in tone that are more pronounced than in A. 1
     (b) Onset and/or cessation that is not abrupt		

B. *Myoclonic seizures*
   Myoclonic jerks
   (single or multiple)
	Polyspike and wave, or sometimes spike and wave or sharp and slow waves	Same as ictal

C. *Clonic seizures*	Fast activity (10 c/s or more) and slow waves; occasional spike-and-wave patterns	Spike-and-wave or polyspike-and-wave discharges

Clinical seizure type	EEG seizure type	EEG interictal expression
D. *Tonic seizures*	Low voltage, fast activity or a fast rhythm of 0–10 c/s or more decreasing in frequency and increasing in amplitude	More or less rhythmic discharges of sharp and slow waves, sometimes times asymmetrical. Background is often abnormal for age
E. *Tonic-clonic seizures*	Rhythm at 10 or more c/s decreasing in frequency and increasing in amplitude during tonic phase, interrupted by slow waves during clonic phase	Polyspike and waves or spike and wave, or, soemtimes, sharp and slow wave discharges
F. *Atonic seizures* (Astatic) (combinations of the above may occur, e.g. B and F, B and D)	Polyspikes and wave or flattening or low-voltage fast activity	Polyspikes and slow wave

III. UNCLASSIFIED EPILEPTIC SEIZURES

Includes all seizures that cannot be classified because of inadequate or incomplete data and some that defy classification in hitherto described categories. This includes some neonatal seizures, e.g. rhythmic eye movements, chewing, and swimming moveents.

IV. ADDENDUM

Repeated epileptic seizures occur under a variety of circumstances:

1. as fortuitous attacks, coming unexpectedly and without any apparent provocation; 2. as cyclic attacks, at more or less regular intervals (e.g., in relation to the menstrual cycle, or the sleep-waking cycle); 3. as attacks provoked by: (a) nonsensory factors (fatigue, alcohol, emotion, etc.), or (b) sensory factors, sometimes referred to as "reflex seizures."

Prolonged or repetitive seizures (status epiletticus). The term "status epilepticus" is used whenever a seizure persists for a sufficient length of time or is repeated frequently enough that recovery between attacks does not occur. Status epilepticus may be divided into partial (e.g. Jacksonian), or generalized (e.g., absence status or tonic-clonic status). When very localized motor status occurs, it is referred to as epilepsia partialis continua.

APPENDIX B

The material in Appendix B is reprinted with the permission of Raven Press Ltd from Commission on Classification and Terminology of the International League against Epilepsy 1989.

INTERNATIONAL CLASSIFICATION OF EPILEPSIES AND EPILEPTIC SYNDROMES

1. Localization-related (focal, local, partial) epilepsies and syndromes
   1.1 Idiopathic (with age-related onset)
   At present, the following syndromes are established, but more may be identified in the future:
   - Benign childhood epilepsy with centrotemporal spike
   - Childhood epilepsy with occipital paroxysms
   - Primary reading epilepsy

   1.2 Symptomatic (Appendix I)
   - Chronic progressive epilepsia partialis continua of childhood (Kojewnikow's syndrome)
   - Syndromes characterized by seizures with specific modes of precipitation (see Appendix II)

Apart from these rare conditions, the symptomatic category comprises syndromes of great individual variability which are based mainly on seizure types and other clinical features as well as anatomic localization and aetiology—as far as these are known.

The seizure types refer to the ICES. Inferences regarding anatomic localization must be drawn carefully. The scalp EEG (both interictal and ictal) may be misleading, and even local morphological findings detected by neuroimaging techniques are not necessarily identical with an epileptogenic lesion. Seizure symptomatology and, sometimes, additional clinical features often provide important clues. The first sign or symptom of a seizure is often the most important indicator of the site of origin of seizure discharge, whereas the following sequence of ictal events can reflect its further propagation through the brain. This sequence, however, can still be of high localizing importance. One must bear in mind that a seizure may start in a clinically silent region, so that the first clinical event occurs only after spread to a site more or less distant from the locus of initial discharge. The following tentative descriptions of syndromes related to anatomic localizations are based on data which include findings in studies with depth electrodes.

• Temporal lobe epilepsies

Temporal lobe syndromes are characterized by simple partial seizures, complex partial seizures, and secondarily generalized seizures, or combinations of these. Frequently, there is a history of febrile seizures, and a family history of seizures is common. Memory deficits may occur. On metabolic imaging studies, hypometabolism is frequently observed [e.g., positron emission tomography (PET)]. Unilateral or bilateral temporal lobe spikes are common on EEG. Onset is frequently in childhood or young adulthood. Seizures occur in clusters at intervals or randomly.

General characteristics

Features strongly suggestive of the diagnosis when present include:

1. Simple partial seizures typically characterized by autonomic and/or psychic symptoms and certain sensory phenomena such as olfactory and auditory (including illusions). Most common is an epigastric, often rising, sensation.
2. Complex partial seizures often but not always beginning with motor arrest typically followed by oroalimentary automatism. Other automatisms frequently follow. The duration is typically >1 min. Postictal confusion usually occurs. The attacks are followed by amnesia. Recovery is gradual.

Electroencephalographic characteristics

In temporal lobe epilepsies the interictal scalp EEG may show the following:

1. No abnormality.
2. Slight or marked asymmetry of the background activity.
3. Temporal spikes, sharp waves and/or slow waves, unilateral or bilateral, synchronous but also asynchronous. These findings are not always confined to the temporal region.
4. In addition to scalp EEG findings, intracranial recordings may allow better definition of the intracranial distribution of the interictal abnormalities.

In temporal lobe epilepsies various EEG patterns may accompany the initial clinical ictal symptomatology, including (a) a unilateral or bilateral interruption of background activity; and (b) temporal or multilobar low-amplitude fast activity, rhythmic spikes, or rhythmic slow waves. The onset of the EEG may not correlate with the clinical onset depending on methodology. Intracranial recordings may provide additional information regarding the chronologic and spatial evolution of the discharges.

Amygdalo-hippocampal (mesiobasal limbic or rhinencephalic) seizures. Hippocampal seizures are the most common form; the symptoms are those described in the previous paragraphs except that auditory symptoms may not occur. The interictal scalp EEG may be normal, may show interictal unilateral temporal sharp or slow waves, may show bilateral sharp or slow waves, synchronous or asynchronous. The intracranial interictal EEG may show mesial anterior temporal spikes or sharp waves. Seizures are characterized by rising epigastric discomfort, nausea, marked autonomic signs, and other symptoms, including borborygmi, belching, pallor, fullness of the face, flushing of the face, arrest of respiration, pupillary dilatation, fear, panic, and olfactory-gustatory hallucinations.

Lateral temporal seizures. Simple seizures characterized by auditory hallucinations or illusions or dreamy states, visual misperceptions, or language disorders in case of language dominant hemisphere focus. These may progress to complex partial seizures if propagation to mesial temporal or extratemporal structures occur. The scalp EEG shows unilateral or bilateral midtemporal or posterior temporal spikes which are most prominent in the lateral derivations.

● Frontal lobe epilepsies

Frontal lobe epilepsies are characterized by simple partial, complex partial, secondarily generalized seizures or combinations of these. Seizures often occur several times a day and frequently occur during sleep. Frontal lobe partial seizures are sometimes mistaken for psychogenic seizures. Status epilepticus is a frequent complication.

General characteristics

Features strongly suggestive of the diagnosis include:

1. Generally short seizures.
2. Complex partial seizures arising from the frontal lobe, often with minimal or no confusion.
3. Rapid secondary generalization (more common in seizures of frontal than of temporal lobe epilepsy).
4. Prominent motor manifestations which are tonic or postural.
5. Complex gestural automatisms frequent at onset.
6. Frequent falling when the discharge is bilateral.

A number of seizure types are described below; however, multiple frontal areas may be involved rapidly and specific seizure types may not be discernible.

Supplementary motor seizures. In supplementary motor seizures, the seizure patterns are postural, focal tonic, with vocalization, speech arrest, and fencing postures.

Cingulate. Cingulate seizure patterns are complex partial with complex motor gestural automatisms at onset. Autonomic signs are common, as are changes in mood and affect.

Anterior frontopolar region. Anterior frontopolar seizure patterns include forced thinking or initial loss of contact and adversive movement of head and eyes, with possible evolution including contraversive movements and axial clonic jerks and falls and autonomic signs.

Orbitofrontal. The orbitofrontal seizure pattern is one of complex partial seizures with initial motor and gestural automatisms, olfactory hallucinations and illusions, and autonomic signs.

Dorsolateral. Dorsolateral seizure patterns may be tonic or, less commonly, clonic with versive eye and head movements and speech arrest.

Opercular. Opercular seizure characteristics include mastication, salivation, swallowing, laryngeal symptoms, speech arrest, epigastric aura, fear, and autonomic phenomena. Simple partial seizures, particularly partial clonic facial seizures, are common and may be ipsilateral. If secondary sensory changes occur, numbness may be a symptom, particularly in the hands. Gustatory hallucinations are particularly common in this area.

Motor cortex. Motor cortex epilepsies are mainly characterized by simple partial seizures, and their localization depends on the side and topography of the area involved. In cases of the lower prerolandic area there may be speech arrest, vocalization or dysphasia, tonic-clonic movements of the face on the contralateral side, or swallowing. Generalization of the seizure frequently occurs. In the rolandic area, partial motor seizures without march or jacksonian seizures occur, particularly beginning in the contralateral upper extremities. In the case of seizures involving the paracentral lobule, tonic movements of the ipsilateral foot may occur as well as the expected contralateral leg movements. Postictal or Todd's paralysis is frequent.

Kojewnikow's syndrome. Two types of Kojewnikow's syndrome are recognized, one of which is also known as Rasmussen's syndrome and is included among the epileptic syndromes of childhood noted under symptomatic seizures. The other type represents a particular form of rolandic partial epilepsy in both adults and children and is related to a variable lesion of the motor cortex. Its principal features are (a) motor partial seizures, always well localized; (b) often late appearance of myoclonus in the same site where somatomotor seizures occur; (c) an EEG with normal background activity and a focal paroxysmal abnormality (spikes and slow waves); (d) occurrence at any age in childhood and adulthood; (e) frequently demonstrable aetiology (tumour, vascular); and (f) no progressive evolution of the syndrome (clinical, electroencephalographic or psychological, except in relation to the evolution of the causal lesion). This condition may result from mitochondrial encephalopathy (MELAS).

NOTE: Anatomical origins of some epilepsies are difficult to assign to specific lobes. Such epilepsies include those with pre- and postcentral symptomatology (perirolandic seizures). Such overlap to adjacent anatomic regions also occurs in opercular epilepsy.

In frontal lobe epilepsies, the interictal scalp recordings may show (a) no abnormality; (b) sometimes background asymmetry, frontal spikes or sharp waves; or (c) sharp waves or slow waves (either unilateral or frequently bilateral or unilateral multilobar). Intracranial recordings can sometimes distinguish unilateral from bilateral involvement.

In frontal lobe seizures, various EEG patterns can accompany the initial clinical symptomatology. Uncommonly, the EEG abnormality precedes the seizure onset and then provides important localizing information, such as: (a) frontal or multilobar, often bilateral, low-amplitude fast activity, mixed spikes, rhythmic spikes, rhythmic spike waves, or rhythmic slow waves; or (b) bilateral high amplitude single sharp waves followed by diffuse flattening.

Depending on the methodology, intracranial recordings may provide additional information regarding the chronologic and spatial evolution of the discharges; localization may be difficult.

• Patrietal lobe epilepsies

Partial lobe epilepsy syndromes are usually characterized by simple partial and secondarily generalized seizures. Most seizures arising in the parietal lobe remain as simple partial seizures, but complex partial seizures may arise out of simple partial seizures and occur with spread beyond the parietal lobe. Seizures arising from the parietal lobe have the following features: Seizures are predominantly sensory with many characteristics. Positive phenomena consist of tingling and a feeling of electricity, which may be confined or may spread in a Jacksonian manner. There may be a desire to move a body part or a sensation as if a part were being moved. Muscle tone may be lost. The parts most frequently involved are those with the largest cortical representation (e.g. the hand, arm, and face). There may be tongue sensations of crawling, stiffness, or coldness, and facial sensory phenomena may occur bilaterally. Occasionally, an intra-abdominal sensation of sinking, choking, or nausea may occur, particularly in cases of inferior and lateral parietal lobe involvement. Rarely, there may be pain, which may take the form of a superficial burning dysaesthesia, or a vague, very severe, painful sensation. Parietal lobe visual phenomena may occur as hallucinations of a formed variety. Metamorphopsia with distortions, foreshortenings, and elongations may occur, and are more frequently observed in cases of nondominant hemisphere discharges. Negative phenomena include numbness, a feeling that a body part is absent, and a loss of awareness of a part or a half of the body, known as asomatognosia. This is particularly the case with nondominant hemisphere involvement. Severe vertigo or disorientation in space may be indicative of inferior parietal lobe seizures. Seizures in the dominant parietal lobe result in a variety of receptive or conductive language disturbances. Some well-lateralized genital sensations may occur with paracentral involvement. Some rotatory or postural motor phenomena may occur. Seizures of the paracentral lobule have a tendency to become secondarily generalized.

• Occipital lobe epilepsies

Occipital lobe epilepsy syndromes are usually characterized by simple partial and secondarily generalized seizures. Complex partial seizures may occur with spread beyond the occipital lobe. The frequent association of occipital lobe seizures and migraine is complicated and controversial. The clinical seizure manifestations usually, but not always, include visual manifestations. Elementary visual seizures are characterized by fleeting visual manifestations which may be either negative (scotoma, hemianopsia, amaurosis) or, more commonly, positive (sparks or flashes, phosphenes). Such sensations appear in the visual field contralateral to the discharge in the specific visual cortex but can spread to the entire visual field. Perceptive illusions, in which the objects appear to be distorted, may occur. The following varieties can be distinguished: a change in size (macropsia or micropsia), or a change in distance, an inclination of objects in a given plane of space and distortion of objects or a sudden change of shape (metamorphopsia). Visual hallucinatory seizures are occasionally characterized by complex visual perceptions (e.g. colourful scenes of varying complexity). In some cases, the scene is distorted or made smaller, and in rare instances, the subject sees his own image (heautoscopy). Such illusional and hallucinatory visual seizures involve epileptic discharge in the temporoparieto-occipital junction. The initial signs may also include tonic and/or clonic contraversion of eyes and head or eyes only (oculoclonic or oculogyric deviation), palpebral jerks, and forced closure of eyelids. Sensation of ocular oscillation or of the whole body may occur. The discharge may spread to the temporal lobe, producing seizure manifestations of either lateral posterior temporal or hippocampoamygdala seizures. When the primary focus is located in the supracalcarine area, the discharge can spread forward to the suprasylvian convexity or the mesial surface, mimicking those of parietal or frontal lobe seizures. Spread to contralateral occipital lobe may be rapid. Occasionally the seizure tends to become secondarily generalized.

1.3 Cryptogenic
Cryptogenic epilepsies are presumed to be symptomatic and the aetiology is unknown. This category thus differs from the previous one by the lack of aetiological evidence (See definitions).

2. Generalized epilepsies and syndromes
2.1 Idiopathic (with age-related onset—listed in order of age)
- Benign neonatal familial convulsions
- Benign neonatal convulsions
- Benign myoclonic epilepsy in infancy
- Childhood absence epilepsy (pyknolepsy)
- Juvenile absence epilepsy
- Juvenile myoclonic epilepsy (impulsive petit mal)
- Epilepsy with grand mal (GTCS) seizures on awakening
- Other generalized idiopathic epilepsies not defined above
- Epilepsies with seizures precipitated by specific modes of activation

2.2 Cryptogenic or symptomatic (in order of age)
- West syndrome (infantile spasms, Blitz–Nick–Salaam Krämpfe)
- Lennox–Gastaut syndrome
- Epilepsy with myoclonic-astatic seizures
- Epilepsy with myoclonic absences

2.3 Symptomatic
2.3.1 Non-specific aetiology
- Early myoclonic encephalopathy
- Early infantile epileptic encephalopathy with suppression burst
- Other symptomatic generalized epilepsies not defined above

2.3.2 Specific syndromes
- Epileptic seizures may complicate many disease states. Under this heading are included diseases in which seizures are a presenting or predominant feature

3. Epilepsies and syndromes undetermined whether focal or generalized
3.1 With both generalized and focal seizures
- Neonatal seizures
- Severe myoclonic epilepsy in infancy
- Epilepsy with continuous spike-waves during slow wave sleep
- Acquired epileptic aphasia (Landau–Kleffner-syndrome)
- Other undetermined epilepsies not defined above

3.2 Without unequivocal generalized or focal features. All cases with generalized tonic-clonic seizures in which clinical and EEG findings do not permit classification as clearly generalized or localization related, such as in many cases of sleep-grand mal (GTCS) are considered not to have unequivocal generalized or focal features.

4. Special syndromes
4.1 Situation-related seizures (Gelegenheitsanfälle)

- Febrile convulsions
- Isolated seizures or isolated status epilepticus
- Seizures occurring only when there

is an acute metabolic or toxic event due to factors such as alcohol, drugs, eclampsia, nonketotic hyperglycaemia.

REFERENCES

Annegers J F, Hauser W A, Shirts S B, Kurland L T 1987 Factors prognostic of unprovoked seizures after febrile convulsions. New England Journal of Medicine 316: 493–498

Browne T R, Penry J K, Porter R J, Dreifuss F E 1974 Responsiveness before, during, and after spike-wave paroxysms. Neurology 24: 659–665

Charleton M H (ed) 1975 Myoclonic seizures. Exerpta Medica, Amsterdam

Commission for the Control of Epilepsy and Its Consequences: Plan for Nationwide Action on Epilepsy 1978 Vol 1. DHEW Publication (NIH). US Department of Health Education and Welfare, Washington, DC, p 78–276

Commission on Classification and Terminology of the International League Against Epilepsy 1981 Proposal for revised clinical and electroencephalographic classification of epileptic seizures. Epilepsia 22: 489–501

Commission on Classification and Terminology of the International League Against Epilepsy 1985 Proposal for classification of epilepsies and epileptic syndromes. Epilepsia 26: 268–278

Commission on Classification and Terminology of the International League Against Epilepsy 1989 Proposal for revised classification of epilepsies and epileptic syndromes. Epilepsia 30: 389–399

Delgado-Escueta A V, Treiman D M 1987 Focal Status Epilepticus: Modern Concepts. In: Luders H, Lesser R P (eds) Epilepsy: electroclinical syndromes, p 347–391

Delgado-Escueta A V, Greenberg D, Maldonado H et al 1988 JME-6 Genotype: Clinical phenotypes and EEG traits. Epilepsia 29: 706

Devinsky O, Sato S, Kufta C V et al 1989 Electroencephalographic studies of simple partial seizures with subdural electrode recordings. Neurology 39: 527–533

Efron R 1961 Post-epileptic paralysis: Theoretical critique and report of a case. Brain 84: 381–394

Elwes R D C, Chesterman P, Reynolds E H 1985 Prognosis after a first untreated tonic-clonic seizure. Lancet 2: 752–753

Elwes R D C, Reynolds E H 1988 Should people be treated after a first seizure? Archives of Neurology 45: 490–491

Engel J Jr 1989 Seizures and Epilepsy. F A Davis, Philadelphia

Escueta A V, Bacsal F, Treiman D 1981 Complex partial seizures on closed-circuit television and EEG: A study of 691 attacks in 79 patients. Annals of Neurology 11: 292–300

Gastaut H 1968 Semeiologie des myoclonies et nosologie analytique des syndromes myocloniques. In: Bonduelle M, Gastaut H (eds) Les Myoclonies. Masson, Paris, p 1–30

Gastaut H 1973 Dictionary of Epilepsy. World Health Organization, Geneva

Gastaut H, Broughton R 1972 Epileptic seizures: clinical and electrographic features, diagnosis and treatment. Charles C. Thomas, Springfield, Ill

Glaze D G, Hrachovy R A, Frost J D, Kellaway P, Zion T E 1988 Prospective study of outcome of infants with infantile spasms treated during controlled studies of ACTH and prednisone. Journal of Pediatrics 112: 389–396

Gloor P, Olivier A, Ives J 1980 Loss of consciousness in temporal lobe seizures: Observations obtained with stereotaxic depth electrode recordings and stimulations. In: Canger R, Angeleri F, Penry J K (eds) Advances in epileptology: XIth epilepsy international symposium. Raven Press, New York, p 349–353

Gloor P 1984 Electroencephalography and the role of intracerebral depth electrode recordings in the selection of patients for surgical treatment of epilepsy. In: Porter R J, Mattson R H, Ward Jr A A, Dam M (eds) Advances in epileptology: the XVth epilepsy international symposium. Raven Press, New York, p 433–437

Gloor P 1986 Consciousness as a neurological concept in epileptology: a critical review. Epilepsia 27(supple 2): S14–S26

Hallett M 1986 Myoclonus. In: Handbook of clinical neurology: extrapyramidal disorders. Amsterdam: Elsevier, Amsterdam, Vol 49, p 609–625

Harper M, Roth M 1962 Temporal lobe epilepsy and the phobic anxiety-depersonalization syndrome. Part I: A comparative study. Comprehensive Psychiatry 3: 129–151

Hauser W A 1981 The natural history of febrile seizures. In: Nelson K B, Ellenberg J H (eds) Febrile seizures. Raven Press, New York, p 5–17

Hauser W A 1986 Should people be treated after a first seizure. Archives of Neurology 43: 1287–1288

Hauser W A, Anderson V E, Loewenson R B, McRoberts S M 1982 Seizure recurrence after a first unprovoked seizure. New England Journal of Medicine 307: 522–528

Holmes G L, McKeever M, Adamson M 1987 Absence seizures in children: Clinical and electroencephalographic features. Annals of Neurology 21: 268–273

Hopkins A, Garman A, Clarke C 1988 The first seizure in adult life. Lancet 1: 721–726

Howe J G, Gibson J D 1982 Uncinate seizures and tumors: A myth reexamined. Annals of Neurology 12: 227

Hrachovy R A 1982 Infantile spasms. In: Classification of the epilepsies: age related syndromic seizure types. State of the science in EEG and epilepsy. Annual meeting of the American EEG Society and the American Epilepsy Society, Phoenix

Janz D 1985 Epilepsy with impulsive petit mal (juvenile myoclonic epilepsy). Acta Neurologica Scandinavica 72: 449–459

Janz D, Christian W 1957 Impulsiv-Petit mal. Deutsche Zeitschrift fur Nervenheilkunde 176: 346–386

Kellaway P, Hrachovy R A, Frost J D, Zion T 1979 A precise characterization and quantification of infantile spasms. Annals of Neurology 6: 214–218

Kelly E C 1939 John Hughlings Jackson. Medical Classics 3: 915

Marsden C D, Hallett M, Fahn S 1982 The nosology and pathophysiology of myoclonus. In: Marsden C D, Fahn S (eds) Neurology 2: movement disorders. Butterworths, London, p 196–248

Mizrahi E M, Kellaway P 1987 Characterization and

classification of neonatal seizures. Neurology
37: 1837–1844

Niedermyer E 1976 Immediate transition from a petit mal
absence into a grand mal seizure: Case report. European
Neurology 14: 11–16

Oller-Daurella L 1974 The confusional states (absence
status). Acta Neurologica Belgica 74: 265–275

Penfield W, Jasper H 1954 Epilepsy and the functional
anatomy of the human brain. Little Brown, Boston

Penry J K, Dreifuss F E 1969 Automatisms associated with
the absence of petit mal epilepsy. Archives of Neurology
21: 142–149

Penry J K, Porter R J, Dreifuss F E 1975 Simultaneous
recording of absence seizures with video tape and
electroencephalography: A study of 374 seizures in 48
patients. Brain 98: 427–440

Plum F, Posner J B 1980 The diagnosis of stupor and coma,
3rd edn. F A Davis, Philadelphia

Porter R J 1986 Recognizing and classifying epileptic seizures
and epileptic syndromes. In: Porter R J, Theodore W H
(eds) Neurologic clinics: epilepsy. Saunders, Philadelphia

Porter R J 1989 Epilepsy: 100 elementary principles, 2nd
edn. Saunders, London

Porter R J 1990a Epilepsy: prevalence, classification,
diagnosis and prognosis. In Apuzzo M L J. Am Assoc of
Neurol Surgeons. (in press)

Porter R J 1990b Disorders of consciousness and associated
complex behaviors. In Devinsky, O. (in press)

Porter R J, Sato S 1982 Secondary generalization of epileptic
seizures. In: Akimoto H, Kazamatsuri H, Seino M, Ward Jr
A A (eds) Advances in epileptology: XIIIth epilepsy
international symposium. Raven Press, New York, p 47–48

Riikonen R 1982 A long-term follow-up study of 214 children
with the syndrome of infantile spasms. Neuropediatrics
13: 14–23

Sato S et al 1983 Long-term follow-up of absence seizures.
Neurology 33: 1590–1595

Spencer S S, Spencer D D, Williamson P D, Sass K, Novelly
R A & Mattson R H 1988 Corpus callosotomy for epilepsy:
seizure effects. Neurology 38: 19–24

Stefan H 1982 Epileptische Absencen: Studien zur
Anfallsstruktur, Pathophysiologie und zum klinischen
Verlauf. Thieme, Stuttgrat

Taylor J (ed) 1958 Selected writings of John Hughlings
Jackson, Vol 1: On epilepsy and epileptiform convulsions.
Hodder and Stoughton, London 1931; 1958 Reprint: Basic
Books, New York

Theodore W H, Porter R J, Penry J K 1983 Complex partial
seizures: Clinical characteristics and differential diagnosis.
Neurology 33: 1115–1121

Volpe J J 1981 Neurology of the newborn. W B Saunders,
Philadelphia

Weinberger J, Lusins J 1973 Simultaneous bilateral focal
seizures without loss of consciousness. Mount Sinai
Medical Journal 40: 693–696

Wolf P 1985 The classification of seizures and the epilepsies.
In: Porter R J, Morselli P L (eds) The epilepsies.
Butterworths, London, p 106–124

2. Epidemiology of epilepsy

W. A. Hauser   J. F. Annegers

INTRODUCTION

Over the past 50 years there has been an increasing appreciation of the value of epidemiological studies to enhance understanding of medical conditions. Before discussing the 'epidemiology' of epilepsy, it is first appropriate to define epidemiology. Unlike the clinician whose interest is the individual, the epidemiologist is interested in the study of the distribution of disease within the population.

Unfortunately, many clinicians still equate 'epidemiology' with the useful but rather mundane concept of prevalence, a measure basic to our perception of the current burden of the disease in the community, but of uncertain value otherwise. The applications of epidemiological techniques in the field of epilepsy have extended well beyond these simple 'nose counting' techniques. We have progressed beyond the descriptive studies necessary for hypothesis generation to a series of additional types of studies. These include but are not limited to 1. cohort and case control studies to identify risk factors for epilepsy and to estimate the effect of potential interventions, 2. longitudinal studies to determine the overall prognosis for seizure control and the identification of factors which may modify this prognosis, 3. co-morbidity studies to assess risk for other conditions in both the patient as well as in relatives, and 4. experimental studies which evaluate interventions including drug trials.

The current discussion will include a selective review summarizing recent descriptive studies of epilepsy, a review of factors associated (and not associated) with an increased risk for epilepsy, a brief review of epilepsy-related outcomes, many of which are covered in greater detail in other sections of this volume, and a review of other co-morbidity and mortality. A comprehensive review of most of the topics is available elsewhere (Hauser & Hesdorffer 1990a).

DEFINITIONS OF SEIZURES AND EPILEPSY FOR EPIDEMIOLOGICAL STUDIES

While all people with epilepsy experience seizures, not all individuals with seizures have epilepsy. Unfortunately, there has been wide variation in definitions of epilepsy used in epidemiological studies of epilepsy. To assure completeness, investigators generally start by identifying individuals with seizures of any type or, at times, individuals with alteration of consciousness for any reason. From, this group a subset with epilepsy is then identified. This strategy has been used in the population based studies of epilepsy in Rochester, Minnesota (Hauser et al 1991b) and we have provided some rationale for our classification in another publication (Annegers & Hauser 1984).

Once an individual has been identified as experiencing a seizure, the event can be categorized in one of the following mutually exclusive categories.

Acute symptomatic (or provoked) seizure

Included in this category are seizures which occur in close temporal association and as a direct consequence to an acute systemic, metabolic, or toxic insult or in association with an acute insult to the central nervous system and presumed to be an acute manifestation of the insult. The definition of 'close' varies with the nature of the insult. A unique subgroup of acute symptomatic seizures are those associated only with febrile illness. We have separately categorized cases in this latter group both because of the high frequency within the population (2–8% of children in some studies) and because of the unique age group in which these occur. This group is probably synonymous with those categorized as 'situation-related seizures and epilepsies' in the latest revision of the ILAE Classification of epilepsy and epileptic syndromes (Commission on Classification and Terminology 1989).

Unprovoked seizure

Included here is a seizure occurring without an identified proximate precipitant (although some may have experienced a 'remote' insult associated with an increased risk for epilepsy). This excludes seizures associated only with an acute insult to the central nervous system or a generalized systemic metabolic disturbance. We have again assigned cases into two mutually exclusive categories as follows.

Single unprovoked seizure

This category included individuals who are 'potential' patients with epilepsy. Such cases may have the social restrictions of an individual with epilepsy and may be receiving antiepileptic medication. These individuals may be appropriate for inclusion in aetiological studies.

Epilepsy

Epilepsy has been defined as a condition characterized by recurrent unprovoked seizures. There may be some debate as to what constitutes 'recurrent'. Studies have required at least two unprovoked seizures, others have required at least three (Hauser & Hesdorffer 1990a; Beran et al 1985).

Unfortunately some investigators have included all cases identified with seizures as 'epilepsy' or have provided inconsistent definitions. Acute symptomatic seizures as a group are the most frequently occurring single class of seizure and their

occurrence is associated with a distinctly different prognosis than of unprovoked seizure. Inclusion of such cases as epilepsy will clearly modify the apparent distribution of cases in descriptive studies and the apparent outcome in prognostic studies. In our own studies we have included as epilepsy only individuals who have experienced recurrent (two or more) unprovoked seizures and we shall try to provide comparisons with this group wherever possible.

Virtually all studies attempt to categorize cases by aetiology, although definitions are seldom provided, and in some studies categories are included which have not as yet been established as clear antecedents from an epidemiological standpoint. In general there has been some attempt to categorize cases by seizure type based upon one of the ILAE classifications (Commission on Classification and Terminology 1981).

DESCRIPTIVE STUDIES OF EPILEPSY

Three basic measures of disease frequency are used in descriptive studies of epilepsy and will be discussed: incidence, prevalence and cumulative incidence. Each measure has specific uses, but the clinical literature interchanges these measures and uses them incorrectly. For example, prevalence, useful only for determination of current health care needs, is frequently used in place of cumulative incidence or of incidence estimates of risk.

Incidence studies

Incidence is a measure of the frequency with which new cases of epilepsy occur in a population. To determine incidence, one ideally should identify individuals at the time of onset of an illness. From a practical standpoint, conditions such as epilepsy are seldom identified at the onset of symptoms, but only after a defined constellation of symptoms and signs are identified which allow a definitive diagnosis to be made. For a patient with epilepsy, the interval between onset and definitive diagnosis is, on the average, 2 years.

Incidence cohorts are of great value for several reasons. They are more representative of the spectrum of cases with epilepsy than prevalence cohorts because they include mild cases as well as cases who will die shortly after diagnosis. This allows evaluation of a wider spectrum of severity in the search for antecedents or the identification of factors which will influence course. As with most conditions, the closer the interval between onset of symptoms of epilepsy and case identification, the more reliably one can identify causal associations. Incidence cases are usually identified at an earlier point in the course of their illness, and thus a time closer to the occurrence of presumed aetiological factors. They are more likely to provide reliable information regarding potential antecedents.

Incidence studies require ongoing surveillance of a population of adequate size over a period of time sufficiently long to assure stable estimates of frequency. Because of this, incidence studies are expensive, and there are relatively few reports for total populations available in the literature. In many reports incidence data is available for selected age groups and these more detailed studies provide confirmation and further understanding of data from the total population.

Total population studies

In total population studies, defining epilepsy as recurrent unprovoked seizures, age adjusted incidence rates vary from 24 to 53 per 100 000 person years (Hauser & Kurland 1975, Brewis et al 1966, Granieri et al 1983, De Graaf 1974, Joensen 1986, Loiseau 1987). Studies which include individuals with either a single seizure or with recurrent unprovoked seizures provide somewhat higher estimates of incidence. Estimates range from 26 to 70 per 100 000 person years (Loiseau 1987, Gudmundsson 1966, Zielinski 1974a,b, Crombie et al 1960, Juul-Jensen & Foldspang 1983, Stanhope et al 1972). The higher estimates are similar to those from Rochester, Minnesota, where the comparable (combined) rate for isolated seizures and for epilepsy range from 72.2 to 86.1 per 100 000 patient years over the study period (Hauser & Kurland 1975). Given methodological differences, rates seem remarkably consistent across geographic areas.

There are a number of studies reporting incidence in populations defined by specific age groups. These are generally divided into studies dealing with children alone (Van den Berg & Yerushalamy 1969, Ellenberg et al 1984, Doose & Sitepu 1983, Benna et al 1984, Tsuhoi 1988, Shamansky & Glaser 1979), adults alone (Keranen et al 1989, Forsgren 1990), or in the elderly (Luhdorf et al 1986a). In general these provide information complementary to and consistent with the total population studies when age specific rates are evaluated.

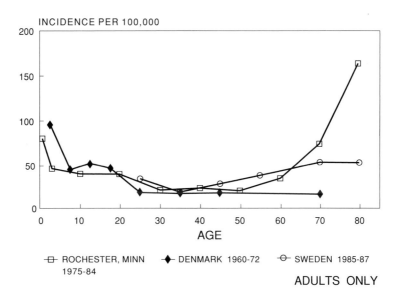

Fig. 2.1 Age-specific incidence of epilepsy in selected studies.

Age-specific incidence rates

Contrary to popular belief, epilepsy is a condition which affects all ages but with the highest incidence at the extremes of life (Fig. 2.1). Age-specific incidence rates are consistently high in the youngest age groups with highest rates occurring during the first few months of life, although most studies of children (Van den Berg & Yerushalamy 1969) include as epilepsy children with neonatal seizures and children with a single unprovoked seizure in their rates (for a review see Hauser & Nelson 1989). Incidence rates in the youngest age group in total population studies are in general similar to those reported in studies limited to children. Age-specific rates are consistently lowest during the adult years, and several recent studies show an increasing incidence—at times dramatic—in the elderly (Hauser & Kurland 1975, Zielinski 1974, Keranen et al 1989, Forsgren 1990, Luhdorf et al 1986a, Loiseau 1990a,b). In Rochester, Minnesota, the incidence rates for epilepsy are actually higher among people over age 70 than during the first 10 years of life (Hauser et al 1984a). In the community-based study in Rochester, only about 50% of cases of epilepsy start in childhood or the teen aged years. The importance of the elderly is stressed in a British study in which almost 25 % of newly identified seizures (not epilepsy) were accounted for by those age 60 and over (Sander et al 1990).

Gender

In all studies reporting gender-specific incidence rates for epilepsy or for first unprovoked seizure, the incidence is higher in males compared to females. Although the male/female ratio varies from 1.1 to 1.7, for most studies, these gender specific differences in incidence are not statistically significant and the differences are less marked if only 'idiopathic' seizures are considered. None the less, the consistency of this difference across studies suggests that males are at higher risk to develop unprovoked seizures.

Aetiology

Several total population studies provide incidence data by aetiology. Although virtually none of these studies define inclusion criteria for various categories of remote symptomatic epilepsy, the proportion of incidence cases with an identified antecedent is relatively consistent, ranging from 23% to 39% (Hauser & Kurland 1975, Brewis et al 1966, Granieri et al 1983, De Graaf 1974, Gudmundsson 1966). In the study of adults in Sweden, a presumed aetiology was identified in 50% (Forsgren 1990). In children epilepsy associated with neurological deficits from birth seems to be the most important single aetiology while cerebrovascular disease is the most commonly identified cause among adults (Sander et al 1990).

Seizure type

Incidence rates or proportions of incidence cases with specific seizure type based upon the International classification of Seizures (Hauser et al 1991b) are provided in three recent total population studies. In studies in Rochester, Minnesota (Hauser & Kurland 1975) based upon seizure description alone and in the Faroes (Joensen 1986) based upon seizure description and electroencephalographic findings, slightly more than 50% of cases were classified as partial. This contrasts with the findings in Copparo, Italy where, based upon seizure description alone, only 32% of cases were partial (Granieri et al 1983). In the study of adults from Sweden, 70% of cases experienced partial seizures. This is not inconsistent with the population data from Rochester in which about O of new cases of adult-onset epilepsy experienced partial seizures.

Race

Virtually all total population incidence studies have been performed in white populations of European extraction. Racial differences have been examined only in incidence or cohort studies in children. Rates for afebrile seizures did not differ by race through age 7 in the National Collaborative Perinatal Project (NCPP) (Nelson & Ellenberg 1986). Using similar definitions, age specific incidence rates in Tokyo through age 14 are similar to those in the predominantly Caucasian population of Rochester, Minnesota (Hauser & Kurland

1975, Tsuboi 1988). Only the incidence study performed in New Haven, Connecticut shows differences in incidence by race (Shamansky & Glaser 1979). Using referrals to electroencephalographic laboratories, the incidence of epilepsy through age 15 was 1.7 times greater in blacks than in whites. The study in New Haven is also the only incidence study to provide information on social class. Making comparisons based upon the mean socioeconomic level of the neighbourhood in which cases resided, rates are significantly higher in lower socioeconomic classes, even after controlling for race.

The incidence of epilepsy syndromes

There are many clinical series which, after thorough clinical evaluation, report the proportion of cases with specific epilepsy syndromes (Commission 1989). In contrast there is limited data on the incidence of specific epilepsy syndromes. The only total population study to provide data on the incidence of seizure syndromes is that from southwestern France (Loiseau et al 1990a,b) but this report fails to provide age adjustment or age specific rates for any specific syndrome.

The crude incidence for epilepsy was about 25/100 000, about half that in Rochester, Minnesota at the same time period. The incidence of idiopathic localization related epilepsy was 1.7/100 000 (7% of all cases). An additional 13.6/100 000 (56% of all cases) had symptomatic localization related epilepsy. Thus about 60% of cases would be classified as partial seizures by the criteria used in most other studies. About 1% had juvenile myoclonic epilepsy, and 1% awakening grand mal. About 1% had West syndrome and 2% had absence epilepsy. The rate of non-febrile situation rated epilepsy was about 30/100 000, a frequency of roughly twice that in Rochester. Isolated unprovoked seizures occurred at a rate of 18/100 000, similar to that in Rochester.

The incidence of specific epilepsy syndromes

West syndrome. There are a few reports of incidence of epilepsy syndromes in other studies. The incidence of West syndrome seems consistent across studies. In Rochester (Hauser et al 1991a) and in Iceland (Olafsson et al 1991) the incidence was about 3/10 000 live births. The overall incidence of West syndrome in the Faroes was 0.9/100 000 but a similar rate of 2–3/10 000 live births may be projected (Joensen 1986). The incidence in Japan was about 2.3/10 000 based upon the number of children examined at age 3 (Tsuboi 1988). The prevalence (in this situation presumably incidence in the first year of life and survivorship to age 1) in those age 1 and under in Oklahoma was 2.2/10 000 (Cowan 1989).

Lennox–Gastaut syndrome. In the incidence study in the Faroes, four individuals (2% of cases) were diagnosed as Lennox–Gastaut syndrome (Joensen 1986). Overall incidence was 0.9/100 000. Presumably, these cases did not have preceding West syndrome. In Japan, two cases of Lennox–Gastaut syndrome were identified—a frequency of 1.1/10 000 children (Tsuboi 1988). In Modena, Italy, 3.2% of cases in children had this diagnosis and the overall incidence was about 4/100 000 (Cavazzuti 1980). This is again probably comparable to the incidence in total population studies.

Severe myoclonic epilepsy of infancy (Dravet syndrome). Based upon one case identified in the NCPP (54 000 live births), and on five cases identified from clinics in west Texas, the cumulative risk through age 7 has been suggested to be about 1 in 40 000 (Hurst 1990).

Childhood and juvenile absence epilepsy. These two categories are reported as a combined group for Rochester and for the Faroes (Joensen 1986). The incidence of absence epilepsy in the Faroes was 0.7/100 000, and this diagnosis accounted for about 1.5% of cases. In Rochester, about 3% of all cases fell into this category and the incidence was 1.3/100 000. In Italy the combined incidence of 'simple' and 'complex' absence was 4.6/100 000. As in Rochester, all cases were identified in the first two decades, so this group comprises 10 to 15% of all incidence cases in children. Seven cases of absence epilepsy were identified in Tokyo for a cumulative risk of 4/100 000 through age 14. This frequency would probably be similar to that in the Faroes and in Rochester if converted to total population rates.

Juvenile myoclonic epilepsy. The incidence

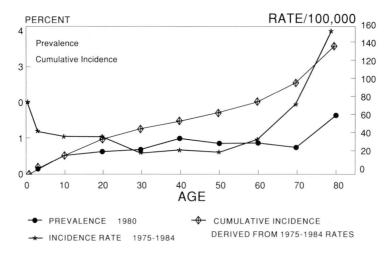

ROCHESTER, MINNESOTA

Fig. 2.2 Prevalence, cumulative incidence and incidence rates of epilepsy.

of JME in the Faroes was 1.1/100 000 per year and this syndrome accounted for about 2.5% of cases. This seems greater than that reported from Bordeaux (0.2/100 000) but numbers are small in both series so wide variation may be expected.

Idiopathic localization related epilepsies. Data is available only for benign rolandic epilepsy. This syndrome comprised about 24% of cases of epilepsy in children between age 4 and 15 in an Italian study (Cavazzuti 1980).

Time trends

Information on time trends is provided only in the studies from Copparo and Rochester, Minnesota (Hauser & Kurland 1975, Granieri et al 1983). In the former study, decreasing rates over three time intervals from 1964 to 1978 may be related to less complete case ascertainment in the later years. This is accounted for by the interval between onset of seizures and diagnosis. The Minnesota study shows stable rates of overall incidence from 1935 to 1979, although a significant fall in the incidence of epilepsy over time in those under age 10 is counter-balanced by an increasing incidence of epilepsy in those over age 60 over the same time interval. In this latter study, the incidence in those over age 60 was higher than the incidence in the first 10 years of life. When an aetiology was

identified, the most frequent antecedent was cerebrovascular disease, but no clear aetiology was identified in almost 50% of cases in this age group (Hauser et al 1984a).

Cumulative incidence

The cumulative incidence is the risk of developing epilepsy by a specific age or over a specific period of time. Epidemiological studies have thus far failed to identify any substantial increase in mortality in epilepsy cohorts, and the cumulative incidence at any age should be a close approximation to the prevalence of a history of epilepsy. Cumulative incidence is the appropriate comparison measure of expected frequency of illness studies of familial aggregation.

The cumulative incidence of epilepsy was determined in two total population studies. The risk of developing epilepsy through age 80 was 1.3% in Denmark (Juul-Jensen & Foldspang 1983). The cumulative incidence of epilepsy for ages 8–80 in Rochester was more than 4% and more than 5% for all unprovoked seizures (Hauser & Annegers 1988). The difference in these two studies is explained by the considerably higher age-specific incidence in the elderly in the Minnesota study. As would be expected from the age-specific incidences rates, cumulative incidences of epilepsy in Japan and in Rochester are almost identical.

Studies of the prevalence of epilepsy

Prevalence is the proportion of individuals within a population affected with a disease at a particular point in time. For epilepsy, prevalence at a minimum should include individuals who have had a diagnosis of epilepsy and who at the time of prevalence determination are having seizures or who require limitations of activity because of the condition (usually by virtue of use of antiepileptic medication). In our own studies prevalence by this definition has been termed 'active prevalence'. 'Life time prevalence' includes all individuals identified with a history of epilepsy at any time, a measure obviously biased by recall. As with all studies of epilepsy, one needs to pay attention to definitions (if provided). In many studies, individuals with single seizures or with provoked seizures are included as prevalence cases.

Because of the relative ease in obtaining information about prevalence compared to incidence, many prevalence studies of epilepsy from diverse populations have been reported. Comparison of prevalence may allow rough estimates of the relative frequency of an illness across populations which vary by race, geographic area and socioeconomic status, but such comparisons must be made with caution. In general, variation in rates can be attributed more to differences in the method of case identification than differences associated with biological factors.

Prevalence represents a complex interaction among obvious factors such as incidence, death, or remission of illness. Prevalence may also be affected by less obvious factors such as selective in or out migration from a community or selective drop out from medical care. Prevalence is as much a reflection of survivorship and severity or chronicity of illness as it is of frequency. The study of prevalence cases will give little information regarding aetiology or prognosis and is of value primarily for health planning purposes.

Prevalence in total population surveys

Age-adjusted prevalence per 1000 population varies widely, from 2.7 to more than 40, although for most studies the range is from 4 to 8 per 1000 (Hauser & Hesdorffer 1990a, Hauser & Kurland 1975, Osuntokun et al 1982). Even when the same investigators have used similar protocols, definitions of epilepsy, and methodologies, the prevalence of 'active' epilepsy ranges from a low of 3.6 to a high of 41.3 (Osuntokun et al 1982, Bharucha 1988). The differences are related to changes in definitions of 'active prevalence'.

The majority of point prevalence rates range from 4 to 8 per 1000 population (Hauser & Kurland 1975, Granieri et al 1983, Joensen 1986, Stanhope et al 1972, Maremmani 1991, Gudmundsson 1966, Osuntokun et al 1987, Haerer et al 1986, Zielinski 1974 a,b, Goodridge & Shorvon 1983). Somewhat higher rates (ranging from 14 to 57 per 1000) have been observed in pilot studies using a standardized WHO protocol in Panama, Ecuador, Columbia, and Venezuela (Gracia et al 1990, Cruz et al 1985, Ponce Ducharne 1986, Pradilla-Ardila et al 1984). On the other hand, using the same protocol in large scale population surveys yielded low prevalence rates in India (Bharucha 1988, Koul et al 1988) and in China (Li et al 1985).

The high prevalence reported in central and south America may be a reflection of the pilot methodology. Prevalence rates in rural Ecuador using the ICEBERG protocol (8.6/1000) were lower than those reported in a pilot study by investigators in the same country using the WHO protocol (Placencia 1989). The latter prevalence estimates may be more realistic since case verification methodology was more stringent and the population studied was considerably larger. A recent population survey in a village in rural Mexico also revealed a prevalence of active epilepsy of 5.9/1000 age-adjusted to the 1980 US population (Hauser et al 1990a).

As with the study of incidence, there are a number of studies providing information on prevalence within specific age groups (Cowan et al 1989, Cavazzuti 1980, Tsuboi 1988, Keranen et al 1989). Many were performed in association with incidence studies. As with the incidence studies, prevalence in selected age groups is consistent with age-specific prevalence reported from total population studies.

Age-specific prevalence

Epilepsy is a condition which is acquired through-out life but the patterns of age-specific prevalence seem not to reflect this pattern. In Rochester, Minnesota, after 1940, there is a consistent pattern of increasing prevalence in each subsequent age group with highest prevalence in the elderly (Hauser et al 1991b). Most other studies report the highest prevalence in the second and third decades of life, with lower rates in the elderly, although several recent studies from European countries and the Faroes report a relatively constant prevalence in the adult age group after the teenage years (Fig. 2.2). In many cases age-specific estimates are unstable because of small numbers within age groups (Joensen 1986, Keranen et al 1989, Wagner 1983).

Several prevalence studies have been performed in selected age groups. Studies reporting the active prevalence of recurrent unprovoked seizures in Italian children using school children as an opportunistic sample report prevalence rates generally ranging from 4 to 5/1000 (Cavazzuti 1980, Pisani 1987). Higher rates were reported (6 to 9/1000) in Kentucky which also screened the institutionalized population (Bauman et al 1977, 1978). Medical record studies of children under age 15 in Tokyo (Tsuboi 1988) and to age 20 in Oklahoma (Cowan et al 1989) report prevalence rates of about 4.7.

As with the general prevalence studies, the prevalence of epilepsy in children is reported to be considerably higher in studies from South America. The (presumably active) prevalence of epilepsy through age 20 in Bogota was 2% (Gomez et al 1978) and in Chile, 2.1% (Chiofalo 1979). A prevalence of 1.8% was reported among children in Mexico (Garcia-Pedroza et al 1983).

European studies of adult patients tend to report somewhat higher prevalence than the studies of children, ranging from 4.3 to 7.6.

While it is possible that the differences in age-specific prevalence in the oldest age groups in Rochester when compared with other studies, particularly those from Asia, Africa, South America and Mexico, are explained by under reporting of cases in the elderly in these other communities, it is also possible that the causes of epilepsy in the adult in the United States and Europe either do not exist or are fatal in these less industrialized countries. The differences in age-specific patterns of incidence and of prevalence remain an intriguing problem.

Gender

As is the case with incidence studies, most studies of prevalence report a higher prevalence in males compared to females. The studies at variance to this are from Nigeria and from the pilot study in rural Ecuador. Studies in Norway and in Iceland report equal prevalence in males and females despite a higher incidence in males in both studies. The largest discrepancy in gender-specific prevalence seems to be in studies from Asia. Prevalence in Rochester, Minnesota, in 1980 is higher in females than males, but this was a deviation from data from other prevalence studies. In general the prevalence data suggest a higher risk for epilepsy or at least better identification of epilepsy in males.

Aetiology

As with incidence cases, when aetiological categorization is provided, most prevalence studies fail to provide definitions for inclusion into aetiological categories. For all total population studies providing information, the majority of cases (55–89%) are idiopathic, with most studies reporting rates ranging around 65% (Hauser & Kurland 1975, Stanhope et al 1972, Gudmundsson 1966, Granieri et al 1983, Osuntokun et al 1987, Haerer et al 1986). In studies reporting both incidence and prevalence, the proportion of cases categorized as idiopathic and as remote symptomatic is similar for both measures (Hauser & Kurland 1975, Granieri et al 1983). There seems to be little variation in the proportion of cases with an identified aetiology in studies dealing with adults when compared with children.

In some prevalence studies, the difference by gender was accounted for by a higher prevalence of remote symptomatic epilepsy among males (Haerer et al 1986, Keranen et al 1989). This was not the case in Rochester where the prevalence of idiopathic and remote symptomatic epilepsy were similar in males and females. In this study approximately 75% of prevalence cases were idiopathic. Epilepsy attributable to cerebrovascular disease was the most important single identified aetiology of epilepsy, accounting for 8% of prevalence cases. This was followed by epilepsy associated with neurological deficits from birth (mental retardation or cerebral palsy) and accounted for 5% of all cases. It could be argued that most of these cases have epilepsy of unknown aetiology from an epidemiological standpoint. Cerebrovascular disease was the most frequently identified aetiology in the elderly. Neurological deficit from birth was the most frequently identified cause in children, while head injury and infection of the central nervous system were most frequently identified as the cause in the middle aged adult age group.

Seizure type

As with incidence, most total population studies of prevalence report the majority of patients to have partial seizures. In studies of specific age groups, studies in children tend to show a predominance of generalized seizures (Cowan et al 1989, Tsuboi 1988). The exception to this observation is the study of Otohara which also includes single seizures. Studies limited to adults tend to report an excess of partial seizures. The studies in Rochester note that 60% of prevalence cases in 1980 had partial seizures. Consistent with the age-limited studies, generalized onset seizures were the most frequent seizure type in young children, the ratio between generalized and partial seizures was about 50/50 in adults while partial seizures were considerably more frequent in the elderly.

Prevalence of epilepsy syndromes

The prevalence of seizure syndromes may be less important than the incidence. As with the incidence studies, there is limited data available on this topic. The prevalence of West syndrome in studies limited to children was 1.4 and 1.9/10 000 in the studies of Otohara et al (1981) and Cowan et al (1989) respectively. In total population studies, the prevalence was 2/200 000 in Coporro

(Granieri et al 1983) and 9/100 000 in the Faroes (Joensen 1986).

Lennox–Gastaut syndrome prevalence was 3/10 000 in the childhood study of Otohara et al (1981) and 1.3/10 000 in the study of Cowan (1989). This compares with a prevalence of 6/100 000 and 2/100 000 in Coporro (Granieri et al 1983) and in the Faroes (Joensen 1986) respectively. The prevalence of idiopathic localization related epilepsy was 2.4/10 000 (accounting for 4% of all cases) in Coporro (Granieri et al 1983) and accounted for 8% of all cases (4/10 000 population) in Tuscany (Maremmani 1991), although this amounted to 24% of cases in children. The prevalence of JME is available only from the study in the Faroes and was 3/10 000. This syndrome accounted for about 2.5% of prevalence cases. Presumably no cases were identified in Coporro or Tuscany.

Race

There are few prevalence studies in which racial differences can be compared directly. Preliminary reports from studies of inner city Black communities provide prevalence estimates of 12 to 14 per 1000 (Hauser et al 1986b, Lampert et al 1984). In their studies, the age-specific prevalence in children was similar to that found in Caucasian communities in which similar definitions were used, but age-specific prevalence was considerably higher in Blacks than Caucasians in the 20–59-year-old age group. In prevalence studies in the United States in which more than one racial group has been evaluted at the same time and using the same methodology, the prevalence of epilepsy has been higher in Blacks than Whites (Cowan 1989, Haerer et al 1986, Hollingsworth 1978) or in Hispanics (Lampert et al 1984).

Race is invariably tied to geographic area, but even when the same protocol is used (such as studies using the WHO neurological disease protocol) it is difficult to make comparisons because of variation in methodology. Further, cultural issues may be associated with differential completeness of patient identification within age groups, or for the total population. In countries such as China or India (where epilepsy continues to have considerable stigma attached impinging upon educational and marital opportunities), there may be considerable denial of illness leading to substantial underreporting in general or within specific age groups (Lai 1990). Even in areas where less social stigma is perceived, there is considerable denial of illness. At face value, these studies are consistent with a prevalence of epilepsy which is high in Native American Indians of South America and in Blacks in the United States and in Africa. Prevalence rates are intermediate in Caucasian populations studied in the United States and in Europe, and low in Asians based upon studies in China and in India. In Japan, total population studies report an exceedingly low prevalence although the incidence and prevalence study of children reported by Tsuboi demonstrates incidence and prevalence similar to that in the United States and Europe.

Racial studies of the incidence or prevalence of epilepsy in minority populations are inexorably confounded by socioeconomic status. There are few studies which attempt to address the relationship of socioeconomic status and the prevalence of epilepsy. In Ecuador, the prevalence of epilepsy was inversely correlated with community ranking by socioeconomic class (Placencia 1989). Unfortunately, it is not clear whether low socioeconomic class is a risk factor for or the consequence of epilepsy. While the prevalence cases of epilepsy identified in the general practice survey of Pond tented to be of lower socioeconomic standing than the study population, the socioeconomic standing was also lower than that of siblings of those with epilepsy suggesting that low socioeconomic status was a consequence rather than a risk factor for epilepsy (Pond et al 1960). In Bogota, the prevalence of epilepsy in children was higher in lower socioeconomic classes (Gomez et al 1978). In the United States, studies in prison populations and in inner city populations have identified a high prevalence of epilepsy, but the findings are confounded by race (Whitman et al 1984).

Time trends

Three studies provide data at independent points in time (Gudmundsson 1966, Maremmani 1991, Hauser & Kurland 1975). The studies in Italy and in Iceland cover only a brief period of time and show some slight reduction in prevalence— probably related to incomplete identification. In Rochester, prevalence steadily increases, more than doubling over a 40-year period. The increase was attributed to more complete case ascertainment in the latter years of the study rather than any substantial change in prevalence.

RISK FACTORS FOR EPILEPSY

One of the main objectives of epidemiology is to identify causative factors in order to develop preventive strategies, either for the disease itself (primary prevention), or for the consequences of the disease (secondary prevention). To accomplish these ends one must understand who is at risk for the illness and what factors seem to increase this risk.

Types of causal associations

The number of analytic studies of aetiological factors of epilepsy are few when compared with those available for conditions such as cancer or cardiac disease, and our knowledge of potential risk factors is less exhaustive. None the less, from the standpoint of causation, several levels of association have been identified. There are factors such as head injury or infection of the central nervous system for which a clear and substantial increase in risk for epilepsy has been established and for which it is biologically plausible to assume a direct causal relationship. At this same level, but possibly more important, have been studies of factors suspected to increase the risk for epilepsy (such as immunization or of adverse pre and perinatal events) which *fail* to demonstrate causal associations despite adequate power.

At another level, there are factors such as febrile seizures or the presence of a neurological handicap at birth (mental retardation or cerebral palsy) which are also clearly associated with an increased risk for epilepsy but for which the association is best explained by common (but frequently unidentified) antecedents. Factors such as asthma or hypertension have been associated with an increased risk for epilepsy in exploratory studies but have no ready explanation based upon current biological theory.

Epidemiological measures of risk or association

In epidemiological studies, the level of risk (or protection) imparted by a particular exposure (or disease) is measured as the ratio of the frequency of the exposure in question (such as epilepsy) among those exposed to that in those unexposed. Of necessity, the determination of these 'risk ratios' requires a comparison population. A risk ratio of 1 implies no association. Ratios greater than 1 suggest a causal association while ratios less than 1 suggest a protective effect. While epidemiologists consider risk ratios of 3 to 4 to be substantial, most of the aetiologies identified in clinical studies of epilepsy and considered to be causal carry relative risks of 5 to 20. On the other hand, some factors frequently assumed by clinicians to be important in the development of epilepsy have not been established as risk factors in rigorous epidemiological studies.

Postnatally acquired brain insults

There are a number of insults to the central nervous system which are associated with an increased risk for epilepsy in survivors. A summary of the increase in risk above that expected in the general or non-exposed population (relative risk) for many of those conditions is presented in Figure 2.3. For all of these conditions, the risk for epilepsy is highest shortly after the occurrence of

the insult, although for most, the risk for epilepsy remains elevated for many years after the insult.

Cranio-cerebral trauma

The age-specific incidence of head injury with brain involvement has a trimodal pattern, with a peak in young children, a second peak in the teenager and young adult, and a third peak in the elderly (Annegers et al 1980b, Cooper et al 1983). Males are affected almost twice as frequently as females. All head injury with evidence of brain involvement is associated with a 3-fold increase in risk for epilepsy. This risk increases with severity of injury (Annegers et al 1980a). There is no detectable increase in risk for individuals with mild head injury (amnesia or loss of consciousness of less than half an hour). The risk is elevated about 5-fold for individuals with moderate head injury (loss of consciousness from 30 minutes up to 24 hours), although this risk is probably not increased beyond the first 5 years following the injury. Among the survivors of severe head injuries in civilian populations (intracranial mass lesions and/or unconsciousness more than 24 hours) approximately 10% will develop epilepsy, a risk 20–30 times that expected in the general population. Roughly 50% of survivors of penetrating military head injuries will develop epilepsy (Salazar et al 1985). In this severely head-injured group, risk continues to be elevated 15 to 20 years following the injury.

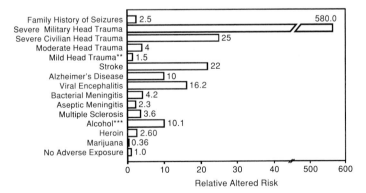

Fig. 2.3 Factors associated with an altered risk for epilepsy relative to people without these adverse exposures. **Not statistically significant. ***One pint of 80° proof alcohol, 2.5 bottles of wine. Reproduced with permission from Hauser & Hesdorffer 1990b. © 1990 Epilepsy Foundation of America.

There are factors which seem to increase the risk for subsequent epilepsy within the brain injured group. In the military studies metal fragments increased the risk. Approximately 3–5% of brain injured individuals will experience one or more seizures at the time of the head injury (early or acute symptomatic seizures) (Annegers et al 1980a, Salazar et al 1985). For brain injured adults but not children, these early seizures also are a risk factor for subsequent epilepsy (Annegers et al 1980a).

Cerebrovascular disease

The incidence of cerebrovascular disease increases with advancing age and in those over age 80 more than 1% of the population previously free of stroke will suffer a cerebrovascular insult annually. Individuals with cerebrovascular disease have a 20-fold increase in risk to develop epilepsy. About 15% of individuals will experience unprovoked seizures within 5 years following a first clinically identified cerebrovascular insult (Hauser et al 1984b, Olsen et al 1987, Viitanen et al 1988). As with severe head injury, the risk of epilepsy remains significantly elevated for at least 20 years following the insult. As might be expected, cerebrovascular insults involving the brain stem have not shown an association with epilepsy. Early seizures, which occur in 5–10% of patients with a stroke, are associated with a further increase in risk within the stroke group. It is possible that unsuspected cerbrovascular disease is associated with some of the 'idiopathic' epilepsy in the elderly. In a case control study, newly diagnosed adults with epilepsy were more likely to have evidence of lesions on computerized axial tomography (CT) examination than a control group (Roberts et al 1988) and a case control study of newly identified people with stroke demonstrated an increased frequency of prior epilepsy (Shinton et al 1987).

Central nervous system infections

The incidence of central nervous system infections is highest in children although a second peak in incidence is noted in the elderly (Nicolosi et al 1986). In the first decade of life, approximately 1% of children can be expected to have experienced an infection of the CNS. Survivors of an infection of the CNS have a 3-fold increase in risk for epilepsy (Annegers et al 1988). This risk is independent of age at infection but does vary by type of infection. There is no discernible increase in risk for epilepsy for those with aseptic meningitis. For those with bacterial meningitis, the risk is increased about 5-fold although most of this risk occurs in the first 2 years following the infection. Increased risk may be limited to the first 5 years following the infection. For those with a viral encephalitis, the risk is increased 10-fold and this increased risk persists at least 15 years following the infection.

As with head trauma and stroke, about 5% of individuals will have seizures at the time of the CNS infections. The occurrence of acute symptomatic seizures during the infection is associated with an additional increase in risk for epilepsy.

Brain tumours

A newly identified seizure disorder, particularly among adults, invariably raises a concern about a brain tumour as a potential causal mechanism. About 30% of patients with brain tumours will present with seizures as an initial symptom (Foy et al 1981, Franceschetti 1988). Brain tumours as an assigned aetiology account for a substantial proportion of individuals included in epilepsy case series in the elderly, but as yet there is no quantification of risk (Dam et al 1985, Roberts et al 1982, Luhdorf et al 1986b). For most individuals with seizures caused by a primary central nervous system neoplasm, the diagnosis will be made at the time of first evaluation for the seizures. These seizures may be more appropriately categorized as acute symptomatic since the lesion is presumably progressive and the appropriate therapy relates to removal of the neoplasm. For tumours of glial origin, subsequent seizures are frequently related to recurrence or expansion of the original lesion and as such are again not truly unprovoked. Only a small proportion of cases will have subsequent seizures which can truly be construed as unprovoked.

More difficult to categorize are cases in which cerebral neoplasms are identified in individuals with longstanding epilepsy. Prior to the availability of CT or of magnetic resonance imaging (MRI), case series of patients undergoing surgery for intractable epilepsy reported unsuspected neoplasms to be identified at surgery in 15–45% of patients (Blume et al 1982, Spenser et al 1984, Mathieson 1975). In historical cohort studies cases which may have been considered 'idiopathic' at diagnosis are generally categorized as related to the neoplasm. Even so, clinically manifest brain tumours account for only a small proportion of all epilepsy in epidemiological studies, even in the elderly.

Degenerative diseases of the central nervous system

In children primary degenerative disease of the central nervous system are frequently inherited as a Mendelian trait and are associated with seizures in a high proportion of cases. Such cases account for only a small proportion of cases with epilepsy. The incidence of other 'degenerative conditions' of the central nervous system increases with advancing age, and may account for a substantial proportion of the cases with epilepsy. The most frequent of these conditions, Alzheimer disease, affects 1–2% of the population over age 60 and the incidence increases with advancing age (Sayetta 1986, Kokmen et al 1988, Evans et al 1989). It is associated with a 10-fold increase in risk for epilepsy (Hauser et al 1986a, Romanelli et al 1990). By 10 years following diagnosis, roughly 10% of survivors will have provoked seizures.

Based upon findings of animal experiments, it has been suggested that Parkinson's disease may be associated with an improvement in control of seizures in those with epilepsy who develop the disease and may be protective for the development of epilepsy in those previously seizure free. This hypothesis has been confirmed in epidemiological studies of epilepsy and in fact a modest (but not significant) increase in risk for epilepsy in patients with Parkinson disease has been identified.

Individuals with demyelinating disease appear to be at increased risk for epilepsy. In clinical series, up to 5% of patients with multiple sclerosis are reported to have seizures or epilepsy—at least a 10-fold increase over that expected. In the only study quantifying risk, epilepsy occurred at the time of or following the diagnosis of multiple sclerosis in 1.8% of patients, a risk 3.4 times that expected (Kinnunen & Wikstrom 1986).

Alcohol

Rougly 10% of the adult population can be considered to drink heavily, based upon volume and frequency criteria (Hauser 1990). While debate continues as to the relationship of alcohol use and abuse and brain degeneration, individuals who drink heavily on a chronic basis not only have risk for seizures with abrupt reduction or discontinuation of alcohol ingestion (withdrawal seizures), but they also have a 3-fold increased risk for epilepsy (Ng et al 1988). A threshold effect for alcohol use has been identified. There is no increase in risk for seizures in those who drink less than 50 grams of alcohol daily (about two drinks). The risk increases with increasing daily alcohol intake. For those who drink 300 grams of alcohol or more daily, the risk is increased more than 20-fold.

Family history

Familial aggregation is consistent with both a common environmental exposures as well as a genetic tendency for epilepsy. The genetics of epilepsy is discussed elsewhere in this volume. If looked upon as an epidemiological risk factor, siblings of patients with epilepsy are at a 2.5-fold increased risk to develop epilepsy, and the risk may be somewhat higher in offspring (Annegers et al 1982, Beck-Mannagetta et al 1989, Hauser & Anderson 1986, Jimenez 1989).

Factors associated with, but not necessarily causal for, the development of epilepsy

Mental retardation and cerebral palsy

The association between neurological handicaps presumed present from birth, as manifest by some individuals with mental retardation (MR) and cerebral palsy (CP), is well recognized. Approximately 3–6/1000 live births will be affected with CP or moderate or severe MR, and one-third of those affected will subsequently develop epilepsy. While CP has been demonstrated to occur with an increased frequency with some adverse perinatal events, by far the majority of these cases occur in individuals with no identified risk factors. Thus these conditions, as is the case with epilepsy, are in most situations 'idiopathic'.

In the National Collaborative Perinatal Project (a cohort of more than 50 000 births followed prospectively to their seventh birthday), epilepsy occurred in 33% of those with motor handicaps (Nelson & Ellenberg 1986). Conversely, CP was present in 19% of children with epilepsy.

In a study of the frequency of seizures and epilepsy at a referral centre for the developmentally disabled (but not epilepsy) in the Bronx (New York), the frequency of epilepsy was evaluated separately in those with MR alone, with CP alone, and when both conditions coexisted (Benedetti et al 1991). In those with moderate (IQ 50–70) or severe (IQ<50) mental retardation but without motor handicap, about 10% had developed epilepsy. Similarly, in those with cerebral palsy alone but with IQ above 70, about 10% developed epilepsy. While these proportions represent a substantial increase over that expected in the general population (10-fold or more), it was considerably less than the proportion with epilepsy among children with both MR and CP (50%). Studies from a Kaiser-Permanente birth cohort followed in Oakland also reported a higher frequency of epilepsy in children with MR and CP than in children with either condition alone. Epilepsy developed in 32% of children diagnosed as having CP, 29% of children with MR (not defined) and in 50% of children with both conditions (Van den Berg & Yerushalamy 1969). The risk for epilepsy in these children with neurological handicaps presumed present from birth is highest in the first few years of life, but the risk remains elevated at least through the second decade of life (Goulden 1991).

Neither CP nor MR are causal for epilepsy, but both should be considered 'markers' for underlying brain abnormalities which are responsible for both the neurological handicap and the epilepsy. For both conditions, the majority of cases have no readily identifiable aetiology, and as yet little insight in either the basic mechanisms or preventative strategies for epilepsy is provided by the MR/CP group.

Febrile seizures

Because of the increased risk for epilepsy in individuals who have experienced febrile seizures this condition is frequently assumed to be a cause of epilepsy. Depending upon clinical features, cohort studies have identified an increased risk over that expected in the general population ranging from less than 3 to 50 (Annegers et al 1987). Case control studies have identified febrile seizures as a risk factor for all forms of epilepsy (Rocca et al 1987a,b,c). As with MR and CP, febrile convulsions and epilepsy should be considered independent outcomes of a common antecedent.

When type of epilepsy is assessed (generalized versus partial onset), different predictors emerge (Annegers et al 1987). For those who develop generalized onset epilepsy after febrile convulsions, genetic factors are the major predictors of increased risk (Rich et al 1987). Conversely, for those who develop partial epilepsy following febrile convulsions, there is usually evidence of localized brain dysfunction at the time of the first febrile seizure. While it is possible that prolonged febrile seizures can lead to neuronal damage or death with residual Ammon's Horn sclerosis (Falconer 1971), such prolonged events are exceedingly rare in the general population (less than 0.5% of all febrile seizures). For most cases of complex partial epilepsy following febrile seizures, it is likely that brain pathology antedated both conditions.

Risk factors with no established or suspected mechanism

Exploratory epidemiological studies have identified a number of other factors associated with an increased risk for the development of epilepsy. For many of these, the causal sequence and underlying mechanism are not identified. Drug abuse, specifically heroin abuse, is associated with a 3-fold increase in risk for epilepsy (Ng et al 1990). A history of asthma may carry an increased risk for epilepsy independent of that associated with acute attacks and or medication (Ng et al 1985). Hypertension, independent of cerebrovascular disease, may be associated with an increased risk for epilepsy. Age alone appears to increase the risk for epilepsy independent of factors such as head trauma, cerebrovascular disease, or factors such as drug or alcohol abuse. Whether this represents an effect of aging alone or the accumulated effect of repeated exposure to environmental insults which in themselves would not increase the risk for epilepsy remains to be clarified. A maternal history of mental retardation, a maternal history of seizures during the pregnancy, and the presence of central nervous system congenital malformations are also associated with an increased risk for epilepsy.

Factors frequently assumed to be causal for the development of epilepsy which lack substantiation in epidemiological studies

Adverse pre- and perinatal events

There is a general perception that adverse pre- and perinatal events are associated with an increased risk for epilepsy. Most clinical series include cases of epilepsy ascribed to a variety of events occurring during pregnancy or at the time of delivery. While an association seems inherently plausible, recent epidemiological studies fail to confirm an association of such events with epilepsy after controlling for cerebral palsy (Nelson & Ellenberg 1984, Rocca et al 1987a,b,c) (Fig. 2.4). The erroneous assumptions of causality probably stem from the association of some of these factors with cerebral palsy and the high frequency of epilepsy.

Immunization

There has been considerable concern regarding the risk of encephalopathy and the subsequent development of epilepsy, following immunization. While postvaccination encephalopathies have been reported for virtually all vaccines, pertussis vaccine has come under particular scrutiny as an antecedent of some of the more severe childhood epileptic syndromes (Stewart 1977). In Great Britain, concern became so widespread that the childhood immunization programmes were severely curtailed. Less than 70% of children received pertussis vaccine in the late 1970s resulting in epidemics of pertussis (Griffith 1989). Concurrent product liability litigation has brought vaccine manufacture to a standstill in the United States.

To address the question of childhood encephalopathy and the role of pertussis immunization specifically, a nationwide case control study of children with acute neurological syndromes was initiated in Great British in 1976 and follow-up of affected children was instituted (Miller et al 1981, 1982). When all cases of acute encephalopathy, including those associated with viral encephalitis and Reye's syndrome were compared, the investigators found an increased risk for an acute neurological syndrome (but not necessarily seizures) within the week following pertussis immunization. They estimated an excess above base rates of about 1/100 000 vaccinations, but less than 1 in 300 000 vaccinations in children felt to be

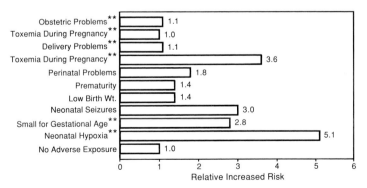

Fig. 2.4 Perinatal factors possibly associated with an increased risk of epilepsy relative to people without these adverse exposures **Not statistically significant. Reproduced with permission from Hauser & Hesdorffer 1990b. © Epilepsy Foundation of America.

previously normal. This study has been subject to inordinate scrutiny and the conclusions challenged on both clinical and epidemiological grounds. Two of the 11 children died, nine had 'developmental delay' at 1 year following the brain syndrome, but only one was handicapped at last follow-up. No recognizable syndrome could be identified and none had late epilepsy. When cases were examined from a clinical standpoint, a ready explanation for the clinical picture independent of the immunization was apparent in most cases (Ross & Miller 1986). If these cases are excluded from case and control series, no identifiable increase in risk for encephalopathy could be identified.

Several recent studies have specifically addressed the role of pertussis immunization and the subsequent development of seizures. In a study of the relationship between immunization and seizures among births to a Health Maintenance Organization in Seattle (Walker 1988), an increased risk for a febrile seizure within 1 month of the immunization was identified, but there was no increase in risk for unprovoked seizures. A retrospective study among two Danish cohorts characterized by different timing of immunization and different strength of vaccine was undertaken to evaluate timing of onset of febrile and afebrile seizures (Shields et al 1988). No relationship between vaccination schedule and the onset of epilepsy was identified, although the age of onset of first febrile seizure was significantly different. No association could be identified in a study of medicaid recipients in Tennessee (Griffin et al 1989). These studies suggest that the incidence and timing of unprovoked seizures is unaffected by vaccination. If such a phenomenon does exist, the frequency can be no more than one in several million. Adequate power to detect a causal association as rare as this would require a study of all births in the United States for several years.

The incidence of febrile seizures is also unaffected, although there may be a shift in the timing of first febrile seizure associated with immunization. Pertussis vaccine is a pyrogen, and many children develop a low grade fever in the first 24 hours after immunization, usually within 2–7 hours (Griffith 1974). Thus the fever may trigger a febrile seizure in a susceptible child as NCPP data suggest (Hirtz et al 1983).

In a Nigerian case control study a history of vaccination was found to be protective for epilepsy (Ogunniyi 1987). This most likely reflects educational and possibly socioeconomic factors associated with immunization status in developing countries.

PROGNOSIS OF PATIENTS WITH EPILEPSY

Prognosis may cover a number of concepts. The clinician dealing with the patient is interested in prognosis for seizure control since this is the most obvious basis for assessing success or failure. There are a number of additional areas which become important topics for prognosis. This includes mortality, co-morbidity for other disease, and intellectual and social function.

Prognosis for seizure control

It is generally understood today that the prognosis for most people with epilepsy is excellent in terms of expected seizure control, remission, and medication withdrawal. This represents a major departure from attitudes in the past, and the change is largely related to epidemiological studies undertaken in the past two decades. It is important that we understand the natural history of epilepsy to better evaluate the role of interventions and to target specific groups for more aggressive therapy. Studies of prognosis are reviewed in other sections of this book so the review here will not be exhaustive and will primarily address the epidemiological aspects of the question.

There are several times in the clinical course of epilepsy at which estimates of ultimate prognosis may be attempted. These include the time of the first seizure, the time of the first diagnosis of epilepsy, the time of achieving seizure control, and on attempt at medication withdrawal after seizure control. These estimates of overall remission and the identification of factors associated with altered likelihood of remission are invariably based upon prior probability and therefore cannot be applied with certainty to an individual patient. The studies provide estimates of the frequency of remission of epilepsy in groups defined by specific clinical characteristics. Even though these characteristics are at times inexactly defined, there is some consistency in the predictors of remission. Obviously, inconsistent definition of these variables may preclude direct comparisons across studies.

Likelihood of remission from the time of the first seizure

Epilepsy is defined as a condition in which there is a tendency to experience recurrent unprovoked seizures. A person with one seizure does not by definition have epilepsy but is clearly different from the general population in terms of risk to develop epilepsy. Before one can evaluate remission from epilepsy, there must be additional unprovoked seizures so that criteria for epilepsy are met. There is wide variation in the prediction of risk for seizure recurrence after a first seizure (Hopkins et al 1988, Camfield et al 1985, Ewles et al 1985). While much of this variation appears due to study design, prospective follow-up studies of individuals identified from the day of the first seizure suggest that only about 25% will experience a second episode within the next 2 years (Shinnar et al 1990, Hauser et al 1990b), considerably less than that reported in retrospective studies. It is also clear that there is considerable clinical heterogeneity in the study populations, and that in the same study, recurrence risk at 2 year varies from less than 15% in those with no currently identified risk factors to 100% in those with some combinations of risk factors.

The most consistent and most powerful risk factor for seizure recurrence is the history of an antecedent brain insult (aetiology), but seizure type, abnormal EEG, family (sibling) history of *epilepsy*, prior acute seizures including febrile seizures, the occurrence of status epilepticus, or the presence of a Todd's paralysis all are associated with an increased likelihood of having a second seizure. The risk for seizure recurrence is also increased when antiepileptic drugs are prescribed (not necessarily used), even after controlling for these other identified risk factors. It is reassuring (but not surprising) that in a clinical trial, antiepileptic drugs taken in doses to obtain adequate serum levels reduced the proportion of cases who experienced a seizure recurrence after a first seizure (Mussico et al 1989).

Predictors of remission at the time of diagnosis

The majority of individuals with epilepsy (60% or more) will have experienced multiple seizures at the time of first medical contact for epilepsy (Hauser & Kurland 1975). About 70% of these patients will ultimately go into remission of their seizures. Clinically, this situation is quite different from that of the first seizure and a different spectrum of predictors might be expected. None the less, a know aetiology, seizure type (partial) and (abnormal) EEG findings, particularly a generalized spike-and-wave EEG pattern, are associated with reduced likelihood of remission (Annegers et al 1979, Shafer et al 1988). In addition, age at diagnosis, number of seizures prior to diagnosis, and duration of seizures prior to diagnosis are inversely proportional to the likelihood of remission.

Predictors of remission after diagnosis, during the course, but prior to remission

There are a few factors which may provide a 'mid course assessment' of prognosis for remission (Elwes et al 1984, Collaborative Group 1988). The interval required to achieve seizure control after diagnosis is inversely correlated with likelihood of remission. Control on a single drug and the drug under which control is achieved are also predictors of ultimate remission. Each of these factors is interrelated. The occurrence of a generalized seizure at any time during the course of the condition is associated with a reduced likelihood of remission.

Predictors of successful withdrawal after remission is achieved

From 60 to 70% of patients diagnosed as having epilepsy will enter remission, and in the majority of these seizure-free individuals, antiepileptic drugs can be successfully withdrawn (Juul-Jensen 1964, Overweg et al 1987, Shinnar et al 1985, Arts et al 1988, Callaghan et al 1988, Todt 1984, Medical Research Council 1991). Factors associated with successful (or failed) withdrawal are familiar. Known aetiology for the epilepsy and/or abnormal neurological examination, seizure type (multiple or partial), age at onset, more than a single drug to achieve control, low serum levels of drugs used to obtain control, number of seizures prior to control, and a prolonged interval between onset of seizures and initial seizure control all suggest a poor outcome. In addition, lack of improvement in EEG over time, a brief duration of seizure freedom prior to attempted withdrawal, and the occurrence of generalized tonic-clonic seizures as part of the pattern of epilepsy are associated with an increased risk for seizure recurrence.

Mortality in patients with epilepsy

There are potential biases in all studies of mortality in patients with epilepsy. It is impossible to determine a referent population for autopsy studies, and the bias associated with this method of study seems obvious. Studies using death certificates have little value in the study of mortality in epilepsy. Less than 10% of patients with epilepsy will have the condition mentioned anywhere on the death certificate much less in a place from which the diagnosis can be retrieved from data routinely collected for statistical purposes (Hauser & Kurland 1975). Those certificates which appropriately identify patients with epilepsy disproportionately identify deaths in institutionalized individuals or in individuals with other neurological handicap. Further, for many individuals with seizures or epilepsy recorded on a death certificate, no evidence of a convulsive disorder can be identified when medical record review is possible. These are individuals who may have manifest convulsive activity in association with a terminal event. The misclassification makes death certificate data virtually useless for anything beyond simple hypothesis generation. People with life insurance are likely to be in higher socioeconomic strata and actuarial data regarding insured people with epilepsy deal with individuals unrepresentative of the general population with epilepsy. Studies of clinic populations are likely to include people with more severe epilepsy and low socioeconomic status. These individuals are again unrepresentative of a general epilepsy population and the mortality is likely to be overestimated. When mortality data from epilepsy clinics is compared with life insurance actuarial data (with survivorship which is even better than the general population), a further inflation of apparent mortality might be expected. Population-based cohort studies relying on medical records for both diagnosis of epilepsy and for outcome will provide the most accurate estimates of mortality but are generally hampered by small numbers.

Despite differences in populations studied and in measures used to examine the mortality of individuals with epilepsy, results are generally consistent. When compared to the general population or an insurance population, mortality is increased in patients with epilepsy (Henriksen et al 1970, Hauser et al 1980, Zielinski 1974a,b, Brorson & Wranne 1987, Preston & Clarke 1966, Singer & Levinson 1976). The excess risk is greater in men than women, is seen in all age groups, and is greatest in individuals with remote symptomatic epilepsy. In younger age groups, the excess mortality is seen in those with epilepsy who also have MR, CP, or congenital malformations of the central nervous system. In older age groups, epilepsy is associated with brain tumours or cerebrovascular disease. Thus much of the excess mortality is related to the underlying cause of the epilepsy rather than factors attributable to the epilepsy per se.

When survivorship analysis is limited to those with idiopathic epilepsy, there is still an increased risk of mortality, although no increase has been identified in idiopathic cases with onset under the age of 20. Mortality is increased in those with generalized tonic-clonic seizures and with myoclonic seizures, but not in those with absence seizures or with idiopathic complex partial epilepsy. Increased severity of epilepsy as measured by seizure frequency may be associated with an increased mortality. In Denmark, mortality was greater in those with 'moderate or severe' epilepsy when compared with seizure-free or with 'infrequent' seizures. In Rochester, mortality was not increased among those with a single idiopathic seizure.

In Rochester, altered mortality varied with duration of the condition. Among idiopathic cases, standardized mortality ratio (SMR) was highest in the first year following diagnosis

(Hauser & Kurland 1975, Hauser et al 1980), and could be identified for only the first 10 years following diagnosis. Mortality in those with idiopathic epilepsy did not exceed that in the general population after that time.

Specific causes of death in patients with epilepsy were examined in the Rochester cohort (Hauser et al 1980). Death due to heart disease was not increased in those with epilepsy when compared with the local population. There was an increased mortality attributable to neoplasms even after exclusion of brain tumours although in most cases the malignancy had been identified prior to the diagnosis of epilepsy. Consistent with other studies, there was an increased risk of death attributed to accidents. Drowning has come under particular scrutiny as a cause of death in people with epilepsy although this cause of death may also be related to underlying neurological handicaps associated with the development of epilepsy (Davis et al 1985).

Patients with epilepsy may have an increased risk for suicide. The highest risk for suicide has been reported from clinical or surgical series of 'temporal lobe' epilepsy, followed by studies of institutionalized individuals, followed by studies of patients from general hospitals (Matthews & Barabas 1981, Barraclough 1987). The population based study in Rochester, Minnesota found no evidence of an increased risk for suicide among people with epilepsy. There may be increased risk among selected subgroups of patients which represent a small proportion of the general population with epilepsy.

Sudden death and epilepsy

Clinical impressions and several autopsy studies have suggested that individuals with epilepsy are at an increase in risk from sudden death (Jay & Leestma 1981, Neuspiel & Kuller 1985, Leestma et al 1984, Leestma 1990). Tachycardia or cardiac arrhythmia may be identified at the time of seizures although there is no evidence that patients with epilepsy have an increased frequency of spontaneous arrhythmia (Keilson et al 1987, Blumhardt et al 1986). Despite this, it has been suggested that sudden death can be attributed to cardiac arrhythmia associated with seizures or with reduction in antiepileptic drugs.

Heart disease mortality and incidence and, more specifically, the frequency of sudden death in patients with epilepsy has been explored in Rochester (Annegers et al 1984). The US White population served as the comparison group for heart disease mortality, while the Rochester population was used for ischaemic heart disease and sudden death. All comparisons were adjusted for age, sex, and temporal changes in rates of disease or death. The risk for mortality attributable to heart disease was elevated up to age 65 in the whole epilepsy cohort. The incidence of ischaemic heart disease as a cause of death was increased over that expected in subjects with remote symptomatic epilepsy. The risk for sudden death was more than doubled in the whole epilepsy group. This risk was accounted for by the group with remote symptomatic epilepsy—primarily those with epilepsy attributed to cerebrovascular disease. Sudden death did not occur with greater frequency in the group with idiopathic epilepsy when compared to the general Rochester population.

Other co-morbidity

It has been suggested that repeated seizures may lead to intellectual deterioration. Results of psychological testing in children with afebrile seizures were compared with those of siblings in the NCPP (Ellenberg et al 1986). No significant difference in mental performance could be identified.

A number of studies have raised the question of an increased risk for neoplasms in patients with epilepsy. The questions have been more related to potential carcinogenic effects of antiepileptic medication rather than a direct effect of the epilepsy. Clinical studies have reported an increased frequency of lymphoproliferative disorders in individuals exposed to antiepileptic medication, and case control studies have raised the question of an increase risk for central nervous system neoplasms associated with barbiturate exposure. Studies in Rochester found an increased risk for CNS neoplasms but not from other tumour types (Shirts et al 1986). It is likely that the neoplasms were a cause rather than a consequence of epilepsy.

REFERENCES

Annegers J F, Hauser W A 1984 Epidemiologic measures of occurrence and association for the study of convulsive disorders. In: Porter R J, Mattson R H, Ward A A, Dam M (eds) Advances in epileptology: the XVth epilepsy international symposium. Raven Press, New York, p 521–529

Annegers J F, Hauser W A, Elveback L R 1979 Remission of seizures and relapse in patients with epilepsy. Epilepsia 20: 729–737

Annegers J F, Grabow J D, Groover R V, Laws E R, Elveback L R, Kurland L T 1980a Seizures after head trauma: A population study. Neurology 30: 683–689

Annegers J F, Grabow J D, Kurland L T, Laws E R 1980b The incidence, causes, and secular trends of head trauma in Olmsted County, Minnesota, 1935–1974. Neurology 30: 912–919

Annegers J F, Hauser W A, Anderson V E, Kurland L T 1982 The risks of seizure disorders among relatives of patients with childhood onset epilepsy. Neurology 32: 174–179

Annegers J F, Hauser W A, Shirts S B 1984 Heart disease mortality and morbidity in patients with epilepsy. Epilepsia 25: 699–704

Annegers J F, Hauser W A, Shirts S B, Kurland L T 1987 Factors prognostic of unprovoked seizures after febrile convulsions. New England of Medicine 316: 493–498

Annegers J F, Hauser W A, Beghi E, Hauser W A, Kurland L T 1988 The risk of unprovoked seizures after encephalitis and meningitis. Neurology 38: 1407–1410

Arts W F M, Visser T H, Loonen M C B et al 1988 Follow-up of 146 children with epilepsy after withdrawal of antiepileptic therapy. Epilepsia 29: 244–250

Barraclough B M 1987 The suicide rate of epilepsy. Acta Psychiatrica Scandinavica 76: 339–345

Baumann R J, Marx M B, Leonidakis M G 1977 An estimate of the prevalence of epilepsy in a rural Appalachian population. American Journal of Epidemiology 106: 42–52

Baumann R J, Marx M B, Leonidakis M G 1978 Epilepsy in rural Kentucky: Prevalence in a population of school age children. Epilepsia 19: 75–80

Beck-Mannagetta G, Janz D, Hoffmeister U, Behl I, Schulz G 1989 Morbidity risk for seizures and epilepsy in offspring of patients with epilepsy. In Beck-Mannagetta G, Anderson V E, Doose H, Janz D (eds) Genetics of the epilepsies. Springer-Verlag, Berlin, p 119

Benedetti M D, Hauser W A, Shinnar S. Frequency of seizures among children with cerebral palsy and/or mental retardation. I. The frequency of epilepsy in children with cerebral palsy and/or mental retardation.(submitted)

Benna P, Ferrero P, Bianco C et al 1984 Epidemiologic aspects of epilepsy in the children of a Piedmontese district (Alba-Bra). Pan Med 26: 113–118

Beran R G, Hall L, Michelazzi J 1985 An accurate assessment of the prevalence ratio of epilepsy adequately adjusted for influencing factors. Neuroepidemiology 4: 71–81

Bharucha N E, Bharucha E P, Bharucha A E et al 1988 Prevalence of epilepsy in the Parsi community of Bombay. Epilepsia 29: 111–115

Blume W T, Girvin J P, Kaufmann J C E 1982 Childhood brain tumors presenting as chronic uncontrolled focal seizure disorders. Annals of Neurology 12: 538–541

Blumhardt L D, Smith P E M, Owen L 1986 Electrocardiographic accompaniments of temporal lobe epileptic seizures. The Lancet May 10: 1051–1055

Brewis M, Poskanzer D C, Rolland C, Miller H 1966 Neurologic disease in an English city. Acta Neurologica Scandinavica 42(suppl 24): 9–89

Brorson L O, Wranne L 1987 Long-term prognosis in childhood epilepsy: Survival and seizure prognosis. Epilepsia 28: 324–330

Callaghan N, Garrett A, Googin T 1988 Withdrawal of anticonvulsant drugs in patients free of seizures for two years. New England Journal of Medicine 318: 942–946

Camfield P R, Camfield C S, Dooley J M, Tibbles J A R, Fung T, Garner B 1985 Epilepsy after a first unprovoked seizure in childhood. Neurology 35: 1567–1660

Cavazzuti G B 1980 Epidemiology of different types of epilepsy in school age children of Modena Italy. Epilepsia 21: 57–62

Chiofalo N, Kirschbaum A, Fuentes A et al 1979 Prevalence of epilepsy in children of Melipilla, Chile. Epilepsia 20: 261–266

Collaborative Group for the study of Epilepsy 1988 Prognosis of Epilepsy in newly referred patients: a multicenter prospective study. Epilepsia 29: 236–243

Commission on Classification and Terminology of the International League Against Epilepsy 1981 Proposal for revised clinical and electroencephalographic classification of epileptic seizures. Epilepsia 22: 489–501

Commission on Classification and Terminology of the International League Against Epilepsy 1989 A revised proposal for the classification of Epilepsy and Epileptic Syndromes. Epilepsia 30: 268–278

Cooper K D, Tabaddor K, Hauser W A et al 1983 The epidemiology of head injury in the Bronx. Neuroepidemiology 2: 70–81

Cowan L D, Bodensteiner J B, Leviton A, Doherty L 1989 Prevalence of the epilepsies in children and adolescents. Epilepsia 30: 94–106

Crombie D L, Cross K W, Fry J et al 1960 A survey of the epilepsies in general practice: A report by the research committee of the college of general practitioners. British Medical Journal 2: 416–422

Cruz M E, Schoenberg B S, Ruales J et al 1985 Pilot study to detect neurologic disease in Equador among a population with high prevalence of endemic goiter. Neuroepidemiology 4: 108–116

Dam A M, Fuglsang-Frederiksen A, Svarre-Olsen U, Dam M 1985 Late-onset epilepsy: Etiologies, types of seizures, and value of clinical investigation, EEG, and computerized tomography scan. Epilepsia 26: 227–231

Davis S, Ledman J, Kilgore J 1985 Drownings of children and youth in a desert state. Western Medical Journal 143: 196–201

De Graaf A S 1974 Epidemiological aspects of epilepsy in Norway. Epilepsia 15: 291–299

Doose H, Sitepu B 1983 Childhood epilepsy in a German city. Neuropediatrics 14: 220–224

Ellenberg J H, Hirtz D G, Nelson K B 1984 Age at onset of seizures in young children. Annals of Neurology 15: 127–134

Ellenberg J H, Hirtz D G, Nelson K B 1986 Do seizures cause intellectual deterioration? New England Journal of Medicine 314: 1085–1088

Elwes R D C, Johnson A L, Shorvon S D, Reynolds E H 1984 The prognosis for seizure control in newly diagnosed epilepsy. New England Journal of Medicine 311: 944–947

Elwes R D C, Chesterman P, Reynold S E H 1985 Prognosis after a first untreated tonic clonic seizure. Lancet ii: 752–753

Evans D A, Funchenstein H H, Albert M S et al 1989 Prevalence of Alzheimer's disease in a community population of older persons: Higher than previously reported. Journal of the American Medical Association 262: 255–256

Falconer M 1971 Genetic and related aetiologic factors in temporal lobe epilepsy. A review. Epilepsia 12: 13–31

Forsgren L 1990 Prospective incidence study and clinical characterization of seizures in newly referred adults. Epilepsia 31: 292–301

Foy P M, Copeland G P , Shaw M D M 1981 The incidence of postoperative seizures. Acta Neurochirurgica 55: 252–264

Franceschetti S, Battagha G, Lodrini S, Avanzini G 1988 Relationship between tumors and epilepsy. In: Broggi G (ed) The rational basis of the surgical treatment of epilepsies. John Libbey, London

Garcia-Pedroza F, Rubio-Donnadieu F, Garcia Ramos G et al 1983 Prevalance of epilepsy in children: Tlalpan, Mexico City, Mexico. Neuroepidemiology 2: 16–23

Gomez J G, Arciniegas E, Torres J 1978 Prevalence of epilepsy in Bogota, Columbia. Neurology 28: 90–94

Goodridge D M G, Shorvon S D 1983 Epileptic seizures in a population of 6000. I. Demography, diagnosis and classification, and role of hospital services. British Medical Journal 287: 641–644

Goulden K S, Shinnar S, Koller H, Katz M, Richardson S 1991 Epilepsy in children with mental retardation: A cohort study. Epilepsia 32: 690–697

Gracia F, Loo de Lar S, Castillo L, Larreategui M, Archbold C, Brenes M M, Reeves W 1990 Epidemiology of epilepsy in Guaymi Indians from Bocas del Toro Province, Republic of Panama. Epilepsia 31: 718–724

Granieri E, Rosati G, Tola R et al 1983 A descriptive study of epilepsy in the district of Copparo, Italy, 1964–1978. Epilepsia 24: 502–514

Griffith A H 1974 Petrussis vaccine and convulsive disorders of childhood. Proceedings of the Royal Society of Medicine 67: 372–374

Griffith A H 1989 Permanent brain damage and pertussis vaccination: is the end of the saga in sight? Vaccine 7: 199–210

Griffin M R, Ray W A, Mortimer E A, Fenichel G M, Schaffner W 1990 Risk of seizures and encephalopathy after immunization with the diphtheria-tetanus-pertussis vaccine. Journal of the American Medical Association 263: 1641–1645

Gudmundsson G 1966 Epilepsy in Iceland. A clinical and epidemiologic investigation. Acta Neurologica Scandinavica 43:(suppl 25): 1–124

Haerer A F, Anderson D W, Schoenberg B S 1986 Prevalence and clinical features of epilepsy in a biracial United States population. Epilepsia 27: 66–75

Hauser W A 1990 Epidemiology of alcohol use and of epilepsy. The magnitude of the problem. In: Porter R J, Mattson R H, Cramer J A, Diamond I (eds) Alcohol and seizures. F A Davis, Philadelphia, p 12–21

Hauser W A, Anderson V E 1986 Genetics of epilepsy. In: Pedley T A, Meldrum B S (eds) Recent advances in epilepsy. Churchill Livingstone, Edinburgh

Hauser W A, Annegers J F 1989 Epidemiologic measurements for the determination of genetic risks. In

Beck-Mannagetta G, Anderson V E, Doose H, Janz D (eds) Genetics of the epilepsies. Springer Verlag, Berlin

Hauser W A, Hesdorffer D H 1990a Epilepsy: frequency, causes and consequences. Demos Press, New York

Hauser W A, Hesdorffer D H 1990b Facts about epilepsy. Demos Publications, New York

Hauser W A, Kurland L T 1975 The epidemiology of epilepsy in Rochester, Minnesota, 1935 through 1967. Epilepsia 16: 1–66

Hauser W A, Nelson K B 1989 Epidemiology of epilepsy in children. Cleveland Clinical Journal of Medicine 56(suppl 2): S185–194

Hauser W A, Annegers J F, Elveback L R 1980 Mortality in patients with epilepsy. Epilepsia 21: 339–412

Hauser W A, Annegers J F, Kurland L T 1984a The incidence of epilepsy in Rochester, Minnesota 1935–79. Epilepsia 25: 666

Hauser W A, Ramirez-Lassepas M, Rosenstein R 1984b Risk for seizures and epilepsy following cerebrovascular insults. Epilepsia 25: 666

Hauser W A, Morris M L, Heston L L, Anderson V E 1986a Seizures and myoclonus in patients with Alzheimer's disease. Neurologica 36: 1226–1230

Hauser W A, Ng S, Marc L, Brust J C M 1986b Prevalence of epilepsy in a black inner-city community—a telephone survey. Neurology 36(Suppl 1): 108

Hauser W A, Ortega R, Zarelli M 1990a The prevalence of epilepsy in a rural Mexican Village. Epilepsia 31: 604

Hauser W A, Rich S S, Annegers J F, Anderson V E 1990b Seizure recurrence after a first unprovoked seizure: An extended follow-up. Neurology 40: 1163–1170

Hauser W A, Annegers J F, Gomez M 1991a The incidence of West Syndrome in Rochester, Minnesota. Epilepsia 32 (53): 83

Hauser W A, Annegers J F, Kurland L T 1991b Prevalence of epilepsy in Rochester, Minnesota; 1940–1980. Epilepsia 32: 429–445

Henriksen B, Juul-Jensen P, Lund M 1970 The mortality of epileptics. In: Brackenridge R D C (ed) Proceedings of the 10th International Congress of Life Assurance Medicine. Pitman, London

Hirtz D G, Nelson K B, Ellenberg J H 1983 Seizures following childhood immunization. Journal of Pediatrics 102: 14–18

Hollingsworth J S 1978 Mental retardation, cerebral palsy, and epilepsy in Alabama: a sociological analysis. University of Alabama Press

Hopkins A, Garman A, Clarke C 1988 The first seizure in adult life. Lancet 1: 721–726

Hurst D L 1990 Epidemiology of severe myoclonic epilepsy of infancy. Epilepsia 31: 397–400

Jay G W, Leestma J F 1981 Sudden death in epilepsy: A comprehensive review of the literature and proposed mechanisms. Acta Neurologica Scandinavica 82 [suppl]: 1–66

Jimenez I 1989 A case control study of epilepsy in Columbia. Presented at the 18th Epilepsy International, Oct 20, New Delhi, India

Joensen P 1986 Prevalence, incidence and classification of epilepsy in the Faroes. Acta Neurologica Scandinavica 76: 150–155

Juul-Jensen P 1964 Frequency of seizure recurrence after discontinuance of anticonvulsant medication in patients with epileptic seizures. Epilepsia 5: 352–363

Juul-Jensen P, Foldspang A 1983 Natural history of epileptic seizures. Epilepsia 24: 297–312

Keilson M J, Hauser W A, Magrill J P, Goldman M 1987 ECG abnormalities in patients with epilepsy. Neurology 37: 1624–1626

Keranen T, Reikkinen, P, Sillanpaa M 1989 Incidence and prevalence of epilepsy in adults in Eastern Finland. Epilepsia 30: 412–421

Kinnunen E, Wikstrom J 1986 Prevalence and prognosis of epilepsy in patients with multiple sclerosis. Epilepsia 27: 729–733

Kokmen E, Chandra V, Schoenberg B S 1988 Trends in incidence of dementing illness in Rochester Minnesota in three quinquannial periods 1960–1974. Neurology 38: 975–980

Koul R, Razdan S, Motta A 1988 Prevalence and pattern of epilepsy (Lath/Mirgi/Laran) in rural Kashmir, India. Epilepsia 29: 116–122

Lai C W, Huang X S, Lai Y H 1990 Survey of public awareness understanding, and attitudes toward epilepsy in Henan Province, China. Epilepsia 31: 182–187

Lampert D I, Locke G E, Hauser W A et al 1984 Prevalence of epilepsy in an urban minority population. Epilepsia 25: 665

Leestma J E, Kalelkar M B, Teas S S et al 1984 Sudden unexpected death associated with seizures: Analysis of 66 cases. Epilepsia 25: 84–88

Leestma J E, Walczak T, Hughs J R, Kalelkar M B, Teas S S 1989 A prospective study on sudden unexpected death in epilepsy. Annals of Neurology 26: 195–203

Li S, Schoenberg B S, Wang C et al 1985 Epidemiology of epilepsy in urban areas of the People's Republic of China. Epilepsia 26: 391–394

Loiseau P 1987 Incidence et evolution a 1 an des syndromes epileptiques en Gironde. These No 338, Universite de Bordeaux II

Loiseau J, Loiseau P, Duche B, Guyot M, Dartigues J, Aublet B 1990a A survey of epileptic disorders in southwest France: Seizures in elderly patients. Annals of Neurology 27: 232–237

Loiseau J, Loiseau P, Guyot M, Duche B, Dartigues J, Aublet B 1990b Survey of seizure disorders in the French Southwest. I. Incidence of epileptic syndromes. Epilepsia 31: 391–396

Luhdorf K, Jensen L K, Plesner A M 1986a Epilepsy in the elderly: incidence, social function, and disability. Epilepsia 27: 135–141

Luhdorf K, Jensen L K, Plesner A M 1986b Etiology of seizures in the elderly. Epilepsia 27: 458–463

Maremmani C, Rossi G, Bonuccille U, Murri L 1991 Descriptive epidemiologic study of epilepsy syndrome in a district of Northwest Tuscany, Italy. Epilepsia 32: 294–298

Mathieson G 1975 Pathologic aspects of epilepsy to the surgical pathology of focal cerebral seizures. Advances in Neurology 8: 107–138

Matthews W S, Barabas G 1981 Suicide and epilepsy: A review of the literature. Psychosomatics 22: 515–524

Medical Research Council Antiepileptic Drug Withdrawal Group 1991 Randomized study of antiepileptic drug withdrawal in patients in remission. Lancet 337: 1175–1180

Miller D L, Ross E M, Alderslade R, Bellman M H, Rawson N S B 1981 Pertussis immunization and serious acute neurological illness in children. British Medical Journal 282: 1595–1599

Miller D L, Alderslade R, Ross E M 1982 Whooping cough and whooping cough vaccine: The risks and benefits debate. Epidemiologic Review 1–24

Mussico, Massimo, First Italian Multicenter study on first seizure treatment 1989 The effect of drug treatment on the risk of recurrence after a first unprovoked tonic clonic seizure. An Italian multicenter trial. Neurology 39 (S1): 148

Nelson K B, Ellenberg J H 1984 Obstetric complications as risk factors for cerebral palsy or seizure disorders. Journal of the American Medical Association 251: 1843–1848

Nelson K B, Ellenberg J H 1986 Antecedents of seizure disorders in early childhood. American Journal of Diseases of Childhood 40: 1053–1061

Neuspiel D R, Kuller L H 1985 Sudden and unexpected natural death in childhood and adolescence. Journal of the American Association 254: 1321–1325

Ng S K, Hauser W A, Brust J C M, Healton E B, Susser M W 1985 Risk factors for adult-onset first seizures. Annals of Neurology 18: 153

Ng S K C, Hauser W A, Brust J C M, Susser M 1988 Alcohol consumption and the risk of new onset seizures. New England Journal of Medicine 319: 666–673

Ng S K C, Hauser W A, Brust J C M, Susser M 1990 Illicit drug use and first onset seizures. American Journal of Epidemiology 132: 147–153

Nicolosi A, Hauser W A, Beghi E, Kurland L T 1986 Epidemiology of central nervous system infections in Olmsted County, Minnesota, 1950–1981. Journal of Infectious Diseases 154: 399–408

Ogunniyi A, Osuntokun B O, Bademosi O et al 1987 Risk factors for epilepsy: Case-control study in Nigeria. Epilepsia 28: 280–285

Olsen T S, Hogenhaven H, Thage O 1987 Epilepsy after stroke. Neurology 37: 1209–1211

Osuntokun B O, Schoenberg B S, Nottidge V A et al 1982 Research protocol for measuring the prevalence of neurologic disorders in developing countries: Results of a pilot study in Nigeria. Neuroepidemiology 1: 143–153

Osuntokun B O, Adeuja A O G, Nottidge V A et al 1987 Prevalence of the epilepsies in Nigerian Africans: A community based study. Epilepsia 28: 272–279

Otohara S, Ishida S, Oka R, Yamatogi Y, Ohtsuka Y, Miuake S, Iuoda K 1981 Epilepsy and febrile convulsions in Okayama prefecture A neuroepidemiologic study. In: Fukuyama Y et al (eds) Proceedings of the IVDP commemorative international symposium on developmental disabilities. Elsevier, Amsterdam, 376–382

Overweg J, Binnie C D, Oosting J, Rowan A J 1989 Clinical and EEG prediction of seizure recurrence following antiepileptic drug withdrawal. Epilepsy Research 1: 373–383

Pisani F, Trunfio C, Oteri G et al 1987 Prevalence of epilepsy in children of Reggio Calabria, Southern Italy. Acta Neurologica (Napoli) 9: 40–43

Placencia M 1984 Main epidemiologic findings in the communitary management of epilepsy, Ecuador, 1986–1989. Presented at Epilepsy International Delhi India, October 20

Ponce Ducharne P L et al 1986 Estudios neuroepidemiologicos en Venezuela. Ministerio de Sanidad. See Cruz M E, Barberis P, Schoenberg B S. Epidemiology of Epilepsy. In Poeck K, Freund H J, Ganshirt H (eds) Neurology. Springer-Verlag, Heidelberg, 129

Pond D A, Bidwell B H, Stein L 1960 A survey of epilepsy in fourteen general practices. I. Demographic and medical data. Journal of Neurology, Neurosurgery and Psychiatry 63: 217–236

Pradilla-Ardila G, Puentes F, Rivera R et al 1984 Estudio Neuroepidemiologico Piloto. Neurologia en Columbia 8: 103–130

Pradilla-Ardila G, Pardo C A, Mendez I R, Zafra C I, Restrepo J A, Blanco S 1991 Estudio Neuroepidemiologico en la commeded rural del el Wato-Santander, Medicas VIS 5: 181–187

Preston T W, Clarke R D 1966 An investigation into the mortality of impaired lives during the period 1947–63. J Inst Act 92: 27–74

Rich S S, Annegers J F, Hauser W A, Anderson V E 1987 Complex segregation analysis of febrile convulsions. American Journal of Human Genetics 41: 249–257

Roberts M A, Godfrey J W, Caird F I 1982 Epileptic seizures in the elderly. I. Aetiology and type of seizure. Age and Ageing 11: 24–28

Roberts R C, Shorvon S D, Cox T C S, Gilliatt R W 1988 Clinically unsuspected cerebral infarction revealed by computed tomography scanning in late onset epilepsy. Epilepsia 29: 190–194

Rocca W A, Sharbrough F W, Hauser W A, Annegers J F, Schoenberg B S 1987a Risk factors for absence seizures: A population-based case-control study in Rochester, Minnesota. Neurology 37: 1309–1314

Rocca W A, Sharbrough F W, Hauser W A, Annegers J F, Schoenberg B S 1987b Risk factors for complex partial seizures: A population-based case-control study. Annals of Neurology 21: 22–31

Rocca W A, Sharbrough F W, Hauser W A, Annegers J F, Schoenberg B S 1987c Risk factors for generalized tonic-clonic seizures: A population-based case-control study in Rochester, Minnesota. Neurology 37: 1315–1322

Romanelli M F, Morris J C, Ashkin K, Coben L A 1990 Advanced Alzheimer's disease is a risk factor for late onset seizures. Archives of Neurology 47: 847–850

Ross E M, Miller D L 1986 Risk and pertussis vaccine. Archives of Disease of Childhood 61: 98–99

Salazar A M, Jabbari B, Vance S C et al 1985 Epilepsy after penetrating head injury. I. Clinical correlates: A report of the Vietnam Head Injury Study. Neurology 35: 1406–1414

Sander J W A, Hart Y M, Johnson A L, Shorvon S D 1990 National general pratice study of epilepsy: newly diagnosed epileptic seizures in a general population. Lancet 336: 1267–1271

Sayetta R B 1986 Rates of senile dementia—Alzheimer's type in the Baltimore longitudinal study. Journal of Chronic Disease 39: 271–286

Shafer S, Hauser W A, Annegers J F, Klass D W 1988 EEG and other early predictors of later epilepsy remission: a community study. Epilepsia 29: 590–600

Shamansky S I, Glaser G H 1979 Socioeconomic characteristics of childhood seizure disorders in the New Haven area: an epidemiologic study. Epilepsia 20: 457–474

Shields W D, Neilsen C, Buch D et al 1988 Relationship of pertussis immunization to the onset of neurologic disorders: A retrospective epidemiologic study. Prediatrics 113: 801–805

Shinnar S, Vining E P G, Mellits E D et al 1985 Discontinuing antiepileptic medication in children with epilepsy after two years without seizures. New England Journal of Medicine 313: 976–980

Shinnar S, Berg D, Moshe S L et al 1990 The risk of seizure recurrence following a first unprovoked seizure in childhood: A prospective study. Pediatrics 85: 1076–1085

Shinton R A, Gill J S, Zezulka A V, Bevers D G 1987 The frequency of epilepsy preceeding stroke: Case control study in 230 patients. Lancet i: 11–12

Shirts S B, Annegers J F, Hauser W A, Kurland L T 1986 Cancer incidence in a cohort of patients with seizure disorders. Journal of the National Cancer Institute 77: 83–87

Sigurdardottir S, Ludvigsson P, Olafsson E 1991 West syndrome. A 10 year population study in an island population in Iceland. Epilepsia 32(53): 57

Singer R D 1976 Neuropsychiatric Disorders. In: Singer R D, Levinson L (eds) Medical risks: patterns of mortality and survival. Lexington Books, Toronto, p 248–249

Spenser D D, Spenser S S, Mattson R H, Williamson P D 1984 Intracerebral masses in patients with intractable partial epilepsy. Neurology (Cleveland) 34: 432–436

Stanhope J M, Brody J A, Brink E 1972 Convulsions among the Chamorro people of Guam, Mariana Islands. I. Seizure disorders. American Journal of Epidemiology 95: 292–298

Stewart G T 1977 Vaccination against whooping cough: efficacy versus risks. Lancet 1: 234–237

Todt H 1984 The late prognosis of epilepsy in childhood: results of a prospective follow-up study. Epilepsia 25: 137–144

Tsuboi T 1988 Prevalence and incidence of epilepsy in Tokyo. Epilepsia 29: 103–110

Van den Berg B J, Yerushalamy J 1969 Studies on convulsive disorders in young children. I. Incidence of febrile and nonfebrile convulsions by age and other factors. Pediatric Research 3: 298–304

Viitanen M, Erickssson S, Asplund K 1988 Risk of recurrent stroke, myocardial infarction and epilepsy during long-term follow-up after stroke. European Neurology 28: 227–231

Wagner A L 1983 A clinical and epidemiological study of adult patients with epilepsy. Acta Neurologica Scandinavica suppl 94: 63–72

Walker A M, Jick H, Perera D R et al 1988 Neurologic events following diptheria-tetanus-pertussis immunization. Pediatrics 81: 345–349

Whitman S, Coleman T E, Patmon C et al 1984 Epilepsy in prison: Elevated prevalence and no relationship to violence. Neurology 34: 775–782

Zielinski J J 1974a Epidemiology and medical-social problems of epilepsy in Warsaw. Psychoneurological Institute, Warsaw

Zielinski J J 1974b Epilepsy and mortality rate and cause of death. Epilepsia 15: 191–201

3. Genetics

V. E. Anderson   W. A. Hauser

INTRODUCTION

There is convincing evidence that genetic factors are involved in the development of seizures and epilepsy. The application to clinical practice is not simple, however, since it may be difficult to determine the relative contribution of genetics to the epilepsy in an individual patient

Recent developments are clarifying the basic issues and can be expected to have an impact on clinical work in the near future (Beck-Mannagetta et al 1989a, Anderson et al 1991). The genetic loci for three epilepsy syndromes have been mapped to specific chromosomes and others will soon be added. Ion channels and membrane receptors are high on the list of candidate gene defects, their genes are being cloned, and our understanding of their molecular structure is progressing rapidly. Single locus mutations in the mouse provide critical model systems for identifying genes involved in the epilepsies, and transgenic mice can be used to study human gene mutations. Seizures themselves are known to alter the expression of specific genes.

For clinical work with epilepsy patients a basic understanding of genetics along four lines will be useful:

1. Genetic heterogeneity
2. Differential diagnosis
3. Treatment and prognosis and
4. Genetic counselling.

Genetic heterogeneity

We cannot expect to find a single mechanism causing seizures. Animal models for epilepsy present firm evidence that genetic factors can influence the hypersensitivity of neurones, but many different aetiological pathways appear to be involved. Furthermore, about 160 Mendelian traits in the human carry an increased risk of seizures. These conditions include disturbances of amino acids, enzymes and hormones, and vascular changes and neoplasms in the brain. In other syndromes the mechanism of seizure enhancement is not yet apparent. Obviously, there are many different genetic pathways leading to epilepsy.

Another argument for genetic heterogeneity in seizure mechanisms comes from the fact that the optimum for neuronal excitability is intermediate between two extremes (hyperexcitability and unresponsiveness). It is generally observed that systems with an intermediate optimum (such as blood clotting and blood glucose) are complex, and involve a number of mechanisms under independent genetic control. Thus, we might expect to find heterogeneity in the epilepsies as well.

Finally, basic research studies show that seizures may result if there are defects in any of the following steps: neuronal inhibition, inactivation of excitatory neurotransmitters, feedback control, and the control of spread of the seizure state. Each of these can be affected by genetic variation, with the result that some individuals may have a reduced ability to handle the effects of environmental insults.

Differential diagnosis

When multiple malformations are encountered in a seizure patient, the possibility of a chromosome problem should be considered. Essentially all of the detectable changes in chromosomes have some effect upon the nervous system, usually in the form of mild to severe mental retardation and, less often, seizures.

Only a small proportion of patients with epilepsy (perhaps 1–2%) will have a diagnosable Mendelian trait or chromosomal abnormality, but for these few cases the distinction may be important for treatment and prognosis.

Treatment and prognosis

Family medical history and other genetic information may sometimes influence patient seizure management. In some, but not all, of the Mendelian traits manifesting seizures, the treatment of the underlying genetic problem may also alleviate the seizures.

A family history may be important as a predictor of prognosis, although findings have not been consistent. Among 149 patients with a first unprovoked idiopathic seizure, having a sibling with epilepsy was associated with a 2-fold increase in risk for seizure recurrence (Hauser et al 1990). In a similar study of seizure occurrence after a first seizure in children, family history was an important predictor only in those with an abnormal EEG (Shinnar et al 1990). Other studies of first seizures have not found family history important, but the analyses were not limited to first degree relatives or to epilepsy (Hirtz et al 1984, Hopkins et al 1988). Family history could not be shown to be a predictor of remission in general patients with epilepsy (Shafer et al 1989) and, conversely, the offspring of individuals with a protracted course of their epilepsy do not have a higher risk of developing epilepsy than those who go into remission.

Genetic counselling

The goal of genetic counselling is to provide individuals and families with the information and understanding they need in order to make informed choices about future reproduction (Blandfort et al 1987). In the case of epilepsy, close teamwork is required between neurologist and geneticist, with the former evaluating the seizure history and EEG patterns and the latter helping to detect any genetic syndrome and estimating risks for siblings or children.

Whenever a Mendelian or chromosomal syndrome is diagnosed, the sibling risk for the syndrome itself, with or without seizures, is used. In other situations, empiric risks are estimated from family studies, as presented in a later section.

GENETIC APPROACHES

The methods of genetic study range from the level of molecules to that of populations and thus provide a way to integrate the insights from other disciplines. In this section our purpose is to review some of the genetic approaches of particular relevance to epilepsy and to list selected references for any who may wish further details.

The general principles are covered in textbooks on medical genetics (Sutton 1988, Thompson & Thompson, 1986). More specialized sources address genetics in neurology (Baraitser 1990), behavioural genetics (Plomin et al 1990) and molecular genetics (Rosenberg 1985, Rowland et al 1989).

Mendelian traits

In the evaluation of a new patient with seizures, it is essential to consider the possibility of one of the Mendelian traits that increase the risk of seizures. An understanding of these traits is of obvious importance for the clinical evaluation and treatment of seizure patients (Baraitser 1990, Anderson & Hauser 1990).

Mendelian traits are thus named because each is thought to be controlled by two or more alleles at a single genetic locus. McKusick's ninth edition (1990) provides information on 4937 such traits, and 160 of these increase the risk of seizures (Table 3.1). The three common modes of inheritance are described in the following paragraphs.

Autosomal dominant

In autosomal dominant traits, only one of the pair of alleles at a locus needs to be defective for the disorder to occur. These disorders are often found in several generations, since the defective allele is transmitted from affected persons to offspring with a 50% probability. The genetic basis for such conditions is more easily detected and this fact

Table 3.1 Mendelian traits associated with seizures, with and without mental retardation

	Total number*	Seizures and retardation		Seizures only		Total seizures	
		No.	%	No.	%	No.	%
Autosomal dominant	3047	19	0.6	24	0.8	43	1.4
Autosomal recessive	1554	79	5.1	19	1.2	98	6.3
X-linked recessive	336	15	4.5	4	1.2	19	5.7
Totals	4937	113	2.3	47	1.0	160	3.2

* From McKusick 1990.

explains in part why over half of all traits in McKusick's index are inherited in this way.

Dominant traits are usually less severe and have later onset than recessive traits; relatively few lead to seizures. Dominants often affect cell surface phenomena (such as receptors) or structural proteins (such as collagen), rather than enzymes. Furthermore, a dominant gene may sometimes be transmitted through an individual without showing any effect (described as lack of penetrance).

Autosomal recessive

Autosomal recessive traits result when both alleles at a locus are defective. They tend to be more severe and have earlier onset. A large proportion of the traits manifesting seizures (Table 3.1) have this mode of inheritance, particularly those also causing retardation. Often an enzyme defect is involved. In almost all cases, both parents are heterozygous carriers and there is a 25% risk for each sibling of an index case being affected.

If the trait is rare in the population, an individual is unlikely to receive a mutant gene from both parents unless the parents are related. Therefore, when consanguinity is noted, the possibility of autosomal recessive inheritance should be considered. Parents and other presumed carriers also should be examined for clinical signs of heterozygosity whenever such tests are available.

X-linked recessive

Recessive traits carried on the X chromosome are generally seen only in males, since genes on the single X chromosome of the male are readily expressed, while females (with two X chromosomes) are much more likely to be heterozygous. The characteristic pedigree pattern (transmitted through unaffected females and expressed only in males) makes recognition of the genetic basis for such traits relatively easy. In X-linked traits serious enough to limit reproduction, however, the possibility of new mutations must be considered in genetic counselling.

Genetic mapping of the X chromosome is relatively advanced, with Duchenne muscular dystrophy (Rowland 1988, Kunkel et al 1989) serving as a prototype.

Mendelian disorders involving seizures

Generally, when a Mendelian disorder is diagnosed, medical attention turns to means of treatment for the underlying condition. As a result, the pathways leading to the seizures are seldom explored, and we lose the opportunity to gain more insight into the aetiology of seizures. It is likely that genetic mutations may be as useful in discriminating among various physiological explanations for seizures as they have been for the explication of enzyme pathways.

For each of these conditions we need thoughtful attention to these questions:

1. Why do seizures occur at all in this syndrome?
2. Why do seizures occur in some, but not all, of the affected individuals?
3. What variability is observed within families that might be ascribed to environmental variables, modifying genes, sex and age?
4. What is the distribution by age at onset of seizures?
5. What types of seizures are observed?
6. What variations in EEG patterns have been found?

7. Which antiepileptic drugs are most effective and least effective in controlling the seizures associated with this trait?

Multifactorial (polygenic) inheritance

Many of the more common medical conditions (such as congenital malformations of the heart or central nervous system) do not fit any of the Mendelian inheritance patterns. In such conditions it is assumed that a number of genetic and environmental factors (each with only a small effect) contribute to an underlying liability. In order to facilitate calculations the liability is assumed to take a normal (bell-shaped) distribution. The liability curves for close relatives are assumed to shift to an extent proportional to the heritability (the fraction of liability that is genetically determined).

The relation between population and sibling risks can be expressed in graph form (Fig. 3.1). Point A represents data for febrile convulsions (FC) in Rochester, Minnesota, while point B represents FC data from Tokyo. Both the population and sibling risks differ sharply between these two populations, but the estimates of the heritability of liability are quite similar. Thus, if we assume that FC follows multifactorial inheritance, about two-thirds of the variation in liability is genetic.

In contrast, for an autosomal recessive trait the line for sibling risk would run straight across the graph at 25%, with little relation to the population rate. It will be noted that for common traits the distinction between single-locus and multifactorial inheritance becomes more difficult since the lines converge.

The epidemiological data from Rochester concerning FC in general are consistent with a polygenic mode of inheritance. Rich et al (1986) used complex segregation analysis on these data and found that all the genetic models involving a single major locus were rejected. The most likely hypothesis was polygenic inheritance with significant heritability of liability (68%).

However, in the small subgroup, in which the proband had three or more FC episodes, the evidence favoured a single major locus. An enlarged sample will be needed to verify this tentative finding, but there are two important implications:

1. Samples of FC may be more heterogeneous than has been suspected.
2. A small subgroup may follow an autosomal dominant pattern of inheritance, while the majority are polygenic, thus suggesting a resolution to former controversies.

Other patterns of inheritance

A maternal inheritance pattern (from an affected mother to most of her children) is found with mutations of mitochondrial genes (DiMauro et al 1991, Harding 1991). Mitochondria have a ring chromosome with 13 structural genes, all coding for components of the respiratory chain. These mitochondria are transmitted through the ova, thus accounting for the maternal inheritance pattern. The number of mutant mitochrondria in a given cell is variable, however, with the result that the expression in children is also variable. Furthermore, it must be understood that the mitochondrial enzyme complexes are formed from subunits, some of which are encoded by mitochrondrial genes and others by nuclear genes.

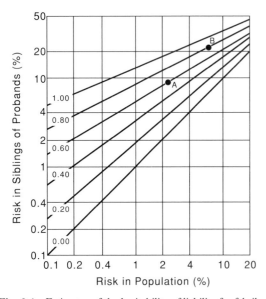

Fig. 3.1 Estimates of the heritability of liability for febrile convulsions in population samples from Minnesota (A) and Japan (B). Based on data from Tsuboi (1982) and Hauser et al (1985). Graph adapted from Smith (1970). Reproduced with permission from Anderson et al 1986.

As a result some mitochondrial enzyme defects will map to nuclear genes and will not follow a maternal inheritance pattern.

Another phenomenon which produces distinctive family patterns is genome imprinting (Hall 1990). An imprintable allele will be transmitted in a Mendelian manner to half of the offspring, but the expression of the gene will be determined by the sex of the transmitting parent. The Angelman syndrome, for example, is expressed when the maternal genes in a short segment of the long arm of chromosome 15 are deleted, while Prader–Willi syndrome involves deletion of the paternal genes in the similar area. (The seizures in Angelman syndrome will be described later in this chapter.)

Multiplex families

If there is marked heterogeneity, a search for biochemical causes in a routine clinical series of epilepsy cases will be ineffective, since a potentially significant finding in a few individuals will be lost in the data for the total group. On the other hand, the study of multiplex families (each with several affected siblings) will pick out families with a greater likelihood of genetic aetiology for their seizures and will permit the detection of biochemical deviations that appear in only one or a few families. This approach is recommended for wider use (Haines et al 1986).

Comparable population rate

When a family is given an estimate of the risk for seizures in another child, they should have for comparison an estimate of the risk for the general population. Adequate genetic counselling requires both family and population data, such as those provided by studies of Rochester, Minnesota and the surrounding county (Hauser & Annegers 1989). In this situation we need the *cumulative incidence* (or cumulative risk)—the chance that persons of a given age will have been affected by that age. In a study of probands having onset of *idiopathic* epilepsy (recurrent seizures without acute precipitating central nervous system insult) before 15 years of age, 3.6% of the siblings developed epilepsy by the age of 40, as compared with a cumulative incidence rate of 1.7% in the general

population (Fig. 3.2). When febrile and other acute symptomatic seizures are added, the rates by the age of 40 are 11.6% for siblings and 5.1% for the population.

Risk ratios

Epidemiological studies measure the effect of a particular exposure in terms of *risk ratios* (Hauser & Annegers 1991). This is the ratio of the frequency of the outcome of interest in an exposed group to that of an unexposed group. In genetic studies of epilepsy, 'exposure' may be defined as the presence of seizures or epilepsy in a specific class of relatives. The frequency of epilepsy is then compared with that expected in a non-exposed population (which is matched or adjusted for age, sex or other relevant variables). The term *relative risk* may be used in prospective studies which compare the incidence of epilepsy in an exposed and unexposed group. The *standardized morbidity ratio* (SMR) may be a more appropriate statistic for studies such as those in Rochester, Minnesota, which compare the incidence in the exposed group (those with positive family history) to the incidence in the general population including those exposed. This will tend to underestimate slightly the size of the effect.

The use of risk ratios allows comparison of the size of an effect across populations which may

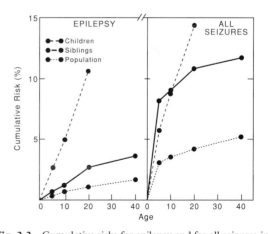

Fig. 3.2 Cumulative risks for epilepsy and for all seizures in the general population of Rochester, Minnesota and in the siblings of probands with initial diagnosis of idiopathic epilepsy before 15 years of age. Based on data from Annegers et al 1982.

have very different base population rates. Thus, in studies of familial risks for febrile seizures (Table 3.1), the 20.7% risk for febrile seizures among siblings of febrile seizure probands in Tokyo (Tsuboi 1982) seems much higher than the comparable sibling risk of 8.0% in Rochester, Minnesota (Hauser et al 1985). On the other hand, the population frequency of febrile seizures is also very different in the two populations (6.7% versus 2.3% respectively), so the SMR of 3 is similar in both populations.

Twin studies

The overall concordance rate for epilepsy in six major twin studies was 60% for monozygotic (MZ) pairs and 13% for dizygotic (DZ) pairs (Tsuboi & Okada 1985). In addition, there have been a number of reports of one or a few twin pairs concordant for specific types of epilepsy.

One population-based twin study involved a follow-up of all twins born in Denmark in the years 1870–1910 (Harvald & Hauge 1965). Among the MZ pairs, 10 out of 27 (37%) were concordant for epilepsy. Among the DZ pairs (pooling same-sex and opposite-sex) 10 out of 100 (10%) were concordant.

A series of twins identified through clinical practice was studied carefully by Lennox & Lennox (1960). Where clinical examination suggested a brain lesion in the epilepsy proband, concordance was seen in four out of 37 (10.8%) MZ pairs, and in five out of 67 (7.5%) DZ pairs. Where there was no evidence of a structural brain lesion in the epileptic proband, however, concordance was 33 out of 47 (70.2%) MZ pairs as contrasted with three out of 54 (5.6%) DZ pairs, suggesting a genetic influence.

In a smaller series, Inouye (1960) identified 40 twin pairs from out-patients and in-patients. In re-analysing the data, we excluded a pair with ichthyosis and mental retardation, a pair with phenylketonuria, a pair with tuberous sclerosis, and a pair first identified at 79 years of age. Furthermore, we did not count febrile convulsions alone as epilepsy. Among 24 MZ pairs, 12 were concordant for epilepsy. Among the 12 MZ discordant pairs, the co-twin had abnormal EEG in seven cases; among 12 DZ pairs, none were

concordant for epilepsy, although one co-twin had febrile seizures and two showed abnormal EEGs.

Finally, twins can be used to explore variability in specifically defined types of epilepsy (Anderson et al 1989). MZ pairs that are concordant for epilepsy will share any major susceptibility genes plus modifying genes and thus should show greater similarity in seizure types and EEG patterns than concordant DZ pairs. In an ongoing Australian study Berkovic et al (1990) found that nine out of 13 MZ pairs were concordant for seizures, and in each of the nine pairs both co-twins showed exactly the same 'subsyndrome'. Two of eight DZ pairs were concordant for seizures, and these two pairs showed less clinical similarity.

Gene mapping

The most notable advance since the last edition of this book is that three linkage relationships have been identified between an epilepsy gene and genetic markers. A gene for benign familial neonatal convulsions has been mapped to the long arm of chromosome 20 (Leppert et al 1991), a gene for juvenile myoclonic epilepsy and related idiopathic generalized epilepsies has been mapped to the short arm of chromosome 6 (Delgado-Escueta et al 1991), and a gene for progressive myoclonus epilepsy in Finnish families has been located on the long arm of chromosome 21 (Lehesjoki et al 1991). These conditions will be discussed in more detail later.

Whenever a gene for an epilepsy syndrome can be mapped to a specific chromosome the genetic contribution to the trait is verified (Leppert 1990). It then becomes possible to identify all those who carry the gene and thus to study the variability in its expression. The question of genetic heterogeneity can be answered by determining whether all families with the same clinical picture map to the same chromosomal locus.

Gene mapping studies require informative families and selected gene markers. Clinicians play a most important role in identifying the families and in careful documentation of the seizure histories. Each relative must be classified as *affected* (with a clear history of seizures), *unaffected* (with good evidence of being seizure-free), or *unknown* (no seizures reported, but evidence weak).

The markers can be *candidate genes* (if hypotheses as to pathogenetic mechanisms are available) or *anonymous probes* selected to cover the chromosomes systematically. Genes for ion channels, membrane receptors, and enzymes are high on the candidate lists, and remarkable progress is being made in mapping and cloning these genes.

It must be remembered that these DNA markers are only tracers. Without other information from the general population and the specific family they cannot be used for diagnosis or genetic counselling. The next steps, the exact determination of the physical location of the gene and the cloning and the sequencing of the seizure susceptibility genes, involve more stringent requirements (Leppert et al 1991). Fortunately, powerful new techniques for producing high density linkage maps will assist in the task (Evans 1991).

Cellular and molecular mechanisms

Many different mechanisms associated with seizures have been postulated and studied (Wasterlain et al 1985, Delgado-Escueta et al 1986). Pathological changes may be observed in hippocampal structure, intermediate metabolism, the lipid constituents of membranes, calcium levels and protein synthesis. Among the amino acids, glutamate and aspartate are excitatory, while GABA and glycine are generally inhibitory; catecholamines and cyclic nucleotides also are involved. It is difficult, however, to distinguish causes of seizures from their effects and to understand paradoxical findings in different areas of the brain and under varying circumstances.

Within the past few years, however, the use of recombinant DNA and other new techniques has led to significant advances in the understanding of brain structure and function, as indicated by the breadth of coverage in the 55th symposium held by Cold Spring Harbor Laboratory (1991). Many aspects of this work have clear implications for epilepsy research.

There may be as many as 30 000 genes expressed in the brain, and many of these may be exclusive to, or highly enriched in, brain. It is now possible to identify those genes whose expression is limited to a subset of CNS neurones, to detect the products of the genes, and to analyse their functions (Sutcliffe et al 1991). Furthermore, transgenic technology can be used to produce animal models for further study of gene function in vitro.

Ganetzky (1991) has studied neuronal membrane excitability in *Drosophila* by identifying the genes that affect the structure, function, and regulation of ion channels. Both sodium and potassium channels have been well characterized and, by manipulating the number of such genes, their effects on neuronal membrane excitability can be observed. The mechanisms by which *Drosophila* neurones generate and propagate electrical signals turn out to be fundamentally similar to those in vertebrates. The *opisthotonos* gene in the mouse appears to involve a potassium channel (Tempel et al 1990). Potassium channel genes have been mapped to human chromosome 12 (Wilhelmsen et al 1990), and a human sodium channel gene is located on chromosome 2 (Litt et al 1989). One member of the family of mammalian potassium channel genes produces a dendrotoxin binding protein (Newitt et al 1991). Further study of the structure and function of this product may help in the search for pharmacological agents that can alter convulsive behaviour. Popko (1991) has characterized genes that affect myelination in the mouse, and finds that subtle variations in gene expression can lead to profound alterations of the phenotype.

Altered genes can lead to seizures, but an effect in the reverse direction is also possible. Seizure activity itself stimulates alterations in neuronal gene expression which could lead to changes in levels of excitability and hence to changes in the susceptibility to further seizures (Gall et al 1991). The influence of limbic seizures on the expression of nerve growth factor, related factors and neuropeptides could lead to both short- and long-term changes in regional excitability.

Within the next few years studies along these lines can be expected to make further significant contributions. More candidate genes will be mapped to specific chromosomal locations, and the mechanisms by which mutations can lead to seizures will be clarified. The function of ion channels, receptors, and transporters will be related to the specific structure of gene products.

Animal models

The evidence for heterogeneity also influences the expectations and interpretations of experimental and animal models of epilepsy. Some models are rejected on the basis that they do not faithfully copy the features of human seizures. In this context Wasterlain et al (1984) stated: 'Since the diversity of the epilepsies must be emphasized, and a unitary mechanism is unlikely, we need models not to imitate a human illness too complex for current methods, but to simplify it and to permit precise testing of specific hypotheses.' Thus, the parallelism should be sought at the level of gene action rather than phenotypic consequences. A model is useful if it permits the careful exploration of a specific mechanism for seizures to the point that the role of that mechanism can be demonstrated or excluded in other models and in human epilepsy patients.

Audiogenic seizures (AGS) in the mouse involve severe seizures (often leading to death by respiratory paralysis) in response to a specific sound. These seizures show a number of similarities to certain convulsive disorders in humans (Seyfried & Glaser 1985). AGS appear to involve abnormalities of the brainstem as do absence (petit mal) seizures. There is a characteristic age-dependent incidence pattern with the highest susceptibility at juvenile ages. AGS are sensitive to a number of antiepileptic drugs. The distinct advantage, of course, is that detailed biochemical studies and genetic analyses are possible.

Seyfried & Glaser (1985) used recombinant inbred mouse lines which started with a cross between parents that were resistant and susceptible to AGS, followed by intercrosses which shuffled the chromosome combinations and, later, the establishment of new inbred lines. This strategy, followed by a more extensive genetic analysis using a congenic strain and backcrosses (Neumann & Seyfried, 1990) has led to the following conclusions:

1. Juvenile-onset and adult-onset AGS can be caused by different genetic mechanisms.
2. There is a significant association between a low-affinity Ca^{2+} adenosine triphosphatase (ATPase) activity in the brainstem and AGS susceptibility.

3. Most of the variation between the susceptible and resistant strains results from allelic differences at two loci, a gene with major effect (Asp-1) on chromosome 12, and a minor gene (Asp-2) on chromosome 4. (ASP indicates 'audiogenic seizure prone'.)

The seizures in El (epileptic) mice are inherited as an autosomal dominant trait and are considered a model for human temporal lobe epilepsy or complex partial seizures with secondary generalization (Seyfried & Glaser 1985). These seizures occur spontaneously or can be induced by vestibular stimulation (produced by shaking). The analysis of crosses between El mice and two seizure-resistant strains (Rise et al 1991) indicates that El seizures result in large part from the actions of a major gene on chromosome 9 (El-1) and another gene (El-2) on chromosome 2. Furthermore, there was evidence suggesting the effect of a gene on chromosome 4 (possibly the same as Asp-2 described above for audiogenic seizures). This raises the interesting possibility that variations at a specific locus can have an effect on several different seizure types.

Noebels (1991) has followed the different, and very informative, approach of identifying a mutation, and then assessing its effects in the developing organism at the molecular and cellular levels. When several mutants can be isolated, each producing a similar disease phenotype by blocking different cellular mechanisms, these variants comprise a *model system*. Through this strategy one can identify: 1. models of human disease at the molecular, if not phenotypic, level or 2. different mechanisms which nonetheless lead to identical seizure patterns.

The *tottering* mutation, on chromosome 8, leads to generalized spike-wave epilepsy and behavioural arrest in adolescent homozygous mice. (Mutations at four other independent loci, on chromosomes 2, 9, 10 and 15, produce nearly identical seizure phenotypes.) Earlier work had shown that the *tg\tg* homozygote shows a diffuse noradrenergic (NE) axon terminal hyperinnervation in forebrain target regions innervated by the pontine locus coeruleus, and that the generalized cortical seizures can be prevented by selectively reducing the abnormal NE projection at birth

(Noebels 1991). Current research is directed toward a systematic exploration of alternative mechanisms that might explain these findings and then to formulate new strategies to correct these and other epileptogenic defects prior to seizure onset (Noebels 1991).

GENETIC EVALUATION OF PATIENTS

The factors involved in the genetic evaluation of epilepsy patients are generally well known to physicians, but some specific details may deserve comment.

Family history

The patient who is the focus of a genetic study is known as the 'proband'. In the absence of information about specific aetiological mechanisms, the major source of data about possible genetic factors comes from the reported history of epilepsy and seizures in near relatives. It is important, however, to keep the information about the several types of relatives separate. Siblings of probands, for example, are at increased risk for any of the modes of inheritance, whether autosomal, X-linked or mutifactorial. Affected parents or offspring may represent dominant or multifactorial patterns of inheritance, but seldom recessive ones. Therefore, a note in a patient's chart stating only that the family history is negative (or positive) is of little value for patient care or for research.

Specific questions should be directed toward the presence or absence of seizures in parents and siblings, with a more general enquiry about seizures in other relatives. If a relative is reported to have seizures, record should be made of the similarities and differences in seizure history as compared with the features observed in the proband.

If there is a presumed precipitating cause (such as trauma) for the seizures in the index case, but a close relative (such as one parent) also has a seizure history, then the possibility of an underlying genetic predisposition should be considered.

Age at onset

The epilepsies involve a number of age-related phenomena. Many of the seizure types and abnormal EEG patterns show characteristic age patterns rising to a peak at a certain age and falling thereafter, often similar within families.

In family studies the sibling risk for seizures for the most part is inversely related to the age at onset in the proband. It is likely that very early onset (say in the first 6 months of life) results mainly from nongenetic events (Hauser & Annegers 1991). In a study of epilepsies with primarily generalized minor seizures the sibling risk for any seizure was 3.5% for probands with onset in the first year of life, as compared with 10–12% for later onset (Doose & Baier 1987). With this exception, however, the predicted relationship appears to hold. In data from the Minnesota Epilepsy Clinical Research Program the sibling risk for epilepsy by age 40 was 5.5% for probands with onset of seizures at 0–9 years, 3.8% for onset 10–24 years, and 1.9% for onset 25–39 years (Fig. 3.3). For probands with onset at age 25 or later, the sibling risk is close to the population rate, unless one of the parents has a seizure history (Anderson & Hauser 1990). Genetic analysis, therefore, will be most productive when the probands are limited to those with younger age at onset.

The age-at-onset effect may occur in either of two ways. Under a heterogeneity hypothesis, those subtypes of epilepsy that are more strongly genetic may have an earlier age at onset. Alternatively, under a multifactorial hypothesis, those probands with early onset of seizures may have a higher genetic liability reflected in a higher sibling risk. The relationship between age and seizure manifestations may reflect the importance of developmental changes in the nervous system, such as alterations (in neuronal networks) of recurrent excitation and maturation of inhibitory processes (Shinnar & Moshe 1991).

Seizure type

A system for classifying seizure type must meet several different, and sometimes conflicting, functions. For clinical purposes, one needs a system that will provide guidance for prescribing treatment and assessing prognosis, but such a system does not necessarily represent discrete

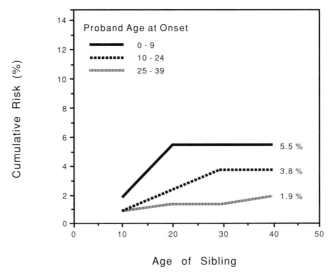

Fig. 3.3 Cumulative risks for epilepsy among siblings by age at onset of seizures in the probands. Reproduced with permission from Anderson & Hauser 1990.

aetiological classes. The *ILAE classification of seizures* (Commission on classification and terminology 1981) combines ictal EEG and clinical manifestations as well as interictal EEG manifestations to categorize individual seizures.

Individuals with epilepsy may have several different seizure types. A tentative scheme for the classification of the epilepsies has been proposed by the ILAE (Commission on classification and terminology 1989). Individuals with epilepsy characterized by partial seizures are included under the rubric of 'localization related' epilepsies and syndromes, while those characterized by generalized onset seizures are characterized as generalized epilepsies or syndromes. Syndromes are categorized as idiopathic (implying no antecedent other than a genetic predisposition), symptomatic (related to an identified insult or lesion) and cryptogenic (related to a presumed but unidentified lesion). The classification depends heavily on phenotypic seizure manifestation which is frequently age dependent; and family history is included as part of the definition of some of the syndromes even though the genetic influence is frequently poorly established.

It must be recognized that some of the presumed unique seizure syndromes discussed in the literature are not different entities, but are age-specific variations in the manifestations of seizure predisposition. Thus, a given individual may show distinct seizure syndromes at different ages. Age-related changes in seizure type appear to reflect the complex interaction of: 1. the nature and likelihood of specific antecedent factors, 2. the developmental maturation of the nervous system, and 3. genetic variation influencing the structure and biochemistry of the developing brain.

EEG characteristics

Genetic factors seem important in the manifestation of general features of the electroencephalogram. In monozygotic (MZ) twins, studies of basic EEG characteristics such as frequency spectrum and spatial wave form distribution suggest that a substantial proportion of interindividual variation may be genetically determined (Vogel 1970, 1986). If EEG recordings in MZ twins are compared, the variation between co-twins (within pairs) is no greater than that of sequential recordings in the same individual. Patterns during maturation, the rate of maturation of the EEG, and age-specific manifestations of specific patterns are also similar in MZ pairs, as are quantitative EEG analyses (Stassen et al 1986). This is true even if the MZ siblings are reared apart (Juel-Nielsen & Harvald 1958). In older MZ pairs, the degree of slowing of dominant rhythms, and increase of temporal theta are also concordant (Stassen et al 1986). Sleep patterns (Zung & Wilson 1967) and responses to activation procedures and alcohol (Propping 1977) are also similar in MZ pairs.

Nonepileptiform patterns such as alpha variants and some beta patterns also may be under genetic control. When present, low voltage fast EEG patterns tend to show a bimodal distribution within families, and segregation analysis suggests a single major locus with dominant mode of inheritance (Vogel 1986). Although rare on a population basis, *slow alpha variant* patterns have shown concordance both for occurrence and for persistence in MZ pairs and also have been observed in siblings. The pattern of inheritance of the slow alpha variant (if any is involved) remains elusive (Heintel et al 1986). Some beta patterns also may be genetically determined (Vogel 1989).

Generalized spike and wave

Based upon family and twin studies, Lennox (1951) suggested that the risk of manifesting a generalized spike and wave EEG pattern (GSW) was in part genetic. He reported an 84% concordance for GSW in MZ and no concordance in DZ pairs. The tendency for these patterns to aggregate in families was further analysed by Metrakos & Metrakos (1961, 1970). All of the probands in these studies had epilepsy and there

was no distinction between the GSW pattern and the photoparoxysmal pattern which now are felt to be phenotypic manifestations of independent genetic traits.

It is possible that there are major population differences in the frequency of the GSW pattern. In European children with no history of neurological difficulties, waking records with activation by hyperventilation show GSW in from 0.3% to 1.8% of children (Gerken & Doose 1973). The frequency of abnormalities in the waking state may be much higher in nonepileptic French Canadian populations (10%) although GSW and PPR were not categorized separately (Metrakos & Metrakos 1970). The age at time of recording must be taken into consideration, since the manifestation of GSW seems to be age dependent (Fig. 3.4). In normal German children on waking and hyperventilation activated records, the peak prevalence of GSW (2.8%) was noted in the 7–8-year-old age group. In studies of normal children which included sleep (Eeg-Olofsson et al 1970, Tsuboi 1986), 7.9% of normal Swedish children and 16.3% of Japanese children are reported to demonstrate GSW. These proportions in fact may not be different. Japanese children were recorded only at age 3, whereas the Swedish study includes children from age 1 to 15. In Sweden, 15% of 3- and 4-year-old children demonstrated GSW during sleep. Thus studies limited

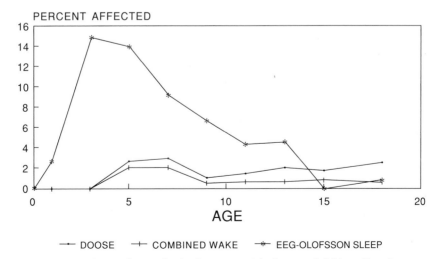

Fig. 3.4 Prevalence of generalized spike-wave activity in normal children. Data from Gerken & Doose (1972) and Eeg-Olofsson et al (1971).

to other age groups may be expected to report different frequencies of abnormalities, and the age distribution of a total population must be taken into account when interpreting summary percentages.

Photoparoxysmal response

Another EEG pattern of interest is the appearance of generalized epileptiform discharges during stimulation with intermittent light (photoparoxysmal response or PPR) (Doose et al 1969). Morphologically this EEG pattern is similar to the GSW pattern, which occurs spontaneously. PPR has attracted a good deal of attention since it is the most common stimulus-sensitive brain phenomenon thus far identified in the human (in most other species an auditory stimulus is the most effective in producing such changes).

Between 8% and 9% of children with no history of brain disease will demonstrate such responses (Vogel 1989, Doose & Gerken 1973). In the teenage years females are much more likely to be affected than males; over 20% of normal females will demonstrate this pattern compared with 10% of males. In a study of siblings of probands with PPR (most probands with epilepsy), Doose found that 25% of siblings also had PPR (Doose & Gerken 1973). Age-specific trends in the distribution of PPR in siblings of PPR probands were similar to those observed in normal children, although the prevalence was greater in each age group.

While dominant inheritance of PPR has been suggested in some Japanese populations (Takayaski & Tsukahara 1976), other patterns of inheritance have been suggested by others (Doose & Gerken 1973). If epilepsy is considered as an outcome in siblings of probands with epilepsy and PPR, the familial patterns are most consistent with a single major locus (Rich et al 1985).

Theta waves

Studies by Doose and his co-workers in Kiel, Germany have shown a strong family occurrence for certain specific EEG patterns. A theta EEG pattern (bilateral, synchronous, monomorphous waves of 4–7 Hz) seen maximally in the parietal area is found most often in children aged 2–6

years (Doose & Gundel 1982). Among 3–4-year-old siblings of probands with this theta pattern, up to 30% will show the same EEG pattern. Doose & Gundel argue that theta waves may serve as an indicator of a genetic predisposition for seizures.

It is clear that Doose is aware of the similarities between hypnagogic patterns in children and parietal theta rhythms, and he has required that the patients be clearly alert at the time that these patterns occur. No other investigators have systematically searched for this pattern to confirm or refute Doose's observation and his hypothesis of a relationship between these patterns and generalized spike and wave (GSW) patterns.

Implications

The family studies of epilepsy probands have established the importance of thorough EEG evaluation, not only for diagnostic purposes but also for genetic counselling. Hyperventilation and photic stimulation should be used routinely within those age groups which are potentially responsive (about 3–19 years). Sleep should also be used when possible in order to increase the probability of eliciting a spike-wave pattern. The EEG response under each of these conditions should be recorded separately, since the possibility of heterogeneity has not yet been explored fully.

Antecedent factors

There are many antecedent factors which predispose individuals to epilepsy (Hauser & Annegers 1991). While there are differences in the proportion of cases with epilepsy attributed to specific causes within age strata, the majority of cases of epilepsy fall into an idiopathic or cryptogenic category in all age groups, even the elderly. A distinction must be made between predisposing factors which increase the risk for developing an epileptogenic state such as history of infection of the central nervous system or severe head (brain) injury, and factors which directly trigger the seizure episode such as systemic metabolic derangement or the immediate consequences of brain insult. At the time of some acute insults such as febrile illness, a family history of epilepsy or of febrile seizures may increase the likelihood of a seizure. There is as yet no clear evidence that family history of epilepsy is associated with an increase in risk for epilepsy following specific brain insults.

MENDELIAN DISORDERS INVOLVING SEIZURES

It must be emphasized that there seldom is a one-to-one correspondence between seizures and any Mendelian disorder. In few of these disorders are seizures found in all of the affected individuals; nor is it yet clear whether a comprehensive review of the Mendelian traits will provide insight into aetiological pathways involved for the manifestation of seizures in general. Nevertheless, some points of clinical and genetic interest can be illustrated by reference to a few selected conditions.

Progressive myoclonus epilepsy

Norio & Koskiniemi (1979) reviewed the data for 74 Finnish families with progressive myoclonus epilepsy of the Baltic (or Unverricht-Lundborg) type and calculated the risk for siblings of probands to be 26%, an excellent fit to the hypothesis of autosomal recessive inheritance. Most cases developed signs in the age range of 8–13 years and there were no Lafora bodies in cases coming to autopsy. This condition is characterized by severe, incapacitating stimulus-sensitive myoclonus and tonic-clonic seizures.

Recently the gene locus has been mapped to the terminal sub-band q22.3 of the long arm of chromosome 21 (Lehesjoki et al 1991). This finding was based on studies of 68 individuals in 12 Finnish families, including 26 affected patients. The maximum multipoint lod score was 10.08. Now it will be possible to study families in other populations and also to test the hypothesis that Ramsay Hunt syndrome is caused by mutations at the same locus. Meanwhile, presymptomatic and prenatal diagnosis can now be offered to those families in which linkage to chromosome 21 is well established.

Benign familial neonatal convulsions

Benign familial neonatal convulsions (BFNC) are characterized by early onset of frequent brief seizures with normal condition between seizures and with other known causes of neonatal seizures excluded (Rett & Teubel 1964, Bjerre & Corelius 1968, Quattlebaum 1979, Zonana et al 1984). The pattern of inheritance is autosomal dominant with about 85% penetrance.

The developmental history is unique in that onset is in the first week of life in 80% cases, with peak onset on the third day. The seizures stop by 4 months in 35% of cases, by 1 year in 70%, and by 2 years in 85%. Recurrent seizures after age 5 are seen in 15%. The seizure pattern is variable, including motor and other clinical manifestations.

The gene locus for BFNC has been mapped to the long arm of chromosome 20 (Leppert et al 1989, 1991). Joint analysis of BFNC and two DNA markers gave a lod score of 5.64, with no obligate recombinants. Additional families have been tested with informative markers and the total lod score is now over 15 (Leppert, personal communication). This syndrome appears to meet the qualifications for cloning the gene by means of reverse genetics.

BFNC should be considered in the differential diagnosis of neonatal seizures. Genetic counselling includes information about the relatively benign course of the disease, and also the high risk (40–45%) for subsequent pregnancies.

Tuberous sclerosis and neurofibromatosis

Tuberous sclerosis and neurofibromatosis are autosomal dominant traits that share a number of other interesting features.

1. Series of cases are often identified through hospitals and clinics, and thus tend to miss those with milder manifestations; hence, the population prevalence will be underestimated and the proportion with seizures will be overestimated.
2. A careful examination of relatives is essential to identify those with minimal signs.
3. Genetic counselling must take into account the clinical findings and the possibility of new mutations.

There are two population-based studies of tuberous sclerosis. The prevalence for children under 5 years old was 15.4 per 100 000 for the

Oxford, England, area (Hunt & Lindenbaum 1984) and 23.5 per 100 000 in Rochester, Minnesota (Wiederholt et al 1985). The true rates may be higher. In the Oxford series, it was estimated that 50–75% of 68 cases were new mutations, as compared with 70–86% in an earlier review (Bundey & Evans 1969). Four out of eight cases in Rochester developed seizures (all with onset before the age of 2), and two of these were mentally retarded. There were no neurological abnormalities in those free of seizures. Tuberous sclerosis has been identified as an important cause of infantile spasms, in 25 of 195 (13%) in the series investigated by Charlton & Mellinger (1970) and 14 of 54 (26%) in the study by Pampiglione & Pugh (1975). The importance of careful examination of siblings is emphasized by the report of seven cases in which hypopigmented maculae of the skin developed at varying intervals after birth (Oppenheimer et al 1985). Two separate genetic loci have been identified for tuberous sclerosis on chromosomes 9 and 11 (Janssen et al 1990), and the evidence indicates that the frequency of seizures is similar for cases mapped to the two loci (Sandkuyl et al 1990).

Neurofibromatosis (NF) has a population frequency of about one in 3000 and about half of the cases are isolated (presumably new mutations). Two clinically distinct subtypes have been clearly defined (and there may be others as well). NF-1 (von Recklinghausen or peripheral type) involves cafe-au-lait spots and fibromatous skin tumours, and the gene maps to chromosome 17. NF-2 (the bilateral acoustic or central type) involves tumours of the eighth cranial nerve, meningiomas, neurofibromas, ependymomas, and acoustic neuromas, and the responsible gene is on chromosome 22 (Rouleau et al 1987). More recently the gene for NF-1 has been isolated and cloned, and the various mutations are under intensive examination (Wallace et al 1990, Cawthon et al 1990). Seizures have been reported in 6–13% of NF cases (Carey et al 1979), presumably mainly in NF-1.

Homocystinuria

Homocystinuria is an autosomal recessive metabolic disease with interesting features. A deficiency of cystathionine ß-synthase leads to increased plasma homocysteine and methionine and decreased cysteine. The major complications are mental retardation, dislocation of the lens, skeletal abnormalities and a tendency to thromboembolic episodes. Mudd et al (1985) reviewed questionnaires and published reports for 629 cases. Among 55 detected on newborn screening and treated, one developed seizures; of those detected at older ages, 21% had seizures, which may have contributed to their recognition as affected. (It is possible that some of the seizures were secondary to cerebrovascular accidents.) Among 19 patients with EEG records, 10 showed mild diffuse nonspecific slowing of the background (Del Giudice et al 1983). In nine cases with abnormal EEGs, treatment with pyridoxine was followed by change to a normal EEG in three. The gene for homocystinuria has now been mapped to chromosome 21q22.3 (Munke et al 1988).

Mitochondrial encephalopathies

The mitochondrial enzyme complexes are formed from subunits, some of which are encoded by mitochondrial genes and some from nuclear genes. Disorders of the mitochondrial enzyme complexes involved in the respiratory chain, therefore, can result from mutations in nuclear or mitochondrial genes, or in defects of communication. As a result some mitochondrial enzyme defects will be inherited in regular Mendelian patterns while others will follow a maternal inheritance pattern.

The frequency of epilepsy in these disorders has been reviewed by DiMauro et al (1991). Epilepsy is included by definition in myoclonus epilepsy with ragged-red fibres (MERRF), but there is considerable variability within families. In one large pedigree with clear maternal inheritance, four out of eight relatives of the proband lacked seizures although they carried a specific point mutation in a transfer RNA gene (Shoffner at al 1990). Such variability may result from heteroplasmy (different relative amounts of mutant and wild-type mitochondrial genomes in different tissues) or differences in rate of growth, metabolism, or energy requirements of various tissues. In mitochondrial encephalomyopathy, lactic acidosis, and stroke-like episodes (MELAS)

62 of 66 patients (94%) had seizures (DiMauro et al 1991). Seizures are rare in Kearns–Sayre syndrome (KSS), but are seen in 31% of patients with Leigh syndrome.

CHROMOSOMAL ABNORMALITIES

Down syndrome

In a survey of 1654 hospitalized Down syndrome patients around London and in south-east England, Veall (1974) found a prevalence of epilepsy of 5.8%. In the age group from 0 to 19, the prevalence of epilepsy was 1.9%. In the age groups from 20 to 59 there was some variation, but the average prevalence was 6.5%. In the much smaller sample, from the age of 60, the prevalence was 15.4%.

In a study of 111 patients with Down syndrome in a hospital serving the city of Glasgow, there were 11 (8.1%) with epilepsy (MacGillivray 1967). In general, their seizures were milder than those of other retarded patients. In another series of 128 patients in a hospital in Lancaster, England, there were 13 (10.2%) with a history of epilepsy; only five of these had onset of seizures prior to the age of 25 (Tangye 1979).

Alzheimer disease

A gene for familial Alzheimer disease (AD) has been mapped to chromosome 21 in some families but not in others (St. George-Hyslop et al 1990, Schellenberg et al 1990). AD is associated with a 10-fold increase in risk for epilepsy over that expected in the general population (Hauser et al 1986, Romanelli et al 1990), and by 10 years following diagnosis roughly 15% of survivors will have developed epilepsy (Hauser et al 1986, Romanelli et al 1990). This high frequency of seizures should not be surprising since disorders of grey matter are in general characterized by seizures. The pathology in aging Down syndrome and in patients with Alzheimer disease is similar, which may explain in part the high frequency of seizures in older Down syndrome patients.

Ring chromosome 14

The diagnosis of tuberous sclerosis was at first entertained for an infant girl with mental retardation and seizures associated with scattered vitiliginous spots and multiple hyperpigmented spots (Schmidt et al 1981). The presence of dysmorphic features of the head and face, however, led to a chromosome study which showed a ring chromosome 14. A review of this and six previously reported cases with a ring 14 showed that seizures occurred in six out of seven. These were generalized tonic-clonic seizures and myoclonic jerks which were fully controlled with antiepileptic treatment.

Inverted duplicated 15

Occasionally, chromosomal changes are found without associated dysmorphology. A high frequency of seizures is found in patients with an extra inverted duplicated chromosome 15 (Schreck et al 1977, Wisniewski et al 1979, Maraschio et al 1981). Of the 28 cases reported in these three papers, 21 (75%) had seizures, but there were no major physical abnormalities.

Ring chromosome 20

Epilepsy has been seen in seven of 12 patients with a ring (20) chromosome (Back et al 1989). The epilepsies were characterized by complex partial seizures, sometimes evolving secondarily into generalized tonic-clonic seizures. The seizures were poorly controlled or were resistant to medical treatment. Other features included mental retardation, microcephaly, and behavioural disorders.

Fragile X syndrome

Seizures are a common manifestation of the fra(X) syndrome (Hecht 1991). The seizures can begin neonatally and do not require a detectable environmental event as a trigger. The clinical features and EEG pattern appear to resemble those seen in benign childhood epilepsy with centrotemporal spikes (Musumeci et al 1991). Further study of these points would be desirable in view of the relatively high frequency of this syndrome.

Angelman syndrome

The Angelman syndrome (also known as the

happy puppet syndrome) is characterized by jerky limb movements, prominent lower jaw and wide mouth, unprovoked bursts of laughter, seizures, and mental retardation. Other features which help to make this diagnosis in infants include profound global developmental delay, postnatal-onset microcephaly, hypotonia, hyper-reflexia, hyperkinesis, choroidal pigment hypoplasia, and hypopigmentation as compared to relatives (Fryburg et al 1991). The EEG pattern includes very large amplitude slow spike-wave activity, posterior discharges facilitated by eye closure, and large amplitude rhythmic 4–6/s intermediate slow activity, and is said to be sufficiently specific to aid in the diagnosis (Boyd et al 1988). The risk of this syndrome in siblings of probands is only about 4% (Willems et al 1987).

In many cases of the Angelman syndrome the maternal genes in a short segment of the long arm of chromosome 15 are deleted, while Prader Willi syndrome involves deletion of the paternal genes in the same, but not necessarily identical, area (Magenis et al 1990, Imaizumi et al 1990). Deletion cases may involve genome imprinting, a phenomenon in which an imprintable allele is transmitted in a Mendelian manner, but the expression is determined by the sex of the transmitting parent (Williams et al 1990).

GENETICS IN SPECIFIC EPILEPSIES

Generalized onset epilepsy

The electroencephalographic hallmark of the generalized epilepsies is the interictal GSW (generalized spike and wave). Thus, studies of the generalized epilepsies are by definition studies of GSW, but GSW may occur also in individuals who have other forms of epilepsy or, for that matter, in asymptomatic individuals. Patients having generalized epilepsies with GSW, therefore, must be considered highly selected groups, and the results from studies of such patients cannot be generalized to all individuals with GSW.

The study carried out by Metrakos & Metrakos (1970) has served as a benchmark for comparison with later studies and deserves an extended discussion. The probands were identified at the Montreal Children's Hospital and thus had onset in childhood. The classification of probands followed the proposal by Penfield & Jasper (1954) which placed seizures into three main groups (localized, unlocalized and centrencephalic) depending upon the presumed origin of the epileptic discharge. Gastaut (1964) suggested that the term 'centrencephalic' be replaced by 'epilepsy of subcortical origin', while Gloor (1968) preferred the term 'cortico-reticular epilepsy'.

Based on the EEG tracings, the probands were divided into those with typical and atypical patterns (Metrakos & Metrakos 1961). The prevalence rates of convulsions among near relatives of these two categories of probands were not different and thus the data were pooled.

The probands had either recurrent absence (petit mal) seizures or grand mal seizures (presumably 'tonic-clonic' in current terminology) (not tabulated separately) with no obvious neuropathology which would account for their seizures. The EEGs for the probands and relatives were considered positive for a GSW pattern, whether such a pattern occurred during the resting period, during hyperventilation or during photic stimulation. The category of spike-wave abnormalities referred to all types of generalized paroxysmal abnormalities, both epileptiform and nonepileptiform (Andermann 1982).

Control probands were collected by examining every twentieth admission to the same hospital and selecting those who had never had a convulsion, whose illness was not considered to be neuropathological and whose EEG was within normal or borderline normal limits. The history of seizures among siblings of the probands and controls is shown in Table 3.2.

The information about EEG abnormalities among siblings was also evaluated carefully. Follow-up EEG studies were done on 94 of the siblings (Metrakos & Metrakos 1974). At the time of the first EEG, the mean age was 7.6 years and 29% had generalized spike and wave EEGs. The mean age at the time of the second EEG was 15.3 years, and at that time 28% had the EEG trait. However, 45% had the trait in their first and/or second EEG. These data were used to support the hypothesis of an autosomal dominant inheritance for the EEG trait which is thought to underlie the seizures. Recently, Andermann (1991) has reviewed these Montreal data.

Table 3.2 Risk of epilepsy or any seizure in siblings of probands with primary generalized epilepsy

Seizure type in proband	Total No. siblings	With epilepsy %	Total with seizures %
Absence and/or grand mal (GSW*)			
Metrakos & Metrakos 1961, 1966	519	8.0	12.7
Control	322		4.7
Absence (with or without grand mal) (GSW)			
Matthes 1969	240	3.7	10.0
Doose et al 1973	448		6.7
Absence first symptom with onset after 5 years (GSW)			
Baier & Doose 1985	131		14.5
Myoclonic-astatic (akinetic)			
Matthes 1969	131	3.8	6.8
Doose 1985	154		16.0
Impulsive petit mal (Juvenile myoclonic)			
Tsuboi & Christian 1973	705	4.4	

* GSW = generalized spike and wave EEG pattern

Doose et al (1973) found lower sibling risks for seizures among absence probands than did Metrakos & Metrakos, and they also listed separately the data for probands with GSW occurring spontaneously and the data for those with GSW occurring only during PCR. The results suggest that a GSW in the EEG at rest or during hyperventilation may be genetically different from GSW occurring only during photic stimulation.

Doose et al (1973) studied 252 epileptic children who at some time had shown absences with generalized 3/s spike-waves. Among 448 siblings there were 30 (6.7%) who had one or more seizures (Table 3.2). This rate was higher for sisters than brothers (9.1% versus 3.9%). Among 242 siblings for whom EEG tracings were available there were 54 (22.3%) with GSW and/or PCR. Of these, 15 showed GSW only, 33 PCR only, and six showed both.

A later report was restricted to probands whose epilepsy started after the fifth year of life with absences as the first symptom and whose EEGs showed typical 3/s spikes and waves (Baier &

Doose 1985). This limitation was based on evidence that early infantile epilepsies with absences seem to run a worse course and have different sex ratios of affected relatives than diseases of later onset. Nineteen patients from the earlier study (Doose et al 1973) were included in the total of 77 probands. Among 131 siblings, 19 (14.5%) developed seizures and 20 (15.3%) reported migraine (Table 3.2).

Doose (1985) reported studies on probands with myoclonic-astatic petit mal (Table 3.2). The onset is usually in the third and fourth year of life, and the course of the disease is generally unfavourable. Among 154 siblings there were 16% with a history of seizures.

Matthes (1969) carried out similar studies (Table 3.2). Among 240 siblings of probands with absence epilepsy and 3/s GSW there were nine (3.8%) with epilepsy and 15 (6.3%) with childhood convulsions, for a total of 10.0%. Among 131 siblings of probands with akinetic seizures (but with a slow generalized spike and wave complex) there were five (3.8%) with epilepsy and an additional four (3%) with childhood convulsions, for a total of 6.9%. While these rates are generally lower, strict comparisons require age adjustments.

Additional information is provided by EEGs on the siblings themselves. Doose et al (1984) studied 294 probands with primary generalized minor seizures (myoclonic-astatic or absence epilepsy with or without tonic-clonic seizures). The highest seizure rate was found in siblings with

Table 3.3 Risk of any seizure by EEG findings in siblings of epilepsy probands with primary generalized minor seizures (Doose et al 1984)

EEG findings in siblings	Siblings No.	With any seizure No.	%	
Photosensitivity without other patterns	43	3	7.0	⎫ 9.0
Theta rhythms without spikes and waves	24	3	12.5	⎭
Spike waves without other patterns	20	7	35.0	⎫ 34.0
Spike waves with photosensitivity and/or theta rhythms	27	9	33.3	⎭
Normal EEG	123	5	4.1	

spikes and waves during rest and hyperventilation (34%), as compared with 9.0% in siblings with only photosensitivity or theta rhythms, and 4.1% in siblings with normal EEGs (Table 3.3).

An interesting parallel comes from the work of Cavazzuti et al (1980). EEGs were recorded in 3726 school children, from 6 to 13 years of age, who were neurologically normal and had no history of epileptic seizures. In 41 (1.1%) there were generalized discharges on the EEG and, upon follow-up over an 8–9-year period, five out of 35 (14.3%) developed epileptic seizures. Another 90 (2.3% of the total) showed other epileptiform EEG patterns at the outset, and two out of 65 (3.1%) developed epileptic seizures during the follow-up period.

Juvenile myoclonic epilepsy

In this discussion of generalized onset epilepsy, special attention must be given to juvenile myoclonic epilepsy (JME), as described by Janz (Janz & Christian 1957, Janz 1989). In a large, comprehensive study by Tsuboi & Christian (1973) the majority of the probands were aged 10 to 20 years at onset. Among 705 siblings there were 31 (4.4%) who had developed epilepsy (Table 3.2).

The inheritance of JME is consistent with either a single dominant or recessive gene, or a two-locus model with one gene dominant and the other recessive (Delgado-Escueta et al 1989). Some

relatives have JME itself, but more show absence, other myoclonic, and other generalized seizures, but rarely partial seizures (Delgado-Escueta et al 1991, Beck-Mannagetta & Janz 1991).

Analysis of JME families, with relatives classified as affected if they presented with JME or other generalized epilepsy or had the characteristic EEG pattern associated with JME, produced evidence for linkage to the HLA region on the short arm of chromosome 6, regardless of the mode of inheritance (Delgado-Escueta et al 1991). Linkage with the HLA region has been confirmed in a different set of families from Berlin using HLA typing (Weissbecker et al 1991) and DNA markers (Durner et al 1991).

It is reasonable to conclude that JME is a defined epilepsy syndrome which is part of a larger genetic entity, and that a gene locus affecting the development of JME and related epilepsies is in or near the HLA region of chromosome 6. Linkage studies using additional markers will further define the susceptibility locus and provide insight into the pathogenesis of this form of seizure activity.

Implications for genetic counselling

The basic information about sibling risks is summarized in Figure 3.5. The risks to siblings are for *any epilepsy*, since parental concern is not limited to seizures of the same type found in the proband.

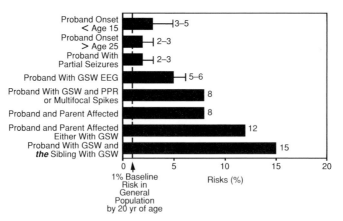

Fig. 3.5   Sibling risk for epilepsy. (EEG = electroencephalogram, GSW = generalized spike-wave, PPR = photoparoxysmal response). Modified with permission from Hauser & Hesdorffer 1990. © 1990 Epilepsy Foundation of America.

The 1% baseline risk was derived from the cumulative risk of epilepsy in the Rochester-Olmsted County population to age 20 (Annegers 1991) as being the period of greatest concern to parents. Some of the risks are given as ranges to reflect the varying estimates from different studies. It will be noted that the risks are lower when the epilepsy proband has only a generalized spike-wave (GSW) EEG than when a GSW is combined with other patterns. The highest sibling risk is found when the epilepsy proband has a GSW EEG pattern and the sibling also has a GSW pattern.

It may be noted that the estimates for sibling risks generally will be lower than the families may have feared. With the exception of the rarer genetic syndromes, sibling risks seldom will exceed 10%, as compared with a population base rate of 1–2%.

Table 3.4 Risk of epilepsy or any seizure in siblings of probands with partial (localization-related) epilepsy

Seizure type in proband	Siblings Total no.	With epilepsy %	With any seizure %
Benign childhood epilepsy with centro-temporal spikes			
Heijbel et al 1975	52		15.6
Morikawa et al 1979	76	1.3	11.8
Partial seizures with focal sharp wave EEG			
Gerken et al 1977	157		1.9
Surgically treated partial epilepsy (mostly temporal)			
Jensen 1975	171	2.9	4.7
Andermann 1982	229	1.3	4.8
Controls	458		(3.9)

Partial (localization related) epilepsies

The term 'partial' (or focal) can be applied either to seizure manifestations or to EEG findings. Some of the cases of focal epilepsy may result from a structural epileptogenic focus such as a scar or mass. Others, however, may be more closely related to the primary generalized epilepsies and syndromes, and may share a genetic predisposition (Metrakos & Metrakos 1970).

Bray & Wiser (1964, 1965) studied 40 probands with focal epilepsy whose EEGs showed paroxysmal sharp waves or spikes in the mid-temporal area, either unilateral or bilateral. Pedigree analysis was reported to show transmission as an autosomal dominant trait, although the details are not presented (except for a note that in 12 of the families at least one close relative had seizures associated with a focal temporal central spike abnormality on the EEG).

From the clinical EEG descriptions, many of the cases studied by Bray & Wiser appear similar to those studied by Heijbel et al (1975). The probands in the latter study had seizures and also Rolandic discharges on the EEG recording. Among the siblings at each age level, one-third showed Rolandic discharges (Table 3.4). The patients described in these two series probably fall under the category of localization related idiopathic epilepsy termed benign childhood epilepsy with

centrotemporal spikes. This epileptic syndrome is said to account for 15–20% of all childhood epilepsies in European series (Blom et al 1972), but seems less frequent in the United States. In addition to the localized spikes which have a unique field distribution (Blom & Heijbel 1975), these children frequently demonstrate generalized spike and wave EEG patterns. Their siblings also demonstrate a high frequency of generalized spike and wave pattern when sleep is obtained (Degen & Degen 1990). It seems that this form of epilepsy may represent a transition between generalized and partial epilepsies.

A larger series of 203 children with various forms of epilepsy was studied by Gerken et al (1977). They were selected for having shown focal sharp waves in the EEG (some in the Rolandic area) at least once. The sibling risk for seizures was considerably lower than in families of probands with spike-wave absences.

One of the most carefully studied series is based on 60 patients with focal cerebral seizures (mostly temporal) who underwent surgical treatment for their epilepsy (Andermann 1982). There was no significant increase in history of seizures among siblings as compared to control relatives (Table 3.4). There was, however, a significant increase in the prevalence of total EEG abnormalities. Upon review of the data, using stricter criteria for EEG classification, the frequency of generalized, but not focal, epileptiform EEG abnormalities was significantly elevated in the relatives of focal probands (Andermann & Straszak 1982).

A larger series of 74 patients who underwent unilateral temporal lobectomy for control of seizures was studied by Jensen (1975). Among 171 siblings there were five with epilepsy, and eight with other convulsions, for a total of 13 (7.6%) with seizure history (Table 3.4). The claim is made that the epilepsy rate among siblings is five to six times higher than expected in the general population, but this most likely results from the improper use of population prevalence values.

Implications

The risk of seizures is about 15% for siblings of probands with benign childhood epilepsy with centro-temporal spikes. For other localization-related epilepsies the risk for siblings by the age of 40 appears to be somewhat higher than population rates, perhaps 3% for epilepsy and 5% for any seizure (excluding febrile). There was no difference in the risk for epilepsy in offspring of epilepsy probands with generalized onset seizures when compared with offspring of probands with partial seizures in a study from Rochester, Minnesota (Ottman et al 1989).

Febrile convulsions (FC)

Convulsions associated with febrile illness are one of the common acute neurological disturbances seen in childhood (Hauser 1981). In the United States one-third of the patients with one FC will experience a recurrence of febrile seizures. Furthermore, patients with febrile seizures have a 3- to 6-fold increase in the risk of epilepsy when compared with the general population. The detailed studies on FC have provided clear evidence for an increased risk for both FC and epilepsy among siblings of probands (Hauser et al 1985).

Several twin studies also have been reported. Lennox-Buchthal (1971) analysed the data for the twin series collected by W. G. Lennox and found 13 out of 19 pairs (68%) concordant for febrile convulsions. It was noted, however, that these twins had a higher proportion with a severely abnormal birth history and with subsequent epilepsy than did the population-based series studied by Frantzen et al (1970).

Schiøttz-Christiansen (1972) searched the records for twins born in the Copenhagen area from 1950 to 1965. The incidence of febrile convulsions among all twin-born individuals was estimated at 30%. There were 63 participating index pairs with at least one having febrile convulsions. Among the MZ pairs eight out of 26 (31%) were concordant, while among the DZ pairs five out of 37 (14%) were concordant. The case-wise risk of febrile convulsions was 44% for monozygotic co-twins of probands and 20% for dizygotic co-twins. The MZ–DZ differences were not statistically significant, and the results have been cited as evidence against genetic factors. It seems more reasonable to conclude that the results were indefinite (because of the relatively small sample size) and that both genetic and non-genetic factors were involved. This interpretation is strengthened by Tsuboi's (1982) report of concordance rates of 46% (25/54) for MZ pairs and 13% (12/89) for DZ pairs in his study. In a recent analysis of the Virginia and Norwegian Twin Panels, Corey et al (1990) calculated the proband-wise concordance for febrile convulsions to be 0.33 for MZ pairs and 0.11 for DZ pairs. The MZ concordance for epilepsy as a whole was 0.21 and the DZ concordance was 0.06.

Hauser et al (1985) analysed the data for 1046 siblings of 421 FC probands in Rochester, Minnesota. The general population rate for FC was 2.4%; the sibling FC risk was 5.5% when neither parent had a history of FC, 21.7% when one parent had FC and 55.6% with both parents affected. This effect of parental FC history is seen also in the two Japanese studies.

The Minnesota/Japan contrast for FC risk is sharpest in the families in which neither parent has had a history of FC. When one or both parents are affected, the sibling risks are similar in the United States and Japan. It is possible that a large proportion of the Japanese cases might represent a dominant mode of inheritance, similar to that hypothesized earlier for the smaller Rochester subgroup.

Table 3.5 Risk of febrile convulsions (FC) among siblings of probands

FC in parent(s)	Number of FCs in probands			Overall sibling	Population rate
	1	2	3+ risk		
Rochester				8.0%	2.4%
Yes	10.8%	22.7%	31.9%		
No	3.1%	8.4%	10.9%		
Tokyo				24.9%	6.7%
Yes	37.6%	36.7%	38.8%		
No	19.4%	21.5%	25.6%		

With this question in mind, a further comparison is reported in Table 3.5 for the Rochester data (Rich, personal communication) and the Tokyo data (Tsuboi, personal communication). If anything, this analysis tends to intensify the problem rather than to resolve it. If the Rochester/Tokyo differences arose from more Japanese FC probands having affected parents and/or more FC episodes, the sibling risks within comparable cells should have become more alike.

At this point we may consider the possibility that spike-wave EEG abnormalities are indeed more common in Japanese FC probands and that the GSW serves as an indicator of dominant inheritance. There are now reports from at least seven independent groups of investigators suggesting that generalized spike and wave (GSW) patterns occur with a high frequency in children with FC. Tsuboi (1982), Frantzen et al (1968), and Doose et al (1966) have done serial EEG recordings on children following FC. Between 25 and 40% of children have been reported to show GSW in these studies. None reports GSW at the time of FC. Thorn (1981) and Metrakos & Metrakos (1970) did EEG recordings following

FC (not serial). They reported GSW in 35% of probands.

One further observation from the Rochester study deserves comment. The relative risk of epilepsy (Table 3.6) was the same for 967 siblings of probands with FC only (2.4) as for 552 siblings of probands with unprovoked seizures (2.5), but was twice as high for the 79 siblings of those probands who had FC followed by epilepsy (5). These results emphasize the complexity of the familial relationship between epilepsy and FC.

Implications

For the purposes of genetic counselling, febrile convulsions deserve a separate treatment. In the United States, 2–4% of all children will experience a FC prior to age 5, and siblings have a 3-fold increased risk of FC (Hauser et al 1985). Furthermore, both the FC probands and their siblings have elevated risks for subsequent epilepsy. When one parent also has a history of FC, the risk of FC to siblings of a proband is increased to 22%; when both parents have such a history, the sibling risk is further increased to 56% (Anderson et al

Table 3.6 Risk for febrile convulsions (FC) and unprovoked seizures in siblings of probands (Hauser et al 1985)

Proband seizure type	Total no. siblings	Sibling seizure type			
		Febrile		Unprovoked*	
		Observed	Relative[†] risk	Observed	Relative[†] risk
Febrile only	967	74 (7.7%)	3.5	28 (2.9%)	2.4
Unprovoked* only	552	25 (4.5%)	2.0	16 (2.9%)	2.5
Febrile followed by unprovoked*	79	9 (11.4%)	7.5	5 (6.3%)	5.0

* Single or recurrent unprovoked seizures
[†] All relative risks are significantly greater than 1.9 (P <0.05)

1990). In Japan the FC rate is 8% in the general population and 25% in siblings of FC probands (Table 3.5), significantly different from the risks elsewhere.

Post-traumatic seizures

There is a persistent impression that individuals who have seizures following head trauma may do so because they have a genetic predisposition for seizures (Caveness et al 1979), but data to support this contention are scanty and contradictory. The proportion of cases with post-traumatic seizures was greater in patients with a family history of seizures in the studies of Caveness (1963) and Jennett (1975), but the difference was not significant in either study. Phillips (1954) reported a family history of epilepsy in 12.6% of patients with seizures following closed-head trauma. He concluded that this was no higher than expected among any group of epileptic patients, but presented no comparable information from the general population or from a head trauma cohort. Evans (1962) reported a family history of seizures in 7% of trauma patients with seizures, and in only 2% of trauma patients without seizures. The only study which has rigorously studied family history of seizures and of epilepsy to date is the follow-up of 421 head injured Vietnam veterans (Salazar et al 1985). In this study, information regarding seizures and epilepsy for each class of relative was obtained for those with and without epilepsy. In these severely injured individuals family history had no effect on seizure occurrence.

Risks in offspring

It is difficult to obtain a satisfactory sample of children of probands for analysis. Ideally, the proband should have been identified a generation ago to permit following the offspring to an age reasonably through the risk period.

Tsuboi & Endo (1977) analysed their data about epilepsy and other seizures in children of probands from several points of view. The results are comparable with those from other studies of children and follow the trends demonstrated for siblings.

1. The risk is higher when the probands had

idiopathic (as compared with symptomatic) epilepsy.
2. The risk is higher for children of affected mothers than for children of affected fathers.
3. The risk is higher when the proband developed epilepsy at younger age.
4. The risk is higher when the proband has an affected parent or sibling.
5. Finally, the risk of seizures is considerably higher for those children who themselves showed a specific EEG abnormality.

An important study in progress in Berlin is beginning to yield information about offspring of epileptic probands (Beck-Mannagetta et al 1989b). The Rochester, Minnesota, data have also been studied from this perspective (Annegers et al 1978). These studies are compared with more data from Tsuboi & Okada (1985) in Table 3.7.

Implications

In most studies, children have not been followed far into adulthood. Hence the available data may underestimate the risks, unless appropriate age corrections are used. The risks for children appear to be the same as, or higher than, those for siblings. The data in Figure 3.6 provide reasonable guides for genetic counselling. The maternal effect appears clearly. When the higher risk asso-

Table 3.7 Risk of epilepsy or febrile convulsions in offspring of probands with epilepsy

Study, seizure type in proband	Total no. offspring	With epilepsy %	With FC %
Tsuboi & Christian 1973	275	4.4	
Annegers et al 1978	687	1.9	2.6
Beck-Mannagetta et al 1989b	840	4.6	4.5
Tsuboi & Okada 1985			
Any epilepsy	817	2.4	8.4
Awaking grand mal	208	4.8	11.1
Grand mal during sleep	157	2.0	2.0
Diffuse grand mal	64	6.3	1.6
Myoclonic petit mal	27	14.8	7.4
Absence	30	6.7	10.0
Psychomotor epilepsy	156	0.6	5.1
Focal seizure	28	0	3.6

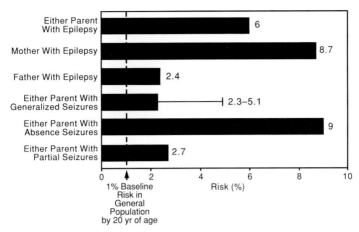

Fig. 3.6 Offspring risk for epilepsy. Modified with permission from Hauser & Hesdorffer 1990. © 1990 Epilepsy Foundation of America.

ciated with absence epilepsy is treated separately, the risk with other generalized epilepsies is similar to that with partial epilepsies (Ottman et al 1989).

Effects of antiepileptic drugs on the fetus

In the process of providing genetic counselling for women with epilepsy, it is important to consider the possibility that a fetus may be affected by genetic factors associated with the mother's predisposition for seizures or by the antiepileptic drugs that she may be taking (Commission on Genetics, Pregnancy and the child 1989). In the Rochester, Minnesota, population-based study the rate of major malformations was 2.4% for children born to mothers with epilepsy not taking antiepileptic drugs during pregnancy, 10.7% for children of mothers who took antiepileptic drugs during pregnancy and 3.8% among the children of men with epilepsy (Annegers et al 1978). In a retrospective study at the Montreal Neurological Hospital, the proportion of viable offspring having major congenital malformations was 15.9% for mothers taking antiepileptic medication, as compared with 6.5% for mothers not taking medication (Dansky et al 1982).

Of particular interest for this chapter is the evidence that genetic variation in the fetus may affect various types of teratogenic expression (Lindhout 1989). Furthermore, fetal genetic variation in the enzyme epoxide hydrolase may affect susceptibility to phenytoin-influenced birth defects (Buehler

& Delimont 1985, Strickler et al 1985). More recent evidence suggests that measurement of epoxide hydrolase activity in amniocytes from pregnancies at risk may be useful in predicting which fetuses will develop malformations (Buehler et al 1990).

While there seems to be a high correlation between exposure to antiepileptic drugs in utero and malformations, patients taking these drugs during pregnancy may be different from those not on such medication. Thus, one could not exclude the possibility that the effect could be due in part to the presence of epilepsy in the mother rather than to the antiepileptic drugs (see also Janz 1982, Annegers et al 1983).

Clefting disorders are among the most frequent major malformations identified in offspring of probands with epilepsy. It has been suggested that epilepsy and clefting may in some way be linked genetically, but epidemiological studies of siblings of probands with epilepsy demonstrated no increase in the frequency of clefting over that expected (Friis et al 1986), and epilepsy occurred no more frequently than expected among descendants of nonepileptic parents of probands with clefting (Hecht et al 1989).

Finnell (1981) studied mice of several inbred strains and also an autosomal recessive locus that produces a spontaneous clonic seizure disorder. The occurrence of fetal defects was correlated with maternal serum concentrations of phenytoin, but not with the maternal or fetal genotype or the presence of a seizure disorder. The maternal serum phenytoin level and not the maternal seizure disorder appears to be the agent responsible for the malformations (Finnell & Chernoff 1982). Further studies in mice add evidence that neither seizure disorder nor antiepileptic treatment in the father leads to an increased incidence of congenital malformations (Finnell & Baer 1986).

Implications

It is beyond the scope of this chapter to review the literature about possible teratogenic effects of the various antiepileptic drugs (the subject is dealt with in more detail in later Chapters). In general, genetic counselling for epileptic women should consider three points:

1. In most types of epilepsy, the risks for epilepsy or other seizures are higher for offspring of female than of male epilepsy patients (Ottman et al 1985).
2. The possible teratogenic effects of antiepileptic drugs should be discussed, using the best available information.
3. As new evidence emerges, fetal genetic variation in response to teratogenic agents can be considered.

The clinician as researcher

In epilepsy clinics, the research possibilities would be enhanced by attention to certain aspects of the family history.

1. We would urge that such clinics keep a running record of those families in which two or more siblings have seizures. These multisib families would provide an excellent panel for extensive biochemical, clinical or other laboratory studies.

2. A similar record should be maintained for patients who are twin-born. Both concordant and discordant pairs can be very useful, although for different questions. In the near future we would envisage that twin studies might focus on specific rare clinical patterns. In such an event it would be extremely important and necessary to have a basis for collaboration among various institutions.

3. We would also urge that special note be made of families in which a number of individuals have a seizure history. Kindreds with five or more affected persons can be reviewed to determine which are likely to be informative for linkage studies.

FUTURE PROSPECTS

The many new strategies being developed for analysing brain structure and function will permit a much clearer description of individual variation in underlying pathology among epilepsy patients. With the use of molecular techniques for assessing neurotransmitters and membrane receptors, family studies will become more informative. Specific biochemical genetic hypotheses can be framed and tested more explicitly. To this end it is fortunate that large, carefully documented series of epilepsy families are already available for exploration.

New genetic methods include a rapidly expanding array of DNA markers for gene mapping, powerful techniques for producing high density linkage maps, and methods for cloning neural genes based on differences in regional mRNA patterns. As human gene mutations are isolated, their phenotypic effects can be examined in transgenic mouse models. Eventually, these approaches can be expected to contribute to a better definition of genetic entities and thus to improved diagnosis and treatment of the epilepsies.

REFERENCES

Andermann E 1982 Multifactorial inheritance of generalized and focal epilepsy. In: Anderson V E, Hauser W A, Penry J K, Sing C F (eds) Genetic basis of the epilepsies. Raven Press, New York, pp 355–374
Andermann E 1991 Genetic studies of epilepsy in Montreal. In: Anderson V E, Hauser W A, Leppik I E, Noebels J L, Rich S S (eds) Genetic strategies in epilepsy research.

Epilepsy Research (suppl 4). Elsevier, Amsterdam, p 129–137
Andermann E, Straszak M 1982 Family studies of epileptiform EEG abnormalities and photosensitivity in focal epilepsy. In: Akimoto H, Kazamatsuri H, Seino M, Ward A (eds) Advances in epileptology: XIII Epilepsy International Symposium, p 105–112
Anderson V E, Hauser W A 1990 Genetics. In: Dam M,

Gram L (eds) Comprehensive epileptology. Raven Press, New York, p 57–76

Anderson V E, Hauser W A, Rich S S 1986 Genetic heterogeneity in the epilepsies. In: Delgado-Escueta A V, Ward Jr A A, Woodbury D M, Porter R J (eds) Advances in Neurology, vol 44. Raven Press, New York, p 59–75

Anderson V E, Wilcox K J, Rich S S, Leppik I E, Hauser W A 1989 Twin studies in epilepsy. In: Beck-Mannagetta G, Anderson V E, Doose H, Janz D (eds) Genetics of the epilepsies. Springer, Berlin, p 145–155

Anderson V E, Hauser W A, Olafsson E, Rich S S 1990 Genetic aspects of the epilepsies. In: Sillanpää M, Johannessen S I, Blennow G, Dam M (eds) Paediatric epilepsy. Wrightson Biomedical Publishing, Petersfield, England, p 37–56

Anderson V E, Hauser W A, Leppik I E, Noebels J L, Rich S S (eds) 1991 Genetic strategies in epilepsy research. Epilepsy Research (suppl 4). Elsevier, Amsterdam

Annegers J F 1991 The use of analytic epidemiologic methods in family studies of epilepsy. In: Anderson V E, Hauser W A, Leppik I E, Noebels J L, Rich S S (eds) Genetic strategies in epilepsy research. Epilepsy Research (suppl 4). Elsevier, Amsterdam, p 139–146

Annegers J, Hauser W, Elveback L, Anderson V, Kurland L 1978 Congenital malformations and seizure disorders in the offspring of parents with epilepsy. International Journal of Epidemiology 7: 241–247

Annegers J F, Hauser W A, Anderson V E 1982 Risk of seizures among relatives of patients with epilepsy: families in defined population. In: Anderson V E, Hauser W A, Penry J K, Sing C F (eds) Genetic basis of the epilepsies. Raven Press, New York, p 151–159

Annegers J, Kurland L, Hauser W 1983 Teratogenicity of anticonvulsant drugs. In: Ward Jr. A A, Penry J K, Purpura D (eds) Epilepsy. Raven Press, New York, p 239–248

Back E, Voiculescu I, Brunger M, Wolff G 1989 Familial ring (20) chromosomal mosaicism. Human Genetics 83: 148–154

Baier W, Doose H 1985 Petit mal-absences of childhood onset: familial prevalences of migraine and seizures. Neuropediatrics 16: 80–83

Baraitser M 1990 The genetics of neurological disorders, 2nd edn. Oxford University Press, New York

Beck-Mannagetta G, Janz D 1991 Syndrome-related genetics in generalized epilepsy. In: Anderson V E, Hauser W A, Leppik I E, Noebels J L, Rich S S (eds) Genetic strategies in epilepsy research. Epilepsy Research (suppl 4). Elsevier, Amsterdam, p 105–111

Beck-Mannagetta G, Anderson V E, Doose H, Janz D 1989a Genetics of the epilepsies. Springer-Verlag, Berlin

Beck-Mannagetta G, Janz D, Hoffmeister U, Behl I, Scholz G 1989b Morbidity risk for seizures and epilepsy in offspring of patients with epilepsy. In: Beck-Mannagetta G, Anderson V E, Doose H, Janz D (eds) Genetics of the epilepsies. Springer-Verlag, Berlin, p 119–126

Berkovic S F, Howell R A, Hopper J L, Hay D A, Andermann E 1990 A twin study of the epilepsies. Epilepsia 31: 813

Bjerre I, Corelius E 1968 Benign familial neonatal convulsions. Acta Paediatrica Scandinavica 57: 557–561

Blandfort M, Tsuboi T, Vogel F 1987 Genetic counseling in the epilepsies. I. Genetic risks. Human Genetics 76: 303–331

Blom S, Heijbel J 1975 Benign epilepsy of children with centro-temporal EEG foci. Discharge rate during sleep. Epilepsia 16: 443–440

Blom S, Heijbel J, Bergfors P G 1972 Benign epilepsy of childhood with centrotemporal EEG foci. Prevalence and follow-up study of 40 patients. Epilepsia 13: 609–619

Boyd S G, Harden A, Patton M A 1988 The EEG in early diagnosis of the Angelman (Happy Puppet) syndrome. European Journal of Pediatrics 147: 508–513

Bray P F, Wiser W C 1964 Evidence for a genetic etiology of temporal-central abnormalities in focal epilepsy. New England Journal of Medicine 271: 926–933

Bray P F, Wiser W C 1965 Hereditary characteristics of familial temporal-central focal epilepsy. Pediatrics 36: 207–211

Buehler B A, Delimont D 1985 Epoxide hydralase activity: a direct assay for prediction of potential dilantin teratogenesis. Proceedings of the Greenwood Genetic Center 4: 92–93

Buehler B A, Delimont D, van Waes M, Finnell R H 1990 Prenatal prediction of risk of the fetal hydantoin syndrome. New England Journal of Medicine 322: 1567–1572

Bundey S, Evans K 1969 Tuberous sclerosis: a genetic study. Journal of Neurology, Neurosurgery and Psychiatry 32: 591–603

Carey J C, Laub J M, Hall B D 1979 Penetrance and variability in neurofibromatosis: a genetic study of 60 families. Birth Defects: Original article series 15(5B): 271–281

Cavazzuti G B, Cappella L, Nalin A 1980 Longitudinal study of epileptiform EEG patterns in normal children. Epilepsia 21: 43–55

Caveness W F 1963 Onset and cessation of fits following craniocerebral trauma. Journal of Neurosurgery 20: 570–582

Caveness W F, Meirowsky A M, Rish B L et al 1979 The nature of posttraumatic epilepsy. Journal of Neurosurgery 50: 545–553

Cawthon R M, Weiss R, Xu G et al 1990 A major segment of the neurofibromatosis type I gene: cDNA sequence, genomic structure, and point mutations. Cell 62: 193–201

Charlton M H, Mellinger J F 1970 Infantile spasms and hypsarrhythmia. Electroencephalography and Clinical Neurophysiology 29: 413

Cold Spring Harbor Laboratory 1991 The brain. Cold Spring Harbor Laboratory Press, Plainview, New York

Commission on classification and terminology of the International League against Epilepsy 1981 Proposal for revised clinical and electroencephalographic classification of epileptic seizures. Epilepsia 22: 489–501

Commission on classification and terminology of the International League Against Epilepsy 1989 Proposal for revised classification of epilepsies and epileptic syndromes. Epilepsia 30: 389–399

Commission On Genetics, Pregnancy, and the Child, International League Against Epilepsy 1989 Guidelines for the care of epileptic women of childbearing age. Epilepsia 30: 409–410

Corey L, Berg K, Pellock J, Nance W, DeLorenzo R 1990 Seizure syndrome in Virginia and Norwegian twin kindreds. Epilepsia 31: 814

Dansky L, Andermann E, Andermann F 1982 Major congenital malformations in the offspring of epileptic patients: Genetic and environmental risk factors. In: Janz D, Dam M, Richens A, Bossi L, Helge H, Schmidt D (eds)

Epilepsy, pregnancy, and the child. Raven Press, New York, p 223–233

Degen R, Degen H-E 1990 Some genetic aspects of Rolandic epilepsy: Waking and sleep EEGs in siblings. Epilepsia 31: 795–801

Delgado-Escueta A V, Ward Jr A A, Woodbury D M, Porter R J (eds) 1986 Advances in Neurology, vol 44. Raven Press, New York

Delgado-Escueta A V, Greenberg D A, Treiman L et al 1989 Mapping the gene for juvenile myoclonic epilepsy. Epilepsia 30: S8–S18

Delgado-Escueta A V, Greenberg D A, Weissbecker K et al 1991 The choice of epilepsy syndromes for genetic analysis. In: Anderson V E, Hauser W A, Leppik I E, Noebels J L, Rich S S (eds) Genetic strategies in epilepsy research. Epilepsy Research (suppl 4). Elsevier, Amsterdam, p 147–159

Del Giudice E, Striano S, Andria G 1983 Electroencephalographic abnormalities in homocystinuria due to cystathionine synthase deficiency. Clinical Neurology and Neurosurgery 85: 165–168

DiMauro S, Ricci E, Hirano M, De Vivo D C 1991 Epilepsy in mitochondrial encephalomyopathies. In: Anderson V E, Hauser W A, Leppik I E, Noebels J L, Rich S S (eds) Genetic strategies in epilepsy research. Epilepsy Research (suppl 4). Elsevier, Amsterdam, p 173–180

Doose H 1985 Myoclonic astatic epilepsy of early childhood. In: Roger J, Dravet C, Bureau M, Dreifuss F E, Wolf P (eds) Epileptic syndromes in infancy, childhood and adolescence. John Libbey Eurotext, London, p 78–88

Doose H, Baier W K 1987 Genetic factors in epilepsies with primarily generalized minor seizures. Journal of Pediatric Neurobiology, Neurology and Neurosurgery 18, Supplement I: 1–64

Doose H, Gerken H 1973 On the genetics of EEG-anomalies in childhood. IV. Photoconvulsive reaction. Neuropädiatrie 4: 162–171

Doose H, Gundel A 1982 Rhythms of 4 to 7 CPS in the childhood EEG. In: Anderson V E, Hauser W A, Penry J K, Sing C F (eds) Genetic basis of the epilepsies. Raven Press, New York, p 83–91

Doose H, Volzke E, Peterson C E, Herzberger E 1966 Fieberkrämpfe und epilepsie II. Elektrencephalographische Verlaufsuntersuchungen bei sogenannten Fieber-oder Infektkrämpfen. Archiv für Psychiatri und Nervenkrankheiten 208: 413–432

Doose H, Gerken H, Hein-Volpel K F, Volzke E 1969 Genetics of photosensitive epilepsy. Neuropädiatrie 1: 56–73

Doose H, Gerken H, Horstmann T, Volzke E 1973 Genetic factors in spike-wave absences. Epilepsia 14: 57–75

Doose H, Baier W, Reinsberg E 1984 Genetic heterogeneity of spike-wave epilepsies. In: Porter R J, Mattson R H, Ward Jr A A, Dam M (eds) Advances in epileptology: XVth Epilepsy International Symposium. Raven Press, New York, p 515–519

Durner M, Sander T, Greenberg D A et al 1991 Localisation of idiopathic generalized epilepsy on chromosome 6p in families of juvenile myoclonic epilepsy patients. Neurology 41: 1651–1655

Eeg-Olofsson O, Petersen I, Sellden U 1970 The development of the electroencephalogram in normal children from the age of 1 through 15 years. Neuropädiatrie 2: 375–404

Evans J H 1962 Post traumatic epilepsy. Neurology 12: 665–674

Evans G A 1991 Recent advances in genetics. In: Anderson V E, Hauser W A, Leppik I E, Noebels J L, Rich S S (eds) Genetic strategies in epilepsy research. Epilepsy Research (suppl 4). Elsevier, Amsterdam, p 189–198

Finnell R H 1981 Phenytoin-induced teratogenesis: a mouse model. Science 211: 483–484

Finnel R H, Baer J F 1986 Congenital defects among the offspring of epileptic fathers: role of the genotype and phenytoin therapy in a mouse model. Epilepsia 27: 697–705

Finnell R H, Chernoff G F 1982 Mouse fetal hydantoin syndrome: effects of maternal seizures. Epilepsia 23: 423–429

Frantzen E, Lennox-Buchthal M, Nygaard A 1968 Longitudinal EEG and clinical study of children with febrile convulsions. Electroencephalography and Clinical Neurophysiology 24: 197–212

Frantzen E, Lennox-Buchthal M, Nygaard A, Stene J 1970 A genetic study of febrile convulsions. Neurology 20: 909–917

Friis M L, Holm N V, Sindrup E H, Fogh-Andersen P, Hauge M 1986 Facial clefts in sibs and children of epileptic patients. Neurology 36: 346–350

Fryburg J S, Breg W R, Lindgren V 1991 Diagnosis of Angelman syndrome in infants. American Journal of Medical Genetics 38: 58–64

Gall C, Lauterborn J, Bundman M, Murray K, Isackson P 1991 Seizures and the regulation of neurotrophic factor and neuropeptide expression in brain. In: Anderson V E, Hauser W A, Leppik I E, Noebels J L, Rich S S (eds) Genetic strategies in epilepsy research. Epilepsy Research (suppl 4). Elsevier, Amsterdam, p 225–245

Ganetzky B 1991 Genetic analysis of ion channels in *Drosophila*. In: Anderson V E, Hauser W A, Leppik I E, Noebels J L, Rich S S (eds) Genetic strategies in epilepsy research. Epilepsy Research (suppl 4). Elsevier, Amsterdam, p 247–261

Gastaut H 1964 A proposed international classification of epileptic seizures. Epilepsia 5: 297–306

Gerken H, Doose H 1973 On the genetics of EEG anomalies. III. Spikes and waves in the resting record and/or during hyperventilation. Neuropädiatrie 4: 88–97

Gerken H, Kiefer R, Doose H, Volzke E 1977 Genetic factors in childhood epilepsy with focal sharp waves I: Clinical data and familial morbidity for seizures. Neuropädiatrie 8: 3–9

Gloor P 1968 Generalized cortico-reticular epilepsies. Epilepsia 9: 249

Haines J L, Panter S S, Rich S S, Eaton J W, Tsai M Y, Anderson V E 1986 Reduced plasma haptoglobin and urinary taurine in familial seizures identified through the multisib strategy. American Journal of Medical Genetics 24: 723–734

Hall J G 1990 Genomic imprinting: review and relevance to human diseases. American Journal of Human Genetics 46: 857–873

Harding A E 1991 Neurological disease and mitochondrial genes. Trends in Neurological Sciences 14: 132–138

Harvald B, Hauge M 1965 Hereditary factors elucidated by twin studies. In: Neel J V, Shaw M W, Schull W J (eds) Genetics and the epidemiology of chronic diseases, Public Health Service Publication No. 1163, Washington DC, p 61–76

Hauser W A 1981 The natural history of febrile seizures. In:

Nelson K B, Ellenberg J H (eds) Febrile seizures. Raven Press, New York, p 5–17

Hauser W A, Annegers J F 1991 Risk factors for epilepsy. In: Anderson V E, Hauser W A, Leppik I E, Noebels J L, Rich S S (eds) Genetic strategies in epilepsy research. Epilepsy Research (suppl 4). Elsevier, Amsterdam, p 45–52

Hauser W A, Annegers J F 1989 Epidemiologic measures for genetic studies. In: Beck-Mannagetta G, Anderson V E, Doose H, Janz D (eds) Genetics of the epilepsies. Springer-Verlag, Berlin, p 7–12

Hauser W A, Hesdorffer D C 1990 Facts about epilepsy. Demos Publications, New York

Hauser W A, Annegers J F, Anderson V E, Kurland L T 1985 The risk of seizure disorders among relatives of children with febrile convulsions. Neurology 35: 1268–1273

Hauser W A, Morris M L, Anderson V E, Heston L L 1986 Seizures and myoclonus in patients with Alzheimer Disease. Neurology 36: 1226–1230

Hauser W A, Rich S S, Annegers J F, Anderson V E 1990 Seizure recurrence after a 1st unprovoked seizure: An extended follow-up. Neurology 40: 1163–1170

Hecht F 1991 Seizure disorders in the fragile X chromosome syndrome. American Journal of Medical Genetics 38: 509

Hecht J T, Annegers J F, Kurland L T 1989 Epilepsy and clefting disorders: Lack of evidence of a familial association. American Journal of Medical Genetics 33: 244–247

Heijbel J, Blom S, Rasmuson M 1975 Benign epilepsy of childhood with centrotemporal EEG foci: a genetic study. Epilepsia 16: 285–293

Heintel H, Schalt E, Vogel F 1986 The 4–5 c/s rhythm—changes in time. European Archives of Psychiatry and Neurological Sciences 235: 299–300

Hirtz D B, Ellenberg J H, Nelson K B 1984 The risk of recurrence of nonfebrile seizures in children. Neurology 34: 637–641

Hopkins A, Garman A, Clarke C 1988 The first seizure in adult life. Lancet 1: 721–726

Hunt A, Lindenbaum R 1984 Tuberous sclerosis: a new estimate of prevalence within the Oxford region. American Journal of Medical Genetics 21: 272–277

Imaizumi K, Takada F, Kuroki Y, Naritomi K, Hamabe J, Niikawa N 1990 Cytogenetic and molecular study of the Angelman syndrome. American Journal of Medical Genetics 35: 314–318

Inouye E 1960 Observations on forty twin cases with chronic epilepsy and their co-twins. Journal of Nervous and Mental Disease 130: 401–416

Janssen L A J, Sandkuyl L A, Merkens E C et al 1990 Genetic heterogeneity in tuberous sclerosis. Genomics 8: 237–242

Janz D 1982 Antiepileptic drugs and pregnancy: altered utilization patterns and teratogenesis. Epilepsia 23 (Suppl 1): S53–S63

Janz D 1989 Juvenile myoclonic epilepsy. Epilepsy with petit mal. Cleveland Clinical Journal of Medicine 56 (suppl part I): S23–S33

Janz D, Christian W 1957 Impulsive-petit mal. Deutsche Medizinische Wochenschrift Zeitschrift für Nervenheilkunde 19: 155–182

Jennett B 1975 Epilepsy after non-missile head injuries. Heinemann, Chicago

Jensen I 1975 Genetic factors in temporal lobe epilepsy. Acta Neurologica Scandinavica 52: 381–394

Juel-Nielsen N, Harvald B 1958 The electroencephalogram in monovular twins brought up apart. Acta Genetica 9: 57–64

Kunkel L M, Beggs A H, Hoffman E P 1989 Molecular genetics of Duchenne and Becker muscular dystrophy: emphasis on improved diagnosis. Clinical Chemistry 35: B21–B24

Lehesjoki A, Koskiniemi M, Sistonen P et al 1991 Localization of a gene for progressive myoclonus epilepsy to chromosome 21q22. Proceedings of the National Academy of Science 88: 3696–3699

Lennox W G 1951 The heredity of epilepsy as told by relatives and twins. Journal of the American Medical Association 146: 529–536

Lennox W G, Lennox M A 1960 Epilepsy and related disorders. Little Brown, Boston

Lennox-Buchthal M 1971 Febrile and nocturnal convulsions in monozygotic twins. Epilepsia 12: 147–156

Leppert M F 1990 Gene mapping and other tools for discovery. Epilepsia 31 (suppl 3): S11–S18

Leppert M, Anderson V E, Quattlebaum T et al 1989 Benign familial neonatal convulsions linked to genetic markers on chromosome 20. Nature 337: 647–648

Leppert M, Anderson V E, White R 1991 The discovery of epilepsy genes by genetic linkage. In: Anderson V E, Hauser W A, Leppik I E, Noebels J L, Rich S S (eds) Genetic strategies in epilepsy research. Epilepsy Research (suppl 4). Elsevier, Amsterdam, p 181–188

Lindhout D 1989 Genetic variability in fetal response to anticonvulsants. In: Beck-Mannagetta G, Anderson V E, Doose H, Janz D (eds) Genetics of the epilepsies. Springer-Verlag, Berlin, p 175–183

Litt M, Luty J, Kwak M, Allen L, Magenis R E, Mandel G (1989) Localization of a human brain sodium channel gene (SCN2A) to chromosome 2. Genomics 5: 204–208

MacGillivray R C 1967 Epilepsy in Down's anomaly. Journal of Mental Deficiency Research 11: 43–48

Magenis R E, Toth-Fejel S, Allen L J et al 1990 Comparison of the 15q deletions in Prader–Willi and Angelman syndromes: specific regions, extent of deletions, parental origin, and clinical consequences. American Journal of Medical Genetics 35: 333–349

Maraschio P, Zuffardi O, Bernardi F et al 1981 Preferential maternal derivation in inv dup (15). Analysis of eight new cases. Human Genetics 59: 349–350

Matthes A 1969 Genetic studies in epilepsy. In: Gastaut H, Jasper H, Bancaud J, Waltregny A (eds) Genetic studies in epilepsy. Charles C Thomas, Springfield, Illinois, p 26–35

McKusick V A 1990 Mendelian inheritance in man, 9th edn. The Johns Hopkins University Press, Baltimore

Metrakos K, Metrakos J D 1961 Genetics of convulsive disorders II. Genetic and electroencephalographic studies in centrencephalic epilepsy. Neurology 11: 474–483

Metrakos J D, Metrakos K 1966 Childhood epilepsy of subcortical ('centrencephalic') origin. Clinical Pediatrics 5: 536–542

Metrakos J D, Metrakos K 1970 Genetic factors in epilepsy. Modern Problems of Pharmacopsychiatry 4: 71–86

Metrakos K, Metrakos J D 1974 Genetics of epilepsy. In: Magnus O, Lorentz de Haas A M (eds) Handbook of Clinical Neurology, vol 15. The epilepsies. North Holland Publishing, Amsterdam, p 429–439

Morikawa T, Osawa T, Ishihara O, Seino M 1979 A reappraisal of 'benign epilepsy of children with centrotemporal EEG foci'. Brain and Development 1: 257–265

Mudd S H, Skovby F, Levy H K et al 1985 The natural history of homocystinuria due to cystathionine ß-synthase deficiency. American Journal of Human Genetics 37: 1–31

Munke M, Kraus J P, Ohura T, Francke U 1988 The gene for cystathionine ß-synthase (CBS) maps to the subtelomeric region on human chromosome 21q and to proximal mouse chromosome 17. American Journal of Human Genetics 42: 550–559

Musemeci S A, Ferri R, Elia M, Colognola R M, Bergonzi P, Tassinari C A 1991 Epilepsy and fragile X syndrome: a follow-up study. American Journal of Medical Genetics 38: 511–513

Neumann P E, Seyfried T N 1990 Mapping of two genes that influence susceptibility to audiogenic seizures in crosses of C57BL/6J and DBA/2J mice. Behavior Genetics 20(2): 307–323

Newitt R A, Houamed K M, Rehm H, Tempel B L 1991 Potassium channels and epilepsy: evidence that the epileptogenic toxin, dendrotoxin, binds to potassium channel proteins. In: Anderson V E, Hauser W A, Leppik I E, Noebels J L, Rich S S (eds) Genetic strategies in epilepsy research. Epilepsy Research, (suppl 4). Elsevier, Amsterdam, p 263–273

Noebels J L 1991 Mutational analysis of spike-wave epilepsy phenotypes. In: Anderson V E, Hauser W A, Leppik I E, Noebels J L, Rich S S (eds) Genetic strategies in epilepsy research. Epilepsy Research (suppl 4). Elsevier, Amsterdam, p 201–212

Norio R, Koskiniemi M 1979 Progressive myoclonus epilepsy: genetic and nosological aspects with special reference to 107 Finnish patients. Clinical Genetics 15: 382–398

Oppenheimer E Y, Rosman N P, Dooling E C 1985 The late appearance of hypopigmented maculae in tuberous sclerosis. American Journal of Diseases of Childhood 139: 408–409

Ottman R, Hauser W A, Susser M 1985 Genetic and maternal influences on susceptibility to seizures. American Journal of Human Genetics 122: 923–939

Ottman R, Annegers J F, Hauser W A, Kurland L T 1989 Seizure risk in offspring of parents with generalized versus partial epilepsy. Epilepsia 30: 157–161

Pampiglione G, Pugh E 1975 Infantile spasms and subsequent appearance of tuberous sclerosis syndrome. Lancet 2: 1046

Penfield W, Jasper H H 1954 Epilepsy and the functional anatomy of the human brain. Little Brown, Boston

Phillips G 1954 Traumatic epilepsy after closed head injury. Journal of Neurology, Neurosurgery and Psychiatry 17: 1–10

Plomin R, DeFries J C, McClearn G E 1990 Behavioral genetics: A primer, 2nd edn. W H Freeman, New York

Popko B 1991 Molecular characterization of the murine mutation myelin deficient. In: Anderson V E, Hauser W A, Leppik I E, Noebels J L, Rich S S (eds) Genetic strategies in epilepsy research. Epilepsy Research (suppl 4). Elsevier, Amsterdam, p 275–282

Propping P 1977 Genetic control of ethanol action on the central nervous system. Human Genetics 33: 309–334

Quattlebaum T G 1979 Benign familial convulsions in the neonatal period and early infancy. Journal of Pediatrics 95: 257–259

Rett A, Teubel R 1964 Neugeborenenkrämpfe im Rahmen einer epileptisch belasteten Familie. Weiner Klinische Wochenschrift 76: 609–613

Rich S S, Hauser W A, Anderson V E 1985 The electroencephalogram and the search for major genes in the inheritance of epilepsy. Epilepsia 26: 546

Rich S S, Annegers J F, Hauser W A, Anderson V E 1986 Complex segregation analysis of febrile convulsions. American Journal of Human Genetics 41: 249–257

Rise M L, Frankel W N, Coffin J M, Seyfried T N 1991 Genes for epilepsy mapped in the mouse. Science 253: 699–673

Romanelli M F, Morris J C, Ashkin K, Coben L A 1990 Advanced Alzheimer's disease is a risk factor for late onset seizures. Archives of Neurology 47: 847–850

Rosenberg R N 1985 Neurogenetics: principles and practice. Raven Press, New York

Rouleau G A, Wertelecki W, Haines J L et al 1987 Genetic linkage of bilateral acoustic neurofibromatosis to a DNA marker on chromosome 22. Nature 329: 246–248

Rowland L P 1988 Clinical concepts of Duchenne muscular dystrophy: the impact of molecular genetics. Brain 111: 479–495

Rowland L P, Wood D S, Schon E A, DiMauro S 1989 Molecular genetics in diseases of brain, nerve, and muscle. Oxford University Press, New York

St. George-Hyslop P H, Haines J L, Farrer L A et al 1990 Genetic linkage studies suggest that Alzheimer's disease is not a single homogeneous disorder. Nature 347: 194–197

Salazar A M, Bahman J, Vance S C, Grafman J, Amin D, Dillion J D 1985 Epilepsy after penetrating head injury. I. Clinical correlates: a report of the Vietnam Head Injury Study. Neurology 35: 1406–1414

Sandkuyl L A, Janssen L A J, Lindhout D et al 1990 Linkage studies in tuberous sclerosis: evidence for genetic heterogeneity. Epilepsia 31: 818

Schellenberg G D, Pericak-Vance M A, Wijsman E M et al 1991 Linkage analysis of familial Alzheimer disease, using chromosome 21 markers. American Journal of Human Genetics 48: 563–583

Schitz-Christensen E 1972 Genetic factors in febrile convulsions. Acta Neurologica Scandinavica 48: 538–546

Schmidt R, Eviatar L, Nitowsky H M, Wong M, Miranda S 1981 Ring chromosome 14: a distinct clinical entity. Journal of Medical Genetics 18: 304–307

Schreck R R, Breg W R, Erlanger B F, Miller O J 1977 Preferential derivation of abnormal human G-group-like chromosomes from chromosome 15. Human Genetics 36: 1–12

Seyfried T N, Glaser G H 1985 A review of mouse mutants as genetic models of epilepsy. Epilepsia 26: 143–150

Shafer S Q, Hauser W A, Annegers J F, Klass D W 1989 EEG and other early predictors of epilepsy remission: A community study. Epilepsia 29: 590–600

Shinnar S, Moshe S L 1991 Age specificity of seizure expression in genetic epilepsies. In: Anderson V E, Hauser W A, Leppik I E, Noebels J L, Rich S S (eds) Genetic strategies in epilepsy research. Epilepsy Research (suppl 4). Elsevier, Amsterdam, p 69–85

Shinnar S, Berg A T, Moshe S L et al 1990 The risk of seizure recurrence following a first unprovoked seizure in childhood: A prospective study. Pediatrics 85: 1076–1085

Shoffner J M, Lott M T, Lezza A M S, Seibel P, Ballinger S W, Wallace D C 1990 Myoclonic epilepsy and ragged-red fiber disease (MERRF) is associated with a mitochondrial DNA tRNA^{Lys} mutation. Cell 61: 931–937

Smith C 1970 Heritability of liability and concordance in monozygous twins. Annals of Human Genetics 34: 85–91

Stassen H H, Lykken D T, Propping P, Bomben G 1986 Genetic determination of the human EEG. Survey of recent results on twins reared together and apart. Human Genetics 80: 165–176

Strickler S M, Dansky L V, Miller M A, Seni M, Andermann E, Spielberg S P 1985 Genetic predisposition to phenytoin-induced birth defects. Lancet 2: 746–749

Sutcliffe J G, Travis G H, Danielson P E, et al 1991 Molecular approaches to genes of the CNS. In: Anderson V E, Hauser W A, Leppik I E, Noebels J L, Rich S S (eds) Genetic strategies in epilepsy research. Epilepsy Research (suppl 4). Elsevier, Amsterdam, p 213–223

Sutton H E 1988 An introduction to human genetics, 4th edn. Harcourt Brace Jovanovich, New York

Takahashi T, Tsukahara Y 1976 Influence of color on the photoconvulsive response. Electroencephalography and Clinical Neurophysiology 41: 124–136

Tangye S R 1979 The EEG and incidence of epilepsy in Down's syndrome. Journal of Mental Deficiency Research 23: 17–24

Tempel B L, Adams L, Newitt R A et al 1990 Potassium channel genes in mice. Epilepsia 31: 818

Thompson J S, Thompson M W 1986 Genetics in medicine, 4th edn. W B Saunders, Philadelphia.

Thorn I 1981 Prevention of recurrent febrile seizures: intermittent prophylaxis with diazepam compared with continuous treatment with phenobarbital. In: Nelson K B, Ellenberg J H (eds) Febrile seizures. Raven Press, New York, p 119–126

Tsuboi T 1982 Febrile convulsions. In: Anderson V E, Hauser W A, Penry J K, Sing C E (eds) Genetic basis of the epilepsies. Raven Press, New York, p 123–134

Tsuboi T 1986 Seizures of childhood. A population-based and clinic-based study. Acta Neurologica Scandinavica 74 (suppl 110): 1–237

Tsuboi T, Christian W 1973 On the genetics of the primary generalized epilepsy with sporadic myoclonias of impulsive petit mal type. Humangenetik 19: 155–182

Tsuboi T, Endo S 1977 Incidence of seizures and EEG abnormalities among offspring of epileptic patients. Human Genetics 36: 173–189

Tsuboi T, Okada S 1985 The genetics of epilepsy. In: Sakai T, Tsuboi T (eds) Genetic aspects of human behavior. Igaku-Shoin, Tokyo, p 113–127

Veall R M 1974 The prevalence of epilepsy among mongols related to age. Journal of Mental Deficiency Research 18: 99–106

Vogel F 1970 The genetic basis of the normal human electroencephalogram (EEG). Humangenetik 10: 91–114

Vogel F 1986 Grundlagen und Bedeutung genetisch bedingter Variabilität des normalen menschlichen EEG. Zeitschrift füer EEG/EMG 17: 173–188

Vogel F 1989 Genetic variation of the normal human EEG. In Beck-Mannagetta G, Anderson V E, Doose H, Janz D (eds) Genetics of the epilepsies. Springer-Verlag, Berlin, p 85–94

Wallace M R, Marchuk D A, Andersen L B et al 1990 Type 1 neurofibromatosis gene: identification of a large transcript disrupted in three NF1 patients. Science 249: 181–186

Wasterlain C G, Morin A M, Fando J L 1984 Cholinergic kindling, protein phosphorylation, calcium, and epilepsy. In: Fariello R G, Lloyd K G, Morselli P L, Quesney L F, Engle Jr J (eds) Neurotransmitters, seizures, and epilepsy II. Raven Press, New York, p 23–26

Wasterlain C G, Morin A M, Dwyer B 1985 The epilepsies. In: Lajtha A (ed) Handbook of neurochemistry, vol. 10: Pathological neurochemistry, Plenum, New York, p 339–419

Weissbecker K A, Durner M, Janz D, Scaramelli A, Sparkes R S, Spence M A 1991 Confirmation of linkage between juvenile myoclonic epilepsy locus and the HLA region of chromosome 6. American Journal of Medical Genetics 38: 32–36

Wiederholt W C, Gomez M R, Kurland L T 1985 Incidence and prevalence of tuberous sclerosis in Rochester, Minnesota, 1950 through 1982. Neurology 35: 600–603

Wilhelmsen K C, Tempel B, Gilliam C 1990 Cloning, mapping and sequencing of the human 'shaker' gene family. Epilepsia 31: 819

Willems P J, Dijkstra I, Brouwer O F, Smit G P A 1987 Recurrence risk in the Angelman ('happy puppet') syndrome. American Journal of Medical Genetics 27: 773–780

Williams C A, Zori R T, Stone J W, Gray B A, Cantu E S, Ostrer H 1990 Maternal origin of 15q11-13 deletions in Angelman syndrome suggests a role for genomic imprinting. American Journal of Medical Genetics 35: 350–353

Wisniewski L, Hassold T, Heffelfinger J, Higgins J V 1979 Cytogenetic and clinical studies in five cases of inv dup (15). Human Genetics 50: 259–270

Zonana J, Silvey K, Strimling B 1984 Familial neonatal and infantile seizures: An autosomal dominant disorder. American Journal of Medical Genetics 18: 455–459

Zung W, Wilson W P 1967 Sleep and dream patterns in twins: Markow analysis of a genetic trait. Recent Advances in Biological Psychiatry 9: 119–130

4. Seizures in children

S. J. Wallace

DEVELOPMENTAL ASPECTS

The clinical features, aetiology and prognosis of childhood seizure disorders are closely related to cerebral maturation. In particular, abnormal cerebral development can increase the risk of seizures and the effects of seizures themselves may vary with the state of cerebral maturation. Drug effects can also differ in relation to age. Thus, it is relevant briefly to review the developmental neuro-anatomy and neurophysiology of the infant and young child.

Early neuroanatomy

Dorsal induction of the neural plate is the first major event in the developing nervous system and is followed by ventral induction at 5–6 weeks of gestation. Neuronal proliferation, migration, organization and myelination follow in an orderly sequence (Volpe 1987). In the interests of simplicity these developmental stages will be considered singly. However, it is important to recognize that the timings of the main events overlap considerably, and that non-neuronal cells, such as astrocytes and oligodendroglia, which have important structural, supportive and metabolic roles, must also undergo normal development if an optimal cerebral state is to be attained.

Neuronal proliferation

Neuronal proliferation is at its peak in the forebrain at 2–4 months gestation and in the cerebellum from 5 months gestation to 1 year or more postnatally. During neuronal proliferation, cells which are destined to be either neuroblasts or glioblasts move from the outer part of the ventricular zone to the inner surface, divide and move out to the periphery again before migrating to form the cortical plate.

Abnormal neuronal proliferation. Children with abnormal neuronal proliferation resulting in microcephaly are not usually affected by seizures. On the other hand, some of the disorders of neuronal proliferation associated with macrocephaly, in particular tuberous sclerosis and unilateral macrocephaly, are complicated by seizures which may be intractable (Volpe 1987).

Migration

Migration of the neurones occurs at 3–5 months gestation. Radial movement of cells from their site of origin in the subventricular and ventricular zones leads to the formation of the cortex and deep nuclear structures. Some tangential movement of cells over the external surface of the cerebral cortex also occurs. In the cerebellum, the roof nuclei and the Purkinje cells become established following radial migration; tangential migration is responsible for the development of the external granular layer from which the cells later migrate inwards to form the internal granular layer of the cerebellar cortex. Fatty acid oxidation in peroxisomes and mitochondria; cell adhesion molecules and polyamines are involved in the migratory process (Barth 1987). Of the developmental stages, migration is the most critical in relation to the later presence or absence of epilepsy (Lancet 1990b).

Abnormal neuronal migration. Abnormalities of migration are frequently associated with early neurological disorder and in particular with seizures (Volpe 1987). There is failure of normal development of the gyri which at its most severe leads to schizencephaly. Lissencephaly describes the appearance of the brain when virtually no gyri develop. Pachygyria is characterized by a paucity of gyri with those present being broad and associated with abnormal thickness of the cortical plate, and in polymicrogyria an excessive number of small gyri are formed. Polymicrogyria may be generalized or focal. The least severe form of aberrant migration results in neuronal heterotopias. These may or may not be associated with clinical neurological disorders and seizures (Livingston & Aicardi 1990). The absolute quantity of heterotopic material is thought to determine the clinical manifestations (Volpe 1987). Agenesis of the corpus callosum is frequently associated with other disorders of neuronal migration. Lissencephaly type I (agyria/pachygyria) occurs either as a feature of the Miller–Dieker syndrome or as an isolated anomaly, and in both circumstances is likely to be associated with the very early onset of seizures, usually infantile spasms (de Rijk-Van Andel et al 1990). Seizures are less common in the various subgroups of lissencephaly type II, which are all inherited in an autosomal recessive manner, and in which hydrocephalus, retinal dysplasia and disorders of muscle coexist with smoothness of the hemispheric surfaces (Dobyns et al 1985). Microgyria are found in the peroxisomal disorders, Zellweger syndrome and neonatal adrenodystrophy; and in Bloch–Sulzberger syndrome and Fukuyama cerebromacular dystrophy (Lancet 1990b). Very small 'hernations' of the second into the first neocortical layer, occurring most commonly in the frontal and Rolandic areas, have been reported in association with multiple acyl-CoA dehydrogenase deficiency (Barth 1987). Neuronal heterotopia are also found in tuberous sclerosis and hypomelanosis of Ito (Barth 1987). Disordered neuronal migration, often referred to as microdysgenesis, has been reported in neuropathological studies in infantile spasms with or without other features of Aicardi syndrome; severe myoclonic epilepsy of infancy; Lennox–Gastaut syndrome; partial epilepsy of temporal lobe origin and primary generalized epilepsies (Lancet 1990b). Major disturbances of migration can be identified on ultrasound (USS) or computed tomography (CT) scans, but magnetic resonance imaging (MRI) and positron emission tomography (PET) may detect lesions not shown on USS or CT scanning (Lancet 1990b).

Organization

In the nervous system, organization occurs maximally from 6 months gestation to the postnatal age of several years. During organization the cortical neurones become aligned, orientated and layered; dendritic and axonal ramifications appear, synaptic contacts are established and there is glial proliferation and differentiation (Volpe 1987). Programmed cell death, axonal pruning and synaptic elimination, which occur during late gestation and in the early postnatal period, are important components of organization.

Abnormal organization. It is believed that defective dendritic development may be responsible for a high proportion of those mentally defective children where no specific cause is identified (Volpe 1987). Huttenlocher (1974) has demonstrated such abnormalities in children with severe mental retardation and infantile myoclonic seizures with hypsarrhythmia on the electroencephalogram. In addition, the brains of children with trisomy 21, trisomy 13–15, Rubinstein Taybi syndrome, congenital rubella and phenylketonuria have been shown to have defects of organization (Volpe 1987). Since birth occurs during the period of maximal organization it is theoretically possible that perinatal insults might also lead to abnormalities in neuronal organization. Definitive confirmation of such an association is lacking in the human.

Myelination

Myelination begins in the phylogenetically oldest parts of the brain at about 3 months gestation and continues at specific times in specific regions of the brain throughout infancy and childhood and into adulthood. Myelination occurs most actively in the greatest number of regions during the first postnatal year (Volpe 1987).

Abnormal myelination. Hypoplasia of the cerebral white matter has been found in a group of infants with severe, but apparently non-progressive, neurological deficits in whom seizures were prominent in the neonatal period (Chattha & Richardson 1977). On the other hand, with the exception of Canavan's disease, in the progressive leucodystrophies such as metachromatic leucodystrophy and Alexander's disease, seizures rarely present until the disorder is well advanced. Disturbance of myelination contributes to the neuropathological findings in disorders of amino acid and organic acid metabolism. This could be related to failure of normal synthesis of myelin proteins but, at least with phenylketonuria, it might partly be a consequence of previous abnormal neuronal organization (Volpe 1987). In the human, birth occurs during the period of maximal myelination. Animal studies suggest that both undernutrition in the latter part of pregnancy and early postnatal life, and acute perinatal insults may be important causes of suboptimal myelination (Volpe 1987).

Conclusions

Disorders of neuronal proliferation, organization and, in particular, migration are important causes of seizure disorders which start early in life and may be intractable.

Developmental neurophysiology

Physiological changes in the developing brain can be reviewed most readily by examining the electroencephalograph (EEG) throughout infancy into childhood. The maturation of conduction in peripheral nerves and evoked responses is of lesser relevance to childhood epilepsy, but awareness of the changing values for these parameters throughout infancy may be helpful in determining whether or not a disorder in which seizures occur is confined to the cerebral hemispheres.

Electroencephalography

Maturation of the EEG in both the waking and sleeping states has been comprehensively described by Niedermeyer (1987). Since small infants spend most of the day asleep, the sleep EEG is the one usually examined in premature babies and in those aged up to a few months old.

Before 28 weeks. In the very premature infant, the EEG is much the same during sleeping and waking. It is characterized by discontinuity of the background activity, which consists of bursts of mixed frequencies lasting for a few seconds, interspersed by periods of almost complete inactivity which may last for several seconds. During the bursts slow delta (0.3 to 1 Hz) activity predominates but scattered sharp waves and spikes can also be identified, even in recordings from a normal preterm infant. These bursts are usually synchronous in right and left hemispheres.

Between 28 and 36 weeks. The greater maturity of the infant's brain and the development of recognizable sleep patterns with increasing gestational age is reflected in the EEG. Between 28 and 36 weeks gestation, the periods of relative EEG inactivity gradually decrease and records in various states of alertness and sleep become clearly recognizable. By 36 weeks gestation, the EEG in quiet, non-REM (rapid eye movement) sleep is characterized by 'tracé alternant', i.e. bursts of delta and theta waves lasting about 1 to 5 seconds with associated high frequency, low amplitude activity. Between the bursts, relative inactivity persists. In contrast, during active (REM) sleep and when awake, the EEG pattern is continuous and consists of mixed frequencies, though those in the slower frequencies predominate.

The full-term neonate. When the full-term infant is awake or in active (REM) sleep, the EEG shows continuous mixed delta and theta activity with possibly more delta during active sleep than in the awake neonate. During quiet (non-REM) sleep tracé alternant is observed but in contrast with younger infants low voltage theta waves are continuous between the bursts of more spectacular activity.

EEG maturation after the perinatal period. Tracé alternant disappears at about 44 weeks gestation. After the neonatal period, in keeping with the longer periods of wakefulness, EEGs tend to be recorded with the child awake. There is gradual increase in the dominant frequencies of the background activity throughout childhood. In the first year of life, 3–4 Hz rhythms predominate. Theta activity can be identified at 5–9 months and alpha rhythms seen at about 2 years (Pampiglione 1965). At 3–5 years the maximal activity is in the

4–6 Hz range and at about 8–10 years 8–10 Hz alpha rhythms start to predominate. There is often slight interhemispheric asymmetry. The young child's EEG is much less stable under provocation by hyperventilation than that of the adult. Decreasing tendencies with age to slowing on overbreathing are further indications of increasing cerebral maturation. The EEG often has features of immaturity until well on into the teens.

Biochemical aspects

In early life the main function of neurotransmitters is considered to be trophic (Hamon et al 1989). 5-hydroxytryptophan and other monoamines, and neuropeptides, including substance P, are reported to have such effects, with their role as neurotransmitters becoming more clearly defined as synaptic contacts increase. Thus substances which in adults may interfere with synaptic transmission, could lead, in the infant, to suboptimal brain growth.

At 32 weeks gestation a sudden increase in membrane lipids in the forebrain coincides with rapid synaptogenesis. Myelinogenesis follows just before term and throughout the first year of life is a swiftly maturing process. In contrast to that formed in fetal animals, the myelin in the brain of the human infant is of almost the same chemical composition as that in the adult. There is, however, a tendency for the concentrations of phospholipids, including plasmalogens, and gangliosides to decrease in the myelin found in older children (Martinez 1989). Seizures occur in disorders involving either plasmalogens or gangliosides.

Effects of drugs and hormones on the developing brain

Little is known of the cellular pathology of the effects of drugs and hormones on the developing human brain. Experimental work on animals has shown that the changes which these substances may cause can be critically related to the stage of cerebral maturation at the time of exposure, and there is good reason to assume that comparable periods of vulnerability exist also in humans. Such concepts are clearly important in the consideration of both the aetiology and the treatment of seizure disorders in childhood.

A review of the literature on the mechanisms of drug action on the developing brain records that cell division is adversely affected by barbiturates, corticosteroids, chlorpromazine, alcohol, reserpine and sex hormones; cell migration is altered by alcohol ingestion; and the formation of neurones and synapses, i.e. organization, is related to the presence of sex hormones and corticosteroids and may be disturbed by morphine/methadone, antiepileptic drugs and alcohol (Swaab & Mirmiran 1984). In the context of human brain development, since abnormalities of cell migration and organization are those most likely to be associated with later seizure disorders, drug exposure or hormonal imbalance occurring between about 3 and 8 months gestation may be of aetiological importance in childhood epilepsy. Since antiepileptic drugs are among those implicated in disorders of cerebral maturation, it is obviously important that they are used in late pregnancy and early infancy only when definite indications exist.

RISK FACTORS FOR CHILDHOOD SEIZURES

Examination of the data collected in the National Collaborative Perinatal Project (NCPP) suggests that only three major significant risk factors for epilepsy can be identified: congenital malformation, family history of motor or mental retardation and/or epilepsy, and neonatal seizures (Nelson & Ellenberg 1986). Nevertheless seizures are symptomatic of a very wide range of childhood disorders. These can be most readily considered as pre-, peri- or postnatal in timing and influence.

Family history of epilepsy

In epilepsies in general the risk of a seizure disorder is increased 3-fold (Ottman et al 1989). A maternal, rather than paternal, history of epilepsy is more important. Parents who have had absences confer the greatest risk of epilepsy to their children. Benign familial neonatal convulsions are inherited in an autosomal dominant manner, and the risk to children of an affected parent is therefore one in two.

Neurodermatoses

Ninety per cent of patients with tuberous sclerosis have epilepsy (Gomez 1987). In most cases seizures begin in childhood, often starting with infantile spasms. Inheritance of tuberous sclerosis is autosomal dominant, but about 50–60% of cases are the result of new mutations.

Approximately 10% of those who have neurofibromatosis I suffer from epilepsy. Other conditions in which melanocytic and neuronal migration are abnormal, i.e. incontinentia pigment and hypomelanosis of Ito, are associated with seizures in a high percentage of patients.

Inherited disorders of metabolism

Seizures can be symptomatic of very many heritable disorders of metabolism. In particular, amino acidopathies in which myelination has been interrupted; peroxisomal disorders, where microgyra have been reported; organic acidurias; and lysosomal storage disorders. The metabolic disorders which occur in association with progressive myoclonus epilepsy have been comprehensively reviewed by Berkovic & Andermann (1986).

Chromosomal abnormalities

Of patients where the sex chromosomes are abnormal, seizures occur in about 30–40% of males with fragile X (Musumeci et al 1988), 18% of institutionalised boys with XXY and 15% of those with XYY chromosomes (Bird 1987). XXXY and XXXXY karyotypes also carry an increased risk of epilepsy (Kunze 1980). When the chromosomal abnormality is a trisomy, epilepsy is reported in up to 9% of children with Down syndrome (Bird 1987), and in up to 50% of those with trisomies 8, 13, 18 or 22 (Kunze 1980, Bird 1987). In trisomy 12p the ictal EEG discharge is 3 c/s spike-wave (Guerrini et al 1990). Epilepsy is invariable in the Miller–Dieker syndrome, when there is partial monosomy 17 p 13 (Dobyns et al 1983), and occurs frequently in Angelman's syndrome where a microdeletion in chromosome 15 is inherited from the mother (Knoll et al 1989). Where there is a ring chromosome 14, epilepsy is almost always found and commonly presents in association with ring chromosomes 4, 17, 20, 21 and 22 (Kunze 1980).

Prenatal infection

Viral infections during gestation can produce epileptogenic lesions. Epilepsy is reported in 20% of children with congenital rubella (Volpe 1987), and infantile spasms can be symptomatic of prenatal cytomegalovirus infection (Riikonen 1978). Approximately 25% of those who have congenital toxoplasmosis infections later have epilepsy (Volpe 1987).

Other prenatal factors

Extra- and intracranial vascular lesions, excessive alcohol intake, poor weight for gestational age and congenital malformations of the brain are other predisposing factors for epilepsy. Seizures have been reported in 48% of children with shunt-treated hydrocephalus (Saukkonen et al 1990).

Perinatal/intrapartum factors

In the NCPP, epilepsy supervened significantly more often than expected if the fetal heart rate was recorded at less than 60 beats per minute (Nelson & Elleberg 1986). The only other perinatal factor which was significantly related to later epilepsy in the NCPP was the occurrence of neonatal seizures. If the latter are secondary to hypoxic-ischaemic encephalopathy or to congenital cerebral malformations continuing epilepsy is usual. Remediable biochemical disorders such as hypocalcaemia have a much more favourable outlook.

Postnatal factors

Head injuries

Approximately 7% of patients who suffer head injuries in civilian accidents later have epilepsy (Annegers et al 1980). The severity of the brain trauma correlates with the development of a seizure disorder. There is evidence to suggest that the release of blood into the brain is an important factor in epileptogenesis (Willmore 1990).

Infection

In a recent comprehensive report on the sequelae of bacterial meningitis in children, although 31%

had seizures during the acute phase, only 7% of 185 patients had one or more afebrile seizures after the initial hospitalization (Pomeroy et al 1990). Almost all of those with later seizures had suffered *Haemophilus influenza* meningitis and for almost half, antiepileptic therapy failed to control all the attacks. Epilepsy may also be symptomatic of chronic infections such as tuberculomata and cystocercosis, and may follow viral encephalitis. A study of the prevalence of Toxocara infection has found that there is a significant association between anti-Toxocara canis seropositivity and childhood epilepsy, particularly in those aged less than 5 years (Arpino et al 1990).

Tumours

In younger children, who tend to have tumours predominantly in the posterior cranial fossa, seizures are only rarely symptomatic of a space occupying lesion. In the later years of childhood, when supratentorial tumours are commoner, epilepsy may be a presenting symptom, particularly when the lesion is relatively indolent (Lee et al 1989).

Degenerative disorders

Seizures are early symptoms of degenerative disorders which affect primarily the cerebral gray matter, e.g. ceroid lipofuscinoses; and occur in the later stages of white matter diseases. They occur in about 75% of girls with Rett syndrome, in which, even in those with no clinical attacks, there is a high prevalence of EEG abnormalities (Bader et al 1989).

CLASSIFICATION AND PREVALENCE OF EPILEPTIC SEIZURES AND SYNDROMES

The International League Against Epilepsy (ILAE) has produced revised classifications of both seizures (Commission on Classification and Terminology of the ILAE 1981) and epileptic syndromes (Commission on Classification and Terminology of the ILAE 1989). Although the results of considerable deliberation, there are limitations to these classifications. By no means all seizures are classifiable and not all epilepsies fit readily into syndromes. Nevertheless, for childhood seizure disorders, the syndromic approach is useful.

The problem of inter-observer variability in the interpretation of childhood seizures has been addressed by Bodensteiner et al (1988). One senior neurologist and three neurology residents classified 2219 seizures on the basis of verbatim descriptions of their manifestations. The overall agreement between observer pairs was poor (k = 0.24–0.38), but somewhat improved by exclusion of unclassified seizures. There was particularly poor agreement on atypical absences, partial seizures with secondary generalization and generalized motor seizures. To some extent this must explain the fairly wide differences between the proportions of partial and generalized seizures reported from the studies of Bodensteiner et al (1988) and Eslava-Cobos & Nariño (1989). The former found that, of 2219 seizures, 24% were partial (secondary generalized in 8%); 45% generalized; 1% mixed; 2% infantile spasms; 5% neonatal; and 22% unclassified (Bodensteiner et al 1988): whereas the latter, (Eslava-Cobos & Nariño 1989), reported that of 222 seizures in 182 children, 58% were partial (secondary generalized in 42%); 37% generalized; and only 5% unclassified or 'other'. Clearly, further studies of interobserver agreement on seizure classification are required.

The overall prevalence of the epilepsies in childhood and adolescence is 4–6 per 1000 (Ross et al 1980, Doose & Sitepu 1983, Cowan et al 1989), the peak prevalence is in the 1–4-year age range. Childhood absence epilepsy and photosensitivity are commoner in females. The majority of other syndromes, particularly those presenting in the first year of life, occur more frequently in males; with a few syndromes, such as benign familial neonatal convulsions, presenting equally in the sexes. Cowan et al (1989) examined the seizure types in 1159 children and reported prevalence rates for types of epilepsy, but did not adhere closely to the ILAE's scheme with the result that only for absences, 2.4%; infantile spasms 2.3%; and, the Lennox–Gastaut syndrome (LGS) 2.1% is the relative frequency of defined syndromes apparent. For infantile spasms and LGS these percentages are marginally higher than those reported by Eslava-Cobos & Nariño (1989);

whereas the latter authors found childhood absence epilepsy in 2% of 182 patients with epilepsy. Partial syndromes which were idiopathic with age-related onset occurred in 1.6%; and those considered symptomatic were found in 65% of the 182 patients. Of the syndromes with generalized seizures juvenile myoclonic epilepsy (JME) has been recorded in between 0.7 (Alving 1979) and 3.8% (Viani et al 1988, Eslava-Cobos & Nariño 1989) of patients, but the prevalence is strictly age-related since this syndrome rarely presents before the second decade.

NEONATAL SEIZURES

Seizures in the newborn can take several clinical forms. They are more likely to be symptomatic than in later childhood and the child's outlook is closely related to the underlying cause. There is evidence from animal experiments that seizure activity can impair brain growth (Wasterlain & Dwyer 1983), and from observations in human infants that it may be associated with the creation of cerebral metabolic demands which outstrip the energy supply with resultant long-term neurological sequelae (Younkin et al 1986). The selective vulnerability of neuronal subpopulations during development has been emphasized by Wasterlain et al (1990).

Incidence of seizures

The figures available for the frequency of neonatal seizure disorders usually refer to attacks which have been witnessed clinically. However, with the increasing use of continuous EEG monitoring in infants in the special care baby units, it is apparent that subclinical seizures are common events in the sick newborn (Eyre et al 1983a, Hellström-Westas et al 1985, Bridgers et al 1986, Connell et al 1989a, Hakeem & Wallace 1990). Estimates of the incidence of clinically observed seizures vary from as high as 30% (Fenichel 1980) to as low as 0.5% (Mellits et al 1981).

Seizure types

Seizures in the young infant can take a number of clinical forms. In the past neonatal seizure types were classified as subtle, clonic, tonic or myoclonic (Volpe 1987). It has now become clear that not all such clinical events are consistently associated with EEG charges, and that some are probably nonepileptic in origin (Kellaway & Mizrahi 1990).

Following clinical investigation of 420 neonates in whom EEG/polygraphic/video data were obtained, these authors concluded that of 100 infants in whom seizures were suspected only one-third had clinical events with a consistent electrocortical correlate. Of the other two-thirds, 60% had clinical changes which were not associated with a consistent electrocortical pattern, 5% had electrical seizures without clinical changes and 2% infantile spasms. The clinical seizures with a consistent electrical correlate were as follows:

1. Focal clonic
2. Focal tonic
3. Myoclonic
4. Apnoea.

When a consistent electrical correlate was not present the attacks were myoclonic, generalized tonic or consisted of motor automatisms. The latter were further itemized as oro-buccolingual, ocular, pedalling, stepping, rotary arm movements and complex purposeless movements. Scher & Painter (1990) have also correlated clinical changes with EEG findings. They found only 14 of 85 EEGs confirmed clinical impressions that epileptic seizures were present. The highest correlation between clinical and EEG findings was for clonic attacks in which eight out of 18 had electrical as well as clinical seizures. Tonic and myoclonic attacks were only very rarely (one of 12, and one of 16 respectively) accompanied by specific EEG changes. In contrast to the report of Kellaway & Mizrahi (1990), Scher & Painter (1990) found buccolingual automatisms and eye deviation were sometimes associated with electrical seizures.

Clonic seizures

Concomitant EEG and/or polygraphic recordings of seizures have demonstrated that clonic attacks are always unilateral at the onset and, even if they become clinically bilateral, they are always electrically asynchronous.

Focal clonic seizures. In focal clonic seizures, the jerking is usually well localized and consciousness is usually retained (Volpe 1987). Persistent clonic movements which are localized to the same part of the body are suggestive of a focal structural abnormality, but metabolic encephalopathies and other generalized cerebral disturbances can also be associated with focal clonic attacks.

Multifocal clonic seizures. In multifocal clonic seizures, the clonic movements appear in an apparently unrelated manner in different parts of the body. Full-term infants are more likely than pre-terms to have multifocal clonic seizures (Volpe 1987).

Hemiconvulsive clonic seizures. The only justification for considering these seizures as a separate clinical entity is that they might give rather stronger evidence of a focal structural cerebral abnormality.

Tonic seizures

Tonic attacks occur particularly in association with intraventricular haemorrhage, when decerebrate posturing is more likely than truly epileptic seizures. Of the seizures with consistent electrocortical correlates only one-sixth are likely to be tonic, and these are either asymmetrical involving the trunk, or associated with eye deviation (Kellaway & Mizrahi 1990).

Myoclonic seizures

Kellaway & Mizrahi (1990) found that, of their cases with consistent EEG correlates, one-eighth had either generalized or focal myoclonic features. On the other hand, only one-fifth of their infants with myoclonic seizures had consistent EEG changes. Myoclonic seizures may be the forerunners of later infantile spasms (Volpe 1987). They can be seen in both premature and full-term infants and are significantly related to mental retardation.

Epileptic syndromes in the newborn

Four epileptic syndromes have been characterized in neonates (Aicardi 1990, Dulac et al 1985, Plouin 1985, Ohtahara 1984).

Benign neonatal convulsions

Two syndromes of benign neonatal convulsions have been identified (Plouin 1985).

Benign idiopathic neonatal convulsions— 'fifth day fits'. Details of 182 cases which appear in the literature have been reviewed by Plouin (1985), and a further 94 infants have been reported by North et al (1989). Overall about 4% of all neonatal convulsions are examples of this condition; but North et al (1989) described a sudden rise in the incidence from 1972 to 1982 for which there is no obvious explanation. A total of 62% of the infants involved are boys; 95% of the convulsions occur between the ages of 3 and 7 days; and 80% between the fourth and sixth days. The convulsions are usually partial, always clonic and are repeated frequently, leading to status epilepticus over periods of between 2 hours and three days (mean about 20 hours). At the onset of the seizures the infants are neurologically normal between fits, but they become hypotonic and drowsy as the status progresses. They revert to normality after the status, but may take several days to do so.

In the cases where EEGs have been recorded, bursts of theta rhythms mainly in the Rolandic areas are common interictally, and rhythmic spikes and rhythmic slow waves have been seen during convulsions. However, these changes are not specific for benign idiopathic neonatal con-vulsions. Usually there is a favourable outcome but the diagnosis is largely one of exclusion and may not become unquestionably apparent until after a period of follow-up. In the study of North et al (1989), some infants, who in the neonatal period seemed to have this syndrome, were later developmentally delayed and neurologically other than normal.

Benign familial neonatal convulsions. Details of 14 families in which 87 individuals have had benign neonatal convulsions have been reviewed by Plouin (1985). Details of another four families are now available (Shevell et al 1986, Leppert et al 1989, Webb & Bobele 1990). Where the appropriate details have been documented, delivery and birth weight have been normal and convulsions have commenced after an interval, usually of 2–3 days. The seizures are clonic, brief and repeated frequently for up to 7 days.

EEG changes are not specific to the condition. Although other seizure types may develop later in infancy or childhood, other aspects of development are unaffected. Inheritance is by autosomal dominant transmission. Leppert et al (1989) have mapped the gene for benign familial neonatal convulsions to the long arm of chromosome 20. They suggest that additional families need to be tested to examine whether there are mutant genes: one for the typical neonatal course with no further seizures; and, one in which the typical neonatal course is followed later by non-febrile seizures.

Early myoclonic encephalopathy

Twenty-nine cases of early myoclonic encephalopathy have been reviewed (Aicardi 1990). A further infant has been described by Otani et al (1989). In the neonatal period fragmentary or partial erratic myoclonus, massive myoclonias and/or partial motor seizures occur. The EEG is devoid of normal background activity and, in both waking and sleeping, consists of a suppression-burst pattern in which the bursts are complexes of irregularly intermingled spikes, sharp waves and slow waves. The infants are always neurologically very abnormal. Death occurred during the first year of life in more than half the cases reviewed. In at least some cases the underlying cause is non-ketotic hyper-glycinaemia (Seppalainen & Smila 1971).

Early infantile epileptic encephalopathy (EIEE)

EIEE is often referred to as Ohtahara syndrome (Ohtahara 1984). In clinical and EEG respects it is similar to early myoclonic encephalopathy (Aicardi 1990). However, the seizures are characteristically tonic spasms rather than myoclonias (Ohtahara 1984, Clarke et al 1987, Otani et al 1989). Nevertheless, separation of early myclonic and early infantile epileptic encephalopathies primarily on the basis of differing seizure types may not be justifiable.

Differential diagnosis in neonatal seizures

Jitteriness, i.e. a high-frequency low-amplitude tremor present particularly on stimulation, is the most common alternative diagnosis. It can be distinguished from seizures by the absence of abnormalities of gaze or extra-ocular movement and its cessation on passive flexion (Volpe 1987). Temporal and spatial summation, irradiation and arrest by restraint are features of reflex behaviour, but not of epileptic seizures (Kellaway & Mizrahi 1990).

It is probable that not all episodic attacks of extension are epileptic seizures. Tonic seizures without EEG epilepti form activity are better explained as 'brainstem release' phenomena.

Neonatal tetanus may sometimes be confused with seizures.

Aetiology of convulsions in the neonate

Convulsions in the neonatal period can be symptomatic of any serious central nervous system disorder. The eventual outcome is closely linked to the underlying pathology.

Prenatal causes of seizures

Prenatal causes are rarely remediable unless a biochemical defect that can be corrected is present. Dennis (1978) coined the useful phrase 'fetus with a problem' to embrace the infants whose suboptimal prenatal histories suggested that cerebral development had probably been abnormal prior to delivery. The prenatal causes of neonatal seizures can be classified as follows:

1. Cerebral dysmorphism—major malformations; abnormalities at a cellular level
2. Prenatal vascular occlusion—porencephalic cysts
3. Prenatal infection
4. Maternal drug ingestion
5. Inborn errors of metabolism—pyridoxine dependency, non-ketotic hyperglycinaemia
6. Heritable disorders of unknown aetiology—benign familial neonatal convulsions.

Cerebral dysmorphism. Abnormalities of cerebral development account for approximately 10% of neonatal convulsions. Major malformations of the cerebrum are often incompatible with survival and seizures are not necessarily the most significant of the neurological signs. Abnormalities at a cellular level are more important. In tuberous sclerosis and some types of macro-cephaly, there are disorders of neuronal proliferation. In lissencephaly, pachygria, polymicrogyria and agenesis of corpus callosum abnormalities of neuronal migration are associated with the early development of seizures. Defective dendritic development such as can occur in trisomy 21, congenital rubella or maternal hyperphenyl-alaninaemia, may also be associated with early seizure development. Huttenlocher (1974) has described abnormal cerebral organization in infants with severe developmental delay and the early onset of myoclonic seizures. On the whole, abnormalities of myelination are not associated with the early development of convulsions, but Chattha & Richardson (1977) reported a group of infants with seizures in the neonatal period who had hypoplasia of the cerebral white matter.

Prenatal vascular occlusion. With more frequent ultrasound and CT scanning in the investigation of neonatal seizures, there is increasing evidence of prenatal vascular occlusion with the formation of porencephalic cysts. These may act as foci of seizure activity.

Prenatal infections. Approximately 4% of infants with convulsions in the newborn period have evidence of prenatal infection. Toxoplasmosis, rubella and cytomegalovirus can cause encephalitis in the fetus, which may lead to abnormalities in cerebral maturation and a subsequent liability to convulse in the neonatal period. Congenital syphilis is now a very unusual cause of fits in the first 2 weeks of life, but a recent increase in incidence has been reported from the United States of America (Dorfman & Glaser 1990).

Maternal drug ingestion. Maternal drug ingestion has the potential to predispose the neonate to seizures by two mechanisms. Firstly, drugs acting on the central nervous system may affect the sequence of normal brain maturation. In a review article, Swaab & Mirmiran (1984) list the possible implications for the developing brain of exposure to hormones and drugs affecting neuro-transmission, e.g. alpha-methyldopa, propranolol, chlorpromazine and barbiturates. Although neonatal seizures might be expected to be consequences of the abnormalities of cell division, migration and organization associated with the use of these drugs, Swaab & Mirmiran do not comment on the incidence of seizures in the new-born of mothers treated with these substances.

On the other hand, there seems to be no doubt that neonates born to mothers who have been addicted to narcotics can have withdrawal seizures in the first few days of life. Between 1.2% and 3% of infants with neourological symptoms related to heroin withdrawal have seizures (Herzlinger et al 1977, Zelson et al 1971). Withdrawal of barbiturates (Bleyer & Marshall 1972) and of alcohol (Pierog et al 1977) can also precipitate convulsions in the neonate.

Inborn errors of metabolism. Inherited biochemical disorders account for 2.5–4.5% of neonatal seizure disorders. Urea cycle defects with hyperammonaemia, maple syrup urine disease, proprionic acidaemia and other organic acidaemias, diseases predisposing to hypoglycaemia (e.g. galactose-1-phosphate-uridyl-transferase deficiency) and disorders of mitochondrial function are those conditions most commonly reported. Early myoclonic encephalopathy/early infantile epileptic encephalopathy may be symptomatic of non-ketotic hyperglycinaemia (Aicardi 1990).

Abnormal central nervous system gamma-aminobutyric acid (GABA) metabolism can also be associated with neonatal seizures (Jaeken et al 1990). Pyridoxine-dependent convulsions occur in the presence of a glutamic acid decarboxylase (GAD) defect which prevents normal GABA synthesis (Yoshida et al 1971). Convulsions occur in the first few days of life in GABA-transaminase deficiency (Jaeken et al 1990).

Although some authors include neurolipidoses and other neurodegenerative disorders among the aetiological possibilities for neonatal seizures, it is extremely rare for these conditions to present at such an early age.

Maternal illness. The infants of mothers who have hyperparathyroidism may present with convulsions associated with hypocalcaemia. Where the mother has poorly controlled diabetes the neonate may have convulsions associated with hypogylcaemia.

Intrapartum causes

Intrapartum causes of neonatal seizures are as follows:

1. Hypoxic-ischaemic encephalopathy
2. Intracranial haemorrhage
3. Birth trauma
4. Infection
5. Local anaesthetic intoxication.

Hypoxic-ischaemic encephalopathy. Deficiencies in oxygen to the brain cause impairments of brain energy metabolism which lead to the irreversible structural deficits characteristic of this condition. The pathological changes are preceded by regional alterations in high energy compounds; accumulation of extracellular potassium; intracellular acidosis; and alterations in neurotransmitter metabolism; and can be identified both clinically and electrophysiologically before structural abnormalities are apparent (Volpe 1987).

Fetal hypoxaemia may predate perinatal hypoxic-ischaemic encephalopathy and can be recorded with fetal monitoring equipment. Even when attempts are made to maximize the available oxgen, approximately 10% of infants with prenatal asphyxia and 25% of those who are hypoxic at birth have seizures and other serious neurological deficits (Low et al 1977). In 89 infants who had asphyxial seizures after delivery in Dublin hospitals in the early 1980s, there were significant associations with antenatal complications, primiparity and prolonged pregnancy (Curtis et al 1988).

Cerebral infarcts. These follow arterial occlusion, which is usually secondary to ischaemic or haemorrhagic lesions, and can be the underlying pathology in neonatal seizures (Aso et al 1990).

Intracranial haemorrhage. Subdural haemorrhage is virtually always secondary to trauma. It may present acutely with signs of raised intracranial pressure and brainstem compromise rather than seizures. However, if the haemorrhage has localized over the cerebral convexities focal seizures are common and usually associated with dysfunction of muscles innervated by the ipsilateral third nerve (Volpe 1987).

Primary subarachnoid haemorrhage can present with seizures in otherwise apparently well babies. In the 1987 cohort of neonates with seizures at Texas Children's Hospital 3% had subarachnoid haemorrhages (Kellaway & Mizrahi 1990). On clinical grounds, it may be difficult to distinguish a haemorrhage confined to the subarachnoid space from blood extravasation from other intracranial sources. Intracranial haemorrhages may, in addition, be secondary to coagulation defects, vascular anomalies or haemorrhagic infarction (Volpe 1987).

Periventricular-intraventricular haemorrhage is almost exclusively a condition of premature infants. The incidence increases with decrease in gestational age.

Intraventricular haemorrhages are precipitated by hypoxia, which increases cerebral blood flow and leads to inadequacy of vascular autoregulation, increased venous pressure and endothelial injury. In addition, increased fibrinolytic activity has been reported in the periventricular region in the pre-term newborn. Periventricular-intraventricular haemorrhage can be catastrophic and associated with generalized tonic-clonic seizures; stupor progressing to coma; respiratory disturbance; decerebrate posturing; brain stem compromise; and flaccid quadriparesis; or can be saltatory when repeated, less severe bleeding occurs and seizures are then a usual clinical feature (Volpe 1987).

Birth trauma. Intracranial haemorrhage can be secondary to direct or indirect trauma during delivery. Cerebral contusion may also occur and can be a cause of seizures which are often focal; it is considered an uncommon neonatal problem (Volpe 1987). In keeping with improved obstetric care, the incidence of trauma as the aetiological factor in neonatal seizures has fallen significantly.

Infections. Both intracranial and extracranial infections may be associated with neonatal seizures. Intracranial infections are present in 12–17% of neonatal fits (Volpe 1987, Kellaway & Mizrahi 1990). Bacterial meningitis is usually a complication of bacteraemia involving organisms acquired from the mother's birth canal. Thus, *Escherichia coli*, *Listeria monocytogenes* and Group B β-haemolytic streptococci are the most common infecting agents. If the onset is early and fulminating, seizures are not a prominent symptom. In cases which present with a more insidious clinical course late in the neonatal period, seizures occur in 75%. The later complications of bacterial meningitis, i.e. hydrocephalus, subdural effusion and intracerebral abscess, may also be associated with seizures.

Of the non-bacterial intracranial infections, herpes simplex is the most likely to be acquired during passage through an infected birth canal. Presentation is towards the end of the first week of life with symptoms of general ill health, complicated in about half the cases by stupor, irritability and seizures. Although enteroviruses, particularly Coxsackie B and echoviruses, may cause encephalitic illnesses in the neonatal period, seizures appear to be relatively rare (Volpe 1987).

The classical febrile convulsion is very rare in the neonate, but extracranial infections, acquired during delivery, may also be associated with seizures. In these cases, the seizures are commonly related to electrolyte imbalance or hypoxia secondary to the severity of the illness.

Local anaesthesia intoxication. Volpe (1987) emphasized that seizures were a prominent feature of intoxication with local anaesthetics in the neonate. In such cases, a local anaesthetic had usually been inadvertently injected into the infant's scalp during a maternal paracervical or pudendal block. The seizures were usually tonic, occurred in the first 6 hours after birth, and were associated with depressed Apgar scores, bradycardia, apnoea, hypertonia, dilated pupils which did not respond to light and absence of the oculocephalic reflex.

Causes of seizures in the early postnatal period

Conditions which are acquired after birth are rather less likely to be the aetiological agents in neonatal seizures than those determined pre- or intranatally.

Metabolic disorders. Hypoglycaemia is most likely to be complicated by seizures if it is prolonged and treatment delayed.

Early transitional-adaptive hypoglycaemia is seen in term babies who are large for gestational age such as those born to mothers with diabetes.

Secondary hypoglycaemia occurs in both appropriate-for-gestational-age and small-for-gestational-age infants who are moderately or severely unwell with symptoms largely referrable to the central nervous system, e.g. illness secondary to asphyxia, intracranial haemorrhage or bacteraemia. In this context it is difficult to separate out the effects of the hypoglycaemia.

Nevertheless, seizures themselves cause changes in cerebral glucose and energy metabolism. The regional cerebral metabolic rate for glucose increases during and decreases between serial seizures, and there is evidence to suggest that, in the neonate, seizures may exacerbate cerebral compromise by increasing metabolic demands above the energy supply (Delivoria-Papadopoulus et al 1990). Thus maintenance of blood glucose is of critical importance.

Classical transient neonatal hypoglycaemia, which used to occur predominately in small-for-gestation infants who had been undernourished in utero, is now usually avoided by early and appropriate feeding of at risk infants.

Severe recurrent hypoglycaemia can be symptomatic of hormonal deficiencies, hormonal excess and inborn errors of carbohydrate, amino acid or organic acid metabolism and should be regarded as an alerting sign for potentially serious underlying biochemical disorders.

Disturbances of calcium, phosphorus and magnesium are frequently interrelated. In almost 80% of cases the serum level of more than one mineral is abnormal with hypocalcaemia/hypomagnesaemia/hyperphosphataemia; hypocalcaemia/hypophosphataemia; and hypocalcaemia/hypomagnesaemia being the most common combinations. Isolated hypocalcaemia presents in 19% of cases and isolated hypomagnesaemia in only 3% of cases.

In those newborns with primary disturbance of calcium, phosphorus or magnesium metabolism related to a high dietary intake of phosphate in milk, the peak incidence of the first convulsion is on the sixth day of life and presentation in the first 48 hours or after the tenth day is very rare. The seizures are usually focal or multifocal clonic in type. It is unusual for them to be associated with cyanosis and the infant is usually hyperalert.

Most infants who have seizures in association with primary hypocalcaemia are full-term and delivered uneventfully by the vertex. However, there is a tendency for them to be delivered to low social class mothers of relatively high parity towards the end of the winter and to be fed on non-human milk (Roberts et al 1973). In a minority of infants, hypocalcaemia occurring between 5 and 10 days of life may be secondary to hyperparathyroidism or untreated coeliac disease in the mother; or, in the infant, congenital hypoparathyroidism, intestinal malabsorption of calcium or magnesium, or renal failure with hyperphosphataemia (Volpe 1987).

Hypocalcaemia in the first 2 days of life is particularly associated with prematurity, asphyxia and maternal diabetes (Volpe 1987). The affected infant is likely to be stuporous and hypotonic, and seizures are much less common than in late (5–10-day) onset hypocalcaemia (Roberton & Smith 1975). Disorders of magnesium absorption can lead to hypomagnesaemia and fits in the neonatal period (Tsang 1972).

Transient hyperammonaemia may complicate respiratory distress in the pre-term infant (Ballard et al 1978). Clinically, stupor/coma accompanied by seizures and fixed dilated pupils present between 4 and 48 hours after birth. The pathogenesis of the condition is unknown. It does not appear to be genetically determined. Hyperammonaemia secondary to defects of enzymes necessary to the urea cycle is of much greater significance. Seizures are accompanied by vomiting and stupor or coma (Volpe 1987).

Seizures can also be symptomatic of maple syrup urine disease, nonketotic hyperglycinaemia, methionine malabsorption, congenital lysine intolerance, hyperbeta-alaninaemia, carnosinaemia, propionic acidaemia, methylmalonic acidaemia and pyruvate dehydrogenase complex deficiency. Multiple carboxylase deficiency and glutaric acidaemia type II may also be associated with seizures (Volpe 1987). In addition, disorders of the metabolism of gamma-amino butyric acid can present with neonatal seizures (Jaeken et al 1990).

Hypo- or hypernatraemia may be associated with neonatal seizures, the former is most commonly seen when there is inappropriate antidiuretic hormone (ADH) secretion secondary to bacterial meningitis or intracranial haemorrhage (Volpe 1987).

Infection. Although neonatal bacterial meningitis is usually secondary to intrapartum infection, postnatal infections can also occur. In these cases the onset of symptoms is usually later than 7 days and the physical signs are likely to be those of meningitis rather than septicaemia or respiratory illness (Volpe 1987).

Of the non-bacterial infections which can be acquired in the early postnatal period, herpes simplex is the one most commonly associated with encephalitis and thus with seizures.

Exogenous toxins. The antiseptic hexchlorophane can be absorbed if it comes into contact with the neonate's skin and may cause a toxic encephalopathy with seizures (Brown 1973).

Unknown causes of seizures. In Volpe's series (1987) only 10% of infants with seizures in the neonatal period had neither a definite nor a highly presumptive aetiological agent.

Timing of neonatal seizures

Since the various causes of seizures can be effective at different times in the neonatal period, the timing of the onset can be helpful in narrowing down the likely aetiology. Onset before birth is recognized only rarely but may be apparent in pyridoxine dependency. If they commence within 3 days of birth seizures are likely to be associated with:

— perinatal asphyxia
— intracranial haemorrhage
— birth trauma
— cerebral dysmorphism
— prenatal vascular occlusion
— hypoglycaemia: 'primary'
— hypoglycaemia: secondary to perinatal asphyxia etc
— hyperammonaemia: secondary to urea cycle defects and organic acidurias
— amino acid disorders: non-ketotic hyperglycinaema
— pyridoxine dependency
— maternal ingestion of short acting drugs
— benign familial neonatal convulsions.

Seizures with onset from 3 to 10 days are usually associated with:

— meningitis
— encephalitis
— hypocalcaemia due to primary disorders of mineral metabolism
— hypoglycaemia secondary to galactosaemia, etc
— amino acid disorders: maple syrup urine disease, methionine malabsorption, hyperbeta-alaninaemia etc

— hyperammonaemia secondary to urea cycle defects and organic acidurias
— transient neonatal hyperammonaemia
— cerebral dysmorphism
— prenatal vascular occlusion
— maternal ingestion of long-acting sedative drugs
— benign idiopathic neonatal convulsions (fifth day fits).

Seizures with onset between 10 and 28 days are most likely to be secondary to either infective or metabolic causes.

Pathophysiological aspects

It is reasonable to postulate that hypoxia, ischaemia and hypoglycaemia will interfere with energy production, reduce the available adenosine triphosphate (ATP) and secondarily lead to failure of the sodium–potassium pump; that hypocalcaemia and hypomagnesaemia will alter membrane permeability allowing greater movement of sodium ions; and that pyridoxine dependency will produce a relative excess of excitatory neurotransmitter (Volpe 1987). In addition, sustained seizures are associated with neuronal necrosis secondary to the action of excitotoxic amino acids, e.g. glutamic and aspartic acids (Ingvar & Siesjo 1990).

There are problems in extrapolating from animal work when considering the special problems of the neonatal brain, since, in many species, the level of cerebral maturity at birth is much greater than in the human neonate. In neonatal rats there is a fall in the brain glucose concentration during sustained seizures even if the plasma glucose is normal or raised; this suggests that the neonatal rat brain has difficulty in maintaining energy supplies during seizures (Wasterlain & Dwyer 1983). Evidence for failure to meet the energy demands during seizures in the human neonate has now become available (Delivoria-Papadopoulos et al 1990). Rats which had seizures during a critical period between 2 and 11 days postnatally, later had significant reduction in the total brain DNA, RNA and cholesterol. These findings suggest that reduction in cell numbers is related to repeated seizures when these occur at specific stages in cer-

ebral development (Wasterlain & Dwyer 1983). In addition, neonatal seizures are probably associated with suboptimal establishment of cell-to-cell connections.

Clinical assessment

The clinical features associated with seizures may assist in identifying the underlying cause.

Family history

A history of previous infants with congenital malformation would lead to the consideration of cerebral dysmorphism. The presence of parental consanguinity, or of death from neurological disease in infancy of siblings, suggests an inborn error of metabolism. Benign syndromes such as that of 'fifth day fits' may be diagnosed if there is a clear history of similar convulsions in parents or prior-born siblings.

Perinatal history

Seizures in premature infants can be associated with any other cause, but those related to intracranial haemorrhage are more common in the pre-term than in the full-term infant. It is important to be aware of potentially asphyxiating or traumatic episodes in babies of any gestation. Prolonged rupture of the membranes prior to delivery is a potential precursor of neonatal meningitis.

Neurological examination

Poor feeding, vomiting and/or lethargy progressing to stupor or coma prior to the onset of seizures suggest a metabolic disorder. Extreme irritability and jitteriness may indicate withdrawal from maternal narcotics. The infant who has cerebral dysmorphism is likely to have an abnormally sized or shaped head. When a porencephalic cyst is present, bulging of the cranium overlying the cyst is common. Hemisyndromes suggest focal structural lesions. An alert well-looking baby with jitteriness and seizures commencing towards the end of the first week of life who has very hyperactive tendon reflexes is most likely to be hypocalcaemic.

General features

The small-for-gestational-age infant is liable to hypogycaemia, as is the very large infant of the mother who has had poorly-controlled diabetes during pregnacy. Specific facies may be present as, for example, in the fetal alcohol syndrome. The presence of an intracranial malformation may be suspected if other dysmorphism is present. In particular, congenital malformations of the optic nerve or other intraorbital structures may be alerting signals for abnormalities of the brain.

It is clearly important to examine the infant in detail so that clues to the aetiology of the neonatal seizures can be appreciated fully.

Investigation

General information

In the neonatal period it is particularly important to ensure that the blood pH and gases, urea and electrolytes are normal. The blood glucose, calcium, phosphate and magnesium should also be measured in all newborns who convulse. Unless there is another obvious reason for seizures, lumbar puncture should be performed as a matter of urgency so that meningitis, which may not be clinically apparent, can either be diagnosed with a minimum of delay or be excluded.

Specific investigations

Biochemical. If there is any reason to suspect, on clinical grounds, that a serious inborn error of metabolism could be present, specimens of blood for ammonia and quantitative amino acid levels, and of urine for amino and organic acids should be obtained at the time of the seizures. If possible, cerebrospinal fluid (CSF) amino acid levels should be measured. Even if the amino and organic acid levels cannot be estimated immediately, the serum, urine or CSF should be obtained and frozen for later estimations.

Ultrasound scans. Ultrasounds scans obtained through the fontanelle can demonstrate subependymal and intraventricular haemorrhages and enlargement of the ventricular system. Intracranial cysts secondary to prenatal vascular occlusions may also be visible but primarily cortical abnormalities, such as lissencephaly and agyria, cannot be readily diagnosed by ultrasound.

Skull X-rays. Straightforward skull X-rays rarely demonstrate any pathology since, even in conditions such as cerebral toxoplasmosis, calcification usually develops later.

CT scans. Computerized axial tomography (CT scanning) can usefully identify intracranial haemorrhage and will demonstrate subdural collections not visualized by ultrasound. In addition, cortical and other malformations can be delineated by CT scanning.

When normal appearances in infants at different gestational ages have been defined, magnetic resonance imaging will probably provide even more information about the cerebral structural abnormalities associated with seizure disorders. PET and SPECT can be helpful in the localization of lesions (Chugani et al 1988, Andersen 1990).

Electroencephalography. The predominant features of the normal neonatal EEG change with increasing gestational age. Normal and abnormal findings have been comprehensively reviewed by Dreyfus-Brissac (1979). Nevertheless, the limits of normality remain imprecisely defined. Normal parameters have recently been defined for premature infants (Connell et al 1987). From 26 to 37 weeks gestation the dominant frequency increases from between 0.5 to 1 Hz to 1 to 3 Hz and the activity is always symmetrical. A number of conditions should be satisfied if maximal information is to be acquired. In particular, the exact gestational age of the infant must be known. Most abnormalities appear during quiet (non-REM) sleep necessitating recordings which are of greater duration than would be usual when recording older children or adults. Where possible, continuous EEG recording with either compressed spectral analysis or storage on tape, e.g. by using Medilog recording apparatus (Oxford Medical Systems), should be obtained. Such recordings allow subtle seizures to be recognized more readily, and interictal and ictal patterns can be identified over longer periods (Eyre et al 1983a, 1983b, Aziz et al 1986, Bridgers et al 1986, Connell et al 1987, 1989a). Responses to therapy can also be monitored by using continuous EEG recordings (Connell et al 1989b, Hakeam & Wallace 1990).

Harris & Tizard (1960) itemized the abnormalities in the neonatal EEG that are related to seizures as follows: rhythmic slow waves; persistent focal sharp waves; spikes; repeated stereotyped sharp waves or wave complexes; gross asymmetry; small amplitude sharp waves during episodic sleep activity; and fast activity. Dreyfus-Brissac (1979) has reviewed reports on the abnormalities to be found in certain pathological states. In primary or late onset hypocalcaemia the interictal EEG is entirely normal. Conversely, when hypocalcaemia occurs early and is secondary to perinatal asphyxia the interictal EEG is abnormal. Seizure discharges may be seen to commence with the appearance of focal sharp waves which may spread throughout the same hemisphere or become alternatively bi- and unilateral. If hypocalcaemia is the major cause of the seizures, normalization of the EEG occurs once the plasma calcium has been restored.

Although abnormalities of the EEG may be found in hypoglycaemia they are non-specific. In other transient metabolic disorders, diffuse or localized spikes and sharp waves or other paroxysmal changes reflect the alterations in electrical activity but are not pathognomonic for any particular condition. Where the disorder is more severe, e.g. in such conditions as the organic acidurias where convulsions are often associated with interictal coma, the record may be periodic and the bursts characterized by high-voltage sharp waves or sharp complexes followed by slow waves with superimposed rapid rhythms. 'Comb-like rhythms', in association with other EEG abnormalities, are sometimes considered diagnostic of maple syrup urine disease. Complexes of sharp high-voltage slow waves which are mainly frontal and associated with Rolandic, occipital or generalized bursts of alpha rhythms have been described in non-ketotic hyperglycinaemia. Dreyfus-Brissac (1979) has suggested that, when a periodic EEG is seen in a neonate delivered normally after a normal pregnancy, an inborn error of metabolism should be suspected.

The EEG changes in seizures secondary to bacterial infections are non-specific. In herpes meningoencephalitis, a periodic EEG abnormality progresses to inactivity unless the infection can be controlled.

In cerebral dysmorphism, when there is a serious lack of cerebral tissue, such as in hydranencephaly, very low voltage recordings may be obtained with superimposed seizure discharges.

It has been suggested that positive sharp Rolandic waves are particularly associated with intraventricular haemorrhage in the premature infant but, in the most severe cases where seizures are likely to be prominent, slow or rapid spikes, or sharp wave discharges are usually recorded. Subclinical seizure discharges are commonly visible in infants with extensive intracranial haemorrhages.

When the seizures are symptomatic of hypoxic-ischaemic encephalopathy, in the mildest cases the EEG fails to show characteristic sleep patterns. In more severely affected babies seizure discharges, suppression-burst or total inactivity may be observed.

In infants with benign convulsive syndromes the EEG patterns usually consist of a background of low-voltage theta rhythms with bursts of asynchronous or synchronous high-voltage theta activity.

The EEG is an important tool in both the management and prognosis of neonatal seizures. It should be available, preferably as part of the continuous monitoring, for all infants with convulsions.

Treatment

Neonates with seizures should be kept as well oxygenated as possible and their general biochemical status retained in as normal a state as practicable.

Specific management

Where hypoglycaemia, hypocalcaemia, hypomagnesaemia, hypo- and hypernatraemia are the cause of convulsions, the appropriate treatment is obvious and correction of the metabolic disorder is relatively easy. The more complicated changes associated with disorders of amino or organic acids are much more difficult to rectify and discussion of their treatment is beyond the scope of this text. Transient hyperammonaemia responds to aggressive intervention by exchange transfusion and peritoneal dialysis (Ballard et al 1978).

Seizures secondary to pyridoxine dependency respond dramatically to Vitamin B6. It may be better initially to give this intravenously and under EEG control so that the necessity for B6 and confirmation of the diagnosis can be made with greater certainty.

Only in the unusual cases of acute subdural haematoma secondary to birth injury is there a definite place for surgery in the treatment of neonatal seizures, but recent studies which include PET scanning may define other circumstances in which surgery can be helpful (Chugani et al 1988).

Symptomatic management

In the absence of a remediable metabolic disorder, neonatal seizures are treated with antiepileptic drugs. The assessment of their efficacy in the newborn is difficult, since the infants are often generally unwell and frequently paralysed and supported with mechanical ventilation. The recognition of persisting seizures may only be possible by the use of continuous EEG monitoring (Eyre et al 1983b, Connell et al 1989b, Hakeem & Wallace 1990). Initially, the neonate clears drugs slowly and relatively small doses are necessary. Monitoring of drug blood levels is important, so that optimal pharmacological responses may be obtained.

Recent studies using EEG monitoring during periods when antiepileptic therapy is being given for neonatal seizures have suggested that the traditional first lines of treatment, phenobarbitone and phenytoin, are even less effective than had previously been reported (Connell et al 1989b, Hakeem & Wallace 1990). The possibility that benzodiazepines might be used more often as first-line treatment is discussed at length by Painter & Alvin (1990).

Benzodiazepines. Diazepam given by intravenous infusion in doses ranging from 0.7 to 12 mg.kg/day^2 is reported, in papers cited by Painter & Alvin (1990), to be 100% effective in control of seizures. However diazepam, 0.25 mg/kg intravenously as a single dose, was associated with neither clinical nor EEG control in seven neonates reported by Connell et al (1989b). Recurrence of seizure activity at 35 minutes after a bolus dose

of diazepam had been given to one neonate, and complete control in an infant in whom a bolus was followed by a continuous infusion are further reported (Hakeem & Wallace 1990). Early concerns that diazepam might cause oversedation, or, because of protein binding, might lead to kernicterus have not been substantiated.

Other benzodiazepines which have been used are clonazepam (Andre et al 1986, Hakeem & Wallace 1990) and lorazepam (Deshmukh et al 1986). In the study of Andre et al (1986), clonazepam was given to 18 infants whose seizures had failed to respond to phenobarbitone. Ten of the infants received 0.2 mg/kg and eight 0.1 mg/kg by slow intravenous infusion. The infants given 0.1 mg/kg all responded, clinically, immediately and completely, whereas those given 0.2 mg/kg took longer to respond and only six of 10 had their seizures controlled. Andre et al (1986) concluded that the optimal therapeutic response to clonazepam is obtained with 0.1 mg/kg given by slow intravenous infusion. In the single case treated with clonazepam by Hakeem & Wallace (1990) a continuous infusion of 0.01 mg.kg/h^2 was given with permanent remission of the seizures after 3 hours. In neonates who have been previously treated with phenobarbitone, the plasma half-life is between 20 and 40 hours and is apparently unrelated to gestation (Andre et al 1986). There is a rapid distribution half-life, in keeping with the almost immediate onset of clinical effect.

Lorezepam is reported to have been very rapidly effective in seven infants whose seizures were unresponsive to phenobarbiturate and phenytoin (Deshmukh et al 1986). Intravenous lorazepam 0.05 mg/kg was given over 2–5 minutes. In three infants the complete effectiveness was confirmed by EEG monitoring before, during and after the injection and in the others EEG monitoring was available within 24 hours. There was no adverse effect on vital signs, and, in particular, no secondary respiratory depression; but generalized suppression of background EEG rhythms was noted.

There are good reasons for considering a benzodiazepine as the first line of treatment for neonatal seizures, but studies which address this approach on a comparative basis are still awaited. So far as diazepam is concerned, on the available evidence, an infusion appears to be more appropriate than a bolus dose.

Phenobarbitone. Phenobarbitone has been the mainstay of treatment, but, when used intravenously in a bolus dose of 15–20 mg/kg, only one-third of infants have clinically-observed seizures controlled (Lockman et al 1979, Painter et al 1981). On the other hand, complete both clinical and EEG responses to phenobarbitone have been recorded in only two of 31 infants, all but one of whom had serum phenobarbitone levels within the target range (Connell et al 1989b). In addition, in another study, although six of seven infants treated with phenobarbitone had clinical responses, EEG evidence of continued or recurring seizures was present in four (Hakeem & Wallace 1990).

Despite these limitations, phenobarbitone probably still has a place in the treatment of neonatal seizures, and, when used as first choice, the following regime is suggested:

1. Give a loading dose of phenobarbitone 20 mg/ kg intravenously (or intramuscularly).
2. Monitor seizure activity carefully over the next 6 hours. If seizures do not remit give an additional dose of phenobarbitone 10 mg/kg intravenously.
3. If after another 6 hours seizures continue give an inital loading dose of phenytoin 20 mg/kg.
4. Start phenobarbitone maintenance with 3.5 mg/kg per 24 hours, 24 hours after loading is completed.
5. Determine serum phenobarbitone (and if necessary phenytoin) levels daily so that concentrations can be maintained within the optimal range.

Phenytoin. Phenytoin can be used either as a first choice or when phenobarbitone fails to control seizures. If an adequate serum level is to be obtained the dose of phenytoin is 20 mg/kg given slowly by the intravenous route. This should be followed up by maintenance dosage of 3–4 mg/kg/ day. Painter et al (1981) did not use phenytoin alone. They found that the number of infants whose seizures were controlled when phenytoin was added to phenobarbitone was twice that when phenobarbitone was used alone. Albani (1983) who used phenytoin as the antiepileptic drug of

first choice in 10 newborns, and as a second or third choice in six others, reports that 14 of the 16 had their seizures controlled by phenytoin, and Rochefort & Wilkinson (1989), in a randomized controlled trial of phenytoin, phenobarbitone, clonazepam and valproate, found phenytoin to be the most effective.

On the other hand, Connell et al (1989b) have reported that none of six infants had seizures recordable by EEG suppressed by phenytoin, although one showed a clinical response. In the neonate phenytoin, due to its nonlinear elimination kinetics and to immaturity of its metabolism, is not effective if given orally (Dodson & Bourgeois 1990). Albani (1983) gave phenytoin exclusively by the intravenous route and with monitoring serum phenytoin levels, doses as high as 68 mg/kg (mean 54.1 ± 2.6 mg/kg) were given for loading and 14 mg/kg (mean 10.6 ± 2.8 mg/kg) for maintenance therapy. The blood levels were 22.1 ± 4 µg/ml after the first 24 hours, 22.9 ± 7.8 µg/ml after the first 72 hours and 16.4 ± 5.3 µg/ml during the following days. Six of the babies (one-third of the total treated) were unwell in relation to high phenytoin levels; two vomited and six had urinary retention secondary to atonic bladders. Of 10 babies who survived and were followed up, six of those who had responded readily to phenytoin were developing normally at the ages of 9–13 months, suggesting that the large doses of phenytoin used to control their seizures had not had any important long-term effects. In the light of the findings of Connell et al (1989b), the role of phenytoin in the treatment of neonatal seizures requires reappraisal.

Other antiepileptic drugs. Paraldehyde has been given by some workers. When given intravenously, it has been reported to be efficacious in about half of those neonates with severe refractory seizures (Koren et al 1986). Fifteen infants received rectal paraldehyde 0.3 ml/kg or intravenous paraldehyde 1–3 ml.kg/h[2] of 5% intravenous infusion in 5% dextrose in the study of Connell et al (1989b). No infant had complete seizure control. In four the response was equivocal; two continued to have electrographic, but were relieved of clinical attacks; and no clinical or EEG response was obtained in the remaining nine. Painter & Alvin (1990) note that, if paraldehyde is used, it can be given as an intravenous infusion of 200 mg/kg followed by 15 mg.kg.h^2; or 200 mg.kg/h^2 for 2 hours; or 150 mg.kg/h^2 for 2 hours. Paraldehyde should be diluted before being used. In a previous report Painter (1983) suggested that a 10% solution would be appropriate, whereas Connell et al (1989b) used a 5% solution in 5% dextrose. Primidone (20 mg/kg) as an oral loading dose has been used with effect as a third antiepileptic drug in difficult cases (Painter 1983), but its limitations outweigh its usefulness (Painter & Alvin 1990). Valproate has been used infrequently and is reported, as a drug of first choice, to be less effective than phenytoin (Rochefort & Wilkinson 1989). Nevertheless, in infants unresponsive to other agents, valproate appears to have been successful (Gal et al 1988). Lidocaine has also been used when neonatal seizures have failed to respond to more conventional drugs (Radvanyi-Bouvet et al 1990). Control has been reported with the following regimens; in a continuous intravenous glucose infusion (4 mg.kg.h^2 on the the first day, 3 mg.kg/h^2 in the second, 2 mg.kg.h^2 on the third, 1 mg.kg/h^2 on the fourth, then discontinued on the fifth day (Radvanyi-Bauvet et al 1990), or 2 mg/kg as a loading dose, followed by infusion of 6 mg.kg.h^2 (Hellström-Westas et al 1988). Half-dosage should be used for premature infants (Radvanyi-Bouvet et al 1990).

Duration of therapy. The practice in neonatal follow-up clinics is to withdraw antiepileptic drugs during the first 3–6 months of life. On theoretical grounds, the first 6 months of life would be a good time to discontinue drug treatment since the seizure threshold appears to be particularly high at this time. In an investigation into the predictors of success for drug discontinuation following neonatal seizures, Brod et al (1988) examined the fates of 58 neonates. The data was inadequate for 10 infants. In the other 48, medication was tapered off if no seizures had occurred during the previous 3 months. Tapering was considered unsuccessful if seizures recurred or if they persisted despite continued therapy. Successful tapering was achieved in 27 out of 32 with initially normal, and seven of 16 with initially abnormal EEGs (P<0.005); in eight out of nine with initially normal, and 22 of 31 with initally abnormal neurological status (not significant);

and, in all eight infants with normal, and 22 of 36 with abnormal CT scans (P<0.03). Normal follow-up also predicted successful tapering. Brod et al (1988) concluded that initial and later EEGs and the initial CT scan were the most meaningful indicators for successful antiepileptic drug withdrawal.

Prognosis

The later outlook for the neonate who has seizures is closely related to the underlying aetiology. The overall mortality in a study spanning 15 years was 15% and the incidence of sequelae in survivors was 35% (Volpe 1987). Cerebral palsy, mental retardation and epilepsy are the handicaps.

It is obvious that cerebral dysmorphism will be permanent and that any infant whose seizures are symptomatic of malformations of the brain will be liable to continue to suffer seizures and show mental retardation and clinical neurological deficits.

Where prenatal vascular occlusion with the formation of a porencephalic cyst is associated with seizures, a persistent structural abnormality may be expected to lead to continuing convulsions, mental retardation and clinical neurological abnormalities. However, since children with porencephalic cysts represent a very small percentage of most series of neonatal seizures, it is difficult to estimate the incidence of sequelae in this group.

When prenatal infection is the aetiological agent only 10% of children are normal later. On the other hand, withdrawal of drugs, such as occurs when the infant is delivered to a mother who is addicted to sedatives, has a good prognosis. Almost all such infants subsequently develop normally.

Inborn errors of metabolism which present with seizures in the neonate are often difficult to treat. Where the seizures appear on the fifth day or are familial the outlook for later normality is good, though subsequent epilepsy can occur.

When seizures are related to perinatal or intrapartum events there is at least a 50% risk of later abnormality (Volpe 1987). When those with intraventricular haemorrhage are examined separately from those with primary subarachnoid haemorrhage, Volpe (1987) found that less than 10% of infants with intraventricular haemorrhage were later normal but that if the haemorrhage was primary subarachnoid there was a 90% chance of later normality.

When postnatal infection or bacterial meningitis is the underlying cause of convulsions between 25% and 65% of infants make a good recovery (Volpe 1987).

Of the metabolic disorders which may present in the neonatal period with seizures, the outcome is good in 36–50% of infants with early onset hypocalcaemia, in 90–100% of those with late onset hypocalcaemia, in 50–70% of neonates with transient hypoglycaemia and in only 28% of those with persistent hypoglycaemia (Volpe 1987).

In papers which correlated the outcomes in neonatal seizures with prenatal and perinatal events rather than with underlying aetiology Mellits et al (1981) found of those followed up to 7 years of age, 70% developed normally. The 5-minute Apgar score was significantly related to outcome: 48% of infants with 5-minute Apgar scores of less than 7 died, and comparable scores were significantly related to later mental retardation and cerebral palsy, but not to epilepsy. Similarly, resuscitation for more than 5 minutes in infants with subsequent seizures was significantly related to death or later cerebral palsy but not to epilepsy. Of the different seizure types, only tonic and myoclonic seizures appeared prognostically important. Tonic attacks were significantly related to later cerebral palsy, mental retardation and epilepsy, whereas neonatal myoclonic seizures were related only to subsequent mental retardation.

With increasing numbers of days on which seizures occurred, the likelihood of later mental retardation, cerebral palsy and epilepsy rose (Bergman et al 1983, Van Zeben-van der Aa et al 1990). By use of a multivariate analysis of factors associated with outcome (resuscitation after the first 5 minutes of life, birth weight, duration of seizures, number of days of seizures, onset time of seizures and 5-minute Apgar score), Mellits et al (1981) have shown that the prediction of death, mental retardation, cerebral palsy or epilepsy can be correctly performed in between 64% and 83% of cases. Of possible investigations, the EEG is the most consistently useful in prediction of outcome (Radvanyi-Bouvet et al 1987, Andre et al 1988).

FEBRILE CONVULSIONS

A febrile convulsion is most suitably defined as any seizure occurring in association with any febrile illness. Once restrictions such as intracranial infection, presence of chronic neurological disorder, or duration or lateralization of convulsion are placed on the definition it becomes extremely difficult to decide whether a convulsion should be characterized as 'febrile' or not. If all seizures which occur in association with a pyrexia are regarded as potentially symptomatic of acute or acute-on-chronic neurological disorders, the possible immediate and long-term consequences fall more readily into place. Febrile seizures occur almost exclusively between 6 months and 5 years of age with most children having their first febrile convulsion between 12 and 24 months. A comprehensive review of the literature prior to 1988 can be found in Wallace (1988).

Incidence

Between 19 and 41 per 1000 children convulse when feverish. The incidence in males is greater than in females, both in populations of children with febrile convulsions and within sibships where at least one child has had a febrile seizure.

Differential diagnosis

Other causes of acute loss of consciousness or rhythmic involuntary movements in early childhood are: breath-holding attacks; reflex anoxic seizures; syncope; rigors; and tetany.

In both breath-holding attacks and reflex anoxic seizures the episodes are acute reactions to noxious stimuli, which are usually unexpected. Syncope is associated with limpness and bradycardia rather than tonic-clonic movements and a tachycardia. Consciousness is not usually lost during rigors or tetany. Benign paroxysmal vertigo, in which sudden acute episodes of unsteadiness occur is not associated with loss of awareness.

Significance of age and sex

Convulsions which occur in association with febrile illnesses are strongly age-related. In a review of 7000 patients reported in the literature, the first seizure occurred before 6 months in 4%, between 6 months and 3 years in 75% and before the age of 5 years in 95% (Millichap 1968). In the British Births Survey of 1970 50% of 303 children ascertained had their first febrile convulsion during the second year of life (Verity et al 1985a). Girls tend to have their first convulsions at younger ages than boys and it has been suggested that because girls tend to convulse earlier they are more likely than boys to acquire cerebral damage as a result of febrile seizures. In some series those with positive family histories for convulsive disorders tend to have their first seizures later and thus at a less vulnerable time than those children with negative family histories.

Aetiological aspects

In a study conducted when a high proportion of febrile children were admitted to hospital only 11.3% had had convulsions. It is therefore relevant to consider the factors which might predispose to convulsions as well as the possible precipitating events.

Preconceptual factors

Chronic maternal ill health predating the conceptions of children with febrile convulsions has been found significantly frequently. Parental subfertility is common in families where children, particularly males, have seizures when pyrexial. Maternal smoking, maternal motor deficit and mental retardation in an older half-sibling are also reported as increasing the risk for febrile convulsions (Nelson & Ellenberg 1990). Thus in some affected children, the prenatal environment may not be conducive to optimal cerebral development.

Prenatal factors

Vaginal bleeding in either early or late pregnancy is reported more commonly when children later have febrile convulsions. Maternal medication during pregnancy with, in particular, diuretics, antiepileptic drugs, antibiotics, antiemetics and antidepressants has been noted more frequently during pregnancies resulting in children liable to pyrexial seizures than in their siblings and, although not a significant factor, was found to double the risk of febrile convulsions in the study of Nelson & Ellenberg (1990). It will be noted that several of these substances might have adverse effects on the developing nervous system.

Perinatal factors

A study of twins discordant for febrile convulsions failed to find a significant difference between convulsing and non-convulsing twins for birth first or second, presentation, assisted delivery, or any other unspecified abnormality during the perinatal period. Nor, in the analysis of the information gathered during the National Collaborative Perinatal Project (NCPP), did Nelson & Ellenberg (1990) find that any of a large number of factors related to pregnancy, labour and delivery increase the risk for febrile convulsions. On the other hand Verity et al (1985b) reported an excess of breech presentations. When patients were compared with non-convulsing siblings, fetal distress during labour and delivery by Caesarean section were significantly more common (Wallace 1988). When uncorrected birth weight is taken as a comparative measurement, children with febrile convulsions do not seem particularly disadvantaged (Verity et al 1985b) but, if the birth weights are corrected for gestational age, sex, birth order and maternal height, an excess of infants with later convulsions can be shown to be small for gestational age at birth. In one study, 62% of children with febrile convulsions had at least one of a number of pre- and perinatal factors found significantly less commonly in non-convulsing siblings (Wallace 1988).

Later postnatal development

Some authors consider that children with chronic neurological handicaps should be excluded from the possible diagnosis of febrile convulsions. However, since many children who convulse when feverish have difficulties compatible with the description of the minimal cerebral dysfunction syndrome, it is difficult to define a level of severity at which neurological disorder would preclude the use of the term febrile convulsion. Prior to their convulsions in both studies in the general population (unselected) and in hospital patients (selected) children with febrile convulsions have a much higher incidence of delay in motor development or other evidence of neurological suboptimality when compared with the general population or siblings.

Family history of seizures

The incidence of convulsive disorders in parents and siblings is significantly higher than in the general population (Forsgren et al 1990). In about 30% of children with febrile convulsions, careful enquiry will reveal a positive family history. In one study, first-degree relatives with seizures were apparently more common in the families of affected males (Wallace 1988), but an investigation of same-sex twins discordant for febrile convulsions found that genetic factors were more important for females. The conclusions from the NCPP were that a positive family history for seizure disorders makes an important contribution to the risk factors for febrile convulsions, and that febrile seizures in the mother have the greatest influence (Nelson & Ellenberg 1990).

Attempts to sort out the genetics of febrile convulsions and to separate them genetically from epilepsy have not been entirely successful. At the time of the first seizure and 5–7 years later, Frantzen et al (1970) enquired about a family history of epilepsy and of childhood convulsions in a group of 228 children: epilepsy was present in the relatives of 20% and febrile convulsions in 40%; both epilepsy and febrile convulsions were found in the family histories of 10% of the children. After analysis of their data, Frantzen et al concluded that febrile convulsions were inherited by a single dominant gene. They noted that the genetic message to convulse when febrile appeared to be strictly age-related and that the pattern for ages at recurrence differed significantly between family history positive and negative cases.

On the other hand Tsuboi (1977), although agreeing that autosomal dominant inheritance could not be ruled out since incomplete expression is possible, concluded on the basis of a study of 450 children that multifactorial inheritance was probable. A further study, conducted using the linkage of medical records over a period of many decades has also suggested that the inheritance pattern is most consistent with a polygenic mechanism (Hauser et al 1985).

Regardless of the mode of inheritance there is general agreement that genetic factors are amongst those of aetiological importance in febrile convulsions.

Low serum IgA levels

In a study mainly aimed at examining the frequency and importance of viral infections in children with febrile convulsions the serum IgA levels were low in some cases. However, although there may be children who convulse because they are not able adequately to contain viral agents, dissemination of viruses was not greater in the children with low IgA levels. The significance of these finding remains in doubt.

Summary of factors predisposing to febrile convulsions

In the histories of children who convulse when febrile there are excesses of:

— family history positive for seizure disorders, particularly febrile convulsions
— chronic maternal ill health
— parental subfertility
— breech presentation
— delivery by Caesarean section
— small birth weight for gestational age
— developmental delay (usually mild and affecting particularly speech)
— minimal cerebral dysfunction
— low serum IgA levels.

The precipitating event

Febrile convulsions present in children with predisposing factors only when a feverish illness occurs during the critical age period.

Viral infections

Even before the possibility of identification of

actual viruses arose, it was noted that upper respiratory tract infections were most commonly present when a child had a febrile convulsion. The important role of respiratory viruses in the illnesses in which convulsions occur has now been demonstrated. A very detailed analysis of the evidence for viral infection has shown that in 86% a viral illness could be held responsible for the fever with which a convulsion occurred. The viruses involved were not confined to those considered 'respiratory'. Febrile convulsions related to any particular viral infection are most likely to occur when these infecting agents are present in epidemic concentrations in the community.

Intracranial infection

Although many authors exclude children with intracranial infections, (particularly bacterial meningitis) from their series of febrile convulsions, the long-term outcome no longer seems to be more serious than in those children with clear cerebrospinal fluid. Up to 8% of children who present with febrile convulsions will be found to have bacterial or viral meningitis.

Other causes of fever

Gastrointestinal infections, particularly with shigella or salmonella, have been recorded in between 4% and 13% of cases. With current vaccination schedules, convulsions in association with the consequent fever are reported after 0.09 per 1000 doses of combined diphtheria, tetanus and pertussis antigens, 0.6 per 1000 doses of polio vaccine. Only after measles vaccination is there a significant, but very small, risk of a febrile convulsion. The concept of predisposition to convulse with fever is emphasized by the wide range of infecting agents and causes of pyrexia which have been identified in children with febrile seizures.

General consequences of infection

Exogenous pyrogens released during viral and bacterial infections cause an upward setting of the thermoregulatory centres in the hypothalamic/preoptic areas. It has been suggested that the associated release of acetylcholine in the caudal hypothalamus, with subsequent activation of nicotinic receptors concerned in thermogenesis, might be directly related to the precipitation of febrile convulsions. However, recent studies have been unable to confirm that there is a simple relationship between experimental febrile convulsions and the cholinergic system. There is evidence that the brain is especially sensitive to extremes of temperature (Lancet 1989), but the fevers associated with convulsions are usually well below the critical level of 42°C.

There has been considerable interest in whether the rate of rise or the height of temperature is the more important precipitant: both are difficult to monitor. On the whole, height of temperature is more commonly favoured, a view which is supported by simultaneous EEG and temperature monitoring in children who have had febrile convulsions.

Pathophysiological aspects

The pathophysiology of febrile convulsions can be examined on the basis of:

— cerebral development prior to and at the critical age
— cerebral damage at the time of the convulsion
— pathological sequelae.

Cerebral development at the age critical for febrile convulsions

Between the ages of 6 months and 3 years, when febrile convulsions are most common, both organization and myelination are occurring in the child's brain. Since prenatal factors and adverse events in early pregnancy may predispose to febrile convulsions, it is possible that abnormal neuronal proliferation and migration might be contributory events, but there is no pathological evidence to confirm this possibility. There is, however, evidence from single photon emission computed tomography (SPECT) that focal areas of hypoperfusion can be found in a proportion of children with febrile convulsions (Michihiro et al 1989). Such areas are most likely to reflect pre-existing abnormalities, but could be secondary to the seizures.

Cerebral damage in association with febrile convulsions

There is a reasonable amount of circumstantial evidence to suggest that single brief (fewer than 15 minutes) generalized convulsions with fever do not cause recognizable cerebral damage. Biochemical evidence of cerebral hypoxia is lacking when the cerebrospinal fluid pyruvate and lactate levels are measured after brief convulsions with fever. Further evidence that short febrile convulsions are benign is provided by a study of cerebrospinal fluid nucleotides. Hypoxanthine, xanthine and uridine levels were comparable in patients and in febrile controls, both of whom had significantly higher levels than afebrile controls, findings consistent with increased cerebral metabolism during fever. Either prolongation of the seizure for more than 30 minutes or repetition within a 24-hour period is associated with raised cerebrospinal fluid lactate levels and lactate : pyruvate ratios suggesting that cerebral hypoxia had occurred. As correlates to these biochemical studies, reports on the post-mortem findings in children with febrile convulsions, on the radiological findings in some children with prolonged seizures and on the clinical consequences of prolonged unilateral or bilateral seizures with fever are available.

In five children who died during illnesses in which febrile convulsions occurred, neuronal necrosis has been described throughout the cerebral cortex but particularly in the frontal and temporal areas, with variable changes in the basal ganglia and selective loss of Purkinje cells in the cerebellum. The brain of a 5-month-old infant who died after prolonged seizures with fever showed, in all areas of the cerebral cortex, ischaemic nerve cell change and reactive astrocytosis. The frontal and occipital horns were more severely affected than the temporal lobes, but bilateral acute Ammon's horn necrosis, characterized by loss of neurones in the H_1 (Sommer) sector and proliferation of glia in this layer and in the subjacent white matter was noted. There was widespread loss of Purkinje cells in the cerebellum. This picture is typical of the findings in those who die a few days after prolonged convulsions. The changes are non-specific in that they are related to severe interference with cerebral energy metabolism such as occurs in arterial hypotension, cardiac arrest, cerebral ischaemia or severe hypoglycaemia. They are now considered secondary to the presence of excitotoxic amino acids, e.g. glutamic acid and aspartic acid, which tend to accumulate when seizures are prolonged (Ingvar & Siesjo 1990).

Studies on adolescent baboons have further emphasized the importance of the duration of seizures in determining whether or not pathological changes occur. If seizures last under 30 minutes there is no correlation with ischaemic neuronal changes, but if the seizures persist for between 30 and 300 minutes the degree of neuronal damage is related to their duration and to the degree and duration of any pyrexia; the severity and duration of arterial hypotension; and the severity of hypoglycaemia. When the autonomic and motor disturbances of the seizures are eliminated by paralysis and artificial ventilation, the cerebellar pathology is eliminated, but neuronal changes still occur in the neocortex, thalamus and hippocampus, confirming that the increased energy demand of the epileptic discharges themselves is an important factor in the pathological changes.

Pathological sequelae

In children, the gross pathological changes subsequent to prolonged convulsions have been demonstrated radiologically: cerebral swelling is followed by cerebral atrophy. In convulsions of lesser duration or greater localization, gross changes may not be demonstrable radiologically but focal neuronal necrosis may nevertheless occur with resultant sclerosis, such as is found in Ammon's horn (mesiotemporal sclerosis) in those children in whom prolonged unilateral convulsions are followed by temporal lobe epilepsy. Ounsted et al (1966) have emphasized the importance of age in determining the cerebral pathology resulting from prolonged seizures. In children aged less than 1 year, febrile convulsions which last for more than 30 minutes carry a high risk of subsequent mental retardation. Between the ages of 1 and 3 years there is selective hemispheric vulnerability related to the child's sex. Mesiotemporal sclerosis, with subsequent temporal lobe epilepsy, is the more likely sequel to a prolonged febrile seizure in these somewhat older children. Areas of hypoperfusion, suggesting focal cerebral abnormalities, are comparable in children with febrile convulsions to those seen in patients with epilepsy (Michihiro et al 1989).

Factors of importance in the first seizure

Since the age at the first seizure, the duration and the number of seizures which occur during any single febrile illness are relevant to the long-term prognosis, it is important that details are recorded as completely as possible. Understandably, since most first febrile seizures occur unexpectedly, there is considerable panic amongst the attendant adults and it is probable that partial features are not recorded as often as they should be. Even if the parents cannot give a figure for the duration of the seizure, it is possible to arrive at a reasonable estimate by asking them what they did during the length of time that the seizure continued. If the child was still convulsing on arrival in hospital the seizure was almost certainly of more than 15 minutes, if not more that 30 minutes, duration.

Prolonged repeated or partial febrile convulsions

Most authors define a prolonged convulsion as one of at least 30 minutes duration. Others define the critical time as 15 minutes. It may be preferable to take the shorter period since this is likely to produce a greater sense of urgency in termination of the seizure.

At least 20% of patients in hospital series have febrile convulsions lasting 30 minutes or more. Before diazepam became readily available, 13–14% of hospital patients were recorded as having febrile seizures of at least 1 hour's duration. Seizures which are repeated within the same illness have been noted in up to 30% and those which are partial with or without secondary generalization in up to 19% of a hospital series. When the convulsions are defined as 'complex' (of at least 15 minutes' duration, repeated within 24 hours and of focal onset), or 'simple', between one-third and one-tenth of children in population studies have complex initial febrile seizures. As might be expected, children with complex seizures are more likely to be admitted to hospital. Thus hospital

series tend to overestimate the relative frequency of complex initial febrile convulsions.

Predisposition to complex initial seizures has been explored in a number of studies. In some series, females seemed to be more vulnerable. In others there is an excess of males. Where both a positive family history and a perinatal abnormality are present and, in females, when previous neurological suboptimality is suspected, the risk of a complex initial seizure rises significantly. Younger children, up to 12–18 months of age, are at greater risk of an initial complex febrile seizure than those whose first attack occurs after 18 months.

Neither the rate of rise of temperature nor the duration of the pyrexia appears to be important in determining the duration of the seizure.

Management of the febrile convulsions

The management of febrile convulsions can be considered under the following headings:

— attention to the effects of the seizure
— antiepileptic drugs in the acute stage
— identification and treatment of the underlying infection
— recognition of parental anxieties.

Attention to the effects of the seizures

In addition to maintaining the airway and giving oxygen and other supportive therapy as necessary, it is paticularly important in febrile convulsions actively to normalize the body temperature: tepid sponging, cooling with a fan and paracetamol or other antipyretics given as suppositories can be helpful.

Antiepileptic drugs in the acute stage

After a duration of 10 minutes if the convulsion does not terminate spontaneouly it is appropriate to use an antiepileptic drug. Diazepam is the drug of first choice. It acts very rapidly if given in a dose of 0.1 mg/kg body weight intravenously. However, children who are at the peak age for febrile convulsions are often a little plump and intravenous injection can be difficult. Diazepam 0.5 mg/kg body weight given rectally in solution acts almost as rapidly as when the intravenous route is used and is a completely satisfactory alternative. If diazepam is given intramuscularly or in suppositories it is not absorbed sufficiently rapidly to be useful in the acute situation. Should the seizure fail to respond to the first dose of either intravenous or rectal diazepam after 15 minutes, a further comparable dose can be given. If this fails to control the convulsion, the child should be nursed in a unit where intubation and ventilation can be carried out. Further sedation using intravenous phenobarbitone or rectal or intramuscular paraldehyde can then be given under suitable supervision. It is particularly important that facilities for resuscitation are available if phenobarbitone is given after diazepam.

Identification and treatment of the underlying infection

Since a febrile convulsion is always a symptom of a generalized illness, it is clearly important that a good physical examination is performed and that treatment for any remediable condition is instituted. Almost 90% of febrile convulsions are related to viral infections and for these children symptomatic therapy will be appropriate. Of the 10% with bacterial infections it is particularly important to consider, and in most cases exclude by lumbar puncture, bacterial meningitis. Bacteraemia and urinary tract infection are present in small percentages of children with febrile convulsions, are often unsuspected, and should be excluded by blood and urine culture.

Recognition of parental anxieties

The parents of at least 70% of the children believe at the time of the febrile convulsion that their child has died. The parents are also concerned that their child might have meningitis, become mentally retarded or develop epilepsy. Only by recognizing these anxieties and dealing with them truthfully and realistically will unjustified fears be suitably allayed and the likelihood of long-term sequelae be put into perspective.

Laboratory investigation in the acute stage

Tests on blood, urine or cerebrospinal fluid are relevant to the underlying illness, secondary metabolic changes or the seizure itself.

On the whole, although a neutropenia usually related to a viral illness occurs commonly, blood counts are not helpful in management. Hyponatraemia has been reported but seems to be no more than a non-specific response to a febrile illness. Calcium and phosphate levels are normal.

Low serum IgA levels are found in some children and might be of significance in handling the infecting agent but this concept requires further investigation. Active immune responses, which are attributed to the presence of viral antigens within the central nervous system, have been demonstrated by measurement of cerebrospinal fluid immunoglobulins.

Examination of the cerebrospinal fluid in the acute stage has demonstrated some variability in amino acids levels, but the significance of these findings is not apparent (Cremades et al 1989). Investigation of monoamine levels in cerebrospinal fluid has produced varying results. Either there has been no difference from controls (Kimiya et al 1989) or the findings have suggested a reduced turnover (Giroud et al 1990).

Lumbar puncture

Lumbar puncture is at best unpleasant and at worst frankly dangerous. It is the most controversial of the investigations appropriate to the child with febrile convulsions. Particularly in younger children it may be impossible to exclude meningitis on clinical grounds. Although complex seizures are sometimes considered to be indicative of more serious underlying acquired pathology, in a series of children in whom a febrile convulsion was the alerting sign for bacterial meningitis, the convulsions were all under 30 minutes' duration. It is recommended that, provided there are no signs of raised intracranial pressure, lumbar puncture should be performed as a routine procedure in children aged under 18 months at the time of a febrile seizure and in those aged 18 months or more whose recovery from the convulsion seems to be unexpectedly delayed. Where there are signs of raised intracranial pressure or other reasons to suspect that lumbar puncture might be hazardous, before examining the cerebrospinal fluid the child should be transferred to a unit where CT scanning and neurosurgical facilities are available. On very rare occasions it may be justifiable to treat the child empirically for meningitis until such time as the cerebrospinal fluid can be examined under safe conditions.

Radiological and other forms of imaging

Skull X-rays are almost invariably normal and should not be requested routinely. More sophisticated radiological imaging techniques i.e. MRI, PET and SPECT, give further information about underlying pathology such as neuronal heterotopias or other areas of dysgenesis and could lead to a better understanding of the pathological substrates, but none of these investigations would be appropriate as a routine.

Electroencephalography

EEGs recorded during the acute stages of febrile illnesses in which convulsions occur reflect changes related more to the underlying infection than the seizures. During the first week after a febrile convulsion between 50% and 70% of children have normal EEGs. Up to one-third of patients show some slowing of background rhythms. When complex seizures occur in children over 2 years old, the pyrexia exceeds 39°C, the illness lasts more than 36 hours or the underlying infection is gastroenteritis, there is marked slowing in association with young age and long duration of fever. However, when EEG changes are related to changes in temperature over a 24-hour period of continuous recording, no relationship was demonstrated between the frequency of the background rhythm and the height of the pyrexia. During the week following the febrile convulsion, it is unusual to record spikes or other paroxysmal discharges. Even when found, their presence is completely unhelpful in prognosis. During continuous recordings for 24 hours after initial convulsions spikes tend to appear during periods of prolonged high fever, but the exact significance of this finding remains in doubt.

Thus, although EEGs might be expected to give some indication of the likelihood of recurrence of febrile seizures or the later development of epilepsy, to date all studies have suggested that when recorded in the acute phase they do not provide any useful information for prognosis. Nevertheless, they can be helpful in the acute assessment and management of the child with a febrile seizure.

Recurrence of febrile convulsions

In children who do not receive antiepileptic prophylaxis following their first febrile seizure the overall risk of recurrence is about 50% (Wallace 1988, Farwell et al 1990). Approximately one-sixth to one-third of children who have twice had febrile convulsions will have three or more episodes. The recurrence rate is related to the presence or absence of risk factors which can easily be defined.

Risk factors for recurrence

Knudsen (1985) has identified five major risk factors:

1. Age less than 15 months
2. Epilepsy in first degree relatives
3. Febrile convulsions in first degree relatives
4. Complex first febrile seizure
5. Day nursery care.

If three to five of these factors are present there is an 80–100% risk of recurrence of febrile seizures during the following 18 months. The risk falls to 50% if two factors are present, to 25% if one factor is present and to 12% if none are in evidence. These factors are similar but not identical to those defined by Wallace & Aldridge Smith (1981):

1. Seizures in first degree relatives
2. Age less than 20 months
3. Unskilled or unemployed parents.

If all three of these risk factors were present the children invariably had a recurrence. Children with two of these factors were significantly more likely to have recurrences than those in whom no risk factor was identified.

Abnormalities of pregnancy, low birth weight and neurological abnormality have also been cited as important in predisposing to recurrent febrile convulsions. On the basis of these studies there should be no difficulty in identifying children at risk of repeated convulsions with fever. A meta-analysis of 14 previous studies has emphasized that young age, less than 12–15 months, at onset is the most powerful predictor of recurrences (Berg et al 1990).

Significance of recurrent febrile convulsions

Annegers et al (1987) have shown that on long-term follow-up, with increasing numbers of febrile convulsions, the relative risk of subsequent generalized epilepsy rises. In addition, children with recurrent febrile convulsions do not maintain normal intellectual progress (Aldridge Smith & Wallace 1982).

Prevention of recurrent febrile convulsions

Although pyrexia is a necessary precipitant of a febrile convulsion, even detailed antipyretic instruction does not reduce the incidence of further convulsions in subsequent pyrexial illnesses. In children with two or more risk factors for recurrence, prophylaxis with an antiepileptic drug should be prescribed.

Intermittent therapy. Benzodiazepines are the only group of drugs effective in the control of febrile convulsions when given on an intermittent basis. The intermittent use of phenobarbitone or phenytoin is both irrational and ineffective.

The prophylactic treatment of choice is rectal diazepam in solution: 5 mg in children aged less that 3 years or 7.5 mg in children aged 3 or more years. The diazepam is given when the temperature reaches 38.5°C and is repeated every 12 hours on up to a total of four occasions until the temperature falls below 38.5°C. This regimen reduces the incidence of recurrence in children with risk factors to a rate comparable with that in children with no risk factor.

Alternatively, diazepam given in suppositories in a dose of 5 mg every 8 hours while the pyrexia lasts has been found to be as effective in preventing recurrences as continuous phenobarbitone.

Both clonazepam (Martinez et al 1990) and nitrazepam (Vanasse et al 1984) have been used on an intermittent basis during pyrexias. Although effective in prophylaxis, both have tended to cause unacceptable sedation. Nitrazepam has the disadvantage for use in young children with illnesses that oral administration is necessary. Clonazepam can be given rectally in solution at a dose of 0.1 mg/kg, but prolonged sleep and ataxia follow.

Continuous therapy. Some parents find the concept of giving rectal medication unacceptable and in some children there is such a short period of ill health prior to the convulsion that there is no time to give intermittent prophylaxis. In these cases, if risk factors for recurrence are present, either phenobarbitone or sodium valproate should be given until there have been 2 years' freedom from convulsions. The dose of phenobarbitone is 4–5 mg/kg body weight per day. Phenytoin has been found to reduce significantly the recurrence rate only in children aged 3 years or older and, in any case, is difficult to use in small children. Carbamazepine has failed to reduce the recurrence risk, either when used as a first choice or when given after phenobarbitone has failed.

Problems with prophylactic medication. Diazepam may cause some mild drowsiness but this appears to be insufficient to obscure serious underlying infections such as meningitis.

Unacceptable overactivity occurs in 20% of children treated with phenobarbitone for febrile convulsions. However, in those children who are not overtly upset, cognitive development has been shown to proceed normally during treatment with phenobarbitone for periods of up to 35 months. A recent suggestion that phenobarbitone was ineffective and caused intellectual dulling (Farwell et al 1990) has been severely criticised on the bases of the methodologies employed and the poor compliance with therapy (Kohrman et al 1990, Hirsch & Painter 1990).

Sodium valproate has not been reported to cause serious irreversible side-effects when used as prophylaxis for febrile convulsions. When given over a 2-year period it produces significantly fewer behavioural side-effects than phenobarbitone and does not adversely effect cognitive development (Aldridge Smith & Wallace 1982).

Compliance with therapy is often very poor, and intention to treat does not reduce recurrences (McKinlay & Newton 1989).

Epilepsy after febrile convulsions

There is an increased risk of later epilepsy in children who have had febrile convulsions.

Incidence of later epilepsy

In a population study children who had not convulsed with fever had a 0.5% risk of epilepsy at the age of 7 whereas 2% of those who had febrile seizures were found to have epilepsy by the same age. Where the follow-up was up to 30 years and actuarial calculations were made to assess the risk of epilepsy in the general population, children who had had febrile convulsions were just over five times more likely to develop epilepsy than those who had not convulsed when febrile. The cumulative risk of epilepsy was 7% by age 25 years (Annegers et al 1987). When children who have been admitted to hospital for treatment and assessment at the time of their first febrile seizure are followed up, the incidence of later epilepsy is higher than that for the general population. In a personal study, only two-thirds of those with epilepsy when aged 9–14 years had had their first non-febrile seizure before the age of 7. Thus figures for the incidence of later epilepsy probably underestimate the problem unless a truly long-term follow-up into adult life is undertaken.

Seizure types and epileptic syndromes subsequent to febrile convulsions

Generalized tonic-clonic seizures are those most commonly reported once epilepsy becomes established. It is rare for typical absences to be the major seizure type.

When a great deal of care had been taken to characterize the seizure type accurately, the risk for later partial epilepsy was almost twice that for generalized epilepsy in a long-term population study (Annegers et al 1987). Similarly, when analysing the previous histories of patients with partial epilepsy, Danesi (1985) found that almost a quarter had had febrile convulsions. Although many authors report a high incidence of generalized tonic-clonic seizures, there also appears to be a sizeable risk of later partial seizures in children who have had febrile convulsions.

High incidences of myoclonic or minor seizures have also been reported. The syndrome of hemi-convulsion (usually febrile), hemiplegia (usually transient) and later complex partial seizures first reported by Gastaut et al (1960) is now well recognized.

In a review of epileptic syndromes linked with previous febrile seizures, it was noted that childhood absence epilepsy, epilepsy with myoclonic absences, severe myoclonic epilepsy in infancy, myoclonic-astatic epilepsy, the Lennox–Gastaut syndrome, benign partial epilepsies and juvenile myoclonic epilepsy all occur more frequently in patients with a personal, or family, history of convulsions when feverish (Wallace 1991).

It is concluded that many types of epilepsy may be sequelae to convulsions with fever and that, in the past, the categorization has not always been optimal.

Risk factors for epilepsy

The important factors for the later development of epilepsy have usually been examined on the assumption that the antecedents of all types of epilepsy are comparable. In a population study in which children were followed up to the age of 7 years, epilepsy occurred significantly more often in the presence of:

1. Suspect or abnormal development prior to the initial seizure complex
2. Prolonged, repeated, focal features in the initial seizure
3. Seizures when afebrile in a parent or prior born sibling.

In children with one of these factors there was a 1.3% risk of epilepsy at 7 years. If two or three factors were present the risk of epilepsy at age 7 years rose to 9.6%.

When the factors related to the development of partial epilepsy have been looked at separately from those present in generalized epilepsy, it has been found that persisting generalized tonic-clonic seizures occurred significantly more often in children of unskilled or unemployed parents, where there had been adverse perinatal events and persistent neurological abnormalities; whereas the complex partial seizures occurred significantly more often when the first febrile convulsion had been prolonged and partial (Wallace 1988). When the outcome for children with unilateral febrile convulsions of at least 30 minutes' duration was examined complex partial seizures were found most often in children who were particularly young at the time of their febrile convulsions and in females where the initial seizure was right-sided (left hemisphere). The overall likelihood of developing an epileptic syndrome is related to the genetic input (Wallace 1991).

In a study spanning 30 years, Annegers et al (1987) examined factors prognostic of unprovoked seizures. Approximately two-thirds of those who had unprovoked seizures had more than a single attack, and thus suffered from epilepsy. When examined by univariate analysis, the following were considered predictive:

1. Increasing numbers of febrile seizures
2. Age at onset less than 1 year
3. Each of focal, repeated or prolonged (at least 30 minutes) features in the initial seizure.

Multivariate analysis slightly reduced the risks, but focal features, seizures repeated within the initial episode and prolonged seizures remained significant predictors. To assess the cumulative risk, the results of the multivariate model were used. Up to the age of 25 years, the cumulative risks for unprovoked seizures were as follows:

1. No prognostic factors: 2.4%
2. Focal features, no other adverse event: 8%
3. Repeated within the same illness, alone: 6%
4. Long (at least 30 minutes) duration, alone: 6%
5. Focal and prolonged or repeated: 21–22%
6. Focal and prolonged and repeated: 49%.

When the prognosis was examined by type of unprovoked seizure, it was found that there was an excess of the onset of partial epilepsies before the age of 10 years, whereas seizures symptomatic of generalized epilepsies presented throughout the period of observation. For unprovoked partial seizures, focal febrile seizures were the strongest predictors, whereas recurrent (at least three) episodes of febrile convulsions preceded generalized unprovoked seizures significantly often. Thus prognostic factors differ for partial and generalized epilepsies. Annegers et al (1987) further re-

ported that for children who have febrile seizures and a positive family history, the febrile seizure is irrelevant to their outcome, since their risks for epilepsy are comparable to children with positive family histories who have not had febrile convulsions.

One further possible risk factor for later epilepsy had been identified by Pavone et al (1989). These authors found that when children aged 6 years or more presented with what appeared to be febrile seizures, their risk for subsequent epilepsy was 16%.

Longitudinal EEG studies

Long-term EEG studies have been conducted with the aims of clarifying genetic trends and of monitoring the progression, or not, to epilepsy. Bilaterally synchronous spike-waves, photosensitivity and 4–7 cycle/second waves, i.e. patterns considered to be genetically determined, have been found in 81% of children with previous febrile convulsions, from whom EEGs had been recorded up to the ages of 11–13 years. Although it was concluded that the findings support the proposal that febrile convulsions occur as a result of a heterogeneous response to polygenetic inheritance, no correlation was found between the EEG characteristics and the family history.

Spikes on EEGs recorded in middle childhood bear no relation to clinical events, but are sometimes typical of those in benign epilepsy of childhood with centro-temporal spikes (Kajitani et al 1981, Wallace 1991).

On the basis of the information available, it seems that intermittent EEG recording over periods of months or years is unhelpful in clinical management.

Later cognitive development

In children who have been admitted to hospital with their initial febrile seizure, between 6% and 18% have been reported to be mentally retarded (IQ less than 70) on subsequent testing (Wallace 1988). The absolute incidence of frank mental retardation has not been reported for non-hospital populations. However, in children with febrile convulsions recorded in the British Births Survey of 1970, speech problems were significantly more prevalent than expected and tests of design copying and vocabulary at the age of 5 were performed particularly badly by those children whose convulsions had been unilateral or prolonged (Verity et al 1985b).

Although some children are of below average ability, the mean intelligence quotient of any group with febrile convulsions is invariably reported to be within the average range. However, specific learning difficulties do seem to be more common than expected. Problems with logical memory, Weschler digit symbol tests, block design, and Part B of the trail-making test were noted in a study where twins discordant for febrile convulsions were compared (Schiottz-Christensen & Bruhn 1973). Specific reading difficulties occur in 35% of children whose initial convulsion was right-sided (left hemisphere) and either of at least 30 minutes or repeated within the same illness. The overall incidence of specific reading retardation was 19% in a hospital-based population who were tested when aged between 8 and 14 years.

Factors related to suboptimal cognitive ability in children who have had febrile convulsions are:

1. Low social class and perinatal abnormalities
2. Prior or continuing neurological abnormalities
3. Recurrence of febrile convulsions
4. Progression to epilepsy.

Prior treatment with phenobarbitone has no effect on later cognitive or reading abilities.

MYOCLONIC EPILEPSIES

Myoclonic epilepsies of childhood include a series of seizure disorders which are usually, but not invariably, associated with an underlying severe generalized cerebral disturbance. As with all other seizure disorders in childhood, these epilepsies and their implications are most readily understood if the child's age at the time of onset and of assessment are taken into account. As a general rule, the younger the child at the onset of an epilepsy which includes myoclonic seizures the more difficult the seizures are to control and the more serious for the ultimate prognosis. The main syndromes are:

1. Early myoclonic encephalopathy
2. Infantile spasms (West syndrome)
3. Benign myoclonic epilepsy in infants
4. Severe myoclonic epilepsy in infants
5. Myoclonic-astatic epilepsy of early childhood
6. Epilepsy with myoclonic absences
7. Juvenile myoclonic epilepsy
8. Progressive myoclonic epilepsies.

In addition, Kojewnikow's syndrome, which is considered with the partial epilepsies, can be associated with myoclonic seizures.

Early myoclonic encephalopathy

Recognition of epileptic syndromes which include myoclonic seizures and which commence in the neonatal period, or very soon thereafter, is relatively recent and it is not entirely clear from the literature whether early infantile epileptic encephalopathy (Ohtahara 1984) should be considered an entity separate from early myoclonic encephalopathy (Otani et al 1989, Aicardi 1990).

Incidence

The incidence of early myoclonic encephalopathy is unknown. Aicardi (1990) has reviewed the data on 29 cases previously reported in the literature. Information on one further case is also available (Otani et al 1989). This type of epilepsy is extremely rare.

Seizure types

The seizures start with erratic partial myoclonus, which may be restricted to only one part of a limb or may be generalized but which are usually repetitive to the extent of being more or less continuous during both waking and sleep. The appearance of partial seizures follows closely on the onset of the erratic myoclonus and tonic infantile spasms appear somewhat later at about 3–4 months of age.

Differential diagnosis

The differential diagnosis is largely from other causes of myoclonus in very early infancy and from Otahara's syndrome (1984). Otani et al (1989) felt that the two syndromes could be differentiated on the basis of clinical and EEG findings, but Aicardi (1990) feels that distinctions between early myoclonic encephalopathy and early infantile epileptic encephalopathy may not be absolute.

Aetiology

Both non-ketotic hyperglycinaemia and D-glutaric acidaemia present with clinical pictures indistinguishable from early myoclonic encephalopathy (Aicardi 1985). In addition, myoclonic jerking and other seizures occur in association with molybdenum co-factor deficiency (Aukett et al 1988). Other cases have occurred frequently on a familial basis and Aicardi noted the following diagnoses or positive findings in seven of the cases he reviewed: poliodystrophy, minor cortical malformations; Menkes' disease in the same family; progressive cerebral atrophy; severe multifocal spongy changes in the cerebral white matter with PAS-positive perivascular concentric bodies; high levels of proprionic acid in the blood and marked poverty of myelin without spongiosis in the cerebral hemispheres; and hemimegalencephaly with astrocytic proliferation but without disturbance of the cortical architecture.

Although in the majority of cases there was no biochemical or pathological confirmation of the underlying problem or problems in early myoclonic encephalopathy, Aicardi (1990) has emphasized the circumstantial evidence that at least some of the cases may have been secondary to autosomal recessive inheritance.

Clinical findings

In all but two of the 30 cases, the onset of the myoclonias was in the neonatal period and in all 30 the condition was established by the age of 3 months. Males and females were equally represented. Since the seizures started very early in life neurological deterioration was not readily confirmed. Hypotonia was universally present and sometimes accompanied by hypertonicity of the back and neck and later opisthotonic posturing. When measured, head circumferences had been reported to be normal at birth, but failure of head growth with subsequent microcephaly had been noted later. All infants had bilateral pyramidal tract signs and none made any recognizable mental development. Most infants are cortically blind. In one case involvement of the peripheral nerves was recorded.

Investigations

In the absence of clearly defined causes in most cases of myoclonic encephalopathy, it is difficult to outline a plan of investigation. Blood glycine and proprionic acid levels should certainly be measured, since non-ketotic hyperglycinaemia and D-glutaric acidaemia can cause clinically indistinguishable pictures, and raised blood proprionic acid has been described in a further case. On the whole, the clinical picture suggests an underlying biochemical disorder and a full metabolic work-up seems justifiable in the hope that further aetiological agents will be identified.

In most of the patients reviewed, CT scanning was initially normal and in a number it remained normal on repeat examination. In others, progressive cortical and periventricular atrophy was demonstrated (Aicardi 1990).

Electroencephalography. The EEG findings are among the distinctive features of this syndrome. Normal background activity is entirely absent. During both waking and sleeping the record is characterized by complex bursts of spikes, sharp waves and slow waves, irregularly intermingled, lasting 1–5 seconds, and separated by episodes of flattening of the tracing lasting 3–10 seconds. The bursts of activity may occur synchronously or asynchronously over both hemispheres but their individual components are never bilaterally synchronous. Although paroxysmal bursts on the EEG are not synchronous with the jerks of the erratic myoclonus, they may occur in synchrony with massive myoclonus. During partial seizures, spike discharges remain localized to part of one hemisphere and the suppression-burst pattern may persist unchanged. After the age of 3–5 months the pattern may change to atypical hypsarrhythmia or to multifocal paroxysms.

Ohtahara (1984) described a very comparable suppression-burst pattern on the EEGs in his cases of early infantile epileptic encephalopathy. On the basis of the EEG findings it is difficult to regard the syndrome of early myoclonic encephalopathy as different from early epileptic encephalopathy. Further detailed case reports may help to resolve the problem.

Treatment

Conventional antiepileptic drugs, ACTH, cortico-steroids and pyridoxine are ineffective in treatment (Aicardi 1990).

Cognitive outlook

Complete failure to make any developmental progress is reported for all cases. Those who survive infancy do so in a vegetative state.

Prognosis

Of the 29 cases reviewed by Aicardi (1990), 18 had died in early childhood, 12 in the first year of life and 15 before the age of 2. Information on one child was incomplete.

Infantile spasms: West syndrome

Infantile spasms were first described by West (1841) when he observed the condition in his own child. The criteria for the diagnosis of West syndrome have been outlined by Jeavons (1985). Spasms, mental retardation or deterioration and hypsarrhythmia on the EEG constitute typical West syndrome. The presence of atypical cases in which only two of the three components of West syndrome are present, or in which mental retardation and hypsarrhythmia are associated with 'staring seizures' or the Aicardi syndrome, are acknowledged. Jeavons felt that onset after the age of 1 year could not be described as West syndrome.

Incidence

Infantile spasms occur in between 1 in 2400 and 1 in 7800 live births (Lacy & Penry 1976, Riikonen & Donner 1979, Bellman 1983) and are thus a rare form of epilepsy.

Seizure types

The spasms are flexor, extensor or mixed. Flexor spasms may be so brief that, unless the child is under continuous observation, they may not be seen. The neck, trunk and limbs are involved and abduction or adduction of the arms may occur. Extensor spasms involve the neck and trunk with extension, abduction and adduction of the limbs.

Both Kellaway et al (1979) and King et al (1985) have characterized the ictal phenomena in West syndrome by simultaneous EEG and video screening. Kellaway et al (1979) defined a spasm as a brief contraction involving the muscles of the neck, trunk and extremities, bilaterally and symmetrically. The character of the spasm was determined by whether there was maximal involvement of the flexor or extensor muscles. In an analysis of 5042 seizures, 42% were considered mixed, 34% flexor, 22.5% extensor, 0.6% asymmetrical, with the remaining 1% described as 'arrest'. Most of the 24 patients studied had more than one seizure type. King et al (1985) examined the characteristics of 1079 spasms which occurred in 10 patients: while the infants were awake, on average 7.7 spasms were observed per hour; the rate fell to 2.5 spasms per hour if the infants were asleep; 46.6% of the spasms occurred in clusters. King et al described the spasms as myoclonic with or without tonic components and/or arrest of activity. Most commonly the spasms were considered to be myoclonic-tonic (40.3%) or myoclonic alone (36.3%) but, when classified by postural motor phenomena, 41.6% were 'flexor', 16.3% 'extensor', 39% 'mixed' and 3.1% were 'arrest' alone. Simultaneous EEG monitoring showed that the myoclonic contractions were the initial paroxysmal event and that tonic contractions and arrests were associated with suppression of the EEG with or without rhythmic activity.

Recognition of the ictal nature of the attacks is sometimes considerably delayed. The correct diagnosis was made by a primary care doctor in only 12% of the cases reported by Bellman (1983).

Other seizures may occur before infantile spasms. Preceding partial attacks have been reported by Yamamoto et al (1988) and Velez et al (1990). The latter also reported generalized seizures. Early infantile epileptic encephalopathy may also progress to West syndrome (Ohtahara et al 1987).

Differential diagnosis

West syndrome can be differentiated from benign myoclonus of epilepsy on the basis of the EEG (Lombroso & Fejerman 1977). Benign myoclonic epilepsy of infancy and severe myoclonic epilepsy of infancy have distinct and different clinical and EEG patterns. Early myoclonic encephalopathy has a much earlier age of onset and is characterized by suppression burst activity on the EEG.

Aetiology

West syndrome can be primary or cryptogenic; or secondary or symptomatic. With increasing sophistication and thoroughness of investigation, the relative proportion of symptomatic cases has now reached about 70%.

Primary or cryptogenic cases. Primary or cryptogenic cases are those where the cognitive and motor development are normal up to the time of onset of the spasms and in whom there is no evidence of any cerebral disorder.

Secondary/symptomatic cases. Early abnormal development with cognitive and motor retardation or neurological abnormality prior to the onset of spasms are necessary for inclusion in the secondary or symptomatic group. Infantile spasms are now generally recognized as possible symptoms of a wide variety of conditions which have as their common property an ability to cause gross generalized disturbance of cerebral function. The precipitating factors can be divided into prenatal, perinatal or postnatal.

Of the prenatal causes, tuberous sclerosis and other congenital defects are those most commonly identified. Jellinger (1987) found on pathological examination that just over 50% of fatal cases had embryo-fetal lesions, and that two-thirds of these were malformations. Ludwig (1987) and Chugani et al (1990), by radiological and other imaging techniques, have shown that structural abnormalities, some of which are prenatal, are common in infantile spasms. Aicardi's syndrome (absence of the corpus callosum, choroidoretinitis, infantile spasms, female sex, severe retardation)

is but one example of a congenital malformation associated with infantile spasms. Others are immature dendritic development (Huttenlocher 1974), hydranencephaly (Neville 1972) and Down syndrome (Bellman 1983, Pollack et al 1978). Prenatally, i.e. genetically determined, metabolic and degenerative disorders can underlie infantile spasms (Jellinger 1987). Leucodystrophies, Leigh's disease, Alper's disease, phenylketonuria, abnormalities of glycine metabolism, and histidinaemia, and a single patient with hyperornithinaemia, hyperammonaemia and homocitrillinuria have been reported. In addition, Jellinger (1987) commented on cases in which infantile spasms had been symptomatic of Krabbe disease, GM1 and GM2 gangliosidoses and Lafora body disease.

Clearly, in the investigation of infantile spasms, if no definitive cerebral structural abnormality can be defined, a full metabolic work-up is indicated. Prenatal infections may also be associated with the development of infantile spasms. Publications on congenital cytomegalovirus, toxoplasmosis and syphilis are cited by Lacy & Penry (1976).

In Bellman's series (1983) and the review of previous literature by Lacy & Penry (1976) adverse perinatal events were the most commonly identified predisposing factors. Where autopsies have been performed only 30% of cases are attributed to peri- and postnatal lesions alone, and a further 10% to embryofetal and peri- and postnatal abnormalities (Jellinger 1987). Of the perinatal factors, hypoxia or anoxia was most frequently reported. Difficult deliveries, intracranial haemorrhage, hypoglycaemia, severe jaundice and septicaemia were also noted to be of aetiological importance.

Truly postnatal events rarely cause infantile spasms. However, both Bellman (1983) and Lacy & Penry (1976) record West syndrome after bacterial meningitis or viral meningitis or encephalitis. These infections may be precipitating rather than causative events.

Contrary to earlier suggestions there appears to be no causal relationship between immunization or vaccination procedures and the development of West syndrome (Melchior 1977, Bellman 1983).

Pathophysiological considerations

The pathological findings in 214 patients reported

in previous publications were reviewed by Jellinger (1987). He divided them into:

1. Embryofetal lesions
   a. Malformations
   b. Metabolic diseases
2. Peri-postnatal lesions
3. Embryofetal plus peri-postnatal lesions
4. Negative findings
5. Acute lesions or unknown.

Of the cerebral malformations, which account for one-third of all autopsy cases, lissencephaly (agyria-pachygyria) is the commonest, but lesser degrees of abnormality of neuronal migration, including heterotopias and minor cortical dysplasias (Meencke & Gerhard 1985), rare malformations of the midline structures and phacomatoses are also found. Leukodystrophies of the Pelizaeus–Merzbacher type, Krabbe disease, metachromatic leukodystrophy, Van Bogaert–Bertrand–Canavan disease, gangliosidoses, Leigh's disease, mitochondrial cytopathies and amino acid disorders, particularly poorly-controlled phenylketonuria, are amongst the metabolic disorders for which pathological specimens were available.

The peri- and postnatal lesions varied in severity from multicystic encephalopathy with bilateral cavitation and sclerosis of the hemispheric white matter and basal ganglia through hemiatrophy; unilateral or bilateral lobular sclerosis; pseudoporencephalic cysts to ulegyrias which particularly affected the frontal, parietal and occipital lobes (Jellinger 1987). In some cases the lesions were relatively localized and consisted of cysts or scars in the periventricular white matter. Only a few cases showed localized gyral shrinkage.

Combined embryofetal and peri-postnatal lesions are probably under reported (Jellinger 1987). In the series of Meencke & Gerhard (1985) they were found in 42% of the autopsied cases. Infantile spasms secondary to meningitis or meningoencephalitis account for only a small proportion of infants who come to autopsy.

With such a diversity of gross pathological findings it is difficult to postulate the physiological consequences which produce the clinical and EEG characteristics of West syndrome. Huttenlocher (1974) has described marked sparsity of dendritic arborization in the neocortex

of five patients with mental retardation and myoclonic seizures. The relevance of this finding is discussed in some detail by Lacy & Penry (1976). However, using the criteria of Jeavons (1985), at the most only two of the five cases described by Huttenlocher (1974) can be diagnosed as having West syndrome. Elevated levels of excitatory amino acids have been found, but only in symptomatic patients, and cannot be related to or considered a direct cause of infantile spasms (Spink et al 1988).

Clinical features

The peak age of onset is between 4 and 7 months. Males are over-represented. Signs of neurological dysfunction in addition to spasms are common in West syndrome. Microcephaly, various types of cerebral palsy and visual inattention or blindness were reported in more than 50% of the case reports reviewed by Jeavons & Bower (1964). In other publications, despite very full accounts of the nature and frequency of the spasms, there is little to suggest that a thorough search has been made for clues to the underling aetiology. In particular, the skin should be examined both by naked eye and under a Wood's lamp for the ash-leaf-shaped patches of depigmentation most commonly seen on the back of the trunk and legs which would suggest tuberous sclerosis, a condition found in one in 10 of 241 patients with infantile spasms (Riikonen & Simell 1990). The shape of the skull may be such as to suggest an underlying malformation, e.g. porencephalic cyst. Stigmata of metabolic disease, such as failure to thrive, vomiting, skin rashes and unusual-smelling urine should also be sought. Infantile spasms only rarely are likely to be secondary to an intracranial storage disorder, but the size of the liver and spleen should be checked. When the spasms are symptomatic of a mitochondrial cytopathy the infants are extremely hypotonic (Egger et al 1984). Mental retardation is present at the onset in about 95% of cases (Jeavons 1985).

Investigations

Establishment of the aetiology is particularly important from the genetic point of view. Infantile spasms may be symptomatic of any condition which causes a gross generalized cerebral disturbance. So in the absence of a very convincing history of perinatal hypoxia, of definite signs on the CT scan of tuberous sclerosis, or of recognizable abnormalities such as Down syndrome, or the Miller-Dieker syndrome, a full work-up for possible inherited metabolic disease should be undertaken. Screening for disorders of amino acids, urea, carbohydrate and catecholamine metabolism is particularly important. In addition, the serum titres for cytomegalovirus and toxoplasmosis should be measured.

A CT head scan is mandatory in all infants who have West syndrome. Spasms can present as the first sign of tuberous sclerosis and parents will wish to know as soon as possible whether or not they are carriers of this dominantly inherited condition. Other intracranial pathology of aetiologic or genetic importance might also be seen on a CT scan. Magnetic resonance imaging (MRI) is likely to be a more sensitive indicator of prenatal cerebral abnormality than CT, since heterotopic gray matter can be seen clearly (Wagner 1990). As yet no specific study of MRI in infantile spasms has been reported. Positron emission tomography (PET) can demonstrate lesions not visible on CT or MRI (Chugani et al 1990).

Electroencephalography. Hypsarrhythmia, the EEG pattern typically found in infantile spasms, is a grossly chaotic mixture of very high amplitude (more than 200 µV) slow waves at frequencies of 1–7 cycles/second with sharp waves and spikes which vary in amplitude, morphology, duration and site. Modified hypsarrhythmia has a more organized appearance with some bilaterally synchronous discharges. During actual seizures Kellaway et al (1979) identified 11 different patterns. A total of 5042 seizures were monitored: high-voltage frontal-dominant, generalized slow wave transients were followed by voltage attenuation in 38% of attacks; generalized sharp and slow wave complexes in 17.4%; generalized sharp and slow wave discharges followed by attentuation in 13.2%; attentuation only in 11.9%; generalized slow wave transients only in 10.9%; attentuation with superimposed fast activity in 6.9% of spasms; and four various other combinations of fast activity, attentuation and slow waves in less than 1%

of attacks. The significance of these various EEG changes is not entirely obvious, since a close correlation between the EEG and the clinical features of the spasm was not demonstrated.

Hrachovy et al (1984) reviewed 290 24-hour polygraphic records of 64 patients with infantile spasms and concluded that features seen in patients in which hypsarrhythmia was recorded depended on the duration of the recording, the clinical state of the patient and the presence of structural cerebral abnormalities. Considerable variations in the records occurred from time to time in the same infants. Hrachovy et al (1984) identified the following variations on the typical hypsarrhythmia pattern: hypsarrhythmia with increased interhemispheric synchronization; asymmetrical hypsarrhythmia; hypsarrhythmia with episodes of attenuation; and hypsarrhythmia comprising primarily high-voltage slow activity with little sharp wave or spike activity. During sleep, particularly REM sleep, there was marked reduction in and sometimes total disappearance of the hypsarrhythmia pattern. There is no discussion in Hrachovy et al's paper of the possible clinical significance of the EEG findings.

The delta activity in EEGs of patients with infantile spasms has been examined in detail by Parmeggiani et al (1990). Diffuse slow activity appeared mainly in the cryptogenic cases, whereas focal slow activity seemed related to brain lesions and was found in the groups with prenatal abnormalities and cortical tubers in tuberous sclerosis. The diffuse component was considered to be a stereotyped neurophysiological phenomenon which was independent of brain lesions, sex or age.

Treatment

Infantile spasms do not respond to barbiturates, phenytoin or carbamazepine. Variable success is achieved with ACTH (adrenocorticotrophin) or steroids, sodium valproate or benzodiazepines. Vigabatrin has been spectacularly successful in some cases. Immunoglobulins, pyridoxal phosphate, tetrabenazine, methysergide and barbiturate coma have also been tried. Surgery to lesions identified by PET scanning can be successful (Chugani et al 1990).

ACTH and steroids. Corticotrophin was first

used in the treatment of infantile spasms by Sorel & Dusaucy-Bauloye (1950). The success reported by these workers encouraged others to study treatment with oral steroids (Jeavons & Bower 1964). Early reports on the successful control of seizures with subsequent good mental development have not been universally confirmed by subsequent studies. Nevertheless, ACTH or oral steroids retain an important place in the treatment of infantile spasms.

The possible modes of action of ACTH and steroids are comprehensively reviewed by Riikonen (1987). Although Lerman & Kivity (1982) advocated high doses of ACTH (80–100 IU/day), until the seizures come under control, Riikonen (1982) found that daily doses of ACTH of 120–160 IU/day were no more effective than 20–40 IU/day. In a very small number of patients, Hrachovy et al (1980) found that their patients did as well on ACTH 20 IU/day as on 30–40 IU/day. All authors agree that ACTH should be given as a course, and if necessary, the course repeated, rather than as a continued long-term medication. There are strong arguments against treating patients with obvious developmental delay or severe neurological abnormalities prior to the onset of infantile spasms with ACTH or steroids, particularly if the spasms have been preceded by other seizures (Velez et al 1990).

The long-term outlook in these patients is very poor, even if their spasms are controlled, and the side-effects of steroid therapy can be dangerous. On the other hand, there is good evidence that, where spasms occur on a background of neurodevelopmental normality, rapid control of the seizures by steroids/ACTH is associated with an improved outcome (Lerman & Kivity 1982, Riikonen 1982, Jeavons 1985). In those patients who do not have obvious prior neurodevelopmental abnormalities either ACTH 20–40 IU/day or prednisolone 2–3 mg kg/day, with reduction in dosage over a period of 3 months is suggested. Snead (1990a) has suggested that if control is achieved and relapse occurs, return to the previous effective dosage is indicated. Some studies have found that prednisolone may not be as effective as ACTH in the control of the seizures (Kellaway et al 1983).

Sodium valproate. Jeavons (1985) has stated that valproate may reduce the frequency of infantile spasms. A study in which valproate was used in increasing dosage up to 100 mg.kg/day^2 reported control in half the patients, but muscle hypotonia, lethargy and vomiting were commonly present and thrombocytopenia was found in one-third of cases (Siemes et al 1988).

Benzodiazepines. Both clonazepam and nitrazepam can be effective in the control of infantile spasms. However, tolerance usually develops rapidly. Schmidt (1983a) reported that 22% of children with infantile spasms became seizure-free on clonazepam. An initial dose of clonazepam 0.01–0.03 mg.kg/day^2 is suggested, with the subsequent dosage tailored to the individual patient's needs. Rather more than 50% of children with infantile spasms are reported to have responded to nitrazepam (Schmidt 1983a). The dose suggested is initially 0.5 or 1 mg.kg/day^2, with adjustment to the seizure control.

Vigabatrin. Vigabatrin 50–100 mg/kg daily has been given to 42 children with infantile spasms for 4–24 months (Chiron et al 1990). A greater than 50% reduction in spasms was obtained in 30 patients and complete suppression was achieved from the onset of vigabatrin in 16. The effect was particularly striking in symptomatic cases, especially when tuberous sclerosis was the underlying cause. Control tended to be transient in cryptogenic and sustained in symptomatic patients.

Other treatment. When doses of intravenous non-treated immunoglobulin 100–200 mg/kg were given at 2–3-weekly intervals to six patients with cryptogenic and five with symptomatic infantile spasms, all those with cryptogenic and one with symptomatic attacks responded (Ariizumi et al 1987). A small percentage of those treated with pyridoxal phosphate 30–400 mg/day (Ohtsuka et al 1987) or 0.2–0.4 g/kg (Blennow & Starck 1986) will respond. Neither tetrabenazine (Hrachovy et al 1988) nor methysergide and alpha-methylparatyrosine (Hrachovy et al 1989) alter the frequency of infantile spasms. Attempts to cure infantile spasms with barbiturate anaesthesia have also failed (Riikonen et al 1988).

Surgery. Unilateral hypometabolism involving the parieto-occipito-temporal region was found using PET scanning in five of 13 infants (Chugani et al 1990). Guided by intraoperative electro-corticography, four of the five were seizure-free following surgical removal of foci. Follow-up was between 4 and 20 months at the time of reporting. In centres where sophisticated investigative and operative techniques are available surgery could be an option for those with clearly localized lesions.

Prognosis

The long-term outlook is dependent on the underlying condition. When taken as a whole, without regard to aetiology, at most 20% of patients will make a complete recovery (Bellman 1983). Death occurs within 7–12 years in a further 20% (Friedman & Pampiglione 1971). Factors associated with a more favourable outcome than usual are age at onset of 6 months or more, 'primary' aetiology and short duration of spasms (Bellman 1983); or normal development before the onset of spasms (Riikonen 1982). In infants seen very soon after the onset of spasms who are treated immediately with ACTH and whose response is more or less immediate, the likelihood of a good outcome is much greater than for those with preceding neurological abnormality whose spasms have been present for many months prior to treatment.

A poor outcome is predictable if there is developmental slowness before the onset of spasms, the attacks last over a long time period, or the Lennox–Gastaut syndrome supervenes (Riikonen 1982).

Seizures. Up to 64% of survivors have persisting epilepsy. Where seizures remit, 74% of patients are seizure-free by age 5 years (Riikonen 1982). If epilepsy persists partial attacks, often with secondary generalization, are the most common, but myoclonic-astatic seizures can supervene, and the Lennox–Gastaut syndrome follows in somewhat less than 25% of cases (Riikonen 1982).

Neurological handicap. One-third to one-half of children who have had infantile spasms continue to have physical handicaps. Persisting neurological abnormality is not necessarily related to continued seizures. It can be predicted in the presence of delayed development before the onset of spasms, radiological abnormality of the brain, symptomatic aetiology, perinatal asphyxia, low birth weight, neonatal seizures and female sex. Hemiplegia, diplegia or quadriplegia have been reported.

Mental development. Up to 90% of survivors are retarded (Friedman & Pampiglione 1971, Riikonen 1982). Factors predictive of mental retardation and/or poor educability are delayed development before infantile spasms started, neurological handicap, radiological abnormality of the brain, pre- and perinatal abnormalities, evolution to other types of seizures, relapse of seizures and seizures of other sorts before the onset of spasms.

Social handicaps. Many of the survivors have severe behaviour difficulties as well as continuing seizures and physical disabilities. Twenty of 100 patients whose fates were examined after 15 years were found to have made a good recovery from their seizures, but were overactive, clumsy, had temper tantrums, stammered and were echolalic (Thornton & Pampiglione 1979). Aggressive and destructive behaviour, pica, head-banging, gaze-avoidance and excessive hand regard were additional problems.

Benign myoclonic epilepsy in infants

The syndrome of benign myoclonic epilepsy in infants has been characterized by Dravet et al (1985a). It can be distinguished from the other myoclonic epilepsies of infancy by the normality of the interictal neurological examination and EEG and the readiness with which the seizures respond to treatment.

Incidence

The syndrome was first recognized in 1981 and seems to be very uncommon. The incidence was only 7% in a group of 142 patients with various types of myoclonic epilepsy (Dravet et al 1982).

Seizure types

The seizures are brief, generalized and myoclonic. Initially they may be barely noticeable, but later they may become more intense and, if they are still present when the child is able to stand, they may cause loss of balance. The myoclonus involves the axis of the body and the limbs; the head drops suddenly onto the trunk and there is an upwards-outwards movement of the arms accompanied by flexion of the legs; the eyes may roll up. The attacks usually last from 1–3 seconds but may persist for as long as 10 seconds. If repeated jerks occur there may be reduction in alertness but loss of consciousness never occurs. These myoclonic seizures can present at any time of day but are never observed during deep sleep.

Although no other seizure type was observed coincidentally with the myoclonus, two of the reported children had had febrile seizures prior to the onset of the myoclonic epilepsy (Dravet et al 1985a).

Differential diagnosis

Benign myoclonic epilepsy in infants can be distinguished from benign myoclonus of early infancy by the absence of EEG changes in the latter condition (Lombroso & Fejerman 1977). Other myoclonic epilepsies are differentiated by the presence of additional seizure types, more severely abnormal EEGs (particularly during interictal recording), developmental standstill or regression, and their poor response to antiepileptic drug therapy.

Aetiology

Family histories are often positive for other types of seizure disorder and suggest that benign myoclonic epilepsy in infants is a very early expression of primary generalized epilepsy.

Clinical features

The age of onset is between 6 months and 2 years and there is a male preponderance. Clinical examination is normal.

Investigations

In one case who had a pneumoencephalograph and two children who had CT scans the findings were normal.

Electroencephalography. Video and polygraphic recordings have enabled Dravet et al (1985a)

to characterize the attacks in detail. The clinically observed myoclonic seizures were synchronous with a discharge on the EEG of generalized spike-waves or polyspike-waves occurring at 3 cycles/second and of the same duration as a seizure. Between seizures the EEGs were normal for age. In some cases, photic stimulation provoked spike-waves or polyspike-waves but this was always accompanied by myoclonus. Drowsiness and light sleep activated generalized spike-waves but these discharges tended to disappear during slow wave sleep.

Treatment

The treatment of choice is sodium valproate. Barbiturates and benzodiazepines are considered unsuitable.

Prognosis

The myoclonic seizures may persist if left untreated and may be replaced by generalized tonic-clonic seizures in later childhood or at puberty. Both types of seizure respond readily to sodium valproate. The EEG changes resolve as the clinical seizures disappear.

Four of the seven cases of Dravet et al (1985a) later required special education because of behaviour disturbances or learning problems. These difficulties were attributed to delay in instituting appropriate treatment for the myoclonic seizures, to the early age of their onset and to their frequency, but they leave a question mark over whether this epileptic syndrome is completely benign.

Severe myoclonic epilepsy in infancy

Severe myoclonic epilepsy in infancy has been characterized by Dalla Bernardina et al (1982), Dravet et al (1985b) and Hurst (1987). As an entity it has been described in the literature in only 91 cases.

Incidence

The overall incidence is unknown. Only one case was found in a cohort of 40 000 children (Hurst

1990). The 42 patients described by Dravet et al (1982) represented 29.5% of a group of 142 children with various types of myoclonic epilepsy in childhood.

Seizure types

The first seizure for which parents seek advice is almost invariably clonic. Generalized clonic attacks occurred in seven-eighths of cases; in the remainder the attacks were unilateral (Dravet et al 1982). In at least half the children, the initial seizure was of more than 15 minutes duration and in three-fifths a fever appeared to precipitate the attack. Short or long myoclonic attacks had been observed before the initial clonic seizures by a small proportion of parents. Frequent recurrences of clonic attacks, usually with fever, were observed before the onset, between 1 and 4 years of age, of generalized myoclonic seizures. The myoclonic seizures are described as lacking any specific characteristics, recurring several times a day, but not occurring in bouts, though they may be very frequent. Severe seizures may cause the child to fall but milder ones may be difficult to discern unless the child is watched during an activity requiring precise movement. Sometimes the myoclonic jerks may be initiated by varying the ambient light intensity. Coincidentally with the appearance of the myoclonic jerks, partial seizures with either autonomic or atonic components and automatisms were observed in one-third of the patients of Dravet et al (1985b). In some children obtunded states were associated with myoclonias. In the seven cases of Hurst (1987) absences occurred in six, myoclonias in six, complex partial seizures in four, tonic-clonic attacks in two and atonic seizures in two.

Differential diagnosis

Severe myoclonic epilepsy of infancy is differentiated from the other myoclonias in this age group by the previous history of clonic seizures with fever, the normality of children at the onset and the absence of a hypsarrhythmic pattern on the EEG. It is not possible to differentiate this condition from recurrent febrile convulsions until the myoclonic seizures begin.

Aetiology

The aetiology is unknown. A family history of febrile convulsions and/or of epilepsy is present in a quarter of the cases. Dravet et al (1985b) feel that in the absence of known aetiological factors, and in the presence of a high percentage of positive family histories, the initial ictal symptomatology and the photosensitivity, a serious form of primary generalized epilepsy is likely. Abnormalities of neuronal migration have been reported in a single pathological study (Renier & Renkawek 1990).

Clinical features

A slightly higher proportion of males has been noted. In all patients the onset of seizures was in the first year of life with the first convulsion occurring at a mean age of about 6 months. Normal development is universal before the initial seizure. With the appearance of the myoclonic seizures, slowing of language acquisition, ataxia, hyperreflexia and interictal fragmentary and segmental myoclonus appear.

Pathophysiological features

In considering that severe myoclonic epilepsy in infancy was a serious form of primary generalized epilepsy, Dravet et al (1985b) hypothesized that the later changes in neurological characteristics could be explained either by the occurrence of repeated prolonged convulsions with fever or the existence of unfavourable genetic factors which might have caused aggravation of a primary epilepsy.

The findings of Renier & Renkawek (1990) suggest that prenatal mid-gestational factors may be important. Although the brain of a child who died suddenly and unexpectedly was macroscopically normal, there was dysgenesis in the cerebellar vermis; and in the frontal and temporal cortices the laminar stratification was irregular. Some groups of nerve cells were found protruding into the superficial subpial region. It was concluded that the microscopic lesions, particularly in the outer cortical layers, could explain the lack of inhibition, and thus myoclonus. Such lesions do not necessarily exclude the concept that severe myoclonic epilepsy in infancy could be a particularly unfavourable form of primary epilepsy since comparable lesions have been reported in association with absences and other primary generalized seizures (Meencke & Janz 1984).

Investigations

A minority of cases have shown dilatation of the cisterna magna on CT scan (Dravet et al 1985b). Otherwise, with the exception of the EEG, investigation appears to have been unrewarding.

Electroencephalography. Comprehensive details of the EEG findings in this syndrome are given by Dravet et al (1985b). The initial records were normal. During the second year paroxysms of generalized spike-waves or polyspike-waves either in isolation or in brief bursts appeared. These eventually became to some extent lateralized, were influenced by intermittent photic stimulation and increased by drowsiness or slow-wave sleep. Photosensitivity was noted before the age of 2 years in up to one-third of patients. In the long term, the EEGs showed considerable variability though spikes, spike-waves and polyspike-waves, usually localized rather than generalized, persisted.

Treatment

Dravet et al (1985b) reported that the seizures are resistant to all forms of treatment but the therapeutic agents which have been given are not enumerated. Hurst (1987) has suggested that response to valproate is better than that to any other antiepileptic drug, but valproate rarely controls all seizures.

Prognosis

Seizures. The time when seizures are particularly frequent is very variable from patient to patient. Attacks are a continuing problem up to the age of 11 or 12 years in some patients. A reduction in seizure frequency is noted initially during the day with a tendency for nocturnal clonic or tonic-clonic attacks to persist. Coincidentally, the myoclonic jerks appear as very atypical absence seizures with minor disturbances in consciousness, random myoclonus and a tendency to

hypertonia. With these attacks the child may be obtunded and the term 'minor motor status' is applicable.

Neurological handicaps. Dravet et al (1985b) felt that they had not studied neurological states of their patients long enough to draw firm conclusions about the long-term motor deficits but noted adults with severe cerebellar and pyramidal syndromes and myoclonus who had histories suggestive of severe myoclonic epilepsy in infancy.

Cognitive aspects. Death in early childhood occurred in approximately one-sixth of the cases of Dravet et al (1985b). All the surviving children required special education and, where the intelligence had been measured, two-thirds were severely subnormal.

Behavioural problems. Many of the children with this syndrome are very overactive. Their extreme sensitivity to photic stimuli makes them drawn to television screens and other sources of intermittent light, with subsequent abstraction, myoclonic jerking and sometimes tonic-clonic seizures. Constant supervision is usually necessary.

Myoclonic-astatic epilepsy

This epileptic syndrome is characterized by the presence of myoclonic and astatic seizures which may occur either independently or in combination.

Incidence

Myclonic-astatic epilepsy represents 1–2% of all epilepsies in children up to the age of 9 years (Doose 1985).

Differential diagnosis

The most frequent source of confusion is with the Lennox–Gastaut syndrome. Table 4.1 lists the distinguishing features.

Seizure types

All children have myoclonic, astatic or myoclonic-astatic seizures. In addition, absences with myoclonic jerks and irregular myoclonias of the face occur in 62%; febrile convulsions in 28%; generalized tonic-clonic seizures in 75% (in 34% at the

Table 4.1 Distinguishing features of myoclonic-astatic epilepsy and Lennox–Gastaut syndrome

Distinguishing features	Myoclonic-astatic epilepsy (Doose 1985)	Lennox–Gastaut syndrome (Beaumanoir 1985a)
Previous neurological history	Normal in 88%	Prior 'enephalopathy'
Inheritance		No familial cases
Family history of seizure disorder	37%	2.5 to 40%
Seizure types		
Classification	1° generalized	2° generalized
Myoclonic	+	±
Astatic	+	+
Myoclonic: astatic	+	–
Absence with myoclonias and/or atonia	+	–
Generalized tonic-clonic	+	+
Status	36%	common with stupor
Axial tonic	Late only	+
Atypical absence	–	+
Partial	–	+
EEG		
Background abnormal	Not initially	+
Irregular fast spike-waves and polyspike-waves	+	–
2–3 Hz spike-waves	+ in status	+ diffuse
Focal abnormalities	rare	Multifocal +

onset); and status of minor seizures in 36%. Tonic seizures may be present in this syndrome in 30% of cases. A status of minor seizures (minor motor status) produces apathy, stupor and, at worst, an apparent dementia. Irregular twitching of the facial muscles, drooling, aphasia which may or may not be interrupted by more obvious visible, or only palpable, myoclonic jerking may be clinically so non-specific to the uninitiated as to be mistaken for a behaviour disorder. In a single case, myoclonic astatic epilepsy is reported to have followed neonatal sleep myoclonus (Nolte 1989). When associated nocturnal focal or generalized seizures have been prominent, the possibility of a variant of the syndrome has been considered (Deonna et al 1986a).

Aetiology

Myoclonic-astatic seizures usually start on a background of normal neuropsychological development, but Doose (1985) was able to identify a history of 'definite higher risk factors' or developmental retardation in 16% of 117 children with this condition. Otherwise Doose felt that the epilepsy could be classified as primary and that genetic predisposition was the most important aetiological factor. He postulated a polygenic type of inheritance.

Pathophysiological aspects

In the absence of a pathologically-identified aetiology, the physiological consequences are difficult to define. At 2–5 years the peak periods of all aspects of cerebral development have passed, but both organization and myelination are still in progress. This may explain the loss of intellectual skills which occurs in some patients.

Clinical features

The maximal age at onset of the seizures is between 2 and 5 years and boys are more often affected than girls. The children are usually neurologically normal at the onset of the myoclonic-astatic seizures, but in two-thirds of the cases of Doose (1985) the initial episode was either a febrile or an afebrile generalized tonic-clonic seizure.

There is a family history of seizure disorders, but not necessarily of myoclonic-astatic epilepsy, in just over one-third of the patients.

Investigations

The only investigation for which information is available is electroencephalography.

Electroencephalography. Doose (1985) has

given details of the EEGs to be expected as myoclonic-astatic epilepsy evolves. Initially, particularly in those cases where the first seizures are either febrile or afebrile tonic-clonic seizures, monomorphic theta rhythms with parietal accentuation and occipital 4 Hz rhythms blocked by eye opening are the usual EEG findings. Irregular spike-wave activity may also be found exclusively during sleep. Later, bilateral synchronous irregular spikes and waves appear. These may be particularly prominent anteriorly. The EEGs in children whose seizures are mostly myoclonic typically show short paroxysms of irregular spike-waves and polyspikes. In those whose attacks are astatic or myoclonic-astatic the findings are of 2–3 Hz spike-waves or spike-wave variants on a background of 4–7 Hz rhythms or, in the more severe cases, generalized slow activity. Photosensitivity is usual between the ages of 5 and 15 years and spike-waves are very common during sleep. Occasional records show lateralization of the abnormalities but these are not characteristic of this syndrome.

Treatment

No controlled trial of any individual antiepileptic drug has been performed. Valproate is more likely to be helpful in the control of seizures than any other antiepileptic medication.

Prognosis

The prognosis is to some extent related to seizure frequency. However, the possibility that difficulty with control of the seizures might be indicative of a more serious underlying condition cannot be ignored. The following suggest a poor outcome:

1. Frequent tonic-clonic seizures
2. Nocturnal tonic seizures
3. Minor motor status
4. Onset with tonic-clonic seizures before the age of 2 years
5. Continuance of 4–7 Hz rhythms and spike and wave during therapy
6. Failure of development of a stable occipital alpha rhythm.

Seizures. Spontaneous remissions occasionally

occur, but 50% of those who have had myoclonic-astatic epilepsy continue to have seizures. In these cases generalized tonic-clonic and nocturnal tonic seizures are usual.

Neurological handicaps. The presence of continuing neurological disorders is strongly related to unremitting epilepsy. Mild cerebellar ataxia, dysfunction of gross motor ability and clumsiness are reported.

Cognitive aspects. In the cases with an unfavourable prognosis speech disorders become evident and dementia supervenes. A total of 17% of children with myoclonic-astatic epilepsy have developmental retardation.

Behaviour problems. These are related to developmental slowness and dementia. No specific associations with this type of epilepsy have been reported.

Epilepsy with myoclonic absences

This syndrome is characterized by frequent seizures in which clonic jerks are associated with 3 Hz spike-waves on the EEG (Tassinari & Bureau 1985).

Incidence

Myoclonic absences are rare. Only 0.5–1% of a selected population of children with epilepsy had this seizure type (Tassinari & Bureau 1985).

Seizure types

The onset and offset of myoclonic absences are abrupt. Seizures occur frequently throughout the day and are of 10–60 seconds in duration. Consciousness may not be completely lost, though it is thought to be impaired in most instances. The motor component consists of rhythmic jerking of the shoulders, head and arms, and staggering; falls are unusual; arrest or alteration in the respiratory pattern may be observed and some patients are incontinent during the attacks. A tonic contraction may follow the initial myoclonias. Some patients also have generalized tonic-clonic seizures. Hyperventilation will precipitate attacks in about two-thirds of the cases and about half the children are photosensitive. Attacks may also be precipitated by wakening from sleep.

Differential diagnosis

Myoclonic absences should be distinguished from other absences by the prominence of the motor symptomatology. In other syndromes with myoclonias the spike-wave discharges on EEG tend to be of 2 Hz rather than 3 Hz frequency.

Aetiology

Genetic factors appear important. A family history of epilepsy is present in 25% of cases; otherwise, nothing is known of the aetiology. Myoclonic absences may be intermediary between primary generalized and secondary generalized epilepsies.

Clinical findings

Males have epilepsy with myoclonic absences more commonly than females. The attacks may commence at almost any age during childhood. In about half the cases mental retardation precedes the onset of seizures.

Investigation

Electroencephalography. During seizures, the EEG shows rhythmic 3 Hz spike-waves which are bilateral, synchronous and symmetrical. The spike onset of the spike-wave discharge is strictly and constantly related to the myoclonic jerk. Photosensitivity can be demonstrated in about half of the children and attacks are provoked by hyperventilation in about two-thirds.

Treatment

A combination of sodium valproate and ethosuximide may be more likely to control the seizures than other forms of treatment. The novel antiepileptic drug lamotrigine has been found effective in a small number of patients who failed to respond to ethosuximide, valproate or clonazepam (Wallace 1990).

Prognosis

Seizures. The seizures remit in some cases but in others they become complicated by the appearance of tonic attacks and atypical absences such as occur in the Lennox–Gastaut syndrome. The EEG then shows slow spike-wave discharges rather than 3 Hz paroxysms.

Neurological handicaps. Gross disturbances do not usually occur, but most of the affected children are mildly ataxic and some have moderate to severe dyspraxia.

Cognitive aspects. Of the children who are intellectually normal at the onset of the myoclonic absences, about half have later loss of cognitive skills. About 75% of this group of patients are finally intellectually impaired.

Behaviour problems. No specific type of behaviour has been related to myoclonic absences.

Progressive myoclonic epilepsy

Progressive myoclonic epilepsy may be symptomatic of recognizable degenerative disorders of the brain or may occur without a definable underlying cause. The progressive myoclonic epilepsy syndrome is characterized clinically by the presence of:

1. Generalized myoclonus and arrhythmic, asynchronous and asymmetrical, partial or segmental myoclonus
2. Multiple seizure types, usually including generalized tonic-clonic, myoclonic and tonic seizures
3. Progressive mental deterioration with ultimate dementia
4. The development of cerebellar, pyramidal and finally extrapyramidal signs (Roger 1985).

Progressive myoclonic epilepsy associated with identifiable underlying conditions

On reviewing the seizures which occur as symptoms of inborn errors of metabolism Aicardi (1985) emphasized that a prominent myoclonic component in a seizure disorder should always be an alerting sign for an underlying metabolic disorder. The following conditions are regularly complicated by myoclonic seizures (Aicardi 1985, Berkovic & Anderman 1986, Aukett et al 1988):

1. Non-ketotic hyperglycinaemia
2. Early infantile ceroid lipofuscinosis (Santavuori–Hagberg–Haltia)

3. Tay–Sachs and Sandhoff diseases
4. Phenylketonuria variant (biopterin deficiency)
5. Late infantile and juvenile ceroid lipofuscinosis
6. Sialosidoses (mucolipidosis 1, cherry red spot with myoclonus syndrome)
7. Juvenile Gaucher's disease
8. Myoclonus epilepsy with ragged red fibres (mitochondrial myopathy)
9. Sub-acute sclerosing panencephalitis
10. GM$_1$ gangliosidosis
11. Niemann–Pick disease
12. Alpers' disease
13. Molybdenum co-factor deficiency.

In all these disorders myoclonic seizures are associated with neurological and intellectual deterioration and only in biopterin deficiency is the underlying problem amenable to correction. Non-ketotic hyperglycinaemia is of particular interest since glycine has been shown to enhance N-methyl-D-aspartate-mediated responses by potentiating synaptic potentials (McDonald & Johnson 1990).

Progressive myoclonic epilepsy with no identified underlying cause

Although myoclonias are not necessarily the seizures which are symptomatic of other metabolic disorders, it is justifiable, and indeed desirable, that a full screen for inborn biochemical disorders and a CT head scan be arranged in all infants and children who have myoclonic epilepsies.

Dyssynergia cerebellaris myoclonica with epilepsy (Ramsey–Hunt syndrome). This term has been used to embrace a rather heterogeneous collection of patients and is not always considered a disease entity (Berkovic & Andermann 1986). Nevertheless, Roger (1985) considers that a definable disorder can be characterized. The features are recessive inheritance with onset between 6 and 20 years and a myoclonic syndrome or epileptic seizures. Typical action and intention myoclonus may be accompanied by partial myoclonus; the seizures are myoclonic, with or without additional tonic-clonic attacks. They tend to occur less often as the condition evolves and usually respond to antiepileptic drugs. An axial cerebellar syndrome is frequent and may be accompanied by other neurological abnormalities. Intellectual deterioration is common. During evolution of this syndrome the action and intention myoclonus becomes gradually more obvious. The EEG shows a normal background activity and well-organized sleep patterns. Spikes, spike-waves and polyspike-waves are precipitated by intermittent photic stimulation. During REM sleep rapid polyspikes localized to the central and vertex regions are characteristic of this condition.

Baltic myoclonus epilepsy. This is an autosomal recessive condition in which seizures commence at about the age of 10 years. Extensive studies have been conducted by Koskiniemi (1990). Photosensitive, occasionally violent, myoclonus occurs particularly on awakening. It is associated with generalized tonic-clonic seizures and, on occasions, with absences. Some learning difficulties may be present, but dementia is not common unless phenytoin is given. The EEGs show light-sensitive, usually synchronous, spike-wave discharges. EEG changes precede the onset of clinical manifestations. In two patients who died, the autopsy has shown marked loss of Purkinje cells of the cerebellum. Inclusion bodies were absent. The patients are made worse by phenytoin and can be greatly improved by sodium valproate.

Lafora body disease. The characteristics of Lafora body disease have been reviewed by Berkovic & Andermann (1986). Complex carbohydrates are stored in the brain and are seen histologically as typical inclusion bodies. The onset is in late childhood or adolescence with tonic-clonic seizures, myoclonus or behavioural changes. Partial seizures with visual symptomatology may also occur. Progressive cognitive impairment, dysarthria and cerebellar ataxia are additional features. Initially the background activity is normal in the EEG, but slowing occurs later. Generalized fast spike-wave discharges activated by photic stimulation become degraded as the condition progresses.

Juvenile myoclonic epilepsy

Myoclonic seizures commence round about

puberty, are particularly common just after wakening, and are often associated with photosensitivity. Infrequent generalized tonic-clonic seizures present in most cases.

Incidence

In a review article, Wolf (1985a) reported juvenile myoclonic epilepsy occurred in between 3.4% and 5.4% of all patients with epilepsy and that, where video-EEG recordings were obtained from adolescents and adults, this condition accounted for 11.9% of all patients studied and 36% of patients with various forms of generalized minor seizures.

Seizure types

The seizures are bilateral, single or repeated, arrhythmic, irregular myoclonic jerks which predominantly affect the arms; sudden falls with the jerks are unusual; consciousness is usually retained. Generalized tonic-clonic seizures are also present in the majority of cases (Asconapé & Penry 1984, Wolf 1985a, Clement & Wallace 1988, Dreifuss 1989). Both seizure types occur almost exclusively on awakening, particularly in the morning. Some patients are aware of precipitation of the seizures by flicker phenomena. Classical absences occur in a minority of patients.

Differential diagnosis

It is important to differentiate juvenile myoclonic epilepsy from other myoclonic syndromes since most others carry a much more serious long-term prognosis. The relatively late age of onset helps to distinguish this condition from both myoclonic-astatic epilepsy and the Lennox–Gastaut syndrome. In myoclonic absences, the jerking is rhythmic and usually symmetrical.

Aetiology

There is a genetic predisposition to this syndrome. The incidence of a positive family history of a seizure disorder has been given as approximately 25% where most of the affected family members had generalized seizure disorders. Recent evidence suggests that the gene for juvenile myoclonic epi-

lepsy is located at chromosome 6p21.3 (Delgado-Escueta et al 1989).

Pathophysiology

On clinical grounds, no particular underlying lesion or previous event appears consistently to predispose to juvenile myoclonic epilepsy. Microdysgenesis has been reported in the cerebrum of one patient (Meencke & Janz 1984). Since intellectual deterioration does not occur it seems likely that the seizures do not have serious pathological consequences.

Clinical findings

Males and females are equally represented in groups of patients with juvenile myoclonic epilepsy. The age at onset of the myoclonic jerks is in the early–mid-teens. In the series of Asconapé & Penry (1984) and Clement & Wallace (1988) myoclonic seizures always preceded any generalized tonic-clonic attacks. Neurological examination and intelligence are normal virtually always (Wolf 1985a, Asconapé & Penry 1984), but Clement & Wallace (1988) found mild dysfunction in two and severe dyspraxia in another of 10 cases. Sleep deprivation, excessive alcohol intake, emotional stress and menstruation may precipitate seizures.

Investigation

Electroencephalography. The background activity is almost always normal. Ictal changes consist of paroxysmal polyspike-slow wave discharges. These are usually bilaterally synchronous and symmetrical but there may be some interhemispheric asymmetry (Asconapé & Penry 1984). Polyspike-wave complexes also occur interictally but these discharges have fewer spikes prior to the slow waves than when myoclonic jerks are observed. Photosensitivity is demonstrable more commonly in this epileptic syndrome than in any other (Wolf & Gooses 1986). A total of 20% patients also have polyspike-wave discharge on eye closure (Wolf 1985a). Asconapé & Penry (1984) reported one patient whose myoclonic seizures were precipitated by loud unexpected noises.

Treatment

Sodium valproate is the treatment of first choice. For those who are photosensitive instruction in the avoidance of flicker phenomena is important.

Prognosis

Seizures. Although the seizures are usually readily responsive to valproate, they tend to recur if treatment is discontinued. It is now recommended that valproate be maintained for life (Dreifuss 1989).

Neurological and intellectual status. Neither new neurological disability nor intellectual handicap is likely to present in the long-term.

Behaviour problems. Immature personality traits have been highlighted by Reintoft et al (1976). Overt behavioural disturbance characterized by rage outbursts, rudeness and rebelliousness, as well as lack of confidence were reported by Clement & Wallace (1988). Thus poor social adjustment seems commoner than expected.

EPILEPSIES WITH PREDOMINANTLY TONIC SEIZURES

Early infantile epileptic encephalopathy

Ohtahara (1984) regards early infantile epileptic encephalopathy (EIEE) as the earliest form of age-dependent epileptic encephalopathy. He and his colleagues have traced the evolution of EIEE to West syndrome and thence to the Lennox–Gastaut syndrome (Ohtahara et al 1987, 1988). Not all authors agree that EIEE is a separate syndrome, since there are many features which are comparable with those of early myoclonic encephalopathy (Aicardi 1990).

Incidence

EIEE is a very rare condition. Fourteen cases are presented in the most recent publication of Ohtahara et al (1988) and a further 11 are described by Clarke et al (1987). The few other publications all refer to very small numbers of patients.

Differential diagnosis

The main differential diagnosis is from early myoclonic encephalopathy. The main reasons for considering EIEE to be a separate entity relate to the seizure types, the absence of a family history of a similar disorder and the frequency with which brain malformation is the aetiology (Aicardi 1990).

Aetiology

In the fourteen cases reported by Ohtahara et al (1988) there were three for whom no cause was found. The other 11 had porencephaly, microcephaly and/or brain atrophy, Aicardi syndrome or diffuse subacute encephalopathy. In contrast, eight of the 11 cases of Clarke et al (1987) were considered idiopathic, with asphyxia, agenesis of the corpus callosum and non-ketotic hyperglycinaemia accounting for the rest. Thus EIEE seems to be symptomatic of a wide variety of conditions, some of which may also be associated with early myoclonic encephalopathy.

Seizure types

Tonic spasms are invariable (Ohtahara et al 1988). Sometimes they occur in a series. Erratic myoclonus is never seen, but massive myoclonias can occur, as can partial seizures (Aicardi 1990).

Pathophysiological aspects

The diversity of underlying pathologies is strongly supportive of the concept that EIEE is an age-related, rather than an aetiology-related, epileptic syndrome. A recent publication on nonketotic hyperglycinaemia has thrown some light on the possible biochemical mechanisms involved (McDonald & Johnson 1990). Experimental evidence suggests that enhanced activation of the N-methyl-D-aspartate receptors, which may lead to neuronal calcium overload and cytotoxicity can be glycine-related. Only a minority of patients with EEIE have nonketotic hyperglycinaemia, but further investigation of the implications of this disorder might lead to a better understanding of the condition as a whole.

Clinical features

EIEE usually commences in the first month of

life with tonic spasms. Rarely the onset may be in the second or third months. In the series of Clarke et al (1987), four of the mothers thought their infants might have had intra-uterine seizures. The infants are all very handicapped and usually very hypotonic. There is severe motor and cognitive delay. The family history is negative in cryptogenic cases.

Investigation

Considering the wide range of possible aetiologies, full investigation for underlying structural and biochemical disorders is important.

Electroencephalography. At the outset, the EEG always shows a suppression-burst pattern which disappears at 3–6 months. As the clinical picture progresses the tracings may later evolve to become hypsarrhythmic, or to show predominantly focal spike disturbances (Ohtahara 1984). Diffuse slow spike-waves may eventually appear if survival is prolonged.

Treatment

Resistance to antiepileptic drug therapy is the rule. After concluding that no drug was particularly helpful, Clarke et al (1987) reported that phenobarbitone might be more effective than any other. There is, as yet, no information on whether newer antiepileptic drugs, such as vigabatrin or lamotrigine, are useful.

Prognosis

The prognosis is always grave. Death occurs in the first year of life in one-third of cases.

Seizures. Progression to West syndrome occurred in 10 of the 14 cases reported by Ohtahara et al (1987). There was further progression to the Lennox–Gastaut syndrome in two of these 10. Daily seizures continued in seven of nine infants who survived more than 3 months (Clarke et al 1987).

Neurological handicap. All infants remain extremely handicapped, with failure to make even the earliest of motor progress.

Cognitive aspects and social awareness. No cognitive progress is made, and the infants remain socially unaware.

The Lennox–Gastaut syndrome

In a paper called 'Clinical correlates of the fast and slow spike-wave electroencephalogram', Lennox & Davis (1950) first drew attention to this clinical syndrome, which was later more clearly defined by Gastaut et al (1966). The cardinal features are the development in children, who are usually neurologically abnormal, of atypical absences, axial tonic seizures and sudden falls (atonic or myoclonic) associated with interictal diffuse slow spike-waves on the waking EEG (Aicardi & Gomes 1988).

Incidence

Since many authors have included under the heading of the Lennox–Gastaut syndrome children with other epileptic syndromes in which myoclonic seizures occur, it is difficult to be sure how many children strictly have this condition. A minimum estimate is that it is present in 3% of childhood seizure disorders.

Differential diagnosis

When it commences in the first 5 years of life any serious seizure disorder particularly with associated myoclonias may be confused with the Lennox–Gastaut syndrome. Features distinguishing this syndrome from myoclonic-astatic epilepsy are summarized in Table 4.1 (p. 118) Beaumanoir (1985a) has noted that both partial and generalized epilepsies, during which deterioration in neurological status and intellect occurs, may be erroneously considered to be the Lennox–Gastaut syndrome.

Aetiology

There is much emphasis on 'encephalopathy' as a feature which precedes or accompanies the onset of this syndrome. The exact nature of this 'encephalopathy' remains to be determined and the impression given is that a generalized cerebral disorder is being referred to as an encephalopathy for lack of a more specific term. Lagenstein et al (1979) found evidence of cortical atrophy in more than 50% of those cases in their series examined by CT scan and prior neurological abnormality was well documented in 60% of their cases. In a review of neuropathological studies, dysplastic lesions were commonly present (Roger & Gambarelli-Dubois 1988), and abnormalities of the inner layers of the cortex were abnormal in a case reported by Renier et al (1988). Generalized hypometabolism of the cerebrum has been reported to be common when PET scanning has been used (Chugani et al 1987, Theodore et al 1987). When patients with neuroradiologically determined abnormalities are not excluded, focal areas of hypometabolism are found in PET scans in about half the patients (Chugani et al 1987). Thus for some patients the presence of focal abnormalities is confirmed.

At a more clinical level, the aetiologies in 265 cases have been reviewed by Ohtahara et al (1988). Cryptogenic cases with or without prior mental defect accounted for 26%, mental defect secondary to recognizable causes preceded 13%, cerebral palsy with or without mental defect was present in 28%, encephalitis had occurred previously in 12.5%, tuberous sclerosis was recognized in 4% and in 8% West syndrome had been diagnosed earlier. Congenital cerebral malformations were present in 7%. The roles of viral infection and possible immune deficiency remain incompletely determined (Eeg-Olofsson 1988). The family history is almost invariably negative.

Seizure types

Tonic seizures are a necessary component of the Lennox–Gastaut syndrome (Beaumanoir 1985a, Tassinari & Ambrosetto 1988). Such seizures may occur during the day or night and can be axial, axorhizomelic or global; they are brief and loss of consciousness is not necessarily present. If nocturnal, they tend to occur during slow-wave sleep, particularly during the latter part of the night.

Most children also have atypical absences which begin and end gradually. During these, loss of consciousness may be incomplete so that some activities can continue even though the child appears abstracted or obtunded. Loss of tone in the face and neck muscles may cause the child to lean forward with the mouth open and myoclonic twitching of the eyelids and mouth may be observed. Massive myoclonic jerks, myoclonic-atonic attacks and/or atonic seizures are much less frequent manifestations of this epileptic syndrome. Tonic-clonic, clonic or partial seizures, symptomatic of the underlying, though non-specific, cerebral disorder may also occur. Episodes of status epilepticus characterized by clouding of consciousness and repeated atonic, or less often myoclonic-atonic, seizures can last for days, weeks or even months, are resistant to therapy and are often recurrent.

Pathophysiological aspects

The reason why some children with prior neurological defects should develop the Lennox–Gastaut syndrome is obscure. Similarly, the progressive loss of intellectual skills remains unexplained. Persistent seizure activity may interfere with the child's attention but this fails to explain the severe intellectual and behavioural problems usual in children who have had this condition over a number of years. The studies using PET scanning are likely to be a useful base for the greater understanding of this syndrome. In particular, Chugani et al (1987) suggested that four predominant subtypes could be identified, each with a distinct metabolic pattern:

1. Unilateral focal hypometabolism
2. Unilateral diffuse hypometabolism
3. Bilateral diffuse hypometabolism
4. Normal.

A review of neuropathological studies has provided information on 30 post-mortem specimens and nine brain biopsies (Roger & Gambarelli-Dubois 1988). In 16 cases there were dysplastic lesions. Of these nine had major dysplasias. The lesions were diffuse in 15, and focal in one case. Where details of the findings were complete 'selective neuronal necrosis' was reported in almost all specimens. Cerebellar lesions were present in 20 cases, in four of whom no other abnormality was found.

Clinical features

The peak age of onset is between 3 and 5 years

with extremes of the first year and the tenth year. The syndrome is more common in males than females. No specific neurological signs are pathognomonic, though neurological abnormality is common and usually precedes the onset of seizures. A family history of some sort of epilepsy is common. However, there is no known familial case of the Lennox–Gastaut syndrome.

Investigations

Investigation by CT scanning will help to indicate underlying structural cerebral abnormalities but atrophic lesions are usually non-specific. In the search for an underlying cause of the 'encephalopathy' it is justifiable to undertake a full metabolic screen, to investigate in detail the immunological state of the child and to search as thoroughly as possible for a viral infection.

Electroencephalography. In brief, the characteristic interictal EEG findings are of diffuse slow (2–3 Hz) spike-waves when awake and bursts of 10 Hz rhythms during sleep (Beaumanoir 1985a, Blume 1988).

During tonic seizures a discharge of bilateral and mainly frontal or vertical rapid rhythms occurs. Such discharges may be preceded by a short period of flattening of the background rhythms or by a brief discharge of slow spike-waves, but there is no postictal depression of activity. When the tonic seizures pass into an automatic stage the rapid rhythms of the tonic phase are followed by diffuse slow spike-waves which corresponds with the automatic phase.

Atypical absences are accompanied by irregular diffuse 2–2.5 Hz spike-and-waves occurring more or less symmetrically from the hemispheres. When myoclonic seizures or atonic seizures occur as part of the Lennox–Gastaut syndrome slow polyspike-and-waves, diffuse spike-waves or rapid rhythms with anterior predominance may be recorded (Beaumanoir 1985a).

The study of sleep patterns could be helpful in delineating subgroups of the Lennox–Gastaut syndrome (Baldy-Moulinier et al 1988). In some patients reduction in sleep spindle activity, rapid eye movement (REM) sleep duration and in eye movements during REM sleep are observed, whereas in others sleep architecture is normal.

Treatment

The seizures are very resistant to therapy: responses to phenytoin, carbamazepine or phenobarbitone are usually totally disappointing. Sodium valproate is sometimes helpful, particularly if used in higher than usual dosage. Benzodiazepines, particularly nitrazepam or clonazepam, can produce a dramatic cessation of seizures but the effect is usually short-lived. Vigabatrin is sometimes effective in controlling the seizures (Livingston et al 1989). Some children are dramatically helped by being placed on a ketogenic diet (Muller & Lenard 1988). Intravenous therapy with immunoglobulins has been found useful in a few cases (Illum et a 1990). Occasional patients benefit from thyrotropin releasing hormone (Matsumoto et al 1987). The role of callosotomy, which can produce a worthwhile reduction in seizures, has been considered in detail by Andermann et al (1988).

Prognosis

A complete recovery with freedom from seizures and normal neurological and psychological development is very unusual (Beaumanoir 1985a). Approximately 5% of children die within 10 years but death is usually due to associated problems.

Seizures. The epilepsy, which is initially so difficult to control, later becomes less prominent, but the Lennox–Gastaut syndrome can persist into adulthood, when absence, myoclonic, generalized tonic-clonic, generalized tonic and simple and complex partial seizures and drop attacks are observed (Bauer et al 1988).

Neurological handicap. Virtually all patients have continuing disabilities which are related to the underlying pathology. Of those still afflicted in adulthood, one-third have localized hemispheric abnormalities (Bauer et al 1988).

Cognitive aspects. Mental retardation is the rule. Although for most children there is an arrest of learning, for some loss of previously acquired skills is noted. In children whose seizures have remitted, difficulties with the use of language and with organization of movement often persist and become increasingly important as the child grows older.

Social integration. Emotional problems were

noted in about a quarter of the cases persisting into adulthood (Bauer et al 1988). Both neurological handicap and mental retardation make full social integration difficult and overactivity in many of the affected children causes additional problems. When the Lennox–Gastaut syndrome persists into adulthood half of the patients are totally dependent and only one-sixth independent (Bauer et al 1988).

GENERALIZED TONIC–CLONIC SEIZURES

Primary and secondary generalized tonic-clonic seizures

Generalized tonic-clonic seizures are a stereotyped expression of maximal involvement of cerebral neurones. They may be 'primary' or 'secondary'. When primary they are completely generalized from the outset. Partial seizures which later become generalized are referred to as 'secondary generalized' attacks.

Incidence

It is probable that generalized tonic-clonic seizures make up at most 50% of seizures seen in children. Secondary generalized tonic-clonic seizures are probably much more common than primary attacks. However, the exact incidence of each type is unknown, since partial features are often either so brief as to pass unnoticed or relatively inconspicuous when followed by a generalized tonic-clonic convulsion.

Seizure characterization

In generalized tonic-clonic seizures consciousness is lost. The tonic phase lasts from 10 to 20 seconds. It starts with brief flexion followed by a longer period of extension giving way to a tremor which leads into the clonic phase. The clonic phase lasts about 30 seconds and begins when the muscular relaxation completely interrupts the tonic contraction. It is characterized by brief, violent flexor spasms of the whole body. Generalized tonic-clonic seizures are followed by postictal sleep.

Differential diagnosis

Prolonged vasovagal attacks leading to anoxia associated with clonic jerking are sometimes confused with generalized tonic-clonic seizures. Hysterical seizures are more common in adolescent girls than boys or younger children of either sex. They can be differentiated from epileptic seizures by ambulatory EEG monitoring or by estimation of the serum prolactin, which is raised for up to 4 hours after a genuine seizure, but remains normal in simulated attacks.

Aetiology

Primary generalized tonic-clonic seizures are of unknown aetiology; there is a strong genetic predisposition. On the other hand, the aetiology is usually known or suspected in secondary generalized tonic-clonic seizures. In these cases, the seizures are symptomatic of an underlying abnormality of the brain. Almost any cerebral lesion due to any pathological process can be responsible, though diffuse or generalized disorders are more likely to be found than well-localized conditions. If generalized tonic-clonic seizures occur secondary to a focal lesion, the lesion is most likely to be in one or other of the frontal lobes. Generalization is then related to synchronization of the cortical discharges by the reticular formation.

Pathophysiology

Gloor (1980) has emphasized the cortical origin of generalized spike-and-wave discharges, i.e. the EEG pattern found in generalized tonic-clonic seizures. Afferent thalamocortical volleys, which would normally lead to the appearance of spindles on the EEG, produce spike discharges when there is a cortical lesion. These activate a recurrent intracortical inhibitory system which intermittently reduces simultaneously the excitability of many pyramidal neurones of the cortex and is characterized on the EEG by the slow-wave component of the spike-and-wave discharge. There is no evidence that brief (under 15 minutes), single, generalized tonic-clonic seizures lead per se to cerebral damage. On the other hand, generalized tonic-clonic status epilepticus is a life-threatening condition. Once such seizures last for 30 minutes or more there is a risk of permanent neurological sequelae. The areas of the brain most vulnerable are, in the cortex, the occipital, frontal and temporal lobes, in particular the amygdala; in the cerebellum, the Purkinje cells; and the thalamus. The histological changes are indistinguishable from those of hypoxia/ischaemia, but are now thought to be secondary to the excessive amounts of excitotoxic amino acids which accumulate during prolonged seizures. There is considerable evidence that the younger the child and the longer the duration of the seizure, the greater is the likelihood that permanent cerebral damage will result.

Clinical findings

In children who have primary generalized tonic-clonic seizures the neurological examination and intelligence are usually normal. In those where there is underlying neurological abnormality and where the seizures are either secondary generalized tonic-clonic or secondarily generalized after starting as partial attacks, almost any underlying neurological condition can be present. It is clearly important to perform a full examination of all children who have generalized tonic-clonic seizures in order to determine the presence or absence of an accompanying diffuse or localized cerebral disorder. Signs other than those found in the neurological system may give further clues to the aetiology of the seizures. To give just one example: examination of the skin is important in the diagnosis of tuberous sclerosis.

Investigation

The necessity for investigations other than an EEG in children who have generalized tonic-clonic seizures depends entirely on the history surrounding the attack(s) and the physical findings. Where there is good reason to suspect that the child has primary generalized tonic-clonic seizures, biochemical and radiological examinations are not indicated. However, if there are features in the history or examination to suggest that an acquired structural disorder, such as a space-occupying lesion; or an underlying biochemical disorder; or an acute or chronic infection might be present, appropriate neuroradiological, biochemical and/or infection screens should be arranged. Routine examination of the cerebrospinal fluid is not indicated in afebrile children with generalized tonic-clonic seizures.

Electroencephalography. In a child who has primary generalized tonic-clonic seizures the interictal EEG may be entirely normal. Since the seizure is associated with considerable muscular activity it is usually difficult to get an artefact-free EEG during a tonic-clonic seizure. The characteristic ictal discharge is bilateral spike-waves. However, the synchrony and rhythmicity seen in absence seizures is not usually present. High-voltage slow waves are seen in the postictal period; brief bilateral spike-and-wave discharges may be seen in the interictal record. Photosensitivity is frequent in children with primary generalized tonic-clonic seizures.

Treatment

Intermittent generalized tonic-clonic seizures. In children who have had a single generalized tonic-clonic seizure, continuous antiepileptic medication is not indicated unless the seizure can be demonstrated to be secondary to an underlying neurological disorder in which recurrence appears probable.

After two or more generalized tonic-clonic seizures, serious consideration should be given to regular antiepileptic therapy. Controlled trials of first-line treatment for childhood generalized tonic-clonic epilepsy have yet to be reported. Sodium valproate 20–30 mg.kg/day^2, carbamazepine 10–20 mg.kg/day^2, phenytoin 5–8 mg.kg/day^2 (monitored by serum levels) or primidone 10–20 mg.kg/day^2 are probably equally effective in the uncomplicated case.

Generalized tonic-clonic status epilepticus. General measures, which include maintenance of the airway, administration of oxygen, monitoring and correction of rises or falls in blood pressure and normalization of the body temperature, are as important as specific antiepileptic medication. Diazepam is the drug of first choice. Given intravenously diazepam 0.1 mg/kg is usually effective. This dose can be repeated after 15 to 20 minutes. In the young child, intravenous injection may be difficult. As an alternative, rectal diazepam 0.5 mg/kg acts almost as rapidly as the intravenous injection. Diazepam given in suppositories or intramuscularly is absorbed only very slowly and neither of these routes is suitable for the treatment of status. If diazepam does not rapidly control the status, the child should be nursed in a place where intensive therapy is available. Only then is it safe to give additional antiepileptic drugs, such as slow intravenous phenobarbitone 10 mg/kg or intravenous phenytoin 10–15 mg/kg (given very slowly with ECG monitoring). Intramuscular or rectal paraldehyde may also be used, as may intravenous clonazepam, intravenous chlormethiazole or intravenous lignocaine. For the child who has been in prolonged status, dexamethasone or mannitol may be required to reduce cerebral oedema.

Prognosis

Seizures. On the whole, children with primary generalized tonic-clonic seizures, and who are thus neurologically and intellectually normal, have a good prognosis for later freedom from seizures. This is particularly so if their seizures are readily controlled with medication. When the seizures are secondary to neurological abnormalities or are refractory to medication, the prognosis is less good.

Social aspects. Generalized tonic-clonic seizures are the most obvious form of epilepsy and are those potentially causing most danger if a child is swimming, cycling or climbing trees etc. Undue restriction of activities may cause resentment and isolation from peer groups making later social integration difficult. It is thus important that physicians aim to render children seizure-free, thereby encouraging the parents of children with generalized tonic-clonic epilepsy to allow their children as much freedom as possible.

Photosensitive epilepsy

Seizures induced by flickering lights are usually generalized tonic-clonic in nature, though they may be preceded by mild clonic jerking (Jeavons & Harding 1975). Flash frequencies of between 15 and 20 Hz are most likely to be critical for the photosensitive subject. The age at the first seizure is usually in middle childhood with photosensitivity apparently diminishing during the twenties (Jeavons et al 1986, Wolf & Gooses 1986). In more than 90% of patients, stimulation of one eye is less epileptogenic than stimulation of both eyes; 30% of patients with a photoconvulsive response to intermittent photic stimulation are also sensitive to stationary patterns of striped lines (Wilkins & Lindsay 1985). The most epileptogenic patterns are composed of stripes, subtend a large area of the visual fields, have a spatial frequency between 1 and 8 cycles/degree, have a contrast in excess of about 30%, have a high luminance, and are vibrating with a temporal frequency between 5 and 30 Hz in a direction orthogonal to that of the stripes and are viewed with both eyes. Television viewed at close quarters has just these characteristics. Video-games (Maeda et al 1990), card games and draughts (Senanayake 1987) may also precipitate seizures.

The relationship of photosensitivity to epileptic syndromes has been examined in 103 patients from a total cohort of 1044 people with epilepsy (Wolf & Gooses 1986). Of those who were photosensitive, 88% had generalized seizures. Childhood absence epilepsy, juvenile myoclonic epilepsy and epilepsy with generalized tonic-clonic seizures on awakening were found to be significantly associated with photosensitivity. In the 12 patients where partial seizures were associated with photosensitivity, there were three in whom this was found only on drug withdrawal.

Avoidance of seizures induced by intermittent photic stimulation

Television. The following steps are recommended to avoid seizures:

1. If possible watch television with a small screen
2. If watching a large screen sit as far from it as possible (at least 2 m distant)
3. Arrange a remote control system for switching on and off and changing the programme
4. Use 'television glasses'—a sheet of polarizer which enhances the contrast of the picture is placed over the television screen, and the patient wears polaroid spectacles in which one lens has an axis of polarization orthogonal to that of the other, with the result that there is functional monocular occlusion (Wilkins & Lindsay 1985).

Other circumstances. Children sensitive to patterns, sunlight on water and visual stimuli other than the television set should be taught to occlude the vision to one eye as soon as a potential epileptogenic circumstance presents itself. However, many find it difficult to comply with this suggestion. In some there is a compulsion to view the television and other flickering phenomena at close and stimulating quarters, to the extent that fire-setting may result (Meinhard et al 1988). Crossed polaroid spectacles may be helpful but are not always acceptable to the child. When physical methods fail, sodium valproate is the drug of first choice for the control of photosensitive epilepsy.

Other reflex epilepsies

Epilepsy can be precipated by other stimuli, e.g. auditory, olfactory, tactile. 'Reading epilepsy' is well-recognized. A potentially particularly dangerous type of reflex epilepsy is that precipitated by bathing (Shaw et al 1988).

ABSENCE EPILEPSY (PETIT MAL)

Childhood absence epilepsy

Childhood absence epilepsy has been defined as an epilepsy starting before puberty in previously normal children whose initial seizures are absences which are very frequent, are not associated with myoclonus, and are accompanied by synchronous 3 Hz spike-waves on the EEG (Loiseau 1985).

Incidence

The incidence of true absence epilepsy is often difficult to determine from figures in the literature since other types of minor seizures are often confused with absences. Cavazzutti (1980) reported that in school-aged children with epilepsy 8% had absences.

Seizure types

Absences are usually brief, start and finish abruptly, are associated with loss of awareness, with or without other changes, and occur many times, often more than 100 times per day.

Penry et al (1975) have reported on 374 absence seizures that were analysed after simultaneous video and EEG recordings had been obtained from 48 patients. In 85% of patients the absences were of under 10 seconds duration and in all the patients the duration was 45 seconds or less. Individual patients tended to have absences of more or less the same duration. The absences in this study have been classified according to Gastaut (1970). The patients were significantly likely to have the same type of absence.

Absence simple. There is an abrupt onset, with cessation of ongoing activities, complete stillness and loss of awareness, but no loss of posture. The attack ends abruptly and activity is resumed where it left off. Only 9.4% of the attacks were simple absences.

Absence with mild clonic components. The onset is abrupt. During the attack clonic movements may occur in the eyelids, causing 3 per second blinking or, less frequently, in other muscles, leading to rhythmic jerking which is usually bilaterally symmetrical and does not impair posture. A total of 45.5% of the recorded absences had clonic components.

Absence with increase in postural tone. Tonic muscular contraction causing arching of the neck or back, which resolved prior to the end of the seizure, was observed in only 4.5% of absences.

Absence with diminution in postural tone. Diminution in postural tone can lead to drooping of the head, rarely slumping of the trunk; dropping of the arms and relaxation of the grip; buckling of the knees; and, rarely, a fall to the ground. Such changes occurred during 22.5% of absences.

Absence with automatisms. Automatisms were observed in 63.1% of absences and were significantly related to the duration of the seizure. They were very rare in absences lasting under 3 seconds but occurred in 95% of those of more than 18 seconds duration. Automatisms were of two main types. When perseverative, a patient persisted in activity which was ongoing at the start of the seizure. De novo automatisms commenced after the onset of the seizure and were characterized by licking, swallowing, scratching, 'fiddling' and other small-range, sometimes apparently semipurposeful, movements.

Absence mixed. In almost 40% of the absences more than one additional component was noted. However, in the majority of these, two, rather than more, components were observed.

It is usual to refer to absences which are other than simple as complex absences. The high percentage of complex absences has been confirmed by later studies using combined video and EEG recordings (Holmes et al 1987, Panayiotopoulos et al 1989).

Generalized tonic-clonic seizures occur, usually after the onset of absences, in 30–40% patients (Loiseau 1985).

Differential diagnosis

Absences with automatisms may be difficult to distinguish clinically from complex partial seizures (temporal lobe epilepsy). If possible, a seizure should be observed. In the untreated patient, absences can almost invariably be precipitated by hyperventilation, whereas complex partial seizures rarely occur under these circumstances. Post-attack confusion is very unusual after an absence, but is invariably present following a complex partial seizure. If the attacks cannot be distinguished clinically, the EEG, which is characteristic in absences, should clinch the diagnosis. On occasion, ambulatory EEG monitoring is necessary in order to record a seizure.

Children with emotional difficulties who become withdrawn or inattentive and those who are having problems with school work are sometimes suspected of absence epilepsy. Clinical and EEG observation during hyperventilation should resolve the situation.

It is important to distinguish absence epilepsy from myoclonic absences, in which myoclonic jerking of the proximal upper limbs is associated with loss of awareness, and atypical absences which occur in, for example, the Lennox–Gastaut syndrome.

Aetiology

Absences are not usually associated with recog-

nizable focal neurological deficits on clinical examination. However, there is evidence from careful stereo-electroencephalographic work that the convulsive discharges originate in the mesio-orbital gyrus of the frontal cortex and are synchronized in the reticular system (Bancaud & Talairach 1965). There is a family history of seizure disorders in between 15% and 40% of cases (Loiseau 1985). Various modes of inheritance have been suggested, but the exact role of the genetic input has yet to be clarified, particularly in relation to the possible presence of a focal frontal lesion as the primary site of the epileptic discharge. In a population-based case-control study, the only factor found to give a significant risk for absences was prior febrile seizures (Rocca et al 1987a). Fourteen of the 59 cases reported by Hashimoto et al (1989) had had earlier febrile seizures.

Pathophysiology

As discussed above it seems probable that a focal disturbance in the mesio-orbital gyrus of the frontal cortex is the basic pathological problem. It is usually assumed that absence seizures themselves cause no additional pathology. However, using (^{18}F) 2-fluoro-2-deoxy-D-glucose (FDG) and positron computed tomography, Engel et al (1982) have demonstrated that glucose metabolism is increased by 2 to 3.5 times during a period of 10 minutes in which hyperventilation produced many absences. The increase in glucose metabolism was not related to the frequency or duration of the absences. Hyperventilation alone did not produce comparable changes. The ictal glucose utilization was higher in these patients than in any others with seizures (Mazziotti & Engel 1985). It is suggested that the youth of the patients and the lack of a period of postictal suppression may be responsible for this finding. Engel et al (1982) did not demonstrate any area of focal metabolic abnormality, i.e. in the frontal region, but felt that the measurements were not yet sufficiently sophisticated to exclude the presence of such an area. The significance of these acute ictal metabolic changes for long-term cerebral development remains undetermined.

Using a gamma-hydroxybutyrate model in rats

Snead (1990b) has examined the ontogeny of GABAergic enhancement, and has found that absences cannot occur until the thalamo-cortical recruiting mechanisms are sufficiently mature.

Clinical features

Absence epilepsy is more common in girls than boys in a ratio of about 2:1. The seizures usually start in middle childhood between 5 and 10 years of age, but typical childhood absences may appear as early as 3 years and as late as 13 years. Dalby (1969) considered that almost all children with classical absences were neurologically normal. However, careful examination often reveals minor difficulties with fine movement and co-ordination. Virtually all patients with absences are mentally normal. However, if absences are frequent, attentional defects are likely (Browne et al 1974). Using video-EEG with telemetry absences have been shown to be less frequent in the afternoon than in the morning, and to occur less often in sleep (Nagao et al 1990). In REM sleep and stage 1 of non-REM sleep absences were as frequent as during waking, but in stage 2 there were very few and in stages 3 and 4 no absences. Nagao et al (1990) found an inversely significant association between the duration of the absences and their frequency.

Investigation

Electroencephalography. Absences are associated with bilaterally synchronous and symmetrical rhythmic spike-waves. The discharges commence abruptly but cease over a period of seconds. Spike-wave complexes have a frequency of 3 Hz at the onset but may slow to 2.5 to 2 Hz towards the end of the attack. Irregular spike-wave discharges may also accompany childhood absence seizures (Loiseau 1985). Between attacks, the background activity is usually normal, but single or brief discharges may be found without any recognizable clinical accompaniment. Hyperventilation will usually precipitate an attack if the resting record is non-contributory. Generalized rhythmic delta activity has been reported in association with absences in a few cases (Lee & Kirby 1988).

Treatment

Absences are responsive to ethosuximide and to sodium valproate. These drugs are equally efficacious (Callaghan et al 1982, Sato et al 1982b), but ethosuximide is the usual first-choice therapy if absences are uncomplicated by other seizures. If other seizure types are present valproate is indicated.

The starting dose of ethosuximide is 15 mg.kg/day^2 and this can be increased to 40 mg.kg/day^2 if neither the clinical state nor the monitoring of the serum levels suggest that toxicity is occurring. With careful attention to regularity of medication and adjustment of the dosage to ensure optimal serum ethosuximide levels, absences can be controlled for practical purposes in 80% of patients and 60% will become seizure-free (Sherwin 1982). Since ethosuximide has a long half-life, once daily dosage can be used (Dooley et al 1990).

Sodium valproate 20 to 30 mg.kg/day^2 is indicated if generalized tonic-clonic seizures accompany absences or if the attacks fail to respond to ethosuximide. Significant correlations between the plasma valproate concentrations and both reduction in epileptic discharges on the EEG and the clinical response have been reported (Braathen et al 1988). Where monotherapy with neither ethosuximide nor valproate produces adequate control of absences, the use of both drugs together will be more effective than either alone in some patients (Schmidt 1983b).

For the very small group of patients whose attacks remain clinically uncontrolled by ethosuximide and/or valproate, clonazepam can be helpful, but tolerance is likely to develop (Sato et al 1977).

Prognosis

Seizures. It is unusual for absences to persist beyond adolescence. A rapid response to therapy is usually a good prognostic sign. An IQ of at least 90, the absence of generalized tonic-clonic seizures and a negative history for absence status have each been significantly correlated with remission of absences (Sato et al 1982a).

About 40% of children with absences later develop generalized tonic-clonic seizures. Such seizures usually present between 5 and 10 years after the onset of the absences and are usually infrequent and readily controlled by sodium valproate. The factors predisposing to the development of generalized tonic-clonic seizures are: onset of absences after 8 years of age, male sex, poor initial response of absences to therapy, abnormalities of background activity and/or photosensitivity demonstrable on the EEG (Loiseau 1985). If the first seizures are generalized tonic-clonic the outlook for remission is significantly less good than if the epilepsy starts with absences (Dieterich et al 1985a,b).

Cognitive aspects. Although intelligence is usually normal, if absences are inadequately controlled the accompanying attentional deficits can be associated with educational under-functioning.

Behaviour problems. One-third of the patients studied by Loiseau et al (1983) had behaviour problems. These were attributed to frequent attacks, effects of the parents' attitudes to the absences or to therapy.

Juvenile absence epilepsy

In juvenile absence epilepsy the seizures are clinically similar to those in childhood absence epilepsy, but occur infrequently and often sporadically. The age of onset is about puberty and males and females are equally likely to be affected. If generalized tonic-clonic seizures occur they are most common an awakening. Myoclonic seizures may also be present. Spike-wave discharges on the EEG have a frequency greater than 3 Hz (Wolf 1985b).

Response to ethosuximide and/or valproate is not as readily obtained as in childhood absence epilepsy, but higher than usual dosage and combination therapy can be effective, even in adolescents initially considered to be poor responders (Wolf & Inoue 1984).

PARTIAL SEIZURES

By definition, there is clinical or EEG evidence that partial seizures arise from a localized lesion. Nevertheless, it is often difficult to identify the lesion precisely. If the partial seizure spreads to involve neurones throughout both cerebral hemispheres, secondary generalization is deemed to have occurred. Partial seizures account for 40% of childhood seizures (Gastaut et al 1975, Cavazzutti 1980). Childhood partial seizures can be examined in four broad groups:

1. Associated with defined cerebral lesions
2. Complex partial seizures of temporal lobe origin
3. Epilepsia partialis continua (Kojewnikow's syndrome)
4. Benign partial epilepsies.

Partial seizures associated with defined cerebral lesions

Incidence

At least 30% of patients with childhood epilepsy have lesional partial seizures.

Seizure types

The clinical expression of a partial seizure which occurs in relation to a defined cerebral abnormality clearly depends on the localization of the structural changes, so that partial seizures may be primarily motor, sensory, visual, etc. They may be well localized, i.e. involving only a few muscle groups, or sufficiently extensive as to produce a complete unilateral attack. Virtually any intermittent stereotyped alteration in movement or sensation can be some form of partial seizure.

Differential diagnosis

Partial seizures may be confused with hemiplegic migraine and, when the motor component is well localized, with nervous tics. If visual or auditory seizures occur, psychiatric disturbance may be erroneously diagnosed. A localized EEG disturbance is usually helpful in distinguishing partial seizures from other events, particularly if the EEG can be recorded during an attack.

Aetiology

Any insult which might lead to localized brain disturbance can be associated with partial seizures. Prenatal disorders of neuronal proliferation and organization are probably under-diagnosed. Perinatal abnormalities such as intra-ventricular haemorrhage in premature infants and hypoxic ischaemic encephalopathy in the full-term infant, as well as more obvious intrapartum cerebral trauma, may cause localized cerebral scarring with later development of partial seizures. Head injuries such as those secondary to non-accidental injury or road traffic accidents are responsible for the epileptogenic lesions in other children. Other causes of brain abnormalities which may be associated with partial seizures are meningitis, encephalitis, cerebral abscess, vascular anomalies, demyelination (multiple sclerosis), hydrocephalus and cerebral tumours. Although for many parents the possibility that a tumour may be the underlying cause of the child's seizures ranks high in their list of anxieties, seizures are only very rarely the presenting event in childhood space-occupying lesions. However, when true Jacksonian seizures with a well-localized distal onset and a recognizable march proximally occur, a very careful search for a slow-growing tumour should be undertaken. Partial epilepsies other than complex partial seizures sometimes follow prolonged unilateral febrile convulsions.

Pathophysiological aspects

Regardless of the initiating process (e.g. head injury, anoxia), neuropathological studies have shown the epileptogenic focus is characterized by neuronal drop-out, gliosis and distortions in neuronal morphology which include loss of dendritic spines, simplification of dendritic arborization patterns and shrinkage of the entire neurone. Such morphological changes may lead to selective loss of GABA-ergic interneurones, with possible attenuation of postsynaptic inhibitory control on dendrites which in turn could allow the emergence of latent burst properties; and changes in the distribution and density of different ion channels which might affect the relationship between excitatory and inhibitory conductances (Benardo & Pedley 1985). The possible relevance of the subjection of the epileptogenic focus to constantly changing inputs from ascending brain stem projections, the thalamus and other cortical neurones is difficult to quantify

and, in practice, a number of pathophysiological routes may lead to a final common pathway when synchronized cellular bursting occurs. In childhood, and particularly in very young children, the significance of 'acquired' lesions in focal epileptogenesis may be less than disorders of neuronal proliferation or migration.

During the actual seizures, the epileptogenic areas have markedly elevated metabolic rates and blood flow, and associated efflux of potassium and influx of calcium. Reductions in glucose and glycogen content, elevations of lactate, cyclic nucleotides, adenosine, free fatty acids and prostaglandins and inhibition of regional protein synthesis also occur (Chapman 1985). Thus, not only may partial seizures be symptomatic of focal cerebral abnormalities, but the attacks themselves may cause secondary problems if they are sufficiently prolonged.

Clinical features

Since partial seizures are particularly likely to be secondary to a recognizable cerebral lesion it is essential that careful neurological and general systemic examinations are carried out.

Seizures are unusual as the presenting symptoms for space-occupying lesions, but the possibility of an underlying tumour cannot be ignored, particularly when partial seizures occur in association with acquired progressive neurological deficits, headaches, early morning vomiting or other symptoms of raised intracranial pressure. Even in young children, in whom examination of the optic fundi is difficult, it is important to exclude: papilloedema which might be associated with any cause of intracranial hypertension; optic atrophy, which if not related to recognizable perinatal events, might suggest a metabolic cause for the seizures; the scarring of previous choroidoretinitis, such as might follow prenatal toxoplasmosis; retinal pigmentation due to metabolic disorders; and disorders of the macula such as the cherry red spot characteristically found in GM_1 gangliosidosis, Tay–Sachs disease and other neurodegenerative disorders.

Other than the central nervous system, the skin is most likely to give clues to an underlying problem. For example, although the typical rash of tuberous sclerosis may not be evident in the young infant, ash-leaf-shaped patches of depigmentation, seen most commonly on the back and the backs of the legs, are early indications of this condition. The facial haemangioma of Sturge–Weber's disease is a much more obvious lesion. When this involves a frontal region it is often associated with seizures affecting the contralateral side of the body. Patients with the cafe-au-lait spots of neurofibromatosis may have neuronal heterotopias and are at increased risk of intracranial tumours. Enlargement of the liver and spleen may indicate that seizures are symptomatic of a diffuse storage disorder involving the brain.

Investigation

The chief diagnostic aids in the definition of a structural abnormality of the brain are neuro-imaging/radiology and electroencephalography.

Neuroimaging/radiology. Plain X-rays of the skull can show asymmetries of skull size or enlargement of one cranial compartment which may give clues to: the chronicity of the lesion; sutural diastasis, when there is an expanding intracranial lesion present; and intracranial calcification in tuberous sclerosis, congenital toxoplasmosis and some tumours.

CT scanning is indicated whenever partial seizures are associated with abnormal neurological signs during interictal periods; when there is a localized slow-wave abnormality on the EEG; when seizures are refractory to medical treatment; and when there is any suspicion that a space-occupying lesion may be present. Localized or generalized cerebral dysgenesis, porencephalic cysts, localized or generalized cortical atrophy or demyelination, tumours, abscesses, localized encephalitis (e.g. herpes) and moderately-sized vascular malformations can be identified on a CT scan. Up to 70% of children with partial seizures may have lesions demonstrable by CT scanning, with the highest yield coming from those with secondary generalization (Pedersen 1990).

Isotope scanning may be helpful in the early diagnosis of herpes simplex encephalitis and cerebral abscess, both of which are commonly associated with partial seizures.

Ultrasound scanning through the open anterior fontanelle can demonstrate ventricular enlargement, porencephalic cysts and the multiple intra-cerebral cysts seen following neonatal intra-parenchymal haemorrhage, but usually needs to be followed up by CT scanning so that any lesion seen can be more clearly defined. Nevertheless, some disorders of neuronal migration have been identified sonographically (Trounce et al 1986).

Magnetic resonance imaging can detect lesions not readily definable on CT scans. Disorders of neuronal migration and of myelination are particularly well-delineated (Kendall 1988, Curatolo et al 1989, Byrd et al 1989). Close correlation between EEG foci and abnormalities detected by MRI has been demonstrated in tuberous sclerosis (Tamaki et al 1990).

Single photon emission computed tomography (SPECT) has been compared with EEG, CT and MRI findings in children with partial seizures (Vles et al 1990). It was found to be superior to CT and MRI.

Positron emission tomography (PET), which is more complex and very expensive, demonstrates, interictally, focal areas of hypometabolism, and during seizures striking increases in metabolic activity in regions where there is EEG evidence of abnormality.

Angiography is indicated when a vascular abnormality is suspected.

Electroencephalography. When there is a definable structural lesion present, standard EEGs are usually abnormal in the interictal period. However, the absence of an interictal abnormality does not totally exclude the possibility of local pathology. Focal or lateralized non-paroxysmal or continuous abnormalities are particularly suggestive of an underlying lesion and may take the form of changes in the background rhythms, focal slow waves, localized depression of activity, asymmetries or local failure of response to activating mechanisms such as sleep or hyperventilation. Of the unifocal spike-waves seen in partial epilepsies, those that are non-repetitive and of varying morphology, of fixed location, whose frequency does not increase with sleep, and are related to focal slow abnormalities, are suggestive of a structural lesion, as are the multifocal spike-waves which have a constant localization (Revol 1985). When there is a frontal lesion the EEG abnormality may be bilateral spike-waves which predominate in both frontal regions but may not be totally symmetrical.

Ambulatory monitoring is often helpful in allowing a seizure to be recorded electro-encephalographically so that better localization may be obtained. Similarly, sphenoidal or other deeply placed electrodes may give more detailed information on the position of a small lesion.

Simultaneous EEG and video-monitoring can be very helpful in defining the nature of events in which there is doubt as to whether or not epilepsy is present. It is particularly useful when repetitive behavioural changes occur (Duchowny et al 1988).

Computed EEG topography can increase information gained electroencephalographically. In 40 children examined by conventional EEG and by computed EEG topography, the latter was shown to better identify localized dysfunction (De Negri et al 1990).

Other investigations. The indications for biochemical investigations, viral serology, examination of the bone marrow for storage disorder etc, vary from case to case and depend on the type of neurological and/or other disorders found on general examination.

Magnetoencephalography may become more widely used (Lancet 1990a).

Treatment

Partial epilepsy secondary to a defined cerebral lesion may be treated medically or surgically.

When a space-occupying lesion is present the first choice would obviously be surgery, but under almost all other circumstances a trial of antiepileptic drug therapy is indicated. Carbamazepine and phenytoin are both well tried in the treatment of partial seizures. Carbamazepine is preferred since it is less likely to cause side-effects. It should be introduced at a dose of 5 mg.kg/day^2 in two or three divided doses with an increase to 10 mg.kg/day^2 after one week. Subsequent increases up to 20 mg.kg/day^2 may be necessary and in small children, where the elimination rate is high, 30 mg.kg/day^2 given in up to four divided doses may be necessary to acquire constant optimal serum levels throughout 24

hours. If phenytoin is given it can be started at a dose of 5–8 mg.kg/day^2 and given in a single daily dose or two divided doses.

The careful serum monitoring essential to the proper use of phenytoin and the gum hypertrophy, hirsutism and possible interference with cognition are features which make phenytoin less attractive than carbamazepine, but it is undoubtedly effective in many children in whom carbamazepine has failed to control seizures. In a minority of children, the response to combined medication with carbamazepine and phenytoin is better than either drug alone. Recent investigations of the efficacy of valproate suggest that it may also be useful in partial seizures. Primidone sometimes controls such attacks when other anti-epileptic drugs have been ineffective. Vigabatrin 50–80 mg.kg/day^2 can be very effective when other antiepileptic drugs have failed.

If the optimal use of drugs fails to control the seizures and there is a clearly localized lesion, surgery should be considered. Very careful assessment should precede surgical intervention and should include realistic consideration of the most appropriate surgical procedure, the possibility of subsequent unacceptable neurological or psychological deficit and the likely benefit (Flanigin et al 1985). Possible procedures are ablation, i.e. removal of the lesion or its epileptogenic area; disconnection, e.g. cortical undercutting; corpus callostomy; stereotaxic procedures, e.g. the production of thalamic lesions; stimulation procedures, i.e. cerebellar stimulation; and cerebral cooling. Of these, ablative and disconnection procedures are those most commonly considered in childhood. The outcome following surgery depends to some extent on the selection of patients but it is probable that between 60% and 90% achieve worthwhile improvement (Flanigin et al 1985).

Prognosis

Partial attacks associated with definite cerebral lesions are amongst the childhood seizures from which remission and cure are unlikely. Neurological deficits will persist and intellectual problems are common with the exact incidence and type of intellectual defect being dependent on the localization of the lesion and its aetiology. Factors which are associated with a poor prognosis include:

1. Early onset of seizures
2. Associated generalized seizures
3. Frequent seizures
4. Interictal EEG abnormalities and ictal discharges on routine recordings
5. Associated neurological and psychopathological signs (Revol 1985).

Factors considered favourable are:

1. Family history of seizures
2. No generalized seizures prior to partial attacks
3. Low frequency of seizures after therapy for 12 months
4. Short duration of 'active' epilepsy
5. Normal background activity on EEG (Porro et al 1988).

Complex partial seizures of temporal lobe origin

Although complex partial seizures are usually related to discharges arising in one temporal lobe, in some patients the frontal lobe or another area is primarily involved. This section concentrates on epilepsy of temporal lobe origin.

Incidence

Temporal lobe epilepsy accounts for about 25% of the childhood epileptic population (Ounsted et al 1966, Hauser & Kurland 1975)

Seizures

The initial symptom or sign may be loss of consciousness or an aura. The attack may be very brief, as little as under 15 seconds or as long as 8 minutes. Automatisms occur in almost all patients and can be classified as de novo from internal stimuli, de novo from external stimuli and perseverative. Automatisms which occur de novo from internal stimuli include chewing, lip-smacking, swallowing, scratching, rubbing, picking, fumbling, running and undressing. Those which occur de novo from external stimuli include response to pin-prick, drinking from a cup and pushing in

response to a restraint. In perseverative automatisms, the patient continues to perform any complex act initiated prior to the loss of consciousness. Psychic phenomena such as depersonalization, déjà vu sensations, formed hallucinations, illusions and distortions of perception and ideas of a 'presence' may also occur during complex partial seizures. Secondary generalization may follow.

Differential diagnosis

Complex partial seizures are sometimes confused with absences in which automatisms occur. The distinguishing clinical feature is that awareness returns immediately after an absence, whereas confusion is usual for at least a brief period after a complex partial seizure.

Behavioural aberrations may also cause diagnostic difficulties. On the whole they can be differentiated from complex partial seizures by the retention of awareness, their relationship to situations which cause stress and lack of the stereotyped nature of abnormal behaviour. Although in any one patient the sequence of events observed during a seizure may not be completed each time, the onset is usually the same. Video-EEG recordings can be very helpful in distinguishing between epileptic and non-epileptic behavioural changes.

Aetiology

Ounsted et al (1966) found that the cause of temporal lobe epilepsy fell into three categories. The first aetiological category consisted of organic cerebral insults. These included adverse perinatal events, head injury, tuberous sclerosis, tumours and post-meningitic or encephalitic lesions. In the second category an episode of status epilepticus preceded the development of complex partial seizures usually by some years. There remained a third category in which the aetiology never became evident.

The mechanism whereby acute neonatal events may predispose to temporal lobe epilepsy remains obscure. Earlier suggestions related to uncal herniation are now considered untenable. On the other hand there is good evidence that pre- and perinatal events predispose to prolongation and lateralization of febrile seizures (Wallace 1988) and that prolonged unilateral convulsions with fever can be followed by complex partial seizures. Recent pathological reports (Armstrong et al 1987, Hardiman et al 1988) have found that malformative lesions such as foci of dysgenesis are present in a very high percentage of temporal lobes resected for intractable epilepsy. This suggests that the prolonged lateralized febrile seizure which is followed by temporal lobe epilepsy may be symptomatic of a neuronal migrational disorder. The damaging presence of excessive concentrations of excitotoxic amino acids, accumulating during prolonged seizure activity must also have a role. In a series, not confined to childhood, either a difficult birth, febrile convulsions, or both, preceded complex partial seizures in two-thirds of 63 patients in whom hippocampal sclerosis was found on histology (Mathieson 1975). In a population-based case-control study, the significant risk factors for complex partial seizures were: a history of epilepsy or febrile seizures in the mother, febrile seizures, neonatal convulsions, cerebral palsy, head trauma and viral encephalitis (Rocca et al 1987b).

For those whose epilepsy follows an episode of status there is a positive history of seizures, usually when feverish, in 30% of siblings (Ounsted et al 1966). In a detailed study of the genetics of the epilepsies, complex partial epilepsy was found to be only slightly less familial that other types of epilepsy (Ottman 1989).

Pathophysiology

Between seizures, local discharges are thought to be initiated in small columnar units in neo- and palaeocortical structures located mainly in the temporal lobe, where paroxysmal activity consists of depolarization shifts at the centre of the focus and predominantly inhibitory potentials in the surrounding areas. At the onset of a complex partial seizure there is intensification of the local paroxysmal activity and spread via synapses to other areas, where self-sustained discharges arise. Spread is initially through the ipsilateral hemisphere, during which an aura can occur, and later to the opposite hemisphere when memory and

consciousness become disturbed (Goldensohn 1975). The pathology of the lesion cannot be deduced from the clinical features of the seizure (Theodore et al 1986).

In a series of 40 children in whom a temporal lobectomy was performed before the age of 15 years mesial temporal sclerosis was found in 24 (associated with a hamartoma in two), hamartomata alone in seven, tumours in three, viral encephalitis in one and the findings were non-specific in the remaining seven (Davidson & Falconer 1975).

In addition to the presence of lesions such as microdysgenesis, which must be prenatal in origin, evidence of abnormalities with later timing comes from a study which found mossy fibre synaptic terminals to be in excess in the supragranular region and the inner molecular layer in patients with epilepsy (Sutula et al 1989). It has been suggested that this excess is related to anatomical plasticity of the hippocampus, and that the establishment of new synaptic contacts is important in the genesis of complex partial epilepsy (Represa et al 1989).

Clinical features

Of the 100 children with temporal lobe epilepsy examined by Ounsted et al (1966), 63 were males. In only nine were gross neurological abnormalities detected, of whom five had hemiplegias and two monoplegias; 14 of the children had either visual field defects, optic atrophy or disorders of eye movement. Speech was abnormal in 28 of the 100 children. Complex partial seizures started at a median age of 5 years 4 months for the whole group. For those who had had preceding episodes of status epilepticus, the median age at the first seizure was 1 year 4 months and at the onset of complex partial attacks was 4 years 2 months.

On the whole, children with temporal lobe epilepsy have intelligence levels within the normal range. However, when the epilepsy is a symptom of either a perinatal insult or a sequel of status, the intellectual level is likely to be below average. One-quarter of the children in the group studied by Ounsted et al (1966) were hyperkinetic and those affected were almost invariably of subnormal intelligence; 36 of the 100 children had catastrophic rage outbursts. Ounsted et al (1966) also reported that social and schooling difficulties were common and that many children with complex partial seizures failed to reach the educational level expected from their intelligence scores. Only half the children whose first seizure occurred before 3 years completed their education in normal schools. The frequency of complex partial seizures did not influence the outcome for schooling.

Investigation

Biochemical investigation is indicated only when there is evidence from general examination that there is an underlying metabolic disorder.

Neuroimaging/radiology. Skull X-rays will sometimes show asymmetries of the middle cranial fossae, particularly if the underlying lesion is very longstanding. Calcification suggests tuberous sclerosis, a tumour or, occasionally, a vascular malformation which has previously undergone thrombosis.

Even though various scanning devices can give good details of the brain, pneumoencephalography can still add to the delineation of a temporal lesion if atrophy is the major pathological process.

Angiography is indicated when a vascular malformation is suspected and will occasionally demonstrate very small angiomata in temporal lobes which seem to be normal on routine CT scanning.

CT scanning is indicated whenever complex partial seizures commence in a child who has had no history of either perinatal problems or status epilepticus, particularly febrile status. It is also indicated in the 'insult' and 'status' groups when medical treatment is apparently ineffective. In these circumstances, an area of atrophy or another definable structural lesion, which might be amenable to surgery, may be outlined.

Preliminary reports on the use of advanced neuroimaging techniques (PET, SPECT and MRI) suggest that these can be very valuable in the delineation of both the physiological and anatomical characteristics of epileptogenic foci (Mazziotti & Engel 1985). In particular, disorders of neuronal migration and other types of dysgenesis can be seen on MRI, when not visible by CT (Kendall 1988).

Electroencephalography. In pure temporal lobe epilepsy, abnormalities of the EEG are focal and are recorded predominantly from one or both temporal regions. Spikes, sharp waves or, less frequently, slow waves may be found interictally but are much more likely to be seen if a seizure occurs during the recording. In fact, the record may otherwise be only equivocally abnormal. Repeated standard EEGs are often necessary before a definite focus is seen. When seizures occur several times a week, ambulatory monitoring, which can easily incorporate a sleep recording, allows a greater knowledge of the changes during attacks and can produce information about the origin and spread of the seizure discharge. The insertion of sphenoidal, foramen ovale and other depth electrodes is rarely justifiable in the establishment of the diagnosis, but may be indicated prior to consideration for surgery. Depth electrodes can be connected to the Medilog (Oxford Medical Systems) ambulatory EEG monitor, allowing continuous recordings to be collected from intracranial sites over considerable lengths of time.

Treatment

Treatment may be medical or surgical. In the follow-up of the 100 patients with temporal lobe epilepsy originally reported by Ounsted et al (1966), Lindsay et al (1984) considered the role neurosurgery played in their biographies. For 42 children surgery was not indicated. Of these, 10 had severe intellectual and physical disabilities which were of more serious import than their seizure disorders, and in the other 32, remission of seizures occurred during childhood. Surgery was actually considered in 29 of the other 58 children and performed in 13. However, in only four of the 13 was surgery performed before the age of 16 years, and in three cases the operation was a hemispherectomy rather than a temporal lobectomy. All had periods of freedom from seizures thereafter and Lindsay et al (1984) suggest that surgery might be considered earlier rather than later. However, since in one-third of the cases remission of seizures occurred before adulthood, careful consideration must be given to all aspects of the seizure disorder before submitting the child to surgery.

A group of 27 patients considered by very strict criteria to have complex partial seizures of temporal lobe origin were considered by Kotagal et al (1987) for surgery. Thirteen had temporal lobectomies, and eight were seizure-free 5 years later.

In the series of Davidson & Falconer (1975) children were selected for temporal lobectomy if they had frequent disabling seizures which were resistant to adequate drug therapy, neuroradiological studies appeared to have ruled out a gross space-occupying lesion and EEGs, including a special study using sphenoidal electrodes under intravenous pentothal narcosis, had shown a spike-discharging focus which was prominent in, or confined to, one temporal lobe. Gross mental retardation was considered a contraindication to surgery. Surgery produced the most satisfactory results both in terms of seizure control and amelioration of behaviour when the underlying pathology was mesial temporal sclerosis. The least satisfactory results were obtained when non-specific pathological changes were found in the excised temporal lobes. It is clear that surgery can be beneficial and in some cases curative, but that antiepileptic drugs remain the mainstay of treatment.

There is probably little to choose between the efficacies of phenytoin and carbamazepine in the medical treatment of complex partial seizures, but carbamazepine is the usual first choice since side-effects are less of a problem than with phenytoin. Valproate or primidone may also be helpful in some cases, as may vigabatrin.

Prognosis

The long-term outcome for children with temporal lobe epilepsy has been reported in considerable detail by Ounsted et al (1987).

Seizures. After at least 13 years of follow-up one-third of the patients investigated were free of seizures on no therapy, and self-supporting; one-third were self-supporting, still on antiepileptic drugs but not necessarily seizure-free; rather less than one-third were dependent and 5% were dead. Those whose seizures were secondary to 'birth injury' or to meningitis did poorly. Other adverse factors were an IQ of less than 90, seizures

starting before 2 years 4 months, five or more generalized tonic-clonic seizures, complex partial seizures occurring at least once a day, left-sided foci, the hyperkinetic syndrome, catastrophic rage and special schooling. When three or fewer of these adverse factors were present the outcome was on the whole good and when more than five were present no child became seizure-free. A positive family history of seizures appeared to override adverse factors in some cases. Kotagal et al (1987) reported that after follow-up for 5 years, of a cohort of 29 patients, eight were still having more than one seizure per week, six had one to four seizures per month and 12, of whom eight had had temporal lobectomies, were seizure-free.

Neurological handicaps. The literature contains little information on the long-term neurological status of children who have temporal lobe epilepsy. Some of the children have significant hemiplegias, but for many, motor deficits are minimal, if present at all.

Cognitive aspects. In a comparison of the characteristics of children with well-defined right- or left-sided temporal lobe EEG foci, Camfield et al (1984) failed to find any significant right–left differences for intelligence, neuropsychological traits or clinical features, but one-third of the children were shown to be maladjusted on the Personality Inventory for Children. The maladjusted patients did significantly less well on the neuropsychological testing than those who appeared well adjusted, emphasizing the tendency for suboptimality to be present in more than one sphere. Fourteen (47%) of the patients in the study of Kotagal et al (1987) had school difficulties, including requirement for special education.

Behaviour problems and social integration. Hyperactivity, temper tantrums, rage attacks, antisocial behaviour and sexual acting-out were problems in over half of those in the study of Kotagal et al (1987). One-third of the same group were self-supporting in adulthood, and half totally dependent. When surgery had improved seizure-control, behaviour and social integration were better.

When marriage, parenthood and sexual indifference were considered, slightly less than two-thirds of those deemed marriageable had actually married (Ounsted et al 1987). Trauma or status was the aetiology in most of those who had not married and affected males were much less likely to marry than affected females. Marriage was significantly more common where remission had occurred before puberty and this factor was particularly important for males who, even if they were married, were less likely than females to become parents.

Psychiatric problems had been present during childhood in 85% of the group reported by Ounsted et al (1987), but by adulthood 70% of those who were not seriously mentally retarded were psychiatrically healthy. Nevertheless, overt schizophreniform psychosis was present in 10%, being most common in males with continuing epilepsy with a left-sided focus, where the incidence was 30%.

Kojewnikow's syndrome (Rasmussen's syndrome)

Two types of Kojewnikow's syndrome, or epilepsia partialis continua, have been identified by Bancaud (1985). The first type occurs at any age on the background of a stable neurological deficit and the second, presenting only in children, is associated with progressive neurological and psychological deterioration.

Incidence

Both types I and II of Kojewnikow's syndrome appear to be rare and figures for the incidence are not available.

Seizure type

Bancaud (1985) used two seizure types as necessary criteria for the diagnosis of this syndrome. The first was semi-continuous or permanent muscle jerks, which were localized and usually confined to a small group of muscles. The second was unilateral somatomotor seizures whether or not they were associated with other seizure types. In type I seizures occurred daily at their most frequent, whereas in type II seizures often occurred very many times a day.

Aetiology

There appears to be little argument about the constancy of a definable structural lesion in type I. The aetiology of type II remains a matter for discussion.

Type I. Although a definable lesion is usually present its exact nature may be extremely variable. Infection, vascular abnormalities and tumours have been described (Bancaud 1985).

Type II. This subdivision of Kojewnikow's syndrome is a progressive disorder in which 'encephalitis' is said to be the underlying condition (Rasmussen et al 1958). However with the exception of a recent report on the finding of cytomegalovirus genomic material in surgical specimens (Power et al 1990), no infecting agent has been identified. Examination of the cerebrospinal fluid has shown that the percentage of E-rosette forming cells was much reduced in two patients when compared with controls (Gaggero et al 1990). In one of these patients there was also a raised IgG-index and oligoclonal bands were present. There are thus some suggestions that immunological abnormalities may have a role in this syndrome. Although Juul-Jensen & Denny-Brown (1966) suggested that the lesions were often subcortical, Bancaud (1985) claimed unequivocal evidence of the cortical localization of the pathology.

Differential diagnosis

Behavioural tics may be differentiated from both types of Kojewnikow's syndrome by the absence of neurological and EEG abnormalities and, particularly from type II of the syndrome, by the retention of normal intellect.

Clinical features

In a study of 22 patients with this syndrome of whom five had the features of type I and 17 had the features of type II, Bancaud (1985) found that the onset of the condition could be as early as 8 months and tended to be younger in those patients with type II. In three of the five children with type I and 14 of the 17 with type II, myoclonic jerks followed unilateral seizures within a year. The interval was less than 4 months in 11 of the 17 patients with type II. Of the five patients with type I, one had no neurological deficit, two had localized abnormalities and two had hemiplegias. On the other hand, all 17 patients with type II had hemiplegias which were complicated by other motor deficits in four children. All five children with type I were mentally unimpaired; whereas of the 17 with type II 13 have severe mental impairment, two mild and only two no mental impairment.

Investigation

The search for a surgically remediable lesion is clearly important in this group of patients. In the 22 patients of Bancaud (1985) neuroradiology, not further specified, revealed a cortical-subcortical scar in one of five patients with type I. Relatively localized lesions were identified in two, extensive lesions in eight and bilateral or diffuse lesions in the remaining seven of those with type II.

Electroencephalography. Bancaud (1985) has investigated his group of patients very extensively, using in addition to more conventional recordings, stereo-EEG.

In patients with type I, the interictal EEG almost invariably showed normal background activity (asymmetry was noted in only one case); delta waves were either absent or localized; spikes and/or spike-waves were localized in four of the five patients; and subclinical paroxysmal discharges were not identified. The ictal discharges were localized to the central region in all type I patients.

In the 17 type II patients, interictally, the EEGs showed background activity which was asymmetrical in seven, and absent or very slow in 10; delta waves which were localized in three, widespread in six and diffuse (or bilateral) in eight; spikes and/or spikewaves which were widespread in three and diffuse (bilateral) in 14; and, subclinical paroxysmal discharges, which were evident in all 17 and bilateral in 13. During seizures, the ictal discharge was widespread in 10 and multifocal and/or bilateral in six. Stereo-EEGs allowed identification of the origin of the ictus and it was noted that the end of the intracerebral discharge might not coincide with cessation of the muscle jerks.

Treatment

Since a localized cerebral lesion is usually under consideration, assessment for surgery and subsequent surgical management are the main therapeutic considerations. Bancaud (1985) reported in type I one patient cured by surgery and one whose seizures were reduced to rare localized nocturnal clonic jerks and in type II, four of the 17 patients had operations which were initially successful, but were followed by relapse after between 1 and 8 months.

Prognosis

The patients of Bancaud (1985) with type I Kojewnikow's syndrome did not deteriorate during 12 years of follow-up. Those with type II had evidence of a progressive disorder from the EEG and clinical and neuropsychological examinations.

Benign partial epilepsies

Following the report by Nayrac & Beaussart (1958) of a benign partial epilepsy with spike-wave discharges in the pre-Rolandic area, the various benign partial epilepsies of childhood have become increasingly well recognized. However, the first description of a benign focal epilepsy in childhood should probably be attributed to Rulandus, a sixteenth century medical author (Van Huffelen 1989). Benign partial epilepsy with centrotemporal spikes is the variety most commonly reported, but benign epilepsy with occipital paroxysms, benign partial epilepsy with affective symptoms and partial epilepsy with extreme somatosensory evoked potentials have also been described.

As a group, the benign partial epilepsies are characterized clinically by absence of neurological or intellectual deficits; a positive family history of epilepsy; onset of seizures after the age of 18 months; seizures which are brief, infrequent, respond readily to treatment, are variable in symptomatology, do not cause prolonged deficits in the postictal period; and absence of acquired neurological and psychological deficits throughout the evolution (Dalla Bernardina et al 1985a). The EEGs show normal background activity; normal sleep organization; focal abnormalities such as Rolandic spikes, or sharp waves which increase in frequency during sleep; possibly multifocal abnormalities; possibly brief bursts of generalized spike-wave discharges; and identical ictal patterns during waking and sleep.

A review of partial epilepsy in children who are normal on neurological examination has suggested that a recognizable syndrome can be identified in rather less than 50% even though the outcome may be benign (Deonna et al 1986b).

Benign partial epilepsy with centro-temporal spikes

Lerman (1985) has stated that 15–20% of young people with epilepsy have this form of epilepsy. Seizures usually start in the first decade and cease during the second decade. The age range at onset is 3–13 years with a peak at about 9 years. Males constitute 60% of cases. The incidence of previous febrile convulsions at 7–9% is about twice that in the general population. A close relationship between febrile seizures and benign epilepsy with centro-temporal spikes has been emphasized by Kajitani et al (1981). The children are normal both on neurological and psychological examination. There is a history of seizure disorders or epileptic discharges on the EEG in up to 40% of close relatives and autosomal dominant inheritance with age-dependent penetrance has been suggested (Lerman 1985).

Seizures. The seizures are usually infrequent, but can occur as often as many times per day, particularly at the onset. They may occur in clusters, and are usually brief, perhaps 2 minutes at the most. In about two-thirds of cases they occur only during sleep, in about one-sixth during sleep and in the awake state, and in the remaining one-sixth only while the child is awake.

The seizures are characterized by a somato-sensory onset with unilateral paraesthesias involving the tongue, lips, gums and inner cheeks; followed by unilateral tonic, clonic or tonic-clonic convulsions which involve the face, lips, tongue, pharynx and larynx and lead to speech arrest or anarthria and drooling. Consciousness is preserved. On occasion, the seizure may spread to the arm and more rarely the leg. Diurnal seizures never become generalized, but those occurring during sleep may do so. Prolonged intermittent

drooling and oromotor dyspraxia has been described in a single child who suffered from this syndrome (Roulet et al 1989).

Electroencephalography. Centro-temporal spikes which may be unifocal or bifocal are seen on the interictal EEG. The spikes are typically slow, diphasic and of high voltage. They may recur at short intervals, appear in clusters and be followed by a slow wave. In the 60% of patients where the spikes are unilateral, they are always synchronous in the central and mid-temporal areas. In some patients, occipital spikes occur in addition to, or rather than, centro-temporal discharges and in others generalized spike-wave abnormalities are recorded, but there appear to be no clinical accompaniments. The centro-temporal spikes increase with drowsiness and during sleep.

Treatment. Where seizures are infrequent and exclusively nocturnal, antiepileptic treatment is not essential, since the condition is self-limiting. If the seizures are frequent, especially if they occur during waking hours, they should be treated with carbamazepine or phenytoin, either of which usually produces a rapid remission.

Prognosis. Loiseau et al (1988) reported on 168 patients who had been followed for 7–30 years, and all of whom were over the age of 20 years; 165 of this group were seizure-free. Of these 2% had mild pyramidal difficulties and 17% had mildly reduced intelligence, learning difficulties, inattention, overactivity and/or emotional lability. Thus not all children maintain complete neurological and intellectual normality in the long-term. Sex, type and timing of the seizures and neurodevelopmental status were not important in predicting outcome. The frequency of the seizures was to some extent related to the duration of the period when seizures occurred, but not significantly so. The only independent predictor of the duration of the active period was age at onset with the earlier onset, the longer the duration when seizures were likely to occur ($P < 0.002$). If there have been prior febrile seizures, the centro-temporal spikes appear at 5.5 ± 2.7 years of age and disappear at 7.8 ± 2.9 years; but if there have been no febrile seizures, the spikes appear at 7.8 ± 2.8 years and disappear at 10.7 ± 3.7 years (Nakamuri & Kajitani 1983).

Benign epilepsy of childhood with occipital paroxysms

This epileptic syndrome has been characterized by Gastaut (1985) and Panayiotopoulos (1989). Males and females were equally affected in Gastaut's series, but other authors have found a female preponderance. The age of onset can be up to 17 years but peaks at 7 years. Up to one-third of the patients have a family history of epilepsy, and one-sixth of migraine. In one family not all who had the specific EEG changes suffered from seizures, and it was suggested that there is autosomal dominant inheritance of the EEG abnormalities with age-dependent expression and variable penetrance of the seizure disorder (Kuzniecky & Rosenblatt 1987). Febrile convulsions feature in the previous histories of 14% of cases. Neurological or cognitive abnormalities occur rarely.

Seizures. In keeping with the particular involvement of the occipital regions, there is a prominent, but not exclusive, visual component to the seizures. Gastaut (1985) has listed the visual ictal symptoms in decreasing order of frequency as:

— amaurosis, sometimes preceded by hemianopsia
— elementary visual hallucinations, i.e. phosphenes
— complex visual hallucinations
— visual illusions
— combinations of the individual visual symptoms.

Nonvisual symptoms which may follow the visual disturbances are: hemi-clonic seizures; complex partial seizures with automatisms; generalized tonic-clonic seizures; and, infrequently, other ictal manifestations such as dysaesthesia, adversive seizures, etc. If nocturnal seizures occur they are characterized by tonic deviation of the eyes and vomiting (Panayiotopoulos 1989). Following the seizures, diffuse headaches, occurring in about one-third of the patients, are accompanied by migraine-like nausea and vomiting in about half of those affected.

There are very wide variations in the seizure frequency from patient to patient. Attacks are precipitated in about a quarter of the patients by moving from a dark room to a brightly lit area or vice versa.

Electroencephalography. In interictal periods, the background activity is normal. Paroxysmal activity is characterized by spike-waves or, less frequently, sharp waves, of 200 to 300 μV amplitude, which are recorded over the occipital and posterotemporal regions of one hemisphere, or both hemispheres simultaneously or independently. The paroxysms occur in bursts or trains and are usually rhythmic at 1–3 Hz, but may be isolated and appear at irregular intervals. In almost all cases, the paroxysms disappear abruptly on eye opening and reappear within 1–20 seconds of eye closure. Hyperventilation and photic stimulation do not usually accentuate the abnormality and slow-wave sleep reinforces the changes in only a minority of cases (Gastaut 1985).

During seizures the occipital discharge has been recorded over one or both hemispheres.

Both Newton & Aicardi (1983) and Fois et al (1988) caution against the automatic assumption of a benign outcome if occipital paroxysms are found on EEG. In the series of Newton & Aicardi, 10 of 16 patients had learning difficulties, thus it might be argued that they did not suffer from this syndrome.

Treatment. No special study of the merits of particular antiepileptic drugs has been conducted for this condition. Carbamazepine, phenobarbitone, valproate or benzodiazepines are reported to control seizures in about 60% of the patients (Gastaut 1985).

Prognosis. The typical seizures associated with benign epilepsy of childhood with occipital paroxysms always disappear during adolecence. Other types of recurring seizures may present in adulthood in about 5% of cases (Gastaut 1985).

Benign partial epilepsy with affective symptoms

The cardinal feature of this epileptic syndrome is the presence of sudden fright or terror as the ictal phenomenon. In a study of 26 patients, Dalla Bernardina et al (1985b) found males and females to be equally affected. One-third had a family history of seizures and one-fifth had themselves had febrile convulsions of brief duration. The afebrile seizures had started between 2 and 9 years with an early peak up to 5 years and a later one between 6 and 9 years. All 6 patients had normal CT scans.

Seizures. The seizures are characterized by sudden fright or terror causing the child to rush to cling to the mother or any other person nearby. Chewing or swallowing movements; distressed laughter; arrest of speech with glottal noises, moans or salivation; or autonomic phenomena may accompany the periods of terror. Changes in awareness, but not total loss of consciousness, are usual. The seizures last for about 1–2 minutes and are not followed by any postictal deficit. Brief orofacial fits may occur nocturnally in a minority of the children, but tonic, clonic, tonic-clonic or atonic seizures do not occur. Seizures are often very frequent soon after the onset and oocur in the same form nocturnally as diurnally.

Electroencephalography. In all cases the background activity and sleep organization is normal. During interictal periods slow spikes/slow waves are consistently activated by sleep and are recorded from the fronto-temporal or parieto-temporal areas, either uni- or bilaterally. In some children brief bursts of generalized spike-waves are also recorded.

When the EEG is recorded during a seizure, the seizure discharges are usually clearly localized to the fronto-temporal, centro-temporal or parietal areas. Polygraphic studies show that, although movements of various sorts may occur during the seizures, they are never tonic or clonic.

Treatment. Carbamazepine is the treatment of choice, but phenobarbitone is probably equally effective in the control of the seizures.

Prognosis. Seizures are likely to remit during adolescence and there are no neurological or intellectual sequelae. Although behavioural difficulties can be a problem at times when the seizures are frequent, Dalla Bernardina et al (1985b) found that these resolved on remission of the epilepsy.

Benign partial epilepsy with extreme somatosensory evoked potentials

This epileptic syndrome has been described by Tassinari & De Marco (1985). Affected children pass through four distinct phases of the syndrome. Initially between the ages of 2.5–5.5 years, tapping of the feet during EEG recording produces extreme somatosensory potentials, manifest as spikes of up to 400 μV in amplitude. Later, spon-

taneous focal EEG abnormalities appear during sleep, followed by spontaneous focal EEG abnormalities when awake. The spontaneous abnormalities are strikingly similar to those evoked by foot-tapping. In the final stage, 5 months to 2 years after the appearance of these spontaneous focal discharges, and at ages between 4.5 and 8 years, clinical seizures appear. These are characterized by head and body version in most cases, but generalized tonic-clonic seizures are also observed. Almost half the patients have personal histories of 'simple' febrile convulsions. Neurological and psychological assessments are normal, as are the results of either arteriography or CT scanning. The response of seizures to antiepileptic drugs is unclear but remission is likely within 1 year.

Partial epilepsies with onset in infancy

Although the benign partial epilepsies characteristically have their onsets in middle to late childhood, there are reports that some simple and complex partial epilepsies which start in infancy can remit, and the outcome be generally good (Watanabe et al 1987, Dulac et al 1989, Dravet et al 1989, Oller-Daurella & Oller 1989). The records of patients attending specialized epilepsy clinics in three centres have been perused for children with the onset of partial seizures in the first 3 years of life (Dravet et al 1989, Dulac et al 1989, Oller-Daurella & Oller 1989). All three publications report remission in some patients.

Benign epilepsy of childhood with centro-temporal spikes and 'idiopathic' cases were described by Dravet et al (1989). Of a total of 442 patients who had their first seizure between 8 days and 3 years, Dulac et al (1989) identified 11 who started to have simple, complex or both simple and complex partial seizures between the ages of 15 and 34 months, and in whom the seizures remitted by 8 years. All 11 are reported to have normal mental development. Oller-Daurella & Oller (1989) examined the outlook in relation to the presenting seizure types and underlying causes. They found that where the initial seizures were partial and no cause was found, the prognosis was good; if the first seizure was hemiclonic and subsequent episodes were complex partial, epilepsy was likely to continue; if the initial attack was clonic or myoclonic there was a variable outcome; and the prognosis for remission from partial seizures was least good for children whose initial seizures had been tonic, atonic or generalized tonic-clonic. Nine infants with complex partial seizures were studied by Watanabe et al (1987). The seizures tended to occur in clusters and were characterized by motion arrest, decreased responsiveness and staring with blank eyes, often associated with simple automatisms. Control was easily achieved by either carbamazepine or phenobarbitone, and psychological development was normal. Thus partial seizures commencing in infancy can have a good outlook, but more detailed information is probably necessary before the delineation of a definite syndrome is justifiable.

Not all infants with cryptogenic partial seizures have a good prognosis. Dulac et al (1989) reported 120 cases in whom no cause could be found for partial seizures which persisted and were associated with mental retardation. These authors emphasized that if the age at onset was between 2 and 15 months, rather than later or earlier, the outlook for epilepsy with partial seizures due to unknown causes was poor.

MISCELLANEOUS SYNDROMES

Landau–Kleffner Syndrome

The syndrome of acquired aphasia with convulsive disorder was first described over 30 years ago (Landau & Kleffner 1957). It has been more recently defined as a childhood condition in which acquired aphasia is associated with EEG findings of multifocal spikes and spike-wave discharges, which are not stable in the course of the evolution of the disorder (Beaumanoir 1985b).

Incidence

No incidence figures are available, but males are more commonly affected than females.

Seizures

Seizures are observed clinically in about 70% of cases. They may be single and then tend to present between 5 and 10 years of age. If recurrent, the onset is rather earlier at 4–6 years. Generalized or partial convulsive and non-convulsive seizures may occur. Tonic attacks have been reported (Deonna et al 1987). Complex partial seizures are rare. A single episode of status epilepticus is recorded in a small percentage of the cases (Beaumanoir 1985b).

Differential diagnosis

In the absence of clinical seizures, the acquired aphasia may be confused with elective mutism, deafness or autism. Disorders associated with organic dementia should be excluded.

Aetiology

No cause has been identified. A pre-existing language disorder has been reported in 10% of cases. There is a positive family history of epilepsy in 12% of all cases, and in only 5% of the 30% in whom clinical seizures do not occur (Beaumanoir 1985b). No pathological studies are available for the whole brain, and biopsies have provided miscellaneous results.

Clinical features

The most striking clinical features relate to the language disorder. Initially there is an auditory verbal agnosia which may embrace familiar noises. As a consequence there is inability to attribute semantic value to acoustic signals. Spontaneous verbal expression is reduced and sometimes abolished. There may be stereotypies, perseverations or paraphrasias. Spontaneous speech can be monotonous, interrupted by pauses and hesitations and lacking in intonation and stress (Deonna et al 1987). Overactive behaviour and unspecified personality disorders are common, as are developmental problems other than those associated with language (Beaumanoir 1985b) .

Investigation

Investigations other than EEG are not consistently helpful. CT scans are normal. It is possible that PET and SPECT scans might be of interest, but reports are awaited.

Electroencephalography. There are no EEG changes which are specific to this syndrome. The background activity is usually normal, with superadded repetitive spikes and spike-waves of high amplitude, organized in foci which are variable in space and time. On the conventional EEG the foci are most often found in the temporal or parieto-occipital regions (Beaumanoir 1985b). Spectral mapping of the EEG has shown high powers of delta, theta and alpha frequencies over the fronto-centro-parietal areas, with variable positioning and modes of propagation of accompanying sharp waves and spikes (Nakano et al 1989).

Treatment

So far as the epilepsy is concerned, therapy is not a major problem. Carbamazepine, valporate and various benzodiazepines have been used with effect. It is not known whether complete normalization of the EEG is necessary for return of language function. The language disorder is more difficult to treat. There are recent suggestions that early treatment with corticosteroids in high dosage could be helpful for both the language and the seizure disorder (Marescaux et al 1990). Early intervention with the use of signing to compensate for lack of oral communication is advocated.

Prognosis

Seizures. The epilepsy tends to remit by the second decade, and the EEG is usually normal by 15 years of age (Beaumanoir 1985b).

Cognitive aspects. For many, there are continuing problems with language. Deonna et al (1989) have followed seven cases into adulthood. All have continuing problems. None is able to use written language in a functional manner. Two of the seven had made good recoveries in spoken language, one had normal comprehension, but severe expressive language problems, and the remaining four had absence of language comprehension and lack of expressive speech. Only one of these four was able to use sign language effectively.

Behaviour/social problems. The difficulties with language cause considerable problems with behaviour and social integration. Disorders of personality, which have not been further specified, are reputedly common.

Epilepsy with continuous spike-waves during slow wave sleep

The alternative term for this syndrome is electrical status epilepticus during slow sleep (ESES). The essential component is that spike-waves are recorded on the EEG during no less than 85% of the time of slow wave sleep (Tassinari et al 1985). The incidence is unknown, and the sex ratio, for the small number of reported cases, equal. There is no evidence for a strong genetic input.

Seizures

The epilepsy can start at any time during childhood (Tassinari et al 1985, Morikawa et al 1985). The initial seizures may be unilateral or generalized motor, myoclonic, absence or motor involving the facial muscles with trismus and loss of consciousness. In half the patients the initial seizure occurs during sleep. It is possible to classify the patients on the basis of seizures. Some patients have only motor seizures throughout the time that ESES is recorded. The attacks are infrequent and remit in early adolescence. In those patients where absences appear at the time of discovery of ESES, and whose previous seizures have been unilateral motor or generalized tonic-clonic in nature and in the children in whom rare nocturnal seizures and atypical absences are associated with ESES, remission is likely by the age of 16 years.

Differential diagnosis

On the whole the seizures which occur are recognizable as epilepsy, but some take less usual forms and might initially be confused with pseudo-seizures. Other types of sleep disorders come into the differential diagnosis.

Investigation

Electroencephalography. Before ESES begins the EEG shows, in most cases, fronto-temporal or centro-temporal seizure discharges. In a minority, spike-waves are more or less generalized. During

ESES the interictal pattern while waking is much the same as before ESES, but as soon as the child enters slow wave sleep continuous bilateral and diffuse slow spike-waves are recorded, and they persist throughout this stage of sleep. During rapid eye movement sleep the electrical status disappears (Tassinari et al 1985).

Treatment

No treatment has been found completely effective in abolishing ESES. Benzodiazepines can give temporary relief only, and other antiepileptic drugs rarely make any impact.

Prognosis

Seizures. ESES itself remits roundabout puberty. Clinical seizures also disappear in some patients (Morikawa et al 1985).
Neurological handicap. Neurological abnormalities of varying severity can pre-date ESES. New physical handicaps do not occur as a result.
Cognitive aspects. Intellectual deterioration is a constant feature of ESES. Morikawa et al (1985) measured the intelligence quotients of children before, during and after ESES, and recorded falls in IQ of as much as 56 points. Since the electrical status occurs only during sleep, it must be concluded that the seizure discharges are themselves damaging. Language function may be particularly affected (Tassinari et al 1985).
Behaviour problems. Difficulty with social integration is another invariable complication of ESES. Where it is possible to set a time to the onset of ESES, behaviour problems are recorded as starting simultaneously (Morikawa et al 1985). Reduced attention span, overactivity aggressiveness and occasional psychosis have been reported (Tassinari et al 1985).

COGNITIVE FUNCTIONING

Cognitive functioning has been related to each epileptic syndrome described earlier in this chapter, so far as this is possible. Learning abilities in children with epilepsy can be considered under the following headings:

1. Underlying aetiological features

2. Seizure type or epileptic syndrome
3. Duration of 'active' epilepsy
4. Therapy.

The overall incidence of mental handicap in children with epilepsy is about 20% (Gudmundsson 1966).

Underlying aetiological features

Epilepsy is reported in 44% of 1000 mentally retarded patients assessed by Iivanainen (1990). When the presumed cause was prenatal, 35% of retarded patients had epilepsy and when due to peri- or postnatal or multiple causes, over 50% were affected. Clearly where epilepsy is symptomatic of recognizable brain abnormalities, such as occur in major malformations, tuberous sclerosis or following severe head injuries, associated cognitive disabilities are to be expected. However, even when overt structural abnormalities are not identified children with epilepsy perform less well on intelligence tests than age-matched controls. Farwell et al (1985) found that only in those with absence epilepsy was intelligence as high as expected. In particular, children with 'minor motor' or 'atypical absence' seizures are likely to be of low ability (Farwell et al 1985). These seizures are often symptomatic of prenatal abnormalities such as migrational disorders and both seizures and intellectual problems are likely to have a common origin.

Underlying aetiological determinants for the epilepsy are the most important factors in the intellectual abilities of the child with epilepsy.

Effects of seizure type or epileptic syndrome

Generalized epilepsies

Mental retardation is almost invariable in West syndrome, Lennox–Gastaut syndrome and epilepsy with myoclonic absences, and is constant in early myoclonic encephalopathy and early infantile epileptic encephalopathy. In all of these syndromes, regression and/or arrest of learning skills can occur. Developmental delay can complicate myoclonic-astatic epilepsy, but is unusual in benign familial and non-familial neonatal convulsions, benign myoclonic epilepsy in infants, childhood and juvenile absence epilepsies, juvenile myoclonic epilepsy and epilepsy with grand mal on awakening.

Studies in absence epilepsy have demonstrated that a generalized seizure discharge which lasts for at least 3 seconds is invariably associated with loss of awareness (Goode et al 1970). Despite the frequency of absences, often more than 100 per day, the majority of which are likely to cause interruptions in consciousness, the one group of children with epilepsy who are likely to be of good ability are those with absences (Farwell et al 1985). Thus neither repetitive short generalized epileptic discharges nor frequent lapses in awareness are necessarily associated with diminished intelligence.

On the other hand generalized convulsive status epilepticus can be followed by permanent cognitive deficits. Factors other than seizure discharge may be responsible for alterations in cerebral metabolism secondary to convulsive status, and the roles of hypoxia, hypotension and/or hypoglycaemia can then be difficult to separate from those of the epilepsy itself. In most of the generalized epilepsies where development arrests or regresses there is EEG evidence of almost continuous seizure discharges, and adverse effects of accumulations of excitotoxic amino acids could be postulated as responsible for the cognitive problems. There remains, however, difficulty with an explanation for the cognitive impairment which becomes apparent in epilepsy with myoclonic absences. In this condition, the absences are no more frequent that those in childhood absence epilepsy and the EEG findings are indistinguishable. If the absences are myoclonic, they are much less readily controlled by antiepileptic drugs and are thus likely to persist as a frequent daily problem; but, in typical absence epilepsy even those who as a result of poor compliance do not receive therapy, do not develop long-term cognitive problems.

As a whole, children with epilepsy tend to do less well in academic subjects than children with comparable intelligence (Seidenberg et al 1986). Specific difficulties with both arithmetic and reading have been described. In patients who have generalized seizure discharges without obvious clinical signs transient cognitive impairment has been demonstrated more readily when spatial rather than verbal tasks are presented (Binnie et al 1987). Thus subclinical events could be important in determining the educational outcome. A recent study of reading ability in adolescents with epilepsy has shown that, compared with controls matched for abilities by their schoolteachers, those with epilepsy have comparable scores for accuracy and rate, but comprehend the reading material significantly less well (Clement & Wallace 1990). In this study, the numbers with individual seizure types are very small. Nevertheless, those with absences had better scores than adolescents with generalized tonic-clonic seizures, whether primary or secondary generalized; and those with myoclonic seizures performed particularly poorly. Reductions in arithmetic scores, most marked in children with generalized seizures, are significantly related to the lifetime seizure frequency (Seidenberg et al 1986). The particular problems with arithmetic in children with generalized seizures no doubt correlate with the preferential interference with spatial tasks found in association with generalized discharges (Binnie et al 1987). Children with epilepsy who are of average intelligence make more spelling errors than would be expected (Seidenberg et al 1986, Jennekens-Schinkel et al 1987). This problem does not appear to be related to specific seizure types.

Partial epilepsies

Two major categories of the partial epilepsies should be considered: those in which a structural change can be defined and those considered benign. However, in studies of cognitive functioning in patients with focal epileptiform discharges on the EEG, the distinction between these categories has not always been made. The overall intelligence has been found to be significantly lower in children with partial as compared with generalized epilepsies (Bourgeois et al 1983), but, by definition, children with benign partial epilepsies are of normal intelligence. In a survey of adolescents with epilepsy, those with complex partial seizures had higher scores for reading rate, accuracy and comprehension than those whose seizures were generalized, whether primary or secondary (Clement & Wallace 1990). Thus the heterogeneity of patients with partial epilepsies can make statements on the group as a whole meaningless.

There have been a number of reports on the influences of the lateralization of epileptic foci on specific abilities (Ounsted et al 1966, Piccirilli et al 1988, Binnie et al 1987, Aldenkamp et al 1990, Stores & Hart 1976, Camfield et al 1984, Kasteleijn-Nolst Trenité 1990a, l990b, Aarts et al 1984). When attainments are examined interictally, in a purely clinical sense, reduced verbal abilities in children with left temporal lobe involvement and reduced visuospatial abilities in those with right-sided lesions have been reported (Ounsted et al 1966). On the other hand cognitive testing in children with pure right- compared with pure left-sided temporal EEG foci failed to demonstrate significant differences (Camfield et al 1984). Although academic attainment does not necessarily relate to the site of an EEG focus (Seidenberg et al 1986), and spelling performance could not be correlated with hand preference or the laterality of epileptic activity (Jennekens-Schinkel et al 1987), boys with left hemisphere foci are reported to have a particular tendency to specific reading difficulty (Stores & Hart 1976) and temporal lobe epilepsy seems to definitely be associated with memory deficits (Aldenkamp et al 1990). Piccirilli et al (1988) have provided evidence for lateralization of language mechanisms in the right hemisphere of children with benign partial epilepsies who have left-sided unilateral foci. Thus some of the apparently contradictory data on effects of or associations with lateralized epilepsies may be explained on the basis of cerebral plasticity.

The role of transient cognitive impairment in test results for patients with lateralized seizure discharges has been examined (Aarts et al 1984, Binnie et al 1987, Siebelink et al 1988, Kasteleijn-Nolst Trenité et al 1988, 1990a, b). All these studies show that when spike discharges occur in the left hemisphere there is impairment of performance on verbal tasks as compared with testing in the same patient when spikes are not occurring. Right-sided discharges temporarily impair visuo-spatial tasks (Kasteleijn-Nolst Trenité et al l990a, Binnie et al 1987). Not all discharges interfered with performance of the tasks. Impairment of

visuo-spatial abilities was noted in 50% of sessions in which right-sided discharges occurred (Kasteleijn-Nolst Trenité et al l990a). The effects of subclinical seizure activity on reading and arithmetic were examined by Kasteleijn-Nolst Trenité et al (1990b). Children with left-sided discharges were 2 years, and those with right-sided discharges 1 year, below their expected levels for reading while both groups were approximately 1 year behind in arithmetic. During reading, epileptic discharges in the left hemisphere became relatively less frequent and of shorter duration, when compared with findings from the right hemisphere. These results are considered compatible with the suggestion that cognitive tasks suppress discharges when they activate a part of the brain within the epileptogenic zone; and tend to accentuate discharges from other epileptogenic areas, when these are not directly involved in the tasks (Kasteleijn-Nolst Trenité et al l990b). Although the role of spike discharges in test results is becoming clearer, it remains uncertain whether elimination of the discharges by drugs would improve cognitive functioning.

Duration of 'active' epilepsy

'Active' epilepsy can be defined as a continued tendency to seizures. The early onset of epilepsy is generally considered a poor prognostic factor for cognitive development. This is to some extent explained by survival of infants with severe epileptic syndromes such West syndrome. In a study of 118 children with epilepsy aged 6–15 years Farwell et al (1985) found that the years during which seizures occurred correlated inversely with the IQ ($P<0.0001$). The performance quotient has been reported to be particularly depressed when seizures are poorly controlled (Rodin et al 1986). If generalized seizures start early in life, the later intelligence is lower than if the early seizures are partial (O'Leary et al 1983).

The suggestion that intellectual deterioration is inevitable with prolonged periods of 'active' epilepsy has been challenged by Aldenkamp et al (1990). Forty-five children were retested over a 3-year period during which seizure frequency was high. The same strengths and weaknesses were found in the subtest profiles of the Wechsler

Intelligence Scale for Children (WISC-R), on all three occasions. Nevertheless, Besag (1988) has been able to identify from a population in a special school for epilepsy a small sub-group of children in whom intellectual arrest, rather than deterioration, occurred. No definite predictive features for arrest are reported, but all had severe epilepsy and one of the children suffered a prolonged episode of status epilepticus. Bourgeois et al (1983) found a fall in IQ was most likely to occur if the onset of epilepsy had been early.

Therapy and cognitive functioning

Drug treatment

Lack of appreciation of the close aetiological relationship of intellectual functioning to epilepsy has tended to over-emphasize possible deleterious effects of drug treatment in childhood seizure disorders. Many studies have failed to assess the children before therapy begins. So far as the literature allows, the possible effects of individual antiepileptic drugs are examined.

Phenobarbitone. Most of the studies on phenobarbitone have been conducted in children with febrile seizures. Camfield et al (1979) in a double-blind, placebo-controlled trial found phenobarbitone, given over a 12-month period, was not associated with reduction in scores on any of the five Stanford-Binet subscales. There was, however, a significant negative correlation between the serum levels of phenobarbitone and the memory concentration subscores ($P<0.05$). In a comparison with untreated children, phenobarbitone given over a 2-year period did not cause significant changes in development as measured by the Griffiths scales (Aldridge Smith & Wallace 1982). On the other hand, using data from the NCPP, Farwell et al (1990) concluded that phenobarbitone had deleterious effects on cognitive development if really strenuous efforts were made to find them, and highly sophisticated statistical methods were used in the analysis. Thus, since phenobarbitone is a sedative drug, although adverse effects might be expected, there is little hard evidence that they occur.

Phenytoin. There is only one study of the cognitive abilities of a cohort of children tested before being placed on phenytoin monotherapy and re-tested after some months or years of treatment (Nolte et al 1980). High serum levels of phenytoin were associated with deteriorations in intelligence scores, whereas children with low serum levels were indistinguishable from healthy controls. Cognitive function improved after phenytoin was withdrawn in the groups with both high and low serum levels. Other more indirect evidence for interference with cognitive functioning by phenytoin is available. Significantly, inferior reading skills have been reported in children prescribed phenytoin when compared with those on other antiepileptic drugs (Stores & Hart 1976). However, the same authors found that focal left-sided seizure discharges were also associated with poor reading and no attempt was made to distinguish between the relative contributions of the seizure discharges and phenytoin. In children on multiple drugs, high serum phenytoin levels have been found to be associated with intellectual deterioration, but the exact role of the phenytoin remains problematical (Trimble & Corbett 1980).

Valproate. Forty-six children aged 4–15 years (mean 9 years) were investigated using a very comprehensive battery of tests before and during treatment with either high- or low-dose valproate (Aman et al 1987). No consistent effects on cognitive tests were demonstrated. In children treated with valproate for febrile seizures, developmental quotients after 2 years were comparable with those who received no drugs (Aldridge Smith & Wallace 1982). Thus there is no evidence that valproate when used as monotherapy interferes with cognitive development.

Carbamazepine. Virtually all reports on carbamazepine suggest that it is devoid of adverse effects on cognition. In a study of the effects of carbamazepine in relation to serum concentrations and times of medication a very extensive battery of tests was used (Aman et al 1990). At peak concentrations the children were significantly improved in attention span, motor steadiness and general restlessness as measured by seat movements. It was concluded that carbamazepine in normal dosage does not impair cognitive functioning and might lead to some improvement. In children already receiving carbamazepine motor performance tends to be faster than that found in controls, but accuracy is reduced (Blennow et al 1990).

Ethosuximide. Since ethosuximide is used almost exclusively for typical absence seizures, underlying cognitive impairment is unusual. Treatment of absences with ethosuximide has been reported to improve psychological scores in 50% of patients (Browne et al 1975), but it is not clear whether abolition of the absences was the factor most important in the improvement.

Benzodiazepines. As a rule benzodiazepines are used only for seizures which are persistently resistant to other drugs. The children with such severe epilepsy very often have underlying cognitive deficits and the effects of drugs are difficult to gauge. Drowsiness and difficulties with short-term memory are common in patients treated with benzodiazepines.

Vigabatrin. Studies of possible effects of vigabatrin on cognitive development in children have yet to be reported.

Surgery

Children who are considered for surgery to localized epileptogenic lesions usually have a high seizure frequency. Improvement in cognitive functioning is often reported to parallel postoperative relief of seizures (Lindsay et al 1987, Duchowny 1989, Mizrahi et al 1990). However, systematic scientific studies are still needed, particularly in relation to surgery performed at a very early age (Luders et al 1989, Taylor 1990).

Testing cognitive skills in children with epilepsy

Recognition of difficulties with attention (Stores 1973, Aman et al 1990) and of episodes of transient cognitive impairment (Kasteleijn-Nolst Trenité et al 1988, 1990a, b) has led to suggestions that the cognitive skills of children with epilepsy can easily be underestimated. Thus, although most reports use tests applicable to any children of the age range to be investigated, it has been suggested that computer-aided testing can emphasize particular difficulties in those with epilepsy (Alpherts & Aldenkamp 1990, Rugland 1990).

The neuropsychological assessment of cogni-

tive functioning has been reviewed by Rugland (1990). She points out that the Halstead–Reitan battery of sub-tests is unrelated to educational level, and the more difficult parts of the battery are insensitive to focal or lateralized brain pathology. The Luria–Nebraska battery of neuropsychiatric tests is criticized on the grounds of subjectivity and lack of norms, and the Wechsler Intelligence Scale for Children for its rather narrow emphasis on intelligence. In keeping with the failure of any one battery to give an overall picture, Rugland (1990) comments that experienced neuropsychologists tend to choose tests from several sources, with the result that procedural changes produce inconsistent findings. Rugland (1990) describes the computerized test battery which she has devised for routine use. It includes tests of simple reaction time, choice reaction time, verbal and spatial memory, and verbal and figurative problem-solving. During testing the computer is connected to the EEG machine and the results can be related to the presence or absence of epileptic discharges during testing.

The results of assessment of children with epilepsy aged 8–18 years with IQ levels of above 85, using a computerized system are presented by Alpherts & Aldenkamp (1990).

The battery consisted of measurement of simple reaction time, binary choice reaction time, a tapping task, a computerized visual searching task and a recognition task. The testing is correlated with a simultaneously-recorded EEG. Even the younger children were found to have no difficulties in handling the keyboard. Alpherts & Aldenkamp (1990) comment that their system could be extended to include assessment during recordings from depth or surface electrodes, and note that the development of voice, and language, recognition systems should be possible in future.

Educational placement

The best school placement for the child with epilepsy is that which provides education at a level appropriate for intelligence, while recognizing that specific difficulties with reading and arithmetic may be present in children of good all-round ability. It is important that teachers have a basic understanding of the varieties of seizure types, and their management. All too often excessive restrictions are imposed on children whose seizures are well-controlled, leading to the stunting of social and emotional growth. In addition, teachers should recognize that difficulties with academic subjects are much more likely to be secondary to inherent problems than to effects of medication.

SOCIAL ASPECTS

Much of the social adjustment of the child with epilepsy depends on the attitudes of parents, other relatives, school-teachers, youth-leaders and other adults with whom close contact is made. Nevertheless, there are features of the child which can dictate social incompetence. So far as it is possible associated behaviour problems have been identified for each of the epileptic syndromes described earlier in this chapter. For many children with learning difficulties, failure to learn to behave in a socially acceptable manner is but one facet of their overall problems.

The association of catastrophic rage outbursts with temporal lobe epilepsy has been highlighted by Ounsted et al (1966, 1987). In a study of social integration in adolescents with epilepsy, factors other than the epilepsy were shown to be common determinants of poor peer-group interaction (Freeman et al 1984). In fact epilepsy was never cited by the parents as the main cause of a specific problem.

Mental handicap is present in approximately one-fifth of children with epilepsy (Gudmundsson 1966). In many cases, particularly in the younger children where the prognosis for long-term survival is poor, the handicap is severe or very severe. For these children, personal social integration is always at a very simple level, and the child's family as a whole is likely to suffer as a consequence. Kitamoto et al (1988) found that if children with epilepsy had neurological or mental abnormalities the fathers were rejecting and the mothers anxious and doting. The mothers' reactions were particularly intense if the children were over the age of 12 years and still having seizures.

Many parents think that their child has died when the first seizure occurs (Ward & Bower 1978, Clare et al 1978). The cessation of respiration and loss of consciousness cause particular anxiety, while accompanying noises, salivation, twisting, jerking and eye-rolling also provoke fear (Ward & Bower 1978). In children with benign partial epilepsy with affective symptoms the seizure is associated with extreme fear, and this is frequently transferred to observers. Parents of children who have nocturnal seizures of frontal lobe origin find the penetrating cry at the onset of the attack very disturbing.

At the onset of epilepsy the parents, having found the initial seizure very frightening, may try to deny its occurrence (Hoare & Kerley 1988). They develop fears of intellectual and behavioural deterioration; and worry that there may be a serious aetiological cause such as a tumour. Once medication is introduced, there is a need for realization that the condition is unlikely to remit spontaneously, at least in the short-term; concerns about side-effects of drugs arise; and there are worries about over-dependency on the fate of the child (Hoare & Kerley 1988). Adjustment to the diagnosis of epilepsy takes time and discussions of the implications in terms of educational and social abilities or problems should not be ignored.

Scambler (1990) suggests that children's understanding of epilepsy is related to the explanations and behaviour of teachers and parents. He comments that parents can act as 'stigma coaches' by training their children to feel ashamed and apprehensive about epilepsy, thus producing secrecy by advice or example. Secondary effects of over-protection and denial by the parents may be anger and resentment in their children, with the subsequent development of behavioural and personality problems.

The development of personality has been examined in adolescents with epilepsy by Viberg et al (1987). Most of the patients denied problems related to epilepsy, but regarded their seizures as frightening both for themselves and their relatives, and were not willing to discuss them with their classmates. Compared with controls, the adolescents with epilepsy had poor body and self-images, were more threatened by the unknown and the risk of acting out, had less stable sex identity, and their defence mechanisms were dominated by flight, with poor capacity for adaptation. These features were not influenced by seizure type or control, or by age at onset.

The need for a wider approach to childhood epilepsy than purely control of seizures is emphasized (Hoare & Kerley 1988, Viberg et al 1987, Scambler 1990, Freeman et al 1984, Lewis et al 1990). The involvement of a social worker who could help families come to terms with the diagnosis of epilepsy is advocated by Hoare & Kerley (1988). Scambler (1990) suggests that the physician should encourage co-participation of the parents in all aspects of care; accept an open agenda during physician–patient contacts; use a holistic, rather than biomedical orientation to care; and be prepared to develop counselling skills. A programme designed to enhance the competence of children with epilepsy has been subjected to a randomized trial (Lewis et al 1990). An experimental group of patients were given four sessions with instruction in understanding body messages; controlling seizures with medication; telling others in a matter-of-fact manner; and coping and adapting to balanced life. The control group, who also had epilepsy, were given lectures and question-and-answer sessions. The experimental group gained very significantly in knowledge, behaved significantly better and reported self-perceived improvements in knowledge and social skills; and an increase in normal activities. Lewis et al (1990) concluded that a tailor-made programme is more effective than question and answer sessions.

Remediation through a school-based programme has been demonstrated to be very effective (Freeman et al 1984). A total of 333 adolescents were identified; of these the parents reported behaviour difficulties in 35%, lack of friends 29%, difficulties with peer/sibling relationships 18%, poor parent/child interaction 2%, lack of motivation 13%, lack of self-confidence 14%, psychological problems 17% and substance abuse 6%. The children's teachers felt that for 63% seizures did not interfere with normal activities. A further 13% improved after entry into the programme, leaving 24% in whom normal activities were not possible. However only 16% of the cohort had problems exclusively related to their seizures. Epilepsy and psychosocial difficulties and psychosocial difficulties alone were important determinants of social competence. The remediation programme included intervention in classroom placement and participation in vocational training courses. The employment outcome was much better for children who had been in the programme than for non-epileptic children of similar social backgrounds.

The importance of comprehensive management of the child with epilepsy has been emphasized by Munthe-Kaas (1990). He uses the term habilitation, which underlines the need for anticipation of problems, rather than remediation after they have arisen. Cooperation between members of the professions (e.g. medicine, nursing, psychology, psychiatry, social work) and education is vital if the child is to derive maximum benefit.

REFERENCES

Aarts J H P, Binnie C D, Smit A M, Wilkins A J 1984 Selective cognitive impairment during focal and generalized epileptiform EEG activity. Brain 107: 293–308

Aicardi J 1985 Epileptic seizures in inborn errors of metabolism. In: Roger J, Dravet C, Bureau M, Dreifuss F E, Wolf P (eds) Epileptic syndromes in infancy, childhood and adolescence. John Libbey Eurotext, London, p 73–77

Aicardi J 1990 Neonatal myoclonic encephalopathy and early infantile epileptic encephalopathy. In: Wasterlain C G, Vert P (eds) Neonatal seizures. Raven Press, New York, p 41–49

Aicardi J, Gomes A L 1988 The Lennox–Gastaut Syndrome: clinical and electrographic features. In: Niedermeyer E, Degen R (eds) The Lennox–Gastaut Syndrome. Alan R Liss, New York, p 25–46

Albani M 1983 Phenytoin in infancy and childhood. In: Delgado-Escueta A V, Wasterlain C G, Treiman D M, Porter R J (eds) Advances in Neurology, vol 34: Status epilepticus. Raven Press, New York, p 457–464

Aldenkamp A P, Alpherts W C J, Dekker M J A, Overweg J 1990 Neuropsychological aspects of learning disabilities in epilepsy. Epilepsia 31 (suppl 4): S9–S20

Aldridge Smith J, Wallace S J 1982 Febrile convulsions: Intellectual progress in relation to anticonvulsant therapy and to recurrence of fits. Archives of Disease in Childhood 57: 104–107

Alpherts W C J, Aldenkamp A P 1990 Computerized neuropsychological assessment of cognitive functioning in children with epilepsy. Epilepsia 31(suppl 14): S35–S40

Alving J 1979 Classification of the epilepsies. An investigation of 402 children. Acta Neurologica Scandinavica 60: 157–163

Aman M G, Merry J S, Paxton J W, Turbott S H 1987 Effect of sodium valproate on psychomotor performance in children as a function of dose, fluctuations in concentration, and diagnosis. Epilepsia 28: 115–124

Aman M G, Merry J S, Paxton J W 1990 Effects of carbamazepine on psychomotor performance in children as a function of drug concentration, seizure type, and time of medication. Epilepsia 31: 51–60

Andermann F, Olivier A, Gotman J, Sergent J 1988 Callosotomy for the treatment of patients with intractable epilepsy and the Lennox–Gastaut Syndrome. In: Niedermeyer E, Degen R (eds) The Lennox–Gastaut Syndrome. Alan R Liss, New York, p 361–376

Andersen A R 1990 Single proton and positron emission computerized tomography in infants and young adults with epilepsy. In: Sillanpäa M, Johanessen S I, Blennow G, Dam M (eds) Paediatric epilepsy. Wrightson Biomedical Publishing, Petersfield, p 195–204

André M, Boutroy M J, Dubruc C et al 1986 Clonazepam pharmacokinetics and therapeutic efficacy in neonatal seizures. European Journal of Clinical Pharmacology 30: 585–589

André M, Matisse N, Verte P, Debruille Ch 1988 Neonatal seizures—recent aspects. Neuropediatrics 19: 201–207

Annegers J F, Grabow J D, Grover R V et al 1980 Seizures after head trauma: a population study. Neurology 30: 683–689

Annegers J F, Hauser W A, Shirts S B, Kurland L T 1987 Factors prognostic of unprovoked seizures after febrile convulsions. New England Journal of Medicine 316: 493–498

Ariizumi M, Baba K, Hibio S et al 1987 Immunoglobulin therapy in the West syndrome. Brain and Development 9: 422–425

Armstrong D L, Grossman R G, Zhu Z 1987 Complex partial epilepsy; evidence of a malformative process in the resected anterior temporal lobes of thirty-three patients. Journal of Neuropathology and Experimental Neurology 46: 359

Arpino C, Gattinara G C, Piergili D, Curatolo P 1990 Toxocara infection and epilepsy in children: a case-control study. Epilepsia 31: 33–36

Asconapé J, Penry J K 1984 Some clinical and EEG aspects of benign juvenile myoclonic epilepsy. Epilepsia 25: 108–114

Aso K, Scher M S, Barmada M A 1990 Cerebral infarcts and seizures in the neonate. Journal of Child Neurology 5: 224–228

Aukett A, Bennett M J, Hosking G P 1988 Molybdenum co-factor deficiency: an easily missed inborn error of metabolism. Developmental Medicine and Child Neurology 30: 531–535

Aziz S S, Wallace S J, Murphy J F, Sainsbury C P Q, Gray O P 1986 Cotside EEG monitoring using computerized spectral analysis. Archives of Disease in Childhood 61: 242–246

Bader G G, Witt-Engerström I, Hagberg B 1989 Neurophysiological findings in the Rett syndrome. 1: EMG, conduction velocity, EEG and somatosensory evoked potential studies. Brain and Development 11: 102–109

Baldy-Moulinier M, Touchon J, Billiard M et al 1988 Nocturnal sleep studies in the Lennox–Gastaut syndrome. In: Niedermeyer E, Degen R (eds) The Lennox–Gastaut Syndrome. Alan R Liss, New York, p 243–260

Ballard R A, Vinocur B, Reynolds J W et al 1978 Transient hyperammonemia of the pre-term infant. New England Journal of Medicine 299: 920–925

Bancaud J 1985 Kojewnikow's syndrome (epilepsia partialis continua) in children. In: Roger J, Dravet C, Bureau M, Dreifuss F E, Wolf P (eds). Epileptic syndromes in infancy,

childhood and adolescence. John Libbey Eurotext, London, p 286–298

Barth P G 1987 Disorders of neuronal migration. Canadian Journal of Neurological Sciences 14: 1–16

Bauer G, Benke T, Bohr K 1988 The Lennox–Gastaut syndrome in adulthood. In: Niedermeyer E, Degen R (eds) The Lennox–Gastaut Syndrome. Alan R Liss, New York, p 317–327

Beaumanoir A 1985a The Lennox–Gastaut syndrome. In: Roger J, Dravet C, Bureau M, Dreifuss F E, Wolf P (eds) Epileptic syndromes in infancy, childhood and adolescence. John Libbey Eurotext, London, p 89–99

Beaumanoir A 1985b The Landau–Kleffner syndrome. In: Roger J, Dravet C, Bureau M, Dreifuss F E, Wolf P (eds) Epileptic syndromes in infancy, childhood and adolescence. John Libbey Eurotext, London, p 181–191

Bellman M H 1983 Infantile spasms. In: Pedley T A, Meldrum B S (eds) Recent advances in epilepsy, 1. Churchill Livingstone, Edinburgh, p 113–138

Benardo L S, Pedley T A 1985 Cellular mechanisms of focal epileptogenesis In: Pedley T A, Meldrum B S (eds) Recent advances in epilepsy, 2. Churchill Livingstone, Edinburgh, p 1–18

Berg A T, Shinnar S, Hauser W A, Leventhal J M 1990 Predictors of recurrent febrile seizures: a meta-analytic review. Journal of Paediatrics 116: 329–337

Bergman I, Painter M J, Hirsch R P et al 1983 Outcome of neonates with convulsions treated in an intensive care unit. Annals of Neurology 14: 642–647

Berkovic S F, Andermann F 1986 The progressive myoclonus epilepsies. In Pedley T A, Meldrum B S (eds) Recent advances in epilepsy, 3. Churchill Livingstone, Edinburgh, p 157–187

Besag F M C 1988 Cognitive deterioration in children with epilepsy. In: Trimble M R, Reynolds E H (eds) Epilepsy, behaviour and cognitive function. Wiley, Chichester, p 113–127

Binnie C D, Kasteleijn-Nolst Trenité D G A, Smit A M, Wilkins A J 1987 Interactions of epileptiform EEG discharges and cognition. Epilepsy Research 1: 239–245

Bird T D 1987 Genetic considerations in childhood epilepsy. Epilepsia 28 (suppl): S71–S81

Blennow G, Starck L 1986 High dose B_6 treatment in infantile spasms. Neuropediatrics 17: 7–10

Blennow G, Heijbel J, Sandstedt P, Tonnby B 1990 Discontinuation of antiepileptic drugs in children who have outgrown epilepsy: Effects on cognitive function. Epilepsia 31 (suppl) S50–S53

Bleyer W A, Marshall R E 1972 Barbiturate withdrawal syndrome in a passively addicted infant. Journal of the American Medical Association 221: 185–186

Blume W T 1988 The EEG features of the Lennox–Gastaut syndrome. In Niedermeyer E, Degen R (eds) The Lennox–Gastaut Syndrome. Alan R Liss, New York, p 159–176

Bodensteiner J B, Brownsworth R D, Knapik J R et al 1988 Interobserver variability in the ILAE classification of seizures in childhood. Epilepsia 29: 123–128

Bourgeois B F D, Prensky A L, Palkes H S et al 1983 Intelligence in epilepsy: a prospective study in children. Annals of Neurology 14: 438–444

Braathen G, Theorell K, Persson A, Rane A 1988 Valproate in the treatment of absence epilepsy in children: a study of dose–response relationship. Epilepsia 29: 548–552

Bridgers S L, Ebersole J S, Ment L R et al 1986 Cassette

electroencephalography in the evaluation of neonatal seizures. Archives of Neurology 43: 49–51

Brod S A, Ment L R, Ehrenkranz R A, Bridgers S 1988 Predictors of success for drug discontinuation following neonatal seizures. Pediatric Neurology 4: 13–17

Brown J K 1973 Convulsions in the newborn period. Developmental Medicine and Child Neurology 15: 823–846

Browne T R, Penry J K, Porter R J, Dreifuss F E 1974 Responsiveness before, during and after spike-wave paroxysms. Neurology 24: 659–665

Browne T R, Dreifuss F E, Dyken P R et al 1975 Ethosuximide in the treatment of absence (petit mal) epilepsy. Neurology 25: 515–525

Byrd S E, Osborn R E, Bohan T P, Naidich T P 1989 The CT and MR evaluation of migrational disorders of the brain. 2: Schizencephaly, heterotopia and polymicrogyria. Pediatric Radiology 19: 219–222

Callaghan N, O'Hare J, O'Driscoll D et al 1982 Comparative study of ethosuximide and sodium valproate in the treatment of typical absence seizures (petit mal). Developmental Medicine and Child Neurology 24: 830–836

Camfield C S, Chaplin S, Doyle A B, Shapiro S H, Cummings C, Camfield P R 1979 Side-effects of phenobarbital in toddlers; behavioural and cognitive aspects. Journal of Pediatrics 95: 361–365

Camfield P R, Gates R, Ronen G et al 1984 Comparison of cognitive ability, personality profile, and school success in epileptic children with pure right versus pure left temporal lobe EEG foci. Annals of Neurology 15: 122–126

Cavazzutti G B 1980 Epidemiology of different types of epilepsy in school age children of Modena, Italy. Epilepsia 21: 57–62

Chapman A G 1985 Cerebral energy metabolism and seizures. In: Pedley T A, Meldrum B S (eds) Recent advances in epilepsy, 2. Churchill Livingstone, Edinburgh, p 19–63

Chattha A S, Richardson E P Jr 1977 Cerebral white matter hypoplasia. Archives of Neurology 34: 137–141

Chiron C, Dulac O, Luna D et al 1990 Vigabatrin in infantile spasms. Lancet 335: 363–364

Chugani H T, Mazziotta J C, Engel J Jr et al 1987 The Lennox–Gastaut syndrome: metabolic sub-types determined by 2-deoxy-2(^{18}F) fluoro-D-glucose positron emission tomography. Annals of Neurology 21: 4–13

Chugani H T, Shewmon D A, Peacock W J et al 1988 Surgical treatment of intractable neonatal onset seizures: The role of positron emission tomography. Neurology 38: 1178–1188

Chugani H T, Shields W D, Shewmon D A 1990 Infantile spasms: I PET identifies focal cortical dysgenesis in cryptogenic cases for surgical treatment. Annals of Neurology 27: 406–413

Clare M, Aldridge Smith J, Wallace S J 1978 A child's first febrile convulsion. Practitioner 221: 775–776

Clarke M, Gill J, Noronha M, McKinlay I 1987 Early infantile epileptic encephalopathy with suppression-burst; Ohtahara syndrome. Developmental Medicine and Child Neurology 29: 520–528

Clement M J, Wallace S J 1988 Juvenile myoclonic epilepsy. Archives of Disease in Childhood 63: 1049–1053

Clement M J, Wallace S J 1990 A survey of adolescents with epilepsy. Developmental Medicine and Child Neurology 32: 849–857

Commission on Classification and Terminology of the International League Against Epilepsy 1981 Proposal for revised clinical and electroencephalographic classification of epileptic seizures. Epilepsia 22: 489–501

Commission on Classification and Terminology of the International League Against Epilepsy 1989 Proposal for revised classification of epilepsies and epileptic syndromes. Epilepsia 30: 389–399

Connell J, Oozeer R, Dubowitz V 1987 Continuous 4-channel EEG monitoring: a guide to interpretation with normal values in pre-term infants. Neuropediatrics 18: 138–145

Connell J, Oozeer R, de Vries L et al 1989a Continuous EEG monitoring of neonatal seizures: Diagnostic and prognostic considerations. Archives of Disease in Childhood 64: 452–458

Connell J, Oozeer R, de Vries L et al 1989b Clinical and EEG response to anticonvulsants in neonatal seizures. Archives of Disease in Childhood 64: 459–464

Cowan L D, Bodensteiner J B, Leviton A, Doherty L 1989 Prevalence of the epilepsies in childhood and adolescents. Epilepsia 30: 94–106

Cremades A, Peñafiel R, Monserrat F et al 1989 Free amino acids in the cerebrospinal fluid of children with febrile seizures. Neuropediatrics 20: 129–131

Curatolo P, Pruna D, Cusmai R, Feliciani M 1989 Polymicrogyria: A case detected by MRI. Brain and Development 11: 257–259

Curtis P D, Matthews T G, Clarke T A et al 1988 Neonatal seizures: The Dublin Collaborative Study. Archives of Disease in Childhood 63: 1065–1068

Dalby M A 1969 Epilepsy and 3 per second spike and wave rhythms. A clinical electroencephalographic and prognostic analysis of 346 patients. Acta Neurologica Scandinavica 45: supplement 40

Dalla Bernardina B, Capovilla G, Gattoni M B et al 1982 Epilepsie myoclonique grave de la première année. Revue d'Électroencéphalographic et de Neurophysiologie Clinique 12: 21–25

Dalla Bernardina B, Chiamenti C, Capovilla G, Colamaria V 1985a Benign partial epilepsies in childhood. In: Roger J, Dravet C, Bureau M, Dreifuss F E, Wolf P (eds) Epileptic syndromes in infancy, childhood and adolescence. John Libbey Eurotext, London, p 137–149

Dalla Bernardina B, Chiamenti C, Capovilla G, Trevisan E, Tassinari C A 1985b Benign partial epilepsy with affective symptoms ('Benign psychomotor epilepsy'). In: Roger J, Dravet C, Bureau M, Dreifuss F E, Wolf P (eds) Epileptic syndromes in infancy, childhood and adolescence. John Libbey Eurotext, London, p 171–175

Danesi M A 1985 Classification of the epilepsies: An investigation of 945 patients in a developing country. Epilepsia 26: 131–136

Davidson S, Falconer M A 1975 Outcome of surgery in 40 children with temporal-lobe epilepsy. Lancet i: 1260–1261

De Negri M, Gaggero R, Baglietto M G 1990 Computed EEG topography (CET) and childhood epilepsy: Two years experience. Brain and Development 12: 253–256

Rijk-van Andel J F, Arts W F M, Barth P G, Loonen M C B 1990 Diagnostic features and clinical signs of 21 patients with lissencephaly type I. Developmental Medicine and Child Neurology 30: 707–717

Delgado-Escueta A V, Greenberg D A, Treiman L et al 1989 Mapping the gene for juvenile myoclonic epilepsy. Epilepsia 30 (suppl 4): S8–S18

Delivoria-Papadopoulos M, Younkin D P, Chance B 1990 Cerebral metabolic studies during neonatal seizures with 31-p NMR spectroscopy. In: Wasterlain C G, Vert P (eds) Neonatal seizures. Raven Press, New York, p 181–189

Dennis J 1978 Neonatal convulsions. Aetiology, late neonatal status and long-term outcome. Developmental Medicine and Child Neurology 20: 143–148

Deonna Th, Ziegler A-L, Despland P-A 1986a Combined myoclonic-astatic and 'benign' focal epilepsy of childhood ('atypical' benign partial epilepsy of childhood). A separate syndrome? Neuropediatrics 17: 144–151

Deonna Th, Ziegler A-L, Despland P-A, van Melle G 1986b Partial epilepsy in neurologically normal children: clinical syndromes and prognosis. Epilepsia 27: 241–247

Deonna Th, Chevrie C, Horning E 1987 Childhood epileptic speech disorder: prolonged, isolated deficit of prosodic features. Developmental Medicine and Child Neurology 29: 96–109

Deonna Th, Peter Cl, Ziegler A-L 1989 Adult follow-up of the acquired aphasia-epilepsy syndrome. Report of 7 cases. Neuropediatrics 20: 132–138

Deshmukh A, Wittert W, Schnitzler E, Mangurten H H 1986 Lorazepam in the treatment of refractory neonatal seizures. A pilot study. American Journal of Diseases in Children 140: 1042–1044

Dieterich E, Baier W K, Doose H et al 1985a Long-term follow-up of childhood epilepsy with absences. 1. Epilepsy with absences at onset. Neuropediatrics 16: 149–154

Dieterich E, Doose H, Baier W K, Fichsel H 1985b Long-term follow-up of childhood epilepsy with absences. II Absence-epilepsy with initial grand mal. Neuropediatrics 16: 155–158

Dobyns W B, Stratton R F, Parke J T et al 1983 Miller–Dieker syndrome: lissencephaly and monosomy 17p. Journal of Pediatrics 102: 552–558

Dobyns W B, Kirkpatrick J B, Hittner H M et al 1985 Syndromes with lissencephaly. II: Walker-Warburg and cerebro-oculo-muscular syndromes with a new syndrome with type II lissencephaly. American Journal of Medical Genetics 22: 157–195

Dodson W E, Bourgeois B F 1990 Changing kinetic patterns of phenytoin in newborns. In Wasterlain C G, Vert P (eds) Neonatal seizures. Raven Press, New York, p 269–274

Dooley J M, Camfield P R, Camfield C S, Fraser A D 1990 Once-daily ethosuximide in the treatment of absence epilepsy. Pediatric Neurology 6: 38–39

Doose H 1985 Myoclonic-astatic epilepsy of early childhood. In: Roger J, Dravet C, Bureau M, Dreifuss F E, Wolf P (eds) Epileptic syndromes in infancy, childhood and adolescence. John Libbey Eurotext, London, p 78–88

Doose H, Sitepu B 1983 Childhood epilepsy in a German city. Neuropediatrics 14: 220–224

Dorfman D H, Glaser J H 1990 Congenital syphilis presenting in infants after the newborn period. New England Journal of Medicine 323: 1229–1302

Dravet C, Roger J, Bureau M, Dalla Bernardina B 1982 Myoclonic epilepsies in childhood. In: Akimoto H, Kazamatsuri H, Seino M, Ward A (eds) Advances in Epileptology: VIIIth Epilepsy International Symposium, Raven Press, New York, p 135–140

Dravet C, Bureau M, Roger J 1985a Benign myoclonic epilepsy in infants. In: Roger J, Dravet C, Bureau M, Dreifuss F E, Wolf P (eds) Epileptic syndromes in infancy, childhood and adolescence. John Libbey Eurotext, London, p 51–57

Dravet C, Bureau M, Roger J 1985b Severe myoclonic epilepsy in infants. In: Roger J, Dravet C, Bureau M, Dreifuss F E, Wolf P (eds) Epileptic syndromes in infancy, childhood and adolescence. John Libbey. Eurotext, London, p 58–67

Dravet C, Catani C, Bureau M, Roger J 1989 Partial epilepsies in infancy: a study of 40 cases. Epilepsia 30: 807–812

Dreifuss F E 1989 Juvenile myoclonic epilepsy: characteristics of a primary generalized epilepsy. Epilepsia 30(suppl 4): S1–S7

Dreyfus-Brissac C 1979 Neonatal electroencephalography. In: Scarpelli E M, Cosmi E V (eds) Reviews in Perinatal Medicine, vol 3. Raven Press, New York, p 397–472

Duchowny S 1989 Surgery for intractable epilepsy, issues and outcomes. Pediatrics 84: 886-894

Duchowny M S, Resnick T J, Deray M J, Alvarez L A 1988 Video EEG diagnosis of repetitive behaviour in early childhood and its relationship to seizures. Pediatric Neurology 4: 162–164

Dulac O, Aubourg P, Plouin P 1985 Other epileptic syndromes in neonates. In: Roger J, Dravet C, Bureau M, Dreifuss F E, Wolf P (eds) Epileptic syndromes in infancy, childhood and adolescence. John Libbey Eurotext, London, p 23–29

Dulac O, Cusmai R, de Oliveira K 1989 Is there a partial benign epilepsy in infancy? Epilepsia 30: 798–801

Eeg-Olofsson O 1988 Genetic factors. In: Niedermeyer E, Degen R (eds) The Lennox-Gastaut Syndrome, Alan R Liss, New York, p 65–71

Egger J, Pincott J R, Wilson J, Erdohazi M 1984 Cortical subacute necrotizing encephalomyelitis. A study of two patients with mitochondrial dysfunction. Neuropediatrics 15: 150–158

Engel J Jr, Kuhl D E, Phelps M E 1982 Patterns of human local cerebral glucose metabolism during epileptic seizures. Science 218: 64–66

Eslava-Cobos J, Nariño D 1989 Experience with the International League Against Epilepsy proposals for classification of epileptic seizures and the epilepsies and epileptic syndromes in a pediatric outpatient epilepsy clinic. Epilepsia 30: 112–115

Eyre J, Oozeer R C, Wilkinson A R 1983a Diagnosis of neonatal seizure by continuous recording and rapid analysis of the electroencephalogram. Archives of Disease in Childhood 58: 785–790

Eyre J, Oozeer R C, Wilkinson A R 1983b Continuous electroencephalographic recording to detect seizures in paralysed newborn babies. British Medical Journal 286: 1017–1018

Farwell J R, Dodrill C B, Batzel L W 1985 Neuropsychological abilities of children with epilepsy. Epilepsia 26: 395–400

Farwell J R, Lee Y J, Hirtz D G et al 1990 Phenobarbital for febrile seizures—effects on intelligence and on seizure recurrence. New England Journal of Medicine 322: 364–369

Fenichel G M 1980 Neonatal neurology. Churchill Livingstone, Edinburgh

Flanigin H, King D, Gallagher B 1985 Surgical treatment of epilepsy. In: Pedley T A, Meldrum B S (eds) Recent advances in epilepsy, 2. Churchill Livingstone, Edinburgh, p 297–339

Fois A, Malandrini F, Tomaccini D 1988 Clinical findings in

children with occipital paroxysmal discharges. Epilepsia 29: 620–623

Forsgren L, Sidenvall R, Blomquist H K et al 1990 An incident case-referent study of febrile convulsions in children: genetical and social aspects. Neuropediatrics 21: 153–159

Frantzen E 1971 Spinal findings in children with febrile convulsions. Epilepsia 12: 192

Freeman J M, Jacob S H, Vining E, Rabin C E 1984 Epilepsy and inner city schools: a school based program that makes a difference. Epilepsia 25: 438–442

Friedman E, Pampiglione G 1971 Prognostic implications of electroencephalographic findings of hypsarrhythmia in the first year of life. British Medical Journal 4: 323–325

Gaggero R, Ferraris P C, De Negri M 1990 Csf anomalies in children affected by epilepsia partialis continua (EPC). Neuropaediatrics 21: 143–145

Gal P, Oles K S, Gilman J C, Weaver R 1988 Valproic acid efficacy and pharmacokinetics in neonates with intractable seizures. Neurology 38: 467–471

Gastaut H 1970 Clinical and electroencephalographical classification of epileptic seizures. Epilepsia 11: 103–113

Gastaut H 1985 Benign epilepsy of childhood with occipital paroxysms. In: Roger J, Dravet C, Bureau M, Dreifuss F E, Wolf P (eds) Epileptic syndromes in infancy, childhood and adolescence. John Libbey Eurotext, London, p 159–170

Gastaut H, Poirier F, Payan H et al 1960 HHE syndrome. Hemiconvulsions, hemiplegia, epilepsy. Epilepsia 1: 418–447

Gastaut H, Roger J, Soulayrol R et al 1966 Childhood epileptic encephalopathy with diffuse slow spike-waves (otherwise known as 'petit mal variant') or Lennox syndrome. Epilepsia 7: 139–179

Gastaut H, Gastaut J L, Gonçalves de Silva G E, Fernandez Sanchez G R 1975 Relative frequency of different types of epilepsy: a study employing the classification of International League against Epilepsy. Epilepsia 16: 457–461

Giroud M, Dumas R, Dauvergne M et al 1990 5-Hydroxyindolacetic acid and homovanillic acid in cerebrospinal fluid of children with febrile convulsions. Epilepsia 31: 178–181

Gloor P 1980 Generalized penicillin epilepsy in the cat: The role of excitability changes in cortical neurons in the genesis of spike and wave discharges and their possible relevance as a model for human generalised corticoreticular epilepsy. In: Canger R, Angeleri F, Penry J K (eds) Advances in Epileptology: XIth Epilepsy International Symposium. Raven Press, New York, p 279–284

Goldensohn E S 1975 Initiation and propagation of epileptogenic foci. In: Penry J K, Daly D D (eds) Complex partial seizures and their treatment. Advances in Neurology, Volume II. Raven Press, New York, p 141–162

Gomez M R 1987 Tuberous sclerosis. In: Gomez M R (ed) Neurocutaneous diseases. Butterworths, Boston, p 30–52

Goode D J, Penry J K, Dreifuss F E 1970 Effect of paroxysmal spike-wave on continuous visual-motor performance. Epilepsia 11: 241–254

Gudmundssen G 1966 Epilepsy in Iceland. Acta Neurologica Scandinavica 43(Suppl 25): 72–73

Guerrini R, Bureau M, Mattei M-G et al 1990 Trisomy 12p syndrome: a chromosomal disorder associated with generalised 3-Hz spike and wave discharges. Epilepsia 31: 557–566

Hakeem V F, Wallace S J 1990 EEG monitoring of therapy for neonatal seizures. Developmental Medicine and Child Neurology 32: 858–864

Hamon M, Bourgoin S, Chanez C, DeVitry F 1989 Do serotonin and other neurotransmitters exert a trophic influence on the immature brain? In: Evrard P, Minkowski A (eds) Developmental neurobiology. Nestec Vevey/Raven Press, New York, p 171–181

Hardiman O, Burke T, Phillips J et al 1988 Microdysgenesis in dissected temporal neocortex: Incidence and clinical significance in focal epilepsy. Neurology 38: 1041–1047

Harris R, Tizard J P M 1960 The electroencephalogram in neonatal convulsions. Journal of Pediatrics 57: 501–520

Hashimoto K, Fujita T, Furuya M et al 1989 Absence seizures following febrile seizures. Brain and Development 11: 268

Hauser W A, Kurland L T 1975 The epidemiology of epilepsy in Rochester, Minnesota, 1935 through 1967. Epilepsia 16: 1–66

Hauser W A, Annegers J F, Anderson V E, Kurland L T 1985 The risk of seizure disorders among relatives of children with febrile convulsions. Neurology 35: 1268–1273

Hellström-Westas L, Rosen I, Svenningsen N W 1985 Silent seizures in sick infants in early life. Acta Paediatrica Scandinavica 74: 741–748

Hellström-Westas L, Westgren L, Rosen I, Svenningsen N W 1988 Lidocaine for treatment of severe seizures in newborn infants. I. Clinical effect and cerebral activity monitoring. Acta Paediatrica Scandinavica 77: 79–84

Herzlinger R A, Kandall S R, Vaughan H G 1977 Neonatal seizures associated with narcotic withdrawal. Journal of Pediatrics 91: 638–641

Hirsch R P, Painter M J 1990 Phenobarbital for febrile seizures. New England Journal of Medicine 323: 484

Hoare P, Kerley S 1988 The family's experience of epilepsy. In: Hoare P (ed) Epilepsy and the family. A Medical Symposium on New Approaches to Family Care. Sanofi, Wythenshawe, p 65–72

Holmes G L, McKeever M, Adamson M 1987 Absence seizures in children: clinical and electroencephalographic features. Annals of Neurology 21: 268–273

Hrachovy R A, Frost J D, Kellaway P, Zion T 1980 A controlled study of ACTH therapy in infantile spasms. Epilepsia 21: 631–636

Hrachovy R A, Frost J D, Kellaway P 1984 Hyparrhythmia: variations on a theme. Epilepsia 25: 317–325

Hrachovy R A, Frost J D, Glaze D G 1988 Treatment of infantile spasms with tetrabenazine. Epilepsia 29: 561–563

Hrachovy R A, Frost J D, Glaze D G, Rose D 1989 Treatment of infantile spasms with methysergide and alpha-methylparatyrosine. Epilepsia 30: 607–610

Hurst D L 1987 Severe myoclonic epilepsy of infancy. Pediatric Neurology 3: 269–272

Hurst D L 1990 Epidemiology of severe myoclonic epilepsy of infancy. Epilepsia 31: 497–500

Huttenlocher P R 1974 Dendritic development in neocortex of children with mental defect and infantile spasms. Neurology 24: 203–210

Iivanainen M 1990 Diagnosis of epileptic seizures and syndromes in mentally retarded patients. In: Sillanpää M, Johannessen S I, Blennow G, Dam M (eds) Paediatric epilepsy. Wrightson, Petersfield, p 233–241

Illum N, Taudorf K, Heilmann C et al 1990 Intravenous

immunoglobulin: A single-blind trial in children with Lennox–Gastaut syndrome. Neuropediatrics 21: 87–90

Ingvar M, Siesjö B K 1990 Pathophysiology of epileptic brain damage. In: Wasterlain C G, Vert P (eds) Neonatal seizures. Raven Press, New York, p 113–122

Jaeken J, Casaer P, Haegele K D, Schechter P J 1990 Review: Normal and abnormal central nervous system GABA metabolism in childhood. Journal of Inherited Metabolic Disease 13: 793–801

Jeavons P M 1985 West syndrome: infantile spasms. In: Roger J, Dravet C, Bureau M, Dreifuss F E, Wolf P (eds) Epileptic syndromes in infancy, childhood and adolescence. John Libbey Eurotext, London, p 42–48

Jeavons P M, Bower B D 1964 Infantile spasms. A review of the literature and a study of 112 cases. Clinics in Developmental Medicine, No 15. Heinemann, London

Jeavons P M, Harding G F A 1975 Photosensitive epilepsy. Clinics in Developmental Medicine, Number 56. Heinemann, London

Jeavons P M, Bishop A, Harding G F A 1986 The prognosis of photosensitivity. Epilepsia 27: 569–575

Jellinger K 1987 Neuropathological aspects of infantile spasms. Brain and Development 9: 349–357

Jennekens-Schinkel A, Linschooten-Duikersloot E M E M, Bouma P A D et al 1987 Spelling errors made by children with mild epilepsy: writing-to-dictation. Epilepsia 28: 555–563

Juul-Jensen P, Denny-Brown D 1966 Epilepsia partialis continua. Archives of Neurology 15: 563–578

Kajitani T, Ueoka K, Nakamura M, Kumanomidu Y 1981 Febrile convulsions and Rolandic discharges. Brain and Development 3: 351–359

Kasteleijn-Nolst Trenité D G A, Bakker D J, Binnie C D et al 1988 Psychological effects of subclinical epileptiform EEG discharges in children I: Scholastic skills. Epilepsy Research 2: 111–116

Kasteleijn-Nolst Trenité D G A, Smit A M, Velis D N et al 1990a On-line detection of transient neuropsychological disturbances during EEG discharges in children with epilepsy. Developmental Medicine and Child Neurology 32: 46–50

Kasteleijn-Nolst Trenité D G A, Siebelink B M, Berends S G C et al 1990b Lateralized effects of subclinical epileptiform EEG discharges on scholastic performance in children. Epilepsia 31: 740–746

Kellaway P, Mizrahi E M 1990 Clinical electroencephalographic, therapeutic and pathophysiologic studies of neonatal seizures. In: Wasterlain C G, Vert P (eds) Neonatal seizures. Raven Press, New York, p 1–13

Kellaway P, Hrachovy R, Frost J D, Zion T 1979 Precise characterisation and quantification of infantile spasms. Annals of Neurology 6: 214–218

Kellaway P, Frost J D, Hrachovy R A 1983 Infantile spasms. In: Morselli P, Pippenger C E, Penry J K (eds) Antiepileptic drug therapy in pediatrics. Raven Press, New York, p 115–136

Kendall B E 1988 Magnetic resonance in diseases of the nervous system. Archives of Disease in Childhood 63: 1301–1304

Kimiya S, Seki T, Hara M 1989 Monoamine metabolism in cerebrospinal fluid in febrile convulsions. Brain and Development 11: 273–274

King D W, Dyken P R, Spinks I L Jr, Murvina A J 1985 Infantile spasms: Ictal phenomena. Pediatric Neurology 1: 213–218

Kitamoto I, Kurokawa T, Tomitas S et al 1988 Child–parent relationships in the care of epileptic children. Brain and Development 10: 36–40

Knoll J H M, Nicholls R D, Magenis R E et al 1989 Angelman and Prader–Willi syndromes share a common chromosome 15 deletion but differ in the parental origin of the deletion. American Journal of Medical Genetics 32: 285–290

Knudsen F U 1985 Recurrence risk after first febrile seizure and effect of short term diazepam prophylaxis. Archives of Disease in Childhood 60: 1045–1049

Kohrman M H, Hayes M S, Kerr S L et al 1990 Phenobarbital for febrile seizures. New England Journal of Medicine 323: 484

Koren G, Warwick B, Rajchgot R et al 1986 Intravenous paraldehyde for seizure control in newborn infants. Neurology 36: 108–111

Koskiniemi M 1990 Progressive myoclonic epilepsy. In: Sillanpää M, Johannessen S I, Blennow G, Dam M (eds) Paediatric epilepsy. Wrightson Biomedical, Petersfield, p 137–144

Kotagal P, Rothner A D, Erenberg G et al 1987 Complex partial seizures of childhood onset. A five-year follow-up study. Archives of Neurology 44: 1177–1180

Kunze J 1980 Neurological disorders in patients with chromosomal anomalies. Neuropediatrics 11: 203–230

Kuzmiechky R, Rosenblatt B 1987 Benign occipital epilepsy: a family study. Epilepsia 24: 346–350

Lacy J R, Penry J K 1976 Infantile spasms. Raven Press, New York

Lagenstein I, Kühne D, Sternuwsky H J, Ruthe E 1979 Computerised cranial transverse axial tomography (CTAT) in 145 patients with primary and secondary generalised West syndrome, myoclonic-astatic petit mal, absence epilepsy. Neuropädiatrie 10: 15–28

Lancet Editorial 1989 Endotoxins in heatstroke. Lancet 2: 1137–1138

Lancet Editorial 1990a Magnetoencephalography. Lancet 335: 576–577

Lancet Editorial 1990b Epilepsy and disorders of neuronal migration. Lancet 336: 1035

Landau W M, Kleffner F R 1957 Syndrome of acquired aphasia with convulsive disorder in children. Neurology 7: 523–530

Lee S I, Kirby D 1988 Absence seizures with generalized rhythmic delta activity. Epilepsia 29: 262–267

Lee T K Y, Nakasu, Jefree M A et al 1989 Indolent glioma: a cause of epilepsy. Archives of Disease in Childhood 64: 1666–1671

Lennox W G, Davis J P 1950 Clinical correlates of the fast and slow spike wave electroencephalogram. Pediatrics 5: 626–644

Leppert M, Anderson V E, Quattlebaum T et al 1989 Benign familial convulsions linked to genetic markers on chromosome 20. Nature 337: 647–648

Lerman P 1985 Benign partial epilepsy with centro-temporal spikes. In: Roger J, Dravet C, Bureau M, Dreifuss F E, Wolf P (eds) Epileptic syndromes in infancy, childhood and adolescence. John Libbey Eurotext, London, p 150–158

Lerman P, Kivity S 1982 The efficacy of corticotrophin in primary infantile spasms. Journal of Pediatrics 101: 294–296

Lewis M A, Salas I, de la Sota A et al 1990 Randomized trial of a program to enhance the competencies of children with epilepsy. Epilepsia 31: 101–109

Lindsay J, Ounsted C, Richards P 1987 Hemispherectomy for childhood epilepsy: a 36-year study. Developmental Medicine and Child Neurology 29: 592–600

Livingston J H, Aicardi J 1990 Unusual MRI appearance of diffuse subcortical heterotopia or 'double cortex' in two children. Journal of Neurology, Neurosurgery and Psychiatry 53: 617–620

Livingston J H, Beaumont D, Arizimanoglou A, Aicardi J 1989 Vigabatrin in the treatment of epilepsy in children. British Journal of Clinical Pharmacology 27: 1095–1125

Lockman L A, Kriel R, Zaske D et al 1979 Phenobarbital dosage for control of neonatal seizures. Neurology 29: 1445–1449

Loiseau P 1985 Childhood absence epilepsy. In: Roger J, Dravet C, Bureau M, Dreifuss F E, Wolf P (eds) Epileptic syndromes in infancy, childhood and adolescence. John Libbey Eurotext, London, p 106–120

Loiseau P, Petre M, Dartigues J F et al 1983 Long-term prognosis in two forms of childhood epilepsy: typical absences and epilepsy with Rolandic (centro-temporal) EEG foci. Annals of Neurology 13: 642–648

Loiseau P, Duché B, Cordova S et al 1988 Prognosis of benign childhood epilepsy with centro-temporal spikes: a follow-up study of 168 patients. Epilepsia 29: 229–235

Lombroso C T, Fejerman N 1977 Benign myoclonus of early infancy. Annals of Neurology 1: 138–143

Low J A, Paucham S R, Piercy W N, Worthington D, Karchmar J 1977 Intrapartum fetal asphyxia: clinical characteristics, diagnosis and significance in relation to pattern of development. American Journal of Obstetrics and Gynecology 129: 857–870

Lüders S H, Wyllie E, Rothner D A et al 1989 Surgery of localization-related epilepsies in children. Brain and Development 11: 98–101

Ludwig B 1987 Review: Neuroradiological aspects of infantile spasms. Brain and Development 9: 358–360

McDonald J W, Johnston M V 1990 Nonketotic hyperglycinemia: pathophysiological role of NMDA-type excitory amino acid receptors. Annals of Neurology 27: 449–450

McKinlay I, Newton R 1989 Intention to treat febrile convulsions with rectal diazepam, valproate or phenobarbitone. Developmental Medicine and Child Neurology 31: 617–625

Maeda Y, Kurokawa T, Sakamoto K et al 1990 Electroclinical study of video-game epilepsy. Developmental Medicine and Child Neurology 32: 493–500

Marescaux C, Hirsch E, Finck S et al 1990 Landau–Kleffner syndrome: A pharmacologic study of five cases. Epilepsia 31: 768–777

Martinez J A, Bermejo A M, Gonzales L G et al 1990 Intermittent treatment with clonazepam in single febrile seizures. Brain and Development 12: 274–275

Martinez M 1989 Biochemical changes during early myelination of the human brain. In: Evrard P, Minkowski A (eds) Developmental neurobiology. Nestec Vevey/Raven Press, New York, p 185–200

Mathieson G 1975 Pathology of temporal lobe foci. In: Penry J K, Daly D D (eds) Complex partial seizures and their treatment. Advances in Neurology, Vol 11. Raven Press, New York, p 163–185

Matsumoto A, Kumagai T, Takeuchi T et al 1987 Clinical effects of thyrotropin-releasing hormone for severe epilepsy in childhood: a comparative study with ACTH therapy. Epilepsy 28: 49–55

Mazziotti J C, Engel J Jr 1985 Advanced neuro-imaging techniques in the study of human epilepsy: PET, SPECT and NMR-CT. In: Pedley T A, Meldrum B S (eds) Recent advances in epilepsy, 2. Churchill Livingstone, Edinburgh, p 65–99

Meencke H J, Janz D 1984 Neuropathological findings in primary generalised epilepsy: a study of eight cases. Epilepsia 25: 8–21

Meencke H J, Gerhard C 1985 Morphological aspects of aetiology and the course of infantile spasms (West syndrome). Neuropediatrics 16: 59–66

Meinhard E A, Oozeer R, Cameron D 1988 Photosensitive epilepsy in children who set fires. British Medical Journal 296: 1773

Melchior J C 1977 Infantile spasms and early immunisation against whooping cough. Danish survey from 1970 to 1975. Archives of Disease in Childhood 52: 134–137

Mellits E D, Holden K R, Freeman J M 1981 Neonatal seizures. II Multivariate analysis of factors associated with outcome. Pediatrics 70: 177–185

Michihiro N, Kurosawa Y, Suemitsu T et al 1989 Cerebral blood perfusion in febrile convulsions with N-isopropyl-p-(^{123}I) iodoamphetamine and single photon emission CT. Brain and Development 11: 275

Millichap J G 1968 Febrile convulsions. Macmillan, New York

Mizrahi E M, Kellaway P, Grossman R G, Rutecki P A 1990 Anteriotemporal lobectomy and medically refractory temporal lobe epilepsy of childhood. Epilepsia 31: 302–312

Morikawa T, Seino M, Osawa T, Yagi K 1985 Five children with continuous spike-wave discharges during sleep. In: Roger J, Dravet C, Bureau M, Dreifuss F E, Wolf P (eds) Epileptic syndromes in infancy Childhood and Adolescence. John Libbey Eurotext, London, p 205–212

Müller K, Lenard H G 1988 The Lennox–Gastaut syndrome: therapeutic aspects including dietary measures and general management. In: Niedermeyer E, Degen R (eds) The Lennox–Gastaut syndrome. Alan R Liss, New York, p 341–355

Munthe-Kaas A W 1990 Habilitation of the child with epilepsy. In: Sillanpää M, Johannessen S I, Blennow G, Dam M (eds) Paediatric epilepsy. Wrightson Biomedical Publishing, Petersfield, p 317–326

Musumeci S A, Colognola R M, Ferri R et al 1988 Fragile X syndrome: a particular epileptogenic EEG pattern. Epilepsia 29: 41–47

Nagao H, Morimoto T, Takahashi M et al 1990 The circadian rhythm of typical absence seizures—the frequency and duration of paroxysmal discharges. Neuropediatrics 21: 79–82

Nakamuri M, Kajitani T 1983 Longitudinal study of Rolandic discharges. Brain and Development 5: 183

Nakano S, Okuno T, Mikawa H 1989 Landau–Kleffner syndrome, EEG topographic studies. Brain and Development 11: 43–50

Nayrac P, Beaussart M 1958 Les pointe-ondes pré-rolandiques: expression EEG très particulière. Etude électroclinique de 21 cas. Revue Neurologique 99: 201–206

Nelson K B, Ellenberg J H 1986 Antecedents of seizure disorders in early childhood. American Journal of Diseases of Children 140: 1053–1061

Nelson K B, Ellenberg J H 1990 Prenatal and perinatal

antecedents of febrile seizures. Annals of Neurology 27: 127–131

Neville B G R 1972 The origin of infantile spasms: evidence from a case of hydronencephaly. Developmental Medicine and Child Neurology 14: 644–656

Newton R, Aicardi J 1983 Clinical findings in children with occipital spike-wave complexes suppressed by eye-opening. Neurology 33: 1526–1529

Niedermeyer E 1987 Maturation of the EEG: Development of waking and sleeping patterns. In: Niedermeyer E, Lopes da Silva F (eds) Electroencephalography: basic principles, clinical applications and related fields, 2nd edn. Urban & Schwarzenberg, Baltimore, p 133–158

Nolte R 1989 Neonatal sleep myoclonus followed by myoclonic-astatic epilepsy: a case report. Epilepsia 30: 844–850

Nolte R, Wetzel B, Brugmann G, Brintzinger I 1980 Effects of phenytoin and primidone monotherapy on mental performance in children. In: Johannessen S I, Morselli P L, Pippenger C E et al (eds) Antiepileptic therapy: advances in drug monitoring. Raven Press, New York, p 81–86

North K N, Storey G N B, Henderson-Smart D J 1989 Fifth day fits in the newborn. Australian Paediatric Journal 25: 284–287

Ohtahara S 1984 Seizure disorders in infancy and childhood. Brain and Development 6: 509–519

Ohtahara S, Ohtsuka Y, Yamatogi Y, Oka E 1987 The early-infantile epileptic encephalopathy with suppression-burst: Developmental aspects. Brain and Development 9: 371–376

Ohtahara S, Ohtsuka Y, Yoshinaga H et al 1988 Lennox–Gastaut syndrome: etiological considerations. In: Niedermeyer E, Degen R (eds) The Lennox–Gastaut Syndrome. Alan R Liss, New York, p 47–63

Ohtsuka Y, Matsuda M, Ogino T et al 1987 Treatment of the West syndrome with high-dose pyridoxal phosphate. Brain and Development 9: 418–421

O'Leary D S, Lovell M R, Sackellares J C et al 1983 Effects of age at onset of partial and generalized seizures on neuropsychological performance in children. Journal of Nervous and Mental Disease 171: 624–629

Oller-Daurella L, Oller L F V 1989 Partial epilepsy with seizures appearing in the first three years of life. Epilepsia 30: 820–826

Otani K, Abe J, Futagi Y et al 1989 Clinical and electroencephalographic follow-up study of early myoclonic encephalopathy. Brain and Development 11: 332–337

Ottman R 1989 Genetics of the partial epilepsies: A review. Epilepsia 30: 107–111

Ottman R, Annegers J F, Hauser W A, Kurland L T 1989 Seizure risk in offspring of parents with generalized versus partial epilepsy. Epilepsia 30: 157–161

Ounsted C, Lindsay J, Norman R 1966 Biological factors in temporal lobe epilepsy. Clinics in Developmental Medicine, 22. Heinemann, London

Ounsted C, Lindsay J, Richards P 1987 Temporal lobe epilepsy. A biographical study 1948–1986. Blackwell, Oxford

Overall J C 1970 Neonatal bacterial meningitis. Journal of Pediatrics 76: 499–511

Painter M J 1983 General principles of treatment: status epilepticus in neonates. In: Delgado-Escueta A V, Wasterlain C G, Treiman D M Porter R J (eds) Advances in neurology, vol 34: Status epilepticus. Raven Press, New York, p 385–393

Painter M J, Alvin J 1990 Choice of anticonvulsants in the treatment of neonatal seizures. In: Wasterlain C G, Vert P (eds) Neonatal seizures. Raven Press, New York, p 243–256

Painter M J, Pippenger C, Wasterlain C et al 1981 Phenobarbital and phenytoin in neonatal seizures: metabolism and tissue distribution. Neurology 31: 1107–1112

Pampiglione G 1965 Brain development and the EEG of normal children of various ethnical groups. British Medical Journal 2: 573– 575

Panayiotopoulos C P 1989 Benign childhood epilepsy with occipital paroxysms: A 15-year prospective study. Annals of Neurology 26: 51–56

Panayiotopoulos C P, Obeid T, Waheed G 1989 Differentiation of typical absence seizures in epileptic syndromes. A video EEG study of 224 seizures in 20 patients. Brain 112: 1039–1056

Parmeggiani A, Plouin P, Dulac O 1990 Quantification of diffuse and focal delta activity in hypsarrhythmia. Brain and Development 12: 310–315

Pavone L, Cavazzutti G B, Incorpora G et al 1989 Late febrile convulsions: a clinical follow-up. Brain and Development 11: 183–185

Pedersen H 1990 Cranial CT in children with epilepsy: findings and indications. In: Sillanpää M, Johannessen S I, Blennow G, Dam M (eds) Paediatric epilepsy. Wrightson Biomedical, Petersfield, p 179–184

Penry J K, Porter R J, Dreifuss F E 1975 Simultaneous recording of absence seizures with video tape and electroencephalography. A study of 374 seizures in 48 patients. Brain 98: 427–440

Piccirilli M, D'Alessandro P, Tiacci C, Ferroni A 1988 Language lateralization in children with benign partial epilepsy. Epilepsia 29: 19–25

Pierog S, Chandavasu O, Wexler I 1977 Withdrawal symptoms in infants with fetal alcohol syndrome. Journal of Pediatrics 90: 630–633

Plouin P 1985 Benign neonatal convulsions (familial and non-familial). In: Roger J, Dravet C, Bureau M, Dreifuss F E, Wolf P (eds) Epileptic syndromes in infancy, childhood and adolescence. John Libbey Eurotext, London, p 2–9

Pollack M A, Golden G S, Schmidt R et al 1978 Infantile spasms in Down syndrome: a report of 5 cases and review of the literature. Annals of Neurology 3: 406–408

Pomeroy S L, Holmes S J, Dodge P R, Feigin R D 1990 Seizures and other sequelae of bacterial meningitis in children. New England Journal of Medicine 323: 1651–1657

Porro G, Matricardi M, Guidetti V, Benedetti P 1988 Prognosis of partial epilepsy. Archives of Disease in Childhood 63: 1192–1197

Power C, Polano S D, Blume W T et al 1990 Cytomegalovirus and Rasmussen's encephalitis. Lancet 336: 1282–1284

Radvanyi-Bouvet M-F, de Bethmann O, Monset-Couchard M, Fazzi E 1987 Cerebral lesions in early prematurity: EEG prognostic value in the neonatal period. Brain and Development 9: 399–405

Radvanyi-Bouvet M-F, Toricelli A, Rey E et al 1990 Effects of lidocaine on seizures in the neonatal period: some electroclinical aspects. In: Wasterlain C G, Vert P (eds) Neonatal seizures. Raven Press, New York, p 275–283

Rasmussen T, Olszewski J, Lloyd-Smith D 1958 Focal

seizures due to chronic localised encephalitides. Neurology 8: 435–445

Reintoft H, Simonsen N, Lund M 1976 A controlled sociological study of juvenile myoclonic epilepsy. In: Janz D (ed) Epileptology. Thieme, Stuttgart, p 48–50

Renier W O, Renkawek K 1990 Clinical and neuropathological findings in a case of severe myoclonic epilepsy of infancy. Epilepsia 31: 287–291

Renier W O, Gabreels F J M, Jaspar H H J 1988 Morphological and biochemical analysis of a brain biopsy in a case of idiopathic Lennox–Gastaut syndrome. Epilepsia 29: 644–649

Represa A, Robain O, Tremblay E, Ben-Ari Y 1989 Hippocampal plasticity in childhood epilepsy. Neuroscience Letters 99: 351–355

Revol M 1985 Lesional epilepsies with partial seizures. In: Roger J, Dravet C, Bureau M, Dreifuss F E, Wolf P (eds) Epileptic syndromes in infancy, childhood and adolescence. John Libbey Eurotext, London, p 287–285

Riikonen R 1978 Cytomegalovirus and infantile spasms. Developmental Medicine and Child Neurology 20: 570–579

Riikonen R 1982 A long-term follow-up study of 214 children with the syndrome of infantile spasms. Neuropediatrics 13/14: 23

Riikonen R 1987 Current knowledge of actions of ACTH and steroids. Brain and Development 9: 409–414

Riikonen R, Donner M 1979 Incidence and aetiology of infantile spasms during the period 1960–76. A population study in Finland. Developmental Medicine and Child Neurology 21: 333–343

Riikonen R, Simell O 1990 Tuberous sclerosis and infantile spasms. Developmental Medicine and Child Neurology 32: 203–209

Riikonen R, Santavuori P, Meretoja O et al 1988 Can barbiturate anaesthesia cure infantile spasms? Brain and Development 10: 300–304

Roberton N R C, Smith M A 1975 Early neonatal hypocalcaemia. Archives of Disease in Childhood 50: 604–609

Roberts S A, Cohen M D, Forfar J O 1973 Antenatal factors associated with neonatal hypocalcaemic convulsions. Lancet 2: 809–811

Rocca W A, Sharbrough F W, Hauser W A et al 1987a Risk factors for absence seizures: A population based case-control study in Rochester, Minnesota. Neurology 37: 1309–1314

Rocca W A, Sharbrough T W, Hauser W A et al 1987b Risk factors for complex partial seizures: A population-based case-control study. Annals of Neurology 21: 22–31

Rochefort M J, Wilkinson A R 1989 The safety and efficacy of alternative anticonvulsant regimes to control newborn seizures. Early Human Development 19: 218

Rodin E A, Schmaltz S, Twitty G 1986 Intellectual functions of patients with childhood-onset epilepsy. Developmental Medicine and Child Neurology 28: 25–33

Roger J 1985 Progressive myoclonic epilepsy in childhood and adolescence. In: Roger J, Dravet C, Bureau M, Dreifuss F E, Wolf P (eds) Epileptic syndromes in infancy, childhood and adolescence. John Libbey Eurotext, London, p 302–310

Roger J, Gambarelli-Dubois D 1988 Neuropathological studies of the Lennox–Gastaut syndrome. In: Niedermeyer E, Degen R (eds) The Lennox–Gastaut Syndrome. Alan R Liss, New York, p 73–93

Ross E M, Peckham C S, West P B, Butler N R 1980 Epilepsy in childhood, findings from the National Child Development Study. British Medical Journal 280: 207–210

Roulet E, Deonna T H, Despland P A 1989 Prolonged intermittent drooling and oromotor dyspraxia in benign childhood epilepsy with centrotemporal spikes. Epilepsia 30: 564–568

Rugland A-L 1990 Neurophysiological assessment of cognitive functioning in children with epilepsy. Epilepsia 31(supp l4): S41–S44

Sato S, Penry J K, Dreifuss F E, Dyken P R 1977 Clonazepam in the treatment of absence seizures: a double-blind clinical trial. Neurology 27: 371

Sato S, Dreifuss F E, Penry J K, Kirby D, White B G 1982a Long-term follow-up study of absence seizures. In: Akimoto H, Kazamatsuri H, Seino M, Ward A (eds) Advances in Epileptology: XIIIth Epilepsy International Symposium. Raven Press, New York, p 41–42

Sato S, White B G, Penry J K 1982b Valproic acid versus ethosuximide in the treatment of absence seizures. Neurology 32: 157–163

Saukkonen A-L, Serlo W, Von Wendt L 1990 Epilepsy in hydrocephalic children. Acta Paediatrica Scandinavica 79: 212–218

Scambler G 1990 Social factors and quality of life and quality of care in epilepsy. In: Chadwick D (ed) Quality of Life and Quality of Care in Epilepsy. Royal Society of Medicine Services, Round Table Series No. 23. Royal Society of Medicine, London, p 63–68

Scher M S, Painter M J 1990 Electroencephalographic diagnosis of neonatal seizures: Issues of diagnostic accuracy, clinical correlation, and survival. In: Wasterlain C G, Vert P (eds) Neonatal seizures. Raven Press, New York, p 15–25

Schiottz-Christensen E, Bruhn P 1973 Intelligence, behaviour and scholastic achievement subsequent to febrile convulsions: an analysis of discordant twin-pairs. Developmental Medicine and Child Neurology 15: 565–575

Schmidt D 1983a How to use benzodiazepines. In: Morselli P L, Pippenger C E, Penry J K (eds) Antiepileptic Drug Therapy in Pediatrics. Raven Press, New York, p 271–278

Schmidt D 1983b How to use ethosuximide. In: Morselli P L, Pippenger C E, Penry J K (eds) Antiepileptic drug therapy in pediatrics. Raven Press, New York, p 236

Seidenberg M, Beck N, Geisser M et al 1986 Academic achievement of children with epilepsy. Epilepsia 27: 753–759

Senanayake N 1987 Epileptic seizures evoked by card games, draughts and similar games. Epilepsia 28: 356–361

Seppäläinen A M, Smila S 1971 Electroencephalographic findings in three patients with non-ketotic hyperglycinemia. Epilepsia 12: 101–107

Shaw N J, Livingston J H, Minns R A, Clarke M 1988 Epilepsy precipitated by bathing. Developmental Medicine and Child Neurology 30: 108–111

Sherwin A L 1982 Ethosuximide: relation of plasma concentration to seizure control. In: Woodbury D M, Penry J K, Pippenger C E (eds) Antiepileptic drugs. Raven Press, New York, p 637–645

Shevell M I, Sinclair D B, Metrakos K 1986 Benign familial neonatal seizures: clinical and electroencephalographic characteristics. Pediatric Neurology 2: 272–275

Siebelink B M, Bakker D J, Binnie C D et al 1988 Psychological effects of subclinical epileptiform EEG discharges in children. II: General intelligence tests. Epilepsy Research 2: 117–121

Siemes H, Spohr H L, Michael Th, Nau H 1988 Therapy of infantile spasms with valproate: results of a prospective study. Epilepsia 29: 553–560

Snead O C III 1990a Treatment of infantile spasms. Pediatric Neurology 6: 147–150

Snead O C III 1990b The ontogeny of GABAergic enhancement of the γ-hydroxybutyrate model of generalized absence seizures. Epilepsia 31: 363–368

Sorel L, Dusaucy-Bauloye 1958 A propos de 21 cas d-hypsarhythmie de Gibbs: son traitement spectaculaire par l'ACTH. Acta Neurologica et Psychiatrica Belgica 58: 130–141

Spink D C, Snead O C III, Swann J W, Martin D L 1988 Free amino acids in cerebrospinal fluid from patients with infantile spasms. Epilepsia 29: 300–306

Stores G 1973 Studies of attention and seizure disorders. Developmental Medicine and Child Neurology 15: 376–382

Stores G, Hart J 1976 Reading skills of children with generalised or focal epilepsy attending ordinary school. Developmental Medicine and Child Neurology 18: 705–716

Sutula T, Cascino G, Cavazos J et al 1989 Mossy fiber synaptic reorganization in the epileptic human temporal lobe. Annals of Neurology 26: 321–330

Swaab D F, Mirmiran M 1984 Possible mechanisms underlying the teratogenic effects of medicines on the developing brain. In: Yanai J (ed) Neurobehavioural Teratology. Elsevier, Amsterdam, p 55–71

Tamaki K, Okuno T, Ito M et al 1990 Magnetic resonance imaging in relation to EEG epileptic foci in tuberous sclerosis. Brain and Development 12: 316–320

Tassinari C A, Ambrosetto G 1988 Tonic seizures in the Lennox–Gastaut syndrome: semiology and differential diagnosis. In: Niedermeyer E, Degen R (eds) The Lennox–Gastaut Syndrome. Alan R Liss, New York, p 109–124

Tassinari C A, Bureau M 1985 Epilepsy with myoclonic absences. In: Roger J, Dravet C, Bureau M, Dreifuss F E, Wolf P (eds) Epileptic syndromes in infancy, childhood and adolescence. John Libbey Eurotext, London, p 121–129

Tassinari C A, DeMarco P 1985 Benign partial epilepsy with extreme somato-sensory evoked potentials. In: Roger J, Dravet C, Bureau M, Dreifuss F E, Wolf P (eds) Epileptic syndromes in infancy, childhood and adolescence. John Libbey Eurotext, London, p 176–180

Tassinari C A, Bureau M, Dravet C et al 1985 Epilepsy with continuous spikes and waves during slow sleep. In: Roger J, Dravet C, Bureau M, Dreifuss F E, Wolf P (eds) Epileptic syndromes in infancy, childhood and adolescence. John Libbey Eurotext, London, p 194–204

Taylor D C 1990 Callosal section for epilepsy and the avoidance of doing everything possible. Developmental Medicine and Child Neurology 32: 267–270

Theodore W H, Holmes M D, Dorwart R H et al 1986 Complex partial seizures: cerebral structure and cerebral function. Epilepsia 27: 576–582

Theodore W H, Rose D, Patronas N et al 1987 Cerebral glucose metabolism in the Lennox–Gastaut syndrome. Annals of Neurology 21: 14–21

Thornton E M, Pampiglione G 1979 Psychiatric disorders following infantile spasms. Lancet i: 1297

Trimble M R, Corbett J A 1980 Behavioural and cognitive disturbances in epileptic children. Irish Medical Journal 73: 21–28

Trounce J Q, Fagan D G, Young I D, Levene M I 1986 Disorders of neuronal migration: sonographic appearances. Developmental Medicine and Child Neurology 28: 467–471

Tsang R C 1972 Neonatal magnesium disturbances. American Journal of Diseases in Children 124: 282–293

Tsuboi T 1977 Genetic aspects of febrile convulsions. Human Genetics 38: 169–173

Van Huffelen A C 1989 A tribute to Martimus Rulandus. A 16th-century description of benign focal epilepsy of childhood. Archives of Neurology 46: 445–447

Van Zeben-Van der Aa D M, Verloove-Van Horick S P, den Ouden L et al 1990 Neonatal seizures in very preterm and very low birth-weight infants: mortality and handicaps at two years of age in a nationwide cohort. Neuropaediatrics 21: 62–65

Vanasse M, Masson P, Geoffrey G et al 1984 Intermittent treatment of febrile convulsions with nitrazepam. Canadian Journal of Neurological Science 11: 377–379

Velez A, Dulac O, Plouin P 1990 Prognosis for seizure control in infantile spasms preceded by other seizures. Brain and Development 12: 306–309

Verity C M, Butler N R, Golding J 1985a Febrile convulsions in a national cohort followed up from birth. I Prevalence and recurrence in the first five years of life. British Medical Journal 290: 1307–1310

Verity C M, Butler N R, Golding J 1985b Febrile convulsions in a national cohort followed up from birth. II Medical history and intellectual ability at 5 years of age. British Medical Journal 290: 1311–1315

Viani F, Ettori Beghi M, Atza G, Gulotta M P 1988 Classification of epileptic syndromes: Advantages and limitations for evaluation of childhood epileptic syndromes in clinical practice. Epilepsia 29: 440–445

Viberg M, Blennow G, Polski B 1987 Epilepsy in adolescence: implications for the development of personality. Epilepsia 28: 542–546

Vles J S H, Demandt E, Ceulemans B et al 1990 Single photon emission computed tomography (SPECT) in seizure disorders in childhood. Brain and Development 12: 385–389

Volpe J J 1987 Neurology of the newborn, 2nd edn. W B Saunders, Philadelphia

Wagner A 1990 Magnetic resonance imaging in the diagnosis and treatment of epileptic seizures and syndromes. In: Sillanpää M, Johanessen S I, Blennow G, Dam M (eds) Paediatric epilepsy. Wrightson Biomedical, Petersfield, p 185–193

Wallace S J 1988 The child with febrile seizures. Butterworth, London

Wallace S J 1990 Add-on open trial of lamotrigine in persistent childhood seizures. Brain and Development 12: 743

Wallace S J 1991 Epileptic syndromes linked with previous history of febrile seizures. In: Fukuyama Y, Kamashita S, Ohtsuka C, Suzuki Y (eds) Modern perspectives of child neurology. Japanese Society of Child Neurology, Tokyo, p 175–182

Wallace S J, Aldridge Smith J 1981 Recurrence of convulsions in febrile children on no anticonvulsant. In:

Dam M, Gram L, Penry J K (eds) Advances in Epileptology: XIIth Epilepsy International Symposium. Raven Press, New York, p 499–502

Ward F, Bower B D 1978 A study of certain social aspects of epilepsy in childhood. Developmental Medicine and Child Neurology 20: suppl 39

Wasterlain C G, Dwyer B E 1983 Brain metabolism during prolonged seizures in neonates. In: Delgado-Escueta A V, Wasterlain C G, Treiman D M, Porter R J (eds) Advances in neurology, vol 34: status epilepticus. Raven Press, New York, p 241–260

Wasterlain C G, Hattori H, Yang C et al 1990 Selective vulnerability of neuronal subpopulations during ontogeny reflects discrete molecular events associated with normal brain development. In: Wasterlain C G, Vert P (eds) Neonatal seizures. Raven Press, New York, p 69–81

Watanabe K, Yamamoto N, Negoro T et al 1987 Benign complex partial epilepsies in infancy. Pediatric Neurology 3: 208–211

Webb R, Bobele G 1990 'Benign' familial neonatal convulsions. Journal of Child Neurology 5: 295–298

West W J 1841 On a peculiar form of infantile convulsions. Lancet 1: 724–725

Wilkins A, Lindsay J 1985 Common forms of reflex epilepsy: physiological mechanisms and techniques for treatment. In: Pedley T A, Meldrum B S (eds) Recent advances in epilepsy, 2. Churchill Livingstone, Edinburgh, p 239–271

Willmore L J 1990 Post-traumatic epilepsy: cellular mechanisms and implications for treatment. Epilepsia 31(suppl 3): S67–S73

Wolf P 1985a Juvenile absence epilepsy. In: Roger J, Dravet C, Bureau M, Dreifuss F E, Wolf P (eds) Epileptic syndromes in infancy, childhood and adolescence. John Libbey Eurotext, London, p 242–246

Wolf P 1985b Juvenile myoclonic epilepsy. In: Roger J, Dravet C, Bureau M, Dreifuss F E, Wolf P (eds) Epileptic syndromes in infancy, childhood and adolescence. John Libbey Eurotext, London, p 247–258

Wolf P, Gooses R 1986 Relationship of photosensitivity to epileptic syndromes. Journal of Neurology, Neurosurgery and Psychiatry 49: 1386–1391

Wolf P, Inoue Y 1984 Therapeutic response of absence seizures in patients of an epilepsy clinic for adolescents and adults. Journal of Neurology 231: 225–229

Yamamoto N, Watanabe K, Negoro T et al 1988 Partial seizures evolving to infantile spasms. Epilepsia 29: 34–40

Yoshida T, Tada K, Arakawa T 1971 Vitamin B_6-dependency of glutamic acid decarboxylase in the kidney from a patient with vitamin B_6-dependent convulsion. Tohoku Journal of Experimental Medicine 104: 195–198

Younkin D P, Deliviora-Papadopoulos M, Maris J et al 1986 Cerebral metabolic effects of neonatal seizures measured with in vivo ^{31}P-NMR spectroscopy. Annals of Neurology 20: 513–514

Zelson C, Rubio E, Wasserman E 1971 Neonatal narcotic addiction. Pediatrics 48: 178–189

5. Seizures and epilepsy in adults

D. W. Chadwick

INTRODUCTION

There is considerably less heterogeneity in the epileptic seizures and epileptic syndromes occurring in the adult than in children. While some of the age-related syndromes of childhood may persist into adult life, symptomatic partial epilepsies become predominant in the adult age range. For late onset seizures and epilepsy, determination of aetiology becomes an increasingly important part of management. For this reason, whilst the accepted international classifications of seizures and epileptic syndromes are of continued relevance, greater emphasis may be placed upon classifications that utilize localization and aetiology.

THE INTERNATIONAL CLASSIFICATION OF SEIZURES

This classification, based on clinical and electro-encephalographic features, has been described (Ch. 1). In adults partial seizures with or without secondary generalization become predominant. Late onset epilepsies almost inevitably take this form, and there is frequently a change in both the clinical and electroencephalographic features of seizures of patients with less benign childhood epilepsies so that primary generalized seizures become less frequent and more overt and typical partial seizures become more common as subjects enter adult life. For these reasons it is important to discuss partial seizures, their phenomenology and their localizing value in some detail.

Simple partial seizures

Classical neurological teaching has suggested that motor and sensory phenomena may be used to infer precise localizing value. This has increasingly been questioned as more detailed intracranial recording has become available to correlate with observed clinical phenomena. Thus, the clinical phenomena of seizures reflect not only the site of origin, but also the structures through which seizure discharge spreads during the seizure. This imprecision is illustrated in Figure 5.1 for both sensory and motor components of partial seizures.

Simple partial seizures with motor signs may give rise to clonic or tonic movements involving any part of the body. Clonic seizures most often involve face or hand area, because of the disproportionate amount of the motor cortex occupied by the somatotopic representation of these areas. Whilst clonic seizures involving an arm or a leg may be taken as a reasonably satisfactory indication of seizures involving the motor strip, clonic movements of the eye or facial muscles around the eye can be produced by occipital discharge and clonic movements of the mouth, tongue or pharynx can be caused by temporal discharge (Lesser et al 1987). True Jacksonian 'march' with a slow spread of clonic activity from one muscle group to another is uncommon but when seen does seem to imply relatively specific localization to the pre-central gyrus.

It is evident that tonic motor seizures resulting in adversion or dystonic posturing of limbs have considerably less localizing value than was previously understood. The classical versive seizure with turning of the head and eyes to one side associated with flexion of one arm and possibly extension of the other was originally ascribed by Penfield & Welch (1951) to discharges arising in the pre-motor areas of the frontal lobe. When pronounced such posturing may result in circling

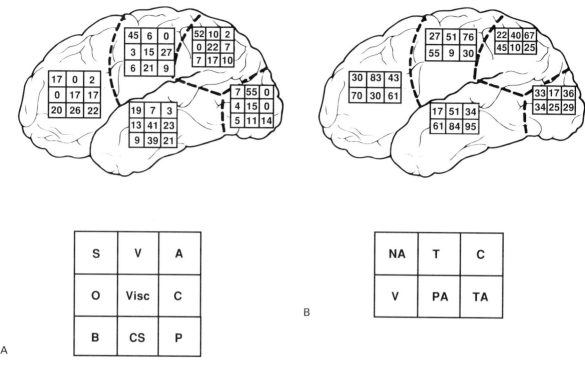

Fig. 5.1 (A) Characteristics of simple partial seizures with sensory symptoms associated with epileptiform EEG abnormalities in various regions of the brain. The numbers in each grid represent the percentage of patients with seizures characterized by the specific features noted in the large grids below each figure. The numbers in each grid may add up to more than 100 because seizures can have more than one feature. Note the relative lack of anatomical specificity for most phenomena. S. somatosensory; V. visual; A, auditory; O, olfactory and gustatory; Visc. visceral; C, cephalic; B, body; CS. complex subjective (emotional, feelings of unreality, discomfort); P, psychic. (B) Characteristics of partial seizures with motor signs associated with epileptiform EEG abnormalities in various regions of the brain. NA, no aura; T, tonic motor; C, clonic motor; V, versive posture; PA, pure automatisms (no other features); TA, total automatisms. As in (A) there is a relative lack of anatomical specificity for most of these phenomena. Reproduced with permission from Engel 1989.

movements. Versive movement, however, can occur in seizures arising in temporal, parietal and occipital lobes as well as in generalized seizures (Ochs et al 1984, Ajmone-Marsan & Goldhammer 1973). Ipsilateral head turning can be as common as contralateral head turning (Ochs et al 1984).

Negative motor phenomena may occur during simple partial seizures. Speech arrest may be the most common manifestation. Whilst speech arrest with a preserved ability to understand speech suggests a seizure in the inferior frontal gyrus (Broca's area) (Geier et al 1977) less specific forms of speech arrest can occur with seizure onset in the supplementary motor areas of the dominant or non-dominant hemisphere (Geier et al 1977). Very rarely, inhibition of movement has been described as part of simple partial seizures (Lesser et al 1987). Postictal paralysis (Todd's

paralysis) seems specific for seizures involving the contralateral motor strip at some point. Versive seizures tend not to be followed by such paralysis.

Sensory seizures

Somatosensory seizures usually arise in the postcentral area. They usually affect the face or hand and may occasionally spread as do Jacksonian seizures. Sensations are usually those of paraesthesiae or numbness (Mauguiere & Courjon 1978). Rarely, disturbing or painful sensations can occur (Young & Blume 1983). Because of the close association between sensory and motor cortex, somatosensory seizures are very frequently associated with motor symptoms. Postictal numbness similar to Todd's phenomena may occur.

Primitive visual symptoms including spots, flashes of light, or patterns in one visual field are most commonly associated with occipital seizures. On occasion occipital seizures may produce visual symptoms that involve both half visual fields. More complex visual hallucinations are less likely to have an occipital onset (see below).

Whilst non-specific 'dizziness' is often described by patients as part of a simple partial seizure, usually it seems that this term is used because of difficulties in describing complex sensory disturbances. True vertigo must be exceptionally uncommon (Smith 1960). Buzzing, hissing, whistling and ringing noises can be experienced most commonly with involvement of the lateral parts of the temporal lobe.

Olfactory and gustatory symptoms are most commonly associated with medial temporal involvement or involvement of the frontal orbital regions. Smells and tastes are usually unpleasant but may be difficult to characterize further than this. Such symptoms are sometimes described as uncinate seizures and whilst it has been suggested that such symptoms are more likely to be associated with temporal tumours, this seems unlikely (Howe & Gibson 1982).

Visceral symptoms form one of the commonest components of simple partial seizures. They are most often associated with involvement of limbic structures of the temporal and frontal lobes. Most common is an epigastric sensation, sometimes described as butterflies or nausea, which tends to rise characteristically into the throat or mouth. More rarely stomach pain, belching or even vomiting can occur (Van Buren 1963). Autonomic signs can include pallor, flushing and sweating, pupillary dilatation and increases in heart rate (Blumhardt et al 1986). Sexual arousal may also occur (Lesser et al 1987). Involuntary micturition or defaecation, whilst not uncommon in seizures associated with loss of consciousness, is extremely rare in simple partial seizures (Maurice-Williams 1974).

Complicated psychic symptoms are not uncommon during simple partial seizures. Again they usually indicate involvement of mesial temporal or frontal limbic structures. Psychic symptoms are often associated with other olfactory gustatory or autonomic disturbances. Dysmnesic symptoms are perhaps the most common with sensations of familiarity (déjà vu) or strangeness (jamais vu). Memory flashbacks or playbacks may occur and may merge into rather non-specific symptoms of dream-like states, unreality and depersonalization on the one hand, and more formed illusions and hallucinations combining visual and auditory aspects on the other. A variety of perceptual changes may occur during seizures with objects appearing larger or smaller or changing in shape or being perseverated (Gloor et al 1982). Emotional experiences are often described, the most frequent being intense fear (Williams 1956). Pleasurable sensations are much rarer but laughter can occur (Gumpert et al 1970). Anger or rage is extremely rare as a true ictal disturbance.

Complex partial seizures

Complex partial seizures in adults are of considerable importance. They are the predominant seizure-type in approximately 40% of patients with epilepsy (Gastaut et al 1975, Juul-Jensen & Foldspang 1983). They tend to be more resistant to antiepileptic drug treatment with at best only 50% of patients attaining long-term remissions (Annegers et al 1979, Turnbull et al 1985). Patients with this seizure type most commonly present additional psychological or psychiatric handicap which greatly adds to the complexity of the management problems that they present (see Ch. 11). Additionally, it is in this group of patients that a surgical approach to the treatment of epilepsy is likely to be most successful (see Ch. 16).

The international classification of seizures emphasizes that complex partial seizures must include some impairment of consciousness. They may or may not be preceded by symptoms of a simple partial seizure and they may or may not be associated with automatism. Complex partial seizures most commonly originate in the medial temporal lobes and the most common electrophysiological correlate is bilateral medial temporal discharge of the hippocampus. However, complex partial seizures may also arise from fronto-orbital regions or more rarely from other extra-temporal sites. It is important to emphasize that complex partial seizures are not identical and synonymous with temporal lobe seizures and that there is no absolute correlation between the phenomenology of complex partial seizures and their site of origin.

By far the most typical form of complex partial seizure will start with an aura or simple partial seizure, usually of the type associated with temporal lobe discharge. There is then an arrest of activity and a motionless stare followed by a phase of stereotyped automatism. Such automatisms occur in a similar fashion in almost all of an individual patient's seizures and most commonly consist of lip smacking, chewing or swallowing or picking at clothes or fidgeting with objects (Delgado-Escueta et al 1982). Walking or running or verbal automatisms are less frequent. Stereotyped automatisms are usually followed by a phase of confusion associated with reactive automatisms. In these, the patient may continue with a previous activity or begin some form of activity that may be considerably influenced by the patients immediate environment. Restraint during this phase of a seizure may sometimes give rise to reactive violent behaviour. It is probable that the majority of such typical complex partial seizures arise from the hippocampus (Delgado-Escueta & Walsh 1985) but by no means all do so (Weiser 1983, Williamson et al 1985).

Complex partial seizures arising from the fronto-orbital regions are more likely to exhibit some of the following phenomena but again there is no absolute correlation. Such seizures are usually frequent, brief and less commonly followed by postictal confusion. The onset of seizures is sudden without any warning and automatisms begin immediately without a preceding motionless stare. Automatisms tend to be bilateral and include thrashing, rolling, kicking or bicycling movements. Sexual automatism with pelvic thrusting may be more common with seizures of frontal onset and complex partial status seems to be more common with fronto-orbital seizures (Williamson et al 1985, Walsh & Delgado-Escueta 1984, Quesney 1986).

A third type of complex partial seizure is sometimes described in which there is a sudden loss of postural tone that has been described as temporal lobe syncope (Caffi 1973).

Partial seizures evolving to secondary generalized seizures

Secondarily generalized seizures are relatively uncommon in adults and may only contribute approximately 9% of seizures in adults compared to approximately 16% in children (Gastaut et al 1975). Furthermore, they are particularly susceptible to antiepileptic drug treatment and the majority of patients developing partial epilepsy in adult life have very few secondarily generalized seizures even though their partial seizures remain a management problem (Turnbull et al 1985). In adults, secondary generalized seizures not infrequently occur during sleep and certainly late onset tonic-clonic seizures occurring during sleep must be regarded as having a focal onset until proved otherwise.

Table 5.1   Classification of myoclonus

Physiological
Sleep myoclonus (hypnic jerks)
Anxiety
Exercise
Hiccough

Essential
Familial
Sporadic
Nocturnal myoclonus

Epileptic
Fragments of epilepsy
  Isolated myoclonic jerks
  Epilepsia partialis continua
  Stimulus-sensitive myoclonus

Childhood myoclonic epilepsies
  Benign myoclonus of infancy
  Infantile astatic epilepsy
  Cryptogenic myoclonic epilepsy
Juvenile myoclonic epilepsy

Symptomatic
Degenerative
  Storage disease (Lafora, Tay–Sachs, Batten's)
  Spinocerebellar degenerations (Ramsay Hunt,
    Baltic myoclonus, Ataxia telegectasia)
  Basal ganglia (Wilsons)
  Dementias (Creutzfeld–Jakob, Alzheimer's)

Acquired
  Viral (SSPE, togavirus encephalitis)
  Metabolic (hepatic, renal, etc.)
  Toxic (heavy metals)
  Physical (post-anoxia, post-traumatic)
  Focal damage (post-CVA, tumour)

Generalized seizures

Primary generalized seizures are relatively uncommon in adult life and will not be discussed in great detail here. Whilst typical absence, myoclonus and primary tonic-clonic seizures may begin in adolescence and early adult life, other forms of generalized seizures such as atypical absence, tonic and atonic seizures are features of age-related childhood epilepsies and therefore, whilst they may persist into adult life, they never commence in adult life. However, many children with severe childhood epilepsies tend to develop more typical partial seizures (particularly complex partial seizures) or may expect remission when they enter adult life (Huttenlocher & Hapke 1990).

Myoclonus does, however, demand some further discussion because of its complex relationship to epilepsy. A classification of myoclonus is included in Table 5.1. The term myoclonus denotes a brief, rapid, jerky movement and as such it has a wide variety of neurophysiological correlates

(Fahn et al 1986). Whilst it may form a distinctive part of age-related epilepsy syndromes of infancy, childhood and adolescence, it will also be seen in a group of conditions that have been termed progressive myoclonic epilepsy in which frequent action myoclonus and occasional tonic-clonic seizures occur on a background of progressive neurological deterioration often associated with specific genetic disorders (Table 5.2).

EPILEPSY SYNDROMES IN ADULT LIFE

A systematic classification of epilepsy syndromes has been proposed (Commission on Classification 1989). Most epilepsy syndromes are age-related and occur in childhood, whilst the majority of the epilepsies of adult life are symptomatic partial epilepsies. For this reason the classification has less relevance to adults in whom accurate localization of the onset of partial seizures and determination of their aetiology is of greater importance (see below). Some reference does, however, need

Table 5.2 The spetrum of progressive myclonic epilepsy

(a) Progressive myoclonus epilepsies	(b) Progressive encephalopathies with myoclonus: disordes where myoclonus is generally overshadowed by other clinical manifestations
Unverricht-Lundborg disease	GM_2 gangliosidoses
Lafora-body disease	GM_1 gangliosidoses
Classical form	Niemann–Pick disease
Late onset form	Krabbe's disease
Neuronal ceroid lipofuscinoses	Neuronal ceroid lipofuscinoses
Late infantile form	Phenylketonuria
Juvenile form	Maple syrup urine disease
Adult form	Non-ketotic hyperglycinemia
Sialidoses	Gaucher disease
Type 1	Menkes disease
Type 2	Alpers disease
Mitochondrial encephalomyopathies	SSPE
Rare syndromes biochemically defined	Progressive rubella encephalitis
Gaucher disease	Alzheimer disease
Biotin-responsive encephalopathy	Jakob–Creutzfeldt disease
Rare syndromes pathologically defined	
Neuroaxonal dystrophy	
Hallervorden–Spatz disease	
Atypical inclusion body disease	
Action myoclonus-renal failure syndrome	
Hereditary dentatorubral-pallidoluysian atrophy	
Rare syndromes clinically defined	
PME and deafness	
PME and lipomas	
Ramsay Hunt syndrome	
Benign familial myoclonus	

Reproduced from Berkovic & Anderman (1986) with permission.

to be made to those specific epilepsy syndromes where seizures have a predilection to continue into adult life.

Idiopathic generalized epilepsies

Childhood absence epilepsy

This syndrome probably accounts for about 8% of epilepsy in school age children (Cavazzuti 1980). It is probably genetic (Metrakos & Metrakos 1972, Hauser & Anderson 1986). The prognosis seems to be excellent with anywhere between 33% (Oller-Daurella & Sanchez 1981) to 80% (Dalby 1969) achieving long-term remission. Figures at the lower range of these estimates include patients followed up for longer periods. Only about 6% of patients with this seizure disorder have absences which persist into adult life (Oller-Daurella & Sanchez 1981). Tonic-clonic seizures, however, commonly develop, usually between 5 and 10 years after the onset of absences (Loiseau et al 1983). Again there may be significant effects of varying lengths of follow-up of patients on the proportion developing tonic-clonic seizures. These may occur in between 40% (Loiseau et al 1983) and 60% of patients (Oller-Daurella and Sanchez, 1981). It may be that tonic-clonic seizures are more likely to develop in subjects whose absences initially respond poorly to appropriate antiepileptic drug therapy (Oller-Daurella & Sanchez 1981).

When tonic-clonic seizures occur in subjects with this syndrome in adult life, they occur without an aura and have a tendency to occur within 1–2 hours of wakening. Sodium valproate is undoubtedly the drug of choice for the treatment of persisting seizures in adults with this syndrome (Loiseau 1985).

The idiopathic epilepsies of adolescence and early adult life

Three specific age-related syndromes share many similarities and may potentially be regarded as different phenotypic presentations of what may be a single genetic disorder. They are juvenile myoclonic epilepsy, juvenile absence epilepsy and epilepsy with tonic-clonic seizures on awakening.

All tend to commence after puberty but rarely commence after the age of 20–25, are strongly associated with spike-wave activity (4–6 Hz) and are characterized by seizures that tend to occur on wakening, often precipitated by sleep deprivation.

Juvenile absence epilepsy. This syndrome is less common than childhood absence epilepsy. Absence seizures begin in the second decade of life but tend to be much less frequent than those of childhood absence epilepsy. A greater proportion (80%) also have tonic-clonic seizures; 75% of these latter seizures occur on awakening (Janz, 1969). Myoclonic seizures can also occur in this syndrome, perhaps in as many as 16% of patients (Wolfe & Inoue 1984). Valproate is again the drug of choice with remission in 85% of patients (Wolfe & Inoue 1984). It seems that the small proportion of patients with only absence seizures will almost certainly be guaranteed remission with appropriate therapy.

Juvenile myoclonic epilepsy. This is a common epilepsy syndrome which was first comprehensively described by Janz & Christian (1957). It is a genetic disorder and up to 25% of patients have a family history (Janz 1969). The gene encoding for this disorder has been shown by linkage analysis to lie on the short arm of the 6th chromosome (Greenberg et al 1988).

It accounts for approximately 6% of the epilepsies. Seizures can begin between the age 8 and 26, but 80% commence between the ages of 12 and 18 (Janz 1969). Myoclonic jerks are usually symmetrical and mostly affect the upper limbs. Myoclonus can on occasion be associated with absence or typical absence seizures can occur independently. Seizures most commonly occur after wakening but there may also be a second peak in seizure susceptibility during the evening. Sleep deprivation appears to be a potent provocative factor for seizures.

A total 90% of patients have generalized tonic-clonic seizures (Janz 1969); 10% of patients may have absence seizures. It is, however, the tonic-clonic seizures that precipitate medical referral and patients may not recognize the important association with jerks which may have preceded the first tonic-clonic seizure by some time. It is therefore important in identifying this syndrome to ask specifically for a history of myoclonus.

The EEG typically shows polyspike and spike wave activity at a more rapid rate than the classic 3 cycle/second spike wave (Janz 1969). Photosensitivity is extremely common and is usually identified in about 30% of patients, though this phenomena may frequently be blocked by treatment with valproate (Goosses 1984). There can be no doubt that valproate is the drug of choice in this syndrome and indeed remission may be uncommon if patients are treated with other antiepileptic drugs (Delgado-Escueta & Enrile-Bascal 1984). However, remissions of this syndrome are drug-dependent and 90% of patients with it will relapse if drugs are withdrawn (Janz et al 1983).

Tonic-clonic seizures on awakening. Tonic-clonic (or clonic-tonic-clonic) seizures predominate in this syndrome though the presence of occasional myoclonus or absence does not preclude the diagnosis. Janz (1962) examined the timing of tonic-clonic seizures in 2825 patients: 33% had tonic-clonic seizures on awakening compared to 44% occurring during sleep and 23% occurring at random. There was a strong association between tonic-clonic seizures occurring on wakening and generalized spike-wave activity in the EEG.

Precipitating factors seem particularly important in this syndrome, where sleep deprivation and alcohol intake again appear important but where sudden arousal from sleep and catamenial seizures are also prominent.

Avoidance of precipitating factors is important in management and valproate is probably the drug of choice for this syndrome. The occurrence of seizures on wakening seems to increase the risk of relapse if drugs are withdrawn after a period of remission (Janz et al 1983, MRC Drug Antiepileptic Withdrawal Study Group 1991).

Symptomatic generalized epilepsies

These childhood epilepsies are frequently malignant (see Ch. 4) and are associated with a significant mortality. However, many children with such epilepsies will survive into the adult age-range. They are frequently mentally handicapped and may also have motor disability (cerebral palsy). In adult life there is often a change in the nature of seizures with myoclonic, tonic, atonic, and complex absence seizures becoming less frequent. More typical simple partial and complex partial seizures become evident. The characteristic of these seizures is often that they appear multi-focal from a clinical and electroencephalographic point of view. Whilst such patients may continue to have severe epilepsy during adult life, seizure frequency tends to be less than in childhood.

Partial (localization-related) epilepsies

The idiopathic age-related syndromes (e.g. Rolandic epilepsy) are not seen in adult life as they have an early age of onset in childhood and a uniformly excellent prognosis. The great majority of partial epilepsies of adult life are likely to be symptomatic. The international classification divides symptomatic epilepsies into frontal, temporal, parietal and occipital lobe epilepsies on the grounds of the site of origin of the seizures. This adds little further help or information to classifying a patient's seizures. It is perhaps more important to consider specific aetiologies for seizures and epilepsy in adult life (see below).

FACTORS PRECIPITATING SEIZURES IN ADULTS

A number of factors may appear to precipitate seizures in susceptible individuals. These may be regarded as either specific sensory stimuli or actions (reflexly induced seizures) or non-specific precipitants.

Reflexly-induced seizures

Whilst the term 'reflex epilepsy' has been widely applied, the validity of the term needs to be questioned as most patients who have reflexly-induced seizures may also have apparently spontaneous seizures occurring at other times. Photically-induced seizures are the most common reflex seizures. About 3% of patients with epilepsy may show visually-induced seizures (Jeavons & Harding 1975) and over half the patients with reflex seizures would appear to be sensitive to visual stimuli (Forster 1977). The crudest visual stimulus to evoke seizures is flicker or flash, a factor that is made use of in the routine recording of most EEGs. This form of sensitivity is most common in childhood and juvenile absence epilepsy and juvenile myoclonic epilepsy and some forms of progressive myoclonic epilepsy. It is a much rarer accompaniment of symptomatic generalized epilepsies and is rarely seen in partial epilepsy. Flicker stimuli may be produced in the environment by television and video games, stroboscopic illumination or sunlight passing through trees or railings or other regularly spaced objects. Most individuals are maximally sensitive between 15 and 20 Hz (Jeavons & Harding 1975). Maximum sensitivity often occurs just after the eyes are closed or when the eyes are open. Stimulation of one eye rather than both eyes reduces sensitivity. The greater the visual field taken up by stimuli and the luminance affect sensitivity and in many individuals patterned flash is a more potent stimulus.

The electrophysiological correlate of photosensitivity is the photoconvulsive response (see Ch. 9). This is most commonly seen in females during childhood and adolescence and may disappear in adult life.

About a third of flash-sensitive patients exhibit sensitivity to patterns, the most potent of which are strong stripes (Wilkins et al 1980). The most important practical implication of pattern sensitivity is television epilepsy. A television picture is created by variations in the brightness of a spot that scans the screen repeatedly from left to right. The pattern that is generated in this way is similar to a vibrating pattern which is a very potent stimulus to pattern-sensitive individuals. Seizures can be prevented in susceptible individuals by maintaining a satisfactory distance from the television set and using a remote control to adjust the picture. More complex methods involve viewing the screen through polarized spectacles so as to produce only monocular stimulation (Wilkins & Lindsay 1985).

Primary reading epilepsy can be viewed as a form of visually-induced epilepsy. The characteristic seizures in this disorder are myoclonic jerks of the jaw which may proceed to tonic-clonic seizures. Both focal and paroxysmal EEG abnormalities have been described in this condition (Wilkins & Lindsay 1985). A number of different mechanisms may be involved in producing seizures with reading. The lines of print may in some patients act as patterns (Mayersdorf & Marshall 1970). In others, eye movements may potentially provoke the seizures (Alajouanine et al 1959). In some patients neither pattern sensitivity nor eye movements appear important and in these comprehension of the written material may be the important provocative factor (Forster 1977).

Some patients may rarely make use of photic sensitivity to induce their own seizures. This may be achieved by waving the fingers of a hand across the forehead or by staring at patterns. A similar stimulus can be delivered by rolling up the eyes and attempting to close the eyelids at the same time (Binnie et al 1980).

Sodium valproate seems to have a particularly potent effect in blocking photo-sensitivity and is the anticonvulsant of choice where drug treatment is necessary for this form of reflexly-induced seizures.

Sudden noise or other startle may give rise to seizures, particularly in mentally handicapped patients (Anderman & Anderman 1986). More complex auditory stimuli can also provoke seizures in musicogenic epilepsy (Critchley 1937, Poskanzer et al 1962). Such seizures are usually complex partial seizures. A variety of other complex reflex epilepsies have been described including eating epilepsy, which causes clonus of the muscles of swallowing, and writing epilepsy, producing jerking of the writing hand. Other cognitive functions such as arithmetic (Ingvar & Nyman 1962) and listening to spoken language (Tsuki & Kasuga 1978) can evoke seizures.

Touch or muscle stretch may occasionally provoke seizures but more commonly evokes myoclonic jerking in patients with progressive myoclonic or post-hypoxic myoclonus. Rarely seizures may be provoked by movement (Lishman et al 1962), though many of the patients described in this paper probably had paroxysmal choreoathetosis.

Non-specific precipitants

The sleep–waking cycle can have a profound influence on the occurrence of seizures in susceptible individuals (Baldy-Moulinier, 1986). Many patients have tonic-clonic seizures only during sleep (Gibberd & Bateson 1974). Sleep may enhance focal epileptogenic discharges and tonic-clonic seizures limited to sleep in the adult should usually be regarded as having a partial onset until proved otherwise (Janz, 1962). However, it must be noted that some patients with generalized epilepsies also exhibit frequent spike wave activity during sleep (Tassinari et al 1985).

Seizures occurring shortly after wakening are common in juvenile myoclonic epilepsy, tonic-clonic seizures on awakening and childhood and juvenile absence epilepsy (see above). Such individuals seem particularly sensitive to sleep deprivation or to sudden rousing from deep sleep.

Many women with epilepsy are subject to catamenial exacerbation of seizures although it is uncommon to see women who only have seizures corresponding to such a pattern (Newmark & Penry 1980). The time of greatest susceptibility seems to be in the few days preceding the onset of menstruation. Whilst it has been suggested that water retention is an important factor in the mechanisms precipitating such seizures, the evidence for this is weak and diuretics seem to have little effect in suppressing such seizures. There is, however, evidence that oestrogens may be potentially epileptogenic and progestogens potentially anticonvulsant (Backstrom 1976). In spite of this, regulation of periods using oral contraceptive preparations has not shown any benefit in suppressing such seizures but where periods are regular the prescription of a benzodiazepine such as clobazam for a number of days around the period of maximum risk can be beneficial (Feely et al 1982). The effects of pregnancy on seizure control in women with epilepsy is unpredictable. In some individuals seizures may increase in frequency, in some they may decrease but in the majority there is no significant change in seizures frequency.

Psychological stress is often quoted by patients as precipitating seizures. Emotional stress precipitated fits in 21% of patients with temporal lobe epilepsy (Curry et al 1971). The mechanisms involved may in some circumstances include alterations in sleep–waking cycle which commonly accompany stress and the role of psychotropic drugs in increasing seizure susceptibility must always be remembered (see below).

CAUSES OF SEIZURES AND EPILEPSY IN ADULTS

The great majority of seizures and epilepsies developing in adult life will be regarded as symptomatic. However, significant numbers of patients may be investigated without those becoming apparent (cryptogenic epilepsies). In The National General Practice Study of Epilepsy, 60% of all patients had no identifiable cause of seizures or epilepsy though a proportion of these may have had a specific (genetically determined) epilepsy syndrome (Sander et al 1990).

It may be useful to differentiate causes of seizures and epilepsy in adult life into acute symptomatic seizures where seizures occur acutely in response to metabolic or cerebral insult, and remote symptomatic epilepsies in which epilepsy develops as a chronic phenomenon in relationship to persisting cerebral lesion or damage. Some aetiologies, e.g. head injury, stroke, intracerebral infections, may cause both acute symptomatic seizures and remote symptomatic epilepsy. The presence of the one does not necessarily determine the other.

Sander et al (1990) found that the commonest remote symptomatic causes of epilepsy were vascular disease (15%) and tumour (6%). Remote symptomatic epilepsy was commonest in the elderly where vascular disease accounted for 49% of cases. Tumour was a rare cause of epilepsy below 30 (1%), but accounted for 19% of cases between 50 and 59 years. Trauma caused 3% of cases, infection 2%. Acute symptomatic seizures occurred in 15%, and alcohol was the commonest cause (6%), its incidence being highest between 30 and 39 years (27%).

Acute symptomatic seizures

This term was suggested by Hauser et al (1982). Such seizures are often associated with an acute encephalopathy and most commonly seizures are of a tonic-clonic type. Patients will often exhibit tremor, asterixis and multifocal myoclonus. Focal seizures are uncommon but can occur and when they do they are usually recognized as focal motor seizures, sometimes as epilepsia partialis continua. It is suggested that complex partial seizures rarely occur as acute symptomatic seizures but one would have to acknowledge that such seizures could be difficult to recognize when accompanied by an acute confusional state or coma. When acute symptomatic seizures occur due to metabolic disorders, drugs, or drug withdrawal, it often appears that they are more related to the rate of metabolic change or drug exposure than to the absolute disturbance.

They are common, accounting for 15% of new cases of seizures overall (Sander et al 1990) and being particularly common in the elderly, where they may account for as much as 77% of the incidence (Loiseau et al 1990).

Whilst such seizures may be suppressed by short-acting antiepileptic drugs (e.g. benzodiazepines) they do not require longer term antiepileptic drug treatment. On occasion acute symptomatic seizures may be resistant to benzodiazepines and other antiepileptic drugs and correction of the underlying metabolic abnormality may be necessary to suppress seizures.

Disorders of fluid and electrolyte balance

Hypernatraemia. This may occur in gastro-enteritis, fever, sweating, burns and diabetes, and due to gross fluid restriction or excessive salt intake. Neurological signs are seen in 50% of patients with serum sodium concentrations above 151 mmol/l (Swanson, 1976). Altered consciousness is common and focal or generalized seizures occur most commonly in patients who are also uraemic or acidotic (Stephenson 1971). They are also seen during rehydration, which should be undertaken cautiously with dextrose-saline solutions (Bruck et al 1968).

Hyponatraemia. This is more common than hypernatraemia and may be seen with congestive cardiac failure, liver disease, nephrotic syndrome and water-overload as well as with renal disease and inappropriate ADH syndromes which are commonly associated with neurological disorders. Focal or generalized seizures occur. Convulsions were noted in 9% of 65 patients with serum sodium concentrations of less than 125 mmol/l

(Arieff et al 1976). Hyponatraemia is associated with a high mortality and too rapid a correction by the over-enthusiastic use of hypertonic saline has been associated with the occurrence of central pontine myelinolysis (Norenberg et al 1982).

Hypocalcaemia. This may be seen in hypoparathyroidism, vitamin D deficiency, acute pancreatitis and pseudohypoparathyroidism. Up to 70% of patients with hypoparathyroidism may have seizures associated with tetany, altered consciousness and abnormal behaviour and dyskinesia (Frame 1976). Both tonic-clonic and focal motor seizures are described.

Hypercalcaemia. This most commonly occurs in disseminated malignant disease and hyperparathyroidism. It results in weakness, drowsiness and confusion and occasionally seizures, which can be generalized (Bauermeister et al 1967) or focal motor seizures (Herishanu et al 1970).

Hypomagnesaemia. This may be seen in inflammatory bowel disease, bowel resection and other malabsorption syndromes. Neurological syndromes may be seen with levels below 1.3 mmol/l and the clinical state may be indistinguishable from hypocalcaemia (Hanna et al 1960), although tetany may be less common (Fishman 1965). Hypomagnesaemic seizures may be resistant to antiepileptic drug therapy and may only respond to the administration of magnesium. This fact should be remembered as hypomagnesaemia may not infrequently accompany hypocalcaemia. Hypomagnesaemia needs to be considered if seizures continue in a treated hypocalcaemic patient.

Hypophosphataemia. Hypophosphataemia may occur in association with long duration, intensive therapy or parenteral feeding. Tonic-clonic seizures may occur with serum phosphate levels below 1 mg/100 ml (Knochel 1977). Most hypophosphataemic patients will also require potassium and magnesium replacement.

Endocrine disorders

Disorders of glucose metabolism. Seizures seem particularly common in association with non-ketotic hyperosmolar coma (Venna & Sabin 1981). They may occur in up to a quarter of patients and focal motor seizures appear particularly common and epilepsia partialis continua can occur. In about 6% of patients focal motor seizures were the initial symptom of the disorder (Aquino & Gabor 1980). Such seizures may be very resistant to antiepileptic drug treatment but seem to respond rapidly to the correction of the hyperglycaemia. In contrast, seizures seem to be extremely rare in ketoacidotic coma (Messing & Simon 1986).

Hypoglycaemia is usually seen in diabetic patients using insulin or hypoglycaemic drugs. It occurs more rarely with insulinoma, other neoplasms or severe liver disease. Seizures, usually tonic-clonic seizures without an aura, may occur in 7% of patients (Malouf & Brust 1985).

Thyroid disease. Seizures appear extremely uncommon in hyperthyroidism but they do occur occasionally (Korczyn & Bechar, 1976). They can accompany an acute or subacute encephalopathy that sometimes precedes other manifestations of thyrotoxicosis (Thrush & Boddie 1974). Seizures appear more common in patients with hypothyroidism and may occur in as many as a quarter of patients with myxoedema coma (Jellinek 1962). Patients would not seem to be at risk of continued seizures after the underlying thyroid abnormality has been corrected.

Porphyria. Seizures may occur in approximately 15% of patients during episodes of acute intermittent porphyria (Reynolds & Miska, 1976). Control of seizures can be a significant management problem as hydantoins, barbiturates and carbamazepine can all induce attacks of porphyria. Benzodiazepines or valproate may be used with caution but it has also been suggested that magnesium sulphate may also be effective in controlling seizures (Taylor 1981).

Liver disease. Seizures appear to be a feature of acute hepatic failure but not of chronic hepatic dysfunction. Seizures may be focal but are more commonly tonic-clonic seizures often preceded by multifocal myoclonus. Their incidence varies greatly in different series. Adams & Foley (1953) reported convulsions in a third of patients but only one of 83 patients reported by Plumb & Posner (1980) had fits. Some differences may arise from the aetiology of hepatic failure, alcohol being much commoner in the former series. Hypoglycaemia complicating acute liver failure may be a further factor affecting its incidence (Plumb & Hindfelt 1968).

Renal failure. Acute uraemic encephalopathy commonly presents with motor excitability including tremors, multifocal myoclonus and tetany. Convulsions occur in as many as a third of

Table 5.3 Drugs associated with seizures

Anaesthetics	Antibiotics	Antipsychotic agents
Ether	Benzylpenicillin	Chlorpromazine
Halothane	Carbenicillin	Lithium
Ketamine	Oxacillin	
Methohexitone	Ampicillin	Radiographic contrast media
Propanidid	Cycloserine	Meglumine carbamate
Althesin	Isoniazid	Meglumine iothalamate
	Nalidixic acid	Metrizamide
	Quinalones	
Analeptics		
Nikethamide	Anticonvulsants	Miscellaneous
Aminophylline	(in overdosage)	D-Penicillamine
Amphetamines	Phenobarbitone	Baclofen
Ephedrine	Phenytoin	Hyperbaric oxygen
	Ethosuximide	Folate
Analgesics		Piperazine
Cocaine	Antidepressants	Cyclosporin
Pethidine	Amitryptiline	Interferon
Dextropropoxyphene	Imipramine	
	Mianserin	
Antidysrhythmics	Maprotiline	
Disopyramide		
Lignocaine		

patients (Raskin & Fishman 1976). Again, most are tonic-clonic seizures but focal motor seizures can occur. Seizures have also been reported during dialysis (dialysis disequilibrium syndrome) and as part of dialysis encephalopathy, a subacute progressive disorder in which speech disorders, dementia and myoclonus are prominent (Lederman & Henry 1978). This disorder seems to be related to levels of aluminium in water used for dialysis medium (Dunea et al 1978).

The use of antiepileptic drugs in patients with chronic renal failure presents some difficulties. Protein-bound antiepileptic drugs such as phenytoin may have relatively high, free, and therefore active, concentrations of phenytoin relative to total estimated plasma levels. Similar problems may exist for carbamazepine which also tends to be excreted in the urine and dosage reduction may be necessary (Bennett et al 1980).

Drug-related seizures. Drugs, and particularly alcohol, are not an uncommon cause of seizures (Chadwick 1983, Messing et al 1984) and many different drugs have been associated with seizures (Table 5.3). The Boston collaborative drugs surveillance programme (1972) reported 26 cases of drug-induced convulsions in approximately 33 000 in-patients (an incidence of 0.08%). The most commonly involved drugs were penicillin, hypoglycaemic drugs, lignocaine and psychotropic agents. Messing et al (1984) reviewed case records of over 3000 patients presenting with seizures and found that they were drug-related in 1.7%, the most common drugs involved being isoniazid, psychotropic drugs, bronchodilators, hypoglycaemic agents, lignocaine and penicillin. The majority of seizures are tonic-clonic seizures but whilst most begin without an aura, there was a simple partial (motor) onset in nine patients.

Seizures may be provoked in two ways: there may be specific CNS excitatory effects for some drugs or alternatively there may be non-specific effects resulting from high doses of drugs often administered during self-poisoning. Most drug-induced seizures are dose related and particular care must be exercised when drugs are administered parenterally or intrathecally. Patients with renal or hepatic failure may be at risk because of inability to metabolize potentially convulsant

drugs and individuals with a previous history of epilepsy or pre-existing brain disease may be particularly at risk.

Antibiotics. Penicillin is a potent epileptogenic substance in animals and has been widely used as a model for both focal and generalized epilepsies. It appears to act as a GABA antagonist and may also bind to benzodiazepine receptors (Antoniadis et al 1980, Curtis et al 1972). Benzylpenicillin is probably the most potent antibiotic in causing seizures but ampicillin and cephalosporins can also have some effect. Newer quinalone antibiotics may similarly interfere with gabergic mechanisms and isoniazid may cause seizures because of its action in antagonizing pyridoxine, a co-enzyme required for the synthesis of GABA (Blakemore 1980).

Psychotropic drugs. Tricyclics are particularly likely to cause myoclonus and convulsions when taken in overdose but seizures may occur in up to 1% of patients taking therapeutic dosages (Lowry & Dunner 1980). Phenothiazines are also associated with a 1–2% incidence of seizures (Logothetis 1967).

Analeptic drugs. Most CNS stimulant drugs are capable of causing seizures. Problems most commonly arise with theophylline and its derivatives which significantly lower seizure threshold possibly by elevating cyclic GMP levels in brain (Walker 1981).

Drugs of abuse. Cocaine, amphetamines and phencyclidine have been associated with seizures (Messing & Simon 1986). They have stimulant actions on the central nervous system and lower seizure threshold (Gawin & Ellinwood 1988).

Withdrawal seizures. Withdrawal of chronically administered sedative drugs which show tolerance is a well recognized cause of seizures and may occur with alcohol, barbiturates, benzodiazepines, glutethimide and meprobamate (Chadwick 1983). The best studied of withdrawal seizures are those that occur with alcohol often as part of the delirium tremens syndrome. There can be no doubt that abuse of alcohol is an important cause of seizures in the community (Sander et al 1990) and that it must be considered in adults developing tonic-clonic seizures for the first time (Hillbom 1980). The risk is clearly related to the dose of alcohol consumed (Ng et al 1988). Whilst the latter group of workers dispute the fact, it does seem that it is abrupt, absolute or relative withdrawal of alcohol that is most commonly responsible for causing seizures. [Alcohol can be shown to have short-term antiepileptic properties in rodents and similar effect has been suggested in man (Mattson et al 1975)]. The suggestion is supported by a study of 10 institutionalized heroin addicts who were given intoxicating quantities of alcohol for periods of up to 3 months. Seizures occurred on abrupt withdrawal but not whilst patients were intoxicated (Isbel et al 1955). The studies of Victor & Adams (1953) and Victor & Brauch (1967) showed a clustering of seizures between 7 and 48 hours after the withdrawal of alcohol. Sixty percent of patients have more than one seizure but status epilepticus occurs in less than 5% of patients. During the withdrawal period photo-myoclonic and photo-convulsive responses may be seen in the EEG.

On occasions seizures do seem to occur in patients whilst intoxicated with alcohol. This has conventionally been explained by suggesting a relative withdrawal of alcohol as being responsible (Simon 1988). Ng et al (1988) cast some doubt on this assertion using complex statistical approaches to the timing of seizures in individuals consuming large quantities of alcohol. An alternative explanation may be that alcohol as a short-term anticonvulsant shares with other anticonvulsant drugs a biphasic action on the central nervous system. A convulsant effect at high dosage similar to that that can be seen with anticonvulsants such as phenytoin and phenobarbitone (Chadwick 1983) could be important.

It is well recognized that non-compliance with antiepileptic drug medication is a common cause of seizures in people with epilepsy and indeed is an important cause of status epilepticus (Aminoff & Simon 1980). Historically, abuse of barbiturates and subsequent withdrawal has been an important cause of seizures. This effect is dose-related and seizures occur with other withdrawal symptoms such as insomnia, tremor, anorexia and autonomic over-activity (Fraser et al 1958). The EEG of patients undergoing barbiturate withdrawal has features of both photo-myoclonic and photo-convulsant responses (Essig 1967). Benzodiazepines have also, on occasion, been associated with presumed withdrawal seizure (Chadwick 1983).

The withdrawal sydrome associated with opiates, however, is unusual in that seizures occur very rarely.

Remote symptomatic causes of epilepsy

It is well recognized that a number of cerebral injuries predispose to the development of epilepsy. Where such insults can lead to acute symptomatic seizures the importance of the latter will be discussed in this section.

Hypoxic/ischaemic cerebral insults

Pre- and perinatal hypoxia. Mental and motor handicap present from birth are commonly associated with seizure disorders. Zielinski (1974) found 20% of the epileptic population to be retarded or dull and Gudmundson (1966) found a similar proportion of mentally handicapped individuals to have epilepsy in Iceland. Cerebral palsy is also strongly associated with epilepsy and as many as 50% of individuals with mental handicap and cerebral palsy have a seizure disorder (Hauser et al 1987). The more severe the mental and physical handicap the higher the risk of epilepsy (Blomquist et al 1981, Gustavson et al 1977, Edebol-Tysk 1989). Pre- and perinatal hypoxia of one form or another seems to be the commonest single cause of mental handicap and cerebral palsy (Forsgren 1990, Nelson & Ellenberg 1986).

The great majority of individuals with mental handicap and cerebral palsy develop seizures early in life but up to 15% of patients may have a seizure disorder that starts after the age of 15 (Forsgren 1990). Whilst primary generalized seizures including myoclonus, tonic and atonic seizures and infantile spasms, as part of a secondary generalized epilepsy are common in such people in childhood, as these individuals mature partial seizures and secondary generalized tonic-clonic seizures predominate (Forsgren 1990). In this population the outcome for epilepsy is worse than would be generally expected, only a third achieving seizure remissions of a year and a third having at least one seizure per month. Early brain damage is one of the strongest factors predicting a poor outcome of epilepsy (Shaffer et al 1988).

Hippocampal sclerosis. Hippocampal sclerosis is the most common pathological lesion in surgically treated patients with complex partial seizures (Babb 1987) and a case controlled study has suggested that complicated febrile seizures during childhood may be the aetiological factor in up to 20% of patients with complex partial seizures (Rocca et al 1987). Falconer (1971) suggested that prolonged febrile seizures produce such damage by leading to hypoxic/ischaemic cell loss in the hippocampus (Meldrum et al 1974). This hypothesis is now widely accepted even though it is well recognized that simple febrile seizures do not seem to be associated with a high risk of late epilepsy (Nelson & Ellenberg 1978).

This aetiological factor is of particular importance in epilepsies in adolescents and young adults in view of the high prevalence of complex partial seizures, their poor response to antiepileptic drug treatment, and their excellent response to surgical treatment (see Ch. 16).

Cerebral hypoxia in adult life. Generalized cerebral hypoxia during adult life seems much less likely to result in seizures. Acute hypoxia is commonly associated with convulsions and multifocal myoclonus (Wardrope et al 1991). In patients with post-hypoxic coma following an anoxic insult, seizures seem to be much rarer (Bates et al 1977) and when they occur they may be associated with an adverse prognosis. Seizures seem to be relatively rare in adults surviving post-hypoxic coma but action myoclonus can be disabling in such individuals (Lance & Adams 1963).

Head injury

The relationship between head injury, acute symptomatic seizures (within the first week of injury) and late post-traumatic epilepsy represents perhaps the best studied of all causes of epilepsy. The relationship between head injury and epilepsy is well known to every member of the public and most patients developing epilepsy will recall a minor head injury sometime before the development of seizures. However, it is clear that only specific types of head injury carry a significant risk of post-traumatic epilepsy.

Although perhaps 2% of all concussive head injuries result in epilepsy (Annegers et al 1980), head trauma was the cause of seizures in 3% of patients registered in the National General Practitioners Survey of Epilepsy (Sander et al 1990). There can be no doubt that the more severe the head injury, the higher the risk of post-traumatic epilepsy (Annegers et al 1980, Jennett 1975).

Missile injuries and epilepsy. Brain injuries caused by missiles provide a well defined and relatively homogenous group of injuries that fortunately are rare in civilian life. They have, however, been very fully studied in cohorts of patients from the First World War through to the Vietnam War. In many, the localization and the extent of the injury are known to be anatomically precise and the relationship between the incidence of epilepsy and factors such as retention of foreign bodies, haematoma, brain infection and the extent of the cerebral injury can be determined. Table 5.4 summarizes a number of series. The varying risks of post-traumatic epilepsy may be influenced by varying periods of follow-up of patients. Overall, it would seem that 50% of patients with such injuries will eventually develop post-traumatic epilepsy and the relative risk of developing such epilepsy will initially be approximately 580 times higher than a general age-matched population during the first year, falling to 25 times higher after 10 years (Salazar et al 1985).

The site of the injury may be important, wounds of the motor and pre-motor cortex having a higher risk of epilepsy than wounds elsewhere (Russell & Witty 1952). There is no doubt that the extent of the cerebral injury and the amount of brain loss, which may also be determined by surgical intervention, is an important factor. Walker & Jablon (1961) found an association

Table 5.4 Incidence of epilepsy following missile injuries

Reference	%	Source of injury
Ascroft (1941)	45	World War I
Russel & Whitty (1952)	43	World War II
Walker & Jablon (1961)	36	World War II
Caveness & Liss (1961)	40	Korean War
Caveness et al (1979)	33	Vietnam War
Salazar et al (1985)	53	Vietnam War

between the risk of epilepsy and the extent of the wound as judged by surface and depth measurements, and most recently a CT scan assessment of the extent of the injury similarly affects the risk of epilepsy (Salazar et al 1985). Almost certainly correlated with the extent of the injury is the presence of persisting neurological deficit which has been consistently associated with a high risk of epilepsy (Russell & Witty 1952, Salazar et al 1985).

Walker & Jablon (1961) did not find that the removal of intracranial metal and bone fragments affected the incidence of epilepsy, though Ascroft (1941) noted a higher incidence of epilepsy when metal had been removed than when it was left indwelling, another possible effect of surgical intervention.

Infection probably exerts an important influence on the incidence of epilepsy. After abscess formation the incidence may rise to 73% (Walker & Jablon 1961) and even higher risks of epilepsy are associated with complicating fungal infections (Caveness et al 1979).

Salazar et al (1985) suggest that 75% of patients develop seizures with a partial onset though 70% have at least one tonic-clonic seizure. Persistence of seizures in the face of treatment was more common in patients with clearly simple partial than complex partial seizures. Seizure frequency during the first year seems to predict the duration and frequency of subsequent epilepsy although the characteristics of the wound and persisting neurological deficit did not seem to determine persistence. Fifteen years after injury 53% of patients with epilepsy had had at least one seizure in the previous 2 years (28% of all head injured subjects—Salazar et al 1985). Only 8% of patients had a single seizure.

Blunt injuries to the head. The most satisfactory unselected population of patients developing post-traumatic epilepsy has been studied by Annegers et al (1980). This study utilized the records-linkage system of the Mayo Clinic to identify 2747 patients with head injuries between 1935 and 1974. The minimal clinical criteria for inclusion in the study was an injury resulting in loss of consciousness, post-traumatic amnesia or evidence of skull fracture. Patients were excluded if they died within 1 month of injury or had epilepsy pre-dating the index head injury. The head injuries were classified as:

1. Severe: brain contusion, intracerebral or intracranial haematoma or 24 hours of unconsciousness or amnesia
2. Moderate: skull fracture or 30 minutes to 24 hours of unconsciousness or post-traumatic amnesia
3. Mild: briefer periods of unconsciousness or amnesia.

The overall risk of early seizures (within the first week) was 2.1%. This was greater in children (2.8%) than adults (1.8%). For severe head injuries the risk of early seizures rose to 30.5% in children and 10.3% in adults. For late seizures the risk in patients with severe injuries was 7.1% at 1 year and 11.5% at 5 years. For moderate injuries the corresponding figures were 0.7% and 1.6%, and for mild injuries 0.1% and 0.6%. The risk of seizures at any time is not significantly different from the general population for the group with mild head injuries. For all cases the risk of late seizures was 2.6 times greater than the expected risk. The relative risk was 12.7 in the first year, 4.4 in the next 4 years and thereafter 1.4.

Early seizures following blunt head injury. There has long been an opinion among clinicians that fits within the first few weeks of an injury do not carry the same prognostic significance as those with later onset. Jennett (1975) studied what might now be termed acute symptomatic seizures occurring in the first week after injury. He found that early seizures after minor injuries are more common in children under the age of 5 than in adults. The severity of the injury as judged by the presence of a fracture, prolonged post-traumatic amnesia, neurological deficit and intracranial haemorrhage was associated with a higher incidence of early seizures. A total of 25% of patients with an intracranial haematoma suffered such seizures. Early seizures are associated with a higher mortality because of this association. Jennett noted that 25% of patients with early seizures developed late epilepsy compared with 3% of those without early seizures. In adults the respective incidences of early and late seizures were 33% and 3% whereas in children they were 17% and 4%.

Annegers et al (1980) confirm the importance of early seizures in predicting post-traumatic epilepsy in adults. In Jennett's series of patients referred to a neurological centre 5% of survivors developed late post-traumatic epilepsy. The most important risk factors were early seizures (see above), depressed fracture with dural tear and intracranial haematoma. Late epilepsy occurred in one-third of patients who survived a haematoma (Jennett makes the important practical point that a seizure was never the only indication of a developing haematoma). Depressed fracture with dural laceration was associated with an incidence of late epilepsy of 24% which doubled in the presence of focal signs or a post-traumatic amnesia exceeding 24 hours. Whilst Phillips (1954) found prolonged post-traumatic amnesia to be associated with a high incidence of post-traumatic epilepsy, Jennett (1975) stressed that the risk of late epilepsy in patients without depressed fracture, intracranial haematoma, or early seizures was less than 2% even when post-traumatic amnesia exceeded 24 hours.

The relative frequency of partial and tonic-clonic seizures (presumably developing due to secondary generalization from a focal onset) following blunt injuries varies in different series. Jennett (1975) states that in 43% of patients with early epilepsy at least some of the fits were 'focal motor' seizures, whilst for late epilepsy 40% of patients had focal seizures at some time. Temporal lobe seizures were often not recognized until later; their complex nature probably militating against their recognition at an earlier stage of recovery.

The prognosis for post-traumatic epilepsy following blunt injuries is variable. In one series with prolonged follow up for at least 15 years, approximately 50% of patients had had no seizures for at least 5 years, 25% were experiencing between one and six seizures per year and the other 25% more than six seizures per year (Walker & Erculei 1968).

Management of post-traumatic epilepsy. The ability to identify patients with a high prospective risk of post-traumatic epilepsy, as well as early uncontrolled reports (Servit & Musil 1981) persuaded many neurosurgeons to recommend prophylactic anticonvulsant drugs after head injuries carrying a high prospective risk of epilepsy (Rapport & Penry 1973). Subsequent prospective randomized studies, however, have failed to show any significant effects of prophylaxis in the longer term (Young et al 1983, Temkin et al 1990) though phenytoin may reduce the incidence of seizures within the first week following a head injury (Temkin et al 1990). These disappointing findings coupled with the difficulty in maintaining compliance in head injured patients given prophylaxis (McQueen et al 1983) mean that routine prophylaxis in head injured patients cannot be recommended with currently available antiepileptic drugs. The debate about prophylactic treatment will, however, continue as it can be argued that those antiepileptic drugs studied to date (phenytoin in particular) do not have significant effects in suppressing kindling in animals. Valproate has some effects in this model of epilepsy and may be a more rational drug with which to attempt prophylaxis (Hauser 1990).

Post-craniotomy seizures and epilepsy

The overall incidence of seizures occurring after supratentorial craniotomy was 17% during a follow-up period of at least 5 years (Foy et al 1981a). The incidence varied from 3% to 92% depending on the condition for which the craniotomy was undertaken.

Approximately one-fifth of patients undergoing aneurysm surgery develop postoperative seizures (Cabral et al 1976a, North et al 1983). The incidence varies according to the site of the aneurysm. Thus, approximate risks may be 7.5% from internal carotid aneurysms, 21% from anterior communicating aneurysms and 39% for middle cerebral artery aneurysms (Cabral et al 1976b, Foy et al 1981a). Additional factors influencing the incidence may be the presence of an intracerebral haematoma, cortical damage, splitting the Sylvian fissure, cerebral swelling and perioperative aneurysmal rupture, and the length of surgery (Foy et al 1981a, 1992). That at least part of the risk of epilepsy associated with aneurysm is associated with a surgical procedure is suggested by the 8.3% incidence in 261 conservatively managed survivors following aneurysmal subarachnoid haemorrhage reported by Storey

(1967). Arteriovenous malformations and spontaneous intracerebral haematoma from other causes carry risks of epilepsy of 50% and 20% respectively and surgical treatment does seem to be an additional risk factor for these conditions (Crawford et al 1986).

The incidence of epilepsy following tumour surgery is more difficult to assess because of the progressive nature of the underlying pathology. However, surgery may play a role as Cabral et al (1976a) found that postoperative seizures only occurred in patients with acoustic neuroma who underwent a transtentorial approach and by the fact that burr hole biopsy carries a lower risk of seizures than craniotomy (Foy et al 1981a).

The incidence of seizures commencing de novo following meningioma surgery is of the order of 20% (North et al 1983, Foy et al 1981a). The incidence is higher for parasagittal lesions than for convexity or basal tumours. Some 44% of patients who have preoperative seizures do not have any further seizures postoperatively. The incidence of seizures following frontal surgery for pituitary adenomas and craniopharyngiomas may be as high as 15% (Cast & Wilson 1981, Foy et al 1992).

Surgery for supratentorial abscess carries a very high risk. With suffiently long follow-up virtually all patients develop epilepsy (Legg et al 1973, Foy et al 1981b). Ventricular shunting procedures can be associated with a 24% risk of seizures (Copeland et al 1982) and multiple shunt revisions and shunt infections significantly increase the risks.

Of all patients who experience postoperative seizures, 37% do so within the first week and 40% of this group continue to have later seizures. By the time 1 year has elapsed 77% of those who will develop seizure disorders will have done so and by 2 years, 92% will have had their first seizure (Foy et al 1981b). The group with the highest continuing risk after 2 years are patients with supratentorial abscesses. In patients with early seizures the risk of developing further seizures is high. Only 5% of patients developing seizures later than 1 week postoperatively have a single seizure (Foy et al 1981b).

The possible effects of prophylaxis in high risk patients has been studied by a number of authors (North et al 1983, Foy et al 1992). There is no evidence that phenytoin or carbamazepine significantly reduce the incidence of post-craniotomy seizures in high risk groups of patients, nor do they seem to effect the likelihood of persistence of the seizure disorder over a period of time. The use of prophylactic antiepileptic drugs can be associated with a high incidence for adverse effects, particularly drug-induced rash (Chadwick et al 1984). For this reason prophylactic treatment does not seem to be justified.

Intracranial tumours and epilepsy

The relationship between intracranial tumours and epilepsy is well-recognized and results in a considerable pressure to investigate all patients presenting with epilepsy. In fact, brain tumours are responsible for late onset epilepsy in only about 10% of cases from many series (Shehan 1958, Raynor et al 1959, Hyllested & Pakkenberg 1963, Juul-Jensen 1964). The incidence of tumours rises steeply where seizures are clearly focal in nature (Raynor et al 1959, Sumi & Teasdall 1963). Tumours of the frontal, parietal and occipital lobes seem to carry the highest risk of epilepsy (Penfield & Jasper 1954, Mauguiere & Courjon 1978). The incidence of tumours causing complex partial seizures is lower (about 15%) (Currie et al 1971). Gastaut found that 16% of 1702 epileptic patients with epilepsy beginning over the age of 20 had tumours on CT scanning (Gastaut 1976).

These early studies can, of course, be criticized as showing a falsely low frequency of tumour epilepsies, having been undertaken in the era before modern neurological imaging. In less selected populations of patients the incidence of tumours found on CT scanning is even lower. They were found in 6% of patients registered with the National General Practice Survey of Epilepsy (Sander et al 1990) and only 3% of patients investigated following a first seizure (Hopkins et al 1988). The combination of focal seizures, focal slowing on the EEG and focal neurological signs predicts the presence of a tumour on CT scanning in a high proportion of cases (Young et al 1982).

In general, about 40% of those with fits due to tumour have seizures as the first symptom (Penfield & Jasper 1954). Very often the interval between the first seizure and the diagnosis of the tumour and the development of further neurological problems is prolonged (Douglas 1971, Smith et al 1991). This reflects the fact that the majority of tumours that present with only epilepsy tend to be benign. Thus, oligodendrogiomas are complicated by epilepsy in 80–90% of cases, meningioma in 40–60% of cases, and astrocytoma in 60–70% of cases, compared to 30–40% of malignant glioma or glioblastoma (Penfield & Jasper 1954, Lund 1952). Indeed, presentation with the first symptom of epilepsy is one of the most powerful prognostic factors indicating a good prognosis with prolonged survival for patients with intracerebral tumours diagnosed on CT scan (Smith et al 1991). Such intracerebral tumours are most commonly shown to be low density, non-enhancing lesions on initial CT scans and to be relatively low grade astrocytomas.

The prognosis for tumour epilepsies is poor. Only 11 of 164 patients achieved a 1 year remission of epilepsy with antiepileptic drug treatment (Smith et al 1991) and 50% of patients with tumour epilepsies in adult life die within 4 years. However, 20–30% show prolonged survival.

Whilst meningiomas should be treated surgically where this is practical and where the patient is not old or infirm, seizures will only be suppressed in about 40% of patients (Foy et al 1981a).

There is a considerable dilemma about the management of intracerebral tumours. Many neurologists find it difficult to recommend aggressive treatment with biopsy or tumour debulking, and radiotherapy in a patient whose only symptom is epilepsy and in whom there is a good prospect of good quality survival for many years. In relatively few instances are tumours fully resectable, though when they are the outcome for both survival and suppression of epilepsy may be excellent (see Ch. 16).

Cerebrovascular disease

Cerebrovascular disease and stroke become an increasingly common cause of epilepsy in the later years of life (Sander et al 1990, Loiseau et al 1990). A community based study of stroke showed an incidence of seizures by 1 year in 4% of patients with infarction (mainly for patients with total anterior circulation syndrome), 18% of patients with intracerebral haemorrhage, and 28% of patients with subarachnoid haemorrhage (Burn et al 1990). Other studies have emphasized that embolic or haemorrhagic stroke carries the highest risk (Lesser et al 1985). However, asymptomatic carotid occlusion (Cocito et al 1982) and cerebral infarction (Shorvon et al 1984) may be found in patients presenting with epilepsy in later life and seizures may also precede a stroke (Shinton et al 1987, Burn et al 1990). It has been estimated that cerebrovascular disease may account for 15% of new cases of epilepsy (Sander et al 1990) and more than 50% of new cases in the elderly.

Fits that follow stroke most commonly occur in the first week as acute symptomatic seizures and such early seizures do not seem highly predictive of later epilepsy.

The incidence of seizures with aneurysmal subarachnoid haemorrhage has already been discussed (see above) but epilepsy is also a common complication of arteriovenous malformations. It may occur in up to 40–50% of patients and most commonly occurs in those that have had episodes of haemorrhage or have been treated surgically (Crawford et al 1986).

Arteritic disorders can be accompanied by seizures as part of stroke-like syndromes or acute encephalopathies. Anywhere between 17% and 50% of patients with systemic lupus erythematosis and CNS involvement have seizures (Bennett et al 1972). Seizures may also complicate, to a lesser degree, involvement in systemic necrotizing vasculitis (polyarteritis nodosa), Behçet's disease and mixed connective tissue disease (Shannon & Goetz 1989). Seizures may also occur in hypertensive encephalopathy and in subacute bacterial endocarditis.

CNS infections and infestations

A wide range of viral, bacterial, opportunistic and parasitic infestations can be associated with seizures. Infections accounted for 3% of seizure disorders in the epidemiological study in Rochester,

Minnesota (Hauser & Kurland, 1975). Annegers et al (1988) examined the risks of unprovoked seizures following common CNS infections in 714 survivors of encephalitis and meningitis. Overall the 20-year risk of developing unprovoked seizures was 6.8%, almost seven times the expected rate. Increased incidence of seizures was highest during the 5 years after a CNS infection but continued to be elevated for as long as 15 years. The risk was highest (22%) for patients with a viral encephalitis associated with acute symptomatic seizures, and 10% for patients with viral encephalitis without early seizures. For bacterial meningitis associated with early seizures the risk was 13% and only 2.4% for patients with bacterial meningitis without early seizures. The risk of seizures for aseptic meningitis was not increased over that of the general population.

Seizures commonly occur during acute viral encephalitis and they may be most common with herpes simplex encephalitis when the seizures are frequently focal in nature. Prenatal infection with cytomegalovirus, rubella and herpes can produce retardation associated with late epilepsy (Forsgren et al 1990). Seizures can also occur with subacute measles encephalitis (Chadwick et al 1982) and subacute rubella encephalitis. Seizures complicate other 'slow virus infections' including subacute sclerosing panencephalitis and Creutzfeld–Jacob disease, but in both these conditions myoclonus tends to dominate the picture. More recently it has been recognized that infection with HIV can be associated with seizures not only because of an increased risk of opportunistic infections, but also because of the direct neurotropic effects of the virus (Wong et al 1990). Bacterial infections causing meningitis are occasionally associated with seizures, particularly if the meningitis is complicated by cortical venous thrombosis, venous sinus thrombosis or cerebral abscess (see above). Chronic meningitis due to tuberculosis may present with seizures and in the Indian subcontinent tuberculomas may be a common cause of epilepsy associated with disappearing ring-enhancing CT lesions (Goulatia et al 1987). Other causes of chronic meningitis are not infrequently associated with seizures, e.g. cryptococcus, candida. Perhaps the commonest infestation associated with seizures is cysticercosis (Sotelo 1987).

Other cause of symptomatic seizures and epilepsy

Neurodegenerative disorders can be associated with epilepsy. In Alzheimer disease seizures occur usually late in the illness in up to 15% of patients (Romanelli et al 1990). Myoclonus is also evident, particularly in patients with familial Alzheimer disease (Jacob 1970) and with Alzheimer change complicating Down syndrome. In contrast, seizures appear rare in Pick disease.

Several authors have noted an increased incidence of seizures in association with multiple sclerosis, the usual figure being quoted as around 5% of cases (Muller 1949). It may be that seizures are particularly likely to occur as an acute symptomatic phenomenon related to plaque formation and longer-term epilepsy seems to be rare.

THE DIAGNOSIS OF EPILEPSY

The diagnosis of epilepsy in the adult is clinical and is based on a detailed description of events experienced by the patient before, during and after a seizure, and, more importantly, on an eye witness account. In view of the social and economic implications diagnostic errors need to be avoided. Thus, the first basic rule about diagnosing epilepsy is never to make the diagnosis without incontrovertible clinical evidence. If there is any doubt, the clinician should resist the temptation to attach a label and should rely on the passage of time and the further description of symptomatic events to reach a firm conclusion. Hardly anyone with epilepsy will come to any harm from a delay in diagnosis whereas a false-positive diagnosis is gravely damaging.

However, it is not enough simply to decide that a patient's attacks are epileptic in nature. Other considerations must be addressed. Are the seizures related to an acute encephalopathy or are they due to epilepsy? If the seizures are thought to be part of an epilepsy, an adequate classification of seizures and of the epilepsy syndrome must be attempted because this can have important prognostic, therapeutic, and aetiological implications. It may also be necessary to determine whether there is an identifiable and independently treatable aetiology for an individual's epilepsy.

The clinical diagnosis

The events at the start of attacks must be determined. Do they occur without warning or are they preceded by symptoms of an epileptic aura or by faintness and syncope? Specifically, epileptic symptoms include involuntary tonic or clonic movements lateralized to one side of the body, olfactory or gustatory hallucinations, and the complex perceptual changes associated with temporal lobe seizures—'it is indescribable'. Symptoms recorded by the patient after recovery of consciousness are also important. The presumptive diagnosis of a seizure may be secure when an individual wakes in a wet bed with a bitten tongue suffering from a headache and muscular aches and pains.

Most eye witnesses will be able to give a reasonable description of a tonic-clonic (grand mal) seizure. However, it may be harder to get a satisfactory description of more minor seizures. Here, direct questioning may become important, particularly to elicit the characteristic features associated with complex partial seizures—a first fixed motionless stare with subsequent automatisms that may include fidgeting repetitive movements with the hands or chewing or swallowing movements of the mouth and face. Documentation of post-ictal confusion by an eye witness is often of great importance.

Having acquired as much clinical information as possible, certain judgements may at this stage be possible.

Is it epilepsy?

The first test will be to differentiate seizures from other events. Syncope and pseudoseizures are most frequently mistaken as epilepsy. Once it is accepted that seizures have occurred, it is important to determine whether they are acute symptomatic events (not necessarily requiring antiepileptic drug treatment) or spontaneously occurring seizures indicating a truly epileptic disorder. Causes of acute symptomatic seizures include alcohol and other drugs and metabolic disturbance (see above). The hallmark of almost all these conditions is that they usually occur in patients with an acute encephalopathy who have an associated confusional state or systemic disturbance that often outlasts the seizures themselves. The presence of other associated symptoms and signs commonly indicates the correct diagnosis for which specific treatment will be required.

Once a definite diagnosis of epilepsy is accepted, the patient must be counselled about the effects of the disorder on driving, employment, schooling and leisure activities and advised about treatment and prognosis.

What kind of epilepsy?

Although a diagnosis of a specific epileptic syndrome may require confirmation from interictal or ictal EEG recordings (Ch. 9), clinical information will sometimes be sufficient to allow a presumptive diagnosis. In an adolescent the development of myoclonic jerking on awakening with occasional tonic-clonic seizures points to a juvenile myoclonic epilepsy. Seizures associated with a specific epileptic aura indicate a localized onset and therefore imply a greater likelihood of a symptomatic epilepsy caused by a localized cerebral lesion.

What is the aetiology of the epilepsy?

In up to 60–70% of people who have epilepsy no specific cause can be determined. The cause may, however, be readily apparent from clinical information alone. Epilepsy may complicate virtually any neurological condition that affects the cerebral hemispheres. A previous neurological disorder may often be the cause of the seizures. Thus the history must include direct questions about early perinatal events and development, severe head injury (especially those that are complicated by prolonged post-traumatic amnesia, depressed skull fracture, or intracerebral haematoma) and previous central nervous system infection. A family history of epilepsy may suggest a genetic cause when seizure disorders develop in individuals aged 5 to about 25.

Investigations

What value is the electroencephalogram? (see Ch. 9)

The EEG provides valuable information that may:

a. add weight to the clinical diagnosis; b. aid the classification of epilepsy, and c. show changes that may increase the suspicion of a structural lesion.

The EEG as a diagnostic aid

Routine interictal EEG recording is one of the most abused investigations in clinical medicine and is unquestionably responsible for great human suffering. The diagnostic value of an interictal EEG is widely misunderstood. EEGs are often requested either to exclude or to prove a diagnosis of epilepsy—something that can seldom, if ever, be done. Erroneous interpretation of the EEG is probably the commonest reason for non-epileptic events being diagnosed as seizures.

Classification of epilepsy

The EEG is especially important in two clinical settings. In patients with seizures occurring without an aura that are characterized by a brief period of absence with or without automatism, it may be difficult to differentiate typical absence seizures from complex partial seizures. The finding of generalized spike wave or focal spike activity, respectively, will clarify the diagnosis. The differentiation has important implications for treatment and prognosis. In patients with tonic-clonic seizures without an aura, especially when these occur during sleep, the EEG can again differentiate between primary generalized epilepsies characterized by generalized spike wave and seizures with a focal onset in which there may be localized abnormalities.

Detecting structural brain lesions

The EEG may, by demonstrating the presence of focal slow-wave abnormalities, suggest the presence of structural lesions as a cause for a patient's epilepsy. Such focal delta activity increases the chances of detection of a cerebral tumour on computed tomographic (CT) scanning in patients who present with epilepsy (Young et al 1982, Dam et al 1985).

Neurological imaging in the diagnosis of epilepsy

In practical terms imaging means CT or MR scanning. The frequency of abnormalities in CT scans of patients with epilepsy varies greatly. In surveys of patients with established epilepsy from specialist centres, 60–80% may have abnormal CT scans but most of these abnormalities are atrophic in nature (Gastaut 1976). Tumours may be identified in approximately 10% of patients. In patients who present with either a first seizure or early epilepsy the incidence is lower—abnormalites are detected in less than 20% of cases—but again atrophic abnormalities predominate. CT scan abnormalities are very strongly predicted by the presence of focal rather than generalized seizures, focal neurological signs and focal EEG abnormalities (Young et al 1982). Where all three are present CT abnormalities may be found in up to 70–80% of cases.

CT scanning is indicated in a group of patients with epilepsy of later onset who have focal seizures (especially simple partial seizures) with or without neurological signs and focal EEG abnormality. An algorithm for selection of patients for CT scanning is shown in Figure 5.2. It may be more important to offer CT scanning to patients whose epilepsy is unresponsive to antiepileptic drug therapy than to pursue a policy of indiscriminate CT scanning of all patients at the presentation of their epilepsy.

The development of magnetic resonance imaging will undoubtedly have a major impact on the investigation of patients with epilepsy. Magnetic resonance imaging seems considerably more sensitive for almost all cerebral pathologies that may be associated with epilepsy with the exception of calcification which is not well demonstrated by this modality. To date its major applications have been in the demonstration of pathology in patients being investigated for surgical treatment of temporal lobe epilepsy. MRI was more sensitive in detecting both medial temporal tumours and degrees of medial temporal gliosis and temporal atrophy than was CT scanning (Triulzi et al 1988, Kuzniecky et al 1987, Schorner et al 1987). The place of MRI in less selected populations of patients remains uncertain. Particularly in the elderly, MRI shows a high incidence of lesions, the clinical relevance of which may be difficult to determine.

Other technologies that produce 'functional'

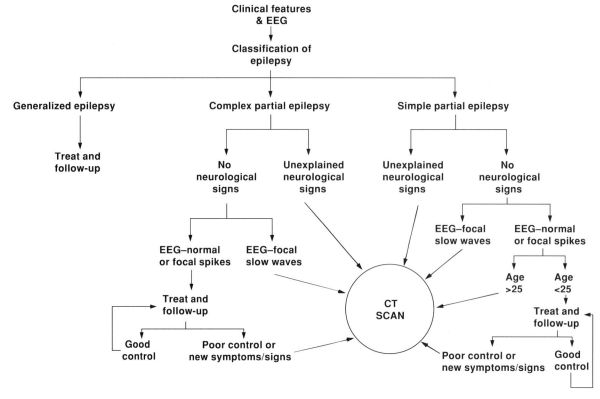

Fig. 5.2   Guidelines for the use of CT scanning in the investigation of epilepsy. Reproduced with permission from Chadwick et al 1989.

imaging such as positron emission tomography (PET), single photon emission computerized tomography (SPECT) and magnetic resonance spectroscopy are largely experimental and to date have usually been used in the assessment of patients for surgical treatment of their epilepsy (see Chapter 16).

Are other investigations indicated as a routine?

In the past skull radiographs were routinely obtained in patients presenting with epilepsy. They provide little useful information and patients who require neurological imaging tests should undergo CT scanning. Similarly, the routine screening of haematological and biochemical indices provides an extremely low yield of clinically useful information. Such tests may be indicated in certain circumstances, e.g. in patients with alcohol-related seizures, but routine use of such investigations is no substitute for adequate clinical appraisal.

The differential diagnosis of epilepsy

Syncope

Syncope is common and occurs for a wide variety of reasons (see Table 5.5). The majority of people who faint are young and have no underlying pathology. Such vaso-vagal fainting is usually precipitated by unpleasant sights or sounds, prolonged standing, standing after a lengthy period of recumbency or squatting, or after exposure to heat, hunger, dehydration and alcohol excess.

The subject usually gets a feeling of warmth with a dry mouth and a desire for fresh air or a drink of water. Nausea can develop quite quickly along with deep, sighing respiration, blurring of vision with spots in front of the eyes and loss of colour vision, noises in the ears, vertigo and depersonalization. The onset of these symptoms is usually gradual and eye-witnesses comment on pallor and sweating. The subject will collapse if they remain standing, and whilst most individuals are flaccid when they do so, there may be some

Table 5.5   Causes of syncope

Reflex syncope
  Postural
  'Psychogenic'
  Micturition syncope
  Cough syncope
  Valsalva
  Swallow syncope
  Glossopharyngeal neuralgia
Cardiac syncope
  Dysrhythmias (heart block, tachycardias, etc.)
  Valvular disease (particularly aortic stenosis)
  Atrial myxoma
  Cardiomyopathies
  Shunts
  Pulmonary hypertension
Perfusion failure
  Hypovolaemia
  Syndromes of autonomic failure
  Subclavian steal
Related to head-posture
  Carotid sinus sensitivity
  Atlanto-axial subluxation
  Syringomyelia/bulbia

Table 5.6   The differences between syncope and seizures

	Syncope	Seizures
Posture	Upright	Any posture
Pallor and sweating	Invariable	Uncommon
Onset	Gradual	Sudden/aura
Injury	Rare	Not uncommon
Convulsive jerks	Rare	Common
Incontinence	Rare	Common
Unconsciousness	Seconds	Minutes
Recovery	Rapid	Often slow
Postictal confusion	Rare	Common
Frequency	Infrequent	May be frequent
Precipitating factors	Crowded places	Rare
	Lack of food	
	Unpleasant	
	circumstances	

rigidity and a few coarse jerks of the limbs which often falsely raise the spectre of epilepsy for the inexperienced. Frank convulsions (reflex anoxic seizures) may occur if individuals faint and are maintained in an upright position by either collapsing between a wall and toilet or being supported by well-meaning bystanders.

Loss of consciousness is usually brief and on recovery the subject is usually nauseated and tremulous with continued pallor and sweating. They are rarely confused.

Cardiac causes of syncope may have somewhat different characteristics as onset is usually rapid and often instantaneous (Ross 1988). Syncope in progressive autonomic failure develops slowly over several minutes. The usual pallor, sweating and bradycardia may be absent. Rarer forms of syncope have been associated with a variety of physiological reflexes (cough and micturition), and a number of pathologies, e.g. atherosclerosis in carotid sinus syncope, oesophageal carcinoma in swallow syncope and syncope associated with glossopharyngeal and trigeminal neuralgia.

No single feature will categorically allow a clinical differentiation between syncope and epileptic seizures of one kind or another. The major differences are summarized in Table 5.6. A carefully taken history is the most important step and it

must always be regarded as unwise to diagnose epilepsy where there is evidence of any of the precipitating factors that are so strongly associated with syncope.

Psychogenic attacks

Pseudoseizures. Whilst on occasion the clinical diagnosis of pseudoseizures may be difficult (King et al 1982), particularly when they occur in patients who also have a history of true epileptic seizures, when they are witnessed by experienced personnel there is usually little possibility of confusion. However, no single clinical feature differentiates pseudoseizures from epilepsy but a number of factors may be of value (Table 5.7). The most frequently useful is resistance to eye opening in pseudoseizures and the presence of pupilary dilatation which is an invariable feature of tonic-clonic seizures. Failure to differentiate between pseudoseizures and epilepsy can have significant consequences. Pseudostatus epilepticus is probably as common as true status epilepticus in Regional Neurological Centres and is a condition with significant morbidity (Howell et al 1989).

The temporal pattern of attacks should particularly alert the clinician to the possibility of pseudoseizures. Pseudoseizures tend to be refractory to anticonvulsant therapy in contrast to epilepsy, where convulsive seizures in particular are highly likely to be well controlled. Failure to control tonic-clonic seizures in a patient who develops attacks after the first decade of life, in whom

Table 5.7   The differences between epileptic seizures and pseudoseizures

	Epileptic seizure	Pseudoseizure
Onset	Sudden	May be gradual
Retained consciousness in prolonged seizure	Very rare	Common
Pelvic thrusting	Rare	Common
Flailing, thrashing, asynchronous limb movements	Rare	Common
Rolling movements	Rare	Common
Cyanosis	Common	Unusual
Tongue biting and other injury	Common	Less common
Stereotyped attacks	Usual	Uncommon
Duration	Seconds or minutes	Often many minutes
Gaze aversion	Rare	Common
Resistance to passive limb movement or eye opening	Unusual	Common
Prevention of hand falling on to face	Unusual	Common
Induced by suggestion	Rarely	Often
Postictal drowsiness or confusion	Usual	Often absent
Ictal EEG abnormality	Almost always	Always never
Postictal EEG abnormal (after seizure with impairment of consciousness)	Usually	Rarely

there is no identifiable cerebral disease and in whom interictal EEG recordings have never shown epileptiform abnormalities, should raise serious suspicions about the diagnosis of epilepsy.

Pseudoseizures most commonly occur in women, with onset most commonly in the second or third decades of life (Roy 1979, Howell et al 1989). Such individuals often have a significant history of self-poisoning and self-injury. Previous episodes of unexplained neurological dysfunction with a possible hysterical basis are common.

Hyperventilation. Hyperventilation is common and the bulk of cases may go unrecognized but a significant number may be misdiagnosed as epilepsy (Riley 1982). Common manifestations include dizziness, detachment, blurred vision, tingling, muscle spasm, tetany, palpitation, dyspnoea and chest pain, heartburn, epigastric pain, muscle cramps and fatigue. Some form of alteration in consciousness is common and up to 15% of patients may lose consciousness during attacks (Pincus 1978). The wide variety of symptoms experienced by patients with hyperventilation will most commonly be confused with complex partial seizures.

The most useful fact which allows differentiation is that hyperventilation attacks are commonly precipitated by stressful circumstances and the fact that they lack a stereotype nature with different types of symptoms referable to different systems occurring on different occasions. A simple diagnostic test is asking the patient to re-breathe from a paper bag held over the mouth and nose during attacks.

Panic attacks. Panic attacks can easily be mistaken for complex partial seizures (Harper & Roth 1962). They commonly encompass abdominal discomfort, a choking feeling, fear, autonomic symptoms and sometimes even loss of consciousness. The episodes, however, are usually clearly precipitated and often more prolonged than seizures. Panic attacks are most likely to occur in association with phobic anxiety states and patients usually have considerable insight into the nature of their attacks.

Rage outbursts (episodic dyscontrol). There are common misconceptions that violence commonly accompanies seizures, particularly complex partial seizures. In fact it is extremely rare. In spite of this it is common for individuals who describe sudden outbursts of violent behaviour with minimal provocation, often with some associated patchy amnesia, to be referred for neurological evaluation with a presumptive diagnosis of a seizure disorder. The issues are always somewhat complicated by the EEG, as non-specific abnormalities are extremely common in psychopathic individuals (Stafford-Clark & Taylor 1949). Strict guidelines must be applied before ever accepting that aggressive or violent behaviour is part of a seizure disorder (Treiman & Delgado-Escueta 1983).

An epileptic basis to such attacks should only be

accepted where definite seizures occur at other times and where violent behaviour is a consistent feature of that individual's seizures. Violence can only be accepted as epilepsy-related where it is brief and poorly directed.

Fugue states. Such states of psychogenic wandering are prolonged, usually with sudden recovery of awareness. It is usually impossible to obtain a clear account of behaviour during such attacks but this usually appears to have been quite normal. Subjects have a dense amnesia for the period for time concerned and individuals usually have an associated depression and the need to escape from some stressful life situation (Stengel 1943). Such episodes may be confused with complex partial status or other forms of non-convulsive status epilepticus (Mayeux & Lender 1978, Mayeux et al 1979)

Focal cerebral ischaemia

It may sometimes be difficult to differentiate between focal seizures and focal ischaemia due to either migraine or thromboembolic disease.

Transient ischaemic attacks (TIAs) will rarely be confused with seizures because they develop more slowly and last for longer. They are virtually never accompanied by altered consciousness, and motor and sensory phenomena that comprise them are almost uniformly negative. Whilst rarely focal seizures may be accompanied by predominantly negative motor or sensory problems (Lesser et al 1987), the greatest difficulties may occur in rare haemodynamic TIAs in which weakness may be accompanied by some shaking and tremor (Yanagihara et al 1985).

Migraine occurring in a younger population is more likely to lead to confusion with seizures. Loss of consciousness is not uncommon in migraine though usually it takes the form of syncope associated with nausea and hypotension. The complex relationship between migraine and epilepsy has been reviewed (Andermann 1987). On occasions migrainous episodes may induce frank seizures and similarly focal lesions such as arteriovenous malformations may cause both seizures and migraine-like phenomena. It does seem that migraine and benign Rolandic and occipital epilepsies co-exist in the same individual more fre-

quently than can easily be attributed to chance (Andermann 1987).

Transient global amnesia

The syndrome of transient global amnesia (TGA) describes an abrupt onset of amnesia usually accompanied by repetitive questioning, in an individual who remains alert and communicative (Fisher & Adams 1958). The amnesia lasts for hours and attacks rarely recur. The aetiology of this syndrome remains controversial but it is highly likely that it has different causes which might include thromboembolic disease, migraine and epilepsy (Hodges & Warlow 1990). The latter authors suggest that up to 7% of patients with TGA are likely to have an epileptic basis to their attacks and these can usually be identified by attacks that last for less than an hour and which are recurrent over a short period of time. Sometimes such individuals will also describe some features at the start of the attacks which would support focal seizure onset, e.g. olfactory hallucination.

Sleep phenomena

A number of sleep phenomena may be confused with seizures. Hypnic jerks (Oswald 1959) are usually single jerks that occur in the very early stages of sleep. They usually lead to arousal and may be accompanied by a feeling of falling, a cry or some other kind of brief sensory disturbance. They occur in 60–70% of normal subjects and are so characteristic that they should not easily be confused with nocturnal seizures. Periodic movements of sleep are rhythmic and repetitive leg movements more commonly seen in later life. They usually consist of jerking movements, usually dorsiflexion of the foot and extension of the toes that can occur repetitively during non-REM sleep (Coleman et al 1980). It was probably this phenomenon that Symmonds (1953) described as nocturnal myoclonus and suggested that it could be some form of epileptic equivalent. There is no evidence to support this view.

Sleep walking is a form of automatic behaviour occurring during deep non-REM sleep and is much more common in children than in adults. It usually ceases by the mid-teens (Cirignotta et al

1983). It is more common for children not to walk but to sit up in bed, making repetitive purposeful movements and perhaps to talk. Walking may sometimes occur, usually with the eyes open, avoiding familiar objects. The individual can usually be led back to bed without waking. When sleep walking does occur in adults there is usually a clear preceding history of it having occurred during childhood. In adults it must be distinguished from postictal automatism following sleep seizures or from complex partial seizures resulting in automatic behaviour (Pedley & Guilleminault 1977).

Abnormalities of sleep can also lead to confusion with seizures because of daytime disturbances. Narcolepsy itself in which there are frequent episodes of irresistable sleep should not lead to significant confusion. However, cataplexy in which there may be sudden collapse with loss of postural tone triggered by emotion or startle or loud noise could potentially be confused with atonic drop attacks. However, the age of onset of such episodes precludes real confusion as atonic seizures most commonly occur during the first decade of life and symptoms of the narcoleptic syndrome rarely begin before the second or third decades of life (Parkes 1982). Some subjects with narcolepsy can also exhibit automatic behaviour when they appear to be only half awake. The individual appears drowsy and absent-minded, though may be capable of carrying on relatively complex tasks for which they are subsequently amnesic.

Sleep apnoea which is most commonly obstructive in nature and associated with obesity and night-time snoring leads to day time drowsiness. Occasionally episodes of day time sleepiness may be associated with respiratory obstruction and jerks that can lead to referral with the suggestion of a seizure disorder.

Movement disorders

Some unusual movement disorders may on occasion cause confusion with seizures. Paroxysmal kinesogenic choreoathetosis is a rare disorder in which short-lasting tonic spasms with writhing movements, usually affecting an arm or a leg occur (Kertesz 1967). The onset is usually in adolescence; it is probably a familial condition with an autosomal dominant pattern inheritance. The attacks are precipitated by sudden movement after a period of rest and are often preceded by a peculiar sensation in the limb before the movement commences. The attacks can be quite frequent but they respond readily to antiepileptic drugs, though there is no evidence to suggest that they are epileptic in nature as EEGs are quite normal. The syndrome is so striking that it should not easily be confused with a seizure disorder although rarely some patients with movement induced seizures and abnormal ictal EEGs have been described (Whitty et al 1964).

Similar tonic spasms induced by movement can also occur in multiple sclerosis, as may paroxysmal episodes of dysarthria and ataxia (Matthews 1975).

Another negative motor phenomenon that may sometimes be confused with epilepsy is so-called cryptogenic or benign drop attacks seen in middle-aged women (Stevens & Mathews 1973). These result in a sudden fall, usually onto the knees, without any clouding of consciousness. The episodes tend to be infrequent and overall outcome seems to be quite benign.

Hypoglycaemia

Hypoglycaemia is most commonly seen in diabetics receiving insulin or oral hypoglycaemic agents. Diabetics may be particularly sensitive to hypoglycaemia and experience symptoms at higher blood glucose levels than non-diabetic subjects. As blood sugar falls, pallor, sweating and tachycardia develop associated with confusion, collapse and occasionally coma. True seizures may occur during the course of hypoglycaemia further complicating diagnosis. Hypoglycaemia must always be considered in the differential diagnosis of epilepsy in the diabetic population but perhaps the greatest diagnostic difficulty will arise in the rare cases of insulin-secreting tumours in non-diabetic patients. Here, hypoglycaemia is most likely to occur during the course of the night and may then be associated with seizures. The confused behaviour of hypoglycaemia may be difficult to differentiate from complex partial seizures occurring during sleep.

THE PROGNOSIS OF EPILEPSY

Table 5.8 summarizes remission rates in those studies reviewed by Rodin (1968) and some important subsequent studies. Many problems exist in the interpretation of these data, not least the varying minimum period required as a definition of remission, and the period of follow-up; Bridge (1949) having emphasized that success in control of seizures is inversely proportional to the length of follow-up.

The majority of studies have been hospital based, which has an adverse effect on outcome, patients with more severe and refractory epilepsy being more likely to be referred to specialist centres. In this respect the study of Annegers et al (1979) is of particular importance in being community rather than hospital based: 457 patients identified in Rochester, with a history of two or more non-febrile seizures were followed for at least 5 years, and in the case of 141 for 20 years. The probability of being in a remission lasting for 5 years or more was 61% at 10 years, and as high as 70% at 20 years (Fig. 5.3). This large study is supported by a smaller one of 122 patients drawn from a general practice population (Goodridge & Shorvon 1983). By 15 years after onset of seizures, 80% had achieved a 2-year remission, and only 38% were still taking antiepileptic drugs. Some further support for such high rates of remission is obtained from studies of patients followed prospectively from diagnosis and the

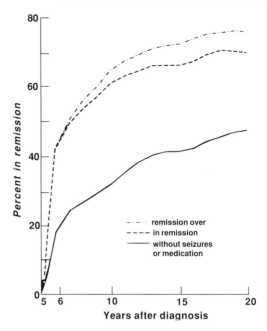

Fig. 5.3 Actuarial percentage of patients in remission of 5 years following diagnosis of epilepsy. Reproduced with permission from Annegers et al 1979.

commencement of therapy, which show that between 50% and 77% of such patients are 'controlled' depending on how control is defined (Turnbull et al 1985, Reynolds 1987).

The majority of hospital-based studies are striking in that remission rates are consistent at between 20% and 30% despite the fact that they include periods before the advent of modern

Table 5.8 Prognosis for remission

Author	No. patients	Min duration remission (years)	% Remitted
Habermaas (1901)	937	2	10
Turner (1907)	212	2	33
Grosz (1930)	91	10	11
Kirstein (1942)	174	3	22
Alstroem (1950)	897	5	22
Kiorboe (1961)	130	4	22
Strobos (1959)	228	1	38
Probst (1960)	83	2	31
Trolle (1961)	799	2	37
Juul-Jensen (1963)	969	2	32
Lorge (1964)	177	2	34
Rodin (1968)	90	2	32
Annegers et al (1979)	457	5	70
Sofijanov (1982)	512	2	50
Jap. study (1981)	1868	3	58

anticonvulsant therapy. Turner recorded a 2-year remission rate in 1907, identical to that reported by Rodin in 1968! This might suggest that remission in epilepsy largely reflects the natural history of the disease rather than the influence of anticonvulsant medication, a suggestion which receives some support from Annegers et al (1979) who were unable to show major changes in remission rates in patients diagnosed with epilepsy between the years of 1935 and 1959 and those diagnosed between 1960 and 1974.

These figures then at least illustrate that a significant number of patients will attain a remission of seizures sufficient to raise the question of whether antiepileptic drugs should be withdrawn. However, a number of factors influence prognosis.

The age of onset of epilepsy is perhaps one of the most important. There is general agreement that the commencement of seizures within the first year of life (when it is usually symptomatic of cerebral pathology), carries an adverse prognosis (Kiorboe 1961, Hedenstroem & Schorsch 1963, Strobos 1959, Sofijanov 1982). The Group for the study of the prognosis of epilepsy in Japan (1981) emphasized the poor prognosis for seizures beginning before the age of 1 compared with those commencing between the ages of 1 and 10. However, apart from this exception they found that childhood epilepsy is more likely to remit than adult onset epilepsy. Annegers et al (1979) found that both partial and generalized epilepsies had a better prognosis should they start before the age of 20.

Whatever the age of onset, the duration of the epilepsy prior to treatment is an important prognostic factor. Gowers (1881) stated that 83% of patients would have their seizures arrested if treated within 1 year. Annegers et al (1979) showed that most patients who achieve remission do so early during the course of treatment. With continuing seizures it becomes progressively less likely that an individual patient will enter remission (Reynolds 1987). Thus there is a plateau in the number of patients in remission 15–20 years after the onset of epilepsy. Similar findings have been reported with shorter-term follow-up in children (Sofijanov 1982). Rodin (1968) also emphasized that the fewer and the less frequent the seizures, the better the prognosis for remission.

The possible importance of the early course and treatment of epilepsy in its long-term outcome has been discussed in detail by Reynolds (1987). He has analysed data from a number of sources which show that the frequency of both partial and tonic-clonic seizures prior to treatment has an adverse effect on outcome and also that intervals between seizures may decrease progressively. As Hauser et al (1982) have also shown that the risk of subsequent seizures increases from the first to the second and third seizures, it can be argued that these observations indicate that early and effective antiepileptic drug treatment may be capable of preventing the onset of chronic epilepsy. This view, however, remains controversial and could only be proved by a prospective randomized study of the use of antiepileptic drugs after first seizures and early epilepsy.

Seizure classification is of major importance in determining outcome. Remission rates range from approximately 60% to 80% for patients with only tonic-clonic seizures to between 20% and 60% in patients with complex partial seizures (Yahr et al 1952, Trolle 1961, Juul-Jensen 1963, Reynolds et al 1981, Turnbull et al 1985). The combination of complex partial seizures with secondary generalized tonic-clonic seizures may have a particularly adverse prognosis (Rodin 1968, Group for study of prognosis of epilepsy in Japan 1981). In such patients it is common to find that whilst tonic-clonic seizures come under good control with anticonvulsant therapy, partial seizures remain resistant to drug therapy (Rodin 1968, Reynolds et al 1981, Turnbull et al 1985). Other generalized epilepsies of childhood carry varying prognoses. Between 70% and 80% of patients with typical absences (petit mal) are likely to enter remission (Group for the study of prognosis of epilepsy in Japan 1981, Sofijanov 1982). Atypical absences show a lesser remission rate (33–65%), and in patients with the West or Lennox–Gastaut syndromes remission rates may be as low as 35–50%.

Epilepsy of unknown aetiology has a better prognosis than symptomatic epilepsy (Juul-Jensen 1963, Group for the study of prognosis of epilepsy in Japan 1981, Annegers et al 1979). In keeping with this, epilepsy complicated by an associated neurological or psychiatric deficit carries an adverse prognosis (Sofijanov 1982, Shorvon & Reynolds 1982).

Rodin (1968) drew attention to the adverse prognosis associated with the occurrence of injuries during seizures, and the clustering of attacks in close temporal association.

There is a considerable volume of literature on EEG findings and their prognostic value. This is well reviewed by Rodin (1968). This evidence provides no clear indication that any specific EEG abnormalities either in historical EEGs or at a particular point in time when prognosis is to be predicted are of great value.

The evidence about the factors affecting the prognosis of epilepsy does not allow any very satisfactory qualification and assessment of the varying weights that prognostic factors carry. Some of these difficulties have recently been addressed by Shaffer et al (1988). This group examined the prognosis of 306 patients diagnosed between 1935 and 1978 and used Cox's proportional hazards model to investigate those factors determining the likelihood of achieving a 5-year seizure-free period and a 5-year seizure-free period off drugs. They calculated the risk ratios and 95% confidence limits for a number of factors. Those of importance are presented in Table 5.9. It can be seen that no individual factor is very strongly predictive of remission but those that are include the absence of early brain damage, never having had a tonic-clonic seizure, and the absence of generalized spike-wave from a number of EEGs. Similar factors were also predictive of 5-year seizure-free periods off anti-

epileptic drugs. It can be seen that the risk ratio for any of these factors is relatively small and confidence limits wide, emphasizing the variability of outcome in apparently homogenous groups of patients with epilepsy. It is clear from this that very large groups of patients have to be studied in order to further refine predictions of good or adverse outcome.

The prognosis of a (first) seizure

A common clinical problem is the patient who presents with a single, apparently unprovoked seizure. Is this a purely isolated event that needs no treatment or is it the first event of the developing epilepsy? The practical implication of this question is whether antiepileptic drug treatment should be commenced after the first seizure. This is not the practice in the United Kingdom (Hopkins et al 1988) but the majority of patients with single seizures are treated in the United States (Hauser et al 1990).

There is no doubt that some patients experience a single isolated seizure during their life and never develop epilepsy. The recurrence rate for patients seen at a time when they have a history of a single seizure may vary depending on the population studied and the time that elapsed between the first seizure and the time at which the patient was registered for the study (Cleland et al 1981, Hauser et al 1982, Elwes et al 1985, Hauser 1986, Hopkins et al 1988, Hart et al 1990).

The studies of single seizures of Hauser et al (1982) and Hopkins et al (1988) included both untreated and antiepileptic drug treated patients,

Table 5.9 Factors affecting prognosis of epilepsy (Shaffer et al 1988)

Factor	5 years seizure free Relative risk* (95% CL)	5 years seizure free and off medication Relative risk (95% CL)
Age <16 at first fit	1.09 (0.82, 1.44)	1.88 (1.23, 2.8)
No early brain damage	2.15 (1.22, 3.78)	4.27 (1.35, 13.47)
No known aetiology	1.5 (1.05, 2.13)	2.64 (1.45, 2.84)
Never had a tonic-clonic fit	1.37 (1.03, 1.82)	2.19 (1.48, 3.24)
No generalized spike-wave in third year EEG	3.47 (1.37, 8.8)	2.36 (0.56, 10.16)

* Univariate Cox regression estimate of relative risk from 298 patients.

though not on a randomized basis. The differences in the long-term risk of further seizures was small.

There have been considerable problems identifying those factors which adversely affect recurrence rates after a single seizure. This difficulty almost certainly is due to the small numbers of patients in individual series and also to a lack of sophistication in the techniques used to identify prognostic factors. The most satisfactory in this respect are those of Hauser et al (1990) and Hart et al (1990). This first group studied 208 patients from the day of their first unprovoked seizure. A Cox's proportional hazards model was used and in the group as a whole the presence of a known remote aetiology for a first seizure, a Todd's paresis following the first seizure and a family history of seizures as well as the presence of generalized spike-wave in an EEG had a significant adverse effect on outcome. In the group of patients without an obvious aetiology for seizures the presence of generalized spike-wave in the EEG became more important in predicting outcome whereas in the group of patients with a remote aetiology for seizures previous acute seizures greatly increased the risk of subsequent epilepsy (e.g. seizures acutely related to head injury, encephalitis etc.).

Hart et al (1990) identified 564 patients presenting for the first time to general practitioners with seizures and epilepsy. Seizures in patients with a neurological deficit recurred in 100% of cases, but seizures occurring within 3 months of an acute brain insult (stroke or head injury) carried the lowest risk (40% by 12 months). Recurrence was highest at the extremes of life (83% by 3 years under the age of 16 years and over the age of 59 years). Partial seizures were more likely to recur (94% by 3 years) than were tonic-clonic seizures (72% by 3 years).

Prognosis for the withdrawal of antiepileptic drugs

One factor that complicates the assessment of the prognosis of epilepsy is that many patients continue to take antiepileptic drugs for many years after seizures cease to occur. It is therefore difficult to know in how many patients the remission is dependent on continued antiepileptic drug treatment.

The fact that antiepileptic drugs have been associated with various acute idiosyncratic and dose-related adverse reactions and increasingly well documented chronic toxic and teratogenetic effects, as well as more subtle effects on behaviour and cognitive function (Schmidt 1982), is a potent argument for exploring the possibility of withdrawing drugs in patients who achieve remissions lasting 2, 3 or more years. Against this are the dangers of a recurrence of seizures, which may have important consequences for driving and employment as well as self esteem.

Advice offered to patients on this subject varies widely. Paediatricians and paediatric neurologists suggest a trial withdrawal of antiepileptic drugs in most children attaining remission, as they are concerned about the impact of drugs on cognitive function and learning and are impressed by the high expectation of success. Adult neurologists tend to be much more circumspect, expressing concern over the possible effects of further seizures on driving and employment. In the United Kingdom, if not elsewhere, however, most patients attaining prolonged remission are unlikely to receive any advice from a neurologist or other physician with an interest in the treatment of epilepsy because they will have been discharged from regular follow-up. Of 122 patients with a history of epilepsy drawn from general practice, 49 had stopped treatment, most of them on their own initiative (Goodridge & Shorvon 1983).

The few studies that have been undertaken to determine the success of withdrawing drugs and the factors that identify patients likely to remain free of seizures have recently been reviewed (Chadwick 1985, Pedley, 1988). Comparison of the available studies is difficult because there is often little information about the patients, a lack of uniformity in the length of remission before withdrawal of the antiepileptic drugs, and no information about the period over which withdrawal occurred and for how long patients were subsequently followed up (Tables 5.10 and 5.11). Quoted incidence rates for relapse tend to be crude figures after follow-up for an arbitrary period. Actuarial figures are more valid. Further-

Table 5.10 Relapse after withdrawal of antiepileptic drugs (studies in children)

Authors	n	Duration of remission (years)	Relapse %	Duration of follow up (years)
Zenker et al (1957)	117	>0.5	21	
Holowach et al (1972)	148	>4	24	5-12
Tudor et al (1973)	82	>1	15	
Forster & Schmidberger (1978)	114	>1	31	
Rodin & John (1980)	32	>1.75	6	2
Emerson et al (1981)	68	>4	26	0.5–6
Nalin et al (1982)	457		17.5	
Thurston et al (1982)	148	>4	28	15-23
Todt (1984)	433	>2	36.3	>3 (mean 5)
Shinnar et al (1985)	88	>2	25	0.5–5
Visser et al (1987)	166	>2	24	2–10
Bouma et al (1987)	116	>2	20	0.75–10
Arts et al (1988)	146	>2	25.5	1.4–9
Maitricarde et al (1989)	425	>2	11.8*	1.6–12

* Excludes patients with recurrence during dose reduction.

Table 5.11 Relapse after withdrawal of antiepileptic drugs (studies mainly including adults)

Reference	n	Duration of remission (years)	Relapse %	Duration of follow up (years)
Yahr et al (1952)	26	>2	46	
Merritt (1958)	89	>3	44	
Strobos (1959)	41	>2	46	
Juul-Jensen (1968)	196	>2	40	5
Janz & Sommer-Burkhardt (1976)	253	>2	49	>5
Oller-Daurella et al (1976)	317	>5	17	0.5–27
Heycop Ten Ham (1980)	151	>5	32	2
Janz et al (1983a,b)	232	>1	62	
Prococcianti et al (1987)	100	>2	34	1
Tsai & Schmidt (1987)	96	>2	76	3–23
Pestre et al (1987)	272	>5	50	5–10
Overweg et al (1987)	62	>3	66	
Callaghan et al (1988)	92	>2	34	0.5–5
MRC AED Withdrawal group (1991)	510	>2	43	1–5

more, the numbers of patients in the studies tend to be small, which means that important subgroup analysis may be difficult.

One question that has not been considered is the relative risk of recurrence on withdrawal of antiepileptic drugs compared to continued treatment. The MRC AED Withdrawal Group (1991) studied this in a randomized study. The risk of relapse on continued treatment was approximately 10% per annum, but was greater in the group withdrawing treatment for up to 2 years after commencing withdrawal (Fig. 5.4).

Prognostic factors for relapse

Overall, relapse rates for studies that have included adults are approximately 40–50% whilst those for children are more likely to be of the order of 20%. Such overall figures are, however, of little value to the clinician or his patient as within the population there may be groups of patients with relatively low or relatively high risks of relapse following antiepileptic drug withdrawal. It is therefore important to determine which prognostic factors might define groups of patients with the least risk of seizure relapse.

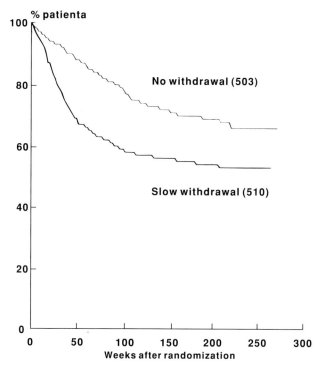

Fig. 5.4 Actuarial percentage of patients remaining seizure-free under continued treatment and slow withdrawal of antiepileptic drugs. Reproduced with permission from MRC Antiepileptic Drug Withdrawal Group 1991.

The most striking observation which emerges from studies is that the prospect for successful withdrawal of medication is better in children than in adults; only Callaghan et al (1988) disagree. The relapse rate in children has varied between 6 and 36%. This is approximately half the relapse rate in adult studies with a relapse rate between 17 and 76%. This finding makes it important to examine children and adults separately when considering other prognostic factors.

Classification of seizures and epilepsy. According to Janz (1987) the classification of epilepsy has no great prognostic significance. However, this view may have arisen by inappropriately combining the experience of adult and childhood epilepsies. In children, most authors find a more favourable prognosis in the primary generalized epilepsies, though Janz stresses the unfavourable prognosis in adolescents with juvenile myoclonic epilepsy.

When considering individual seizure types there is general agreement that the prognosis for typical absence (petit mal) is very good. However, it is also clear that the rather unsatisfactory prospects for drug withdrawal in adult patients with complex partial seizures may not be shared by children. Indeed, Shinnar et al (1985) found that complex partial seizures in children had the best prognosis of all. There is agreement that patients with more than one seizure type have a higher relapse than those with only one seizure type, whether in children or in adults.

Duration of epilepsy. Several authors studying both adults and children suggest that the duration of epilepsy before the onset of remission has a significant influence on subsequent relapse rate, the longer the illness the higher the relapse rate. Janz (1987) emphasizes this in his review and quotes the experience of Oller-Daurella et al (1976) to support this contention. Similarly, the number and frequency of seizures prior to remission and the duration of treatment (MRC AED Withdrawal Group 1991) has an adverse effect on prognosis (Callaghan et al 1988, Todt 1984).

Additional handicaps. Most authors who have examined this question find at least a trend if not a significant adverse influence of brain lesions, neurological signs and intellectual impairment on relapse rate in both children and adults.

The electroencephalogram (EEG). This is perhaps the most controversial issue of all and no statements can be made with confidence. Some authors report an adverse influence of epileptiform abnormalities in the EEG prior to withdrawal or if such abnormalities persist or emerge during withdrawal. Others find no relationship to relapse rates. For example, although the findings in children by Shinnar et al (1985) are impressive and in agreement with those of Todt (1984), Thurston et al (1982) found no influence of the EEG on outcome. Overweg et al (1987) support the latter finding in adults. Overall, there is some dichotomy between adult and childhood studies, the EEG appearing to be of greater prognostic significance in children than in adults.

Duration of remission. It is difficult to compare data from different studies that have required different periods of remission for the recruitment to the study. There is, however, considerable evidence that the longer that remission has lasted the better the outcome of drug withdrawal (MRC AED Withdrawal Group 1991, Todt 1984). This must be expected as not all patients who achieve a 2-year remission of seizures will necessarily remain in remission for a full 5 years, even if their therapy is continued. Selection of a group of patients with longer remissions may simply select a group of patients with more benign epilepsy rather than identifying an effect of prolonged treatment.

Rate of antiepileptic drug reduction. There is a suspicion that more rapid rates of reduction are associated with higher relapse rates. The low relapse rate in the large adult study reported by Oller-Daurella et al (1976) may have been due to the very slow rate of drug reduction employed in this study. Overweg et al (1987) however, did not find this to influence relapse and a minimum 6-month period of drug withdrawal in a largely adult population did not seem to result in lesser rate of recurrence (MRC AED Withdrawal Group 1991).

Duration of follow-up. It is generally agreed that over 50% of relapses occur during the phase of antiepileptic drug withdrawal or within a few months thereafter. Some 70–80% of relapses occur within 1 year of withdrawal. Nevertheless, occasional relapses continue for years after withdrawal and therefore duration of follow up will influence overall relapse rates. In the longest study to date, Thurson et al (1982) re-examined the fate of 148 children originally reported by Holowach et al (1972). In the original study the later authors reported a relapse rate of 24% at 5–12 years of follow up. Ten years later Thurston et al (1982) found that only five further patients had relapsed, increasing the relapse rate from 24% to 28%. Such late relapses may be more frequent in adults (Tsai & Schmidt 1987).

Several authors have tried to assess the relative contribution of several prognostic factors to the prognosis after withdrawal of drugs. Emerson et al (1981) found that a normal EEG before withdrawal and a history of only a few tonic-clonic seizures were of greatest importance. Thurston et al (1982), again in children, found that the most important adverse factors were a long duration of epilepsy, the presence of focal motor seizures, or a combination of seizure types, and the presence of neurological deficit. Shinnar et al (1985) found that the EEG, seizure type and age of onset were the major determinants of outcome. Callaghan et al (1988) found that the EEG and seizure type were the most important prognostic factors.

The most detailed assessment of prognostic factors has been undertaken in the MRC AED Withdrawal Study (1991). Here 1013 patients were randomized to continue treatment or slow withdrawal. A relatively few clinical factors influenced the risk of recurrence in both groups (Table 5.12). These include the length of seizure remission, taking more than one AED, the presence of tonic-clonic or myoclonic seizures and the duration of treatment.

Two further issues deserve consideration. Firstly, it is often assumed that if relapse occurs following drug withdrawal then reinstitution of therapy will promptly control the epilepsy as before. Whilst this is probably true of the great majority of cases, Todt (1984) reported that 14% of his patients with relapses had a 'problematic' course after treatment was reinstituted. Secondly,

Table 5.12 Influence of prognostic factors on relative risk of seizure recurrence (1013 in MRC Antiepileptic Drug Withdrawal Study—1991)

	Relative risk[*]	(95% CL)
Partial seizures only, no generalized tonic seizures	2.51	(1.0, 6.3)
History of myoclonic seizures	1.85	(1.09, 3.12)
History of any tonic-clonic seizure	3.40	(1.48, 7.84)
Seizures occurring after starting treatment	1.57	(1.10, 2.24)
Taking more than one antiepileptic drug	1.79	(1.34, 2.39)
Period seizure free (years)		
2.5–3	0.94	(0.67, 1.32)
3–<5	0.67	(0.48, 0.93)
5–<10	0.47	(0.32, 0.69)
>10	0.27	(0.15, 0.48)
Duration of AED treatment (years)		
3–<5	0.85	(0.56, 1.30)
5–<10	0.92	(0.56, 1.41)
10–<20	1.35	(0.72, 2.51)
>20	1.61	(0.73, 3.54)

[*] From multivariate Cox model.

if relapse does occur, especially during or soon after withdrawal, is this a recurrence of the original epilepsy demanding further therapy or simply withdrawal seizure requiring no immediate intervention? Todt (1984) describes 14 patients (seven with paroxysmal EEG activity) in whom he did not reinstate therapy and in whom no further attacks occurred during the following 3 years.

REFERENCES

Adams R D, Foley J M 1953 The neurological disorder associated with liver disease. In: Merritt H H, Hare C C (eds) Metabolic and toxic liver disease of the nervous systems. Williams and Wilkins, Baltimore, 198–237

Ajmone-Marsan G, Goldhammer L 1973 Clinical ictal patterns and electrographic data in cases of partial seizures of frontal-central-parietal origin. In: Brazier M A B (ed) Epilepsy, its phenomenon in man. Academic Press, New York, p 235–258

Alajouanine T, Nehil J, Gabersek V 1959 A propos d'un cas d'épilépsie déclenche par la lecture. Revue Neurologique (Paris) 101: 463–467

Alstroem C H 1950 A study of epilepsy, its clinical, social and genetic aspects. Munksgaard, Copenhagen

Aminoff M J, Simon R P 1980 Status epilepticus: causes, clinical features and consequences in 98 patients. American Journal of Medicine 69: 657–666

Anderman F 1987 Migraine-epilepsy relationships. Epilepsy Research 1: 213–226

Anderman F, Andermann E 1986 Excessive startle syndromes: Startle disease, jumping and startle epilepsy. In: Fahn S, Marsden C D, Van Woest M (eds) Advances in Neurology, Vol. 43

Annegers J F, Hauser W A, Elverback L R 1979 Remission of seizures and relapse in patients with epilepsy. Epilepsia 20: 729–737

Annegers J F, Grabow J D, Groover R V, Laws E R, Elveback L R, Kurland L T 1980 Seizures after head trauma: A populations study. Neurology 30: 683–689

Annegers J F, Hauser W A, Beghi E, Nicolosi A, Kurland L T 1988 The risk of uprovoked seizures after encephalitis and meningitis. Neurology 38: 1407–1410

Antoniadis A, Mueller W E, Wollert U 1980 Benzodiazepine receptor interactions may be involved in the neurotoxicity of various penicillin derivatives. Annals of Neurology 8: 71–73

Aquimno A, Gabor A J 1980 Movement-induced seizures in nonketotic hypoglycaemia. Neurology 30: 600–604

Arieff A I, Llach F, Massry S G 1976 Neurological manifestations and morbidity of hyponatraemia: Correlation with brain water and electrolytes. Medicine 55: 121–129

Arts W F M, Visser L H, Loonen M C B et al 1988 Follow-up of 146 children with epilepsy after withdrawal of antiepileptic therapy. Epilepsia 29: 244–250

Ascroft P B 1941 Traumatic epilepsy after gunshot wounds of the head. British Medical Journal 1: 739–744

Babb T L, Brown W J 1987 Pathological findings in epilepsy. In Engel Jr J (ed) Surgical treatment of the epilepsies. Raven Press, New York, p 511–540

Backstrom T 1976 Epileptic seizures in women related to plasma oestrogen and progesterone during the menstrual cycle. Acta Neurologica Scandinavica 54: 321–347

Baldy-Moulinier M 1986 Inter-relationships between sleep and epilepsy. In: Pedley T A, Meldrum J (eds) Recent advances in epilepsy, Vol 3: Churchill-Livingstone, Edinburgh, p 37–57

Bates D, Caronna J J, Cartlidge N E F et al 1977 A prospective study of non-traumatic coma: methods and results in 310 patients. Annals of Neurology 2: 211–220

Bauermeister D, Jennings E R, Cruse D, Sedgwick De Mott V 1967 Hypercalcaemia with seizures. A clinical paradox. Journal of the American Medical Association 201: 132–134

Bennett R, Hughes G R V, Bywaters E G L, Holt P J L 1972 Neuropsychiatric problems in systemic lupus erythematosis. British Medical Journal 4: 342–344

Bennett W M, Muther R S, Parker R A et al 1980 Drug therapy in renal failure. Dosing guidelines for adults. Annals of Internal Medicine 93: 286–325

Berkovie S F, Andermann F 1986 The progressive myoclonus epilepsies. In Pedley T A, Meldrum B S (eds) Recent advances in epilepsy, Vol. 3: Churchill Livingstone, Edinburgh, p 157–188

Binnie C D, Darby C E, de Korte R A, Wilkins A J 1980 Self-induction of epileptic seizures by eye closure: incidence and recognition. Journal of Neurology, Neurosurgery and Psychiatry 43: 386–389

Blakemore W F 1980 Isoniazid. In: Spencer P S, Schaumburg H H (eds) Experimental and clinical neurotoxicology. Williams and Wilkins, Baltimore, p 476–489

Blomquist H K, Gustavson K H, Holmgren G 1981 Mild mental retardation in children in northern Swedish county. Journal of Mental Deficiency Research 25: 169–186

Blumhardt L D, Smith P E M, Owen L 1986 Electrocardiographic accompaniments of temporal lobe epileptic seizures. Lancet 1: 1051–1055

Boston Collaborative Drug Surveilllance Program 1972 Drug-induced convulsions. Lancet 2: 677–679

Bouma P A D, Peters A C B, Arts R J H M, Stijnen T, Rossum J Van 1987 Discontinuation of antiepileptic therapy: A prospective study in children. Journal of Neurology, Neurosurgery and Psychiatry 50: 1579–1583

Bridge E M 1949 Epilepsy and convulsive disorders in children. McGraw-Hill, New York

Bruck E, Abal G, Aceto T Jr 1968 Therapy of infants with hypertonic dehydration due to diarrhoea. American Journal of Diseases of Childhood 115: 281–301

Burn J P S, Sandercock P A G, Bamford J, Dennis M S, Warlow C P 1990 The incidence of epileptic seizures after a first ever stroke. Journal of Neurology, Neurosurgery and Psychiatry 53: 810

Cabral R J, King T T, Scott D F 1976a Incidence of postoperative epilepsy after a transentorial approach to acoustic nerve tumours: Journal of Neurology, Neurosurgery and Psychiatry 39: 663–665

Cabral R J, King T T, Scott D F 1976b Epilepsy after two different neurological approaches to the treatment of ruptured intracranial aneurysm. Journal of Neurology, Neurosurgery and Psychiatry 39: 1052–1056

Caffi J 1973 Zur frage klinischer anfallformen bei psychomotorischer epilepsie. Schweiz medizinische wochenschrift 103: 469–475

Callaghan N, Garrett A, Goggin T 1988 Withdrawal of antiepileptic drugs in patients free of seizures for two years. A prospective study. New England Journal of Medicine 318: 942–946

Cast I P, Wilson P J E 1981 Pituitary tumours (abst). Journal of Neurology, Neurosurgery and Psychiatry 44: 371

Cavazzuti G B 1980 Epidemiology of different types of epilepsy in school-age children of Modena, Italy. Epilepsia 21: 57–62

Caveness W F, Liss H R 1961 Incidence of post-traumatic epilepsy in Korean veterans as compared with those from World War I and World War II. Epilepsia 2: 123–129

Caveness W F, Meirowsky A M, Rish B C et al 1979 The nature of posttraumatic epilepsy. Journal of Neurosurgery 50: 545–553

Chadwick D 1983 Drug-induced convulsions. In Rose F C

(ed) Research progress in epilepsy. Pitman, London, p 151–160

Chadwick D 1985 The discontinuation of antiepileptic therapy. In: Meldrum B M, Pedley T A (eds) Recent advances in epilepsy, vol 2. Churchill Livingstone, Edinburgh

Chadwick D, Martin S, Buxton P H, Tomlinson A H 1982 Measles virus and subacute neurological disease: an unusual presentation of measles inclusion body encephalitis. Journal of Neurology, Neurosurgery and Psychiatry 45: 680–684

Chadwick D, Shaw M D M, Foy P, Rawlins M D, Turnbull D M 1984 Serum anticonvulsant concentrations and the risk of drug induced skin eruptions. Journal of Neurology, Neurosurgery and Psychiatry 47: 642–644

Cirignotta F, Zuconni M, Mondini S, Lenzi P L, Lugaresi E 1983 Enuresis, sleep walking and nightmares: an epidemiological survey in the republic of San Marino. In: Guilleminault C, Lugaresi E (eds) Sleep/wake disorders, natural history, epidemiology and long-term evolution. Raven Press, New York, p 237–241

Cleland P G, Mosbue R J, Steward W P, Fosta J B 1981 Prognosis of isolated seizures in adult life. British Medical Journal 283: 1364

Cocito L, Favle E, Reni L 1982 Epileptic seizures in cerebral arterial occlusive disease. Stroke 13: 189–195

Coleman R M, Pollak C P, Weitzman E D 1980 Periodic movements in sleep (nocturnal myoclonus): relation to sleep disorders. Annals of Neurology 8: 416–421

Commission on classification and terminology of the International League Against Epilepsy 1989 Proposal for revised classification of epilepsies and epileptic syndromes. Epilepsia 30: 389–399

Copeland G P, Foy P, Shaw M D M 1982 The incidence of epilepsy after ventricular shunting operations. Surgical Neurology 17: 279–281

Crawford P M, West C R, Chadwick D W, Shaw M D M 1986 Cerebral arteriovenous malformations and epilepsy: factors in the development of epilepsy. Epilepsia 27: 270–275

Critchley M 1937 Musicogenic epilepsy. Brain 60: 13–27

Currie S, Heathfield K W G, Henson R A, Scott D F 1971 Clinical course and prognosis of temporal lobe epilepsy. Brain 94: 173–190

Curtis D R, Game C J A, Johnston G A R, McCulloch R M, MacLachlan R M 1972 Convulsant action of penicillin. Brain Research 43: 242–245

Dalby M A 1969 Epilepsy and 3 per second spike and wave rhythms. A clinical, electroencephalographic and prognostic analysis of 346 patients. Acta Neurologica Scandinavica 45: suppl 40

Dam A M, Fuglsang-Frederiksen A, Svarre-Olsen U, Dam M 1985 Late-onset epilepsy: etiologies, types of seizure, and value of clinical investigation, EEG, and computerized tomography scan. Epilepsia 26: 227–231

Delgado-Escueta A V, Enrile-Bacsal F 1984 Juvenile myoclonic epilepsy of Janz. Neurology 34: 285–294

Delgado-Escueta A V, Walsh G O 1985 Type I complex partial seizures of hippocampal origin: Excellent results of anterior temporal lobectomy. Neurology 35: 143–154

Delgado-Escueta A V, Enrile Bascal F, Treiman D M 1982 Complex partial seizures on closed-circuit television and EEG: A study of 691 attacks in 79 patients. Annals of Neurology 11: 292–300

Douglas D B 1971 Interval between first seizure and

diagnosis of brain tumour. Diseases of the Nervous System 32: 255

Dunea G, Mahurkar S D, Mamdani B, Smith E C 1978 Role of aluminium in dialysis dementia. Annals of Internal Medicine 88: 502–504

Edebol-Tysk K 1989 Epidemiology of spastic tetraplegic cerebral palsy in Sweden. I. Impairments and disabilities. Neuropediatrics 20: 41–45

Elwes R D C, Chesterman P, Reynolds E H 1985 Prognosis after a first untreated tonic-clonic seizure. Lancet 2: 752–753

Emerson R, D'Souza B J, Vining E P, Holden K R, Mellits E D, Freeman J M 1981 Stopping medication in children with epilepsy. New England Journal of Medicine 304: 1125–1129

Engle J 1989 Seizures and epilepsy. F A Davis, Philadelphia

Essig C F 1967 Clinical and experimental aspects of barbiturate withdrawal convulsions. Epilepsia 8: 21–30

Fahn S, Marsden C D, Van Woert M H 1986 Definition and classification of myoclonus. In: Fahn S, Marsden C D, Van Woert M (eds) Advances in Neurology, Vol 43. Raven Press, New York, p 1–6

Falconer M A 1971 Genetic and related aetiological factors in temporal lobe epilepsy: A review. Epilepsia 12: 13–31

Feeley M, Calvert R, Gibson J 1982 Clobazam in catamenial epilepsy: a model for evaluating anticonvulsants. Lancet ii: 71

Fisher C M, Adams R D 1958 Transient global amnesia. Transactions of the American Neurological Association 83: 143–146

Fishman R A 1965 Neurological aspects of magnesium metabolism. Archives of Neurology 12: 562–569

Forsgren L, Edvinsson S-O, Blomquist H K, Heijbel J, Sidenvall R 1990 Epilepsy in a population of mentally retarded children and adults. Epilepsy Research 6: 234–248

Forster F M 1977 Reflex epilepsy, behavioural therapy and conditional reflexes. Thomas, Illinois

Forster C, Schmidberger D 1978 Prognose der epilepsie in kindesalte nach absetzen der medikation. Monatschreift. Kinderheilk 30: 225–228

Foy P M, Copeland G P, Shaw M D M 1981a The incidence of postoperative seizures. Acta Neurochirurgica 55: 253–264

Foy P M, Copeland G P, Shaw M D M 1981b. The natural history of postoperative seizures. Acta Neurochirurgica 57: 15–22

Foy P M, Chadwick D W, Rajgopalan N, Johnson A L, Shaw M D M 1992 Do prophylactic anticonvulsant drugs alter the pattern of seizures following craniotomy? Journal of Neurology, Neurosurgery and Psychiatry (in press)

Frame B 1976 Neuromuscular manifestations of parathyroid disease. In Vinken P J, Bruyn G W (eds) Handbook of clinical neurology, Vol 27. Elsevier North-Holland, Amsterdam, p 283–320

Fraser H F, Wikler A, Essig C F, Isbell H 1958 Degree of physical dependence induced by secobarbital or pentobarbital. Journal of the American Medical Association 166: 126–129

Gastaut H 1976 Conclusions: computerized transverse axial tomography in epilepsy. Epilepsia 17: 337–338

Gastaut H, Gastaut J L, Gonclaves e Silva G E, Fernandez Sanchez G R 1975 Relative frequency of different types of epilepsy: A study employing the classification of the International League Against Epilepsy. Epilepsia 16: 457–461

Gawin F H, Ellinwood E H 1988 Cocaine and other stimulants. New England Journal of Medicine 318: 1173–1182

Geier S, Bancaud J, Talairach J, Bonis A, Szikla G, Enjelvin M 1977 The seizures of frontal lobe epilepsy. Neurology 27: 951–958

Gibberd F B, Bateson M C 1974 Sleep epilepsy: its pattern and prognosis. British Medical Journal 2: 403–405

Gloor P, Olivier A, Quesney L F, Andermann F, Horowitz S 1982 The role of the limbic system in experential phenomena of temporal lobe epilepsy. Annals of Neurology 12: 129–144

Goodridge D M G, Shorvon S D 1983 Epileptic seizures in a population of 6000: II—treatment and prognosis. British Medical Journal 287: 645–647

Goosses R 1984 Die beziehung der fotosensibilitat zu den verschiedenen epileptischen syndromen. Thesis, University of West Berlin

Goulatia R K, Verma A. Mishra N K, Ahuja G K 1987 Disappearing CT lesion in epilepsy. Epilepsia 28: 523–527

Gowers W R 1881 Epilepsy and other chronic convulsive diseases. Churchill, London

Greenberg D A, Delgado-Escueta A V, Widelitz H et al 1988 Juvenile myoclonic epilepsy (JME) may be linked to the BF and HLA loci on human chromosome 6. American Journal of Medical Genetics 31: 185–192

Grosz W 1930 Ueber den Ausang der genuinen Epilepsie: auf Grund katamnestischer Erhebungen. Archiv fur Psychiatrie und Nevervenkrankheiten 90: 765–776

Group for the study of the prognosis of epilepsy in Japan 1981 Natural history and prognosis of epilepsy: report of a multi-institutional study in Japan. Epilepsia 22: 35–53

Gudmundsson G 1966 Epilepsy in Iceland. Acta Neurologica Scandinavica 43 (Suppl 25): 72–73

Gumpert J, Hanisota P, Upton A 1970 Gelastic epilepsy. Journal of Neurology, Neurosurgery and Psychiatry 33: 479–483

Gustavson K H, Holmgren G, Jonsell R, Blomquist H K 1977 Severe mental retardation in children in a northern Swedish county. Journal of Mental Deficiency Research 21: 161–180

Habermaas F 1901 Ueber die Prognose der Epilepsie. Zeitschrift fur Psychiatrie 58: 243–253

Hanna S, Harrison M, MacIntyre I, Fraser R 1960 The syndrome of magnesium deficiency in man. Lancet 2: 172–176

Harper M, Roth M 1962 Temporal lobe epilepsy and the phobic anxiety-depersonalization syndrome. Part 1. A comparative study. Comprehensive Psychiatry 3: 129–151

Hart Y M, Sander J W A S, Johnson A L, Shorvon S D 1990 National general practice survey of epilepsy: recurrence after a first seizure. Lancet 336: 1271–74

Hauser W A 1986 Should people be treated after a first seizure? Archives of Neurology 43: 1287–1288

Hauser W A 1990 Prevention of post-traumatic epilepsy. New England Journal of Medicine 323: 540–541

Hauser W A, Anderson V E 1986 Genetics of epilepsy. In: Pedley T A, Meldrum B S (eds) Recent advances in epilepsy, vol 3. Churchill Livingstone, Edinburgh, p 21–36

Hauser W A, Kurland L T 1975 The epidemiology of epilepsy in Rochester, Minnesota, 1935 through 1967. Epilepsia 16: 1–66

Hauser W A, Anderson V E, Loewenston R B, McRoberts S M 1982 Seizure recurrence after a first unprovoked seizure. New England of Medicine 307: 522–528

Hauser W A, Shinnar S, Cohen H, Inbar D, Benedetti M D 1987 Clinical predictors of epilepsy among children with cerebral palsy and/or mental retardation. Neurology 37 (Suppl 1): 150

Hauser W A, Rich S S, Annegers J F, Anderson V E 1990 Seizure recurrence after a first unprovoked seizure: an extended follow-up. Neurology 40: 1163–1170

Hedenstroem I, Schorsch G 1963 Ueber thereapierestente epileptiker. Archiv fur psychiatrie und nervenkrankheiten 204: 579–588

Herishanu Y, Abramsky O, Lavy S 1970 Focal neurological manifestations in hypercalcaemia. European Neurology 4: 283–288

Heycop Ten Ham M W 1980 Complete recovery from epilepsy? Huisants en Wetenshap 23: 309–311

Hillbom M E 1980 Occurrence of cerebral seizures provoked by alcohol abuse. Epilepsia 21: 459–466

Hodges J R, Warlow C P 1990 Syndromes of transient amnesia: towards a classification. A study of 153 cases. Journal of Neurology, Neurosurgery and Psychiatry 53: 834–843

Holowach J, Thurston D L, O'Leary J 1972 Prognosis of childhood epilepsy. New England Journal of Medicine 286: 169–174

Hopkins A, Garman A, Clarke C 1988 The first seizure in adult life. Lancet i: 721–726

Howe J G, Gibson J D 1982 Uncinate seizures and tumours, a myth re-examined. Annals of Neurology 12: 227

Howell S J L, Owen L, Chadwick D W 1989 Pseudostatus epilepticus. Quarterly Journal of Medicine 266: 507–519

Huttenlocher P R, Hapke R J 1990 A follow-up study of intractable seizures in childhood. Annals of Neurology 28: 699–705

Hyllested K, Pakkenberg H 1963 Prognosis in epilepsy of late onset. Neurology 13: 641–644

Ingvar D H, Nyman G E 1962 Epilepticus arithmetices. A new psychologic trigger mechanism in a case of epilepsy. Neurology 12: 282–287

Isbell H, Fraser H F, Wikler A, Belleville R E, Eisenman A J 1955 An experimental study of the aetiology of 'rum fits' and delirium tremens. Quarterly Journal for the Study of Alcoholism 16: 1–33

Jacob H 1970 Muscular twitchings in Alzheimer's disease. In: Wolsteholme G E W, O'Connor M (eds) Alzheimer's disease and related conditions. J & A Churchill, London, p 75–89

Janz D 1962 The grand-mal epilepsies and the sleeping–waking cycle. Epilepsia 3: 69–109

Janz D 1969 Die Epilepsien. Thieme, Stuttgart

Janz D 1987 When should antiepileptic drug treatment be terminated? In: Wolf P, Dam M, Janz D, Dreifuss F E (eds) Advances in epileptology, vol 16, Raven Press, New York, p 365–372

Janz D, Christian W 1957 Impulsiv-petit mal. Journal of Neurology 176: 346–386

Janz D, Sommer-Burkhardt E M 1976 Discontinuation of antiepileptic drugs in patients with epilepsy who have been seizure-free for more than two years. In: Janz D (ed) Epileptology. Thieme-Verlag, Stuttgart, p 228–234

Janz D, Kern A, Mossinger H-J, Puhlmann U 1983a Ruckfall-prognose nach reduktion der medikamente hei epilepsiebehandlung. Nervenarzt 54: 525–529

Janz D, Kern A, Mossinger H J, Puhlmann H U 1983b Ruckfallprognose wahrend und nach reduktion der medikamente bei epilepsie behandlung. In: Remschmidt H,

Rentz R, Jungmann J (eds) Epilepsie 1981. Thieme: Stuttgart, p 17–24

Jeavons P M, Harding G F A 1975 Photosensitive epilepsy. Heinemann, London

Jellinek E H 1962 Fits, faints, coma and dementia in myxoedema. Lancet 2: 1010–1012

Jennet W B 1975 Epilepsy after non-missile head injuries, 2nd end, Heinemann Medical Books, London

Juul-Jensen P 1963 Epilepsy, a clinical and social analysis of 1020 adult patients with epileptic seizures. Munksgaard, Copenhagen

Juul-Jensen P 1964 Epilepsy. A clinical and social analysis of 1020 adult patients with epileptic seizures. Acta Neurologica Scandinavica 40(suppl 5): 1–285

Juul-Jensen P 1968 Frequency of recurrence after discontinuance of anticonvulsant therapy in patients with epileptic seizures. A new follow-up study after 5 years. Epilepsia 9: 11–16

Juul-Jensen P, Foldspang A 1983 Natural history of epileptic seizures. Epilepsia 24: 297–312

Kertesz A 1967 Paroxysmal kinesigenic choreoathetosis. Neurology 17: 680–690

King D W, Gallagher B B, Murvin A J et al 1982 Pseudoseizures: diagnostic evaluation. Neurology 32: 18–23

Kiørobe E 1961 The prognosis of epilepsy. Acta Psychiatrica Scandinavica 36(suppl 150): 166–178

Knochel J P 1977 The pathophysiology and clinical characteristics of severe hypophosphataemia. Archives of Internal Medicine 137: 203–220

Korczyn A D, Bechar M 1976 Convulsive fits in thyrotoxicosis. Epilepsia 17: 33–34

Kuzniecky R, De La Sayette D, Ethier R et al 1987 Magnetic resonance imaging in temporal lobe epilepsy: pathological correlations. Annals of Neurology 22: 341–347

Lance J W, Adams R D 1963 The syndrome of intention or action myoclonus as a sequel to hypoxic encephalopathy. Brain 86: 111–136

Lederman R J, Henry C E 1978 Progressive dialysis encephalopathy. Annals of Neurology 4: 199–204

Legg N J, Gupta P C, Scott D F 1973 Epilepsy following cerebral abscess: A clinical and EEG study of 70 patients. Brain 96: 259–268

Lesser R P, Luders H, Dinner D S, Morris H H 1985 Epileptic seizures due to thrombotic and embolic cerebrovascular disease in older patients. Epilepsia 26: 622–630

Lesser R P, Luders H, Dinner D S, Morris H H 1987 Simple partial seizures in epilepsy: In: Luders H, Lesser R P (eds) Electroclinical syndromes. Springer-Verlag, London; p 223–278

Lishman W A, Symonds P, Whitty C W M, Willison R G 1962 Seizures induced by movement. Brain 85: 93–108

Logothetis J 1967 Spontaneous epileptic seizure and electroencephalographic changes in the course of phenothiazine therapy. Neurology (Minneap) 17: 869–877

Loiseau P, Pestre M, Dartigues J F, Commenges D, Barbeger-Gateau C, Cohadon S 1983 Long-term prognosis in two forms of childhood epilepsy; typical absence seizures and epilepsy with rolandic (centrotemporal) EEG foci. Annals of Neurology 13: 642–648

Loiseau J, Loiseau P, Duche B, Guyot M, Dartigues J F, Aublet B 1990 A survey of epileptic disorders in southwest France: seizures in elderly patients. Annals of Neurology 27: 232–237

Loiseau P 1985 Childhood absence epilepsy. In: Roger J, Dravet C, Bureau M, Dreifuss F E, Wolf P (eds) Epileptic syndromes in infancy, childhood and adolescence. John Libbey, London, p 106–120

Lorge M 1964 Epilepsie und Lebensschicksal: Ergebnisse katamnestischer Untersuchungen. Psychiatrica et Neurologica (Basel) 147: 360–381

Lowry M R, Dunner F J 1980 Seizures during tricyclic therapy. American Journal of Psychiatry 137: 1461–1462

Lund M 1952 Epilepsy associated with intracranial tumours. Acta Psychiatrica Neurologica Scandinavica Suppl 81

McQueen J K, Blackwood D H, Harris P, Kalbag R M, Johnson A L 1983 Low risk of late post-traumatic seizures following severe head injury: implications for clinical trials of prophylaxis. Journal of Neurology, Neurosurgery and Psychiatry 46: 899–904

Malouf R, Brust J C M 1985 Hypoglycaemia: Cause, neurological manifestations and outcome. Annals of Neurology 17: 421–430

Matricardi M, Brinciotti M, Benedetti P 1989 Outcome after discontinuation of antiepileptic drug therapy in children with epilepsy. Epilepsia 30: 582–589

Matthews W B 1975 Paroxysmal symptoms in multiple sclerosis. Journal of Neurology, Neurosurgery and Psychiatry 36: 617–623

Mattson R H, Sturman J K, Gronowski M L, Goico H 1975 Effect of alcohol intake in non-alcoholic epileptics. Neurology 25: 361–362

Mauguiere F, Courjon J 1978 Somatosensory epilepsy: A review of 127 cases. Brain 101: 307–332

Maurice-Williams R M 1974 Micturition symptoms in frontal tumours. Journal of Neurology, Neurosurgery and Psychiatry 37: 431–436

Mayersdorf A, Marshall C 1970 Pattern activation in reading epilepsy: a case report. Epilepsia II: 423–426

Mayeux R, Lender H 1978 Complex partial status epilepticus: case report and proposal for diagnostic criteria. Neurology 28: 957–961

Mayeux R, Alexander M P, Benson D F, Brandt J, Rosen J 1979 Poriomania. Neurology 29: 1616–1619

Medical Research Council Antiepileptic Drug Withdrawal Study Group 1991 A randomized study of antiepileptic drug withdrawal in patients in remission of epilepsy. New England Journal of Medicine 337: 1175–1180

Medrum B S, Horton R W, Brierley J B 1974 Epileptic brain damage in adolescent baboons following seizures induced by allylglycine. Brain 97: 407–418

Merritt H 1958 Medical treatment in epilepsy. British Medical Journal 1: 666–669

Messing R O, Simon R P 1986 Seizures as a manifestation of systemic disease. Neurological Clinics 4: 563–584

Messing R O, Closson R G, Simon R P 1984 Drug-induced seizures: A 10-year experience. Neurology 34: 1582–1586

Metrakos J D, Metrakos K 1972 Genetic factors in the epilepsies. In: Alter R, Hauser W A (eds) The epidemiology of epilepsy: a workship. NINDS Monograph, no. 14: US Government Printing Office, Washington DC, p 97–102

Muller R 1949 Studies on disseminated sclerosis with special reference to symptomatology, course and prognosis. Acta Medica Scandinavica 133 (Suppl 222): 1–124

Nalin A, Galli V, Ferrari P, Ciccarone V 1982 Interruzione della terapia anticomizale in una popualazione con epilepsia ad escordia infantile. Boll. Lega. Intal Epil. 39: 113–114

Nelson K B, Ellenberg J H 1978 Prognosis in children with febrile seizures. Paediatrics 61: 720–727

Nelson K B, Ellenberg J H 1986 Antecedents of cerebral palsy, multivariate analysis of risk. New England Journal of Medicine 315: 81–86

Newmark M E, Penry J K 1980 Catamenial epilepsy: A review. Epilepsia 21: 281–300

Ng S K C, Hauser W A, Brust J C M, Susser M 1988 Alcohol consumption and withdrawal in new-onset seizures. New England Journal of Medicine 319: 666–673

Norenberg M D, Leslie K O, Robertson A S 1982 Association between rise in serum sodium and central pontine myelinolysis. Annals of Neurology 11: 128–135

North J B, Penhall R K, Hanieh A, Frewin D B, Taylor W B 1983 Phenytoin and postoperative epilepsy: a double blind study. Journal of Neurosurgery 58: 672–677

Ochs R, Bloor P, Quesney F, Ives J, Oliver A 1984 Does head-turning during a seizure have lateralising or localising significance? Neurology 34: 884–890

Oller-Daurella L, Sanchez M E 1981 Evolucion de las ausencias tipicas. Rev Neurol (Barcelona) 9: 81–102

Oller-Daurella L, Pamies R, Oller L 1976 Reduction or discontinuance of antiepileptic drugs in patients seizure-free for more than 5 years. In: Janz D (ed) Epileptology. Thieme-Verlag, Stuttgart, p 218–227

Oswald I 1959 Sudden bodily jerks on falling asleep. Brain 82: 92–103

Overweg J, Binnie C D, Oosting J, Rowan A J 1987 Clinical and EEG prediction of seizure recurrence following antiepileptic drug withdrawal Epilepsy Research 1: 272–283

Parkes J D 1982 Narcolepsy. In: Riley T L, Roy A (eds) Pseudoseizures. Williams & Wilkins, Baltimore, p 62–82

Pedley T A, Guilmeniault C 1977 Episodic nocturnal wanderings responsive to anticonvulsant drug therapy. Annals of Neurology 2: 30–35

Pedley T A 1988 Discontinuing antiepileptic drugs. New England Journal of Medicine 318: 982–984

Penfield W, Welch K 1951 The supplementary motor area of the cerebral cortex. Archives of Neurology and Psychiatry 66: 289–317

Penfield W, Jasper H 1954 Epilepsy and the functional anatomy of the human brain. Little Brown, Boston

Pestre M, Loiseau P, Larrieu E, Dartigues J F, Cohadon S 1987 Withdrawal of antiepileptic drug therapy in adolescent epileptic patients. In: Wolf P, Dam M, Janz D, Dreifuss F E (eds) Advances in Epileptology, vol. 16. Raven Press, New York, p 395–400

Phillips G 1954 Traumatic epilepsy after closed head injury. Journal of Neurology, Neurosurgery and Psychiatry 17: 1–10

Pincus J H 1978 Disorders of conscious awareness: hyperventilation syndrome. British Journal of Hospital Medicine 19: 312–313

Plum F, Hindfelt B 1968 The neurological complications of liver disease. In Vinken P J, Bruyn G W (eds): Handbook of clinical neurology, Vol 27, Part 1, Elsevier North-Holland, Amsterdam, p 349–377

Plum F, Posner J B 1989 The diagnosis of stupor and coma, 3rd edn. F A Davis, Philadelphia

Poskanzer D C, Brown A E, Miller H 1962 Musicogenic epilepsy caused only by a discrete frequency band of church bells. Brain 85: 77–92

Probst C 1960 Ueber den Verlauf von hirnelektrisch strummen Epilepsien. Schweizer Archives fur Neurologie, Neurochirurgie und Psychiatrie 85: 357–400

Procaccianti G, Luganesi E, Tinuper P, Serracchiou A, Ripamonti L, Baruzzi A 1987 Antiepiletic drug withdrawal: preliminary results of a prospective study. In: Dam M, Gram L, Penry J K (eds) Advances in Epileptology: XII Epilepsy International Symposium. Raven Press, New York, p 379–382

Quesney L F 1986 Seizures of frontal lobe origin. In: Pedley T A, Meldrum B S (eds) Recent advances in epilepsy, vol. 3. Churchill Livingstone, Edinburgh, p 81–110

Rapport R L II, Penry J K 1973 A survey of attitudes towards the pharmacological prophylaxis of post-traumatic epilepsy. Journal of Neurosurgery 38: 159–166

Raskin N H, Fishman R A 1976 Neurologic disorders in renal failure. New England Journal of Medicine 294: 204–210

Raynor R B, Paine R S, Carmichael E A 1959 Epilepsy of late onset. Neurology 9: 111–117

Reynolds E H, Shorvon S D, Galbraith A W, Chadwick D W, Dellaportas C I, Vydelingum L 1981 Phenytoin monotherapy for epilepsy: a long-term prospective study, assisted by serum level monitoring, in previously untreated patients. Epilepsia 22: 475–488

Reynolds E H 1987 Early treatment and prognosis of epilepsy. Epilepsia 28(2): 97–106

Reynolds N C Jr, Miska R M 1976 Safety of anticonvulsants in hepatic porphyrias. Neurology 31: 480–484

Riley T L 1982 Syncope and hyperventilation. In: Riley T L, Roy A (eds) Pseudoseizures Williams & Wilkins, Baltimore, p 34–61

Rocca W A, Sharbrough F W, Hauser W A, Annegers J F, Schoenberg B S 1987 Risk factors for complex partial seizures: A population-based case-control study. Annals of Neurology 21: 22–31

Rodin E A 1968 The prognosis of patients with epilepsy. Charles C Thomas, Springfield, Illinois

Rodin E A, John G 1980 Withdrawal of anticonvulsant medications in successfully treated patients with epilepsy. In: Wada J A, Penry J K (eds) Advances in Epileptology: XII Epilepsy International Symposium. Raven Press, New York, p 183–186

Romanelli M F, Morris J C, Ashkin K, Coben L A 1990 Advanced Alzheimer's disease is a risk factor for late-onset seizures. Archives of Neurology 47: 847–850

Ross R T 1988 Syncope. W B Saunders, London

Roy A 1979 Hysterical seizures. Archives of Neurology 36: 447

Russel W R, Whitty C W M 1952 Studies in traumatic epilepsy part I—Factors influencing the incidence of epilepsy after brain wounds. Journal of Neurology, Neurosurgery and Psychiatry 15: 93–98

Salazar A M, Jabbari B, Vance S C et al 1985 Epilepsy after penetrating head injury: I. Clinical correlates. Neurology 35: 1406–1414

Sander J W A S, Hart Y M, Johnson A L, Shorvon S D 1990 National general practice study of epilepsy: newly diagnosed epileptic seizures in a general population. Lancet 336: 1267–1271

Schmidt D 1982 Adverse effects of antiepileptic drugs. Raven Press, New York

Schorner W, Meencke H J, Felix R 1987 Temporal-lobe epilepsy: comparison of CT and MR imaging. American Journal of Radiology 149: 1231–1239

Servit Z, Musil F 1981 Prophylactic treatment of post-traumatic epilepsy; results of a long-term follow-up in Czechoslovakia. Epilepsia 22: 315–320

Shaffer S Q, Hauser W A, Annegers J F, Klass D W 1988 EEG and other early predictors of epilepsy remission: A community study. Epilepsia 29: 590–600

Shannon M, Goetz G 1989 Connective tissue diseases and the nervous system. In: Aminoff M (ed) Neurology and general medicine. Churchill Livingstone, New York, p 389–412

Sheehan S 1958 One thousand cases of late onset epilepsy. Irish Journal of Medical Science 6: 261

Shinnar S, Vining E P G, Mellits E D et al 1985 Discontinuing antiepileptic medication in children with epilepsy after two years without seizures. New England Journal of Medicine 313: 976–980

Shinton R A, Zezulka A V, Gill J S, Beevers D G 1987 The frequency of epilepsy preceding stroke. Lancet 1: 11–13

Shorvon S D, Reynolds E H 1982 The early prognosis of epilepsy. British Medical Journal 285: 1699–1701

Shorvon S D, Gilliat R W, Cox T C S, Yu Y L 1984 Evidence of vascular disease from CT scanning in late onset epilepsy. Journal of Neurology, Neurosurgery and Psychiatry 47: 225–230

Simon R P 1988 Alcohol and seizures. New England Journal of Medicine 309: 715–716

Smith B H 1060 Vestibular disturbance in epilepsy. Neurology 10: 465–469

Smith D F, Hutton J L, Sandemann D et al 1991 The prognosis of primary intracerebral tumours presenting with epilepsy: the outcome of medical and surgical management. Journal of Neurology, Neurosurgery and Psychiatry 54: 915–920

Sofijanov N G 1982 Clinical evolution and prognosis of childhood epilepsies. Epilepsia 23: 61–69

Sotelo J 1987 Neurocysticercosis. In: Kennedy P G E, Johnson R T (eds) Infections of the nervous system. Butterworths, London, p 144–154

Stafford-Clark D, Taylor F H 1949 Clinical and electro-encephalographic studies of prisoners charged with murder. Neurosurgery and Psychiatry 12: 325–330

Stengel E 1943 Further studies on pathological wandering (fugue with the impulse to wander). Journal of Mental Science 89: 224–241

Stephenson J B P 1971 Uraemia as a determinant of convulsions in acute infantile hypernatraemia. Archives of Diseases of Childhood 46: 676–679

Stevens D L, Matthews W B 1973 Cryptogenic drop attacks. An affliction of women. British Medical Journal 1: 439–442

Storey P B 1967 Psychiatric sequelae of subarachnoid haemorrhage. British Medical Journal 3: 261–266

Strobos R R J 1959 Prognosis in convulsive disorders. Archives of Neurology 1: 216–225

Sumi S M, Teasdall R D 1963 Focal seizures. A review of 150 cases. Neurology 13: 582–586

Swanson P D 1976 Neurological manifestations of hypernatraemia. In: Vinken P J, Bruyn G W (eds) Handbook of clinical neurology, Vol 28. Elsevier North-Holland, Amsterdam, p 443–461

Symonds C P 1953 Nocturnal myoclonus. Journal of Neurology, Neurosurgery and Psychiatry 16: 166–171

Tassinari C A, Bureau M, Dravet C, Dalla Bernardina B, Roger J 1985 Epilepsy with continuous spikes and waves during slow sleep. In: Roger J, Dravet C, Bureau M, Dreifuss F E, Wolf P (eds) Epileptic syndromes in infancy, childhood and adolescence. John Libbey, London, p 194–204

Taylor R L 1981 Magnesium sulphate for AIP seizures. Neurology 31: 1371–1372

Temkin N R, Dikmen S S, Wilensky A J, Keihm J, Chabal S, Winn H R 1900 A randomized, double-blind study of phenytoin for the prevention of post-traumatic seizures. New England Journal of Medicine 323: 497–502

Thrush D C, Boddie H G 1974 Episodic encephalopathy associated with thyroid disorders. Journal of Neurology, Neurosurgery and Psychiatry 37: 696–700

Thurston J H, Thurston D L, Hixon B B, Keller A J 1982 Prognosis in childhood epilepsy. New England Journal of Medicine 306: 831–836

Todt H 1984 The late prognosis of epilepsy in childhood: results of a prospective follow-up study. Epilepsia 25: 137–144

Treiman D N, Delgado-Escueta A V 1983 Violence in epilepsy: a critical review. In: Pedley T A, Meldrum B S (eds) Recent advances in epilepsy, vol 1. Churchill Livingstone, Edinburgh, p 179–209

Trolle E 1961 Drug therapy in epilepsy. Acta Psychiatrica Scandinavica 36 (suppl 150): 187–199

Truilzi F, Franceschi M, Fazzio F, Del Maschio A 1988 Nonrefractory temporal lobe epilepsy: 1. 5T MR imaging. Radiology 166: 181–185

Tsuki H, Kasuga I 1978 Paroxysmal discharges triggered by learning spoken language. Epilepsia 19: 147–154

Tsai J-J, Schmidt D 1987 Seizure relapse in epilepsy with complex partial seizures. In: Wolf P, Dam M, Janz D, Dreifuss F E (eds) Advances in epileptology, Vol 16. Raven Press, New York, p 405–407

Tudor I, Milea S, Bicescu E, Ivana D 1973 Catamnestic study of childhood epilepsy. Rev. Roum. Neurol. 10: 341–352

Turnbull D M, Howell D, Rawlins M D, Chadwick D 1985 Which drug for the adult epileptic patient: phenytoin or valproate? British Medical Journal 290: 815–819

Turner W A 1907 Epilepsy, a study of the idiopathic disease. Macmillan, London

Van Buren J M 1963 The abdominal aura: A study of abdominal sensations occurring in epilepsy and produced by depth stimulation. Electroencephalographic and Clinical Neurophysiology 15: 1–19

Venna N, Sabin T D 1981 Tonic focal seizures in non-ketotic hyperglycaemia of diabetes mellitus. Archives of Neurology 38: 512–514

Victor M, Adams R D 1953 The effect of alcohol on the nervous system. Research Publications of the Association for Nervous and Mental Diseases 32: 526–573

Victor M, Brausch C 1967 The role of abstinence in the genesis of alcoholic epilepsy. Epilepsia 8: 1–20

Visser L H, Arts W F M, Loonen M C B, Tjiam A T, Stuurman P M 1987 Follow-up of 166 children with epilepsy after withdrawal of anticonvulsant therapy: XII Epilepsy International Symposium. Raven Press, New York, p 401–404

Walker J E 1981 Effect of aminophylline on seizure thresholds and brain regional cyclic nucleotides in the rat. Experimental Neurology 74: 299–304

Walker A E, Jablon S 1961 A follow-up study of head wounds in World War II. V. A. Medical Monographs, U S Government Printing Office, Washington DC

Walker A E, Erculei F 1968 Head-injured men 15 years later. Charles C Thomas, Springfield

Walsh G O, Delgado-Escueta A V 1984 Type II complex partial seizures: Poor results of anterior temporal lobectomy. Neurology 34: 1–13

Wardrope J, Ryan F, Clark G, Venable G, Courtney Crosby A, Redgrave P 1991 The Hillsborough tragedy. British Medical Journal 303: 1381–1385

Whitty C W M, Lishman W A, Fitzgibbon J P 1964 Seizures induced by movement: a form of reflex epilepsy. Lancet 1: 1403–1405

Wieser H G 1983 Electroclinical features of the psychomotor seizure. G Fisher/Butterworths, Stuttgart

Wilkins A, Lindsay F 1985 Common forms of reflex epilepsy: physiological mechanisms and techniques for treatment. In: Pedley T A, Meldrum B S (eds) Recent advances in epilepsy, Churchill Livingstone, Edinburgh, p 239–272

Wilkins A J, Binnie C D, Darby C E 1980 Visually-induced seizures. Progress in Neurobiology 15: 85–117

Williams D 1956 The structure of emotions reflected in epileptic experiences. Brain 79: 29

Williamson P D, Spencer D D, Spencer S S, Novelly R A 1985 Complex partial seizures of frontal lobe origin. Annals of Neurology 18: 497–504

Wolf P, Inoue Y 1984 Therapeutic response of absence seizures in patients of an epilepsy clinic for adolescents and adults. Journal of Neurology 231: 225–229

Wong M C, Suite N D A, Labar D R 1990 Seizures in human immunodeficiency virus infection Archives of Neurology 47: 640–642

Yahr M D, Sciarra D, Carter S, Merritt H H 1952 Evaluation of standard anticonvulsant therapy in 319 patients. Journal of the American Medical Association 150: 663–667

Yanagihara T, Piepgras D G, Klass D W 1985 Repetitive involuntary movements associated with episodic cerebral ischaemia. Annals of Neurology 18: 244–250

Young G B, Blume W T 1983 Painful epileptic seizures. Brain 106: 537–554

Young A C, Bog Costanzi J, Mohr P D, Forbes W 1982 Is routine computerised axial tomography in epilepsy worthwhile? Lancet ii: 1446–1447

Young B, Rapp R P, Norton J A, Haack D, Tibbs P A, Bean J R 1983 Failure of prophylactically administered phenytoin to prevent late post-traumatic seizures. Journal of Neurosurgery 58: 236–241

Zenker C, Groh C, Roth G 1957 Probleme und erfahrungen beim abentzen anticonvulsiver therapie. Neue ossterrich zeitschrift fur kinderheilkunde 2: 152–163

Zielinski J J 1974 Epidemiology and medicosocial problems of epilepsy in Warsaw. Final report on research program No. 19-P-58325-F-01. Psychoneurological Institute, Warsaw,

6. Status epilepticus

D. M. Treiman

INTRODUCTION

The term 'status epilepticus' first appeared in medical writings in Babylonian times in a treatise on epilepsy which was part of a medical diagnostic series known as *Sakikku*, or 'All Diseases' (Wilson & Reynolds 1990). Subsequent references to status epilepticus appear in Roman (Temkin 1971) and early European (Roger et al 1974) writings but it was not until the early part of the last century that a detailed description of status epilepticus was first written (Calmeil 1824). Although the definition and classification of various types of status epilepticus have been refined by successive investigators, the fundamental mechanisms which allow a single seizure, normally a short duration self-limited event, to occur repetitively or to persist for an extended period of time are still poorly understood. Nonetheless, significant advances have been made in understanding the clinical presentation and treatment of various types of status epilepticus, and these advances will be outlined in this chapter.

DEFINITION

The operational definition of status epilepticus accepted by most neurologists is two or more seizures without full recovery of consciousness between seizures or recurrent epileptic seizures for more than 30 minutes. From this operational definition it follows that any type of epileptic seizure which occurs so frequently that the patient is unable to recover to a normal level of functioning between seizures can be considered status epilepticus. Thus status epilepticus may present as repeated generalized convulsive seizures with residual postictal confusion between seizures, as nonconvulsive seizures which produce a continuous 'epileptic twilight state' or as repeated simple partial seizures manifested as focal motor convulsions, focal sensory deficits or even speech arrest not associated with any impairment of consciousness.

CLASSIFICATION

Status epilepticus can be classified in the same manner as individual seizures using the International Classification of Epileptic Seizures (Commission 1981). In this classification the fundamental distinction is between seizures which are generalized from onset and those which are partial in onset which may or may not secondarily generalize. The implication of this classification is that partial onset seizures originate from a single cortical focus and then spread to a greater or lesser extent from that focus, whereas seizures which are generalized from onset engage all areas of the cortex simultaneously. This same distinction also applies in status epilepticus, except that the frequently repetitive seizures which define status alter the underlying neurochemical and physiological substrates of the brain and thus may modify clinical expression of the seizure activity as the episode of status progresses.

As is true with single seizures, status epilepticus characterized by seizures generalized from onset occurs most frequently in children whereas partial onset status epilepticus, most commonly expressed as secondarily generalized convulsive status, may occur at any age and accounts for the overwhelming majority of adult cases of status epilepticus. The classification of status epilepticus has been reviewed in detail by Gastaut (1967, 1983) and Roger et al (1974).

Partial onset status epilepticus

Generalized convulsive status epilepticus

At least 70% of all cases of generalized convulsive status epilepticus are partial in onset with secondary generalization (Roger et al 1974). Such episodes of status are symptomatic of previous or acute cerebral insult and in the majority of cases the underlying aetiology, if not the acute precipitating cause, can be identified. Such episodes of status usually begin with clinically recognizable discrete or continuous tonic and/or clonic convulsive seizures with identifiable progression of sequential patterns of convulsive moments associated with an alteration of consciousness. However, in secondarily generalized convulsive status epilepticus the convulsive activity need not be bilaterally symmetrical and may be quite asymmetrical in onset or progression. The electroencephalogram, however, will show some degree of bilateral involvement and the patient will exhibit at least some alteration of consciousness during and between seizures. If the patient does not fully recover to his pre-seizure mental state before the next seizure occurs he is considered to be in status epilepticus. It is this impairment of consciousness which differentiates generalized convulsive status epilepticus with only partial or unilateral convulsive activity from simple partial status epilepticus which, by definition, has no impairment of consciousness during or between the seizures.

There has been considerable confusion regarding the proper classification of patients in status epilepticus who exhibit only partial or subtle signs of convulsive activity, even though the seizures are associated with a marked impairment of consciousness and bilateral ictal discharges on the EEG. Treiman et al (1984) used the term 'subtle generalized convulsive status epilepticus' to describe such patients. They consider this a presentation of generalized convulsive status epilepticus which occurs in patients with severe encephalopathies caused by underlying systemic illnesses, primary brain lesions such as massive cerebral infarctions or infections, or prolonged

uncontrolled overt generalized convulsive status epilepticus. Subtle generalized convulsive status epilepticus is characterized clinically by the occurrence of mild motor movements (nystagmus, clonic twitches) which may be limited to one side of the body and are intermittent, brief, and without sequential pattern but are associated with marked impairment of consciousness and usually continuous bilateral ictal patterns on the EEG. Gastaut (1983) used the term 'somatomotor status epilepticus' to describe this type of status when it is seen accompanying severe brain insults in nonepileptic patients. Celesia et al (1988) described 19 patients with what they called 'generalized status myoclonicus'. These patients also had characteristics similar to those of Treiman's subtle generalized convulsive status epilepticus patients. Thus subtle generalized convulsive status epilepticus is part of a continuum of clinical expression of convulsive activity in generalized convulsive status epilepticus which ranges from overt bilaterally symmetrical generalized tonic-clonic seizures at one end of the continuum to progressively subtle and finally only electrical seizure activity at the other end of the spectrum.

When generalized convulsive status epilepticus is allowed to progress without successful treatment for a sufficiently prolonged period of time that the status episode itself causes a progressively severe encephalopathy, or when status occurs in the presence of a severe underlying encephalopathy, an 'electromechanical dissociation' occurs such that, in spite of the presence of bilateral ictal discharges on the EEG, the encephalopathic brain is unable to successfully transmit appropriate messages from the seizing cortex to muscles in the trunk and extremities to allow full clinical expression of an overt generalized convulsion.

In addition to a progressive evolution in the clinical expression of generalized convulsive status epilepticus from overt generalized tonic-clonic seizures to progressively subtle motor phenomena, there is also a predictable sequence of progressive EEG changes (Figs 6.1–6.5) which occurs in generalized convulsive status epilepticus (Treiman et al 1990). Initially discrete electrographic seizures are seen which coincide temporally with overt clinical convulsions. If generalized convulsive status epilepticus is allowed to progress without

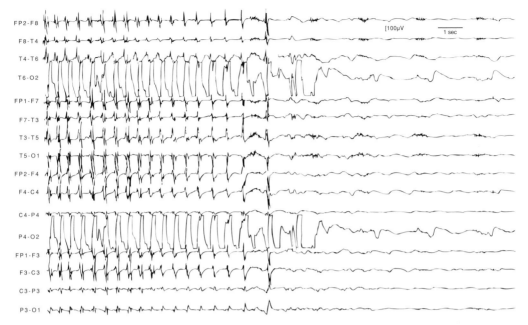

Fig. 6.1 Discrete generalized tonic-clonic seizures with interictal slowing, recorded prior to treatment in a 39-year-old man. Example shows end of clonic phase of the seizure and the appearance of postictal slowing. Reprinted with permission from Treiman et al 1990.

adequate treatment these discrete seizures merge together to produce a waxing and waning ictal pattern on the EEG. This waxing and waning pattern becomes progressively uniform to produce a pattern of continuous ictal discharges on the EEG. Eventually the continuous discharges are punctuated by periods of relative flattening on the EEG which become longer as the ictal discharges become shorter until ultimately the record is one of periodic epileptiform discharges on a relatively flat background. Current evidence suggests that periodic epileptiform discharges in this context represent an ictal EEG pattern, rather than being only an indicator of postictal injury (Handforth & Treiman 1989, Treiman et al 1990). Therefore the patient in status whose EEG exhibits only periodic epileptiform discharges should still be treated aggressively in order to prevent progressively severe epileptic brain damage in excess to that caused by the underlying encephalopathy

Complex partial status epilepticus

In complex partial status epilepticus, like individual complex partial seizures, the spread of ictal activity from the cortical focus involves both cerebral hemispheres but is not sufficiently widespread to produce generalized convulsive activity. Thus the patient exhibits an alteration of consciousness and automatic behaviour but does not have generalized tonic-clonic seizure activity. Complex partial status epilepticus usually begins as a series of discrete complex partial seizures. The patient is considered to be in status epilepticus when he no longer completely recovers consciousness between seizures or does not regain full memory function between seizures. As complex partial status epilepticus becomes more prolonged the patient's contact with his environment becomes progressively impaired between seizures.

When fully developed, complex partial status epilepticus is characterized by an epileptic twilight state in which there is cyclical variation between periods of partial responsiveness and episodes characterized by a motionless stare and complete unresponsiveness and at times by automatic behaviour (Delgado-Escueta et al 1974, Belafsky et al 1978). The EEG is likewise characterized by alternation between relatively normal patterns of background activity, which become progressively

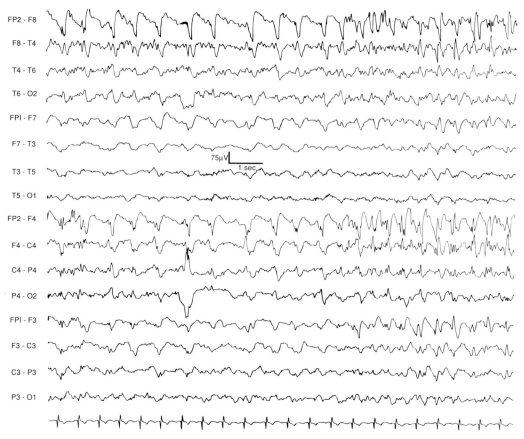

Fig. 6.2 Merging of discrete seizures, recorded prior to treatment in a 64-year-old man. Ictal discharges are continuous, but with waxing and waning of frequency and amplitude. An increase in frequency and amplitude can be seen beginning on the right side of the recording. Reprinted with permission from Treiman et al 1990.

slow as the episode of status persists, and focal rhythmic ictal patterns seen during the unresponsive periods of the cycle.

Complex partial status epilepticus is relatively rare, though probably under-recognized—particularly in the elderly. Since it was first described by Gastaut et al in 1956 only about 60 possible cases have been reported. Complex partial status epilepticus should be distinguished from subtle generalized convulsive status epilepticus. In subtle generalized convulsive status epilepticus the EEG exhibits bilateral ictal discharges which are continuous rather than present in a cyclical fashion and are widespread over both cerebral hemispheres, although the discharges may be asymmetrical. Consciousness is markedly impaired and the convulsive activity, although subtle, is simple and repetitive in contrast to more complex

automatisms sometimes seen in complex partial status epilepticus. Other entities which should be considered in the differential diagnosis of complex partial status epilepticus are listed in Table 6.1. Complex partial status epilepticus has been reviewed in detail by Treiman & Delgado-Escueta (1983) and by Delgado-Escueta & Treiman (1987).

Simple partial status epilepticus

Simple partial status epilepticus refers to focal seizures which are continuous or repetitive over at least 30 minutes without any impairment of consciousness. The clinical manifestation of the focal seizures is dependent on the location of the epileptic focus. Thus there may be focal motor convulsions, focal somatosensory deficits or focal special sensory deficits. The recently described

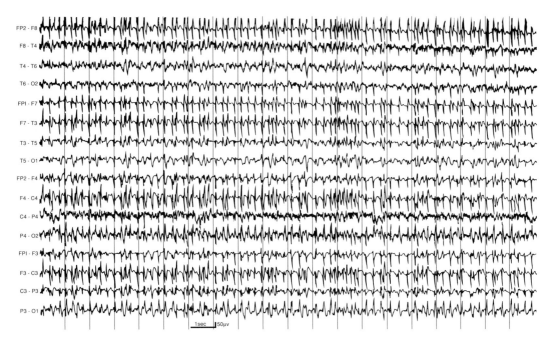

Fig. 6.3 Continuous ictal discharges recorded prior to treatment in a 53-year-old man. Continuous ictal activity persisted more than 3.5 hours despite vigorous treatment with diazepam, lorazepam, phenytoin and phenobarbital. Reprinted with permission from Treiman 1990.

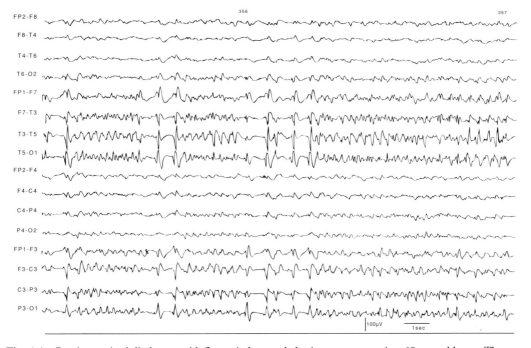

Fig. 6.4 Continuous ictal discharges with flat periods recorded prior to treatment in a 68-year-old man. The seizure focus is clearly in the left hemisphere, but spread of ictal activity to the right hemisphere can be seen as well. Reprinted with permission from Treiman et al 1990.

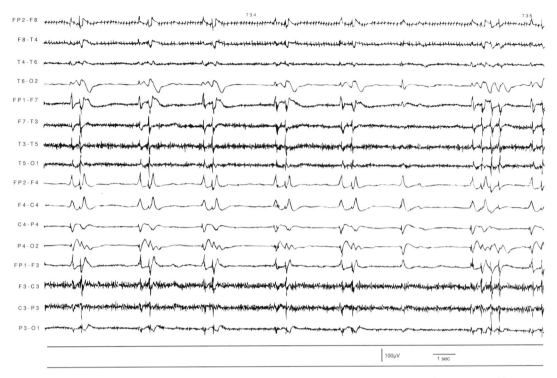

Fig. 6.5 Periodic epileptiform discharges on a flat background recorded prior to treatment in a 64-year-old man. Reprinted with permission from Treiman et al 1990.

entity, epileptic aphasia, is an example of simple partial status epilepticus (Gastaut 1979, Racy et al 1980, Dinner et al 1980, Marrosu et al 1983). In this situation the patient experiences speech arrest but remains fully conscious although unable to speak or sometimes unable to understand language. The EEG during simple partial status epilepticus may exhibit rhythmical ictal discharges which remain focal and unilateral or may not show any abnormalities, even while the patient is actively convulsing, because the area of cortical seizure activity is so small. Simple partial status epilepticus has been reviewed by Delgado-Escueta & Treiman (1987).

Primarily generalized status epilepticus

Primarily generalized tonic-clonic status epilepticus

Although most cases of generalized tonic-clonic status epilepticus are secondarily generalized, in some series up to 30% of these cases are generalized from onset. Such cases occur in two situations: 1. when patients with primary generalized epilepsy develop status epilepticus and 2. when patients develop status epilepticus as a complication of a severe metabolic insult. However, many cases with metabolic encephalopathies exhibit secondarily generalized convulsive status

Table 6.1 Differential diagnosis of complex partial status epilepticus

1. Absence status epilepticus or spike-wave stupor
2. Subtle generalized convulsive status epilepticus
3. Other 'epileptiform' causes of confusion
   Prolonged postictal confusion
   Delirium in cerebral infarction
   Poriomania
4. Organic encephalopathies
   Toxic-metabolic encephalopathies, especially
     hypoglycaemia
   Alcohol and other drug intoxication or withdrawal
   Transient ischaemic attacks
   Transient global amnesia
   Post-traumatic amnesia
5. Psychiatric syndromes
   Dissociative reactions
   Hysterical conversion reactions
   Acute psychotic reactions

Modified from Treiman & Delgado-Escueta (1983).

epilepticus because the metabolic disturbance unmasks a previous cortical insult which serves as a seizure focus. Primarily generalized tonic-clonic status epilepticus is characterized by bilaterally symmetrical tonic and/or clonic seizure activity associated with bilaterally symmetrical ictal discharges on the EEG. When generalized tonic-clonic status epilepticus persists long enough the generalized tonic-clonic seizures become progressively attenuated until they are only tonic in nature (Roger et al 1974).

The EEG, like that of individual primarily generalized tonic-clonic seizures, is characterized by flattening and intense desynchronization of the basic rhythm at the start of the seizure followed by a tonic phase characterized by spikes with a frequency of approximately 10 per second which gradually increase in amplitude. This has been called a recruiting epileptic rhythm. Progressively slower waves of 200–500 milliseconds then interrupt this recruiting rhythm during the clonic phase (Roger et al 1974). The ictal discharges terminate abruptly at the end of the clonic phase of the seizure which is then followed by bilaterally symmetrical low voltage postictal slowing. A period of postictal cortical extinction, which occurs in all isolated primarily generalized tonic-clonic seizures, was absent in 46% of the cases of primarily generalized tonic-clonic status epilepticus

studied by Roger and colleagues (1974). It is not yet known whether untreated primarily generalized tonic-clonic status epilepticus exhibits the same sequence of progressive EEG changes described by Treiman et al (1990) in secondarily generalized tonic-clonic status.

Absence status epilepticus

Absence status epilepticus (petit mal status, spike wave stupor) has been reviewed in detail by Porter & Penry (1983). This form of status epilepticus, along with complex partial status epilepticus, has been termed nonconvulsive status epilepticus. Clinically these two forms of status may be difficult to differentiate without electroencephalographic evaluation. However, in absence status there is a continuous alteration of consciousness of varying degrees of intensity that does not show the cyclical variation between levels of responsiveness and unresponsiveness that is characteristic of complex partial status epilepticus. The EEG exhibits prolonged, sometimes continuous, generalized, synchronous 3 Hz spike-wave complexes rather than the focal ictal discharges seen during the unresponsive phase of complex partial status epilepticus. Table 6.2 presents a comparison between these two forms of nonconvulsive status epilepticus.

Table 6.2 Clinical characteristics of prolonged twilight states

Petit mal status		Complex partial status
Clinical		
Prolonged state of one attack rather than repeated attacks		Continuous series of repeated attacks
Present	Phase of responsiveness with confusion disorientation, speech arrrest, amnesia and automatisms	Present
Absent	Phase of total unresponsiveness stereotyped automatisms	Present
EEG		
Continuous or noncontinuous diffuse irregular 1.5–4 Hz multi-spike-wave complexes; no patterns are time-locked with automatisms	Phase of partial unresponsiveness and reactive automatisms	1. Low-voltage fast activities with bursts of diffuse slow waves, or 2. Rhythmic bilateral diffuse spikes or slow waves or both most evident anteriorly, or 3. Anterior temporal sharp waves with normal background
	Phase of total unresponsiveness and stereotyped automatisms	1. Correlates with bimedial temporal waves or lateralised 8–20 Hz spikes

From Belafsky et al (1978).

Generalized myoclonic status epilepticus

True myoclonic status epilepticus is rare. This presentation of status epilepticus, which represents a complication of primary generalized epilepsy, is limited most exclusively to children and to adolescents. These patients exhibit massive bilateral myoclonic jerks repeated at irregular intervals which often occur in clusters. The EEG, which is bilaterally symmetrical, exhibits polyspike-wave discharges which coincide with the myoclonic jerks. Consciousness is preserved throughout the attack. Gastaut (1983) was able to identify only five reports of true myoclonic status epilepticus (Janz 1963, Roger et al 1967, Gruneberg & Helmchen 1969, Schneemann et al 1969, Ohtahara et al 1979). He also described a different presentation of myoclonic status epilepticus which occurs in children with secondary generalized epilepsy. This form of myoclonic status is much more frequent than myoclonic status in primary generalized epilepsy. It is characterized by myoclonic jerks which, although bilateral, are often asymmetrical, asynchronous and of smaller amplitude. Clouding of consciousness dominates the clinical picture and the EEG exhibits arrhythmically repeated spike-waves interspersed with high amplitude delta rhythms mixed with bursts of theta waves and epileptic recruiting rhythms.

The term 'myoclonic status epilepticus' should not be used when a patient with a severe encephalopathy exhibits repetitive myoclonic jerks which are not accompanied by ictal discharges on the EEG. Gastaut (1983) has also suggested that the myoclonic syndrome which is seen in acute or subacute encephalopathy of metabolic, toxic, viral or degenerative disorders, where the EEG signs are those of the underlying disorder, should not be regarded as status epilepticus. However, when a severe encephalopathy gives rise to ictal EEG patterns such as those which have been described by Treiman et al (1990) for various stages of generalized convulsive status epilepticus, such patients should be considered to be in generalized convulsive status epilepticus, even when the clinical manifestations are extremely subtle.

Clonic status epilepticus

Generalized clonic status epilepticus is seen almost exclusively in infants and very young children. Nonetheless, it is surprisingly common, representing 50–80% of the cases of generalized status epilepticus in children (Aicardi & Chevrie 1970, Congdon & Forsythe 1980). About half of the cases of generalized clonic status epilepticus occur in normal children and are frequently associated with fever. In one-quarter of the cases clonic status epilepticus is the initial presentation of an acute encephalopathy and in the other quarter is a consequence of chronic encephalopathy (Gastaut 1983). In generalized clonic status epilepticus the jerks are of low amplitude and appear bilaterally but are often arrhythmic, asymmetrical and asynchronous.

Tonic status epilepticus

Generalized tonic status epilepticus also occurs almost exclusively in children and is also relatively common. Ohtahara et al (1979) reported that tonic status epilepticus accounted for approximately half of their cases of status epilepticus in children. Almost all cases of tonic status epilepticus occur in children or adolescents with secondary generalized epilepsy such as the Lennox–Gastaut Syndrome. In such children intravenous benzodiazepines may precipitate tonic status epilepticus (Tassinari 1972, Tassinari et al 1971, 1972, Prior et al 1972, Waltregny & Dargent 1975, Amand & Evrard 1976, Bittencourt & Richens 1981). In contrast to adults with generalized tonic-clonic status epilepticus the seizures in tonic status epilepticus are much more numerous but considerably less intense. They may be so subtle as to require EEG confirmation by observing the accompanying generalized electrodecremental event or burst of recruiting epileptic rhythms. Such episodes of status may last days to weeks but the outcome is considerably less severe than prolonged generalized tonic-clonic status in the adult (Gastaut 1983).

EPIDEMIOLOGY

Status epilepticus is much more common than is generally recognized. Hauser (1990) recently estimated that 50 000 to 60 000 cases of status epilepticus occur in the United States each year, divided roughly between one-third with status epilepticus as the presenting symptom in patients with a first unprovoked seizure or with epilepsy, one-third in patients with established epilepsy, and one-third in individuals with no history of epilepsy where status epilepticus occurs as a complication of a severe encephalopathy. These figures probably represent an underestimate of the true incidence of status epilepticus because cases of nonconvulsive and simple partial status epilepticus frequently are not recognized. Nonetheless, if these figures are extrapolated worldwide it becomes apparent that over one million cases of status epilepticus occur throughout the world each year. Because status epilepticus is a neurological emergency which requires immediate vigorous and effective treatment to prevent residual neurological complications or even death, status epilepticus poses a substantial risk to a large number of patients throughout the world.

Mortality rates as high as 50% (Binswanger 1886) were reported at the end of the last century. There has been a progressive decline in mortality as more effective treatment of status has become available and modern series have reported acute mortality rates ranging from 3% to 27% (Hauser 1990). When vigorous treatment is instituted early most of the poor outcome following status can be attributed to the underlying disorder and not to the episode of status itself (Maytal et al

1989). When effective treatment is administered the two most important predictors of outcome following status epilepticus are aetiology and duration of the episode of status (Yager et al 1988, Dunn 1988).

AETIOLOGY

As indicated above, status epilepticus may either be a presentation of epilepsy, a complication of epilepsy, or a complication of an underlying encephalopathy. Specific aetiologies of status epilepticus in a number of case series are presented in Table 6.3. The high incidence of cerebral neoplasm observed by Janz (1961) and by Oxbury & Whitty (1971) has not been observed in other series. Janz (1983) has emphasized that when status epilepticus is symptomatic of focal brain pathology the most common localization is one or other frontal lobe. Recent series have reported an increasing incidence of cases of status epilepticus precipitated by illicit drug abuse and by CNS infection, including HIV infection (Aminoff & Simon 1980, Holtzman et al 1989).

PATHOPHYSIOLOGY AND CONSEQUENCES OF STATUS EPILEPTICUS

Abundant evidence from animal studies (Walton

Table 6.3 Aetiology of status epilepticus

Aetiology	Whitty & Taylor 1949	Hunter 1959	Janz & Kautz 1964	Rowan & Scott 1970	Aicardi & Chevrie 1970	Oxbury & Whitty 1971	Celesia 1976	Meier & Ketz 1976	Delgado-Escueta & Bascal 1983	Hauser 1983	Maytal et al 1989	Total
Idiopathic	3	8	31	9	59	20	15	0	0	42	46	233
Trauma	13	0	30	11	2	7	7	31	4	23	—	128
Tumour	4	4	35	2	0	19	3	18	3	4	2	94
Vascular	0	0	9	4	0	13	9	16	12	17	—	80
CNS infection/ inflammatory	3	4	9	4	29	9	1	7	6	19	15	106
Febrile	—	—	—	—	67	—	—	—	—	7	46	120
Toxic–metabolic	0	0	5	4	—	2	8	0	16	—	—	35
Congenital	1	3	5	7	20	4	4	2	0	—	45	91
Degenerative	0	3	1	1	—	0	4	0	4	—	—	13
Unknown or other	1	8	13	0	62	12	9	36	5	20	39	205
Total	25	30	138	42	239	86	60	110	50	132	˙193	1105

Modified from Treiman & Delgado-Escueta (1980).

& Treiman 1988a,b) and from older human case studies (Calmeil 1824) suggest that untreated or ineffectively treated status epilepticus is frequently fatal. The mortality from status epilepticus is not only due to systemic complications but also to the progressive neuronal damage which occurs during the course of status epilepticus. Pathological changes have been recorded in the brains of children and adults dying shortly after an episode of status epilepticus (Fowler 1957, Scholtz 1959, Norman 1964, Corsellis & Bruton 1983, DeGiorgio et al 1992) and in the brains of animals after prolonged status epilepticus, even in paralysed and artificially ventilated animals (Meldrum et al 1973). This observation suggests that although such systemic complications as hypoxia, hypoglycemia, lactic acidosis and especially hyperpyrexia may exacerbate the neuronal damage which occurs as a result of an episode of status epilepticus (Simon 1985a), the continuing seizure activity itself contributes substantially to the neuronal damage (Meldrum & Horton 1973, Meldrum & Brierley 1973, Meldrum 1983, 1986, Söderfeldt et al 1983).

There is now a growing consensus that the epileptic brain damage which occurs during the course of prolonged status epilepticus is at least partially due to the action of excitatory amino acid neurotransmitters. Rothman & Olney (1987) proposed two mechanisms for this excitotoxic effect. First, activation of excitatory amino acid receptors, particularly the N-methyl-D-aspartate receptor, results in an influx of calcium to the neuronal cytoplasm. Excess calcium acts as an intracellular toxin and may unleash a cascade of destructive neurochemical events. Excitotoxins, on the other hand, may promote a flux of water and cations into neurons which results in osmotolysis and cell destruction.

Although most studies of the consequences of status epilepticus have dealt with results of generalized convulsive status epilepticus it is now clear that prolonged complex partial status epilepticus may also produce neuronal damage, presumably as the result of the primary effect of the seizure activity itself. Long-term memory losses following prolonged complex partial status epilepticus have been reported by several authors (Engel et al 1978, Treiman et al 1981, Treiman & Delgado-Escueta 1983). Engel et al (1983) reported a prolonged visual field deficit following an episode of complex partial status epilepticus from an occipital lobe focus. Thus the current view is that abnormal neuronal discharges play a major role in the development of neurological deficits following both convulsive status epilepticus and at least some forms of nonconvulsive status epilepticus.

DIAGNOSIS

The diagnosis of status epilepticus should be made whenever a patient has two or more recurrent seizures without full recovery of mental status to pre-seizure baseline. Sometimes however a patient will have a single generalized convulsion and then persist in a long period of impaired consciousness even though another overt seizure does not occur. In this situation, an EEG should be obtained and if ictal discharges like those described by Treiman et al (1990) are observed, the diagnosis of status epilepticus should be made and treatment initiated. Sometimes the EEG pattern is difficult to interpret. Particularly when the patient exhibits continuous ictal discharges it may be difficult to differentiate this pattern from that of a metabolic encephalopathy. However, if the alteration of consciousness has been preceded by an overt seizure, subtle generalized convulsive status epilepticus should be suspected and the EEG should be examined closely for evidence of rhythmicity of repetitive, morphologically similar discharges occurring synchronously in at least several adjacent channels.

In nonconvulsive status (complex partial status or spike wave stupor) there may be no history of overt seizures, but rather the patient may present clinically in an epileptic twilight state. In this situation, variation of the patient's behaviour between the twilight state and episodes of complete unresponsiveness strongly suggests the diagnosis of complex partial status epilepticus. The EEG usually becomes more rhythmic and sharper at times of the episodes of complete unresponsiveness and may exhibit phase reversing repetitive spikes or sharp waves from one or another temporal lobe. In the case of spike-wave stupor diffuse bilaterally symmetrical spike-wave discharges are seen over both hemispheres. Although initially such discharges may be very regular and exhibit 3 Hz frequencies, as spike-wave stupor becomes more prolonged the frequency of the spike waves may become more variable and tend to slow.

In the case of simple partial status epilepticus the diagnosis is made on the basis of observing continuous or nearly continuous focal epileptiform discharges for a period of 30 minutes or more. However, the EEG is not always abnormal, even at the time of convulsive activity in simple partial focal motor status. If the area of the epileptiform discharge is sufficiently small all of the cortical electroencephalographic activity may be attenuated by the skull and scalp.

TREATMENT

Treiman (1983) has suggested the following goals and general principles in the management of status epilepticus:

1. Terminate electrical and clinical seizure activity as soon as possible, preferably within 30 minutes.
2. Prevent recurrence of seizures.
3. Ensure adequate cardiorespiratory function and brain oxygenation.
4. Correct any precipitating factors such as hypoglycemia, electrolyte imbalance or fever.
5. Stabilize metabolic balance by prevention or correction of lactic acidosis, electrolyte imbalance and dehydration.
6. Prevent or correct any other systemic complications.
7. Evaluate and treat any possible causes of the episode of status.

Both clinical and electrical seizure activity should be terminated as soon as possible. There is abundant evidence from both clinical and animal literature (summarized by Treiman 1983, Simon 1985b, Lothman 1990) that the longer an episode of status epilepticus continues the more likely it is to result in permanent neuronal damage. Furthermore, clinical experience suggests that the longer an episode of status epilepticus is allowed to continue the more refractory to treatment it will be. Walton & Treiman (1988b) have confirmed this clinical impression using an experiment model of status epilepticus in the rat.

The management of status epilepticus is best carried out with the use of a predetermined protocol. Although a number of drugs have been shown to be effective in the management of status epilepticus, a common error is that drugs, which would be effective if used appropriately, are given in inadequate doses over too long a period of time. For most drugs, serum concentrations above the usual therapeutic range for the management of chronic epilepsy are necessary in order to successfully terminate status epilepticus. Drugs used for the management of status epilepticus should always be given intravenously. Absorption after intramuscular injection is too slow to achieve peak concentrations adequate to stop status. Furthermore, some drugs, such as phenytoin and diazepam, are erratically absorbed from intramuscular sites.

Table 6.4 presents a protocol which is effective in the management of status epilepticus. Treatment should be initiated by the establishment of an intravenous line kept open with normal saline. Blood samples should be drawn for hematology studies, serum chemistries and antiepileptic drug levels. The patient should then be given 100 mg of thiamine followed by 50 ml of 50% glucose by slow intravenous push if hypoglycaemia is suspected. A cardiac monitor should be established and blood pressure checked to make sure the patient is not hypotensive before initiating treatment. Rectal temperatures should be monitored from the beginning of treatment and vigorous efforts should be made to correct hyperthermia as quickly as possible because hyperpyrexia is one of the major factors that contribute to the neurological consequences of status epilepticus (Simon 1985a).

The treatment of status should be monitored with simultaneous EEG recording although treatment should never be delayed in order to obtain an EEG. If necessary, the recording can be initiated after treatment is already underway. If coma persists after convulsive activity is stopped, EEG monitoring should be continued until the record is free from all ictal activity (including periodic epileptiform discharges as discussed above) for at least 30 minutes. EEG monitoring is of considerable importance in patients in whom status appears refractory to intravenous drug therapy

Table 6.4 Treatment protocol for generalized convulsive status epilepticus

---

Make diagnosis by observing one additional seizure in patient with history of recent seizures or impaired consciousness, or continuous seizure activity for more than 30 minutes

Call EEG technician and start electroencephalogram as soon as possible, but do not delay treatment while waiting for the EEG unless necessary to verify diagnosis

Establish intravenous catheter with normal saline

Draw blood for serum chemistries, haematology studies, and antiepileptic drug concentrations

Administer 100 mg thiamine followed by 50 ml of 50% glucose into the intravenous line if hypoglycaemia is suspected

Administer lorazepam, 0.1 mg/kg by intravenous bolus (< 2 mg/min)

If status does not stop, start phenytoin, 20 mg/kg by slow intravenous bolus (< 50 mg/min) directly into port closest to patient. Monitor blood pressure and electrocardiogram closely during infusion.

If status does not stop after 20 mg/kg phenytoin, give an additional 5 mg/kg and, if necessary, another 5 mg/kg to a maximum dose of 30 mg/kg

If status persists, intubate patient and give phenobarbital, 20 mg/kg, by intravenous push (< 100 mg/min)

If status persists, start barbiturate coma. Give pentobarbital, 5 mg/kg, slowly as initial intravenous dose to induce an EEG burst–suppression pattern. Continue 0.5–2 mg.kg/h^2 to maintain burst–suppression pattern. Slow rate of infusion every 2–4 hours to see if seizures have stopped. Monitor BP, ECG, respiratory function closely.

Modified from Treiman (1990).

in appropriate dosage, where the possibility of 'pseudostatus' must be considered in order to avoid iatrogenic complications of intensive therapy (Howell et al 1989).

CHOICE OF DRUGS

A variety of drugs have been used successfully in the management of status epilepticus (Delgado-Escueta et al 1983, Fröscher 1979, Simon 1985b, Treiman 1989, 1990). Table 6.5 summarizes the clinical parameters and pharmacological properties of six of these drugs.

Benzodiazepines as a class are highly potent and effective drugs for the management of status epilepticus. Efficacy has been reported in 39–100% of the patients studied in 47 clinical trials of lorazepam, diazepam or clonazepam. Overall,

lasting control was achieved in 79% of these 1455 patients (Treiman 1989). All three of these drugs cause a transient depression of consciousness after intravenous injection but lorazepam is most likely to cause transient amnesia (George & Dundee 1977, Dundee et al 1979).

Lorazepam is considered by some authors to be the drug of choice for the initial treatment of both generalized convulsive and nonconvulsive status epilepticus. Treiman and his colleagues (1992) found lorazepam (0.1 mg/kg) effective in stopping generalized convulsive status epilepticus in 77% of the cases in which it was used as the first drug in a series which included many patients whose status was due to a severe structural or metabolic encephalopathy. Lorazepam enters the brain nearly as rapidly as diazepam but effective concentrations in brain are maintained much longer than for diazepam (Walton & Treiman 1990). Because of a significantly smaller volume of distribution—12 l/kg for lorazepam compared to 133 l/kg for diazepam (Greenblatt & Divoll 1983)—it does not rapidly redistribute to body fat with the resultant precipitous drop in brain concentrations (Booker & Celesia 1973, Kaplan et al 1973, Celesia et al 1974, Ramsay et al 1979, Greenblatt & Divoll 1983) and consequent recurrence of status (Bamberger & Matthes 1969, Prensky et al 1967) which have been described for diazepam.

The incidence of breakthrough seizures is small, even when no other drug is given within the first 24 hours (Treiman et al 1992). Therefore, once status is stopped a loading dose of phenytoin can be given slowly or the patient's chronic maintenance antiepileptic therapy can be resumed. Respiratory depression may occur in about 10% of the patients in status who are treated intravenously with clonazepam, lorazepam or diazepam. With all three drugs the risk of respiratory depression is increased when the patient has already been treated with barbiturates (Bell 1969, Prensky et al 1967). Hypotension may also occur occasionally with any of these drugs, perhaps because of the propylene glycol solvent (Mattson 1972).

If lorazepam fails to stop the episode of status epilepticus then phenytoin should be given at a loading dose of 20 mg/kg. Many patients, however, require higher doses to stop generalized

Table 6.5 Drugs of importance in treating status epilepticus: clinical parameters and pharmacological properties. The doses given are for adults.

	Diazepam	Clonazepam	Lorazepam	Phenytoin	Phenobarbital	Chlormethiazole
Intravenous loading dose	150–250 µg/kg	20–70 µg/kg	100 µg/kg	20 mg/kg	20 mg/kg	5–13 mg/kg
Maximum rate of administration	5 mg/min	500 µg/min	2 mg/min	50 mg/min	100 mg/min	32 mg/min
Effective serum concentration in SE	200–800 µg/l	5–100 µg/l	100–200 µg/l	25–35 mg/l	20 mg/l	10 mg/l
Time to stop status	1–3 min	1–3 min	6–10 min	~10–30 min	20–30 min	5–20 min
Effective duration against status	15–30 min	> 24 hours	>24 hours	>24 hours	>24 hours	6–12 hours
Elimination half-life	30 hours	8–15 hours	14 hours	~24 hours	4–6 days	4–12 hours
Protein binding	97–99%	47–82%	85–93%	87–93%	45–50%	60–69%
Volume of distribution	1–2 l/kg	2–4 l/kg	0.7–1.0 l/kg	0.5–0.8 l/kg	0.7 l/kg	4–16 l/kg
Potential side effects:						
Depression of consciousness	10–30 min	Several hours	Several hours	None	Several days	Several hours
Respiratory depression	1–5 min	1–5 min	Occasional	Occasional	Intubate before administration	Occasional
Hypotension	Occasional	Occasional	Occasional	Frequent in patients with heart disease	Occasional	Occasional
Cardiac arrhythmias						

Modified from Treiman (1983).

convulsive status epilepticus (Gunawan & Treiman 1987). Therefore, if status persists the initial 20 mg/kg phenytoin should be followed with an additional 5 or 10 mg/kg before switching to a third drug.

Phenytoin should be given by slow intravenous push directly into a line containing normal saline and administered as close to the vein as possible in order to avoid microcrystallization. None-the-less, phenytoin should be administered through a filter needle. Infusion rates no faster than 50 mg/min are necessary to avoid hypotension.

Hypotension occurs most frequently in elderly (Cranford et al 1978) or severely ill patients or when the duration of status is prolonged before treatment (Simon 1985b). Blood pressure should be checked at least every 5 minutes during the infusion. If blood pressure falls below 90/60, infusion should be slowed or stopped until blood pressure stabilizes. At times, when status occurs in severely ill patients, it may be necessary to support blood pressure with dopamine or other pressor agents in order to complete the infusion. The electrocardiogram should be monitored closely and the rate slowed if the Q-T interval widens or arrhythmias appear. Phenytoin is contraindicated in patients with existing cardiac disease, especially

when conduction abnormalities are present. Both cardiac arrhythmias and hypotension are more likely to occur in patients over 40 years of age (Cranford et al 1978). Respiratory depression may also occur as a complication of phenytoin infusion.

Treiman and colleagues (1992) have reported that most cases of generalized convulsive status epilepticus (80%) respond to either lorazepam, phenytoin, or a combination of these two drugs. In 20% of the cases status is medically resistant and requires further therapy. If clinical and/or electrical seizure activity persists after completion of the lorazepam and phenytoin infusion, an endotracheal tube should be inserted for respiratory support and intravenous phenobarbital started. There are few data regarding the appropriate dose of phenobarbital for the treatment of status epilepticus in the adult. Shaner et al (1988), in the only published prospective controlled study of phenobarbital in adult status epilepticus, reported that patients successfully treated with phenobarbital monotherapy had a mean serum concentration of 18.3 µg/ml. Walton & Treiman (1989), using a rodent model of secondarily generalized tonic-clonic status epilepticus, found that serum levels of phenobarbital greater than

21 μg/ml always stopped both behavioural and electrical seizure activity.

If these data from experimental status in the rat are extrapolated to humans with appropriate adjustments for pharmacokinetic differences between species, the data suggest a loading dose of 15 mg/kg should be effective in the initial treatment of status epilepticus in humans. However, when phenobarbital is used as the third drug in the management of medically intractable status, very high loading doses may be necessary. Walton & Treiman (1989) found in their rat model that serum phenobarbital levels in excess of 75 μg/ml are likely to be necessary before electrographic normalization is produced in refractory status. Crawford et al (1988) have reported successful

treatment of refractory status epilepticus in children with serum concentrations ranging from 70 to 344 μg/ml following phenobarbital doses of 30–120 mg/kg.

Most patients with medically refractory generalized convulsive status epilepticus respond to the addition of high-dose phenobarbital. However, occasionally it is necessary to induce barbiturate coma either with the use of very high dose phenobarbital or with pentobarbital or thiopental, as outlined in the protocol. Several authors have recently described their experiences in the use of barbiturate coma in patients with medically refractory generalized convulsive status epilepticus (Lowenstein et al 1988, Osorio & Reed 1989, Van Ness 1990).

REFERENCES

Aicardi J, Chevrie J J 1970 Convulsive status epilepticus in infants and children: a study of 239 cases. Epilepsia 11: 187–197

Amand G, Evrard P 1976 Injectable lorazepam in epilepsy. Electroencephalography and Clinical Neurophysiology 6: 532–533

Aminoff M J, Simon R P 1980 Status epilepticus: causes, clinical features and consequences in 98 patients. American Journal of Medicine 69: 657–666

Bamberger P, Matthes A 1966 Eine neue therapiemoglichkeit des status epilepticus in kinde salter mit Valium i.v. Zeitschrift fur Kinderheilkunde 95: 155–163

Bell D S 1969 Dangers of treatment of status epilepticus with diazepam. British Medical Journal 1: 159–161

Belafsky M A, Carwille S, Miller P, Waddell G, Boxley-Johnson J, Delgado-Escueta A V 1978 Prolonged epileptic twilight states: Continuous recordings with nasopharyngeal electrodes and videotape analysis. Neurology 28: 239–245

Binswanger O 1886 Eulenberg's realencyclopadie, Vol. 6. (Cited in Turner W A 1907 Epilepsy. Macmillan, London)

Bittencourt P R M, Richens A 1981 Anticonvulsant-induced status epilepticus in Lennox–Gastaut syndrome. Epilepsia 22: 129–134

Booker H E, Celesia G G 1973 Serum concentrations of diazepam with epilepsy. Archives of Neurology 29: 191–194

Calmeil J-L 1824 De l'épilepsie, étudiée sous le rapport de son siège et de son influence sur la production de l'aliénation mentale. Université de Paris, Paris (thesis)

Celesia G G 1976 Modern concepts of status epilepticus. Journal of the American Medical Association 235: 1571–1574

Celesia G G, Booker H E, Sato S 1974 Brain and serum concentrations of diazepam in experimental epilepsy. Epilepsia 15: 417–425

Celesia G G, Grigg M M, Ross E 1988 Generalized status myoclonicus in acute anoxic and toxic-metabolic encephalopathies. Archives of Neurology 45: 781–784

Commission on Classification and Terminology of the International League Against Epilepsy 1981 Proposal for revised clinical and electroencephalographic classification of epileptic seizures. Epilepsia 22: 489–501

Congdon P, Forsythe W 1980 Intravenous clonazepam in treatment of status epilepticus in children. Epilepsia 21: 97–102

Corsellis J A N, Bruton C J 1983 Neuropathology of status epilepticus in humans. In: Delgado-Escueta A V, Wasterlain C G, Treiman D M, Porter R J (eds) Advances in neurology, vol 34: Status epilepticus. Raven Press, New York, p 129–140

Cranford R E, Patrick B, Anderson C B, Kostick B 1978 Intravenous phenytoin: clinical and pharmacokinetic aspects. Neurology 28: 874–880

Crawford T O, Mitchell W G, Fishman L S, Snodgrass S R 1988 Very-high-dose phenobarbital for refractory status epilepticus in children. Neurology 38: 1035–1040

DeGiorgio C M, Tomiyasu U, Gott P S, Treiman D M 1992 Hippocampal pyramidal cell loss in human status epilepticus. Epilepsia 33: 23–27

Delgado-Escueta A V, Enrile-Bacsal F 1983 Combination therapy for status epilepticus: intravenous diazepam and phenytoin. In: Delgado-Escueta A V, Waterlain C G, Treiman D M, Porter R J (eds) Advances in neurology, vol 34: Status epilepticus. Raven Press, New York, p 477–485

Delgado-Escueta A V, Treiman D M 1987 Focal status epilepticus: modern concepts. In: Lüders H, Lesser R P (eds) Epilepsy: electroclinical syndromes. Springer-Verlag, London, p 347–391

Delgado-Escueta A V, Boxley J, Stubbs N, Waddell G, Wilson W A 1974 Prolonged twilight state and automatisms: a case report. Neurology 24: 331–339

Delgado-Escueta A V, Wasterlain C G, Treiman D M, Porter R J (eds) 1983 Advances in neurology, vol 34: Status epilepticus. Raven Press, New York

Dinner D S, Lueders H, Lederman R, Gretter T E 1981 Aphasic status epilepticus: a case report. Neurology 31: 888–891

Dundee J W, McGowan A W, Lilburn J K, McKay A C, Hegarty J E 1979 Comparison of the action of diazepam and lorazepam. British Journal of Anaesthesia 51: 439–446

Dunn D W 1988 Status epilepticus in children: etiology, clinical features, and outcome. Journal of Child Neurology 3: 167–173

Engel J Jr, Ludwig B E, Fettell M 1978 Prolonged partial complex status epilepticus: EEG and behavioral observations. Neurology 28: 863–869

Engel J Jr, Kuhl D E, Phelps M E, Rausch R, Nuwer M 1983 Local cerebral metabolism during partial seizures. Neurology 33: 400–413

Fowler M 1957 Brain damage after febrile convulsions. Archives of Disease in Childhood 32: 67–76

Fröscher W 1979 Treatment of status epilepticus (translated by H. Lüders). University Park Press, Baltimore

Gastaut H 1967 A propos d'une classification symptômatologique des états de mal épileptiques. In: Gastaut H, Roger J, Lob H (eds) Les états de mal épileptiques. Masson, Paris, p 1–8

Gastaut H 1979 Aphasia. The sole manifestation of focal status epilepticus. Neurology 29: 1638

Gastaut H 1983 Classification of status epilepticus. In: Delgado-Escueta A V, Wasterlain C G, Treiman D M, Porter R J (eds) Advances in neurology, vol 34: Status epilepticus. Raven Press, New York, p 15–36

Gastaut H, Roger J, Roger A 1956 Sur la signification de certaines fugues épileptiques: état de mal temporal. Revue Neurologique 94: 298–301

George K A, Dundee J W 1977 Relative amnestic actions of diazepam, flunitrazepam and lorazepam in man. British Journal of Clinical Pharmacology 4: 45–50.

Greenblatt D J, Divoll M 1983 Diazepam versus lorazepam: relationship of drug distribution to duration of clinical action. In: Delgado-Escueta A V, Wasterlain C G, Treiman D M, Porter R J (eds) Advances in neurology, vol 34: Status epilepticus. Raven Press, New York, p 487–491

Gunawan S G, Treiman D M 1987 Pharmacokinetics of phenytoin and its metabolite p-HPPH, during treatment of Status epilepticus. Neurology 37(suppl 1): 100

Gruneberg F, Helmchen H 1969 Impulsive petit mal—status und paranoide psychose. Nervenarzt 40: 381–385

Handforth A, Treiman D M 1989 Deoxyglucose functional mapping of periodic epileptiform discharges in the lithium-pilocarpine model of status epilepticus. Epilepsia 30: 735

Hauser W A 1983 Status epilepticus: frequency, etiology, and neurological sequelae. In: Delgado-Escueta A V, Waterlain C G, Treiman D M, Porter R J (eds) Advances in neurology, vol 34: Status epilepticus. Raven Press, New York, p 3–14

Hauser W A 1990 Status epilepticus: epidemiologic considerations. Neurology 40 (suppl 2): 9–13

Holtzman D M, Kaku D A, So Y T 1989 New-onset seizures associated with human immunodeficiency virus infection: causation and clinical features in 100 cases. American Journal of Medicine 87: 173–177

Howell S J L, Owen L, Chadwick D W 1989 Pseudostatus epilepticus. Quarterly Journal of Medicine 71: 507–519

Hunter R A 1959 Status epilepticus: history, incidence and problems. Epilepsia 60(suppl 1): 162–188

Janz D 1961 Conditions and causes of status epilepticus. Epilepsia 2: 170–177

Janz D 1963 Die epilepsien, spezielle pathologie und therapie. Georg Thieme Verlag, Stuttgart

Janz D 1983 Etiology of convulsive status epilepticus. In: Delgado-Escueta A V, Wasterlain C G, Treiman D M,

Porter R J (eds) Advances in neurology, vol 34: Status epilepticus. Raven Press, New York, p 47–54

Janz D, Kautz G 1964 The aetiology and treatment of status epilepticus. German Medical Monthly 9: 451–456

Kaplan S A, Jack M L, Alexander K, Weinfeld R E 1973 Pharmacokinetic profile of diazepam following single intravenous and chronic oral administrations. Journal of Pharmaceutical Sciences 62: 1789–1796

Lothman E 1990 The biochemical basis and pathophysiology of status epilepticus. Neurology 40(suppl 2): 13–23

Lowenstein D H, Aminoff M J, Simon R P 1988 Barbiturate anesthesia in the treatment of status epilepticus: clinical experience with 14 patients. Neurology 38: 395–400

Marrosu F, Brundu A, Rachele M G, Marrosu G 1983 Epileptic aphasia as dynamic disturbance. A case report. Acta Neurologica Napoli 5: 43–46

Mattson R H 1972 The benzodiazepines. In: Woodbury D M, Penry J K, Schmidt R P (eds) Antiepileptic drugs. Raven Press, New York, p 497–516

Maytal J, Shinnar S, Moshe S L, Alvarez L A 1989 Low morbidity and mortality of status epilepticus in children. Pediatrics 83: 321–331

Meier H R, Ketz E 1976 Zur atiologie und klinik des status epilepticus. Schweizer Archiv fur Neurologie und Psychiatrie 119: 3–17

Meldrum B S 1983 Metabolic factors during prolonged seizures and their relation to nerve cell death. In: Delgado-Escueta A V, Wasterlain C G, Treiman D M, Porter R J (eds) Advances in neurology, vol 34: Status epilepticus. Raven Press, New York, p 261–275

Meldrum B S 1986 Cell damage in epilepsy and the role of calcium in cytotoxicity. In: Delgado-Escueta A V, Ward A A, Woodbury D M, Porter R J (eds) Advances in neurology, vol 44: Basic mechanisms of the epilepsies. Raven Press, New York, p 849–855

Meldrum B S, Brierley J B 1973 Prolonged epileptic seizures in primates: ischemic cell change and its relation to ictal physiological events. Archives of Neurology 28: 10–17

Meldrum B S, Horton R W 1973 Physiology of status epilepticus in primates. Archives of Neurology 3: 1–9

Meldrum B S, Vigouroux R A, Brierley J B 1973 Systemic factors and epileptic brain damage: Prolonged seizures in paralyzed artificially ventilated baboons. Archives of Neurology 29: 82–87

Norman R M 1964 The neuropathology of status epilepticus. Medicine, Science and the Law 4: 46–51

Ohtahara S, Oka E, Yamatogi Y et al 1979 Non-convulsive status epilepticus in childhood. Folia Psychiatrica et Neurologica Japonica 33: 345–351

Osorio I, Reed R C 1989 Treatment of refractory generalized tonic-clonic status epilepticus with pentobarbital anesthesia after high-dose phenytoin. Epilepsia 30: 464–471

Oxbury J M, Whitty C W M 1971 The syndrome of isolated epileptic status. Journal of Neurology, Neurosurgery and Psychiatry 34: 182–184

Porter R J, Penry J K 1983 Petit mal status. In: Delgado-Escueta A V, Wasterlain C G, Treiman D M, Porter R J (eds) Advances in neurology, vol 34: Status epilepticus. Raven Press, New York, p 61–67

Prensky A L, Raff M C, Moore M J, Schwab R S 1967 Intravenous diazepam in the treatment of prolonged seizure activity. New England Journal of Medicine 276: 779–784

Prior P F, Maclaine G N, Scott D F, Laurance B M 1972 Tonic status epilepticus precipitated by intravenous diazepam in a child with petit mal status. Epilepsia 13: 467–472

Racy A, Osborn M A, Vern B A, Molinari G F 1980 Epileptic aphasia. First onset of prolonged monosymptomatic status epilepticus in adults. Archives of Neurology 37: 419–422

Ramsay R E, Hammond E J, Perchalski R J, Wilder B J 1979 Brain uptake of phenytoin, phenobarbital and diazepam. Archives of Neurology 36: 535–539

Roger J, Lob H, Regis H, Gastaut H 1967 Les états de mal généralisés myocloniques. In: Gastaut H, Roger J, Lob H (eds) Les états de mal épileptiques. Masson, Paris, p 77–84

Roger J, Lob H, Tassinari C 1974 Status epilepticus. In: Vinken P J, Bruyn G W (eds) Handbook of clinical neurology, vol 15. Elsevier, New York, p 145–188

Rothman S M, Olney J W 1987 Excitotoxicity and the NMDA receptor. Trends in Neuroscience 10: 301–304

Rowan A J, Scott D F 1970 Major status epilepticus: a series of 42 patients. Acta Neurologica Scandinavica 46: 573–584

Schneemann N, Brune F, Busch H 1969 Impulsiv petit mal und dammerzustand. Schweizer Archiv fur Neurologie und Psychiatrie 105: 281–292

Scholtz W 1959 The contribution of patho-anatomical research to the problem of epilepsy. Epilepsia 1: 36–55

Shaner D M, McCurdy S A, Herring M O, Gabor A J 1988 Treatment of status epilepticus: a prospective comparison of diazepam and phenytoin versus phenobarbital and optional phenytoin. Neurology 38: 202–207

Simon R P 1985a Physiologic consequences of status epilepticus. Epilepsia 26 (suppl 1): S58–S66

Simon R P 1985b Management of status epilepticus. In: Pedley T A, Meldrum B S (eds) Recent advances in epilepsy, vol 2. Churchill Livingstone, Edinburgh, p 137–160

Söderfeldt B, Kalimo H, Olsson Y, Siesjö B 1983 Histopathological changes in the rat brain during bicuculline-induced status epilepticus. In: Delgado-Escueta A V, Wasterlain C G, Treiman D M, Porter R J (eds) Advances in neurology, vol 34: Status epilepticus. Raven Press, New York, p 169–175

Tassinari C A 1972 Addendum: A paradoxical effect: benzodiazepine-induced status epilepticus. In: Woodbury D M, Penry J K, Schmidt R P (eds) Antiepileptic drugs. Raven Press, New York, p 518

Tassinari C A, Gastaut H, Dravet C, Roger J 1971 A paradoxical effect: status epilepticus induced by benzodiazepines (Valium and Mogadon). Electroencephalography and Clinical Neurophysiology 31: 182

Tassinari C A, Dravet C, Roger J, Cano J P, Gastaut H 1972 Tonic status epilepticus precipitated by intravenous benzodiazepines in five patients with Lennox-Gastaut syndrome. Epilepsia 13: 421–435

Temkin O 1979 The falling sickness, 2nd edn. Johns Hopkins Press, Baltimore

Treiman D M 1983 General principles of treatment: responsive and intractable status epilepticus in adults. In: Delgado-Escueta A V, Wasterlain C G, Treiman D M,

Porter R J (eds) Advances in neurology, vol 34: Status epilepticus. Raven Press, New York, p 377–384

Treiman D M 1989 Pharmacokinetics and clinical use of benzodiazepines in the management of status epilepticus. Epilepsia 30(suppl 2): 4–10

Treiman D M 1990 The role of benzodiazepines in the management of status epilepticus. Neurology 40 (suppl 2): 32–42

Treiman D M, Delgado-Escueta A V 1980 Status epilepticus. In: Thompson R A, Green J R (eds) Clinical care of neurological and neurosurgical emergencies. Raven Press, New York, p 53–99

Treiman D M, Delgado-Escueta A V 1983 Complex partial status epilepticus. In: Delgado-Escueta A V, Waterlain C G, Treiman D M, Porter R J (eds) Advances in neurology, vol 34: Status epilepticus. Raven Press, New York, p 69–81

Treiman D M, Delgado-Escueta A V, Clark M A 1981 Impairment of memory following prolonged complex partial status epilepticus. Neurology 31: 109

Treiman D M, DeGiorgio C M, Salisbury S M, Wickboldt C L 1984 Subtle generalized convulsive status epilepticus. Epilepsia 25: 653

Treiman D M, Walton N Y, Kendrick C 1990 A progressive sequence of electroencephalographic changes during generalized convulsive status epilepticus. Epilepsy Research 5: 49–60

Treiman D M, DeGiorgio C M, Kendrick C L, Walton N Y 1992 A randomized comparison of intravenous phenytoin and lorazepam in the initial treatment of generalized convulsive status epilepticus. Submitted to New England Journal of Medicine

Van Ness P C 1990 Pentobarbital and EEG burst suppression in treatment of status epilepticus refractory to benzodiazepines and phenytoin. Epilepsia 31: 61–67

Walton N Y, Treiman D M 1988a Experimental secondarily generalized convulsive status epilepticus induced by D,L-homocysteine thiolactone. Epilepsy Research 2: 79–86

Walton N Y, Treiman D M 1988b Response of status epilepticus induced by lithium and pilocarpine to treatment with diazepam. Experimental Neurology 101: 267–275

Walton N Y, Treiman D M 1989 Phenobarbital treatment of status epilepticus in a rodent model. Epilepsy Research 4: 216–221

Walton N Y, Treiman D M 1990 Lorazepam treatment of experimental status epilepticus in the rat: relevance to clinical practice. Neurology 40: 990–994

Waltregny A, Dargent J 1975 Preliminary study of parenteral lorazepam in status epilepticus. Acta Neurologica Belgica 75: 219–229

Whitty C W M, Taylor M 1949 Treatment of status epilepticus. Lancet 2: 591–594

Wilson J V K, Reynolds E H 1990 Translation and analysis of a Cuneiform text forming part of a Babylonian treatise on epilepsy. Medical History 34: 185–198

Yager J Y, Cheany M, Seshia S S 1988 Status epilepticus in children. Canadian Journal of Neurological Sciences 15: 402–405

7. Pathology

G. Mathieson

INTRODUCTION

Morphological studies have made a modest but well-defined contribution to our knowledge of the dynamic disorder of epilepsy in humans. With increasing awareness of the focal origin of seizures in many patients and the efficacy of surgical therapy in some, there has been a growing need and opportunity to study the tissue changes associated with seizures of focal onset. In contrast, pathological studies of patients with corticoreticular epilepsy have been rather barren. In a third broad group of patients, those with endogenous metabolic encephalopathies, histopathological investigation has delineated some distinct diseases which are almost invariably associated with some form of epilepsy.

Since there are no specific histopathological criteria to determine definitively whether or not any particular pattern of cerebral lesion will give rise to seizure discharges, our knowledge depends in large part on implication by association. We must therefore distinguish:

1. Lesions which, directly or indirectly, cause epileptic neuronal discharges
2. Lesions which result from repeated seizures, i.e. ictal brain damage. These secondary lesions may in their turn be potentially epileptogenic
3. Lesions sharing an aetiology with epileptogenic lesions but not themselves epileptogenic
4. Incidental lesions in the brains of habitual epileptics not causally related to the seizure tendency

The concept of epileptic threshold, applying to the brain as a whole, and to various structures

and cortical regions in the brain, clearly implies that the patient's morphological lesion is only one factor in determining if and when cerebral seizures will occur. Brain lesions may therefore be regarded as predisposing to epilepsy and determining the site of origin of abnormal discharges in susceptible subjects.

By common consent, the proximate cause of an epileptic event is an abnormal pattern of discharge in a neuronal pool. Structural abnormalities of individual neurones or, more frequently, an alteration in their number and arrangement are observed in some epileptic lesions but, in many patients, non-neural elements dominate the morphological picture—for example, vascular malformations, scars, glial neoplasms. These obscure the neuronal component of the lesion, but indicate, to a first approximation, its pathogenesis. Thus many of the lesions described in this chapter are at least once removed from the essential predisposing mechanism of the patient's epilepsy. Their demonstration, however, is essential in elucidating intermediary pathogenetic steps; they may also provide valuable clues in the clinical and laboratory investigation of patients with epilepsy.

CATEGORIES OF EPILEPTOGENIC LESIONS

A systematic aetiological classification is the ultimate aim of an account of the pathology of epilepsy. Our present knowledge does not as yet allow this. The range of response of the brain to injury is limited so that, in the long term, the results of various noxious processes may be very similar (pathogenetic convergence). The state of maturation of the brain at the time of initial insult is important. In retrospective assessment of an adult epileptic patient, the age at which the presumed causal event occurred is often more reliably ascertained than the exact nature of the event.

The classification of lesions offered here (Table 7.1) is heterogeneous, being based partly on the stage of development at which the initial cerebral insult occurred, and partly on standard pathological concepts of aetiology.

Epileptogenic lesions originating during intrauterine life

Disturbances of the complex sequence of events by which the embryonic neural tube becomes the neonate brain give rise to a wide spectrum of neurological abnormalities. Some are incompatible with extrauterine survival; others, e.g. dysraphic states, do not concern us here. Lilienfeld & Pasamanick (1954) and Pasamanick & Lilienfeld (1955), in a retrospective survey with controls matched for age, and for maternal age, showed that mothers of epileptic patients had a significantly ($p < 0.05$) higher incidence of complications of pregnancy and delivery in general. In particular, the incidence of maternal bleeding and toxaemia of pregnancy was increased over controls. Their epileptic patient records were clinical, and histopathological evidence was not available to them.

The formal origin of some of these developmental abnormalities is known in general terms. Clues to aetiology may be available in the maternal history: placental abnormality, anoxic episodes, radiation, viral infection and undernutrition have all been implicated. An appropriate gestational age at the time of the noxious event appears to be essential for the development of certain anomalies, e.g. polymicrogyria. Diffuse and morphologically more subtle abnormalities may occur with undernutrition during the brain growth spurt (Dobbing & Sands 1973, Dobbing & Smart 1974), but it is speculative whether these increase the liability to the development of life-long epilepsy, as distinct from impaired motor skills and mentation. Our main concern here is with certain distinctive patterns of anomalous development readily recognized histologically and known to be associated with habitual epilepsy. They are listed in Table 7.2.

Heterotopias

Occasional neurones scattered in the subcortical white matter are a common finding of no significance. Large ectopic clusters of neurones and glia forming grey masses occur in two patterns: laminar within the centrum ovale and nodular at the angles of the lateral ventricles (Fig. 7.1). Some people with heterotopias are free from any neurological disability; others have seizures and some degree of mental retardation. The lesions are commonly bilateral and roughly symmetrical. In the unilateral case reported by Layton (1962), there was close correlation between the site of the lesion and its clinical and electrographic manifestations. Cortical gyral pattern and lamination are usually normal. However, cases also occur in which heterotopias are but one component of a complex cerebral maldevelopment. Crome (1952)

Table 7.1   Outline classification of epileptogenic lesions

Lesions originating during intrauterine life
Lesions associated with childbirth
Lesions resulting from febrile convulsions of childhood
Inflammatory lesions and their residua
Lesions resulting from head injury
Acquired vascular lesions of adults
Neoplasms
Subtle dendritic lesions
Endogenous metabolic encephalopathies
Metabolic encephalopathies of extracerebral origin

Table 7.2   Epileptogenic lesions originating during intrauterine life

A. *Disorders of cellular migration and differentiation*
  Heterotopias
  Polymicrogyria
  Megalencephaly
  Focal cortical dysplasia
  Tuberous sclerosis and formes frustes
  Hamartomas
  Meningioangiomatosis
  Neurocutaneous melanosis
  Dermoid and epidermoid cysts
B. *Disorders of vascular organization*
  Cavernous haemangioma
  Arteriovenous malformation
  Sturge–Weber disease

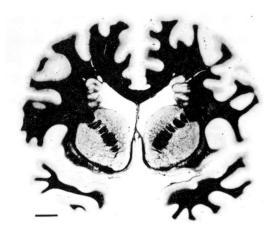

Fig. 7.1 Nodular heterotopias at the angles of the lateral ventricles. From a mildly retarded girl; seizures of varying pattern began in early adolescence; death at 19 years in status epilepticus. Heidenhain's method for myelin. Scale marker 1 cm.

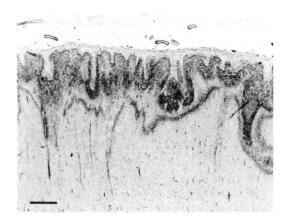

Fig. 7.3 Polymicrogyria. Four-layered cortex in a neonate with disseminated cytomegalovirus infection. Haematoxylin and eosin. Scale marker 1 mm.

has reported occipital heterotopia in a case of extensive polymicrogyria, and Kirschbaum (1947) and Norman (1958) in association with agenesis of the corpus callosum and megalencephaly.

Polymicrogyria

This distinctive lesion is characterized by many small gyrus-like formations without formed sulci. The surface of the involved brain presents rather wide gyri with wrinkled surfaces. The lesion may be fairly extensive and bilateral but, in adults, iso-lated patches of this malformed cortex are more commonly encountered. The opercula of the insula are frequent sites of predilection (Fig. 7.2). Cortical lamination is typically four-layered (Fig. 7.3). Small foci of this lesion may be quite inconspicuous in surgically excised specimens (Fig. 7.4).

Neonates succumbing to cytomegalovirus infection frequently show polymicrogyria in extreme degree (Crome & France 1959, Crome 1961, Bignami & Appicciutoli 1964). It is reasonable to suppose that less severe brain involvement with

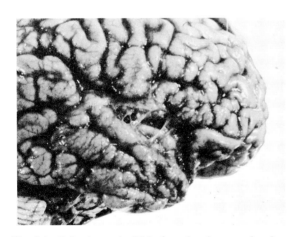

Fig. 7.2 Polymicrogyria. Right frontal and temporal gyri adjacent to the Sylvian fissure are involved.

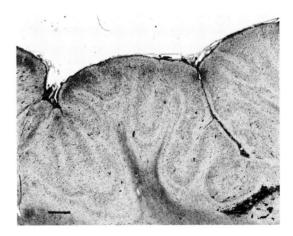

Fig. 7.4 Polymicrogyria. Patient began having seizures characterized by an aura of 'buzzing' followed by automatism at 12 years of age. Left temporal lobectomy at 23 years. Focal polymicrogyria is readily apparent histologically but was inconspicuous on naked eye examination. Luxol fast blue-cresyl violet. Scale marker 1 mm.

survival into adult life may result from intrauterine infection by this and possibly other viruses. A range of nonspecific noxious events, e.g. coal gas poisoning, occurring at a critical stage of cortical maturation, usually in the fifth month of intrauterine life, can produce an identical lesion. Polymicrogyria is, then, generally regarded as resulting from a disturbance of the orderly pattern of differentiation and migration of neuroblasts into the cerebral mantle. An alternative point of view is that the four-layered cortical lamination is due to post-migratory destruction. This has received support from a serial section study (Richman et al 1974) of a 27 week fetus in whom the cell sparse zone of the polymicrogyric cortex was shown to be in continuity with layer V of the intact cortex. The outer cellular layer may thus be formed by layers II, III and IV and the inner cellular layer by layer VI. However, this postmigrational encephaloclastic concept does not account for the abnormality of convolutional pattern. Polymicrogyria may accompany other major malformations. Extensive, usually bilateral, porencephaly was recorded by Dekaban (1965) in 11 patients with profound neurological deficits, including epilepsy; fields of polymicrogyric cortex lay adjacent to these pallial defects. Peach (1965) observed a four-layered cortex type of microgyria in 11 of 20 cases of Arnold–Chiari malformation.

Megalencephaly

The term 'megalencephaly' is properly applied only when the brain is large, not hydrocephalic, and storage diseases such as lipidosis have been rigorously excluded. It is not to be equated with the clinical descriptive term 'macrocephaly'. Essentially, the cerebral cortex is unduly thick and heterotopias are absent. Laurence (1946a) reported a patient with unilateral involvement and persistent seizures leading to death at 5.5 months of age; both neurones and glia contributed to the enlarged hemisphere. In another unilateral example, Bignami et al (1968) using quantitative histochemical techniques showed a three-fold increase in neuronal nuclear volume and suggested heteroploidy as the basic disorder. Laurence (1964b) in a brief review stressed the frequency of seizures in children with this lesion.

Focal cortical dysplasia

This lesion, whole often inconspicuous on naked eye examination, presents prominent histopathological features. Lamination of the involved cortex is lost. Abnormally large neurones are scattered throughout the cortex in a disorderly fashion (Fig. 7.5) and may extend in small clusters into the subjacent white matter (Fig. 7.6). There is an overall reduction in neuronal population in the affected cortex, which is sharply demarcated from adjoining normal cortex. Astrocytes with abundant cytoplasm, lobulated or multiple nuclei, and fibre formation are frequent (Figs 7.7, 7.8).

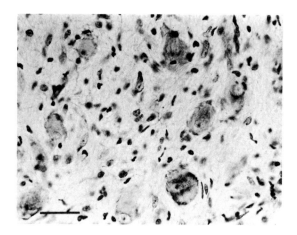

Fig. 7.5   Focal cortical dysplasia. Cortical architecture is disorganized by scattered large neurones and glial proliferation. Luxol fast blue-cresyl violet. Scale marker 50 μm.

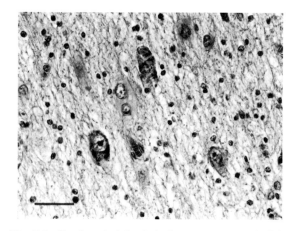

Fig. 7.6   Focal cortical dysplasia. Large neurones and glial cells are clustered in the subcortical white matter. Haematoxylin and eosin. Scale marker 50 μm.

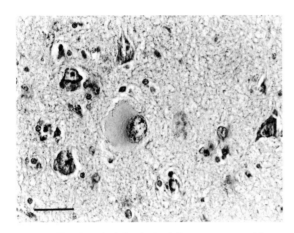

Fig. 7.7 Focal cortical dysplasia. A large astrocyte with voluminous cytoplasm is in the centre of the field. Several small binucleate astrocytes are also present. Haematoxylin and eosin. Scale marker 50 μm.

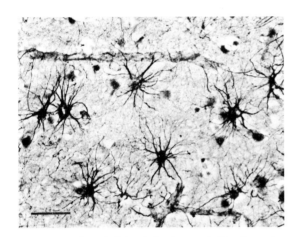

Fig. 7.8 Focal cortical dysplasia. Astrocytic fibre formation in dysplastic cortex. Cajal's gold sublimate impregnation. Scale marker 50 μm. Figures 7.5 to 7.8 are from the second temporal gyrus of a 26-year-old woman whose complex partial seizures began at the age of 15. Her birth and early life were normal and she had no features suggesting tuberous sclerosis.

These features are reminiscent of tuberous sclerosis, but cortical nodularity, calcification, subependymal lesions and the cutaneous and visceral manifestations of tuberous sclerosis do not occur in patients with focal cortical dysplasia.

One of the three cases described by Crome (1957) had an extensive, although unilateral, lesion accompanied by cortico-spinal tract degeneration. His patients were under 3 years of age, and had intractable focal seizures, retarded development and motor deficits. Two were siblings. The patient reported by Cravioto & Feigin (1960), a 21-year-old woman, had seizures with focal onset beginning at 6 months of age. She had permanent interictal neurological deficits but these are not invariable.

The status of this entity was firmly established by Taylor et al (1971) in a detailed account of 10 patients operated upon for intractable seizures; one subsequently died in status epilepticus. These authors give convincing reasons for regarding this disease as distinct from tuberous sclerosis and its formes frustes. A remarkable clinical feature reported by them is the range of age at first seizure of from 2 to 31 years. This latency is interesting in view of the undoubtedly intrauterine developmental origin of the lesion.

Tuberous sclerosis and formes frustes

The pathology of tuberous sclerosis is systematically described by Urich (1976). Our present concern is with patients whose disease is limited, in whom mental retardation and/or cutaneous manifestations are lacking, so that diagnosis is uncertain in the absence of histopathological evidence. Such partial forms of tuberous sclerosis are being increasingly recognized. The three patients reported in detail by Duvoisin & Vinson (1961) were of superior intelligence, although all had radiological evidence of cerebral involvement as well as lesions of tuberous sclerosis elsewhere. Lagos & Gomez (1967) reviewed the records of 71 patients with tuberous sclerosis studied at the Mayo Clinic: 26 of the 69 patients on whom there were records of intellectual capacity had normal intelligence; 18 of these 26 had seizures. Surgical excision of cortical lesions for the relief of seizures in such patients, as carried out by Perot et al (1966), allows histopathological confirmation of the diagnosis. The essential pathological features distinguishing oligosymptomatic tuberous sclerosis from focal cortical dysplasia, which undoubtedly resemble each other, are given in the section above.

Hamartomas

These lesions are tumour-like malformations. On

microscopic examination, many bear a strong resemblance to neoplasms but they lack the property of progressive growth and expansion. Penfield & Ward (1984) directed attention to this lesion as a rare anatomical substrate of temporal lobe seizures. Twenty years later, hamartomas (and closely related lesions) were reported as the essential pathological finding in 22 and 100 consecutive epileptic patients treated by anterior temporal lobectomy (Falconer & Taylor 1968). In the Penfield–Rasmussen–Feindel series from Montreal (reported by Mathieson 1975a), a diagnosis of hamartoma was made in 14 of 202 discrete focal lesions, in a series of 857 patients undergoing surgical excision for epilepsy. This three-fold discrepancy of incidence in the two series may be a consequence of lack of uniform histopathological criteria and terminology, as well as patient selection.

The exact nature of these lesions is thoroughly discussed by Cavanagh (1958), whose paper remains the definitive account and should be consulted for detailed histopathology. Most such hamartomas occur in the amygdaloid nucleus, medial occipitotemporal (fusiform) gyrus or less frequently in the hippocampus. Occurence in the frontal and parietal lobes has been recorded (Mathieson 1975b, Table 5, p. 114). Any combination of astrocytes, oligodendrocytes and neurones may occur. Calcification is frequent.

An interesting clinical correlation of hamartomatous lesions has emerged from Falconer's (1973) review of patients operated on by him. Patients with a psychosis accompanying their epilepsy were statistically more likely to have a hamartoma than an atrophic temporal lobe lesion. Furthermore, although relief of seizures occurred in patients with both types of lesions, aggressive behaviour or a schizophrenia-like illness were more likely to persist in patients who had a pathological diagnosis of hamartoma. The reason for this rather surprising finding remains speculative (Geschwind 1973).

Meningioangiomatosis

Strictly this lesion should be considered under the above heading of hamartoma, for such it is. However, it is non-glial and predominantly composed of cellular elements which normally lie outside the pia mater. Meningioangiomatosis is not to be confused with examples of multiple meningiomas such as sometimes occur in Von Recklinghausen disease, nor with meningioma-enplaque. In meningioangiomatosis a portion of cerebral cortex is replaced by tissue having the structure of meningioma but lacking its propensity to grow. Large neurones are scattered within the lesion (Fig. 7.9). These were present in case 1 of Worster-Drought et al (1937) who gave the first clear account of the lesion and established its association with central neurofibromatosis. This disease probably belongs to that large group of conditions referred to as neurocristopathies by Blonde (1974).

Neurocutaneous melanosis

This striking complex comprises a 'garment type' pigmented lesion of the skin and an excessive accumulation of melanocytes in the leptomeninges. Additionally, in some cases, melanin of both cutaneous and neuronal type is found in neurones, melanocytes and macrophages within certain brain structures. These include the amygdaloid nuclei and dentate nuclei of the cerebellum (Fox et al 1964, Slaughter et al 1969). The development of primary malignant intracranial

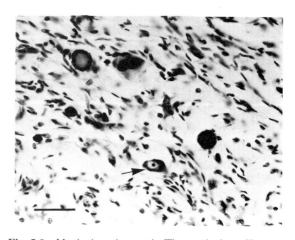

Fig. 7.9 Meningioangiomatosis. The meningioma-like structure contains psammoma bodies and occasional neurones (arrow). From the insular cortex of an adolescent girl with focal cerebral seizures. Haematoxylin and van Gieson. Scale marker 50 μm.

melanomata bring these patients to the attention of pathologists. In some, however, focal seizures clearly arise from causes other than intracranial neoplasm. In a patient studied personally in conjunction with Dr F. Andermann, seizures began at 3 years of age, had a consistent stereotyped pattern and occurred infrequently. Electrophysiological evidence indicated an origin in one amygdaloid nucleus. The appropriate temporal lobe, resected at 26 years of age, showed intense melanosis of the amygdala. There has been no seizure recurrence or evidence of tumour during a 3-year follow up.

Dermoid and epidermoid cysts

The features of dermoid and epidermoid cysts are too well known to require detailed description here. Most are basally situated. Intracerebral examples are most likely to have epilepsy as a prominent, or occasionally the sole clinical feature (Tytus & Pennybacker 1956).

Disorders of vascular organization

The extensive remodelling that the cerebral vasculature undergoes during embryogenesis occasionally results in malformations. Those that concern us here are cavernous haemangioma, arteriovenous malformation and Sturge–Weber disease.

Cavernous haemangiomas are usually static lesions and are certainly not neoplastic despite their terminology. Composed essentially of endothelial lined channels with thick collagenous walls, they often have a surrounding zone of gliosed brain and scattered haemosiderin pigment. Calcification is common. The lesions reported as haemangioma calcificans by Penfield & Ward (1948) in the temporal lobes of five patients with longstanding seizures belong in this category. The frequent incidence of focal motor seizures associated with cavernous haemangiomata in the region of the central fissure is stressed by Russell & Rubinstein (1977). Familial occurence has been reported by Clark (1970).

In contrast, the shunting of arterial blood into much altered venous channels in arteriovenous malformations produces a dynamic lesion with profound local, and occasionally systemic, alterations in cerebral blood flow. Widespread zones of anomalous patterns of epicerebral blood flow and regional cortical blood flow have been demonstrated by Feindel et al (1971). Regional autoregulation of cerebral blood flow is lost. Fluctuating hypoxia of nearby cortex may play a role in the genesis of seizures which occur so commonly in patients with this lesion. An overview of these and related lesions is given by McCormick (1966).

The well-known triad of facial naevus flammeus, seizures and intracerebral calcification which forms Sturge–Weber disease or encephalofacial angiomatosis is the subject of an extensive literature. The monograph by Alexander & Norman (1960) and the systematic account by Urich (1976) should be consulted. The extent of the pial venous angioma varies considerably; cortical atrophy is often more extensive than the vascular abnormality. The site or sites of most active epileptic cortical discharge may be some distance away from the mossy carpet of abnormal pial blood vessels as displayed at operation. Surgical aspects of therapy and the light they shed on pathology are considered by Falconer & Rushworth (1960) and by Rasmussen et al (1972).

Lesions associated with childbirth

By long tradition, birth injury is believed to give rise to lesions causing habitual epilepsy. That prematurity, excessive moulding, precipitate delivery and neonatal asphyxia may give rise to intracranial lesions is not in dispute. Some lesions, such as subependymal cell-plate haemorrhages with secondary ventricular rupture are not compatible with prolonged survival. Others, such as periventricular leukomalacia and basal ganglia lesions are not associated with epilepsy. Lesions identified as being related to habitual epilepsy are listed in Table 7.3.

The early stages of laminar cortical necrosis in neonatal asphyxia are illustrated by Banker (1967) and Friede (1975). The selective involvement of the depths of sulci compared with the crowns of gyri is clear and consistent, but why this pattern should occur remains unknown.

Ulegyria, often in the boundary zones of major cerebral arteries, can readily be visualized as

Table 7.3   Lesions associated with childbirth

Neonatal asphyxia
  Laminar cortical necrosis
  Ulegyria
  Lobular cerebellar sclerosis
Perinatal arterial occlusion
  Cerebral infarct
Excessive moulding
  Medial temporal lobe lesions ('incisural sclerosis')
  Inferior temporal and medial occipital lobe infarction

evolving from these earlier stages by resorption of necrotic tissue and gliosis to form the unmistakable mushroom-like gyri. Hypotension complicating hypoxia is believed to determine the distribution of ulegyria in these cases (Norman et al 1957). In some early accounts of the surgical treatment of epilepsy (e.g. Penfield & Humphries 1940, Penfield & Jasper 1954) these lesions are referred to as focal microgyria, although it is clear from their illustrations that they are entirely different from the lesion termed microgyria by Crome (1952) and described above under the now more customary term of polymicrogyria.

Circumscribed lobular cerebellar sclerosis is discussed and illustrated in a later section of this chapter.

Large, well-defined, destructive lesions occurring in recognized arterial territories in the brains of patients with seizures and often with fixed neurological deficits are readily recognized as old infarcts. Clinical date in some of these patients indicate that the lesion occurred in the perinatal period. The patients with temporal lobe epilepsy and homonymous hemianopia reported by Remilard et al (1974) undoubtedly belong in this category; some of the 85 patients reviewed by Rasmussen & Gossman (1963) under the term 'gross destructive brain lesions' probably had neonatal infarcts; a case is illustrated by Mathieson (1975a). Autopsy accounts in neonates by Clark & Linell (1954) and by Banker (1961) confirmed the occurrence of perinatal arterial cerebral infarcts. In the infantile cases reported by Cocker et al (1965) there was excellent correlation between the regions of brain infarcted and the sites of arterial lesions; these occurred at arterial bifurcations, suggesting lodgement of an embolus. The cause of arterial occlusion is often obscure although in some cases there is evidence of embolism from the placenta, fetal placental veins or mural cardiac thrombus. In patients who develop epilepsy in later infancy or childhood and are found to have a cerebral infarct, the aetiology of the perinatal arterial occlusion usually remains tentative and dependent on analogy with cases studied carefully at an earlier stage of their evolution.

Increasing recognition of the frequency of a temporal lobe origin of habitual seizures and the demonstration of atrophic lesions in therapeutic excisions led Earle et al (1953) to formulate a hypothesis about their origin. In essence, they postulated that transtentorial herniation of medial temporal structures, resulting from excessive moulding of the skull vault during delivery, might compress the anterior choroidal and posterior cerebral arteries with resultant ischaemic lesions in their territories; hence their term 'incisural sclerosis'. With our increasing knowledge of temporal lobe pathology, this mechanicovascular hypothesis has proved to be untenable in the many cases of sclerotic temporal atrophy which are now attributed to other cases. The term 'incisural sclerosis' has thus generally lapsed. The distribution of the temporal atrophy, which could not be mapped in the earlier limited therapeutic excisions, is not consistent with anterior choroidal or posterior cerebral occlusion (Falconer et al 1964, Falconer & Taylor 1968). However, some unusual cases with extensive inferior temporal and medial occipital infarction may be a consequence of posterior cerebral artery compression at the incisura tentorii.

Lesions resulting from febrile illness of childhood

Convulsions due to pyrexial illness, not primarily involving the brain, are reported to accur in from 19 to 48 per 1000 children, mostly between the ages of 6 months and 5 years (Miller et al 1960, Costeff 1965, Schuman & Miller 1966, Van den Berg & Yerushalmy 1969, Rose et al 1973). The tendency for a child to convulse when febrile appears to be genetically determined (Lennox 1949a, Ounsted 1952, Schuman & Miller 1966, Ounsted 1955). Furthermore the evidence indicates that this tendency is inherited in an autosomal dominant fashion (Ounsted et al 1966, Frantzen et al 1970). The tendency becomes manifest only when febrile provocation occurs within the appropriate age range in childhood (Ounsted 1971). The whole subject of febrile convulsions is discussed in detail by Lennox-Buchthal (1973).

During the age of susceptibility to febrile convulsions, the brain is in a phase of active growth and maturation. On general grounds, therefore, it might be supposed that excessive neuronal discharge and hypoxia occurring during prolonged and/or recurrent convulsions might be particularly likely to cause brain damage. The evidence is that this is so. Zimmerman (1938) described cortical neuronal necrosis, sometimes widespread, occasionally laminar, and often most evident in the walls and depths of sulci in 11 children (age range 5 months to 6 years) who died within 1 to 13 days of the onset of severe febrile convulsions. This type of lesion is illustrated in Figure 7.10. Destruction of neurones of Sommer's sector of the hippocampus was prominent in Zimmerman's cases. Cerebellar lesions occurred in some patients. The five patients under 3 years of age reported by Fowler (1957) were previously healthy but, following convulsions associated with fever, had extensive brain lesions with neuronal necrosis and loss. The distribution of lesions included cerebral cortex, hippocampus, amygdaloid nucleus, thalamus and basal ganglia. In one case the hippocampi were normal. Cortical lesions, where

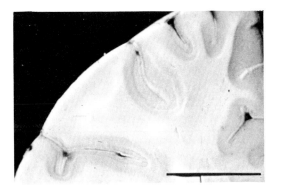

Fig. 7.10 Laminar cortical necrosis. U-shaped involvement of walls and depths of sulci convexity. From an 18-month-old male infant whose persistent febrile convulsions terminated in death on the 3rd day. Scale marker 2 cm.

not complete, tended to be laminar, with layer III most frequently involved. Inflammatory lesions of meninges or brain were not present.

Necropsy studies such as these and others in the literature necessarily describe lethal, and therefore exceptionally severe, instances of insult to the brain. Their relevance to longlasting habitual epilepsy is by extrapolation to patients with lesser degrees of cerebral damage. Thom (1942) quotes figures to indicate that children with a history of febrile convulsions are 12 times more likely to have epilepsy than children without such a history. This theme has been further developed with examples by Lennox (1949b).

Viewed retrospectively, patients with established temporal lobe epilepsy have a greater than normal probability of having had febrile convulsion in early life (Ounsted et al 1966, Ounsted 1967, Mathieson 1975b). Furthermore, patients with temporal lobe epilepsy and a preceding history of febrile convulsions are more likely (at a high degree of statistical significance) to have siblings who have also had febrile convulsions (Ounsted 1967). Of 100 patients treated by temporal lobectomy, those shown histologically to have gliosis of medial temporal structures had a significantly ($p < 0.01$) more frequent onset with status epilepticus than those with other lesions such as hamartomas or cryptic tumours (Falconer & Taylor 1968).

The pathogenetic sequence of events, for which the evidence has been given above, is summarized in Figure 7.11. This is probably not the only aetiology of sclerotic atrophy of the temporal lobe, nor are the lesions resulting from febrile status invariably temporal in distribution. An example of widespread destruction with ulegyria and accentuation in arterial watershed zones is shown in Figure 7.12. The tendency for less severe lesions, especially those in the temporal lobe, to be predominantly unilateral is not yet fully understood; possible operative factors include greater seizure discharge on one side (Aicardi & Chevrie 1970) and a hypothesis regarding differential maturation rates of the cerebral hemispheres (Taylor 1969, Taylor & Ounsted 1971).

Evidence derived from animal experimentation relevant to this problem is discussed in a subsequent section of this chapter.

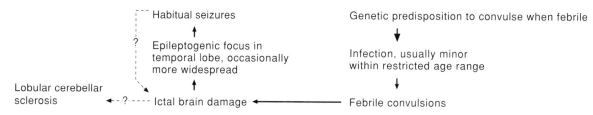

Fig. 7.11   Suggested sequence of events in some patients following prolonged or repeated febrile convulsions. See text for evidence.

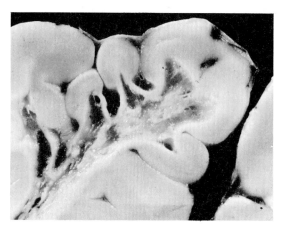

Fig. 7.12 Ulegyria. Birth and early development entirely normal. Severe febrile convulsions at 2 years. Frequent seizures of variable pattern, resistent to medication. Death following epileptic fit at 10 years. Autopsy showed widespread ulegyria mainly in arterial watershed distribution.

Inflammatory lesions and their residua

Established and essentially static epileptogenic lesions may follow bacterial meningitis and cerebral abscess. In some patients with epilepsia partialis continua and progressive neurological deficit an encephalitic histopathology has been found.

In patients with pyogenic meningitis, several pathogenetic mechanisms may be operative. Although fibrinopurulent exudate is usually confined to the leptomeninges, microscopic changes are observed in the superficial cortical layers even in the early stages. These comprise microglial infiltration and astrocytic hypertrophy which may be surmised to affect dendritic arborizations in these layers. Selective neuronal necrosis occurs in some patients (Smith & Landing 1960). More obvious ischaemic lesions, taking the form of patchy infarcts, result from endarteritis obliterans, with or without supervening thrombosis of leptomeningeal vessels, especially in patients who

have received inappropriate or delayed antibiotic therapy and have passed into a subacute phase. A third pathogenetic mechanism, that of convulsions consequent upon fever, may operate in genetically susceptible children of appropriate age. Dodge & Swartz (1965) reported four of 99 patients as having seizures as a late sequel of pyogenic meningitis.

Cerebral abscesses with their attendant granulation tissue, fibrosis and progressive surrounding zone of gliosed brain form potent epileptogenic foci, as a voluminous literature attests. Legg et al (1973) recorded epilepsy as occurring in 51 of 70 patients with supratentorial abscesses, with a mean latency of 3.3 years; latency was shorter in patients with a temporal site than in those with a frontal site. Carey et al (1971) reported a 32% incidence of seizures in 40 patients surviving surgical therapy; seizures in children were more frequent and more resistant to antiepileptic drug therapy than in adults. Morgan et al (1973) found a 55% incidence of seizures in 31 patients with supratentorial abscesses; onset was within 2 years of operation in all but one patient. Other published series confirm that one-third to one-half of patients surviving cerebral abscess develop epilepsy, no matter how treated. These figures bear eloquent witness to the potent epileptogenicity of this lesion.

Seizures are a prominent clinical feature of various forms of encephalitis of known or suspected viral etiology. Of special interest are those patients in whom epilepsia partialis continua or recurrent seizures with focal onset are accompanied by a slowly progressive neurological deficit. A histopathological picture of encephalitis, still apparently active many months after onset, has been described in some such patients by Rasmussen et al (1958) and by Aguilar & Rasmussen (1960).

The syndrome occurs mainly in the first decade of life (Mathieson 1975a). While inflammatory features are impressive, inclusion bodies are rarely found. Serological evidence of viral infection is lacking and attempts to demonstrate virus by electronmicroscopy and culture have not as yet yielded convincing results, despite a number of preliminary published reports, unfortunately unconfirmed. Clinically there is some resemblance to the syndrome of hemiconvulsions, hemiplegia and epilepsy discussed by Gastaut et al (1959) but this latter usually has an abrupt onset and is believed to result from vascular occlusion in most instances, although Coxsackie A9 viral infection causing focal vasculitis or encephalitis has been described (Roden et al 1975, Chalhub et al 1977).

Parasitic infestation of the brain in the form of cysticercosis cerebri is generally limited to certain geographical regions.

Lesions resulting from head injury

Convulsions occurring contralateral to severe head injury have been observed since early times (Hippocrates, cited by Temkin 1971). More recent accounts of post-traumatic epilepsy have been concerned, inter alia, with the probability of its occurrence following varying degrees and types of injury. Caveness & Liss (1961) and Caveness (1963) in studies of Korean war veterans found an incidence ranging from 8.5% after mild closed injury to over 50% after dural and brain penetration. Jennet (1975) in a long-term statistical study of epilepsy following non-missile injuries reported an overall incidence of 5%. This risk was greatly increased by acute intracranial haematoma, by early epilepsy and by depressed skull fracture. In pathological terms, these factors reflect laceration of the brain, as occurs inevitably in penetrating injury. Breach of the pial barrier and mechanical damage to the cortex are therefore important determinants of post-traumatic epilepsy.

Morphologically, the focal residual lesions of trauma comprise saucer-shaped defects with smoothly scalloped borders, occurring most frequently on the crests of the orbital frontal and lateral temporal gyri. Lesions extending into the depths of sulci may result from transient interference with the epicerebral circulation and consequent infarction. Histopathologically, the superficial or all cortical layers are destroyed; a variable amount of collagenous fibrosis intermingled with glial proliferation forms a meningocerebral cicatrix. A narrow bordering zone of partially depopulated cortex is usual.

The more obvious lesions may not be the only important ones. Microscopic lesions, widely scattered throughout the cerebral hemispheres and brain stem, were recorded by Oppenheimer (1968) as occurring in about three-quarters of fatal head injuries; not all brain injuries were severe in the conventional sense, as death in some patients was due to non-neurological causes. Essentially, these lesions seem to stem from stretching and tearing of axons and subsequent cellular reaction. They are considered to be the precursors of the more extensive lesions described by Strich (1956, 1961) in patients with profound neurological deficits following closed head injury. It may be postulated that these predominantly subcortical abnormalities cause partial deafferentation of the cortex and predispose to the development of post-traumatic epilepsy. The evidence from therapeutic cortical resection, however, at least in selected cases of post-traumatic epilepsy (Rasmussen 1969) suggests that the local cortical lesion is of paramount importance in the genesis of seizures; the role of possible subcortical damage in the 33% of patients whose seizures were not ameliorated by cortical excision remains speculative.

Another factor possibly contributing to seizures in head injured patients is anoxic encephalopathy consequent upon systemic hypoxia from thoracic and other injuries.

Acquired vascular lesions of adults

Some patients develop epilepsy following a stroke. Louis & McDowell (1967) recorded seizures in 77 of 1000 patients surviving a cerebral infarct; 29 patients had long term seizures as a sequel of their infarcts. Richardson & Dodge (1954) reported a 12.5% incidence of seizures in a consecutive series of 104 stroke patients. The importance of occlusive cerebrovascular disease in the genesis of epilepsy in the population as a whole is heavily age dependent. In a study of 1008 adult epileptic patients, roughly representative of the population at risk, seizures were attributed to cerebrovascular disease in 8.7%. In patients with onset of seizures after age 40, the proportion attributed to cerebrovascular disease rose to 44.5% (Juul-Jensen 1963).

What determines whether or not a stroke patient develops seizures is unclear. Involvement of the cerebral cortex appears to be essential (Dodge et al 1954). The responsible infarcts are often small and consequent upon small branch occlusion in the epicerebral circulation (Richardson 1958, Waddington 1970). Nevertheless, patients with medium to large infarcts and associated fixed neurological deficits do occasionally have recurrent seizures. The infarcts and the morphological changes in the brain surrounding them differ in no discernible way from those seen in non-convulsing patients. Patients surviving massive stroke rarely have persistent seizures.

Neoplasms

Brain tumours as a cause of adult onset epilepsy are so well known as to require little description here. Some general conclusions can be drawn from the large published series of cases, for example those of White et al (1948), Penfield & Jasper (1954) and Wyke (1959). Almost any supratentorial intracranial tumour can cause brain changes giving rise to seizures. The tendency of different tumours to do so depends partly on their site, but also to a considerable degree on their growth rate as determined by their histopathology. Whether the tumour impinges on the cerebral cortex from without (e.g. meningioma) or infiltrates the brain substance from within (e.g. astrocytoma) appears to make little difference to epileptogenicity. Proximity to the Rolandic motor strip or, more generally, a frontal situation increases the probability of seizures. Chronicity of the lesion is a major factor in epileptogenicity. Thus well-differentiated tumours with low biological growth potential and a course running for several years rather than months are more likely to be associated with epilepsy. Small indolent gliomas with seizures as their sole clinical mani-

festation are sometimes distinguished with difficulty, if at all, from glial hamartomas (Cavanagh 1958, Mathieson 1975b).

In the case of extrinsic tumours, the essential morphological change appears to be an area of pressure atrophy of the cortex characterized by neuronal loss and gliosis. Intrinsic tumours produce a peripheral zone of infiltrated, but incompletely destroyed, brain tissue. This zone, with engulfed but viable neurones, is characteristically prominent in oligodendrogliomas and well differentiated astrocytomas; these lesions are associated with a high incidence of seizures.

For detailed pathological descriptions of nervous system tumours, the reader is referred to standard monographs such as those of Russell & Rubinstein (1977) and Rubinstein (1972).

Subtle dendritic lesions

The arrangement and structure of dendrites are poorly displayed by the staining methods customarily used in light microscopy. Electron microscopy presents difficulties in sampling and the availability of adequately fixed tissue. Morphological observations on dendrites in naturally occurring epileptogenic foci in humans are therefore regrettably sparse, despite the importance of the dendritic tree in the electrophysiological status of neurones. This is in sharp contrast to extensive accounts of dendritic changes in experimental models of epileptogenic foci.

Using Golgi techniques, the Scheibels have described a constellation of dendritic changes in the hippocampal neurones of patients with temporal lobe epilepsy (Scheibel et al 1974, Scheibel & Scheibel 1973). Loss of dendritic spines, nodularity of the dendritic shaft and fusiform swellings of apical dendrites occurred in a patchy fashion in neurones of the pyramidal cell layer. Changes in the neurones of the gyrus dentatus were less consistent but included a 'windswept' appearance of dendrites and narrowing of the dendritic field giving a 'closed parasol' appearance. These changes were not thought to result from deafferentation or remote anoxic injury: in only 50% of the patients reported was there a history of difficult birth or febrile convulsions in childhood. Paucity of dendritic spines has been corroborated by electron microscopic studies, but the fine structure of dendritic nodularity has not been observed (Brown 1973). It is not clear whether the changes described by these investigators form a part of the customary hippocampal sclerosis or are a distinct abnormality selectively involving dendritic spines such as has been described by Marin-Padilla (1972) in infants with established chromosomal anomalies. The authors considered that they constituted a continuing process of neuronal destruction.

Endogeneous metabolic encephalopathies

A host of diseases due to endogenous metabolic abnormality (inborn errors of metabolism) give rise to seizures. They defy brief description. Reference should be made to standard texts, such as that of Blackwood & Corsellis (1976), which give access to primary sources. Some of these diseases are readily recognized clinically and have a chemically characterized storage product and enzymatic deficiency, for example Tay–Sachs disease, GM_2 gangliosidosis and hexosaminidase deficiency. Others, such as neuronal ceroid-lipofuscinosis (Zeman et al 1970, Boehme et al 1971) await full biochemical elucidation. Yet others remain to be segregated from the so-called degenerative diseases.

Clinical manifestations of many endogenous metabolic encephalopathies begin in childhood, but some are asymptomatic until well into adult life, for example, adult ceroid-lipofuscinosis or Kufs disease. Some of the non-gangliosidotic storage diseases may be diagnosed by histochemical and electronmicroscopic examination of sweat glands obtained by skin biopsy (Carpenter et al 1972, Carpenter et al 1973) or of lymphocytes (Noonan et al 1978). Lafora disease, in which myoclonic and generalized seizures are prominent clinical features, may be diagnosed by cerebral biopsy and demonstration of characteristic neuronal inclusions; a detailed description is given by Van Heycop ten Ham (1974). Increasing knowledge of the biochemical abnormalities in the endogenous metabolic encephalopathies should lead to their more precise diagnosis by non-invasive methods.

Metabolic encephalopathies of extracerebral origin

Foremost in frequency and importance amongst these is anoxic encephalopathy which is increasingly encountered among general hospital patients following cardiopulmonary resuscitation. Persistent myoclonic jerks and occasional generalized seizures occur in some patients. Typically at autopsy there is laminar cortical necrosis with accentuation in sulcal depths. An arterial watershed distribution is sometimes encountered or superimposed on a more widespread abnormality.

A morphologically similar encephalopathy may follow profound hypoglycaemia.

ATROPHIC LESIONS OF THE TEMPORAL LOBE

Alike from their frequency, amenability to surgical therapy, and possible prevention, atrophic lesions of the temporal lobe merit our special attention. Sano & Malamud (1953) observed hippocampal sclerosis in 29 of 50 long-term epileptics at autopsy; 16 of the 18 with normal mentation had what we would now term complex partial seizures. Corsellis (1957) reported Ammon's horn sclerosis in 15 of 32 patients. Margerison & Corsellis (1966) found hippocampal sclerosis at autopsy in 36 of 55 unselected epileptic patients. Most early descriptions of temporal lobe pathology stressed hippocampal lesions (see Falconer 1970 for a historical review) but other temporal lobe structures are involved in patients with temporal lobe epilepsy. Neuronal loss and gliosis in the amygdaloid nucleus and uncus of the parahippocampal gyrus occur in a substantial proportion of cases (Meyer & Beck 1955, Margerison & Corsellis 1966). In tabulating severe and often widespread lesions in the temporal lobe, Cavanagh & Meyer (1956) recorded involvement of the fusiform gyrus and the inferior and middle temporal gyri in about half the cases with hippocampal sclerosis. These considerations led Falconer et al (1964) to introduce the term 'mesial temporal sclerosis' as descriptive of the diffuse lesion found in a large proportion of their patients operated upon for temporal lobe epilepsy. In view of the laterally situated lesions in some cases, and the pantemporal atrophy in severe examples, sclerotic temporal atrophy has been suggested as a synonym (Mathieson 1975b).

Niceties of terminology aside, the important fact is that atrophic lesions extend beyond the hippocampus and other mesial structures to involve both cortex and white matter of the temporal convolutions. They lie beyond the territories of irrigation of both choroidal and posterior cerebral arteries and we must look to mechanisms other than impaired circulation in any single vessel for their genesis. Indeed, the laminar cortical cell loss involving mainly the second and third layers with accentuation in the depths of sulci (Meyer et al 1954) is unlikely to be the result of infarction, either arterial or venous. While opinions remain to some extent open, there is a general trend towards the view that most cases of sclerotic temporal atrophy result from severe and/or recurrent febrile convulsions in early childhood; that pre-existing cerebral damage from perinatal asphyxia increases the risk; and that some patients develop this lesion solely as a consequence of birth anoxia. The magnitude of the problem is indicated by the study of Nelson & Ellenberger (1976): 2% of 1706 children who had had one or more febrile convulsions developed epilepsy by the seventh year of life. Children known or suspected of having some neurological abnormality before the febrile convulsive episode had a higher than average incidence of subsequent afebrile seizures. The prophylactic measures indicated are, in principle, clear (Mathieson 1975b, Meldrum 1975). Whether the maturing lesion can be influenced in respect of its potential epileptogenicity following the initiating events is another matter.

The range of severity of lesions found and their histopathological pattern, is illustrated in Figures 7.13 to 7.18.

Lesser degrees of presumed abnormality in resected temporal lobes sometimes make it difficult for the surgical pathologist to give a clear opinion. In patients operated upon in middle life some degree of subpial (Chaslun's) gliosis and perivascular atrophy of the white matter are not unexpected. The gyral pattern of the temporal lobe is variable. Studies by Geschwind & Levitsky (1968), Witelson & Pallie (1973) and Yeni-Komshian & Benson (1976) indicate that there

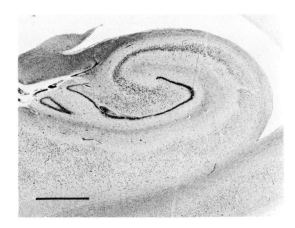

Fig. 7.13 Normal hippocampus. For comparison with Figure 7.14. Cresyl violet. Scale marker 2 mm.

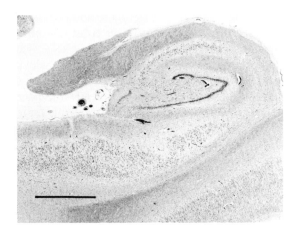

Fig. 7.14 Hippocampal sclerosis. Neuronal loss in H1 Sommer's sector and in end plate. The hippocampus is shrunken. Cresyl violet. Scale marker 2 mm.

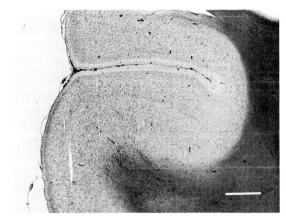

Fig. 7.15 Normal temporal neocortex. For comparison with Fig. 7.16. Luxol fast blue-cresyl violet. Scale marker 2 mm.

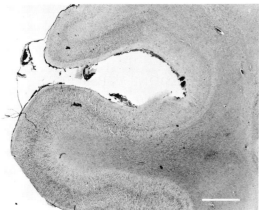

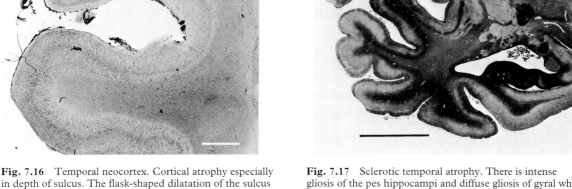

Fig. 7.16 Temporal neocortex. Cortical atrophy especially in depth of sulcus. The flask-shaped dilatation of the sulcus is the most readily apparent feature. From a 42-year-old man who had had focal seizures since 20 years of age. Early history not available. Luxol fast blue-PAS. Scale marker 2 mm.

Fig. 7.17 Sclerotic temporal atrophy. There is intense gliosis of the pes hippocampi and diffuse gliosis of gyral white matter. Cortex of all gyri shows patchy thinning and gliosis, especially in walls and depths of sulci. Long history of temporal lobe epilepsy. Holzer's method for glial fibres. Scale marker 1 cm.

are systemic anatomical differences between right and left temporal lobes. There are thus formidable difficulties in the path of morphometric investigation of resected temporal lobes. Additionally, Crome (1955) has pointed out that many of the histopathological features seen in temporal lobe epilepsy occur in non-epileptic subjects including some of normal intelligence. Equally disturbing are the approximately 20% of therapeutically excised temporal lobes which show little or no morphological abnormality (Mathieson 1975a). Increasing experience suggests that recognition of flask-shaped dilatation of sulci indicating local cortical atrophy will reduce this percentage.

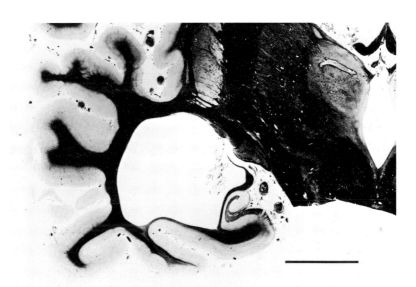

Fig. 7.18 Sclerotic temporal atrophy. Ulegyria of lateral and basal temporal gyri, extending to floor of insula. Hippocampal atrophy. Dilatation of temporal horn of lateral ventricle. Patient had a history of difficult birth and convulsions in infancy. Habitual seizures of varying pattern began at nine years; episodes of status epilepticus; death from unrelated causes at 50 years of age. Heidenhain's method for myelin. Scale marker 1 cm.

Those remaining emphasize the need for studies of dendritic and synaptic morphology and biochemical collabroration.

CEREBELLAR LESIONS IN PATIENTS WITH EPILEPSY

These take the form of either a diffuse cortical atrophy with Purkinje cell loss, gliosis of the molecular layer and sometimes granular cell layer involvement, or a rather well-circumscribed lobular cerebellar sclerosis. This latter lesion (Fig. 7.19) is commonly bilateral and in the posterolateral cerebellar hemispheres suggesting a border zone hypoxia-ischaemic pathogenesis. Lobular cerebellar sclerosis is most often observed in institutionalized patients with severe seizures, making it tempting to assume that the lesion is the cumulative effect of ictal brain damage. While this may be so in some cases, the alternative view that the cerebral epileptogenic foci and the cerebellar lesions both stem from a common episode of perinatal anoxia or febrile convulsions (such as cause ulegyria of watershed distribution) is more attractive. The concepts are not mutually exclusive. The Purkinje and basket cells are known to be selectively vulnerable to hypoxia; boundary zone lesions occur either when there is an abrupt fall in blood pressure or sudden severe hypoxaemia (Brierly et al 1973). Cerebellar le-

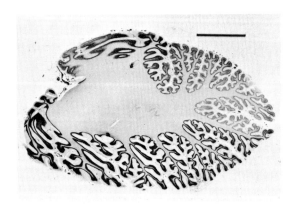

Fig. 7.19   Cerebellum. Lobular cerebellar sclerosis involving posterolateral parts of hemispheres bilaterally. Frequent generalized seizures began at 11 years; early history uncertain; erratic and antisocial behaviour. Death at 25 years due to aspiration pneumonia following seizures. Cresyl violet stain. Scale marker 1 cm.

sions in epileptic patients were recognized before the introduction of phenytion and are probably not attributable to its use.

IATROGENIC LESIONS IN PATIENTS WITH EPILEPSY

The lesions include gingival hyperplasia, a peculiar form of lymphadenopathy and, arguably, cerebellar cortical abnormalities, all relating to phenytoin therapy.

The gum changes, histologically, consist of proliferation of the submucosal connective tissue with plasma cell infiltration and acanthosis of the epithelium (Van der Kwast 1956). Symmers (1978) regards the essential change as hyperplasia of connective tissue, but secondary inflammatory features are usually present.

Hydantoin lymphadenopathy most frequently involves cervical nodes which become enlarged but not matted. Histologically, there is proliferation of reticulum cells, formation of binucleate cells, some loss of nodal architecture, and variable degrees of eosinophilic infiltration and necrosis (Saltztein & Ackerman 1959, Krasznai & Györy 1968, Symmers 1978). The major differential diagnosis is that of Hodgkin disease. Regression of nodal enlargement on withdrawal of the drug is the best demonstration of a benign reactive process. In very rare cases, the lymphadenopathy progresses to malignant lymphoma, even following initial regression (Gams et al 1968).

While an ataxic syndrome is well recognized clinically following phenytoin intoxication, its morphological basis, if any, has proved to be something of a mirage. Purkinje cell loss following phenytoin administration to experimental animals has been described (Utterback 1958 and other investigators) but morphometric studies by Dam (1972) do not confirm any such cell loss in rats, pigs or monkeys. Furthermore, Dam (1970) has shown that a diminished Purkinje cell population in patients with major seizures is related to the frequency of seizures rather than prolonged large doses of phenytoin. Fine structural changes in Purkinje cell dendrites in rats subjected to near lethal doses of phenytoin were described by Del Cerro & Snider (1967), but Nielsen et al (1971) found normal Purkinje cell ultrastructure in rats subject to intoxicating but sublethal doses of this drug.

CONCLUSION

The outstanding feature of any review of the pathology of epilepsy is the range and diversity of lesions which can give rise to seizures. It is clear that the obvious and readily categorized lesions are several steps removed from the essential local abnormality which is causative of seizures. Our inability to find consistent changes in patients with corticoreticular seizures emphasizes this problem. Whether the lesions are discrete and focal, or diffuse and subtle, the abnormal discharges take place in remaining viable neurones. Their environment has been changed not only in structure but also physiologically and biochemically. These aspects are considered in the ensuing chapters of this book.

REFERENCES

Aguilar M J, Rasmussen T 1960 Role of encephalitis in pathogenesis of epilepsy. Archives of Neurology 2: 663

Aicardi J, Chevrie J J 1970 Convulsive status epilepticus in infants and children. A study of 239 cases. Epilepsia 11: 187

Alexander G L, Norman R M 1960 The Sturge–Weber syndrome. Wright, Bristol

Banker B Q 1961 Cerebral vascular disease in infancy and childhood. I. Occlusive vascular disease. Journal of Neuropathology and Experimental Neurology 20: 127

Banker B Q 1967 The neuropathological effects of anoxia and hypoglycaemia in the newborn. Developmental Medicine and Child Neurology 9: 544

Bignami A, Appicciutoli L 1964 Micropolygyria and cerebral calcification in cytomegalic inclusion disease. Acta Neuropatholgica 4: 127

Bignami A, Palladini G, Zappella M 1968 Unilateral megalencephaly with nerve cell hypertrophy. An anatomical and quantitative histochemical study. Brain Research 9: 103

Blackwood W, Corsellis J A N 1976 (eds) Greenfield's neuropathology, 3rd edn. Edward Arnold, Edinburgh

Boehme D H, Cottrell J C, Leonberh S C, Zeman W 1971 A dominant form of neuronal ceroid-lipofuscinosis. Brain 94: 745

Bolande R P 1974 The neurocristopathies. A unifying concept of disease arising in neural crest maldevelopment. Human Pathology 5: 409

Brierly J B, Meldrum B S, Brown A W 1973 The threshold and neuropathology of cerebral 'anoxic-ischemic' cell change. Archives of Neurology 29: 367

Brown W J 1973 In: Brazier M A B (ed) Epilepsy. Its phenomena in man. Academic Press, New York

Carey M E, Chou S N, French L A 1971 Long-term neurological residua in patients surviving brain abscess with surgery. Journal of Neurosurgery 34: 652

Carpenter S, Karpati G, Andermann F 1972 Specific involvement of muscle, nerve and skin in late infantile and juvenile amaurotic idiocy. Neurology 22: 170

Carpenter S, Karpati G, Wolfe L S, Andermann F (1973) A type of juvenile cerebromacular degeneration characterized by granular osmiophilic deposits. Journal of the Neurological Sciences 18: 67

Cavanagh J B 1958 On certain small tumours encountered in the temporal lobe. Brain 81: 389

Cavanagh J B, Meyer A 1956 Aetiological aspects of Ammon's horn sclerosis associated with temporal lobe epilepsy. British Medical Journal 2: 1403

Caveness W F 1963 Onset and cessation of fits following craniocerebral trauma. Journal of Neurosurgery 20: 570

Caveness W F, Liss H R 1961 Incidence of post-traumatic epilepsy. Epilepsia 2: 123

Chalhub E G, Devivo D C, Siegal B A, Gado M H, Feigin R D 1977 Coxsackie A9 focal encephalitis associated with acute infantile hemiplegia and porencephaly. Neurology 27: 574

Clark J V 1970 Familial occurrence of cavernous angiomata of the brain. Journal of Neurology, Neurosurgery and Psychiatry 33: 871

Clark R M, Linell E A 1954 Case report: prenatal occlusion of the internal carotid artery. Journal of Neurology, Neurosurgery and Psychiatry 17: 295

Cocker J, George S W, Yates P O 1965 Perinatal occlusion of the middle cerebral artery. Developmental Medicine and Child Neurology 7: 235

Corsellis J A N 1957 The incidence of Ammon's horn sclerosis. Brain 80: 193

Costeff N 1965 Convulsions in chilhood. Their natural history and indications for treatment. New England Journal of Medicine 273: 1410

Cravioto H, Feigin I 1960 Localized cerebral gliosis with giant neurons histologically resembling tuberous sclerosis. Journal of Neuropathology and Experimental Neurology 19: 572

Crome L 1952 Microgyria. Journal of Pathology and Bacteriology 64: 479

Crome L 1955 A morphological critique of temporal lobectomy. Lancet 1: 882

Crome L 1957 Infantile cerebral gliosis with giant nerve cells. Journal of Neurology, Neurosurgery and Psychiatry 20: 117

Crome L 1961 Cytomegalic inclusion–body disease. World Neurology 2: 447

Crome L, France N E 1959 Microgyria and cytomegalic inclusion disease in infancy. Journal of Clinical Pathology 12: 427

Dam M 1970 Number of Purkinje cells in patients with grand mal epilepsy treated with diphenylhydantoin. Epilepsia 11: 313

Dam M 1972 The density and ultrastructure of the Purkinje cells following diphenylhydantoin treatment in animals and man. Acta Neurologica Scandinavica 48 (suppl 49): 3

Dekaban A 1965 Large defects in cerebral hemispheres associated with cortical dysgenesis. Journal of Neuropathology and Experimental Neurology 24: 512

Del Cerro M P, Snider R S 1967 Studies on Dilantin intoxication. Neurology 17: 452

Dobbing J, Sands J 1973 Quantitative growth and

development of human brain. Archives of Diseases in Childhood 48: 757

Dobbing J, Smart J L 1974 Vulnerability of developing brain and behaviour. British Medical Bulletin 30: 164

Dodge P R, Richardson E P, Victor M 1954 Recurrent convulsive seizures as a sequel to cerebral infarction: a clinical and pathological study. Brain 77: 610

Dodge P R, Swartz M N 1965 Bacterial meningitis—a review of selected aspects. II. Special neurological problems, postmeningitic complications and clinicopathological correlations. New England Journal of Medicine 272: 1003

Duvoisin R C, Vinson W M 1961 Tuberous sclerosis. Report of three cases without mental defect. Journal of the American Medical Association 175: 869

Earle K M, Baldwin M, Penfield W 1953 Incisural sclerosis and temporal lobe seizures produced by hippocampal herniation at birth. Archives of Neurology and Psychiatry 69: 27

Falconer M A 1970 Historical review. The pathological substrate of temporal lobe epilepsy. Guy's Hospital Reports 119: 47

Falconer M A 1973 Reversibility by temporal-lobe resection of the behavioural abnormalities of temporal-lobe epilepsy. New England Journal of Medicine 289: 451

Falconer M A, Rushworth R G 1960 Treatment of encephalotrigeminal angiomatosis (Sturge–Weber diseasse) by hemispherectomy. Archives of Disease in Childhood 35: 433

Falconer M A, Taylor D C 1968 Surgical treatment of drug-resistant epilepsy due to mesial temporal sclerosis. Archives of Neurology 19: 353

Falconer M A, Serafetinides E A, Corsellis J A N 1964 Etiology and pathogenesis of temporal lobe epilepsy. Archives of Neurology 10: 233

Feindel W, Yamamoto Y L, Hodge C L 1971 Red cerebral veins and the cerebral steal syndrome. Evidence from fluorescein angiography and microregional blood flow by radioisotopes during excision of an angioma. Journal of Neurosurgery 35: 167

Fowler M 1957 Brain damage after febrile convulsions. Archives of Diseases in Childhood 32: 67

Fox H, Emery J L, Goodbody R A, Yates P O 1964 Neurocutaneous melanosis. Archives of Diseases in Childhood 39: 508

Frantzen E, Lennox-Buchthal M, Nygaard A, Stene J 1970 A genetic study of febrile convulsions. Neurology 20: 909

Friede R L 1975 Developmental neuropathology. Springer-Verlag, New York

Gams R A, Neal J A, Conrad F G 1968 Hydantoin induced pseudo-pseudolymphoma. Annals of Internal Medicine 69: 557

Gastaut H, Poirier F, Payan H, Salamon G, Toga M, Vigouroux M 1959 HHE syndrome. Hemiconvulsions, hemiplegia, epilepsy. Epilepsia 1: 418

Geschwind N 1973 Effects of temporal lobe surgery on behaviour. New England Journal of Medicine 289: 480

Geschwind N, Levitsky W 1968 Human brain: left–right asymmetries in temporal speech region. Science 161: 186

Jennett B 1975 Epilepsy after non-missile head injuries, 2nd edn. Heinemann, London

Juul-Jensen P 1963 Epilepsy. A clinical and social analysis of 1020 adult patients with epileptic seizures. Acta Neurologica Scandinavica 40 (suppl 5): 1

Kirschbaum W 1947 Agenesis of the corpus callosum and associated malformations. Journal of Neuropathology and Experimental Neurology 6: 78

Krasznai G, Györy Gy 1968 Hydantoin lymphadenopathy. Journal of Pathology and Bacteriology 95: 314

Lagos J G, Gomez M R 1967 Tuberous sclerosis; reappraisal of a clinical entity. Mayo Clinic Proceedings 42: 26

Laurence K M 1964a A case of unilateral megalencephaly. Developmental Medicine and Child Neurology 6: 585

Laurence K M 1964b Megalencephaly (Annotation). Developmental Medicine and Child Neurology 6: 638

Layton D D 1962 Heterotopic cerebral gray metter as an epileptogenic focus. Journal of Neuropathology and Experimental Neurology 21: 244

Legg N J, Gupta P C, Scott D F 1973 Epilepsy following cerebral abscess. A clinical and EEG study of 70 patients. Brain 96: 259

Lennox M A 1949a Febrile convulsions in childhood. A clinical and electroencephalographic study. American Journal of Diseases of Children 78: 868

Lennox M A 1949b Febrile convulsions in childhood: their relationship to adult epilepsy. Journal of Pediatrics 35: 427

Lennox-Buchthal M A 1973 Febrile convulsions. A reappraisal. Electroencephalography and clinical neurophysiology supplement no 32. Elsevier, Amsterdam

Lilienfeld A M, Pasamanick B 1954 Association of maternal and fetal factors with the development of epilepsy. I. Abnormalities of the prenatal and paranatal periods. Journal of the American Medical Association 155: 719

Louis S, McDowell F 1967 Epileptic seizures in nonembolic cerebral infarction. Archives of Neurology 17: 414

Margerison J H, Corsellis J A N 1966 Epilepsy and the temporal lobes. A clinical, electroencephalographic and neuropathological study of the brain in epilepsy with particular reference to the temporal lobes. Brain 89: 499

Marin-Padilla M 1972 Structural abnormalities of the cerebral cortex in human chromosomal aberrations: a Golgi study. Brain Research 44: 625

Mathieson G 1975a Pathologic aspects of epilepsy with special reference to the surgical pathology of focal cerebral seizures. In: Purpura D P, Penry J K, Walter R D (eds) Advances in neurology, vol 8. Neurosurgical management of the epilepsies. Raven Press, New York

Mathieson G 1975b Pathology of temporal lobe foci. In: Penry J K, Daly D D (eds) Advances in neurology, vol II. Complex partial seizures and their treatment. Raven Press, New York

McCormick W F 1966 The pathology of vascular ('arteriovenous') malformations. Journal of Neurosurgery 24: 807

Meldrum B S 1975 Present views on hippocampal sclerosis and epilepsy. In: Williams D (ed) Modern trends in neurology, vol 6. Butterworths, London

Meyer A, Beck E 1955 The hippocampal formation in temporal lobe epilepsy. Proceedings of the Royal Society of Medicine 48: 457

Meyer A, Falconer M A, Beck E 1954 Pathological findings in temporal lobe epilepsy. Journal of Neurology, Neurosurgery and Psychiatry 17: 276

Miller F J W, Court S D M, Walton W S, Knox E J 1960 Growing up in Newcastle upon Tyne: a continuing study of health and illness in young children within their families. Oxford University Press, London

Morgan H, Wood M W, Murphy F 1973 Experience with 88 consecutive cases of brain abscess. Journal of Neurosurgery 38: 698

Nelson K B, Ellenberger J H 1976 Predictors of epilepsy in children who have experienced febrile seizures. New England Journal of Medicine 295: 1029

Nielsen M H, Dam M, Klinken L 1971 The ultrastructure of Purkinje cells in diphenylhydantoin intoxicated rats. Experimental Brain Research 12: 447

Noonan S M, Desousa J, Riddle J M 1978 Lymphocyte ultrastructures in two cases of neuronal ceroid-lipofuscinosis. Neurology 28: 472

Norman R M 1958 Malformations of the nervous system, birth injury and diseases of early life. In: Greenfield J G (ed) Neuropathology. Arnold, London

Norman R M, Urich H, McMenemey W H 1957 Vascular mechanisms of birth injury. Brain 80: 49

Oppenheimer D R 1968 Microscopic lesions in the brain following head injury. Journal of Neurology, Neurosurgery and Psychiatry 31: 299

Ounsted C 1952 The factor of inheritance in convulsive disorders in childhood. Proceedings of the Royal Society of Medicine 45: 865

Ounsted C 1955 Genetic and social aspect of the epilepsies of childhood. Eugenics Review 47: 33

Ounsted C 1967 Temporal lobe epilepsy: the problem of aetiology and prophylaxis. Journal of the Royal College of Physicians of London 1: 273

Ounsted C 1971 In: Gairdner D, Hull D (eds) Recent advances in paediatrics, 4th edn. Churchill, London

Ounsted C, Lindsay J, Norman R 1966 Biological factors in temporal lobe epilepsy. Clinics in developmental medicine no. 22. Heinemann, London

Pasamanick B, Lilienfeld A M 1955 Maternal and fetal factors in the development of epilepsy. 2. Relationship to some clinical features of epilepsy. Neurology 5: 77

Peach B 1965 Arnold–Chiari malformation. Anatomic features of 20 cases. Archives of Neurology 12: 613

Penfield W, Humphreys S 1940 Epileptogenic lesions of the brain. A histologic study. Archives of Neurology and Psychiatry 43: 240

Penfield W, Jasper H 1954 Epilepsy and the functional anatomy of the human brain. Little Brown, Boston

Penfield W, Ward A 1948 Calcifying epileptogenic lesions. Haemangioma calcificans; report of a case. Archives of Neurology and Psychiatry 60: 20

Perot P, Weir B, Rasmussen T 1966 Tuberous sclerosis. Surgical therapy for seizures. Archives of Neurology 15: 498

Rasmussen T 1969 Surgical therapy of post traumatic epilepsy. In: Walker A E, Caveness W F, Critchley M (eds) The late effects of head injury. Thomas, Springfield

Rasmussen T, Gossman H 1963 Epilepsy due to gross destructive brain lesions. Neurology 13: 659

Rasmussen T, Mathieson G, LeBlanc F 1972 Surgical therapy of typical and a forme fruste variety of the Sturge–Weber Syndrome. Schweizer Archiv für Neurologie, Neurochirurgie und Psychiatrie 111: 393

Rasmussen T, Olszewski J, Lloyd-Smith D 1958 Focal seizures due to chronic localized encephalitis. Neurology 8: 435

Remillard G M, Ethier R, Andermann F 1974 Temporal lobe epilepsy and perinatal occlusion of the posterior cerebral artery. Neurology 24: 1001

Richardson E P 1958 Late life epilepsy. Medical Clinics of North America 42: 349

Richardson E P, Dodge P R 1954 Epilepsy in cerebral vascular disease. Epilepsia (3rd series) 3: 49

Richman D P, Stewart R M, Caviness V S Jr 1974 Cerebral microgyria in a 27-week fetus. An architectonic and topographic analysis. Journal of Neuropathology and Experimental Neurology 33: 374

Roden V J, Cantor H E, O'Connor D M, Schmidt R R, Cherry J D 1975 Acute hemiplegia of childhood associated with Coxsackie A9 viral infection. Journal of Pediatrics 86: 56

Rose S W, Penry J K, Markush R E, Radloff L A, Putnam P L 1973 Prevalence of epilepsy in children. Epilepsia 14: 133

Rubinstein L J 1972 Tumours of the central nervous system. Atlas of Tumor Pathology, 2nd Series, Fasicle 6. Armed Forces Institute of Pathology, Washington D C

Russell D S, Rubinstein L J 1977 Pathology of tumours of the nervous system. Arnold, London

Saltzstein S L, Ackerman L V 1959 Lymphadenopathy induced by anti-convulsant drugs and mimicking clinically and pathologically malignant lymphomas. Cancer 12: 164

Sono K, Malamud N 1953 Clinical significance of sclerosis of the cornu Ammonis. Archives of Neurology and Psychiatry 70: 40

Scheibel M E, Crandall P H, Scheibel A B 1974 The hippocampaldentate complex in temporal lobe epilepsy. A Golgi study. Epilepsia 15: 55

Scheibel M E, Scheibel A B 1973 In: Brazier M A B (ed) Epilepsy. Its phenomena in man. Academic Press, New York

Schuman S H, Miller L J 1966 Febrile convulsions in families: findings in an epidemiological survey. Clinical Pediatrics 5: 604

Slaughter J C, Hardman J M, Kempe L G, Earle K M 1969 Neurocutaneous melanosis and leptomeningeal melanomatosis in children. Archives of Pathology 88: 298

Smith J F, Landing B H 1960 Mechanisms of brain damage in H. influenzae meningitis. Journal of Neuropathology and Experimental Neurology 19: 248

Strich S J 1956 Diffuse degeneration of the cerebral white matter in severe dementia following head injury. Journal of Neurology, Neurosurgery and Psychiatry 19: 163

Strich S J 1961 Shearing of nerve fibres as a cause of brain damage due to head injury. Lancet 2: 443

Symmers W StC 1978 In: Symmers, W StC (ed) Systemic Pathology, vol 2, 2nd edn. Churchill Livingstone, Edinburgh

Taylor D C 1969 Differential rates of cerebral maturation between sexes and between hemispheres. Evidence from epilepsy. Lancet 2: 140

Taylor D C, Ounsted C 1971 Biological mechanisms influencing the outcome of seizures in response to fever. Epilepsia 12: 33

Taylor D C, Falconer M A, Bruton C T, Corsellis J A N 1971 Focal dysplasia of the cerebral cortex in epilepsy. Journal of Neurology, Neurosurgery and Psychiatry 34: 369

Temkin O 1971 The falling sickness, 2nd edn. Johns Hopkins Press, Baltimore, p 35

Thom D A 1942 Convulsions of early life and their relation to the chronic convulsive disorders and mental defect. American Journal of Psychiatry 98: 574

Tytus J S, Pennybacker J 1956 Pearly tumours in relation to the central nervous system. Journal of Neurology, Neurosurgery and Psychiatry 19: 241

Urich H 1976 In: Blackwood W, Corsellis J A N (eds) Greenfield's neuropathology. Arnold, London

Utterback R A 1958 Parenchymatous cerebellar degeneration

complicating diphenylhydantoin (Dilantin) therapy. Archives of Neurology and Psychiatry 80: 180

Van den Berg B J, Yerushalmy J 1969 Studies on convulsive disorders in young children. 1 Incidence of febrile and nonfebrile convulsions by age and other factors. Pediatric Research 3: 298

Van der Kwast W A M 1956 Speculations regarding the nature of gingival hyperplasia due to diphenylhydantoin-sodium. Acta Medica Scandinavica 153: 399

Van Heycop ten Ham 1974 Lafora disease. A form of progressive myoclonus epilepsy. In: Vinken P J, Bruyn G W (eds) Handbook of clinical neurology, vol 15. North Holland Publishing, Amsterdam

Waddington M W 1970 Angiographic changes in focal motor epilepsy. Neurology 20: 879

White J C, Liu C T, Mixter W J 1948 Focal epilepsy. A statistical study of its causes and the results of surgical treatment. I. Epilepsy secondary to intracranial tumours. New England Journal of Medicine 238: 891

Witelson S F, Pallie W 1973 Left hemisphere specialisation for language in the newborn. Neuroanatomical evidence of asymmetry. Brain 96: 641

Worster-Drought C, Dickson W E C, McMenemy W H, (1937) Multiple meningeal and perineural tumours with analogous tumours in the glia and ependyma (neurofibroblastomatosis). Brain 60: 85

Wyke B D 1959 The cortical control of movement. A contribution to the surgical physiology of seizures. Epilepsia (4th series) 1: 4

Yeni-Komshian G H, Benson D A 1976 Anatomical study of cerebral asymmetry in the temporal lobe of humans, chimpanzees and rhesus monkeys. Science 192: 387

Zeman W, Donahue S, Dyken P, Green J 1970 The neuronal ceroidlipofuscinoses (Batten–Vogt Syndrome). In: Vinken P J, Bruyn G W (eds) Handbook of clinical neurology, vol 10. North Holland Publishing, Amsterdam

Zimmerman H M 1938 The histopathology of convulsive disorders in children. Journal of Pediatrics 13: 859

8. The pathophysiology of epilepsies

J. G. R. Jefferys

INTRODUCTION

What is the pathophysiology of epilepsy?

Epilepsy is a group of essentially electrical disturbances of brain function. Usually periods of more or less normal EEG activity and behaviour are disrupted by episodes of gross electrical disturbance. The approach in this chapter will be essentially electrophysiological and will explore the cellular basis of epileptic activity, in the belief that the explanation of the characteristic, gross electrical abnormalities in terms of neuronal properties is an essential prerequisite for analyses at the molecular level. Once we have a framework for understanding what epilepsy is at a cellular level, then we can start to make sense of the roles played by risk factors such as traumatic injury, metabolic abnormalities, developmental errors, genetics and environmental hazards. This chapter differs from its predecessor in earlier editions of this book, which concentrated on biochemical and structural correlates of seizure states. The latter certainly are important, and often are the only practical means of studying epilepsy in man. However, in many cases it is difficult to unravel cause and effect within the plethora of abnormalities found following repeated epileptic seizures. The central theme of the present approach is to bridge the gap between epilepsy in the whole organism and abnormalities at the molecular level by a detailed study of the cellular properties and functional circuitry that allow a brain to generate bouts of grossly abnormal electrical activity whilst functioning normally the rest of the time.

Do the epilepsies share common features?

The epilepsies are a remarkably diverse range of diseases, as witnessed by the small industry built up around their classification (Dreifuss 1987). However, there are features common to many of them which offer us real prospects of finding common basic mechanisms. A key feature in nearly all epilepsies is the recurrent episodes of hypersynchronous neuronal activity in one or more of the cortical areas of the brain. Of all the cortical structures, only the cerebellum does not support epileptogenesis, and indeed has been stimulated in attempts to control epilepsies centred on other areas. At the level of the single neuron, epileptic discharges are associated with very rapid bursts of action potentials (see Fig. 8.1 p. 242) (Lockard & Ward 1980), which in turn are associated with abrupt depolarizations of the membrane potential. However, while exploring the properties of single cells is essential to understanding the basic pathophysiology of epilepsies, it is important not to lose sight of the essential feature of epileptogenesis: that neuronal activity has to be hypersynchronous.

Hypersynchrony of cortical neurons even transcends the highest level of classification of the epilepsies into those of focal origin as against those where the initial disturbance has no identifiable localization, the primary generalized seizures. However, in the latter case, the thalamus has a key pacemaker-like role, and the resulting EEG activity and its cellular correlates differ significantly from those of the focal epilepsies, as will be discussed in some detail below.

Developments in understanding the basic mechanisms of the epilepsies

The development of the study of the basic

241

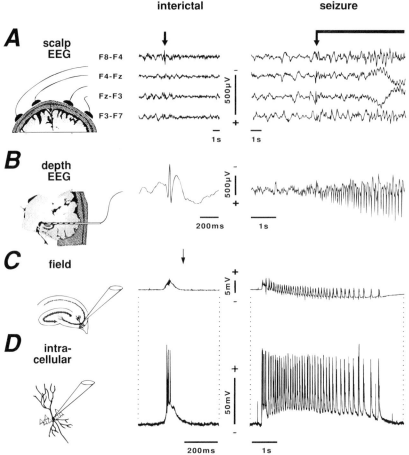

interictal   **seizure**

Fig. 8.1 Electrical events in clinical and experimental focal epilepsies. (A)
Conventional EEG recordings from a patient's scalp (icon, extreme left) show the
contrast between an interictal spike (left column, arrowed on channel F8–F4) and the
much more prolonged seizure discharge (right column, starting at arrow and continuing
for rest of record). The signals are small and noisy because of the volume of tissue
between the source of the currents and the electrodes. (B) Intracranial recordings from
another patient with a mesial temporal epileptic focus also reveals interictal spikes and
seizures initiated locally. The signals are larger and less noisy because the electrodes are
much closer to the source of the electric fields. Similar events can be recorded from a
range of animal models (see Tables 8.1, 8.2). (C), (D). Here are plotted both interictal
(left) and brief seizure or polyspike discharges (right) from brain slices maintained in
vitro after being prepared from a rat that had received an injection of 6 ng tetanus toxin
into its hippocampus 10 days previously. The field potentials (C) are analogous to the
depth recordings obtained in man, except that a greater bandwidth is used than is
typical in clinical work. One key advantage of this kind of experimental preparation is
the ease of intracellular recording (D, recorded simultaneously with the field potentials
in C). They show the classical 'all or none' or 'paroxysmal' depolarization shift found in
many neurons in an epileptic focus. Recordings from humans (A), (B) differ from most
experimental (C), (D) in several technical aspects. They usually are bipolar to help
reduce some sources of interference (voltages compared at two recording sites rather
than with respect to remote reference). They are strongly 'band-pass' filtered, the low
frequency cut (i.e. AC coupled) simplifies the recordings but distorts the signal, so that
the interictal spike in (B) is triphasic rather than the monophasic potential in (C), and
the recording of the seizure (B) cannot show slow potentials such as the negative shift
seen in (C), which probably is due to the accumulation of K^+ in the extracellular space.
More arbitrarily, clinical EEGs conventionally are displayed negative up. Data were
kindly provided by D. Fish and P. Allen of the National Hospital for Neurology and
Neurosurgery (A, B), and by R. Empson from the author's laboratory (C, D).

mechanisms of the epilepsies parallels the development of our concepts of neuronal function in the brain. The very earliest ideas now sound rather naive. Possession by demons does not have much currency in mainstream epileptology today. During the latter part of the last century, concepts of epilepsy started to take recognizable forms. For instance Gowers anticipated much of the debate on the roles of inhibition and excitation with his ideas on 'nerve force' overcoming some endogenous 'resistance' (Gowers 1881). Hughlings Jackson deduced the propagation of epileptic activity across the cortical surface from the clinical observation of what we now call Jacksonian march. However, the modern era really started with the development of new techniques for electrophysiological recording, and other neurosciences, following World War II. This is clearly evident in the first of the large monographs which share the title *Basic mechanisms of the epilepsies* (Jasper et al 1969) where much of the excitement stemmed from the insights from intracellular recordings: the 'Paroxysmal depolarization shift', the role of EPSPs and IPSPs, and the ability of neurons to fire very rapid bursts of action potentials. Developments over the next two decades become clear in the comparison with the second of these monographs (Delgado-Escueta et al 1986). Here, for example, the influence of molecular genetics and molecular biology is prominent, and the electrophysiology and anatomy use a wider repertoire of techniques, including patch clamp and immunocytochemistry, and work on humans now makes extensive use of non-invasive imaging techniques.

It is not surprising that explanations of a disease should use the language of the period. However, the traffic is not all one way. The search for understanding the mechanisms of the various forms of epileptic activity have stimulated much of the progress in our understanding of the fundamental properties of neural tissue; in the memorable subtitle of one monograph, epilepsy indeed provides a 'window on brain mechanisms' (Lockard & Ward 1980). For instance, studies of the basic mechanisms of epilepsies led directly to much of our knowledge on the control of bursts of action potentials in single neurons, on the local circuits in hippocampus and neocortex, and on the functioning of inhibitory and excitatory synapses. This

drive continues today, for instance in work on the roles of gene regulation in the plastic changes caused by repeated epileptic seizures.

Aims and disclaimer

The author's brief here is to write a textbook chapter and not a review, and thus this chapter cannot begin to refer to the massive literature on the subject in any detail. It is the author's hope that those responsible for advances in the field will forgive the inability to give due credit, and that the interested reader will find a gateway to the original work from the limited references included. The following reviews and multi-author works may well help (Prince 1985, Benardo & Pedley 1985, Prince & Connors 1986, Dichter & Ayala 1987, Fisher 1989, Jefferys 1990, Jasper et al 1969, Delgado-Escueta et al 1986).

Fundamental issues

Species affected

Epilepsy is not restricted to humans. It occurs spontaneously in a variety of domestic and wild animals, notably dogs, and some baboons and rodents. Some of these have proved useful experimentally (Delgado-Escueta et al 1986). *Papio papio*, the baboon, is one that has been intensively used by Naquet, Meldrum and others as a naturally occurring seizure susceptible model, which is particularly sensitive to photic stimulation (Meldrum & Wilkins 1984). Other species have needed some selective breeding to provide useful material for research: beagle dogs with spontaneous generalized convulsions, chickens with photic-induced seizures, audiogenic mice and rats, and Mongolian gerbils which respond to stress and to loud noises with generalized convulsions (p. 253).

Selective breeding programmes have also produced novel epileptic strains from standard laboratory animals, particularly mice, and more recently rats. Genetic analysis of these strains is somewhat simplified because many are single gene mutations which can be mapped in some detail (Noebels 1986). The next step, to link the gene mutation to the phenotypic changes that cause the epileptic symptoms is potentially more difficult, although there is encouraging progress in some particular examples, such as the *tottering* mouse which has an excessive growth of noradrenergic axons, and which has evidence of disinhibition in its hippocampus (Noebels & Rutecki 1990). Other epileptic strains appear to have more inhibitory neurons than their non-epileptic relatives, rather paradoxically (Ribak 1986).

Epilepsy, or at least some of its symptoms, can be mimicked ('modelled') in normal animals of more or less any species, by a wide range of experimental methods. This is important because the kinds of investigation needed for studies at the cellular level are very difficult on human tissues. It can be argued that the most commonly used acute convulsant drugs, which block synaptic inhibition, do not provide good models of epilepsy, where repeated seizures are essential for diagnosis, and where inhibition appears to be intact. However, acute convulsants provided the key to understanding how neurons became synchronized during epileptic seizures, as will be made clear below. Experimental models are not identical to epilepsy; their purpose is to make specific aspects of epilepsy accessible to the kinds of technique needed to answer the question posed. In the case of the cellular basis of neuronal synchronization, acute convulsants applied to brain slices in vitro have allowed us to study synchronous neuronal discharges resembling some kinds of epileptic activity using techniques such as: multichannel intracellular recordings, voltage and patch clamp, focal drug application, and modifications of the ionic environment. All of these would be difficult in vivo in experimental animals, and, until recently, impossible in human material.

The clinical relevance of fundamental studies on experimental models must start and finish with the human condition. Many of the key questions were framed decades ago on the basis of recordings made from human epileptic patients from scalp electrodes, and from intracranial electrodes both during and preceding operations to remove epileptogenic tissue. These techniques open novel insights into human epilepsy, and in particular allow us to see how basic processes unravelled in animal models can be applied to clinical problems. They include: the use of brain slices removed during surgery and maintained in vitro

for detailed electrophysiology, through modern variants of the EEG, using advanced computer analysis or novel recording methods such as the MEG, to non-invasive anatomical and biochemical investigations using magnetic resonance imaging, PET and other kinds of imaging (Delgado-Escueta et al 1986).

Cellular features

Typically an epileptic brain behaves normally most of the time, but this is interrupted episodically by abnormal activity, almost always an excessively synchronous discharge of cortical neurons (Fig. 8.1). The transition from irregular, fast, low-amplitude EEG activity to the slower, more rhythmic, high-amplitude EEG of an epileptic discharge was apparent from the earliest EEG recordings. This was interpreted as evidence of increased synchronization, but it was not until intracranial recordings were made from epileptic patients that the correlation of EEG 'spikes' and 'waves' could be made explicitly with the firing of individual neurons. Perhaps one-third to a half of units (single neurons recorded extracellularly) in an epileptic focus can be phase locked to the epileptiform EEG (Ishijimi et al 1975, Babb et al 1987). These unit recordings also showed a second abnormality, that they tended to fire in brief, rapid bursts of action potentials, which has been taken as a signature for 'epileptic' neurons (Ward 1969, Calvin 1980). Bursts of action potentials and synchronization are particularly prominent during seizures, but they can also be seen at other times, as the 'interictal EEG spike' which is often used as a diagnostic for epilepsy (Fig. 8.1). Experimental phenomena resembling the interictal event have played a central role in much of the recent progress in this field.

Primary generalized epilepsies differ from their focal relations in many important respects, but they too exhibit excessively synchronous cortical activity. Their characteristic property is that they do not have an identifiable site of initiation. More specifically, they appear to have a simultaneous onset in the two cerebral hemispheres at least at the time resolution of an EEG recording. The only primary generalized epilepsy which is understood in any detail at the cellular level is absence seizures or 'petit mal'. The extent of the EEG synchronization over the cortex is so large that it led to the hypothesis (Penfield & Jasper 1954) that the cortex was being driven by a hypothetical 'centrencephalic' system somewhere in the upper brain stem and diencephalon. It turns out that this was too simple a view, and that this problem centres on the interaction between the cortex and thalamus as an integrated system (Gloor & Fariello 1988, Steriade & Llinás 1988) as discussed below.

These observations on the 'natural history' of the diverse clinical epilepsies raise important questions on the basic mechanisms. How do neuronal discharges become hypersynchronized to generate the characteristic EEG features of the interictal event, of local (partial) seizures, and of primary and secondary generalized seizures? Why do epileptic discharges occur intermittently? What causes seizures to start? Why do they stop, usually after no more than a few minutes? What factors predispose an individual to epilepsy? What effects do repeated seizures have on brain structure and function?

APPROACHES TO STUDY

There are a bewildering variety of experimental treatments which can cause activity which has something in common with particular aspects of clinical epilepsies. Each has its own merits and limitations. Many of them have recently been reviewed by Fisher (1989). The choice of a particular model depends critically on the nature of the study, the questions posed, and hence the kinds of samples, recordings or observations required. For instance, the requirements for screening potential anticonvulsants (e.g. low cost, technical simplicity, large numbers) are quite different from those of basic studies of cellular mechanisms, where smaller numbers make unit costs less important, and the intensive use of highly skilled personnel is acceptable. I will briefly consider the issues raised by screening for anticonvulsant drugs, where costs are a significant issue, and observations usually are limited to visual and/or EEG recordings. More fundamental studies use a greater variety of more sophisticated recordings to study cellular events, which make quite different demands of experimental models.

Drug screening and drug development

The pharmacological mechanisms of the mainstream anticonvulsants have recently been reviewed in detail (Rogawski & Porter 1990). It is clear that these drugs can operate on many different aspects of neuronal function. Many have multiple cellular effects, which confuses matters, although the issue can be simplified somewhat with careful consideration of clinically relevant doses and specific sites of action in the brain. Some anticonvulsants have as their predominant effect the potentiation of synaptic inhibition mediated by GABA, e.g. the benzodiazepines and barbiturates, which interact with the $GABA_A$ receptor, and the novel anticonvulsant vigabatrin (γ-vinyl-GABA) which blocks the catabolic enzyme GABA-T (GABA transaminase). Others block voltage-dependent ion channels in neuronal membranes, with selectivity either for sodium (e.g. phenytoin, carbamazepine, valproate), or for calcium (e.g. phenytoin, barbiturates, and the anti-absence drug, ethosuximide). Finally, there is a new group of potential anticonvulsants which block receptors to excitatory amino acids which are responsible for most of the fast excitatory synaptic transmission in the brain. Most of these affect the NMDA (N-methyl-D-aspartate) receptor (named after a selective agonist); examples include APV (2-amino-5-phosphonovaleric acid), MK-801, and PCP (phencyclidine).

The search for new anticonvulsants is a major area in its own right, and has recently been reviewed elsewhere (Löscher & Schmidt 1988). In its early stages it depends largely on screening of candidate drugs on a limited number of animal models. Models for drug screening need to be simple and cheap to administer. The most common of these are electroconvulsive shock and systemic injections of pentylenetetrazol (PTZ). Tests based on these two treatments come in a variety of forms. They may use a fixed (usually supramaximal) dose of convulsant or they may estimate the threshold dose of convulsant; they also use a variety of end-points (e.g. onset of clonic seizures, onset of tonic seizures). The various combinations of these conditions provide some selectivity for anticonvulsants acting against the major seizure types, although there is a slightly circular quality to the argument because the specificity of the screening tests often is defined by their sensitivity to the existing major anticonvulsants. Thus subcutaneous PTZ is regarded as a screening test for agents effective against 'petit mal', and maximal electroshock for those against generalized tonic clonic seizures.

Too limited a range of models can reduce the chance of finding really novel drugs; indeed given that the classification of models for screening depends on their sensitivity to existing anticonvulsants, the whole procedure tends to be rather circular. Löscher & Schmidt (1988) considered the problems presented by the search for new antiepileptic drugs in some detail and made specific proposals for the kinds of strategy that should be adopted. For instance they identified marked shortcomings in the screening of drugs active against focal seizures, and proposed the use of the 'kindling' model (see p. 250) to fill this gap. A key issue in the rational development of novel treatments is the identification of the basic mechanisms responsible for epileptiform activity. Two classes of novel antiepileptic drugs which owe something to considerations of basic mechanisms are blockers of GABA inactivation (most notably γ-vinyl GABA or vigabatrin) and the NMDA antagonists, such as APV and MK-801 (Croucher et al 1982). As Löscher & Schmidt (1988) point out vigabatrin, which has some promise clinically, would have failed the classical screening tests, and could have been missed if these had been used in isolation.

Fundamental studies

Drug screening can progress a long way using simple visual observations of the incidence of the motor signs of seizures. Fundamental studies need a much greater variety of recording methods. The technical constraints these present have a considerable impact on the choice of experimental model, which is far more important than considerations of cost or technical difficulty. Some of the preparations and experimental models of epilepsies that are available are described in the following pages.

In vivo and in vitro preparations

Experimental preparations in vivo

Epilepsy is a disorder of whole organisms. The first experimental studies used intact laboratory animals, either under anaesthesia, or freely moving. These preparations in vivo have largely been superseded by preparations in vitro, such as the brain slice, for studies at the level of the single cell or of small populations of cells and local circuits. However, studies in vivo still have important roles, and should not be forgotten in the face of the continuing drive to ever more reductionist explanations. They remain essential for placing more reductionist studies into context. Even the most discrete focal epileptic discharge tends to propagate to other parts of the brain, and indeed may have profound effects on the body as a whole through the motor, autonomic and endocrine systems. In vivo methods also are indispensable for screening new anticonvulsants and studying their toxicity and pharmacokinetics. They are also essential for studying seizure propagation and generalization, the behavioural correlates of seizures, the long-term structural and functional consequences of repeated seizures, and the genetics of epilepsies, where that is a factor. A detailed account of the kinds of technique used is beyond the scope of this chapter. Where the techniques are invasive, the preparation of the animal requires careful consideration of whether to use an anaesthetized animal which will not regain consciousness, or whether the anaesthetic will interfere with the observations or the epileptic activity. If the latter then some kind of chronically implanted electrode, cannula or other measurement system may be the best approach. These kinds of approach demand careful consideration of the animals' welfare, and the associated ethical and legal issues.

In vitro preparations: the brain slice

Tissue slices maintained in vitro have had a long history. They were used by biochemists since

Warburg's work in the 1920s and 30s, but it was not until the late 1950s that their value to electrophysiology became apparent. They now have a central role in fundamental studies of the epilepsies, as will be clear from much of the remainder of this chapter, and indeed they appear to dominate much of neuroscience as a whole (Dingledine 1984).

Techniques such as multichannel intracellular recordings to study local circuits, voltage clamp to study membrane currents, and patch clamp to study individual channels, can only be performed in vitro because of the mechanical stability, access and visibility such preparations provide. In vitro preparations also provide direct control over the extracellular environment, allowing the efficient use of drugs and ions to help unravel cellular mechanisms. Some decades ago in vitro preparations meant invertebrate tissues. This has changed radically with the development of the mammalian brain slice for electrophysiology, which provides the technical advantages of in vitro preparations in tissue which actually generates epileptic activity.

Brain slices are cut from fresh brain, using a razor blade or mechanical slicer (Jefferys 1981a), and quickly put into a suitable, oxygenated artificial cerebrospinal fluid. Usually they are about 400 μm thick, which allows sufficient oxygen to diffuse in, while being thick enough to preserve neurons and many of their local connections. They are kept in slice chambers of varying designs. Usually, but not always, the slice is in contact with a continuously changing, well-oxygenated liquid, the artificial cerebrospinal fluid. The ingredients for this medium are similar in most laboratories, and usually are variations on Krebs solution. They usually contain glucose (ca.10 mM) to support metabolism, and inorganic salts: mostly NaCl (typically 135 mM); $[K^+]$ is at 3–6.5 mM (the author feels that the lower end of the range is more physiological); $[Ca^{2+}]$ at 1.3–2.5 mM (the author uses 2 mM, which probably results in a free Ca^{2+} ion activity in the tissue of about 1.5 mM); other components include Mg^{2+} (1–2 mM), inorganic phosphate (1–2 mM), and bicarbonate (15–25 mM), which buffers the solution at about pH 7.4 when equilibrated with 5% CO_2.

Slices can be maintained in vitro for many hours in solutions of inorganic salts and glucose, as long as they are adequately oxygenated. They can be maintained, as organotypic slice cultures, for weeks in more complex tissue culture media in roller tubes (Thompson & Gähwiler 1989). Often the tissue is irradiated to kill glia which otherwise proliferate. The neurons flatten to a monolayer, which provides a useful combination of clear visualization of and access to the neurons, while they retain many of their connections.

Location of epileptic foci

Not all parts of the brain are equally susceptible to epileptic activity. In general it is the cortex which is most directly implicated, either the neocortex, or phylogenetically older regions such as the hippocampus, entorhinal cortex and piriform cortex. The structure affected determines the kinds of symptoms, the time course and to some extent the cellular substrate for the epileptic activity. Clinically the distinction between neocortical epileptic foci and limbic epilepsies with foci in hippocampus or amygdala, is important, because the latter tend to have profound behavioural consequences.

Neocortex

The neocortex is perhaps the obvious place to start, because it generates the abnormal EEG characteristic of most epilepsies. A wide variety of convulsants will trigger epileptic discharges both in vivo and in vitro, including the full range outlined on page 250. In several of them it appears that the midcortical layers, particularly layer 4–5, are especially sensitive to convulsants, and seem to have a key role in synchronizing epileptic activity.

Epileptic discharges can be induced by a wide variety of agents, including those that block synaptic inhibition, such as penicillin, picrotoxin and bicuculline, those that interfere with potassium channels in neuronal membranes, such as the aminopyridines and tetraethylammonium ions, and those that enhance excitability and EPSPs, such as incubation in media containing low levels of $[Mg^{2+}]_o$. The heterogeneity of the neocortex complicates the analysis of epileptic discharges, at least at a detailed level—for instance there are clear variations in propagation between cortical regions (Chervin et al 1988). On the other hand, it is conveniently accessible to studies in vivo, and works very well as a slice preparation in vitro.

The neocortex is intimately associated with the thalamus, with major reciprocal projections linking the two into what should perhaps be considered the thalamocortical system. On the whole this is disrupted in slices, which may be respons-ible for some of the differences in detail between the propagation of focal epilepsies in vivo and in vitro. More importantly, the whole system has to be present to support the primary generalized epilepsy known as absences.

Hippocampus

The hippocampus is an allocortical structure which occupies a key position in the limbic system. It is often the site of epileptic foci in limbic

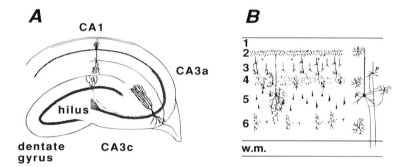

Fig. 8.2 Highly simplified cellular organization of the hippocampus (A) and neocortex (B), two structures that feature prominently in the text. (A) The hippocampus consists of a layer of pyramidal cells with neuropil on either side. There exist a variety of interneurons, not shown here. Most are inhibitory; they represent 5–10% of the total neuronal population; the best understood are the basket cells close to the pyramidal layer, but there are other distinct types towards the distal ends of both the apical and basal pyramidal dendritic fields. The nomenclature used here divides the pyramidal layer into zones CA1–CA4. CA1 is next to the subiculum, which connects to entorhinal cortex and temporal neocortex; it corresponds to Sommers sector or h1 in man, where the pyramidal cells are much more dispersed than they are in this diagram of the rat hippocampus. CA2 is rather variable in rodents, and will be considered as part of CA3 here to simplify matters. CA3 cells project widely to contralateral hippocampus, to ipsilateral CA1, locally, to septum and various subcortical structures. The pyramidal layer merges into the dentate hilus through CA4. The dentate granule cell layer, with the local circuitry in the hilus, act as gate controlling the sensory input to the hippocampus from the entorhinal cortex. (B) The neocortex classically is said to have 6 layers. The predominant neuronal type is again the pyramidal cell (*p*), constituting 80% or more of the population. There are two pyramidal layers, 3 and 5. Layer 5 contains the larger cells which project further afield. In primary sensory cortices layer 4 can be prominent, and contains granule cells, which are excitatory interneurons. The remaining non-pyramidal, or stellate, neurons include both excitatory (usually 'spiny') and inhibitory ('aspiny') types. Most of the neurons in the cortex receive input directly or within 1–3 synapses of the afferent axons in the white matter (WM). Output through the white matter is largely composed of pyramidal cell axons. Local circuitry is complex. Horizontal connections clearly are present and important, linking the vertical columns that have been demonstrated functionally in most cortical areas. Both hippocampus and neocortex lend themselves well to the brain slice preparation. Typically such slices are 400 μm thick, and can be maintained in vitro for many hours. Their mechanical stability, visibility and depth all help electrophysiological recordings greatly, and being an in vitro preparation simplifies studies of drug actions and of the effects of manipulating extracellular ion concentrations.

epilepsies (also known as temporal lobe epilepsy, complex partial seizures). Clinically foci here can present major problems both for medication and for interictal impairments, e.g. of cognitive function. Hippocampal foci constitute a major part of the caseload in surgery for epilepsy.

Many treatments can be used to trigger experimental epileptic activity in the hippocampus, both in vivo and in vitro. In many cases the subregion of the pyramidal layer known as CA3 is the site of initiation of epileptiform discharges (Fig. 8.2). This is the case for all the acute convulsant drugs, including penicillin, picrotoxin, and 4-aminopyridine, as well as for many of the chronic and subacute models such as tetanus toxin and cholera toxin. The other major group of pyramidal cells has been implicated in the synchronous bursts elicited by low $[Ca^{2+}]_o$, and in the prolonged 'ictal' or 'seizure-like' discharges in low $[Mg^{2+}]_o$ and high $[K^+]_o$; these cases all depend on quite distinct mechanisms from those leading to synchrony in CA3.

Piriform cortex and amygdala

The piriform cortex is a phylogenetically old part of the cerebral cortex which receives its major excitatory input from the lateral olfactory tract, and is contiguous with the amygdala. Both structures are particularly sensitive to kindling, and slices including both structures prepared from kindled rats retain epileptic discharges (McIntyre & Wong 1986). These structures are readily made epileptic by a wide range of convulsant treatments, including 4-aminopyridine, bicuculline and low-$[Mg^{2+}]_o$ (Gean & Shinnick-Gallagher 1988, Hoffman & Haberly 1989). The deep prepiriform cortex has been implicated as an intensely epileptogenic area in vivo, and has even been renamed 'area tempesta' (Piredda & Gale 1985). Amygdala foci represent an important group of clinical mesial temporal lobe epilepsies.

Cerebellum

The cerebellum is a major cortical structure, which differs from the other cortices in that the principal neuron, the Purkinje cell, is GABAergic, and thus is inhibitory. This difference may explain why the cerebellum does not support epileptic discharges. However, the synchrony of Purkinje cells can be modulated dramatically by the deep cerebellar nuclei, for instance by drugs such as harmaline, but this never reaches anything as dramatic as an epileptic seizure. Electrical stimulation of the cerebellum through implanted electrodes appears to damp down seizures generated in the neocortex, and this has been used to control seizures in the past, but this procedure is rarely, if ever, used today.

Models

Classification by time course

Experimental models of epilepsies can be divided into three broad categories: acute, chronic and genetic. Acute models typically use convulsant drugs or changes in extracellular ion concentrations (Table 8.1); the epileptogenic activity usually ceases on returning to control conditions. Chronic models typically involve implanted heavy metal compounds, injected toxins, local lesions, or repeated stimulation (Table 8.2). These treatments lead to a prolonged state of increased seizure susceptibility, or to recurrent spontaneous seizures. A permanent change of this kind is clearly chronic. However, there are many models where epileptogenic states persist for a few days or weeks; the precise cut off between acute and chronic is arbitrary, but it can be useful to call some of the briefer (few days) models subacute. Genetic models depend on identifying epilepsy-prone states in natural populations (e.g. photogenic baboon) or artificial selection for epileptic traits in laboratory species (e.g. tottering mouse, genetically epilepsy-prone rat); the underlying phenotypic changes responsible for the susceptibility to epilepsy are varied, and poorly understood in most cases.

Most definitions of epilepsy specifically exclude the single seizure, so it could be argued that acute models can only assess specific symptoms, e.g. interictal spikes or seizures, rather than epileptic states. Chronic models where epileptic discharges recur can be said to resemble more closely epilepsy as a condition. Some of the first experimental models happened to be chronic, e.g. with

Table 8.1 A selection of the more commonly used acute convulsant treatments and their probable major cellular actions. With the exception of high $[K^+]_o$, the alterations of extracellular ions are really only useful in vitro; the other agents are used both in vivo and in vitro.

Convulsant	Likely action
Penicillin	Blocks synaptic inhibition
Picrotoxin	Blocks synaptic inhibition
Bicuculline	Blocks synaptic inhibition
Low $[Cl^-]_o$	Blocks synaptic inhibition
Metrazol, PTZ	Blocks synaptic inhibition (at low doses)
Aminopyridines	Block membrane potassium currents
Tetraethyl ammonium (TEA)	Blocks membrane potassium currents
High $[K^+]_o$	Increases cellular excitability, and perhaps depresses synaptic inhibition
Low $[Mg^{2+}]_o$	Increases excitability, boosts NMDA component of glutaminergic EPSP
Low $[Ca^{2+}]_o$	Increases cellular excitability, promotes nonsynaptic synchronization

intracerebral tetanus toxin (Roux & Borrel 1898) or local freezing (Openchowski 1883). However it was studies of the actions of acute convulsants, such as penicillin, that were responsible for most of the remarkable progress made on the cellular mechanisms of the synchronization of epileptic discharges. In the first studies of convulsant drugs they were applied topically to the brain in vivo, but more recently they have mainly been studied with the brain slice preparation, which has many technical advantages for cellular studies. Over the last few years, several laboratories have started to use brain slices prepared from animals made epileptic with one of the chronic or subacute treatments, which provides the prospect of getting the best of both worlds, albeit with the added problem of distinguishing the initial causes of the epileptic activity from its long-term consequences.

Kindling—a special chronic model

Kindling differs from many of the other chronic

Table 8.2 Some of the more commonly studied subacute, chronic and genetic models of epilepsies. The genetic models usually are primary generalized, absence-type, while the others are focal with secondary generalization. In most cases there are multiple abnormalities at the cellular level, which makes precise identification of mechanisms difficult.

Agent	Cellular action	Gross lesion	Time course
Metals			
Alumina	Gliotic scar; greater loss of inhibitory than excitatory synapses	Yes	Years (primates)
		Yes	3 weeks
Cobalt	Some loss of GABA cells		
Iron salts	Unclear—changes in lipid properties, amino acid metabolism and noradrenergic function		>2 months
Lesions			
Freeze lesion		Yes	variable
Kainic acid	Loss of inhibition; altered intrinsic properties; synaptic remodelling	Yes	3–4 weeks
Toxins			
Tetanus toxin	Blocks synaptic inhibition	Rarely	6 weeks to >7 months
Cholera toxin	Blocks potassium currents	No	5–8 days
Kindling	Loss of inhibition; altered EPSPs; synaptic remodelling; etc.	Usually not	Permanent
Genetic			
Tottering mouse	Hyperinnervation by noradrenergic fibres, ?disinhibition; synaptic remodelling		
Mongolian gerbil	Excessive inhibitory interneurons in dentate area—?disinhibition		
Genetically epilepsy prone rat (GEPR)	Possible increased inhibition in thalamus		
Photosensitive baboon	? Altered inhibition		

experimental epilepsies listed in Table 8.2 in that it does not necessarily involve convulsant drugs. Its essential feature is the repeated presentation of some kind of stimulus. Often this is through electrodes implanted in either the amygdala or hippocampus (Goddard et al 1969). The stimulus can also be a chemical, such as pentylenetetrazol, either injected through an implanted cannula, or given systemically. All that appears to matter is that the stimuli must trigger some kind of after-discharge in one of the susceptible regions, and they must be repeated at a suitable interval, usually once to a few times a day. The definitive feature of kindling is that the electrical and behavioural response to these stimuli progressively increases, so that a constant stimulus which initially can be minimal and clearly non-convulsive response ultimately triggers generalized motor seizures. In most species it is difficult to produce spontaneously recurring seizures. However, the reduction in seizure threshold is more or less permanent.

Interest in kindling stems from several important considerations. First, the phenomenon is independent of any particular kind of stimulus, so that it can be considered a property of the nervous system rather than of any specific convulsant treatment. Second, is the clinical issue of whether kindling can occur in man, which is contentious (Bolwig & Trimble 1989); if it does, then anticonvulsant treatments may be indicated in a number of situations that could result in potentially kindling stimulations (e.g. head injuries, first fits). Third, it has been very influential in ideas of neuronal plasticity and cellular mechanisms of learning and memory. Fourth, kindling-like processes are likely to be involved in all chronic experimental epilepsies because by definition they generate epileptic activity repeatedly.

Epileptogenic treatments that block synaptic inhibition

Acute (topical) convulsants blocking inhibition. Acute convulsants can be broadly divided into those which interfere with synaptic inhibition, and those which do not. While much of the early work studied the topical application of these drugs to the neocortex, hippocampus and other structures in vivo, most of our current understanding of the cellular mechanisms of their actions derives from work on brain slices.

Penicillin was one of the first topical convulsants to be studied (Prince, 1969). It is now clear that it works by blocking synaptic inhibition mediated by the $GABA_A$ receptors. Similar actions have been found with the more specific and potent blockers of $GABA_A$ responses, bicuculline and picrotoxin. The convulsant drug most often used for drug screening, PTZ, probably also works by blocking $GABA_A$ receptors; its other effects on neuronal function tend to require higher doses (Leweke et al 1990). Bathing brain slices in solutions in which chloride has been replaced by impermeant anions has similar effects. The activity found with these disinhibitory models is reminiscent of the interictal spike of the epileptic EEG. This has now been studied in great detail by many laboratories, and has been instrumental in developing the cellular models of epileptic synchronization which are outlined below.

Penicillin is capable of inducing a very different experimental epilepsy when injected systemically or applied to the brain in vivo in very low doses (compared with those used to block inhibition). Under these conditions cats develop a 3 per second spike-and-wave EEG, which models the primary generalized epilepsy, absence or petit mal (Gloor & Fariello 1988). Inhibition appears to be preserved in this 'feline generalized penicillin epilepsy', presumably because of the low concentration of penicillin in the tissue.

Chronic models where inhibition is impaired. There is clear evidence of disrupted synaptic inhibition in at least one chronic experimental epilepsy. That is the chronic focal epilepsy which results from intracerebral injection of tetanus toxin (usually in the rat). The epileptic focus persists for weeks in the hippocampus (Hawkins & Mellanby 1987, Jefferys 1989, Jefferys & Empson 1990), and for months in neocortex (Brener et al 1991). In both cases, IPSPs are severely depressed (Jordan & Jefferys 1992, Brener et al 1991), and in the hippocampus at least this is due to impaired GABA release (Jefferys et al 1991). Impaired release of GABA is consistent with what was known of the toxin's acute actions on the CNS (Collingridge et al

1981), but these impairments outlive the presence of the toxin, which has a half life of the order of days. Inhibitory neurons are still present, in the hippocampus at least (as indeed are the pyramidal cells in most cases), so the toxin disrupts inhibitory function rather than kills inhibitory cell (Najlerahim et al 1992). Interestingly, the interneurons in all subregions of both hippocampi contain increased amount of messenger RNA (mRNA) for the synthetic enzyme for GABA, glutamic acid decarboxylase (GAD) (see also p. 269). However, even in the case of the tetanus toxin model, the relationship between disinhibition and epilepsy is not simple. Thus both hippocampi become epileptic following a single-sided injection of the toxin, but only on the injected side is there a loss of GABA release and a general loss of IPSPs within the focus (Empson & Jefferys 1992); contralaterally GABA release is normal and IPSPs are depressed in some pyramidal cells.

Extensive efforts have been made to find evidence of disrupted inhibition in several other chronic models, mostly using neurochemical and anatomical methods. These include assays for the inhibitory transmitter, GABA, for its receptors, and for its synthetic enzyme GAD. Histological methods include: enzyme histochemistry, immunocytochemical methods for GABA and GAD, radioligand binding for GABA receptors, in situ hybridization for the message for GABA receptors or for GAD, and quantitative electron microscopy for numbers of symmetrical synapses, which are almost always inhibitory. The alumina focus has been studied in some detail. Here there was evidence of a loss of both inhibitory and excitatory synapses and increased glial appositions onto neurons (Ribak 1986). In the centre of the epileptic focus there was a greater loss of ultrastructurally symmetrical (inhibitory) synapses than asymmetrical (excitatory) ones. Surprisingly, the surrounding parafocal tissue, which also plays a significant role in epileptogenesis, had a selective loss of the asymmetrical synapses. This suggests that the story cannot be a simple loss of inhibition analogous to the acute models such as penicillin or bicuculline.

In the case of kindling, there is much evidence on inhibitory function from electrophysiology,

anatomy and neurochemistry. The story is complex and confusing, with different results depending on the type of kindling stimulus, and the site, timing and type of the measurements. Inhibition actually appears to be enhanced in some regions, such as the hippocampal dentate gyrus (Stringer & Lothman 1989). However, it does appear to be disrupted in the CA1 region of the hippocampus (Kapur et al 1989, Kamphuis et al 1988); curiously, there also is a sustained increase in K^+-evoked GABA release here, which has been interpreted as implicating some kind of desensitization process in the physiological impairment of inhibition (Kamphuis et al 1990). The changes in inhibition could be secondary to other changes in the functioning of the local neuronal circuitry, because they appear to depend on NMDA receptor mediated responses to excitatory synaptic transmission (Stelzer et al 1987, Kapur & Lothman 1990), and are associated with reorganization of at least some pathways (Sutula et al 1988). This issue will be discussed in more detail below.

Lesions can lead to epileptic foci. The alumina model mentioned above results in a local loss of neocortical neurons and proliferation of glia, which appear to be necessary for the focus to develop, but not for its continued expression. In contrast, lesions induced in the hippocampal CA3 region by kainic acid have been studied in some detail at the cellular level, and there is evidence of impaired inhibition in the surviving CA1 region (Ashwood & Wheal 1986a, Franck et al 1988, Cornish & Wheal 1989). There are other changes in the kainic acid model, for instance an increased role of NMDA receptors which could be a consequence of the loss of inhibition (Ashwood & Wheal 1986b), and the sprouting of new axons, which probably is not (Tauck & Nadler 1985, Cronin & Dudek 1988); these diverse observations complicate pinpointing the underlying mechanisms of epileptogenesis.

Complications in assessing inhibitory function in chronically epileptic tissues. Overall, the evidence suggests that most chronic experimental epilepsies cannot be simply explained by a loss of inhibition. However, it is important to remember that in the one case where we do have clear evidence of a loss of inhibition, in the tetanus toxin model, most if not all of the neurochemical and histological markers for GABAergic inhibition would be intact. Certainly we know that the mRNA for GAD is still being produced by the same number of cells, indeed they are doing so in larger quantity (see p. 269). This means that the continued presence of a transmitter, such as GABA, or its synthetic enzyme, GAD, or indeed other neurochemical markers, only means the neurons are still present; it does not mean they are functioning normally. Similarly, the kainic acid lesioned hippocampus retains intact many of the neurochemical measures of the GABA system, but still has impaired inhibition (Franck et al 1988, Cornish & Wheal 1989). Conversely the apparent loss of GABA-immunoreactive neurons from the kindled hippocampus did not in fact mean that they had been lost, because they subsequently reappeared (Kamphuis et al 1987); probably it reflected a depletion of GABA due to enhanced release (Kamphuis et al 1990).

Inhibition is a complex process, and it can be disrupted at many other points. For instance in the case of hippocampal kindling, desensitization or down-regulation of GABA receptors has been hypothesized as a corollary of the sustained increase in K$^+$-evoked GABA release (Kamphuis et al 1990). The complexity of the factors controlling inhibitory function has been made clear in a detailed study, in hippocampal slice cultures, of the fading of inhibition with prolonged stimulation (Thompson & Gähwiler 1989). Receptor desensitization, changes in postsynaptic chloride balance, and presynaptic inhibition through GABA$_B$ receptors are amongst the factors involved. None of these is easy to study, and yet a change in any of these processes could contribute to epileptic activity. Although the author might be guilty of some bias, he cannot help concluding that the safest way to assess whether or not inhibition has been disrupted in epileptic tissue is to measure it directly by electrophysiological methods.

Genetic models. There exist many different genetic models of epilepsies. Even where an epileptic trait has been mapped to a single gene, it is usually not at all obvious what the phenotypic implication of that mutation should be. In several cases there have been careful quantitative immuno-cytochemical studies of inhibitory neurons. Surprisingly, none of these have shown a lack of GABAergic neurons. Indeed several appear to have more than their non-epileptic counterparts. This is the case in the hippocampus of the seizure-sensitive Mongolian gerbil, and in the thalamus of the genetic epileptic-prone rat (GEPR) (Ribak 1986). This has been interpreted as indicating that the extra inhibitory neurons may have the effect of inhibiting the inhibitory output to the principal neurons in these regions. While this is an interesting hypothesis, electrophysiological studies are needed to determine whether or not this is the case. An alternative hypothesis, at least in the case of the GEPR is that the stronger recurrent inhibition onto the relay cells would boost their synchronization through the cycle of inhibition and rebound excitation discussed below. Both of these potential mechanisms amplify the point that inhibition and excitation cannot simply be summed algebraically; it is the local circuitry that is the key to what neurons actually do to each other, and hence whether hypersynchronous activity will emerge from a particular population of cells.

Human epilepsy. Work on the chronic experimental epilepsies shows just how difficult it can be to assess the state of inhibition in epileptic tissue. These problems are exacerbated in human tissue by the variability of cases, and by obvious practical and ethical problems in obtaining measurements at an early stage which would not be complicated by the consequences of years of recurrent seizures and medication. In spite of very limited evidence, the idea that inhibition is disrupted in epileptic tissue has often been repeated since its earliest expression (in somewhat different terms) by Gowers (1881).

A coherent case has been put forward by Lloyd et al (1986) on the basis of neurochemical studies of GAD activity and GABA$_A$ binding sites in biopsy samples obtained during surgery for intractable epilepsy. These show a significant drop in both measures in patients with epileptic foci not attributed to tumours, and the authors conclude there is a depression of GABAergic function in 60–70% of this patient group. Some of the uncertainties in the interpretation of this kind of data have been outlined on page 252 on the assessment of inhibition in chronic experimental epilepsies. More information is needed on whether these results for human tissue are due to a loss of neurons. If so, then we need to know whether this is a specific loss of inhibitory neurons, or whether it reflects a generalized loss of neurons at the epileptic focus. If the latter, then the local circuits connecting the remaining cells becomes a key issue. Whatever the interpretation of these kinds of result, the essential question is the functional efficacy of inhibition in epileptogenic tissue. Slices from similar patients seem to have at least some IPSPs as recorded with intracellular electrodes (Schwartzkroin 1986, Avoli & Olivier 1989), although it is possible that inhibition is compromised in more subtle ways, for instance in fading more quickly with repeated use (Masukawa et al 1989).

Implications of inhibition for antiepileptic therapy. While it is difficult to sustain the case that a loss of inhibition causes epilepsy in all cases, that does not invalidate the idea that boosting inhibition might be a good way of controlling seizures. Indeed several drugs, notably the benzodiazepines and barbiturates, do enhance GABAergic function. Drugs that block GABA inactivation, such as vigabatrin, may have special attractions in that they will tend to boost and prolong the effects of endogenous GABA which should be released during seizures, giving a degree of selectivity (Rogawski & Porter 1990).

Experimental epilepsies with intact inhibition

Acute models. Disrupting inhibition may be sufficient to induce epileptic activity, but it certainly is not necessary. Indeed the generally negative results from studies of the GABAergic system in most chronic experimental and human tissues suggest that the more clinically relevant kinds of epileptic activity may well proceed in the face of more or less intact inhibition. Certainly epileptiform discharges can be triggered by a range of agents which do not interfere with synaptic inhibition. These include agents such as the aminopyridines, low extracellular Mg^{2+}, and elevated extracellular K^+. The aminopyridines have a primary action of blocking voltage-dependent K^+ channels, which tends to increase neuronal excitability and to enhance synaptic transmission by prolonging presynaptic depolarization (Ives & Jefferys 1990, Rutecki et al 1987); tetra-ethyl ammonium and related ions have similar effects. Elevated $[K^+]_o$ depolarizes neurons, which increases their excitability and has several other effects, but a total block of inhibition is not one of them (Traub & Dingledine 1990).

Low $[Mg^{2+}]_o$ both increases neuronal excitability by reducing charge screening of membranes by divalent cations, and by promoting a greater contribution to the EPSP from NMDA-type glutamate receptors, which tends to generate a stronger and more prolonged depolarization than the AMPA-type receptor which predominates in most excitatory synaptic transmission in the mammalian brain (Gean & Shinnick-Gallagher 1988, Jones 1989, Jones & Heinemann 1988). The NMDA receptor has several properties that are important in epileptogenesis in general. It admits Ca^{2+} into the cell, which is likely to be a factor in the development of histopathology (Simon et al 1984). It is also blocked by Mg^{2+} ions at resting potential, and not at depolarized potentials. This means it will be unblocked by the PDS, giving a further boost to the epileptic discharge (Ashwood & Wheal 1986b, Herron et al 1985, Thomson & West 1986). As a result NMDA antagonists act as selective anticonvulsants (Coutinho-Netto et al 1981, Croucher et al 1982), although at present they seem to have greatest clinical promise in treatment of stroke (Simon et al 1984).

Chronic models. In most chronic experimental epilepsies the underlying abnormality has yet to be identified. At least part of the problem is that too many changes can be found in most chronic models, and it is extremely difficult to sort out which is cause and which effect. In the case of the subacute focus established by cholera toxin, there is clear evidence of impairments of the intrinsic pyramidal cell properties which cause afterhyperpolarizations and action potential accommodation. The resulting enhancement of burst firing provides a reasonable hypothesis for epileptogenesis (Ives & Jefferys, 1991).

Kindling causes permanent reductions in seizure threshold. As described above, synaptic inhibition is impaired in some regions under some circumstances. Similarly, the kainic acid lesioned hippocampus has impaired inhibition, most prominently during the period of 2–4 weeks when the focus is most active. In both these examples, there are additional factors. Firstly, there is clear evidence of the sprouting of new axons, at least in the dentate area, and probably elsewhere (Tauck & Nadler 1985, Sutula et al 1988, Cronin & Dudek 1988, Ben-Ari & Represa 1990). Secondly there is an increased involvement of the NMDA subtype of glutamate receptor in EPSPs (Mody et al 1988), and there is evidence that NMDA receptor activation can lead to loss of inhibition (Stelzer et al 1987, Kapur & Lothman 1990). Thirdly, K^+ currents appear to be decreased, at least in kindling, perhaps allowing increased Ca^{2+}-mediated bursts (Kiss et al 1990). It is not yet clear whether the sprouting and increased NMDA receptor role in EPSPs are linked causally, but both are forms of plasticity (see p. 268).

Primary generalized epilepsies

In general we know much less about the cellular mechanisms of primary generalized seizures than we know about focal epilepsies. The one notable exception is with absence or 'petit mal' attacks, where several animal models exist which, together with recent advances in our understanding of the electrophysiology of the thalamus, have led to detailed theories on the underlying processes. Absence seizures are especially interesting because of their distinctive clinical, EEG and pharmacological features. They are characterized by: sudden bouts of behavioural unresponsiveness but rather minor motor signs; large, rhythmic, bilaterally synchronous spike-and-wave complexes at about 3 per second; and the drug of choice is valproate or ethosuximide.

The acute systemic administration of γ-hydroxybutyrate or penicillin produces absence-like states in a variety of mammals. Several genetic models also resemble absences in many respects, including the tottering mutant mouse, and genetically epilepsy-prone rats. The thalamocortical system has been implicated from several lines of evidence such as lesion studies, transient inactivation of brain regions with high levels of $[K^+]_o$, intracerebral recordings, and the regional sensitivity to petit mal convulsants and to the selective anti-absence drug, ethosuximide. It seems that the whole system has to be intact to generate the classic spike-and-wave EEG discharges. This has meant that much of the experimental work on absence attacks has had to use intact preparations in vivo (Gloor & Fariello 1988). These studies have been complemented by work on normal thalamus in vitro, either as slices or dissociated cells (Steriade & Llinás 1988, Coulter et al 1989). Together these two distinct approaches have led to a theory of the cellular mechanisms of absences which differs from those for focal epilepsies in many important respects; these will be discussed in more detail on page 262.

SYNCHRONIZATION

Focal epilepsies

The study of the cellular mechanisms of the synchronization of both hippocampal and neocortical neurons into epileptiform discharges has been one of the major successes in the basic mechanisms of the epilepsies. The mechanisms of the interictal discharge have been studied in immense detail in the case of the rodent neocortex and hippocampus, to the extent that the process, in the latter at least, can be simulated in biologically realistic computer models. The selective susceptibility of the CA3 region provided much of the impetus to identify the underlying mechanisms. The following account greatly simplifies and abbreviates a large volume of work. At an early stage, the cellular correlate of the interictal discharge was identified as an all-or-none depolarization of individual neurons, which was named the paroxysmal depolarization shift or PDS. The PDS differs from the EPSP in being much larger and more prolonged, and in being highly stereotyped, so that if it occurs at all, it occurs in its 'full blown' state, which is what is meant by its 'all-or-none' characteristic. The EPSP is smaller and varies smoothly with the number of active afferents (and hence with stimulus size).

One key argument concerned the relative roles of abnormalities at the level of single cells vs those at the level of small populations of cells (the 'epileptic neuron' vs 'epileptic aggregate' controversy

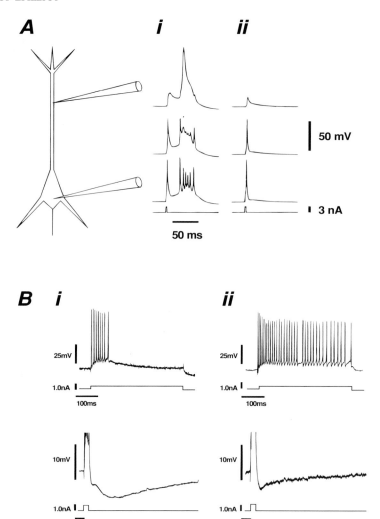

Fig. 8.3 Intrinsic neuronal properties revealed by intracellular recording from hippocampal CA3 pyramidal cells. (A) Computer simulations based on recent voltage clamp data show how the presence of voltage dependent calcium channels on the dendrites leads to a large, slow action potential, or calcium spike, in the dendrites (Ai, top trace), and repetitive firing of the cell body, which can outlast the duration of the intracellular current injection used to trigger this response (Ai, bottom trace). Both features disappear when the calcium channels are blocked (Aii). (B). Calcium entry activates certain potassium channels which limit the neurons ability to discharge in response to sustained depolarization ('accommodation'; Bi), and which lead to the 'afterhyperpolarization' or AHP (Bii). Many transmitters, such as noradrenaline, can modulate these channels through second messenger systems; the records in B were made from slices taken from a rat made epileptic by intrahippocampal cholera toxin 3 days previously. Panel (A) is modified from Traub et al 1991; panel (B) is unpublished data from A. E. Watts in the author's laboratory.

(Dichter & Spencer 1968)). In retrospect this was something of a false distinction. However, it did stimulate much work. There was a major debate on whether the PDS was essentially due to intrinsic mechanisms that could generate all-or-nothing depolarizations or whether it was essentially a giant EPSP. There now is direct evidence to support the latter (Johnston & Brown 1981), but, perhaps inevitably, intrinsic mechanisms do have a role to play, as we will discuss below.

Intrinsic burst mechanisms

Neurons have a remarkably wide repertoire of mechanisms to determine the ways in which they affect other neurons. The classic picture was an oversimplification. Synaptic inputs were ligand-gated ion channels on the dendrites of a neuron. The postsynaptic membrane potential changes were conducted passively to the soma or initial segment, where a weighted sum of all the inputs determined whether or not that cell would discharge action potentials. The action potentials were due to voltage-dependent sodium channels of the kind described by Hodgkin & Huxley in the 1950s, terminated by a combination of a time-dependent inactivation of the sodium channel and a slower voltage-dependent potassium channel which pulled the membrane back to its resting level.

Over the years it has become abundantly clear that there are many more kinds of ion channel in neuronal membranes. For our present purpose we will consider voltage-dependent calcium and potassium channels in general terms. The essential point here is that single neurons, even dissociated neurons which have been physically separated from all other cells, can generate prolonged, regenerative bursts of action potentials in response to brief injections of depolarizing current (Fig. 8.3). A combination of studies with ion substitution and various pharmacological manoeuvres has shown that voltage-dependent calcium currents have a key role in these bursts. In practice there are at least 3 different kinds of voltage-dependent calcium channel, which are distinguished by their thresholds and rates of inactivation. The T-type has a low threshold and inactivates relatively quickly (it is 'transient'); the

L-type has a high threshold and is long-lasting; and the N-type is like neither of these two, and appears to be restricted to neurons (Caterall 1988, Marty 1989, Hille 1989). These three classes of calcium channel may be important in different aspects of epileptogenesis. The Ca^{2+}-mediated bursts usually are terminated by voltage-dependent potassium channels which are activated by the increase in intracellular Ca^{2+} caused by the 'calcium spike'. These calcium activated K^+ channels are important in shaping the cells' output in other ways. They are responsible for 'accommodation', where action potentials driven by a constant depolarization slow down or even cease altogether (Fig. 8.3). Their significance is further underlined by their sensitivity to a wide range of neurotransmitters and neuromodulators, such as noradrenaline, dopamine, acetylcholine, opioid peptides and many more. Potassium channels form a family of at least a dozen closely related channels. In some circumstances, the sequential activity of these Ca^{2+} and K^+ currents can lead to rhythmic pacemaker activity (Carpenter 1982, Steriade & Llinás 1988, McCormick & Pape 1990).

Cortical neurons can be classified according to the presence or absence of intrinsic burst mechanisms, and this correlates well with morphological criteria (Connors et al 1982, Connors & Gutnick 1990, Chagnac-Amitai et al 1990, Mason & Larkman 1990). Intrinsic bursts appear to be particularly common in the subregions most susceptible to epilepsy, layer 4–5 in the neocortex, and CA3 in the hippocampus (Traub 1982, Wong & Prince 1978, Masukawa et al 1982). This reinforced the ideas of epileptic activity being an abnormality of the properties of individual cells. Indeed several convulsant agents interfere with aspects of the intrinsic burst mechanism, for instance the aminopyridines, TEA, and cholera toxin. Furthermore, phenytoin and barbiturates seem to exert some of their anticonvulsant effects by blocking Ca^{2+} channels (Rogawski & Porter 1990); the latter seem to be selective for the N-type Ca^{2+} channel, at least in the hippocampus. Ethosuximide also acts on Ca^{2+} channels, but it is selective for the T-type channels in the thalamus, which is important in its selective effects against absence seizures (Coulter et al

1989). The diversity of Ca^{2+} channels and their regional distribution provides some encouragement for the development of more specific anticonvulsants. However, it should be said that not all regions which are epileptogenic have cells with prominent intrinsic burst mechanisms, such as the piriform cortex, and there is some evidence that high $[K^+]_o$ depresses intrinsic burst mechanisms in hippocampal slices when it makes them epileptic (Traub & Dingledine 1990).

Mutual excitation

Intrinsic burst mechanisms are a common attribute of neurons in epileptogenic tissues, and can generate membrane potentials reminiscent of the PDS. However, a burst in a single neuron does not make an epileptic discharge. The synchronous activity of large numbers of neurons is essential. Furthermore, there is direct evidence for both hippocampus and neocortex that the PDS has many properties of an EPSP, albeit a very large one (Johnston & Brown 1981, Gutnick et al 1982). The picture that has emerged now is that the PDS is caused by what amounts to a positive feedback system mediated by mutual (or 'recurrent') excitation between the principal cells of epileptogenic tissues. This certainly is the case both in the hippocampus, between the pyramidal cells of the CA3 region (MacVicar & Dudek 1980, Miles et al 1984, Wong et al 1986, Christian & Dudek 1988), in the neocortex, between cells in midcortical layers (Szentagothai 1978, Gabbott et al 1987, Kang et al 1988, Takahashi et al 1989), and in the piriform cortex, between layer II pyramidal cells (Hoffman & Haberly 1989).

Disinhibited hippocampus. The CA3 region in the hippocampus receives major inputs from the dentate area, contralateral CA3 and the septum and sends output to the adjacent CA1 region, contralateral CA3 and CA1 and extrahippocampal targets. In the past there seemed to be a reluctance to consider direct connections between the pyramidal cells of either CA3 or CA1, in spite of evidence from the early literature of 'longitudinal association pathways' in CA3. However, the mutual excitation hypothesis of epileptic bursts was outlined some time ago on the basis of studies on denervated CA3 (Ayala et al

1973). More direct and quantitative evidence came from simultaneous intracellular recordings from pairs of pyramidal cells in brain slices obtained from normal (unlesioned) guinea-pigs and rats. These showed that monosynaptic excitatory connections do exist, but that they are not very common, which could explain the difficulty in demonstrating their existence in the past. Monosynaptic connections between CA3 pyramidal cells were found in about 1–2% of the dual intracellular recordings (Miles & Wong 1987). While this appears to be a very low probability of connection, it means that every cell is connected to 99% of the others within five to six synapses (Traub, quoted in Jefferys 1990). All that is required is that the output from each cell must diverge, on average, onto more than one other pyramidal cell, and that individual synapses must be strong enough to drive their postsynaptic cells (reviews in Wong et al 1986, Jefferys 1990). The pyramidal cell–pyramidal cell EPSP in CA3 is relatively large, at about 1 mV (Miles & Wong 1986). While this is not large enough to fire the follower cells, a brief burst of presynaptic action potentials is; the probability of discharging the postsynaptic cell increases from 4% to 30–50% as the number of presynaptic action potentials increases from one to five (Miles & Wong 1986). Intrinsic burst mechanisms may play a crucial role here, in amplifying the output from individual cells to the point that they reliably excite their postsynaptic targets.

It is important to remember that the mutual connections between CA3 pyramidal cells are not there specifically to cause epilepsy. Presumably they have a role in the functions of this region, which appear to involve some aspect of learning, perhaps as a working memory. These kinds of epileptic activity thus are unfortunate consequences of the abnormal operation of the normal circuitry of the region. Indeed the powerful inhibition found in the region most likely has been evolved because it prevents these recurrent excitatory circuits from developing epileptic discharges, and is most effective in this role, given that most animals are not spontaneously epileptic.

Epileptogenic treatments which do not block inhibition in hippocampus. The mechanisms of epileptogenic discharges have been worked out in considerable detail for the hippo-campal slice where inhibition has been blocked, usually by GABA antagonists of some kind. Epileptic activity also results from treatments which clearly do not block inhibition, and indeed may enhance it. Good examples include drugs that block potassium currents, such as the aminopyridines and tetra-ethylammonium ions, and manipulations of extracellular ions, such as reducing $[Mg^{2+}]_o$ or increasing $[K^+]_o$. Epileptic discharges originate from the same subregions as those due to GABA antagonists. However, there may be differences in the fine structure of the burst. In the cases of 4-aminopyridine (Ives & Jefferys 1990), high-$[K^+]_o$ (Traub & Dingledine 1990) and the subacute model induced by cholera toxin (Jefferys & Roberts 1987), the intracellular recordings show slow depolarizations or cascades of EPSPs which precede, by tens to hundreds of milliseconds, the synchronous epileptic bursts seen in the field potential records. This contrasts with the abrupt onset seen with most GABA antagonists. This suggests that the recruitment of individual neurons into the synchronous epileptic burst is more gradual than it is in the disinhibited slice.

The mechanisms of these three models differ in several respects. Aminopyridines block K^+ currents, and in consequence enhance both EPSPs and IPSPs; cholera toxin blocks different K^+ currents, notably the Ca^{2+}-dependent ones that cause accommodation of action potential firing during sustained depolarization, and the subsequent 'afterhyperpolarization'. The high (8 mM) $[K^+]_o$ epileptic activity is associated with increased neuronal excitability, and (hence) an increased incidence of spontaneous EPSPs; inhibition is depressed in this model because the reversal potential for Cl^-, and hence for the fast IPSP, shifts towards the resting potential, but certainly it is not abolished.

Intrinsic bursts appear to be depressed in the high $[K^+]_o$ model, presumably because Ca^{2+} channels are inactivated by the tonic depolarization, and this is thought to retard the spread of excitation through the network of pyramidal cells because it reduces the probability of pyramidal cells discharging their targets (Traub & Dingledine 1990). In contrast there is no evidence of a similar loss of intrinsic bursting in either cholera toxin or 4-aminopyridine. Here we suspect that the presence of inhibition is more important for retarding the spread of activity through the excitatory synaptic network in CA3, and that it also is a factor with the high-$[K^+]_o$ bursts, because their onset becomes highly synchronized when inhibition is blocked.

Hippocampus: an overview. Whether inhibition is present or whether it is absent, the key feature of the synchronization of epileptic bursts in the hippocampus is the mutual, or recurrent, excitatory synaptic connections between the CA3 pyramidal cells, and their ability to depolarize their postsynaptic targets up to the action potential threshold (Fig. 8.4). Normally the 1 mV unitary EPSP is too small to do this, but bursts of presynaptic action potentials lead to summation of the EPSPs, as seen in disinhibited slices, and might be expected with cholera toxin. Tetraethylammonium ions and 4-aminopyridine probably prolong presynaptic action potentials, increasing EPSP amplitude. Low $[Mg^{2+}]_o$ reduces the threshold for postsynaptic action potentials, and enhances EPSPs by unblocking NMDA receptors. Thus, in spite of the diversity of epileptogenic treatments in the hippocampus, we can speculate that they share a common underlying mechanism in enhancing the mutual excitation of CA3 pyramidal cells to the point that each cell is likely to be able to bring its immediate postsynaptic targets to threshold, thus permitting the spread of activity through the whole population. If the safety factor for this mutual excitation is large enough (as with disinhibition), the whole population is recruited within the time it takes to conduct through five or six neurons. If it is comparatively low, then the length of the excitatory chains becomes longer, and the recruitment of the whole population can take hundreds of milliseconds.

Neocortex. The existence of mutual synaptic excitation between neocortical neurons has been accepted for some time (Szentagothai 1978). Such connections have now been demonstrated anatomically, by spike-triggered averaging and, more recently, by dual intracellular recordings (Gabbott et al 1987, Kisvárday et al 1986, Kang et al 1988, Thomson et al 1988). In layer 5 pyramidal cells unitary EPSPs can reach 0.4 mV (Kang et al 1988), and in layer 3 they can reach 2.3 mV (Thomson et al 1988). Layers 4 and 5 appear particularly sensitive to a range of convulsants (Lockton & Holmes 1980, Connors 1984, Ebersole & Chatt 1986, Pockberger et al 1984). Interestingly, this is also the location of most neurons which normally can generate bursts of action potentials by intrinsic (Ca^{2+}-dependent) mechanisms (Connors et al 1982, Chagnac-Amitai et al 1990; Mason & Larkman 1990, Connors & Gutnick 1990). Therefore it seems reasonable to extend the kinds of mechanism outlined for the hippocampus to the neocortex, namely that cortical synchronization depends on mutual excitatory connections between the principal cells, and that these connections are made more effective by intrinsic burst discharges. The neocortex does differ in some respects, particularly in that its neurons tend to have larger resting potentials than those in the hippocampus, and this makes it more difficult for epileptic discharges to occur spontaneously.

The more superficial pyramidal layer, layer 3, appears to be able to sustain epileptic discharges independently of the deeper layers. Optical recording with voltage sensitive dyes have shown that layer 3 generates the maximum all or nothing discharge in neocortical slices exposed to either 3,4-diaminopyridine or bicuculline (Albowitz et al 1990). The laminar sensitivity of the effect of bicuculline is particularly surprising in view of the preferential effect of other blockers of fast IPSPs in layer 5 discussed earlier in this section. However, several studies on penicillin and bicuculline, particularly in vivo, suggest that the issue may not be so clear cut, locating epileptogenesis to layer 4 or a wider range from deep layer 3 to superficial layer 5 (in motor cortex) (Lockton & Holmes 1980, Holmes et al 1987). Superficial neocortical layers have been implicated in other experimental epilepsies, kindling with systemic PTZ (Barkaie & Gutnick, personal communication), and the chronic independent secondary mirror focus induced by neocortical injection of tetanus toxin (in contrast with the primary focus which centres of layers 4–5) (Brener et al 1991).

Both the mid-cortical layers 4–5 and the more superficial layers 2–3 have the apparatus to gen-erate epileptic discharges under suitable conditions. It is likely that there are mutual excitatory synapses between the neurons in both regions (see above, this section). However, intrinsic burster neurons appear to be restricted to layer 5 (Connors et al 1982, Mason & Larkman 1990; Connors & Gutnick 1990), although there is evidence that regular spiking neurons can be transformed into bursters by treatments such as injecting Ca^{2+} chelators (Friedman & Gutnick 1989), so that it is entirely conceivable that neurons can change their intrinsic properties under pathological conditions. Overall it appears that epileptic discharges can be synchronized at two neocortical layers, apparently centred on the superficial pyramidal layer (3) and the deeper pyramidal layer (5). There is evidence that each of these layers can sustain epileptic activity on its own. In other cases the distinction is less clear-cut, perhaps because of the spread across the conventional layers of both the dendritic trees and axonal ramifications of most of the neurons in layers 3 and 5, perhaps because cells are recruited into epileptic discharges from both layers 3 and 5 under many circumstances. Mutual excitation is likely to be a key issue in both layers (Fig. 8.4). However, the role of intrinsic bursting is less clear for layer 3 than it is for layer 5.

Other kinds of synchronization

Mutual excitation between principal neurons is not the only way to synchronize neuronal activity. One of the clearest examples of this was reported by several laboratories within a few weeks of each other (Jefferys & Haas 1982; Taylor & Dudek 1982; Haas & Jefferys 1984). Hippocampal slices bathed in solutions containing levels of $[Ca^{2+}]_o$ low enough to block synaptic transmission, after a delay of tens of minutes, started to generate synchronous discharges. These discharges differed from those seen with more commonly used convulsant treatments in originating most easily from the CA1 region, much more severe conditions being required to elicit them from CA3 or dentate (Snow & Dudek 1984). They also differed in their appearance. They tended to be more prolonged, lasting up to tens of seconds. They invariably had a negative field potential at the pyramidal layer;

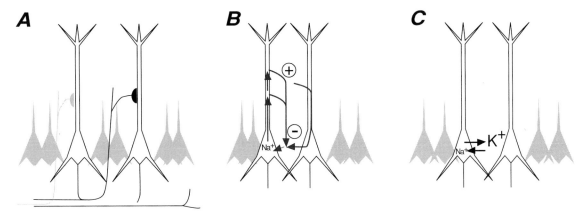

Fig. 8.4 Mechanisms of neuronal synchronization in the hippocampus. (A) Recurrent excitatory collaterals are found between about 1–2% of intracellular recordings made simultaneously from pairs of CA3 pyramidal cells. Simulation studies have shown that this relatively low incidence of monosynaptic connection is sufficient to synchronize epileptic discharges if inhibition is blocked, or if excitatory transmission and/or neuronal excitability are enhanced, e.g. by reducing extracellular magnesium ions ($[Mg^{2+}]_o$), adding aminopyridines, or elevating $[K^+]_o$. The incidence of such connections is probably higher in the neocortex, but each is less effective, and their role in epileptogenesis has yet to be defined quantitatively. (B) Field effects or ephaptic interactions can arise because of the relatively high extracellular current densities and thus potential fields that the hippocampus can generate. These currents tend to depolarize the membranes of adjacent neurons, to threshold if the conditions are suitable (e.g. under low $[Ca^{2+}]_o$, or during a prolonged depolarization). (C) Fluctuations in extracellular ions, especially increased K^+, result from neuronal activity, and tend to depolarize neighbouring neurons and glia. All three mechanisms have roles to play in epileptogenesis. Synaptic mechanisms (A) probably provide the initial synchronization and build up of excitation in most cases; they are effective on the few ms to few hundred ms timescale. Field effects (B) come to the fore when $[Ca^{2+}]_o$ has dropped and $[K^+]_o$ has risen during a seizure, or during metabolic disturbances of ion balance or of osmotic state; they are effective on a fast, ms timescale. Ion fluctuations (C) occur during seizures, and must affect neuronal excitability; they are effective over a slower timescale, of tenths of seconds upwards.

in contrast, synaptically generated bursts had a positive field, essentially due to the large current source driven by the excitatory synapses on the pyramidal cell dendrites (Fig. 8.4).

Two non-synaptic mechanisms were at work in the low $[Ca^{2+}]_o$ field bursts (Fig. 8.4). Fast synchronization (within milliseconds; burst velocities of about 0.1 m/s) is mediated by what we have called electric field effects, while slower synchronization (tens to hundreds of milliseconds; 0.001–0.01 m/s) is mediated through fluctuations in $[K^+]_o$ (Haas & Jefferys 1984, Dudek et al 1986, Konnerth et al 1984). The electric field effects are caused by the extracellular currents generated by the activity of one group of neurons depolarizing the membranes of their neighbours enough to change their excitability. Direct measurements of the sensitivity of populations of hippocampal neurons certainly show that they are sensitive to extracellular currents comparable to those that can be generated by neuronal activity (Jefferys 1981b). This phenomenon has also been termed

ephaptic interaction, although the original definition was limited to interactions between closely apposed neuronal elements, which differs from the situation here where it is the layered arrangement of principal neurons that matters.

The slower form of non-synaptic synchronization also depends on the activity of one set of neurons producing something that can excite their neighbours, in this case $[K^+]_o$ (Konnerth et al 1984). This is analogous to the phenomenon of spreading depression, with the important difference that $[K^+]_o$ stays within a physiological ceiling of 10–12 mM rather than reaching the many tens of millimoles characteristic of spreading depression; perhaps the more controlled K^+ mechanism should be called spreading excitation. The diffusion of ions is slower than the conduction of electric currents in solutions, which explains the slower propagation and onset of K^+-synchronized events.

The essential condition for these kinds of synchronization is that the neurons need to be close to threshold. Experimentally this is achieved by the low (0–0.2 mM) $[Ca^{2+}]_o$, low to normal (1–2 mM) $[Mg^{2+}]_o$ and moderately high (6 mM) $[K^+]_o$. These conditions can arise during seizures (Heinemann et al 1986), so that non-synaptic synchronization may well have a role in the development of a seizure. One factor in the susceptibility of the CA1 region of the rodent hippocampus to this kind of synchronization is the tight packing of the pyramidal cell bodies in stratum pyramidale; the restricted extracellular space reinforces both the electric and ionic mechanisms. Neurons in the human CA1 region are less densely packed, which further argues against nonsynaptic mechanisms triggering epileptic activity, but does not exclude them having a role once such activity has started. They also could be responsible for seizures under some extreme clinical conditions, such as severe water intoxication or gross reductions in free $[Ca^{2+}]_o$.

Primary generalized epilepsies

Role of thalamocortical system

Primary generalized epilepsies differ from focal epilepsies in many respects. In the best studied type, the absence attack, there is a widespread bilateral cortical synchronization of a high amplitude, very regular (typically 3 per second) complex EEG waveform known as spike-and-wave. Cortical neurons do not generate all or nothing PDSs; rather the EEG spikes correlate with a rather variable EPSP with superimposed action potentials, and the EEG wave with a prolonged IPSP (Gloor & Fariello 1988). Inhibition is clearly intact and indeed inhibitory neurons in the thalamus have been implicated in the synchronization of the epileptiform EEG. Studies using lesions or transient inactivation of neurons by high $[K^+]_o$ show that both the thalamus and the cortex are necessary for the expression of absence seizures. There is a high degree of correlation of unit discharges between the thalamic and cortical neurons and the cortical EEG. One theory is that there is a diffuse cortical hyperexcitability, and that this amplifies the otherwise normal thalamocortical circuitry. This would mean that this epilepsy resembles the focal models described

above in representing the abnormal operation of essentially normal neural processes.

Thalamic pacemaker mechanisms

Thalamic neurons have complex intrinsic properties which mean that modest shifts in their resting potentials cause dramatic transitions in discharge patterns when they are stimulated (Steriade & Llinás 1988). Normally thalamic neurons fire in a non-bursting manner, with a sustained train of action potentials in response to a steady depolarizing input; this is the kind of response seen in vivo while animals are awake. However, the same neurons transform into burster neurons (see p. 257) if they are hyperpolarized by 5–10 mV; this corresponds to sleep or to barbiturate anaesthesia in vivo, and is a key factor in the generation of the 'spindles' recorded from thalamus and cortex under these conditions (Steriade & Llinás 1988). Studies on slices and on acutely dissociated cells have shown that thalamic neurons have particularly well-developed 'T'-type Ca^{2+} membrane currents; this is the Ca^{2+} current with a low threshold and relatively rapid inactivation. The spindles seen under physiological conditions depend on an oscillation between the depolarization due this current and a hyperpolarization due to a Ca^{2+} dependent K^+ current which develops as the Ca^{2+} current inactivates. What makes this interesting for epilepsy is that the low threshold Ca^{2+} current is greatly depressed by the specific anti-absence drug, ethosuximide, at clinically relevant doses (Coulter et al 1990).

Inhibition as a mechanism for synchronization

Individual cells generating a rhythmic oscillation do not make an epileptic EEG. That requires synchronization (Fig. 8.5). The thalamus differs from the cortical structures described above in that it appears that synaptic inhibition entrains the cellular discharges. This was first proposed by Andersen & Sears (1964). More recent work has identified the inhibitory neurons involved as the reticular thalamic neurons (Steriade & Llinás 1988), which inhibit the thalamocortical relay neurons, and are excited by both the thalamocortical neurons and by cortical neurons.

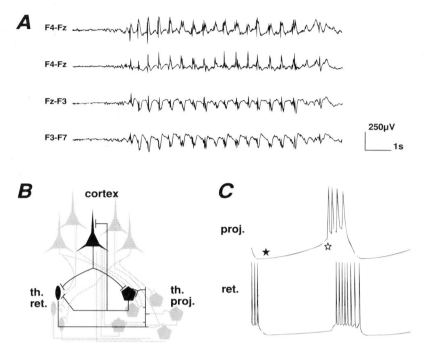

Fig. 8.5 Primary generalized epilepsies are characterized by epileptic EEG activity appearing simultaneously in both hemispheres. Absence attacks have a classical spike and wave pattern (A). (B) The local circuitry between thalamocortical projection neurons (th. proj.), cortical neurons, particularly in layer 6 (cortex), and the highly divergent, inhibitory, GABAergic neurons of the thalamic reticular nucleus (th. ret.) entrain the intrinsic oscillatory properties of the projection neurons (C). The synchronous hyperpolarization of many projection neurons by IPSPs (B: angled synapse; C: filled asterisk) from the reticular neuron input changes the projection neurons' T calcium channels from the inactivated state to the closed, activatable state; they reach threshold as the IPSPs wear off and the membrane potential approaches resting potential (C: open asterisk); the projection neurons burst, activating intrinsic AHP mechanisms, and inactivating the T channels, which tend to stop the burst (Fig. 8.3B), and synaptically exciting both cortex and reticular neurons which then inhibit the projection neurons Thus the T channel provides the 'rebound excitation' postulated many years ago by Andersen & Sears (1964) when they postulated the synchronization through inhibitory circuits. The structure and function of the thalamocortical system is reviewed in Steriade & Llinás (1988). EEG records (A) were kindly provided by D. Fish and P. Allen of the National Hospital for Neurology and Neurosurgery.

If the thalamic relay neurons are in a bursting mode (i.e. they are sufficiently hyperpolarized for the low threshold Ca^{2+} current to be activated), this activates the reticular thalamic neurons both directly and via the corresponding cortical area. These neurons in turn inhibit the relay neurons, helping to terminate the intrinsic burst (along with the intrinsic inactivation of the T channel, and the activation of Ca^{2+} and voltage dependent K^+ channels). The hyperpolarization which results from both the K^+ currents and the inhibition allows the T channels to reverse their inactiva-

tion, so that they reach threshold and initiate another burst as the membrane potential returns to its resting value. However, it is the location of the reticular neurons in the thalamocortical circuit, and the divergence of their output onto the relay neurons that entrains the bursts occurring in the different relay neurons (Steriade & Llinás 1988). The combination of this inhibitory network and the T current, which is the specific cellular mechanism of the 'rebound excitation' described by Andersen & Sears (1964), leads to the synchronous rhythmic oscillations characteristic both of absence seizures and of sleep and barbiturate spindles.

These observations on the cellular mechanisms of absence seizures make an interesting case history of the complementary roles of experiments both in vivo and in vitro and of clinical observation. Thus the detailed analysis of Ca^{2+} currents, and their sensitivity to antiepileptic drugs, depended on the slice preparation, while the role of inhibition in synchronization depended largely on studies in vivo, because of the dispersed anatomy of the systems involved, and the value of the data on ethosuximide rested on its specificity for absence seizures.

LOCAL PROPAGATION OF EPILEPTIC ACTIVITY

If epileptic activity remained localized at the few thousand neurons necessary for its initiation it would be unlikely to cause much trouble to the organism as a whole. But epileptic activity has a considerable tendency to spread, both within the same structure, and over longer distances in the brain.

The spread of epileptic activity has been studied in some detail in both hippocampus and neocortex. In the hippocampus synchronous bursts spread at 0.13–0.15 m/s through CA3, whether parallel or transverse to the long axis of the hippocampus (Knowles et al 1987, Miles et al 1988). Once initiated, discharges seem to propagate smoothly through the pyramidal layer, in either direction. This conduction velocity of the axon collaterals between the CA3 pyramidal cells is about 0.5 m/s (Miles et al 1988). The slower velocity, but longer range, of the epileptic discharge reflects delays in recruiting successive sets of pyramidal cells through the network of excitatory synapses.

Propagation of epileptic discharges through the neocortex also is mediated by axon collaterals, and proceeds at a little under 0.1 m/s in the rat cortical slice exposed to bicuculline (Chervin et al 1988). The precise pattern of propagation is complex. It differs between different cortical areas (primary and secondary visual, somatic sensory and motor), and it is not uniform over distances of the order of 0.1–1 mm, perhaps reflecting varia-

tions in the local interconnections associated with the functional organization of the cortex into columns. These nonuniformities become even more obvious, to the extent that they could block propagation entirely, when very low doses of bicuculline are used, which perhaps only reduce inhibitory synaptic currents by 10% (Chagnac-Amitai & Connors 1989).

Following the propagation of an epileptic discharge with electrodes can be difficult because the variability of the discharge can preclude tracking with a roving electrode, and suitable arrays for simultaneous recording can be difficult to construct, and can compromise slice viability through mechanical damage and obstruction of fluid access. Optical recording methods have real advantages in this kind of study, although they do require the addition of a foreign voltage-sensitive dye. Their spatial resolution is limited only by the microscope used, the density of the photodiode array, and the capacity of the signal acquisition system (usually a computer). They allow simultaneous monitoring of the spread of activity in both axes in the plane of the slice, thus identifying the layers of peak activity as well as the horizontal propagation (Albowitz et al 1990). Horizontal conduction velocities measured this way in slices exposed to two different convulsants, bicuculline and 3,4-diaminopyridine, ranged from 0.01 to 0.14 m/s, comparable to those obtained by electrical recordings from slices.

Epileptic discharges appear to be able to spread faster in vivo than they do in slices. Optical recordings, using voltage-sensitive dyes, have shown that interictal spikes spread at about 0.6 m/s across the cortical surface (London et al 1989); on rare occasions they could appear to spread at several m/s. This reinforces the idea that results from slices need to be interpreted carefully in the context of the whole animal. Several pathways are missing in the slice which could be important for the propagation of epileptic discharges across the cortex. First, horizontal intralaminar connections in the cortex often have a patchy distribution related to the columnar organization, so that axons can project 1–2 mm before ramifying into terminal network, and thus are likely to be disrupted in 400 μm thick slices. Second, the deep white matter carries longer-range cortico-cortical connections which have faster conduction velocities. Third, excitation can spread to the thalamus, both through cortico-thalamic connections from layer 6, and from ectopic action potentials generated in the thalamo-cortical axon terminals in epileptic foci (Leblond & Krnjevic 1989); thalamic activity can then excite wide areas of the neocortex.

SEIZURE ONSET

Seizures vs interictal events

The epileptic phenomenon best understood at a cellular level is the interictal EEG spike. While clinically this is useful for diagnosis, it is not a major problem for patients. Seizures differ from interictal spikes in many ways. They are much more prolonged, lasting tens of seconds or even minutes rather than fractions of a second. They usually involve much larger areas of neural tissue, and may generalize to affect the whole of the cortex, with consequent gross disturbances of behaviour. They may depend on quite different mechanisms of neuronal synchronization. Indeed they may be generated by distinct neural substrates. Finally, they may depend on long range interactions (e.g. mutual excitation) between distant structures in the brain, and thus require quite different analytic techniques from the interictal spike (e.g. whole animals rather than isolated brain slices).

Putative roles of nonsynaptic mechanisms

Seizures present problems for preparations like brain slices in vitro because the amount of tissue that can be used is limited by considerations of oxygen diffusion. However, several groups have now seen events in slices which resemble seizures, in duration at least. Manipulation of the extracellular ion composition seems particularly effective. Thus 'seizure-like' discharges have been seen in hippocampal slices exposed to high $[K^+]_o$ (Korn et al 1987, Jensen & Yaari 1988, Traynelis & Dingledine 1989). While interictal spikes started in CA3, the prolonged discharges originated in CA1, and had a negative field potential at the pyramidal cell body layer. These kinds of seizure-like discharge closely resembled the bursts seen with low-$[Ca^{2+}]_o$ (Jefferys & Haas 1982), and indeed nonsynaptic synchronizing mechanisms probably had major roles to play. The implication of these observations is that seizures differ categorically from interictal events in both their basic mechanisms, and in their substrate neuronal populations.

Exposing hippocampal slices to low-$[Mg^{2+}]_o$ also results in prolonged seizure-like discharges (Wilson et al 1988, Anderson et al 1986b, Schneiderman & MacDonald 1987, Mody et al 1987). In common with the high-$[K^+]_o$ model, there is some evidence that interictal and seizure-like discharges have different neural substrates. Interictal discharges start in CA3 as in most other examples. However, in this case it is the entorhinal cortex that appears to provide the substrate for prolonged, seizure-like activity. GABAergic inhibition in the dentate area seems to control the propagation of this seizure-like activity into the hippocampus, a situation reminiscent of the penicillin-induced entorhinal cortex foci in vivo (see p. 266).

Epileptic discharges lasting several seconds can be generated in the CA3 region of hippocampal slices, for instance following intrahippocampal injection of tetanus toxin (Jefferys 1989). This could constitute the early stages of a seizure. Recordings made in vivo with this model suggested that seizure discharges more prolonged than this always involved both hippocampi (Hawkins & Mellanby 1987). If prolonged seizures depended on propagation to the contralateral hippocampus, or indeed to extrahippocampal structures, such as the cingulate cortex as proposed in this case, then obviously they would not be seen in brain slices. Therefore in this particular chronic experimental epilepsy the suggestion is that the structures that interact to produce seizures are too widely separated to be included in a slice. This underlines the importance of studies in vivo for a complete understanding of epileptogenesis.

Seizure propagation

The propagation of seizures through the brain may well be a key to distinguishing them from interictal events. The dentate area has been identified as a critical structure controlling the propagation of epileptiform activity from foci in the entorhinal cortex in vivo (Collins et al 1983, Jones & Lambert 1990). Recent studies of epileptic bursts induced by low-$[Mg^{2+}]_o$ in slices cut to include both the hippocampus and entorhinal cortex showed that interictal spikes originated in CA3 as expected, but that prolonged bursts started in the entorhinal cortex and usually were damped by the dentate area; when GABAergic inhibition in the dentate was depressed, then seizure-like discharges could propagate through to CA3 (Wilson et al 1988, Rausche et al 1991).

Clearly once epileptic activity has propagated away from the initial focus, its analysis at the cellular level becomes much more difficult, studies in vivo become crucial, and a better understanding of how seizures propagate in man becomes urgent. One structure which has been implicated in the generalization of seizures in several models in vivo is the substantia nigra pars reticulata (Iadorola & Gale 1982). GABAergic inhibition in this midbrain structure appears to control the propagation of seizures, and in particular their motor manifestations. Only with more studies at this level can sensible experiments be designed at the levels of single cells and small populations of cells.

SEIZURE TERMINATION

If seizures last more than 5–10 minutes then severe brain damage or death can result, so that stopping such a prolonged seizure becomes an urgent clinical priority. However, in most cases seizures stop spontaneously within 2 minutes or so. Many systems in the brain can contribute to this rather useful property, and thus could earn the title of 'endogenous anticonvulsant'. Unravelling which is important is no easy matter, largely because of the mass of changes which are induced by excessive excitation over this kind of period.

It is unlikely that seizures stop because the tissue is 'exhausted'. Most studies suggest that the brain tissue continues to be reasonably well supplied with oxygen and other metabolites, at least for the first few minutes. Ion gradients across the neuronal membrane are usually sustained well enough to support action potentials, in marked contrast with the spreading depression phenomenon where gross changes in ion balance across the membrane cause a complete neuronal inactivation. Rather, seizures appear to be terminated by more specific mechanisms. Intrinsic neuronal mechanisms could play a significant role, such as the many voltage and Ca^{2+}-dependent K^+ currents. Ion pumps, notably the Na^+-K^+-Mg^{2+}-ATPase, are activated by the movements of ions caused by the intense neuronal activity during a seizure; however, unequal numbers of ions are exchanged across the membrane, making these pumps electrogenic, so that they hyperpolarize neurons while they restore the ion gradients.

Synaptic mechanisms provide more wide ranging mechanisms to terminate seizures than the intrinsic membrane properties of individual neurons. Synaptic inhibition also is a likely contributor, particularly the slow IPSPs mediated by the $GABA_B$ receptor, and there is some evidence for $GABA_B$ agonists controlling the transition from interictal to seizure like events in hippocampal slices incubated in low-$[Mg^{2+}]_o$ (Jones 1989, Lewis et al 1989). Fast IPSPs mediated by $GABA_A$ are less likely to contribute to the termination of seizures because they tend to fade with repeated use (Thompson & Gähwiler 1989). In contrast there are several neuroactive agents whose release increases with repetitive activation. Peptides are co-localized with 'conventional' transmitters in a large minority of neurons, and are released by trains of presynaptic action potentials (Siggins et al 1986). Interestingly, the behavioural inactivity that follows experimental epileptic seizures in many cases (perhaps analogous to Todd's paresis in man), is sensitive to the opioid peptide antagonist naloxone. Given that the opioids are inhibitory (except in the hippocampus where they selectively inhibit inhibitory interneurons), they are well-placed to boost inhibition when a region comes under the sustained activity of a seizure. Finally, adenosine is an effective endogenous modulator of neuronal excitability. It is released under intense activation, probably by a mixture of Ca^{2+}-dependent and independent mechanisms (i.e. both synaptic and reversed transporter mechanisms), and its analogues are potent antagonists (Chin 1989, Haas & Greene 1988, Stone et al 1990; O'Shaughnessy et al 1988)

The diversity of mechanisms that must be

activated by the intense and prolonged neuronal activity during a seizure means that seizure termination is likely to depend on several factors. Those outlined above are some of the better understood to date. Others are likely to emerge in time, and the particular combination responsible in each case will take some time to determine. Despite these caveats, these endogenous mechanisms do have significant attractions for the development of novel anticonvulsants.

LONG-TERM EFFECTS OF EPILEPTIC DISCHARGES

Most clinical definitions of epilepsy require seizures to recur; a single seizure does not constitute epilepsy. The repeated exposure of neural tissue to intense, hypersynchronous activity is likely to modify neuronal properties in several ways. Indeed the kindling model is entirely based on the long-term changes induced by repeated synchronous discharges. We will consider the kinds of long-term changes caused by epileptic seizures, roughly in descending severity: starting with frank pathology and ending with more subtle functional changes.

Neuropathology

The diverse range of pathologies associated with epilepsy is reviewed in detail in Chapter 7. In some cases they precede the onset of seizures, and act as a risk factor (see p. 252). In others they appear to be a consequence of seizure activity, and indeed long-standing epileptic foci often are associated with local losses of neurons, gliosis and atrophy of the tissue; less severe cases may exhibit distortion and loss of spines on dendrites (Scheibel et al 1974). Here we will restrict our discussion to experimental evidence on the mechanisms of neuronal damage due to seizure activity.

Several factors probably contribute to neuropathology following seizures. Prolonged seizures, i.e. lasting tens of minutes, are particularly likely to kill neurons (Seisjö & Wieloch 1986). This could suggest that the damage is essentially metabolic, e.g. due to anoxia, depletion of glucose, or accumulation of waste products. These could be factors in some cases, although there is

little evidence of anoxia in most experimentally-induced seizures. In at least some cases more specific factors are at work.

An important line of work implicates the build up of excitatory amino acids, such as glutamate, which probably is the neurotransmitter at the majority of fast excitatory synapses, and which certainly accumulates during seizures. Glutamate, and several related agonists, are potent neurotoxins when injected into many parts of the brain. This led to the 'excitotoxic' hypothesis of epileptic pathology (Olney et al 1986, Simon et al 1984). Normally glutamate is removed rapidly from the extracellular space by specific uptake mechanisms in glial and neuronal membranes. This mechanism is thought to be swamped by the continuous release of glutamate during a seizure, with the result that glutamate accumulates; together with the resulting membrane depolarization this activates NMDA receptors, Ca^{2+} ions accumulate inside the neurons, and activate a variety of proteases and other intracellular mechanisms which cause the damage (Meldrum 1986). There is much evidence to support this kind of mechanism. NMDA antagonists such as MK-801, APV and ketamine protect against such damage (though their anticonvulsant effects obviously are relevant), $[Ca^{2+}]_i$ does increase following insults that reliably kill neurons. There are likely to be other factors in cell death, but excitotoxicity is certainly a prominent mechanism.

Epileptic neuropathology is a very variable phenomenon. For instance in the author's work on the rat intrahippocampal tetanus toxin model, the incidence of seizures tends to be quite consistent at any given dose, and prolonged seizures (>2 minutes) are almost unknown at the very low doses used (a few ng protein, or 6–8 mouse LD_{50}). In most cases there is no loss of neurons in these rats. However, in a very small minority there is a clear loss of neurons, usually restricted to CA1, but more widespread in some groups of rats that have additional environmental or genetic risk factors (Jefferys et al 1992).

Gliosis

The proliferation of glia associated with epileptic neuropathology led to the hypothesis that disturbances of $[K^+]_o$ buffering, an important function of glia, might be important in epileptogenesis. However, direct measurements of the K^+ buffering capacity of gliotic scar tissue showed that it was not impaired (Heinemann & Dietzel 1984). The neuronal border to this kind of tissue may well be susceptible for other reasons, for instance, because of changes in the local neuronal circuitry, perhaps as a direct consequence of the denervation following the initial loss of neurons (see p. 252, 270).

Secondary epileptic foci

The idea that epileptic activity originating from one focus can establish independent epileptic foci elsewhere in the brain has a long and troubled history. It was first described in the 1940s (Pope et al 1946). It clearly is implicit in the process of kindling, where the 'epileptic activity' is controlled by the experimenter, and has been described unambiguously in several other chronic experimental epilepsies, including those due to intracerebral tetanus toxin (Jefferys & Empson 1990, Brener et al 1991). The question that causes heated dispute is whether similar events can occur in man, and if so whether there are urgent reasons to give patients prophylactic anticonvulsants following head injury or a single first fit (Bolwig & Trimble 1989). At present we can only conclude that secondary foci could be induced by epileptic activity, and that some caution may be appropriate. What is clear is that such changes do occur in a range of animal models, which means it is prudent to keep this kind of phenomenon in mind. It is possible that a more detailed understanding of the underlying plastic cellular processes, such as are described in the following section, may help make more sense of clinical data on the evolution of epileptic foci.

Plastic changes

The term 'plastic change' in the nervous system covers many mechanisms in which neurons undergo a long-lasting change in their functional properties, or in their interconnections and structure, following some stimulus. Typically this would include the kinds of cellular change respon-

sible for learning new memories, or synaptic reorganisation in response to denervation ('sprouting' or 'reactive synaptogenesis'). Gross losses of neurons, while clearly long-lasting, and not usually considered as plastic changes; in general there is a requirement for some degree of specificity or adaptive value in a 'plastic' response.

Long-term potentiation

Long-term potentiation or LTP is one of the more popular types of synaptic plasticity. It is triggered by stimulus trains which can be as brief as 0.2 seconds, and yet can last for many hours, or even days (Collingridge & Bliss 1987). It has been popular as a model of learning, and indeed there is some evidence that it is related to learning processes in the hippocampus, where it is most commonly studied. LTP is superficially similar to kindling, with a comparatively brief stimulus resulting in a very prolonged functional change. It is likely that LTP is a factor in the evolution of kindling, but it is not the complete story. In particular, kindling continues to evolve long after LTP has reached saturation, has a much more prolonged time course, has a different pharmacological profile, and preferentially affects different parts of the brain (Cain 1989).

Excitatory amino acid neurotransmitters: NMDA receptors

The NMDA receptor for glutamate is involved in many kinds of plastic change, including LTP (Collingridge & Bliss 1987). It differs from the non-NMDA or AMPA receptor in two important respects. Firstly, it is blocked by Mg^{2+} at resting potential, and not at depolarized potentials, so it responds selectively to simultaneous pre- and postsynaptic activity (useful in learning) and also to the intense activity during an epileptic seizure (probably not its primary purpose!). Secondly, it is relatively nonspecific for cations, and admits Ca^{2+} along with Na^+ and K^+; Ca^{2+} can activate a wide range of intracellular processes. This chapter has already mentioned the role of the NMDA receptor in some kinds of acute epilepsy (Ashwood & Wheal 1986b, Herron et al 1985, Thomson & West 1986) and in neuronal death.

The NMDA receptor also takes a greater than normal role in EPSPs in kindled rats (Mody et al 1988). However the availability of selective antagonists, such as APV and MK-801, reveals that blocking NMDA receptors prevents the development of kindling and some of its associated cellular changes, for instance the depression of inhibition (Stelzer et al 1987, Croucher et al 1988, Kapur & Lothman 1990). These two effects, the increase in the EPSP and the depression of inhibition, act together to reduce substantially the seizure threshold in the kindled animals. Particularly important is the observation that NMDA antagonists prevented the progression of the kindling, and thus should be considered as more than simple anticonvulsants; they were acting as antiepileptic drugs.

Sprouting

Sprouting, or reactive synaptogenesis, occurs when new synapses are formed to replace others lost, usually following lesioning. It is an interesting phenomenon which has been characterized in great detail in the hippocampus. Its relevance to epilepsy has become clear as a result of a series of studies which exploited features of the 'mossy fibres', the axons of the granule cells of the hippocampal dentate area. They contain unusually high concentrations of zinc, which can readily be visualized with a sulphide-silver histological method developed by Timm. Mossy fibres normally project to the pyramidal cells of CA3 and to hilar neurons, and do not normally project to the dentate molecular layer above the granule cell body layer. Aberrant, presumably recurrent, projections into the layers containing the granule cell dendrites appeared in at least two chronic epileptic models: kainic acid lesions of CA3 and perforant path kindled rats (Ben-Ari & Represa 1990, Sutula et al 1988, Sutula, 1990). This circuit provides obvious opportunities for abnormal mutual excitation of granule cells. Particularly interesting is that similar aberrant connections have been found in human temporal lobe epilepsies (Sutula et al 1989).

It would be surprising if this effect were restricted to the mossy fibres, but the lack of convenient markers for other pathways makes it much more difficult to demonstrate directly. Sprouting has also been demonstrated in GABAergic axons in the dentate area, alongside that in the mossy fibres (Davenport et al 1990). It is indeed unfortunate that we lack good tools to study the local circuits in other parts of the brain, because 'rewiring', of the kind found with the granule cell and other axons in the dentate area, provides a versatile mechanism for epileptogenesis.

Gene expression

Sustained functional changes associated with epilepsies are likely to be maintained by changes in gene expression. Certainly evidence is accumulating that some of the immediate early genes, such as c-fos and c-jun are switched on by seizures (Morgan et al 1987). Furthermore, the expression of genes directly relevant to neuronal function changes in several experimental epilepsies, for instance that for GAD in the hippocampus after kainic acid lesions and after injection of tetanus toxin (Feldblum et al 1990, Najlerahim et al 1992). It is tempting to speculate that such increases in mRNA for GAD could be associated with the development of new inhibitory synapses, and/or with the growth of new GABAergic axons (Davenport et al 1990). Whatever structural changes might be associated with it, an increased expression of the mRNA for GAD seems a better candidate mechanism for controlling seizures than for sustaining them. Further studies of this kind will, no doubt, soon give us a much clearer picture of the flexibility of the brain's response to epileptogenic insults.

Behavioural changes

The pathophysiology of epilepsy does not necessarily stop with the seizures and other grossly abnormal electrographic events. Limbic foci in particular are associated with a range of cognitive and behavioural problems. Usually they have been attributed to histopathology, which undoubtedly occurs in many cases. However, such behavioural changes can occur in the absence of histopathology, as we have shown in the tetanus toxin model (Brace et al 1985, Jefferys et al 1988), where the underlying mechanism also depressed evoked responses recorded from hippocampal pyramidal cells. Similar changes have been described in man (Meador et al 1987).

WHAT PREDISPOSES PARTICULAR BRAINS TO EPILEPSY?

Epilepsy is perhaps the most common of neurological disorders, but it still does not occur in the vast majority of humans, or indeed other species that have not been specifically selected for epileptic traits. Therefore an important question is why do some individuals succumb to epilepsies (Hopkins 1987)?

Pharmacological insults

Humans are not resistant to the actions of convulsant drugs, although they do not normally encounter them. However, withdrawing a number of commonly used drugs can precipitate seizures, the most obvious being alcohol and barbiturates. Barbiturates are well known both for potentiating GABA receptors, and for the development of tolerance with continued use; their withdrawal therefore is likely to lead to impaired GABAergic function. Ethanol also appears to interact with the GABA receptor, and may act in a similar way.

Gross ionic disturbances in the systemic circulation, such as decreased levels of free Ca^{2+} (which can result from changes in acid–base balance), elevated K^+, and severe water intoxication can lead to seizures, perhaps through some of the mechanisms described above for similar changes in the media bathing brain slices. However such acute symptomatic seizures (see Ch. 5) should not be considered as epilepsy, because the seizures will stop as soon as the underlying problem is resolved.

Injury

Head injuries in man in a minority of cases lead to focal epilepsies in later life. This is perhaps not surprising because several of the chronic experimental models described in this chapter seem to require a histological lesion, such as those caused by alumina, local freezing and kainic acid (Table 8.2). Epileptic discharges appear to originate around the edges of the lesion, perhaps as a consequence of the rewiring that is likely to occur in these neurons which probably have lost many synapses; this kind of rewiring has been shown explicitly in the kainic acid lesioned hippocampus in rats (p. 252). In addition, the experimental epilepsy induced by iron salts raises the prospect that the products of the breakdown of red blood cells after bleeding in the brain could be epileptogenic.

Genetics

There are a multitude of genetic defects that are related to some kind of epileptic disorder (Anderson et al 1986a, Bundey, 1987). At least 140 Mendelian traits have been associated with seizures of one kind or another in man. More significantly in terms of patient numbers is the major role played by inheritance in absences seizures, and some other generalized epilepsies (Gardiner 1990). Inheritance is not an obvious factor in most focal epilepsies, with a notable exception in Rolandic epilepsy.

In those cases where there is definite evidence of a significant role of inheritance, the expression of the epileptic trait is rarely simple, and probably depends on multiple factors, both genetic and environmental. For instance, small abnormalities in amino acid or catecholamine metabolism could predispose an individual to an otherwise innocuous environmental insult with epilepsy (Sherwin & van Gelder, 1986). Another example comes from genetically-linked disorders of neuronal migration, which appear to predispose individuals to epilepsy; these are discussed with other developmental problems in the following section. In general it will not be easy to chart the multiple and diverse factors which cause clinical epilepsies; this will require a combination of the tools of modern genetics with the whole armoury of technology that can be brought to bear on the process of epileptogenesis.

Development

Perinatal problems have been identified as risk factors for epilepsy in later life. One common example is found with febrile convulsions which increase the risk of epilepsy many years later.

However, the fact that only a minority of infants who experience febrile convulsions go on to develop epilepsy implicates other risk factors.

Gross disorders of neuronal migration frequently are associated with early-onset epilepsies. Many of the more obvious examples can be detected with non-invasive techniques such as computed tomography, magnetic resonance imaging or positron emission tomography. At least some of these have a clear genetic basis. However, these are a minority of the overall epileptic population. Much more subtle examples of disordered neuronal migration have been found by histology and morphometry of tissue removed to relieve intractable temporal lobe epilepsy (Hardiman et al 1988, Houser 1990). These more subtle errors of migration were seen as neurons located in the wrong subregion. For instance, foci in temporal neocortex were associated with neurons in the subcortical white matter, and hippocampal foci with dentate granule cells not arranged in their normal tightly-laminar fashion. These abnormalities were relatively common in these patients, who admittedly are a highly selected population coming to surgery; up to 40% of the epileptogenic tissues removed were affected by these abnormalities which are very rare in non-epileptic subjects.

In neither the temporal neocortex nor the hippocampus is it clear why an abnormality present from birth, or shortly after, should predispose an individual to focal epilepsy in later life. It could be that errors in wiring result from the misplacement of these cortical neurons, making the local circuits less tolerant of normal operational fluctuations in synaptic efficiency, or perhaps age-related losses of neurons, which normally would be innocuous, or at least would not be epileptogenic. More detailed studies of the functional implications of these structural abnormalities are needed before we can make specific hypotheses on how hypersynchronous discharges originate. The ideas developed in the search for mechanisms of epileptic synchronization in normal brain tissue exposed to convulsants will provide a key to unravelling the role of the aberrant circuitry in this kind of tissue.

CONCLUDING REMARKS

This chapter should demonstrate that we now know a great deal about the cellular mechanisms of neuronal synchronization and the control of neuronal excitability and firing patterns. We have a more complete understanding of some of the simpler experimental phenomena that are recognizably epileptic, such as the interictal spike and absence seizures, and we are making significant inroads on more complex matters, such as chronic epileptic foci and seizure generation. What these basic studies provide is a framework of ideas to apply to the much more complex issues presented by human epilepsies, with their uncertain and variable clinical and therapeutic histories. The author remains optimistic that by the next edition of this textbook we will have made substantial progress in that direction.

ACKNOWLEDGEMENTS

The author is a Wellcome Trust Senior Lecturer and wishes to thank Professor M. J. Gutnick and Dr R. D. Traub for helpful discussions during the preparation of this manuscript.

REFERENCES

Albowitz B, Kuhnt U, Ehrenreich L 1990 Optical recording of epileptiform voltage changes in the neocortical slice. Experimental Brain Research 81: 241–256

Andersen P, Sears T A 1964 The role of inhibition in the phasing of spontaneous thalamocortical discharge. Journal of Physiology 173: 459–480

Anderson V E, Hauser W A, Rich S S 1986a Genetic heterogeneity on the epilepsies. Advances in Neurology 44: 59–75

Anderson W W, Lewis D V, Swartzwelder H S, Wilson W A 1986b Magnesium-free medium activates seizure-like events in the rat hippocampal slice. Brain Research 398: 215–219

Ashwood T J, Wheal H V 1986a Loss of inhibition in the CA1 region of the kainic acid lesioned hippocampus is not associated with changes in postsynaptic responses to GABA. Brain Research 367: 390–394

Ashwood T J, Wheal H V 1986b Extracellular studies on the role of N-methyl-D-aspartate receptors in epileptiform activity recorded from the kainic acid-lesioned hippocampus. Neuroscience Letters 67: 147–152

Avoli M, Olivier A 1989 Electrophysiological properties and synaptic responses in the deep layers of the human epileptogenic neocortex in vitro. Journal of Neurophysiology 61: 589–606

Ayala G F, Dichter M, Gumnit R J, Matsumoto H, Spencer W A 1973 Genesis of epileptic interictal spikes. New knowledge of cortical feedback systems suggests a neurophysiological explanation of brief paroxysms. Brain Research 52: 1–17

Babb T L, Wilson C L, Isokawa Akesson M 1987 Firing patterns of human limbic neurons during stereoencephalography (SEEG) and clinical temporal lobe seizures. Electroencephalography and Clinical Neurophysiology 66: 467–482

Ben-Ari Y, Represa A 1990 Brief seizure episodes induce long-term potentiation and mossy fibre sprouting in the hippocampus. Trends in Neurosciences 13: 312–318

Benardo L S, Pedley T A 1985 Cellular mechanisms of focal epileptogenesis. In: Pedley T A, Meldrum B S (eds) Recent Advances in Epilepsy. Churchill Livingstone, Edinburgh, p 1–17

Bolwig T G, Trimble M R 1989 The clinical relevance of kindling. John Wiley & Sons, Chichester

Brace H M, Jefferys J G R, Mellanby J 1985 Long-term changes in hippocampal physiology and in learning ability of rats after intrahippocampal tetanus toxin. Journal of Physiology 368: 343–357

Brener K, Chagnac-Amitai Y, Jefferys J G R, Gutnick M J 1991 Chronic epileptic foci in neocortex: in vivo and in vitro effects of tetanus toxin. European Journal of Neuroscience 3: 47–54

Bundey S 1987 The genetic basis of the epilepsies. In: Hopkins A (ed) Epilepsy. Chapman and Hall, London, p 137–149

Cain D P 1989 Long-term potentiation and kindling: How similar are the mechanisms. Trends in Neurosciences 12: 6–10

Calvin W H 1980 Normal repetitive firing and its pathophysiology. In: Lockard J S, Ward A A Jr (eds) Epilepsy: A Window to Brain Mechanisms. Raven Press, New York, p 97–121

Carpenter D O (ed) 1982 Cellular Pacemakers. John Wiley and Sons, New York

Caterall W A 1988 Structure and function of voltage-sensitive ion channels. Science 242: 50–61

Chagnac-Amitai Y, Connors B W 1989 Horizontal spread of synchronized activity in neocortex and its control by GABA-mediated inhibition. Journal of Neurophysiology 61: 747–758

Chagnac-Amitai Y, Luhmann H J, Prince D A 1990 Burst generating and regular spiking layer 5 pyramidal neurons of rat neocortex have different morphological features. Journal of Comparative Neurology 296: 598–613

Chervin R D, Pierce P A, Connors B W 1988 Periodicity and directionality in the propagation of epileptiform discharges across neocortex. Journal of Neurophysiology 60: 1695–1713

Chin J H 1989 Adenosine receptors in brain: Neuro-modulation and role in epilepsy. Annals of Neurology 26: 695–698

Christian E P, Dudek F E 1988 Characteristics of local excitatory circuits studied with glutamate microapplication in the CA3 area of rat hippocampal slices. Journal of Neurophysiology 59: 90–109

Collingridge G L, Bliss T V P 1987 NMDA receptors—their role in long-term potentiation. Trends in Neurosciences 10: 288–293

Collingridge G L Thompson P A, Davies J, Mellanby J 1981 In vitro effect of tetanus toxin on GABA release from rat hippocampal slices. Journal of Neurochemistry 37: 1039–1041

Collins R C, Tearse R G, Lothman E W 1983 Functional anatomy of limbic seizures; focal discharges from medial entorhinal cortex in rats. Brain Research 280: 25–40

Connors B W 1984 Initiation of synchronized bursting in neocortex. Nature 310: 685–687

Connors B W, Gutnick M J 1990 Intrinsic firing patterns of diverse neocortical neurons. Trends in Neurosciences 13: 99–104

Connors B W, Gutnick M J, Prince D A 1982 Electrophysiological properties of neocortical neurons in vitro. Journal of Neurophysiology 48: 1302–1320

Cornish S M, Wheal H V 1989 Long-term loss of paired pulse inhibition in the kainic acid-lesioned hippocampus of the rat. Neuroscience 28: 563–571

Coulter D A, Huguenard J R, Prince D A 1989 Characterization of ethosuximide reduction of low-threshold calcium current in thalamic neurons. Annals of Neurology 25: 582–593

Coulter D A Huguenard J R Prince D A 1990 Differential effects of petit mal anticonvulsants and convulsants on thalamic neurones: Calcium current reduction. British Journal of Pharmacology 100: 800–806

Coutinho-Netto J, Abdul-Ghani A S Collins J F, Bradford H F 1981 Is glutamate a trigger factor in epileptic hyperactivity. Epilepsia 22: 289–296

Cronin J, Dudek F E 1988 Chronic seizures and collateral sprouting of dentate mossy fibers after kainic acid treatment in rats. Brain Research 474: 181–184

Croucher M J, Collins J F, Meldrum B S 1982 Anticonvulsant action of excitatory amino acid antagonists. Science 216: 899–901

Croucher M J, Bradford H F, Sunter D C, Watkins J C 1988 Inhibition of the development of electrical kindling of the prepyriform cortex by daily focal injections of excitatory amino acid antagonists. European Journal of Pharmacology 152: 29–38

Davenport C J, Brown W J, Babb T L 1990 Sprouting of GABAergic and mossy fiber axons in dentate gyrus following intrahippocampal kainate in the rat. Experimental Neurology 109: 180–190

Delgado-Escueta A V, Ward A A Jr, Woodbury D M, Porter R J 1986 Basic mechanisms of the epilepsies. Molecular and cellular approaches. Raven Press, New York

Dichter M A, Ayala G F 1987 Cellular mechanisms of epilepsy: a status report. Science 237: 157–164

Dichter M, Spencer W A 1968 Hippocampal penicillin 'spike' discharge: Epileptic neuron or epileptic aggregate? Neurology (Minneapolis) 18: 282

Dingledine R 1984 Brain slices. Plenum Press, New York

Dreifuss F E 1987 The differential types of epileptic seizures, and the international classification of epileptic seizures and of the epilepsies. In: Hopkins A (ed) Epilepsy, Chapman and Hall, London, p 83–113

Dudek F E, Snow R W, Taylor C P 1986 Role of electrical interactions in sychronization of epileptiform bursts. Advances in Neurology 44: 593–617

Ebersole J S, Chatt A B 1986 Spread and arrest of seizures: The importance of layer 4 in laminar interactions during neocortical epileptogenesis. Advances in Neurology 44: 515–558

Editorial 1990 Epilepsy and disorders of neuronal migration. Lancet 336: 1035

Empson R M, Jefferys J G R 1991 Inhibition in primary and secondary chronic epileptic foci induced by intrahippocampal tetanus toxin. Society for Neuroscience Abstracts 17: 1441

Feldblum S, Ackermann R F, Tobin A J 1990 Long-term increase of glutamate decarboxylase mRNA in a rat model of temporal lobe epilepsy. Neuron 5: 361–371

Fisher R S 1989 Animal models of the epilepsies. Brain Research Review 14: 245–278

Franck J E, Kunkel D D, Baskin D G, Schwartzkroin P A 1988 Inhibition in kainate-lesioned hyperexcitable hippocampi: Physiologic, autoradiographic, and immunocytochemical observations. Journal of Neuroscience 8: 1991–2002

Friedman A, Gutnick M J 1989 Intracellular calcium and control of burst generation in neurons of guinea-pig neocortex in vitro. European Journal of Neuroscience 1: 374–381

Gabbott P L A, Martin K A C, Whitteridge D 1987 Connections between pyramidal cells in layer 5 of cat visual cortex. Journal of Comparative Neurology 259: 364–381

Gardiner R M 1990 Genes and epilepsy. Journal of Medical Genetics 27: 537–544

Gean P-W, Shinnick-Gallagher P 1988 Characterization of the epileptiform activity induced by magnesium-free solution in rat amygdala slices: An intracellular study. Experimental Neurology 101: 248–255

Gloor P, Fariello R G 1988 Generalized epilepsy: some of its cellular mechanisms differ from those of focal epilepsy. Trends in Neurosciences 11: 63–68

Goddard G V, McIntyre D C, Leech C K 1969 A permanent change in brain function resulting from daily electrical stimulation. Experimental Neurology 25: 295–330

Gowers W R 1881 Epilepsy, and other chronic convulsive disorders: Their causes, symptoms and treatment. Churchill, London

Gutnick M J, Connors B W, Prince D A 1982 Mechanisms of neocortical epileptogenesis in vitro. Journal of Neurophysiology 48: 1321–1335

Haas H L, Greene R W 1988 Electrophysiological analysis of effects of exogenous and endogenous adenosine in hippocampal slices. In: Avoli M, Reader T A, Dykes R W, Gloor P (eds) Neurotransmitters and cortical function. Plenum, New York, p 483–494

Haas H L, Jefferys J G R 1984 Low-calcium field burst discharges of CA1 pyramidal neurones in rat hippocampal slices. Journal of Physiology 354: 185–201

Hardiman O, Burke T, Phillips J et al 1988 Microdysgenesis in resected temporal neocortex: incidence and clinical significance in focal epilepsy. Neurology (NY) 38: 1041–1047

Hawkins C A, Mellanby J H 1987 Limbic epilepsy induced by tetanus toxin: a longitudinal electroencephalographic study. Epilepsia 28: 431–444

Heinemann U, Dietzel I 1984 Extracellular potassium concentration in chronic alumina cream foci of cats. Journal of Neurophysiology 52: 421–434

Heinemann U, Konnerth A, Pumain R, Wadman W J 1986 Extracellular calcium and potassium changes in chronic epileptic brain tissue. Advances in Neurology 44: 641–661

Herron C E, Williamson R, Collingridge G L 1985 A selective N-methyl-D-aspartate antagonist depresses epileptiform activity in rat hippocampal slices.

Neuroscience Letters 61: 255–260

Hille B 1989 Ionic channels: evolutionary origins and modern roles. Quarterly Journal of Experimental Physiology 74: 785–804

Hoffman W H, Haberly L B 1989 Bursting induces persistent all-or-none EPSPs by an NMDA-dependent process in piriform cortex. Journal of Neuroscience 9: 206–215

Holmes O, Wallace M N, Campbell A M 1987 Comparison of penicillin epileptogenesis in rat somatosensory and motor cortex. Quarterly Journal of Experimental Physiology 72: 439–452

Hopkins A 1987 The causes and precipitation of seizures. In: Hopkins A (ed) Epilepsy, Chapman and Hall, London, p 115–136

Houser C R 1990 Granule cell dispersion in the dentate gyrus of humans with temporal lobe epilepsy. Brain Research 535: 195–204

Iadorola M J, Gale K 1982 Substantia nigra: site of anticonvulsant activity mediated by γ-aminobutyric acid. Science 218: 1237–1240

Ishijimi B, Hori T, Yoshimasu N, Fukushima T, Hirakawa K, Sekino H 1975 Neuronal activities in human epileptic foci and surrounding areas. Electroencephalography and Clinical Neurophysiology 39: 643–650

Ives A E, Jefferys J G R 1990 Synchronization of epileptiform bursts induced by 4-aminopyridine in the in vitro hippocampal slice preparation. Neuroscience Letters 112: 239–245

Ives A E, Jefferys J G R 1991 Epileptiform activity induced in hippocampal pyramidal cells by cholera toxin. European Journal of Neuroscience Supplement 4: 87

Jasper H H, Ward A A Jr, Pope A 1969 Basic Mechanisms of the Epilepsies. Little, Brown, Boston

Jefferys J G R 1981a The Vibroslice, a new vibrating-blade tissue slicer. Journal of Physiology 324: 2P

Jefferys J G R 1981b Influence of electric fields on the excitability of granule cells in guinea-pig hippocampal slices. Journal of Physiology 319: 143–152

Jefferys J G R 1989 Chronic epileptic foci in vitro in hippocampal slices from rats with the tetanus toxin epileptic syndrome. Journal of Neurophysiology 62: 458–468

Jefferys J G R 1990 Basic mechanisms of focal epilepsies. Experimental Physiology 75: 127–162

Jefferys J G R, Empson R M 1990 Development of chronic secondary epileptic foci following intrahippocampal injection of tetanus toxin. Experimental Physiology 75: 733–736

Jefferys J G R, Evans B J, Hughes S A, Williams S F 1992 Neuropathology of the chronic epileptic syndrome induced by intrahippocampal tetanus toxin in rat: preservation of pyramidal cells and incidence of dark cells. Neuropathy and Applied Neurobiology 18: 53–70

Jefferys J G R, Haas H L 1982 Synchronized bursting of CA1 pyramidal cells in the absence of synaptic transmission. Nature 300: 448–450

Jefferys J G R, Roberts R 1987 The biology of epilepsy. In: Hopkins A (ed) Epilepsy. Chapman and Hall, London, p 19–81

Jefferys J G R, Mitchell P, O'Hara L et al 1991 Ex vivo release of GABA from tetanus toxin-induced chronic epileptic foci decreased during the active seizure phase. Neurochemistry International 18: 373–379

Jensen M S, Yaari Y 1988 The relationship between interictal and ictal paroxysms in an in vitro model of focal hippocampal epilepsy. Annals of Neurology 24: 591–598

Johnston D, Brown T H 1981 Giant synaptic potential hypothesis for epileptiform activity. Science 211: 294–297

Jones R S G 1989 Ictal epileptiform events induced by removal of extracellular magnesium in slices of entorhinal cortex are blocked by baclofen. Experimental Neurology 104: 155–161

Jones R S G, Heinemann U 1988 Synaptic and intrinsic responses of medial entorhinal cortical cells in normal and magnesium-free medium in vitro. Journal of Neurophysiology 59: 1476–1496

Jones R S G, Lambert J D C 1990 The role of excitatory amino acid receptors in the propagation of epileptiform discharges from the entorhinal cortex to the dentate gyrus in vitro. Experimental Brain Research 80: 310–322

Jordan S J, Jefferys J G R 1992 Sustained and selective block of IPSPs in brain slices from rats made epileptic by intrahippocampal tetanus toxin. Epilepsy Research 11: 119–129

Kamphuis W, Huisman E, Dreijer A M C, Ghijsen W E J M, Verhage M, Lopes da Silva F H 1990 Kindling increases the K^+-evoked Ca^{2+}-dependent release of endogenous GABA in area CA1 of rat hippocampus. Brain Research 511: 63–70

Kamphuis W, Lopes da Silva F H, Wadman W J 1988 Changes in local evoked potentials in the rat hippocampus (CA1) during kindling epileptogenesis. Brain Research 440: 205–215

Kamphuis W, Wadman W J, Buijs R M, Lopes da Silva F H 1987 The development of changes in hippocampal GABA immunoreactivity in the rat kindling model of epilepsy: a light microscopic study with GABA antibodies. Neuroscience 23: 433–446

Kang Y, Endo K, Araki T 1988 Excitatory synaptic actions between pairs of neighbouring pyramidal tract cells in the motor cortex. Journal of Neurophysiology 59: 636–647

Kapur J, Lothman E W 1990 NMDA receptor activation mediates the loss of GABAergic inhibition induced by recurrent seizures. Epilepsy Research 5: 103–111

Kapur J, Michelson H B, Buterbaugh G G, Lothman E W 1989 Evidence for a chronic loss of inhibition in the hippocampus after kindling: Electrophysiological studies. Epilepsy Research 4: 90–99

Kiss J, Patel A J, Freund T F 1990 Distribution of septohippocampal neurons containing parvalbumin or choline acetyltransferase in the rat brain. Journal of Comparative Neurology 298: 362–372

Kisvárday Z F, Martin K A C, Freund T F, Magloczky Zs, Whitteridge D, Somogyi P 1986 Synaptic targets of HRP-filled layer III pyramidal cells in the cat striate cortex. Experimental Brain Research 64: 541–552

Knowles W D, Traub R D, Strowbridge B W 1987 The initiation and spread of epileptiform bursts in the in vitro hippocampal slice. Neuroscience 21: 441–455

Konnerth A, Heinemann U, Yaari Y 1984 Slow transmission of neural activity in hippocampal area CA1 in absence of active chemical synapses. Nature 307: 69–71

Korn S J, Giacchino J L, Chamberlin N L, Dingledine R 1987 Epileptiform burst activity induced by potassium in the hippocampus and its regulation by GABA-mediated inhibition. Journal of Neurophysiology 57: 325–340

Leblond J, Krnjevic K 1989 Hypoxic changes in hippocampal neurons. Journal of Neurophysiology 62: 1–14

Leweke F M, Louvel J, Rausche G, Heinemann U 1990 Effects of pentetrazol on neuronal activity and on extracellular calcium concentration in rat hippocampal slices. Epilepsy Research 6: 187–198

Lewis D V, Jones L S, Swartzwelder H S 1989 The effects of baclofen and pertussis toxin on epileptiform activity induced in the hippocampal slice by magnesium depletion. Epilepsy Research 4: 109–118

Lloyd K G, Bossi L, Morselli P L, Munari C, Rougier M, Loiseau H 1986 Alterations of GABA-mediated synaptic transmission in human epilepsy. Advances in Neurology 44: 1033–1044

Lockard J S, Ward A A Jr, 1980 Epilepsy: a window to brain mechanisms. Raven Press, New York

Lockton J W, Holmes O 1980 Site of initiation of penicillin-induced epilepsy in the cortex cerebri of the rat. Brain Research 190: 301–304

London J A, Cohen L B, Wu J-Y 1989 Optical recordings of the cortical response to whisker stimulation before and after the addition of an epileptogenic agent. Journal of Neuroscience 9: 2128–2190

Löscher W, Schmidt D 1988 Which animal models should be used in the search for new antiepileptic drugs? A proposal based on experimental and clinical considerations. Epilepsy Research 2: 145–181

MacVicar B A, Dudek F E 1980 Local synaptic circuits in rat hippocampus: Interaction between pyramidal cells. Brain Research 184: 220–223

Marty A 1989 The physiological role of calcium-dependent channels. Trends in Neurosciences 12: 420–424

Mason A, Larkman A 1990 Correlations between morphology and electrophysiology of pyramidal neurons in slices of rat visual cortex. II. Electrophysiology. Journal of Neuroscience 10: 1415–1428

Masukawa L M, Benardo L S, Prince D A 1982 Variations in electrophysiological properties of hippocampal pyramidal neurons in different subfields. Brain Research 242: 341–344

Masukawa L M, Higashima M, Kim J H, Spencer D D 1989 Epileptiform discharges evoked in hippocampal brain slices from epileptic patients. Brain Research 493: 168–174

McCormick D A, Pape H-C 1990 Properties of a hyperpolarization-activated cation current and its role in rhythmic oscillation in thalamic relay neurones. Journal of Physiology 431: 291–318

McIntyre D C, Wong R K S 1986 Cellular and synaptic properties of amygdala-kindled pyriform cortex in vitro. Journal of Neurophysiology 55: 1295–1307

Meador K J, Loring D W, King D W, Gallagher B B, Gould M J, Smith J R 1987 Limbic evoked potentials predict site of epileptic focus. Neurology (NY) 37: 494–497

Meldrum B S 1986 Cell damage in epilepsy and the role of calcium in cytotoxicity. Advances in Neurology 44: 849–855

Meldrum B S, Wilkins A J 1984 Photosensitive epilepsy in man and the baboon: integration of pharmacological and psychophysical evidence. In: Schwartzkroin P A, Wheal H V (eds) Electrophysiology of epilepsy. Academic Press, London, p 51–77

Miles R, Wong R K S 1986 Excitatory synaptic interactions between CA3 neurones in the guinea-pig hippocampus. Journal of Physiology 373: 397–418

Miles R, Wong R K S 1987 Inhibitory control of local excitatory circuits in the guinea-pig hippocampus. Journal of Physiology 388: 611–629

Miles R, Wong R K S, Traub R D 1984 Synchronized

afterdischarges in the hippocampus: contribution of local synaptic interactions. Neuroscience 12: 1179–1189

Miles R, Traub R D, Wong R K S 1988 Spread of synchronous firing in longitudinal slices from the CA3 region of the hippocampus. Journal of Neurophysiology 60: 1481–1496

Mody I, Lambert J D, Heinemann U 1987 Low extracellular magnesium induces epileptiform activity and spreading depression in rat hippocampal slices. Journal of Neurophysiology 57: 869–888

Mody I, Stanton P K, Heinemann U 1988 Activation of N-methyl-D-aspartate receptors parallels changes in cellular and synaptic properties of dentate gyrus granule cells after kindling. Journal of Neurophysiology 59: 1033–1054

Morgan J I, Cohen D R, Hempstead J L, Curran T 1987 Mapping patterns of c-fos expression in the central nervous system after seizure. Science 237: 192–197

Najlerahim A, Williams S F, Pearson R C A, Jefferys J G R 1992 Increased expression of GAD mRNA during the chronic epileptic syndrome due to intrahippocampal tetanus toxin. Experimental Brain Research (in press)

Noebels J L 1986 Mutational analysis of inherited epilepsies. Advances in Neurology 44: 97–113

Noebels J L, Rutecki P A 1990 Altered hippocampal network excitability in the hypernoradrenergic mutant mouse tottering. Brain Research 524: 225–230

Olney J W, Collins R C, Sloviter R S 1986 Excitotoxic mechanisms of epileptic brain damage. Advances in Neurology 44: 857–877

Openchowski P 1883 Sur l'action localisé du froid, appliqué à la surface de la région corticale du cerveau. Comptes Rendus des Séances et Mémoires de la Société de Biologie 35: 38–43

O'Shaughnessy C T, Aram J A, Lodge D 1988 A1 adenosine receptor-mediated block of epileptiform activity induced in zero magnesium in rat neocortex in vitro. Epilepsy Research 2: 294–301

Penfield W, Jasper H 1954 Epilepsy and the functional anatomy of the human brain. Little, Brown, Boston

Piredda S, Gale K 1985 A crucial epileptogenic site in the deep prepiriform cortex. Nature 317: 623–625

Pockberger H, Rappelsberger P, Petsche H 1984 Penicillin-induced epileptic phenomena in the rabbit's neocortex. II. Laminar specific generation of interictal spikes after the application of penicillin to different cortical depth. Brain Research 309: 261–269

Pope A, Morris A A, Jasper H, Elliott K A C, Penfield W 1946 Histochemical and action potential studies on epileptogenic areas of cerebral cortex in man and the monkey. Research Publications of the Association for Research in Nervous and Mental Diseases 26: 218–233

Prince D A 1969 Microelectrode studies of penicillin foci. In: Jasper H H, Ward A A Jr, Pope A (eds) Basic mechanisms of the epilepsies. Little, Brown, Boston, p 320–328

Prince D A 1985 Physiological mechanisms of focal epileptogenesis. Epilepsia 26(Suppl.1): S1–S14

Prince D A, Connors B W 1986 Mechanisms of interictal epileptogenesis. Advances in Neurology 44: 275–299

Rausche G, Dreyer J, Heinemann U 1991 Slow synaptic inhibition prevents spread of seizure-like activity from the entorhinal cortex to the hippocampus. In: Speckmann E-J, Gutnick M J (eds) Epilepsy and inhibition. Urban & Schwarzenberg, Munich

Ribak C E 1986 Contemporary methods in neurocytology and their applications to the study of epilepsy. Advances in

Neurology 44: 739–764

Rogawski M A, Porter R J 1990 Antiepileptic drugs. Pharmacological mechanisms and clinical efficacy with consideration of promising developmental stage compounds. Pharmacological Reviews 42: 223–270

Roux E, Borrel A 1898 Tétanos cérébral et immunité contre le tétanos. Annals de l'Institut Pasteur 4: 225–239

Rutecki P A, Lebeda F J, Johnston D 1987 4-Aminopyridine produces epileptiform activity in hippocampus and enhances synaptic excitation and inhibition. Journal of Neurophysiology 57: 1911–1924

Scheibel M E, Crandall P H, Scheibel A B 1974 The hippocampal-dentate complex in temporal lobe epilepsy. Epilepsia 15: 55–80

Schneiderman J H, MacDonald J F 1987 Effects of reduced magnesium on hippocampal synchrony. Brain Research 410: 174–178

Schwartzkroin P A 1986 Hippocampal slices in experimental and human epilepsy. Advances in Neurology 44: 991–1010

Seisjö B K, Wieloch T 1986 Epileptic bran damage: pathophysiology and neurochemical pathology. Advances in Neurology 44: 813–847

Sherwin A L, van Gelder N M 1986 Amino acid and catecholamine markers of metabolic abnormalities in human focal epilepsy. Advances in Neurology 44: 1011–1032

Siggins G R, Henriksen S J, Chavkin C, Gruol D 1986 Opioid peptides and epileptogenesis in the limbic system: cellular mechanisms. Advances in Neurology 44: 501–512

Simon R P, Swan J H, Griffiths T, Meldrum B S 1984 N-Methyl-D-Aspartate receptor blockade prevents ischemic brain damage. Science 226: 850–852

Snow R W, Dudek F E 1984 Synchronous epileptiform bursts without chemical transmission in CA2, CA3 and dentate areas of the hippocampus. Brain Research 298: 382–385

Stelzer A, Slater N T, ten Bruggencate G 1987 Activation of NMDA receptors blocks GABAergic inhibition in an in vitro model of epilepsy. Nature 326: 698–701

Steriade M, Llinás R R 1988 The functional states of the thalamus and the associated neuronal interplay. Physiological Reviews 68: 649–742

Stone T W, Connick J H, Bartrup J T 1990 NMDA-receptor-independent effects of low magnesium: Involvement of adenosine. Brain Research 508: 333–336

Stringer J L, Lothman E W 1989 Repetitive seizures cause an increase in paired-pulse inhibition in the dentate gyrus. Neuroscience Letters 105: 91–95

Sutula T P 1990 Experimental models of temporal lobe epilepsy: New insights from the study of kindling and synaptic reorganization. Epilepsia 31 (Suppl. 3): S45–S54

Sutula T, He X X, Cavazos J, Scott G 1988 Synaptic reorganization in the hippocampus induced by abnormal functional activity. Science 239: 1147–1150

Sutula T, Cascino G, Cavazos J, Parada I, Ramirez L 1989 Mossy fiber synaptic reorganization in the epileptic human temporal lobe. Annals of Neurology 26: 321–330

Szentagothai J 1978 The Ferrier Lecture, 1977. The neuron network of the cerebral cortex: a functional interpretation. Proceedings of the Royal Society of London (Biological Sciences) 201: 219–248

Takahashi K, Kubota K, Uno M 1989 Recurrent facilitation in cat pyramidal tract cells. Journal of Neurophysiology 30: 22–34

Tauck D L, Nadler J V 1985 Evidence of functional mossy

fiber sprouting in hippocampal formation of kainic acid-treated rats. Journal of Neuroscience 5: 1016–1022

Taylor C P, Dudek F E 1982 Synchronous neural afterdischarges in rat hippocampal slices without active chemical synapses. Science 218: 810–812

Thompson S M, Gähwiler B H 1989 Activity-dependent disinhibition. I. Repetitive stimulation reduces IPSP driving force and conductance in the hippocampus in vitro. Journal of Neurophysiology 61: 501–511

Thomson A M, Girdlestone D, West D C 1988 Voltage-dependent currents prolong single-axon postsynaptic potentials in layer III pyramidal neurons in rat neocortical slices. Journal of Neurophysiology 60: 1896–1907

Thomson A M, West D C 1986 N-methylaspartate receptors mediate epileptiform activity evoked in some, but not all, conditions in rat neocortical slices. Neuroscience 19: 1161–1177

Traub R D 1982 Simulation of intrinsic bursting in CA3 hippocampal neurons. Neuroscience 7: 1233–1242

Traub R D, Dingledine R 1990 Model of synchronized epileptiform bursts induced by high potassium in CA3 region of rat hippocampal slice. Role of spontaneous EPSPs in initiation. Journal of Neurophysiology 64: 1009–1018

Traub R D, Wong R K S, Miles R, Michelson H 1991 A model of a CA3 hippocampal neuron incorporating voltage-clamp data on intrinsic conductances. Journal of Neurophysiology 66: 635–650

Traynelis S F, Dingledine R 1989 Modification of potassium-induced interictal bursts and electrographic seizures by divalent cations. Neuroscience Letters 98: 194–199

Ward A A, Jr 1969 The epileptic neuron: chronic foci in animals and man. In: Jasper H H, Ward A A, Jr, Pope A (eds) Basic mechanisms of the epilepsies. Little, Brown, Boston, p 263–288

Wilson W A, Swartzwelder H S, Anderson W W, Lewis D V 1988 Seizure activity in vitro: a dual focus model. Epilepsy Research 2: 289–293

Wong R K S, Prince D A 1978 Participation of calcium spikes during intrinsic burst firing in hippocampal neurons. Brain Research 159: 385–390

Wong R K S, Traub R D, Miles R 1986 Cellular basis of neuronal synchrony in epilepsy. Advances in Neurology 44: 583–592

9. Electroencephalography

C. D. Binnie

INTRODUCTION

It may have been more good fortune than prophetic insight which led Hughlings Jackson in 1873 to define epileptic seizures as 'occasional sudden, excessive, rapid and local discharges of grey matter', for half a century was to elapse before it became possible to record such discharges, by means of the electroencephalogram, or EEG. Nevertheless, episodic dysfunction of cerebral neurones, particularly increased and synchronous activity, remains central to current concepts of epilepsy.

Principles of electroencephalography

It is beyond the scope of the present text to explain at length how the electroencephalogram is generated, recorded or interpreted. For the reader wishing to pursue these questions a good starting-point would be *Electroencephalography* by Niedermeyer & Lopes da Silva (1987). There follows a brief summary which may help to elucidate later sections of this chapter.

Physiological basis of the electroencephalogram

The EEG is a record of cerebral electrical activity made with typically some 20 electrodes of roughly 1 cm² surface area applied to the scalp. Cerebral electrical activity can also be registered directly from the surface of the cerebral cortex, as the electrocorticogram (ECoG) by somewhat smaller electrodes inserted at operation. A depth recording, or stereoelectroencephalogram (SEEG), can also be obtained by means of generally more numerous and much smaller electrodes, with a surface area of about 1 mm², inserted into the brain substance. The ECoG and SEEG are recorded in man only in special centres undertaking neurosurgical treatment of epilepsy. All three techniques involve recording from millions of neurones by means of electrodes which are relatively few and large. Consequently, the signals obtained represent only a very crude average of neuronal activity in a relatively large volume of brain tissue. Neurones undergo two main types of electrical change: slow postsynaptic potentials on a time scale of 5–50 ms and much briefer action potentials lasting only of the order of 1 ms. These last do not generate fields recordable far from their site of origin and thus it is virtually only postsynaptic potentials which contribute to the EEG. The fact that the electrodes record the summated signals from many neurones implies that only synchronous activity displayed by many cells simultaneously will be registered. An analogy may be found in the experience of someone listening outside a football stadium. For most of the time he hears but cannot understand the confused shouts of the crowd; however, the general applause when the home team scores a goal and the universal gasp when one is missed are easily recognized. Similarly, electrophysiological recordings with large electrodes reflect only that component of neuronal activity which is synchronous.

Synchronous neuronal activity is, from the point of view of information processing, highly redundant and occurs most readily in drowsiness, sleep and in pathological conditions in which cerebral function is impaired. Conversely, attention is associated with desynchronization of neurones and a reduced amplitude of the EEG. The philosophical implications of a test of cerebral function, which reflects the resting behaviour of neuronal populations not engaged in information processing need not concern us here; abnormal, synchronous neuronal discharge is the hallmark of the pathophysiology of epilepsy and its manifestations in the EEG are the main subject of this chapter.

Although scalp electrodes can in some circumstances pick up widespread electrical fields arising at a distance in the brain, more usually they record the summated activity of the underlying cerebral cortex over an area of about 6 cm² (Cooper et al 1965). The cerebral cortex is a laminar structure and the neurones which contribute most to the EEG are orientated vertically. Changes occurring in membrane potential are usually localized, either to the cell body deep in the cortex or to the dendrites lying more superficially (Fig. 9.1). This will result in the production of a dipole, a potential difference between deep and superficial layers of cortex. The extent to which this electrical field can be registered in the EEG will depend upon the orientation of the dipole with respect to the overlying electrode (more strictly, it depends on the solid angle subtended at the electrode by the generator surface). If the affected cortex is in the wall of a sulcus and the dipole thus orientated tangential to the surface of the brain it may not be detected. The activity of tangential generators can, however, be detected by their magnetic fields, as the magnetoencephalogram, or MEG.

The relations between EEG waves and activity of cerebral neurones are complex and depend on:

1. the nature of the change (increased negativity inside the cell with inhibitory, and decreased negativity with excitatory, postsynaptic potentials)
2. the parts of the neurone where changes in membrane potential are occurring (the soma deep in the cortex or the dendrites more superficially)—thus dendritic EPSPs generally produce negativity in the EEG whereas EPSPs on the soma produce positive EEG changes
3. the rate of spread from one part of the cell to another—during slow changes the surface EEG changes with a polarity opposite to that inside the cell body whereas with more rapid changes the two tend to be in phase (Fig. 9.2).

Fast negative spikes in the EEG may thus reflect cellular excitation and depolarization and surface negative slow waves may occur during hyperpolarization due to inhibition. However, in view of the complexity of the relationships between the EEG and neuronal events, for clinical

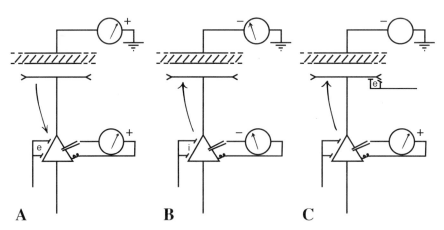

Fig. 9.1 Schematic representation of relationship between surface EEG and activity of cortical neurones. (A) Excitatory post-synaptic potential on cell body (positive-going change inside the cell) produces positive change on the surface. (B) Inhibitory post-synaptic potential on the cell body (negative-going change inside the cell) produces negative surface change. (C) Excitation of dendrites in contrast to (A), produces negative surface change. Large arrow shows direction of current flow.

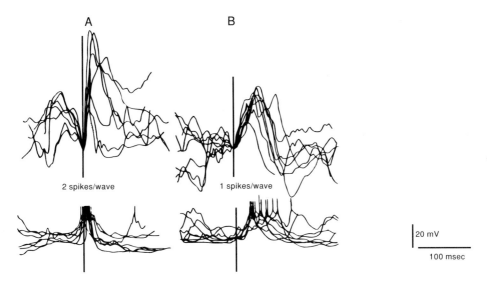

Fig. 9.2 (A) During rapid changes surface potential follows that inside body of cortical neurone. (B) During slower changes surface potentials out of phase with inside of cell body (NB recording convention is negative upwards for EEG and downwards for intracellular tracing). Reproduced with permission from Creutzfeldt et al 1966.

purposes an empirical approach may be more practical than speculation about the underlying physiology.

The clinical EEG

As previously noted, accounts of EEG phenomenology and technology should be sought elsewhere; only a brief summary of essential terms and concepts will be given here. When describing EEGs a distinction is made between more or less continuous 'background' or 'ongoing' activity and episodic transients, and between those phenomena which are generalized or involve large areas of the scalp bilaterally and those which are more localized or 'focal'. Ongoing activity is normally symmetrical and is classified into four frequency bands: delta up to 4 waves per second, theta 4–8/s, alpha 8–14/s and beta above 14/s.

An EEG machine has typically 8–20 channels, each of which writes out on a paper chart a continuous tracing of the potential difference between two points. There are essentially two ways of recording the EEG. One, 'common reference derivation', displays on each channel the potential difference between one electrode on the scalp and a common reference point which is the same for

all channels. The reference may itself be either a particular electrode or an electrical connection inside the EEG machine which corresponds to the average potential of all the electrodes in use. If the reference is appropriately chosen, a localized EEG phenomenon will produce waves on the write out which are largest on the channel recording from the overlying electrode.

An alternative method, which is generally preferred in Europe, is so-called 'bipolar' derivation. This involves connecting rows of electrodes to the EEG machine in such a way that the channels record from consecutive pairs (channel 1: electrodes A and B; channel 2: electrodes B and C; channel 3: electrodes C and D, etc.). This has the effect of highlighting any localized phenomenon, which causes an electrode to assume a potential difference with respect to its neighbours, as this will produce defections in opposite directions on the two channels connected to the affected electrode, so-called 'phase reversal' (Fig. 9.3).

The appearance of the term 'phase reversal' in an EEG report thus signifies merely that a particular method of recording has been used to demonstrate a localized EEG event; it does not necessarily signify that anything abnormal has been found. Examples of both common reference

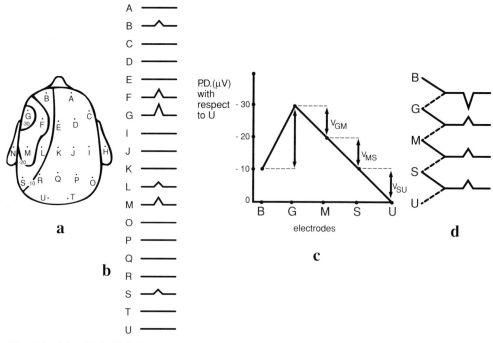

Fig. 9.3   A localized EEG phenomenon in the left frontal region represented (a) as a contour map; (b) on common reference derivation referred to an electrode, H, at a point on the scalp remote from the physiological event in question; (c) as a graph of potential against distance along the line of electrodes B, G, M, S and U on bipolar derivation from the same line of electrodes showing phase-reversal at electrode G. Reproduced with permission from Binnie et al 1982.

and bipolar derivation will be found in various illustrations to this chapter.

THE ICTAL EEG

Depth recording

Intracranial electrodes provide a clearer picture of the electrophysiological events during a seizure than does the scalp EEG. In humans, the occasion to insert intracranial electrodes arises only where there is thought to be a possibility of neurosurgical treatment. An electrode at the site where the seizure commences will typically show at the onset of the attack a high frequency discharge, perhaps of 60/s or faster, reflecting highly synchronized activity within a very restricted volume of surrounding brain. Sometimes seizure onset is characterized by alternating spiky waveforms and slower components (spike-and-wave), more commonly such activity appears only in a later phase of the seizure.

These rhythmic phenomena may sometimes be preceded by a transient event, a DC shift, an isolated sharp wave of 100–200 ms duration or a spike followed by a slower wave (Fig. 9.4). Sometimes, the initial change appears to be a reduction in amplitude of the ongoing background activity or even a cessation of interictal spiky transients which were previously present.

There follows a gradual evolution in both time and space. The picture is very varied, but typically the discharges decrease in frequency and progressively increase in amplitude, changing as they do to discrete spikes falling progressively from a frequency of 20/s to 10/s or less. The spikes generally give way to spike-and-wave activity—short spiky transients alternating with slower waves of some hundreds of milliseconds duration—and the frequency continues to fall progressively over the course of the seizure. The discharges may become irregular before they finally cease, leaving a postictal picture, either of slowing or of a very low amplitude record which gradually gives way to high voltage slow activity. This postictal record in turn shows a progressive rise in frequency and fall

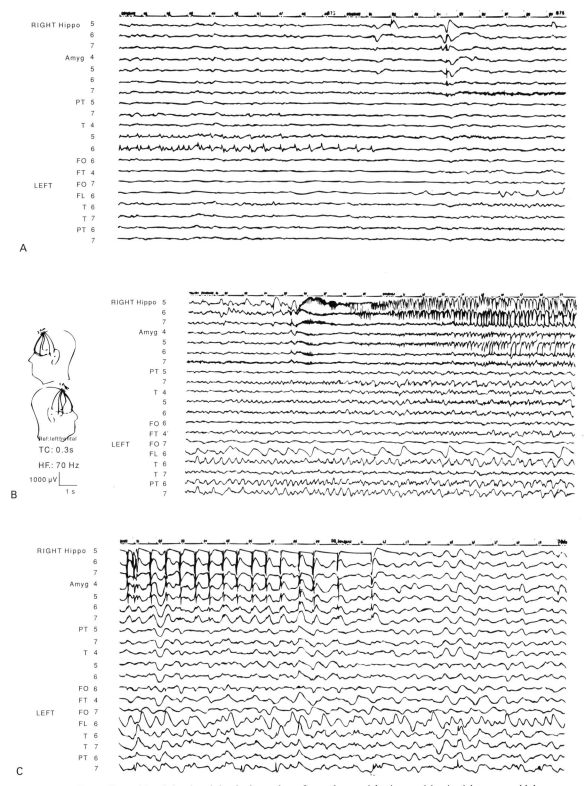

Fig. 9.4 Recording, with subdural and depth electrodes, of complex partial seizure arising in right temporal lobe.

in amplitude until the previous interictal pattern of background activity is restored, minutes or sometimes days later.

The evolution in space of the ictal disturbance will determine the clinical manifestations. The discharge may remain confined within a small volume of tissue close to its site of onset, for instance the amygdala-hippocampus complex on one side. Alternatively, it may spread to involve adjacent cortex within the same hemisphere or, usually abruptly, generalize through the commissural systems to involve the contralateral hemisphere also. Gradual spread through cortex adjacent to the focus will give rise to the classical Jacksonian march; bilateral limbic involvement will produce the impairment of consciousness characteristic of a complex partial seizure, and generalization, involving cortex, thalamus and possibly brainstem structures, will produce a secondarily generalized, usually tonic-clonic, seizure. Depending on the site of onset and the anatomical pattern of spread, various subtly different ictal patterns may be distinguished, as documented by Wieser (1983a). With bilateral hemispheric involvement discharges will generally be synchronous. Residual postictal disturbance may produce a localized neurological deficit (Todd's palsy), if focal, or confusion, if generalized.

Intracerebral ictal recordings in human idiopathic generalized epilepsy have, understandably, rarely been performed. However, Williams (1953) described rhythmic spike-wave activity during absences which was synchronous in thalamus and cortex. Depth electrode studies of experimental generalized epilepsies have usually employed chemical models with varying results. Systemic administration of massive doses of penicillin produces seizures with a diffuse corticothalamic onset with generalized spike-wave activity. By contrast, bicuculline and pentalenetetrazol produce changes which are first apparent in the brain stem reticular formation or the lateral geniculate body consisting of high-frequency multi-unit activity sometimes reaching frequencies of several hundred Hz (Rodin et al 1971, Binnie et al 1985c).

Scalp EEG

Scalp EEG recording involves further loss of in-

formation as compared with depth registration and, in particular, sharply localized ictal events may be undetectable in the conventional EEG. During partial seizures, the EEG presents a picture which may be regarded as a simplification of that obtainable with depth recording. Typically, a similar evolution will be seen from rapid, spiky discharges to spike-wave activity of greater amplitude and lower frequency with eventual postictal reduction of amplitude and/or slowing. Again, typically, the onset of such changes will be focal, roughly overlying the deep focus, and generalization may occur to a greater or lesser degree. However, simultaneous depth and scalp recording show that the initial events found at the depth electrodes may not appear at all on the surface, and the scalp EEG changes may appear only some tens of seconds after the onset of the seizure. High-frequency seizure activity in particular is rarely seen in a scalp recording and the ictal changes in the scalp EEG often commence with spikes, sharp waves or spike-wave activity.

Although localized spiky waveforms due to synchronous discharge are probably an invariable finding in depth recordings of partial seizures (assuming that an electrode is placed at the appropriate site), ictal changes in the scalp EEG in partial epilepsy are not necessarily spiky, focal nor even unilateral. Seizure onset may be heralded by the appearance of an activity not previously present, within the theta, alpha or beta range (Fig. 9.5). The initial, or indeed the only, EEG change may be a reduction in amplitude of ongoing activity (an 'electrodecremental event'). The physiological basis of this is uncertain, but is most probably desynchronization of cortical activity due to corticopetal inputs from the epileptic focus, possibly transmitted through the reticular formation. Rhythmic, non-spiky activities or an electro-decremental event are particularly likely to be generalized and often symmetrical, but even frank spikes or spike-wave discharges may be generalized or show a localization or lateralization which does not reflect the topography of the seizure onset in deep structures. This may be understandable when the evolution of a partial seizure is followed with a combination of depth and subdural electrodes as illustrated in Figure 9.4. This shows the onset of an attack in a patient

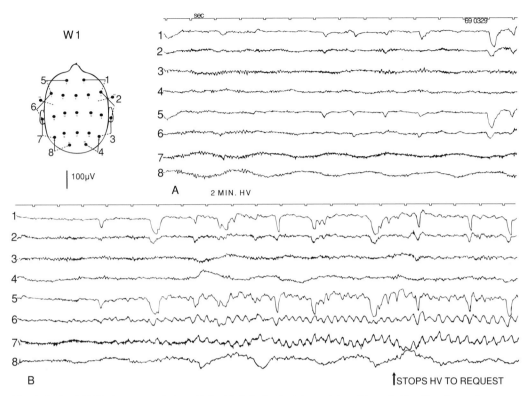

Fig. 9.5 Ictal EEG change consisting of left-sided rhythmic delta activity without 'epileptiform' or spiky phenomena. This picture consistently accompanied the patient's complex partial seizures, induced in this case by overbreathing.

with partial complex seizures which were due to a right mesial temporal sclerotic lesion and ceased when this was removed. The electrographic pattern was consistent and clearly focal in 10 seizures registered with intracranial electrodes. The initial discharge remained localized to deep right temporal structures for some 5–10 seconds. Once the spread to more remote cortical structures occurred, the discharges were bilateral and initially more prominent over the contralateral hemisphere. This gave rise to misleadinq lateralization of the focus in ictal scalp EEGs.

Some partial seizures produce no apparent change in the scalp EEG (Ives & Woods 1980). An absence of ictal change in the scalp EEG in partial epilepsies is most common during simple partial seizures and, indeed, is the usual finding in those with psychic symptomatology (Wieser 1979), or in attacks consisting only of a viscero-sensory aura.

Following a partial seizure, a residual postictal

abnormality may be found in 50–70% of patients, most commonly regional slowing, depression of ongoing activity, or less commonly an increase in epileptiform discharges compared with the preictal state. Kaibara & Blume (1988) reported that the postictal changes were always ipsilateral to the site of seizure onset, but this is contrary to the experience of the present author, particularly in patients where depth recording was used to distinguish the causative focus from the pattern of discharge subsequent to propagation as seen in the scalp EEG (Binnie et al 1990). Similarly, Gloor (1975) points out that postictal changes reflect the region most intensely involved in the seizure, which may not correspond to the site of onset.

The evolution of electrical activity in the EEG during a tonic-clonic convulsion of generalized onset parallels that of many partial seizures but without localizing features (Fig. 9.6). Possibly after a brief electrodecremental event, a rapid

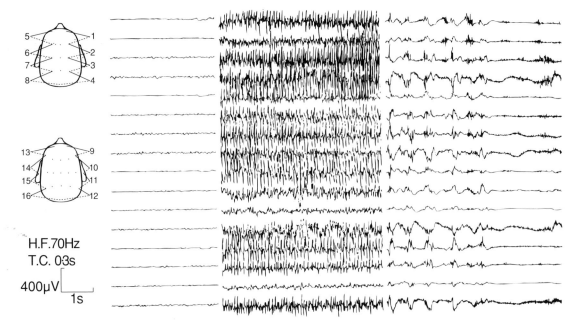

H.F.70Hz
T.C. 03s
400µV
1s

Fig. 9.6 Evolution of EEG during tonic-clonic seizure. (a) pre-ictal pattern; (b) high-frequency spiking intermixed activity with muscle artifact at seizure onset; (c) generalized spike-wave; (d) postictal slowing. (The apparently low amplitude of the EEG before the seizure is due to the use of a low recording sensitivity to accommodate the high voltage ictal discharges.)

build-up of spikes is typically seen followed by generalized spike-wave activity. In the clonic phase, the muscle jerks are synchronous with the spike-wave complexes and, as the seizure ends, both become less frequent and irregular. Marked, generalized postictal slowing is seen, possibly preceded by a period of flattening. The generalized convulsive seizures most convenienty studied in humans are those produced by bilateral ECT, and here the duration of postictal flattening is inversely related to the duration of the convulsive phase (Robin et al 1985). In general, the more severe and prolonged the postictal disturbance in the EEG, the more marked is the clinical symptomatology. However, some patients may show residual slowing and bursts of delta waves, often rhythmic, 24 hours after apparent clinical recovery.

The classical absence seizure of idiopathic generalized epilepsy is accompanied by generalized, fairly symmetrical, regular spike-wave activity of about three per second which commences abruptly, usually 1 or 2 seconds before the onset of apparent clinical manifestations, and which may continue briefly after consciousness has started to return. In absence seizures, spike-wave discharges of under three seconds duration are not usually accompanied by obvious clinical change, although transitory impairment of cognitive function is often demonstrable during shorter discharges. The phenomenology of the absence seizure is in fact very varied. Those attacks in which myoclonic phenomena are prominent are often accompanied by multiple spike and wave activity. As has been pointed out by Binnie & Van der Wens (1986) there is some considerable overlap in clinical and electrical phenomena between absence seizures, which may include involuntary movements and automatisms, and brief complex partial seizures with loss of consciousness at onset. The overlapping clinical pattern probably reflects a common pathophysiology, for both are accompanied by generalized spike-wave activity (Aird et al 1989). It has been claimed that differentiation by the ictal EEG between a complex absence and a brief complex partial seizure may rest on the demonstration of a focal onset of the latter. However, some authors have suggested that the distinction may be somewhat artificial and find that in those patients where this differential diagnosis is difficult, satisfactory therapeutic response is generally obtained only by a combination of drugs usually effective in partial seizures and in absences (Binnie & Van der Wens 1986, Hendrickson 1986, Stefan & Burr 1986).

A lack of apparent ictal EEG change is far less common in generalized than in partial seizures. However, pure atonic seizures without other ictal manifestations may be accompanied only by an electrodecremental event in the scalp EEG (Egli et al 1985). This may be difficult to detect if the EEG is contaminated by artifact as the patient falls.

'EPILEPTIFORM ACTIVITY'

Definitions

A feature of the ictal EEG as described above, whether recorded from the scalp or with intracranial electrodes, is the occurrence of spiky waveforms due to abnormal, synchronous cerebral neuronal activity. Similar discharges, spikes, spike-wave complexes and sharp waves, are also seen in the interictal EEGs of most people with epilepsy. It might therefore seem useful to have a generic term for discharges of this kind, but the question of agreeing a suitable terminology has led to a semantic debate, which in turn has to some extent confused the clinical interpretation of these phenomena.

Such terms as 'epileptic discharge' are not acceptable, as these waveforms are sometimes seen in the EEGs of people who do not apparently have epilepsy. Yet less satisfactory is the American usage 'seizure discharge' as, even in people who do have epilepsy, the discharges are not necessarily ictal. The term 'paroxysmal activity' has been widely used but, strictly speaking, is applicable to any episodic phenomenon as, for instance, a K-complex. Other euphemisms which are used in some European countries include 'irritative activity'. It is not clear whether this implies that the activity is irritating the brain or that it is a manifestation of cerebral irritation, in either case there remains the implication of epileptogenesis. In reality, what is at issue is not

the name but the underlying concept; namely, that these phenomena are typical of, but not specific to, epilepsy. Throughout this text the term 'epileptiform activity' will be used, both recognizing the statistical association with epilepsy and stressing that, as a descriptive EEG term, it refers only to a type of waveform, and not an interpretation.

Numerous terms are listed by the terminology committee of the International Federation of Societies of Electroencephalography and Clinical Neurophysiology (Chatrian et al 1974) to describe the various types of epileptiform activity and many more non-approved expressions are in use. The essential quality of these discharges is their spiky aspect, the steep gradients seen in the EEG tracing and particularly the abrupt change in direction of pen deflection which gives each wave a sharp peak. Those spiky transients which are of less than 80 ms duration are called spikes, those lasting from 80–120 ms are sharp waves. Waves of longer duration than 120 ms and of sharp appearance may also represent epileptiform activity, but there is no official term used to describe them. Published definitions beg the question of how sharp a wave has to be to qualify as a spike or a sharp wave. Moreover, the identification of these waveforms depends in part on the background EEG activity. Continuing rhythmic beta activity may, for instance, be made up of waves every one of which would be regarded as a spike if it occurred against a background from which high frequency components were absent (Fig. 9.7).

Spikes may occur as continuous bursts of activity, the most extreme examples of which are the multi-unit discharges recorded with depth electrodes close to the site of origin of a seizure. Discrete spikes and sharp waves are usually followed by a slower wave and, if this is prominent, the two together are described as a spike-and-wave complex or sharp and slow-wave complex. Often multiple spikes occur with a single slow wave. Spike-wave complexes themselves may be isolated or occur as more or less rhythmic activity. Focal spikes are often polyphasic, but the most prominent component is usually negative, reflecting current flow towards the underlying cortical surface. Positive spikes at 6 or 14/s occur as a normal phenomenon (see below). Otherwise, positive

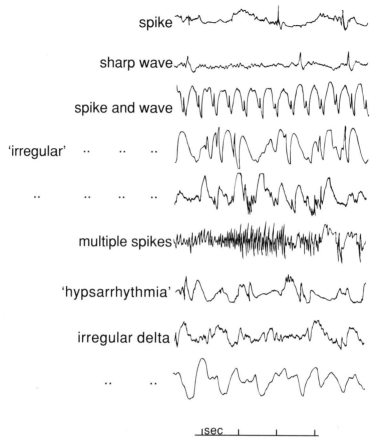

spike

sharp wave

spike and wave

'irregular'

. .   . .   . .

multiple spikes

'hypsarrhythmia'

irregular delta

. .   . .

ₗsec ₗ   ₗ   ₗ

Fig. 9.7   Examples of more or less obvious epileptiform activity.

focal spikes are rare, occur mostly in children and are also seen where a gross cortical defect allows the electrode to record from the deep surface of the cortex in the wall of an adjacent sulcus (Matsuo & Knott 1977). However, the writer has seen one corticographically proven instance of positive spikes arising from the surface of intact, if slightly gliotic, cortex in an adult (Binnie et al 1989b).

Normal epileptiform phenomena

A discussion of definitions and description of the typical waveforms by no means ends the confusion surrounding epileptiform activity. Some spiky waveforms are normal phenomena frequently found in EEGs of healthy subjects and having no significance in relation to epilepsy. They are recognizable, however, by characteristic

morphology and topography, and by occurring under specific circumstances. Some instances will be considered here; for a fuller review see Naquet (1983) and Riley (1983). A good example is provided by so-called '6 and 14 per second positive spikes' (Fig. 9.8).

As the name suggests, these are rhythmic spiky discharges at 6 or 14/s, the most conspicuous component being positive at the surface of the scalp and generally focal towards the posterior temporal region on one or both sides of the head. This is itself an unusual feature as other kinds of focal spikes are predominantly surface negative. This activity occurs in drowsiness and light sleep, and is most often seen in adolescents and young adults where the incidence may be 20% or more. The spikes are of low amplitude and produce widespread electrical fields over the scalp without steep potential gradients and, consequently, are

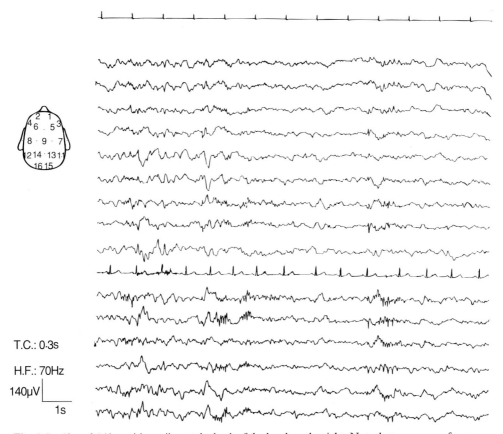

T.C.: 0·3s

H.F.: 70Hz

140μV

1s

Fig. 9.8   6/s and 14/s positive spikes at the back of the head on the right. Note that common reference derivation has been used to display this phenomenon.

more readily detected when common reference methods of EEG derivation are employed than in bipolar montages. It is probably for this technical reason that positive spikes are reported more commonly in North America than in Europe, as in most European countries bipolar methods of recording are used more than common reference. Controlled studies of particular groups of patients, most notably with psychiatric disorders and allergic conditions, show some increase in incidence of positive spikes. However, the association is too weak to be of any clinical significance and in any event epilepsy is not one of those conditions associated with an increased incidence of this phenomenon.

Another example of a spiky waveform without clinical significance is provided by benign epileptiform transients of sleep (BETS). These are spikes or spike-wave complexes of very short duration and stereotyped waveform occurring in the anterior temporal regions during sleep. These, too, are seen frequently in normal subjects, possibly in as many as 50% when appropriate electrode placements are used (White et al 1977). BETS also appear to occur more often in patients than in normal subjects and their clinical significance is disputed (Hughes & Grunener 1984). However, within patient populations they do not appear to discriminate between different diagnostic groups (Gutrecht 1989), and in particular, the finding of BETS does not contribute to the diagnosis of epilepsy. Interestingly, depth recordings in people with partial seizures of temporal lobe origin clearly show BETS, when present, to be independent of the epileptogenic foci from which the seizures themselves arise (Westmoreland et al 1979).

'Mid-temporal rhythmic discharge' consists of rhythmic sharp-waves at about 6/s over the temporal regions. This activity may occur for a few seconds or for hours at a time and may be present in repeated EEGs over many years. It appears to be unaffected by vigilance, attention or overbreathing, and is unresponsive to antiepileptic drugs. During the discharge, no ictal clinical manifestations are seen and no cognitive disturbance is demonstrable. Despite formerly being termed 'psychomotor variant' because of a supposed relationship with temporal lobe epilepsy (Gibbs & Gibbs 1953), it is often seen in patients without evident cerebral disorder and the association with epilepsy is weak (Lipman & Hughes 1969, Hughes & Cayaffa 1973). A similar phenomenon, 'sub-clinical rhythmic epileptiform discharge of adults' (or SREDA), occurs further posteriorly in the parieto-temporal-occipital region and is virtually confined to adults of more than 50 years of age (Naquet et al 1961, Westmoreland & Klass 1981). Again, it appears to have no clinical significance.

To the catalogue of EEG phenomena which may mistakenly be interpreted as evidence for epilepsy, must be added various responses to 'activation procedures' (see below). Hyperventilation is routinely carried out for some 3 min during clinical EEG examination and may induce epileptiform discharges, most dramatically generalized 3/s spike-wave activity in patients with absence seizures. However, young normal subjects respond to this procedure by a slowing of the EEG and, in anyone under the age of 30 who overbreathes vigorously for 3 min, rhythmic bifrontal delta activity at about 3/s may be expected. This normal physiological response is often misinterpreted as evidence of 'cortical instability' and wrongly supposed to support a diagnosis of epilepsy. Sadly, it is not uncommon for healthy children to receive antiepileptic medication for years because of a misinterpreted, normal slow-wave response to overbreathing.

Activation by flashing light, intermittent photic stimulation or IPS, is also routinely performed during EEG examination. The normal response consists of rhythmic activity at the back of the head following the frequency of the flicker. Some patients who are described as 'photosensitive', and generally have epilepsy, respond with clear, generalized epileptiform discharges, a photoconvulsive response or PCR. However, between these extremes a variety of unusual or atypical responses may occur. These include occipital spikes at the frequency of the stimulus, following at sub- or supraharmonics of the flash rate, and the occurrence of theta or delta activity at the back of the head. These various atypical responses are largely genetically determined (Doose & Gerken 1973) and occur in some 15% of normal children. Some indeed have a weak association with epilepsy: nearly half of those exhibiting occipital spikes suffer from seizures and, when the photoconvulsive response is suppressed by effective medication, IPS may continue to elicit occipital spikes or marked harmonic following. It would, however, be misleading to regard any response short of a generalized epileptiform discharge as supportive of epilepsy.

Clinical significance of epileptiform activity

From the above, it should be clear that any statement concerning the clinical predictive significance of 'epileptiform activity' depends firstly on how this term is used. Epileptiform phenomena in the widest sense of spiky waveforms are common in normal people, particularly in the young and during drowsiness or sleep. Any author using the term in this sense may rightly state that epileptiform discharges are common in healthy subjects and are not reliably predictive of epilepsy, nor indeed of any other cerebral disorder. However, this simplistic view misleadingly undervalues the utility of the EEG, because, when the concept of epileptiform activity is applied more narrowly, excluding those spiky waveforms which are known to be normal or unrelated to epilepsy, its clinical significance is greatly enhanced. It is necessary, moreover, to distinguish between the significance of epileptiform activity as evidence of cerebral dysfunction and its specificity to epilepsy. When EEG abnormalities, including epileptiform activity, are found in supposedly healthy volunteers, further enquiry usually reveals that the subjects suffer from, or have a history of, a cerebral disorder (Roubicek et al 1967, Binnie et al 1978). One of the largest studies of normal subjects was performed by Robin et al (1978) in over 7500 airmen: 2% exhibited abnormal epileptiform EEG activity in the narrow sense suggested above. However, of those who were followed up, it transpired that more than half had a history of epilepsy and several of the remainder had been declared unfit for flying duties on neuropsychiatric grounds. In this series, the eventual incidence of epileptiform EEG activity in subjects without evidence of brain dysfunction (after correction for those lost to follow up) was of about 3.4 per 1000.

A different picture emerges when patient populations are considered, not suffering from epilepsy but undergoing EEG examination because of other complaints. Here the incidence of epileptiform EEG activity is some 2–3% overall. In a series of over 6000 patients, Zivin & Ajmone Marsan (1968) found that about one-third of those with EEG discharges had primary disease of the brain. In certain groups the prevalence of epileptiform activity was particularly high: 30% in those with mental handicap, 24% with congenital or perinatal brain damage, 12% after cranial operations and 10% in patients with cerebral tumours. Fourteen percent of patients with discharges later developed epilepsy. Psychiatric patients may represent a group intermediate between neurologically-screened volunteers and other people without epilepsy seen in a general, mixed EEG practice. Bridgers (1987) found epileptiform activity in 2.6% of over 3000 psychiatric patients without epilepsy (and in 37% of those with a seizure history). Psychiatric syndromes with a possible organic aetiology were associated with EEG discharges, notably barbiturate abuse, anorexia nervosa and explosive behaviour in the young. Medication may also have played a role, the prevalence of epileptiform activity being 3.0–3.2% on major tranquillizers, antidepressants or lithium, 0.8% in patients taking benzodiazepines and only 0.7% in those over 25 years of age and taking no drugs. The presence of epileptiform activity is thus of much more value for distinguishing between a person with epilepsy and a healthy volunteer or an unmedicated patient whose symptoms are of psychiatric origin, than for deciding whether or not known brain disease is likely to give rise to seizures.

Variability of the EEG in epilepsy

Epilepsy, although a chronic disorder, is not a static condition. Long, seizure-free, interictal periods are interspersed with brief seizures, which may vary substantially from one attack to the next and which may be preceded by a prodromal phase or followed by a post-ictal state with residual sensory, motor or cognitive deficits, lasting from seconds to days. Outside centres with special facilities for prolonged monitoring, the EEG investigation of epilepsy is concerned almost exclusively with interictal recording. Occasionally, a seizure occurs by chance during EEG registration, or an emergency record can be obtained from a patient during status epilepticus, or in a postictal condition.

Even the interictal EEG is highly variable, and, under apparently constant conditions, epileptiform discharges may be absent in one half-hour period and profuse in the next. It is no wonder then that the findings in 'routine' EEGs of 30–40 min duration even in those centres (few in many countries) which conform to accepted optimum standards are so inconsistent. Some of the variability is apparently random, some is due to circadian rhythms or related to the time interval from the preceding or next seizure, but the most important single factor is sleep and waking (see section below).

EFFECTS OF SLEEP

During sleep the EEG changes dramatically, showing first a loss of the alpha rhythm, and then, with increasing depth of sleep, progressively greater amounts of slow activity. Sleep depth is conventionally classified into four levels according to criteria proposed by Dement & Kleitmann in 1957. There is a further stage of sleep characterized by rapid eye movements (REM) and associated with dreaming. Interictal epileptiform discharges are often very sensitive to changes in the state of awareness. With the onset of drowsiness and stage I sleep, generalized spike-wave activity may either disappear or increase, but focal discharges will generally become more frequent or may appear if absent in the alert state. In light (stage II) sleep the focal epileptiform activity is generally most prominent, whereas generalized discharges may attain a maximum in stage III. REM sleep is usually associated with a reduction or abolition of both generalized (Gastaut et al

1965, Ross et al 1966, Passouant 1967, Billiard 1982) and focal discharges (Batini et al 1963, Perria et al 1966, Angelieri 1974, Daskalov 1975, Manni et al 1990). However, some authors claim an increase of focal temporal discharges in REM sleep (Passouant et al 1965, Epstein & Hill 1966, Mayersdorf & Wilder 1974). Bursts of generalized spike-wave activity may become longer although less numerous during REM (Stevens et al 1971). The increase in discharges during sleep may be dramatic and Tassinari et al (1982) described a group of children who exhibited continuous epileptiform discharges during sleep, although these were generally absent in the waking state.

During all-night sleep recording some patients may show a characteristic distribution of discharges, with maxima shortly after falling asleep, in the middle of the night or towards morning (Kellaway & Frost 1983). Many patients show a circadian pattern of seizure incidence related to sleep and wake which may provide a basis for classifying epilepsy into sleeping, awakening and diffuse forms (Janz 1962). Janz suggested that diffuse epilepsy most often had a lesional basis, whereas wakening epilepsy was usually of the idiopathic generalized type. Others, such as Billiard (1982), do not confirm this. In general, the time of occurrence of the maximum EEG discharge rate corresponds to that of seizure frequency (Martins da Silva et al 1984). Thus, patients with awakening epilepsy tend to show the maximum EEG discharge rates at about the time of wakening from spontaneous, nocturnal sleep.

Conversely, epilepsy and epileptiform discharges affect sleep patterns. REM sleep is variously reported as being normal or reduced, and as occurring earlier or later than in controls (Manni et al 1990). The amount of time spent in light sleep (stages I and II) may increase, and there may be more frequent shifts between sleep stages (Jovanovic 1967, Haiasz and Deveyi 1974, Chemburkar et al 1976, Baldy-Moulinier 1982). Some authors find disruption of sleep continuity to be related to occurrence of interictal discharges or seizures (Bessett 1982, Baldy-Moulinier 1982). Manni et al (1990) found increased awakenings and stage to stage shifts in medicated patients with partial epilepsy, both refractory and seizure-free, although the latter showed no epileptiform discharges. Sleep EEG patterns may themselves be so disrupted that sleep staging by the normal criteria is impossible (Bordas-Ferrer et al 1966, Besset 1982). However, some authors have been unable to confirm any abnormalities of sleep patterns in epilepsy, provided no attack occurred during the night (Delange et al 1962, Angelieri et al 1967, Kazamatsuri et al 1970, Sato et al 1973). The picture is complicated by the effects of antiepileptic drugs. However, Röder-Wanner et al (1985) reported a series of nocturnal sleep studies in untreated patients. Their main finding was an increase of deep sleep in the first part of the night in photosensitive patients with generalized epilepsy. Wolf et al (1985) found specific effects of different antiepileptic drugs on the sleep of previously untreated subjects, but the pattern was complicated by interactions between drugs and various epilepsy syndromes.

THE DIAGNOSTIC EEG SERIES IN EPILEPSY

Many misleading statements have been published concerning 'the EEG in epilepsy', generally emphasizing the poor yield of diagnostically useful information, but ignoring the fact that any single record is a brief sample over a short space of time of a continually fluctuating phenomenon. Ajmone Marsan & Zivin (1970) performed repeated routine waking EEG examinations in a large series of patients with epilepsy. Some 30% showed interictal epileptiform discharges in all recordings; 17.5%, by contrast, were never shown to have interictal discharges even when the EEG was repeated 10 times or more. The remaining 52% exhibited epileptiform activity in some tracings and not in others. From these figures it would be expected that, in a group of patients with epilepsy, a single waking EEG will demonstrate epileptiform activity in approximately 50% and that, with repeated recordings, discharges will be found sooner or later in 85%. There are, of course, various clinical factors which influence the probability of interictal discharges being found; Sundaram et al (1990) reported the yield from a single record to be substantially increased (to 77%) in patients investigated within 2 days after a seizure, and to be much greater in patients with monthly seizures

Table 9.1 Diagnostic EEG investigation of epilepsy (after Binnie 1986)

	Patients with interictal epileptiform activity (EA) present in waking EEG			Cumulative Yield of EA[*]
Patients with epilepsy to be investigated 100	never 15	sometimes 50	always 35	
Wake EEG recorded	15	50	35	
EA present	0	15	35	50
EA absent	15	35	0	
Sleep EEG recorded	15	35	—	
EA present	5	25		80
EA absent	10	10		
Repeated wake and sleep EEGs recorded	10	10		
EA found	2	10		92
Consistently absent	8	0		

[*] EEG investigation of these patients is not necessarily complete: some may require further studies, for instance, for localization of a focus.

(68%) than in those who had been seizure-free for a year (39%).

The yield of diagnostically useful information can, however, be increased by recording during sleep, as this increases the incidence of interictal epileptiform activity. A suitable diagnostic strategy is illustrated in Table 9.1. In half of a typical sample of patients with epilepsy referred for diagnostic EEG investigation, the initial recording will demonstrate epileptiform activity. In some of these, it may be considered that the EEG has provided as much diagnostic information as is required to support the clinical findings, in others, further studies may be needed to address specific problems, for instance to determine whether a focus can be demonstrated during sleep or whether frequent EEG discharges are accompanied by clinical manifestations which have been overlooked. In the 50% in whom the initial EEG failed to demonstrate epileptiform activity, a further recording should be obtained, including a period of sleep. This will increase the yield of diagnostically useful information, partly as a result simply of repeating the EEG and partly because of the emergence of new phenomena, including epileptiform discharges, during sleep. If the findings remain negative and there is a degree of diagnostic uncertainty requiring further investigation, the sleep EEG may be repeated, and many workers would prefer on this occasion to induce sleep by a method which may itself have some activating effect; for instance by previous deprivation of sleep or by drugs which may themselves have some proconvulsive action. Sleep and methods of sleep induction are considered further elsewhere. There will remain some 10% of the original patients with epilepsy in whom no interictal epileptiform discharges have been demonstrated. This group will consist chiefly of patients with infrequent generalized seizures or simple partial seizures, particularly with sensorimotor symptoms only. In many of these patients, the diagnosis of epilepsy appears certain on clinical grounds and further investigation is not justified. However, in perhaps 5% of the original sample a confident clinical diagnosis is not possible and here an attempt may usefully be made by long-term monitoring of the EEG to obtain an ictal recording. There are also a substantial number of patients (about 15% of referrals to one tertiary centre for epilepsy) who have attacks which eventually prove to be non-epileptic in nature. Here too ictal recording may be crucial to establishing the diagnosis.

ACTIVATION PROCEDURES

The yield of epileptiform EEG activity and of

other abnormalities may be increased by the use of various so-called 'activation procedures'. Of these, hyperventilation and intermittent photic stimulation are performed routinely in clinical EEG examination in most departments, irrespective of the reason for referral. Sleep is widely used to increase the yield of diagnostically useful information in epilepsy; other techniques, mostly using chemical convulsant agents, are employed less frequently.

Hyperventilation

The hypocapnia produced by voluntary hyperventilation results in cerebral vasoconstriction and reduced cerebral blood flow. It is probably by this mechanism that the EEG changes on overbreathing are elicited. The degree of response is closely related to the vigour with which overbreathing is performed or, more exactly, to the fall in end-tidal P_{CO_2}. Binnie et al (1969) suggested that the progressive reduction in EEG responses to overbreathing with increasing age could be attributed to a smaller fall in P_{CO_2} in older subjects. The effects are enhanced by hypoglycaemia (Heppenstall 1944).

In the older literature, it was suggested that in various groups of patients, including those with epilepsy, the changes in background activity on overbreathing were enhanced. It may be questioned whether this was in any way attributable to the seizure disorder or merely to the familiarity with the procedure of patients who had undergone many previous EEG investigations. In any event, it is unwise to suppose that a marked but qualitatively normal response to overbreathing is supportive of epilepsy. In many patients with epilepsy, discharges appear or occur more frequently during overbreathing. Both generalized and focal activities may be affected, but those most consistently increased are the generalized spike-wave discharges of about 3/s seen in patients with absence seizures. Indeed 3 min of vigorous overbreathing in such a patient will usually elicit not only a discharge but also an attack. The absence of spike-wave activity after 3 min of overbreathing, performed sufficiently vigorously to produce marked changes in background activity, must cast considerable doubt on a diagnosis of absence sei-

zures; it does not, of course, exclude the possibility that a patient's episodes of unconsciousness are seizures of some other type, such as complex partial.

Photic stimulation

Intermittent photic stimulation (IPS) normally elicits discrete visual evoked responses at low flash rates and rhythmic 'photic following' at frequencies from between 4/s and 10/s up to 20/s or more. These responses are of greatest amplitude at the back of the head and are fairly symmetrical. Gross asymmetry (more than 50% right–left amplitude difference) may reflect cerebral pathology (Kooi et al 1960) and is generally paralleled by a corresponding asymmetry of the alpha rhythm.

As noted above, a variety of atypical responses may also occur. At the back of the head occipital spikes may be seen. These are large, atypical visual evoked responses (Panayiotopoulos et al 1970, 1972, Dimitrakoudi et al 1973) and have a one-to-one relationship to the flashes. They do have a weak association with epilepsy which is present in half the patients showing occipital spikes (Maheshwari & Jeavons 1975). They may be seen in some photosensitive subjects during stimulation at frequencies too low to elicit epileptiform activity, and may persist as a residual abnormality after photosensitivity has been abolished by medication (Harding et al 1978). Other anomalous posterior responses to IPS include runs of theta or delta activity; these are genetically determined but of no clinical significance. Another normal but potentially confusing response consists of spikes synchronous with the flashes and recorded at the front of the head. This is photomyoclonus (Bickford et al 1952) and consists of myogenic potentials due to rhythmic contraction of scalp muscles in time with the flashes. It is a normal finding which can be demonstrated in 50% of volunteers if a sufficiently bright flash is used and if they voluntarily increase their facial muscle tone by grimacing. It has no apparent connection with the photomyoclonus seen in the Senegalese baboon, which is a form of visually-induced myoclonic epileptic seizure.

Most important in the context of epilepsy is the 'photoconvulsive response' (PCR) described by

Bickford et al (1952). This comprises generalized spike-and-wave, or less commonly spike, discharges, which have a repetition rate independent of the frequency of the flashes. The PCR is strongly associated with epilepsy, and must be distinguished from other atypical responses to photic stimulation. Confusion has been caused by the use of the term 'photosensitivity' to describe both the PCR and normal variants of the photic response. A majority of patients showing a PCR are subject to seizures induced by environmental visual stimuli, and the recognition of photosensitivity is therefore often critical to their management. Because of the importance of EEG investigation in this particular group of patients, photosensitive epilepsy is the subject of a later section of this chapter.

Reliable assessment of responses to photic stimulation requires careful technique (Binnie et al 1982). The methods used vary greatly between laboratories and are rarely optimal for demonstrating a PCR. In patients with a history of seizures precipitated by viewing television or by visual patterns, it may be appropriate to assess the EEG responses to these provocative stimuli, using methods similar in principal to those employed for flicker stimulation (Wilkins et al 1979b, Darby et al 1980a). Further details will be found in the section on photosensitive epilepsy.

Auditory stimulation

Rhythmic auditory stimulation enjoyed a brief vogue as an activating method, particularly in patients with seizures of temporal lobe origin. This technique has now been generally abandoned, but possibly deserves to be reconsidered in view of a recent report by Hogan & Sundaram (1989) suggesting that it is almost as effective as photic stimulation in generalized epilepsies.

Sleep induction

The effects of sleep on the EEG in epilepsy and the importance of sleep in diagnostic EEG investigation were noted above. For clinical purposes, it is not often convenient to record during nocturnal sleep and various methods may be used to induce sleep during the working hours of the EEG laboratory. The ideal is probably a restful environment and a relaxed approach to recording which will encourage the patient to sleep spontaneously. The artificial method most often used is administration of sedative drugs, notably quinalbarbitone and chloral hydrate (or its derivatives such as dichloralphenazone). In addition to activating epileptiform discharges, these drugs may provide further diagnostically useful information by virtue of the beta activity which they induce in the EEG. The appearance of beta activity is a normal response to barbiturates in particular and an asymmetry may reflect underlying cerebral pathology.

Other drugs used to induce sleep may have some proconvulsive action in their own right. This is probably the case with methohexitone and possibly with promethazine. Methohexitone has the feature of being administered intravenously, giving a rapid response, saving time and allowing the dose to be titrated accurately. It has the disadvantage that the patient passes rapidly into deep sleep, whereas it is during drowsiness and light sleep in particular that information of diagnostic value in partial epilepsies is most likely to be obtained. It should be given at a rate of about 10 mg per 30 seconds, only by a physician trained in anaesthesia, and with resuscitation equipment on hand. Promethazine may be particularly suitable for inducing sleep in children and is available as a syrup which may be more acceptable than sleeping tablets. Diazepam, given intravenously or by mouth, may seem ill suited as a sleep-inducing agent for investigating epilepsy in view of its antiepileptic action. However, as diazepam selectively suppresses generalized rather than focal discharges, it may be useful for inducing sleep in suspected partial epilepsy where the purpose of the investigation is specifically to attempt to demonstrate a focus (Gotman et al 1982). Thus, where it is suspected that bilateral discharges seen in the waking EEG represent secondary generalization, slow intravenous injection of diazepam may first suppress the generalized activity, unmasking the focus, and then cause the focal discharges to increase as the patient lapses into sleep. A similar result may be obtained with thiopentone, given slowly by intravenous injection, so that the patient does not fall asleep too rapidly (Lombroso & Erba 1970). In light drowsiness, generalized spike-wave discharges are suppressed and focal epileptiform activity may appear. If there is also a depression of barbiturate-induced fast activity at the same site, confidence in localization of the focus is reinforced.

One highly effective method of obtaining sleep during the normal working hours of an EEG laboratory is to arrange for the patient to remain awake all or part of the previous night. This not only produces a fairly natural sleep pattern, uncomplicated by the effects of hypnotic drugs, but also has been claimed to have some activating effect in its own right. This not unreasonable belief is based on the finding that prolonged sleep deprivation can induce seizures, even in persons not ordinarily suffering from epilepsy (Bennett 1962, Bennett et al 1969). However, a difficulty in assessing the yield of diagnostically useful information, both from sleep recording in general and from recording after sleep deprivation in particular, is that the available evidence is mostly derived from uncontrolled studies under conditions of routine clinical practice. The decision to proceed to sleep recording, either drug-induced or after sleep deprivation, generally follows from the failure of the initial EEG to provide the information required. The findings therefore confound the effects of the activation procedures as such with those of simply repeating the EEG. A study by Veldhuizen et al (1983) overcomes this problem: in a group of patients with refractory epilepsy, wake, drug-induced sleep and sleep deprivation records were obtained in random sequence and regardless of the previous findings. There was no evidence of an increased incidence of epileptiform activity in the waking state after 24 hours wakefulness nor was the yield of new information during sleep any greater when this was induced by deprivation rather than by drugs. The findings of Molaie & Cruz (1988) after more than usually prolonged (36 hour) deprivation were in general similar, although they did find, in stage II only, an increase in discharge rate during all night sleep recording. A limitation of both these studies was that they included no children and no patients with idiopathic generalized epilepsy: both groups in which the earlier literature, notwithstanding its methodological deficiencies, claims the greatest yield of activation by sleep deprivation.

A too rigid distinction should not be made between wake and induced-sleep recordings for diagnostic investigation of epilepsy. In partial epilepsies in particular, the yield of new information is likely to be greatest in the early stages of drowsiness, which may be attained during a 'routine' recording if the environment is restful and the approach of the technologist unhurried. This may account for the surprising conclusion, from a major centre for the preoperative assessment of patients with partial epilepsies, that the contribution of recording during drug induced sleep for diagnostic assessment was minimal (Gloor et al 1957).

Antiepileptic drug withdrawal

When the diagnosis of epilepsy is in doubt, clinical considerations will often dictate a trial of antiepileptic drug (AED) withdrawal, to determine the effect, if any, on the seizure frequency. This will also provide the opportunity to reassess the EEG in the absence of medication. It is, however, important to distinguish the results, both clinical and electroencephalographic, of removing the antiepileptic action of the drugs from the proconvulsant effects of acute AED withdrawal. Epileptiform activity not previously present is more likely to be significant if focal or recorded a week or more after the last reduction of medication; whereas generalized discharges, photosensitivity and abnormalities seen in the acute phase of AED withdrawal do not represent evidence of epilepsy (Ludwig & Ajmone Marsan 1975).

Convulsant drugs

Administration of such convulsant drugs as pentylenetetrazol (Metrazol) in normal subjects will induce photosensitivity, spontaneous epileptiform discharges and, eventually, seizures. However, in patients with epilepsy, the dose required to produce these effects may be less and this formed the basis of the 'photometrazol test' (Gastaut 1950), which in clinical practice proved unreliable. Convulsants may also be used in an attempt to activate a focus in a patient undergoing assessment for possible surgical treatment of epilepsy (Kaufman et al 1947). However, comparison of convulsant-induced and spontaneous seizures, with recording from both scalp and depth electrodes, shows that the drug-induced seizures are often generalized and, even if focal, are different both clinically and electrographically from those occurring spontaneously (Bancaud et al 1968, Wieser et al 1979). The localizing value of convulsant-induced focal EEG abnormalities is therefore highly questionable and convulsant activation of the EEG has fallen into disuse, except in some specialized centres for neurosurgical treatment of epilepsy where, it may be assumed, the limitations of the method are appreciated.

Tests of vasomotor lability

As an aid to differential diagnosis between epilepsy and syncope, various manoeuvres may be used to induce postural hypotension by means of a tilt table, or to induce a vasovagal attack by carotid sinus massage or ocular compression. As these manoeuvres often produce hypotensive attacks in normal subjects and negative results in patients who suffer from syncope, their diagnostic reliability is questionable and does not appear to justify the undoubted risks of embolism resulting from massaging a diseased carotid artery or retinal detachment due to eyeball pressure.

THE EEG AND CLASSIFICATION OF EPILEPSY AND SEIZURES

Despite a sustained effort over two decades by the International League against Epilepsy, international conventions on the terminology of epilepsy remain a subject of continuing controversy. The classification of epilepsies by Penfield & Jasper (1954), based on two dimensions (partial versus generalised, idiopathic versus secondary) has survived several revisions (Merlis 1970, Commission on Classification and Terminology 1985, 1989). In its latest form this basic structure is supplemented by a list of epilepsy syndromes which are not mutually exclusive, nor comprehensive. The terms primary and secondary have been renamed, somewhat less ambiguously, idiopathic and symptomatic, and a third category of cryptogenic added. This last allows for the accommodation of epilepsies which are presumed to be

symptomatic, but where the cause has not been established, avoiding the absurdity of describing a Lennox–Gastaut syndrome in a multiply handicapped patient as 'primary' if the cause was not known. Less happily, the term 'partial', with its misleading historical implications of something less than 'genuine epilepsy' has been replaced by 'localization related', in the classification of epilepsies, but is retained in that of seizures. (The present author cannot reconcile himself to this clumsy and meaningless phrase, which must surely disappear with the next revision, and will use the term 'partial' in this text.)

The present text will list mainly the typical EEG features of the four basic groups distinguished since the 1970 classification, noting at the same time some particular syndromes which show special electrographic characteristics.

Generalized and partial seizures

The introductory account in this chapter of the ictal EEG took for granted the traditional distinction between generalized and partial (focal) seizures. This concept, which is fundamental to the classifications of both epilepsies and seizures, has proved useful for descriptive purposes, as an aid to communication and in selecting therapy; however, its physiological basis is suspect. The striking appearance of generalized, bilaterally symmetrical and synchronous discharges led, from the early 1940s, to the concept of a central diencephalic pacemaker (Jasper & Kershman 1941, Jasper & Droogleever-Fortuyn 1947) and hence to the concept of centrencephalic epilepsy formulated by Penfield & Jasper (1954). Experimental data supported this theory: during absence seizures 3/s spike-wave activity had been recorded in the thalamus (Williams 1953) and spike-wave activity or absence-like seizures could be induced by stimulation of the thalamus (Jasper & Kershman 1941, Hunter & Jasper 1949a, Pollen et al 1963, Jasper & Droogleever-Fortuyn 1947) or of the midbrain reticular formation (Weir 1964). Thalamic lesions in kittens are also considered to provide an experimental model of absence seizures (Guerreo-Figueroa & Darros 1963). Some workers never accepted the centrencephalic concept, notably Gibbs & Lennox (Gibbs et al 1937) who regarded generalized epilepsy as a cortical disorder.

An observation by Bennett (1953) in the Gibbs' laboratory, which was subsequently repeated and extended by the Montreal School of Gloor and colleagues (Gloor 1968, 1972) began to undermine this model. The effects of injecting convulsant or anticonvulsant agents into the carotid and vertebrobasilar circulations were studied in humans, in the course of preoperative assessment. From the hypothesis of a diencephalic pacemaker for generalized epileptiform discharges, it would be expected that injection of convulsant drugs into the vertebrobasilar system (the principal blood supply of the diencephalon) should induce generalized discharges, whereas injection of anticonvulsants should inhibit them. This was not found. Conversely, although it might be expected that carotid injections of convulsants or anticonvulsants should have little effect if the primary source of epileptogenesis were diencephalic, the reverse was the case: unilateral carotid amytal injection abolished generalized discharges, and unilateral injection of the convulsant pentylenetetrazol induced generalized discharges and seizures. Clearly, the cortex was at least as important as the diencephalon for the generation of generalized spike-wave activity.

Marcus & Watson (Marcus & Watson 1966, Marcus et al 1968) showed that bilateral topical application to the frontal cortex of metrazol or premarine elicited absence-like seizures and generalized spike-wave activity. These effects persisted after destruction of subcortical grey matter but were abolished by callosal section. Prince & Farrell (1969) showed that parenteral injection of penicillin in the cat would produce generalized spike-wave activity and absence-like seizures; and systemic or topical application of penicillin has formed the experimental model on which much of the subsequent work by the Montreal group has been based. Topical application of penicillin to the cortex, but not to subcortical structures, produces generalized spike-wave activity (Gloor et al 1977). The spike-wave appears first in the cortex and only later in subcortical structures (Fisher & Prince 1977). The initiation of spike-wave activity is closely related to that of spindle formations of the normal EEG (Quesney et al

1977, Kostopoulos & Gloor 1982), and reduction of cortical excitability causes the spike-wave to be replaced by spindles (Gloor et al 1979). The model which thus emerges for 'generalized corticoreticular epilepsies' is thus of a bilaterally hyperexcitable cerebral cortex which responds abnormally with spike-wave activity to afferent impulses from the diencephalon, which are themselves normal and would ordinarily give rise to spindles. This model also helps to explain the marked influence of state of awareness (i.e the activity of the reticular activating system) on seizures and EEG discharges.

However, the model leaves many observations unexplained. If generalized spike-wave activity and seizures are of cortical origin and can be provoked by unilateral carotid injection of a convulsant, then the distinction between generalized discharges and focal discharges with secondary generalization appears to be blurred. Tukel & Jasper (1952) showed that parasaggital lesions could produce bilateral discharges, and Bancaud (1972), using depth recording, found that seemingly symmetrical generalized discharges could arise from a mesial frontal focus. Huck et al (1980) reported the emergence of unilateral foci after callosal section in patients with generalized discharges. Conversely, mesial frontal stimulation can produce bilaterally synchronous spike-wave activity (Bancaud et al 1974). A study by Wilkins et al (1981), using hemifield pattern stimulation in photosensitive subjects, showed that the threshold for inducing spike-wave activity could be markedly asymmetrical between the two hemispheres, implying an asymmetry of the postulated cortical hyper-excitability.

There is also some difficulty in extrapolating from experiments on feline penicillin epilepsy to generalized seizures in humans. Penicillin does not ordinarily cross the blood–brain barrier. Reported experiments on feline penicillin epilepsy have all apparently employed acutely or subacutely implanted electrodes which presumably compromised the blood–brain barrier. Binnie et al (1985c) found in dogs that, if upwards of 3 months were allowed for recovery from electrode insertion, no convulsant effect was obtained with massive parenteral doses of penicillin. Feline penicillin epilepsy may thus be seen as a model, not of generalized, but rather of multifocal epilepsy, the brain being exposed to the convulsant drug wherever electrodes have been placed. When seizures are induced by bicuculline or pentylene-tetrazol, the initial ictal event is high frequency multi-unit activity in brainstem structures, nota-bly the lateral geniculate body, preceding onset of spike-wave discharges in cortex and thalamus; penicillin by contrast induces corticothalamic dis-charges from the start (Rodin et al 1971, 1975, 1977, Binnie et al 1985c). The substantia nigra has also been implicated as a site of chemical epileptogenesis and as a specific target organ for some antiepileptic drugs (Gale 1985, Turski et al 1986), yet nigral stimulation delays amygdaloid kindling and prevents propagation of limbic sei-zures (Morimoto & Goddard 1987). Which of these models is most relevant to generalized seizures in humans remains uncertain.

It is an increasingly widely held view that the distinction between partial and generalized sei-zures is artificial. If a localized area of cortical hyperexcitability is sufficient to produce general-ized seizures in man (as in cats after unilateral application of penicillin), then the difference be-tween generalized and focal seizures may simply be a question of the rate and extent of spread of the physiological disturbance. The more recent view of the Montreal school appears to be that syndromatic classifications are an oversimplifica-tion; they provide practical aids to communication and prognosis, but a neurobiological description of the aetiology and pathophysiology of the seizure disorder in a particular patient allows a more in-dividualized approach (Berkovic et al 1987). This view in turn has been criticized as retrograde, at a time when advances in genetics are at last begin-ning to provide a more robust basis for epilepsy syndromes.

The following didactic account will follow the conventional distinction between generalized and partial epilepsies and seizures, but it should be recognized that these concepts are at best over-simplifications and the physiological models on which they are based are disputed.

Idiopathic generalized epilepsy

The EEG in idiopathic generalized epilepsy is characterized by generalized discharges, most often spike-wave activity, arising against a normal background. In patients with absence seizures, this is rhythmic and has a frequency of 2.5–4/s. If the discharge is of less than 2 or 3 seconds duration, no clinical manifestations may be seen, although psychological testing may reveal transi-tory cognitive impairment. During longer dis-charges, an overt absence may be observed, consciousness being lost within the first 2 seconds and gradually beginning to return some 3 seconds before the end of the discharge. The phenomenon of cognitive impairment during the shorter dis-charges has led some authors to suggest that all the generalized spike-wave activity is ictal or that 'in absence seizures interictal discharges probably do not occur' (Delgado-Escueta 1979). The gen-eralized spike-wave activity is of greatest ampli-tude at the front of the head and may show bifrontal maxima or a single maximum in the midline. It has been suggested by Dondey (1983) that the absence seizures in patients with a single midline maximum are atypical and have a poor prognosis. Minor asymmetries are often present and there appear to be no accepted criteria for determining what degree of asymmetry is accept-able before the question of possible secondary generalization arises. Suspicion will be heightened if the discharges are irregular in form or fre-quency, or are slower than 2.5/s and if the asym-metry is consistent. Onset and termination of the discharge are abrupt but, during a long run of spike-wave activity, the frequency may decrease gradually. Postictal changes are not seen. In those patients whose absence seizures are accompanied by a prominent myoclonus, the spike components are generally multiple.

Less regular generalized spike-wave occurs in the interictal EEGs of patients with tonic-clonic convulsions, as may generalized polyspike dis-charges. These are often activated by sleep, ap-pearing maximally in Stage III. The ictal EEG during a tonic-clonic seizure is characterized by an initial burst of generalized spiking, a tonic phase in which the tracing is usually obscured by muscle artifact and then rhythmic polyspiket-wave dis-charges occurring synchronously with the clonic jerks. As these become irregular and less frequent and eventually cease, so also do the spike-wave complexes. In the postictal state, the EEG may initially be of very low amplitude for some tens of seconds; as activity returns it is usually very slow at first, and the dominant frequency gradually increases to normal values. Just as the rate of clinical recovery is very variable, so is that of the EEG. In some patients there may be only a few seconds of slowing, with no preceding episode of flattening, in others some residual delta activity may be present for up to 2 or 3 days.

Juvenile myoclonic epilepsy is characterized by generalized ictal discharges of multiple, irregular spikes and slow waves, which accompany the seizures and also occur frequently as brief bursts in the interictal recording. Fifty percent of patients with this disorder are photosensitive, and photosensitivity is in general most common in patients with idiopathic generalized epilepsy, having an incidence of some 20% in a typical EEG practice, rising to some 40% in children.

Partial epilepsies

Ictal findings during a partial epileptic seizure have been described above. The interictal EEG may contain normal background activity or exhibit abnormalities reflecting the underlying pathology. These may range from an asymmetry of background activity in a patient with a unilateral chronic lesion such as mesial temporal sclerosis, to a gross delta focus with generalized slowing in a patient with a tumour. For further discussion of the EEG in cerebral lesions the reader is referred to such standard texts as Niedermeyer & Lopes da Silva (1987). Focal epileptiform activity varies greatly in its incidence, both within and between subjects, and is often markedly influenced by state of awareness. It is common for a patient to exhibit no epileptiform activity when tense and apprehensive at the start of a recording, but to show progressively increasing discharges if encouraged to relax as the investigation proceeds. Focal epileptiform activity is found most often over the temporal regions, typically, of course, in patients with seizures of temporal lobe origin. However, central and frontal lesions may also produce focal discharges in the anterior or superior temporal region. Partial epilepsies arising from sites outside

the temporal lobes often produce few interictal focal discharges detectable in the scalp EEG. Thus patients with simple motor or sensory seizures may show no interictal abnormality, and those with seizures of mesial or orbital frontal origin may exhibit only secondarily generalized discharges, or possibly an inconspicuous frontal slow wave focus. In addition to typical spikes, sharp waves and spike-wave complexes, some patients exhibit runs of focal slow activity in the theta or delta range which appear to be related to the 'epileptogenic activity'. Interictal focal epileptiform discharges in partial epilepsy are generally isolated transients or bursts of less than 1 second duration. Sometimes longer discharges occur, lasting some tens of seconds, often with a progressive change in morphology and frequency and without any apparent clinical events. It is tempting to describe those loosely as 'subclinical electrical seizures'. However, it is difficult to establish the absence of clinical manifestations, and one study, using psychological testing during the EEG, showed cognitive disturbances even during extremely brief focal discharges (Aarts et al 1984).

Many patients with partial epilepsy and focal EEG discharges exhibit more than one focus. In most instances the foci appear functionally independent and, indeed, the patient may even exhibit various seizure types which can be shown by ictal recording to arise from different foci. Most often the foci occur over homologous regions of the right and left hemispheres, most typically anterior temporal, and sometimes they may occur synchronously or rather with a small delay between one side and the other. The pathophysiological basis of this EEG picture has not been established and the synchronous foci could reflect either transmission from one hemisphere to the other or simultaneous activation of two independent foci by a common subcortical input. Ralston (1958) found that spikes recorded in the vicinity of an acute experimental lesion tended to be associated with spiky after-discharges and those at a distance did not. Ralston & Papatheodorou (1960) made similar observations in humans, but such discharges are rarely found in human clinical EEGs and do not appear to be of value for locating epileptogenic lesions (Engel et al 1975). Microelectrode studies show discharge rates of neurones in the focus from which seizures arise to be higher than in other foci, with a tendency to firing in bursts (Babb & Crandall 1976). Larger depth electrodes also record higher and more regular discharge rates at the site of seizure onset (Lieb et al 1978).

Serial EEG recordings often show changing patterns of interictal discharge. Foci may be found which were not seen before, and the question arises whether these have always been present, but not previously detected, or whether they have arisen de novo possibly as a consequence of ictal brain damage. Similarly, an established focus may appear to migrate; particularly in children it has been claimed that occipital foci move to the temporal regions (Gibbs et al 1954). Again, it is uncertain whether this reflects a sampling problem or truly represents the evolution of the pathophysiology (Andermann & Oguni 1990, Blume 1990).

One possible explanation of multiple foci over homologous areas of both hemispheres is offered by experimental work on the so-called 'mirror focus' (Morrell 1960). An experimental lesion is created which gives rise to focal EEG spikes and seizures. After an interval ranging from hours to weeks (depending on the site of the focus and the age and species of the animal) a mirror focus of spikes appears over the homologous area of the contralateral hemisphere. At first the two foci are functionally interrelated, the mirror spikes following those in the primary focus, with a delay presumably due to interhemispheric transmission. Later, the secondary focus fires independently. Development of a mirror focus can be prevented by section of interhemispheric connections and by administration of antiepileptic drugs. Removal of the primary focus, or its temporary inactivation by intracarotid barbiturates abolishes the mirror focus if this has not yet become functionally independent. When the firing of the mirror and primary foci is no longer time related, there is an intermediate phase during which ablation of the primary focus will result in a gradual disappearance of the secondary. Finally, the mirror focus achieves full independence, may itself give rise to seizures and will persist, even if the primary is removed; biochemical and microelec-trode studies then show local abnormalities of cortical neurones.

Morrell & Whisler (1980) report a study of patients with well-documented unilateral epileptogenic lesions with bilateral foci. In those patients where intravenous methohexitone suppressed the focus contralateral to the lesion, removal of the latter resulted in relief of seizures. A secondary focus resistant to barbiturate was considered to have attained the stage of independence and operation did not abolish the seizures. In a long-term study, Hughes (1985) found that 40% of unilateral foci eventually became bilateral, particularly where the original focus was left-sided or frontal. Other authors contend that it has not yet been reliably established whether or not the phenomena of the mirror focus and of kindling, seen in experimental animals, actually occur in humans (Goldensohn 1984, Blume 1990). Both models would seem to predict that epilepsy should progressively deteriorate: that the effectiveness of surgical treatment should become less with time as mirror foci become independent, and that kindling should cause an increasing proportion of partial seizures to generalize. Neither prediction appears to be true (Bengzon et al 1968, Wada & Engel 1987). Whatever the physiological basis of interdependence of bilateral foci the second focus often disappears gradually after removal of an epileptogenic lesion (Falconer & Kennedy 1961). In Morrell's terms such foci must presumably have reached the intermediate phase of secondary epileptogenesis.

Focal discharges may spread to a greater or lesser degree not only within one hemisphere or to the homologous region on the other side, but also to produce generalized epileptiform activity (Fig. 9.9). This phenomenon of 'secondary generalization' is seen both in the interictal recording and in the ictal EEG, where it is often associated with the onset of complex symptomatology. Indeed, it is implicit in the 1981 revision of the International Classification of Epileptic Seizures (Dreifuss 1981) that complex symptomatology (i.e. impairment of consciousness) in partial seizures is due to secondary generalization. The fortuitous similarity of the term, 'secondarily generalized discharges' and 'secondary generalized epilepsy' caused much confusion; the mention

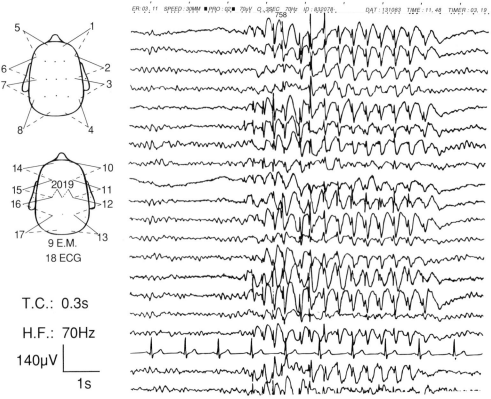

ER: 03, 11   SPEED : 30MM   ■ PRO : 02■   70μV   Q, 3SEC   70Hz   IP : 832078·   DAT : 131083   TIME : 11, 48   TIMER : 03, 19
758

T.C.: 0.3s

H.F.: 70Hz

140μV

1s

Fig. 9.9 Secondary generalization of an initially focal discharge in the left frontal region. The patient's seizures commenced with jerking of the right hand sometimes followed by loss of consciousness. They ceased following removal of a left frontal tumour.

of secondary generalization in an EEG report often caused clinicians to suppose the patient had secondary generalized epilepsy. Possibly the substitution in the latest classification (Commission on Classification and Terminology 1989) of the term 'symptomatic' for secondary will overcome this problem. Secondarily generalized discharges and seizures are common in symptomatic epilepsies, almost always present in the generalized type but often seen in partial epilepsy. Secondary generalization occurs more readily in children than in adults. However, when a patient in whom only generalized discharges have been found exhibits a clear focus with increasing age, it may be impossible to determine whether the focus has always been present but unrecognized due to the generalized activity, or has developed de novo. If this latter were the case, it would suggest that idiopathic generalized epilepsy could evolve to partial, possibly as a result of ictal brain damage.

Idiopathic partial epilepsy

The term 'idiopathic partial epilepsy' is not used, and it was pointed out only comparatively recently by Gastaut (1982) that this niche in the bi-dimensional classification of epilepsies is occupied by the benign epilepsy of childhood. This has not only a very characteristic clinical picture of predominantly nocturnal partial seizures in a child between the ages of 4 and 16, but also produces a striking EEG pattern. Spikes, sharp waves, or spike-wave complexes, of amplitudes often greater than 100 μV are seen, sharply localized, usually over the central region of one or both hemispheres, or sometimes lower in the central coronal plane at a Sylvian or midtemporal site ('Rolandic spikes') (Fig. 9.10). Typically, the spikes produce a dipole electrical field, the negative-going potential in the central region being accompanied by a less obvious positive wave in the mid-frontal area.

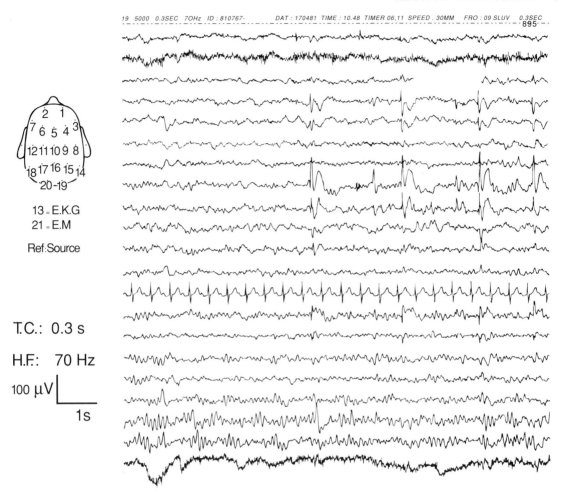

Fig. 9.10   Rolandic spikes in the right centrotemporal region in a 10-year-old with benign childhood epilepsy.

The discharges increase in frequency during sleep and in some patients, particularly shortly after onset of the epilepsy, they may not be detected unless a sleep recording is obtained. Interestingly, despite marked activation, Rolandic spikes do not produce the disruption of sleep patterns usually seen in patients with frequent nocturnal epileptiform discharges (Clemens & Oláh 1987).

The discharges may occur many times a minute and, if not correctly identified, may cause some alarm. However, this epilepsy syndrome is highly sensitive to antiepileptic drugs and disappears by the age of 16 years. Despite the profuse discharges, some children with benign childhood epilepsy may have suffered only one seizure in their lives and Rolandic spikes may be asymptomatic, particularly in siblings of children with overt benign childhood epilepsy. An atypical distribution of the focal discharges is, however, often associated with a different clinical picture and a less favourable prognosis (Wong 1985). Far less common than the typical benign childhood epilepsy of Rolandic origin are temporal and occipital forms. This last is characterized by occipital spike-wave bursts and visual ictal symptoms, including scotomata. Many cases of the occipital form of benign childhood epilepsy are probably misdiagnosed as basilar migraine (Gastaut 1982).

Symptomatic (and cryptogenic) generalized epilepsy

As symptomatic or cryptogenic generalized epilepsy is by definition due to proven or presumed

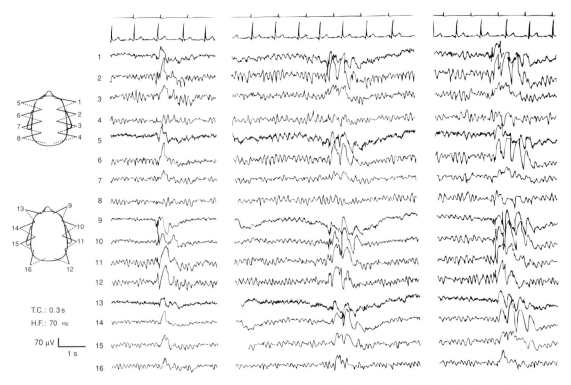

Fig. 9.11 Symptomatic generalized epilepsy. Note slow ongoing EEG activity and multifocal epileptiform discharges of variable morphology and topography with a tendency to generalize.

widespread cerebral pathology, an abnormal background activity may be expected in the EEG. This may range from a slight excess of theta activity to a grossly disturbed picture from which normal rhythms are totally absent. Multiple foci of epileptiform activity are often seen (Fig. 9.11) and this may reflect the multiple seizure patterns often seen in this conditions. The discharges readily become secondarily generalized. The discharges may be very frequent and may indeed occupy more than 50% of the entire recording. In symptomatic generalized epilepsy there is often little correlation between the seizure frequency and the discharge rate, the EEG remaining unimproved even when the patient's attacks are well controlled. Often it is difficult to make a clear distinction between background activity and epileptiform discharges, there being a continuum of waveforms from generalized spike-and-wave activity of greatest amplitude anteriorly, through frontal delta bursts intermixed with sharp components, to intermittent generalized or frontal slow

activity, with no spiky elements. The distinction is not entirely academic, as these patients often show impaired cognition, and EEGs may be requested to distinguish non-convulsive status epilepticus from postictal changes or anticonvulsant intoxication. In view of the inconstant relationship between epileptiform activity and clinical state in this type of epilepsy, such a distinction can often be made reliably only by showing that intravenous benzodiazepines produce suppression of the discharges accompanied by clinical improvement.

Although patients with symptomatic generalized epilepsy often exhibit multiple seizure types, two particular patterns may be noted. Atonic seizures are very characteristic of this form of epilepsy, often causing the patient to fall and suffer injury. The ictal EEG changes are varied but, if the attack consists merely of a loss of muscle tone, the EEG may show only an electrodecremental event (Egli et al 1985). Episodes of impaired awareness, atypical absences, also occur in symptomatic generalized epilepsy and are associated

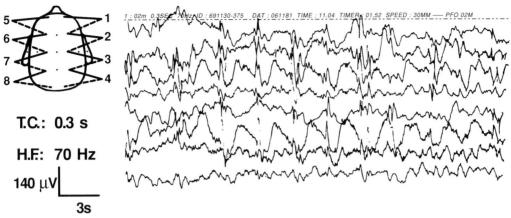

Fig. 9.12 Slow generalized spike wave activity in the interictal EEG of a patient with the Lennox-Gastaut syndrome.

with the very slow spike-wave activity at only 1/s or less (Fig. 9.12) characteristic of the Lennox–Gastaut syndrome. It is rarely necessary to resort to sleep recording to detect epileptiform activity in symptomatic generalized epilepsy. Often the sleeping EEG is characterized by the appearance of profuse, generalized polyspike-wave discharges in stages III and IV (Fig. 9.13).

There exist a large number of, mostly, rare, syndromes of symptomatic or cryptogenic generalized epilepsy in childhood, which are considered in Chapter 4. The Lennox–Gastaut syndrome is mentioned above and one other will be noted here, West syndrome, which is usually associated with a striking EEG picture known as 'hypsarrhythmia' (Fig. 9.14). The record contains

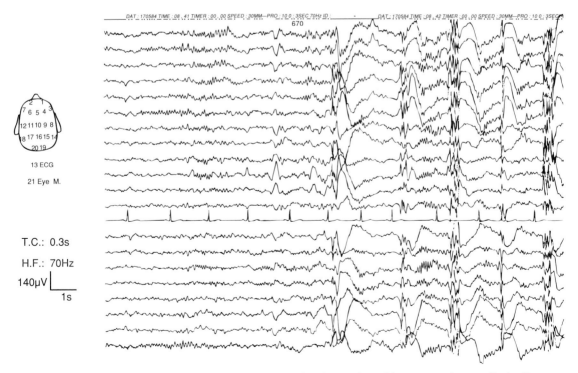

Fig. 9.13 Multiple spikes and slow waves appearing during sleep in a patient with symptomatic generalized epilepsy.

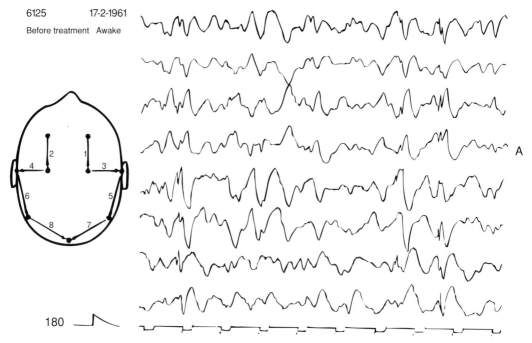

6125   17-2-1961

Before treatment   Awake

A

180

Fig. 9.14   Hypsarryhthmia in a 6-month-old baby with West syndrome. Note chaotic high-amplitude slow activity and epileptiform discharges with no consistent distribution.

multiple epileptiform discharges, both focal and generalized, and displays a grossly disturbed background dominated by slow activity, often interspersed with episodes of reduced amplitude. However, the most striking feature is the chaotic quality, the lack of any consistent organization in either topography or timing of the events. In some patients, the infantile spasms may accompany high voltage generalized epileptiform discharges and the intervening sections of the record are of relatively low amplitude. Often even this degree of consistency is lacking. Atypical forms of the syndrome occur, with unilateral hypsarrhythmia, or with a relatively normal interictal EEG. This last is associated with a better than usual prognosis and may reflect the existence of an idiopathic form of the syndrome. For further details of the EEG investigation of West syndrome see Jeavons & Bower (1964) and Harris (1972).

Unclassifiable epilepsy

Often epilepsy is unclassifiable simply on the basis of lack of clinical information. The electro-encephalographer then asked to classify a patient's epilepsy on the basis of the EEG rapidly finds himself in difficulties. Although the typical clinical and electrographic pictures of partial and symptomatic generalized epilepsy are readily distinguished, the boundary between them is ill-defined. Some patients with diffuse brain disease may nevertheless have a single EEG focus and a single seizure type; some patients have more than one EEG focus, several seizure types and, possibly, multiple cerebral lesions. In both these instances—partial seizures in the context of generalized cerebral disease on the one hand, and multifocal epilepsy on the other—it is difficult to determine whether the appropriate designation is partial or symptomatic generalized epilepsy. The difficulty lies, of course, not with interpretation of the EEG findings but with the classification itself. The recent addition to the international classification of a 'cryptogenic' category may create a demand for EEG evidence as to whether a generalized epilepsy of unknown cause should be classified as idiopathic or cryptogenic; a normal background activity in the EEG in general favours the former.

STATUS EPILEPTICUS

In the early stages of status epilepticus, ictal discharges appropriate to the seizure type are repeatedly seen with incomplete recovery of the postictal disturbance between seizures. With prolonged status involving partial or tonic-clonic seizures the ictal patterns may become progressively less dramatic and the interictal disturbance more severe. Thus, in a prolonged partial status, the EEG may be grossly slowed and asymmetrical, being of lower amplitude on the side of the causative focus. Ictal discharges may be confined to brief runs of spikes or slow waves and, indeed, where there is marked reduction of amplitude on the side of the original focus, ictal spiking may eventually be seen only over the contralateral hemisphere. During prolonged generalized convulsive status epilepticus a progressive evolution is seen in which five stages may be distinguished (Treiman et al 1990):

1. confluent seizures with interictal slowing
2. confluent seizures reflected in continuous but waxing and waning ictal discharges
3. continuous rhythmic sharp or spike-wave discarges
4. continuous discharges interrupted by periods of flattening lasting 0.5 to 8 seconds
5. periodic stereotyped sharp waves against a relatively flat background.

During this evolution the clinical ictal events become less florid and may eventually be unrecognizable without the help of EEG monitoring.

Although status epilepticus with tonic-clonic or simple partial motor seizures may readily be recognized on clinical grounds, status with complex partial or absence seizures may present with psychiatric symptomatology or a fluctuating confusional state. Here the EEG findings may be crucial to diagnosis. Absence status in particular is characterized by irregular spike-wave activity, less well formed than that typical of absence seizures and often waxing and waning in amount rather than showing a clear distinction between ictal and interictal periods. In epileptic patients with frequent EEG discharges and exhibiting confusion or bizarre psychiatric states, the diagnosis of non-convulsive status may be established by the intravenous administration of antiepileptic drugs (usually a benzodiazepine) under EEG control. Improvement in mental state accompanying suppression of EEG discharges may be taken to support the diagnosis.

Drug treatment of status epilepticus has been much improved since the introduction of benzodiazepines, and intractable status is seen less often in epileptological practice than amongst terminally brain-damaged patients in the intensive care unit. Where status does not respond rapidly to treatment, and particularly where it is necessary to resort to anaesthesia and the use of muscle relaxants and artificial ventilation, clinical observation of the attacks becomes difficult and EEG monitoring may be the only satisfactory way of following progress. In this context it may be noted that repeated conventional multichannel EEGs may usefully be supplemented (but not replaced) by continuous registration of ictal events on a slowly moving chart by such devices as the cerebral function monitor (Prior & Maynard 1976).

EPILEPSY MONITORING

One of the great fascinations of epilepsy is the intermittent nature both of the disease and of its electrophysiological manifestations. The full picture can never be grasped by examining the patient at one moment in time or recording the electrical activity of the brain for a few minutes only. The condition is, moreover, profoundly influenced by sleep and waking, vigilance, cognitive function and biorhythms. These considerations led various workers in the 1960s to undertake long-term observations of patients with epilepsy engaged in a variety of everyday activities in, so far as possible, a normal environment. Clinical manifestations were registered first on cine film (Hunter & Jasper 1949b, Schwab et al 1954, Ajmone Marsan & Abraham 1960). However, the advent of video recording provided a far more cost-effective means of recording behaviour over hours or days in order to capture infrequent clinical events of a few minutes' duration (Penin 1968). This technology was combined with EEG registration by radio telemetry, in order to allow the patient greater freedom of movement and a wider range of physical activities than was possible under the conditions of conventional

EEG recording. These early studies were concerned chiefly with the effects of psychological tasks on EEG discharges and seizures (Vidart & Geier 1967, Guey et al 1969) or with documentation of unusual seizure types (Harrison-Covello & De Barros-Ferreira 1975, Dreyer & Wehmeyer 1978). The development of these techniques in a research context led only gradually to the realization of their potential as an aid to the clinical assessment of patients with known or suspected epilepsy. Such facilities existed in only a few dozen centres worldwide in the late 1970s but are now routine, and epilepsy monitoring can be counted one of the most important recent developments of epileptology (So & Penry 1981).

Monitoring technologies

For short, comprehensive reviews of the technologies employed for epilepsy monitoring see Binnie (1990) and Ebersole (1987); a multi-author monograph describing the techniques and experience of many of the world's leading centres is provided by Gotman et al (1985).

EEG monitoring

The possibility of recording the EEG for some hours continuously on a conventional electro-encephalograph is often overlooked, and the development of elaborate telemetry systems seems to have created a myth that an ictal EEG cannot properly be recorded without this technology. The advent of head box preamplifiers, connected to the EEG machine by a cable of 3–5 m, has made it possible to obtain satisfactory recordings from a patient who, while not free to indulge in strenuous activity, can at least sit up and move about within the radius of the cable. This restriction on movement is less than that imposed by many other standard medical procedures, and, indeed, if satisfactory video recordings are to be obtained without multiple cameras and personnel to direct them, it is generally necessary for the patient to be confined within a fairly small area. In practice, monitoring by means of a conventional EEG machine, possibly with some minor modifications such as a miniaturized electrode input box is very acceptable for periods of up to 24 hours, and has

proved very suitable for seizure documentation (Penin 1968, Penry et al 1975, Stefan et al 1981).

A logical extension of this technique, involving further miniaturization of the head box and preamplifiers so that they can be carried on the patient's person, leads to cable telemetry (Ives et al 1976). The signals from the various channels are usually multiplexed (mixed) so that they can be transmitted down a single pair of flexible wires, typically through a cable up to 50 m long which also provides the power supply (Kamp et al 1979). The patient can move freely within this radius, which gives him the run of a typical hospital ward (Binnie et al 1981). If the data acquisition system is located in an EEG laboratory at a distance from the recording area, the signals can with further amplification be transmitted by cable over distances of hundreds of metres around a hospital site (Ives et al 1976). The technology employed for cable telemetry is not necessarily any more costly than that used in conventional EEG machines, and the technical specification can be as high or better in terms of bandwidth, dynamic range, number of channels, etc. The inconvenience to the patient of having to trail a cable about proves, in the event, to be minimal and it is usually the need for close observation and video recording rather than the cable which limits activity.

Greater freedom of movement may, however, be achieved by providing a radio link between the miniaturized amplifiers on the patient and the data acquisition system (Breakell et al 1949, Kamp 1963). The price paid for this increased freedom of movement is considerable, and not only in economic terms. The reliability of radio telemetry is generally lower than that of cable and, while commercially available systems may have a range of 100 m or more in free field, within a steel- and concrete-framed building reception may be erratic, unless multiple antennae are provided (Porter et al 1971). Most decisive in choosing between radio and cable systems are the telecommunications regulations in many countries which limit the range of frequencies which may be used (Manson 1974). This in turn restricts the dynamic range, bandwidth and number of channels of the systems. Power is supplied by batteries, which add to the size and weight of the pack carried by the patient. When EEG monitoring was first introduced, radio transmission was viewed with enthusiasm by most workers and the use of cable derided as not being true telemetry. The position is now reversed: many users prefer cable and manufacturers who originally promoted radio telemetry have found it necessary to provide the options of radio or a hard-wired linkage. Radio telemetry remains the ideal technology for EEG monitoring during physical activity requiring freedom of movement, an application which is more likely to be useful in research than for clinical investigation of epilepsy.

Ambulatory monitoring employs a completely portable data acquisition system carried on the patient's person. This is currently achieved by the use of small cassette recorders which may run either at conventional tape speeds providing up to 1.5 hours continuous recording (Kaiser 1976, Ives 1982a) or, more usually, with a reduced tape speed for up to 24 hours (Ives & Woods 1975). A normal tape speed provides a bandwidth sufficient for recordings of excellent technical quality but the low tape speed systems used to permit continuous registration for 24 hours offer a very limited bandwidth and dynamic range, with a maximum of 10 channels. The cost per channel of ambulatory equipment may be five times greater than than of cable telemetry. Ambulatory monitoring is usually, although not necessarily, performed without simultaneous video registration and most systems provide no means of synchronizing the EEG with video images (see below). The technique comes into its own for investigating the patient in his own natural environment; for instance, to determine how frequently a child suffers absence seizures at school or to test the claim that a patient has seizures at home which cease on admission for observation in hospital.

Because of the considerable capital costs of monitoring equipment, until recently few workers had experience of more than one system and tended therefore to be very partisan in their advocacy of a particular method. Ambulatory monitoring in particular has been overused for applications for which it is not suitable, chiefly because it was the first technique to become widely available commercially. Conversely, the possibilities for monitoring with a conventional EEG machine are often undervalued. An increasing number of workers now have access to all the techniques described above and advocate the selective use of different technologies for various applications (Ives 1982b, O'Kane et al 1982, Gotman et al 1985, Ebersole 1987) (see Table 9.2). Meanwhile the costs themselves have fallen as the technology has improved and the market expanded; one basic video and EEG telemetry system is now marketed for as little as $25 000, less than many EEG machines.

Data acquisition

In ambulatory monitoring, facilities for data acquisition onto magnetic tape form an integral part of the system. When other methods of monitoring are used, EEG data may be collected either directly onto a paper chart or onto magnetic media. The advantage of continuous chart

Table 9.2 Advantages, limitations and uses of available monitoring technologies (after Binnie 1983b).

Conventional EEG recorders
Advantages: high quality recording of many channels; ease of selecting filters, montage etc.
Disadvantage: lack of patient mobility
Application: seizure monitoring for up to 24 hours
Cable telemetry
Advantages: high quality recording of many channels at low cost; less susceptible to artifact than most EEG machines
Disadvantage: limited mobility range of up to 50 m
Application: all forms of intensive monitoring in hospital except during physical exercise.
Radio telemetry
Advantages: excellent mobility, particularly out of doors
Disadvantage: high cost; limited range within buildings; limited bandwidth, number of channels and dynamic range
Application: all forms of intensive monitoring close to laboratory including sporting activities etc.
Cassette recorders (normal tape speed)
Advantages: as cable but with greater mobility
Disadvantage: recording duration limited to 90 min between tape changes; cannot easily be time indexed to video record
Applications: EEG monitoring during tasks of short duration; seizure recording (if combined with buffer memory).
Cassette recorders (low tape speed)
Advantages; excellent mobility, 24 hours recording between cassette changes
Disadvantages: few channels, poor dynamic range and high frequency response; cannot be time indexed to video record; high cost; more expensive than telemetry
Applications: prolonged monitoring, remote from laboratory, of known, preferably generalized, EEG phenomena. Rarely suitable except as preliminary screening procedure for differential diagnosis of epileptic and pseudoseizures; unsuitable for focus localization.

recording is that it is immediately accessible so that prompt action can be taken to correct technical problems or to respond to clinical events; and the chart itself may easily be annotated with information about behaviour, administration of drugs etc. Moreover, a permanent, easily readable record is provided directly without the need for off-line transcription of magnetic media. The obvious disadvantages are in terms of cost, both of paper (1 km/24 h at reasonable chart speeds), storage of the records and the requirement for the continuous presence of personnel to check the chart transport and the paper and ink supplies.

Magnetic recording may use reel-to-reel instrumentation recorders but, if simultaneous video registration is also undertaken, there may be considerable advantages in storing the EEG signals on video tape, together with the images of the patient. A split-screen video picture allows the EEG to be displayed together with the accompanying behaviour, including seizures. With present video standards it is not possible to show more than 16 channels with reasonable clarity in this way and the quality of the EEG is barely adequate for detailed assessment. However, the EEG can also be stored digitally with the video signals themselves. This used a standard feature of modern video cassette recorders, intended for hi-fi sound. This last method gives a high quality recording and the possibility of recovering the original signals for subsequent write-out on chart, computer analysis etc. Re-usable optical discs are currently undergoing rapid development, and seem certain to replace magnetic media in the next generation of telemetry systems.

All the present methods of magnetic registration (with the exception of the use of the hi-fi channel os a video recorder) permit rapid replay for scanning the recorded signals to find particular events of interest. Split-screen video images can simply be scanned in fast picture search mode. Both ambulatory monitoring and the reel-to-reel tape systems provide options for fast replay either as an image which pans continuously across the screen, or in page-turning mode where some 10 seconds of EEG are momentarily presented for about 1 second each. Optical discs will be much more convenient, providing immediate 'random access' to any part of the recording, without the delays of several minutes required for tape positioning.

In many applications, only a small section of the registration encompassing a particular clinical event is of interest. Here it may be possible to economize on recording media by storing only those few minutes of the record which are required. As the initial EEG events in a seizure are of particular importance, it is too late to commence registration only after clinical changes have been detected. Some form of buffer memory is therefore needed so that, when an event of interest is detected, a permanent registration can be made of the signals, commencing some seconds or minutes before the detection and continuing until after the event of interest. This was achieved by Ives et al (1976) using a computer disc as a buffer memory. Such a system may be usefully combined with automatic detection of epileptiform discharges (Gotman et al 1979) or of seizures (Gotman 1981, 1982, 1990). However, the available technology is changing rapidly: digital recording on video-tape provides temporary mass storage at low cost, and the required material can be easily identified with the help of nursing records, patient's reports and alarm signals logged by the telemetry system. Consequently, selective data logging with the use of a buffer memory, which was once almost a practical necessity, may now appear a less satisfactory option.

Stand-alone systems for recognizing and counting ictal and interictal epileptiform events have been used for data reduction (Quy et al 1980, Zetterlund 1982) but, except in the case of spike-wave activity (Principe et al 1985), have not yet achieved any high level of reliability in distinguishing epileptiform events from the artefacts which are invariably present in telemetric records from active subjects. Such systems may reduce the labour of visual assessment by carrying out preliminary data reduction. If this allows the human operator to inspect only a selected 20 minutes out of a 24-hour recording, it is of little consequence if a large proportion of the events detected are artifactual. Moreover, in this author's experience, automatic seizure detection, using the method of Gotman (1982), often identifies important events, particularly at night, which are not reported by the patient or nursing staff.

Documentation of behaviour

Fully to document the clinical events of any but the simplest seizure requires a permanent record which can be replayed repeatedly and preferably at reduced speed. For this purpose, video recording is ideal. Depending on the application and the funds available, the system used may range from a single camera with a wide-angle lens and a home video recorder, to multiple cameras covering an entire hospital ward with remote control facilities and broadcast quality video tape equipment. For many purposes it is essential to be able accurately to relate clinical events to the EEG at the same moment in time, and for this purpose some method of synchronizing the video image with the EEG is required. The simplest and most widely used method is to record EEG and the image of the patient together, either as a split-screen display or by superimposing the EEG on the video picture. If the video registration is time indexed by a standard time-date generator, this latter can be linked to a microcomputer to write out time indexing simultaneously on the EEG chart (Ives 1982c).

The sensitivity of clinical observation may be further enhanced by engaging the subject in structured, continuous activity, the performance of which can be measured. This may permit detection of momentary lapses of cognitive function during subclinical EEG discharges (see below).

Applications

The distinction between the clinical and research applications of monitoring is often blurred, as providing a routine service often yields data of scientific value. However, the principle indications proposed in various evaluation studies of epilepsy monitoring are summarized in Table 9.3.

Differential diagnosis

As noted earlier, in some 5% of persons with epilepsy, conventional clinical and EEG assessment fail to establish the diagnosis with any certainty. Diagnostic problems also exist in some 15% of new referrals to specialist epileptological practice, who eventually prove to be suffering from episodic

Table 9.3 Suggested indications for epilepsy monitoring and yield of useful information in nine evaluation reports (after Binnie 1987)

Indications for epilepsy monitoring	Refs*
Differential diagnosis	1 2 3 4 5 6 7 8 9
Subjective complaints	3 5 7
Pseudoseizures?	2 4 5 6 8
Enuresis	4 5
Nocturnal restlessness/apnoea	3 4 5
Cardiac disorder/syncope?	2 3 6
Diurnal sleepiness	3
Episodic behavioural disturbances	4 7 8 9
Hyperventilation?	8
EEG correlates of known seizures	1 2 3 4 5 6
Classification	1 3 5 6
Focus localization	3 5
Clinical correlates of EEG discharge	2 4 5
Transitory cognitive impairment	2 4 5
Seizure frequency	2 3 4 5 9
Seizure precipitants	1 3 5 8
Reflex epilepsy	5
Self-induction	5
Situational factors	3

* Authors and yield of clinically useful information
1 Bowden et al (1975)   88%   6 Sindrup (1980) 50%
2 Stålberg (1976)   65%   7 Holmes (1982) 89%
3 Vignaendra et al (1979) 47%   8 Smith (1982)?
4 Bruens & Kniiff? (1980)   9 Ramsay (1982) 11%
5 Binnie et al (1981)   72%

events which are not epileptic in origin. In both groups of patients, prolonged observation by means of monitoring may offer the most effective means of established the true diagnosis. The differential diagnosis of epilepsy is considered elsewhere but, in the present context, it should be noted that monitoring of the EEG, together with other appropriate physiological variables, may assist the identification of syncope, cardiac dysrhythmias, sleep apnoea, narcolepsy and the parasomnias. However, the chief differential diagnosis for which EEG and video monitoring are required is to distinguish between epileptic and pseudoseizures. The problems addressed by monitoring can rarely be resolved by the capture of interictal discharges; attacks presenting difficulties of differential diagnosis often occur in people who have epilepsy, or at the least exhibit interictal epileptiform activity. However, in so far as it may be useful to screen the EEG for the presence of interictal discharges it should be noted that these will be found in most persons with epilepsy undergoing monitoring during the first hour of spontaneous sleep (Bridgers et al 1987), and if they are not seen in this period, there is little chance of finding them by examining a prolonged recording in its entirety.

Clinical studies of pseudoseizures (Gross 1983, Riley & Roy 1982) tend to concentrate on background psychiatric and psychological factors and accounts of the ictal phenomenology are mostly confined to emphasizing the more bizarre and histrionic features. However, many patients with pseudoseizures also suffer from epilepsy and their factitious attacks may closely mimic their habitual epileptic seizure pattern (Roy 1977). Moreover, it has only recently been realized that partial epilepsies of mesial frontal origin in particular can give rise to a florid symptomatology previously thought to typify pseudoseizures, including bilaterally symmetrical flapping movements, arc de circle, and obscene or aggressive utterances. Binnie & Van der Wens (1986) attempted to classify the clinical manifestations of 105 video-recorded pseudoseizures, as if they were true epileptic attacks according to the international classification (Dreifuss 1981). Most of the attacks fell well within the range of known epileptic phenomenology. The pseudoseizures in patients who also had epilepsy differed little from those of the patients who did not. There was, indeed, a tendency for pseudoseizures in nonepileptic patients to be more bizarre, whilst attacks resembling absences or complex partial seizures occurred mostly in people with epilepsy. It has been pointed out, for instance by Pedley (1983), that some details of clinical seizure pattern may distinguish pseudo- from epileptic seizures. For instance, a true absence is of abrupt onset and an attack with a prodromal phase of gradual loss of consciousness cannot be an absence. Conversely, any but the shortest complex partial seizure ends with a fairly gradual return of consciousness and, if the patient abruptly awakens and demands to know what has happened, it is unlikely to have been a complex partial seizure. Monitoring attacks thus assists the differential diagnosis of epileptic and pseudo-seizures, not only by providing EEG information, but also by permitting accurate documentation of the clinical events.

However, obtaining an ictal EEG by no means invariably provides a solution to the differential diagnosis of pseudo- and epileptic seizures. The occurrence of ictal EEG changes appropriate to the seizure type is, of course, conclusive in establishing at least that the observed attack was epileptic in nature. The conclusion sometimes comes as a considerable surprise to those concerned with the patient's management, particularly in the case of partial complex seizures of mesial frontal origin, where the attacks may be so grotesque as to invite a psychiatric interpretation. Moreover, patients with this problem often have also psychosocial difficulties which have not been helped by the insistence of their medical advisers that their attacks were psychogenic.

The problem of the negative ictal EEG has been noted previously and when interpreting the findings in the context of the differential diagnosis of pseudoseizures it is essential to consider the EEG in relation to the clinical manifestations. If the seizure is of a type which invariably, if epileptic, produces ictal EEG change and the recording is of sufficient technical quality to establish that no change occurred, one may confidently conclude that the seizure was not epileptic. If the clinical manifestations fall, however, within the range of those seizure types which do not usually produce changes in the scalp EEG, the only possible conclusion is that the findings do not resolve the differential diagnosis and are certainly compatible with an epileptic origin. In the early literature of epilepsy monitoring, the absence of ictal EEG change during an epileptic seizure is often recognized as a theoretical possibility, but disregarded as a practical consideration. It should be stressed that, in certain types of seizure, a negative ictal EEG is not merely possible but is the expected finding. In patients who only have such seizures, telemetry may not be worth undertaking. This problem arises more often than might perhaps be expected, as pseudoseizures are often seen in patients with refractory partial epilepsy when, after many years of failure, effective drug control is achieved. The patient, whose habitual epileptic seizures commenced with a prodromal event, such as a rising epigastric sensation or feeling of derealization, continues to report such episodes which no longer proceed to a fully developed complex partial seizure. Such attacks fall within the classification of simple partial seizures with special sensory or psychic symptomatology and these are types which usually fail to produce changes in the scalp EEG. In undertaking monitoring of such a patient, the most one can hope is that epileptiform activity will nevertheless be found in some of the attacks, establishing an epileptic basis, or conversely that the patient may sometimes display impaired consciousness (complex symptomatology) without ictal EEG change, suggesting, but not conclusively proving, that the attack was non-epileptic.

Evaluation of the ictal EEG

In patients where the diagnosis of epilepsy is not in doubt, an ictal EEG may be required, either as an aid to classification of the seizures or for purposes of focus localization prior to possible surgical treatment.

Seizure classification is claimed as a valuable clinical application of monitoring (Porter et al 1977, Sutula et al 1981). Typically, the argument runs that therapy resistance may be due to the use of inappropriate medication and that correct classification of the seizures is essential to determine the appropriate drugs. In support of this claim, the differential diagnosis of brief partial complex seizures and absence attacks is most often cited. An analysis of 273 monitored seizures from therapy-resistant patients presenting this problem showed the issue to be more complex than had been suggested (Binnie & Van der Wens 1986). There was a considerable overlap in both clinical and EEG phenomenology between absence seizures and brief complex partial seizures presenting as transitory impairment of awareness. Where the clinical manifestations (complex automatism etc.) clearly fell outside the range of absence symptomatology or where the ictal EEG changes were predominantly focal, the diagnosis could readily be determined. However, in the remainder, more than half of this group of patients, there was no consistent association between EEG and clinical features which could form a basis for classifying these absence-like attacks. In practice, patients showing these features do not respond satisfactorily to monotherapy, either with drugs used for absence seizures (sodium valproate, ethosuximide) nor with those appropriate to partial seizures (phenytoin, carbamazepine) and a combination of drugs from both categories is often required (Binnie & Van der Wens 1986, Hendrickson 1986, Stefan & Burr 1986).

In conclusion, while monitoring to determine seizure type may provide useful insights into a patient's problems, it is overoptimistic to suppose that it will often lead to the choice of appropriate medication in a patient who is therapy resistant.

Seizure frequency

It is often important to establish seizure frequency, notably in assessing the effects of medication (Penry et al 1971, Dreifuss et al 1975, Stefan et al 1980). Such studies may usefully be combined with monitoring of antiepileptic drug levels (Rowan et al 1979). It may also sometimes be important to establish how often seizures occur under particular circumstances; for instance, the frequency of absence attacks at school in a child with learning difficulties. Absences can occur several hundred times per day, and estimates of their frequency by patients and other observers are often very unreliable (Browne et al 1974a). Less commonly, brief partial seizures may be difficult to identify or may be reported by the patient more frequently than they are observed by relatives or nursing staff. In these circumstances, monitoring provides a valuable means of assessing seizure frequency. Clearly, it is applicable only where the suspected seizure frequency is so high that a reasonable number of attacks may be expected within an acceptable period of monitoring. It will be noted that this is an application for which ambulatory cassette recorders are particularly suitable and are indeed the only means of monitoring seizure frequency in the patient's own natural environment outside the hospital.

Clinical correlates of known EEG phenomena

The first and second applications above largely concern the study of the EEG during recognizable clinical events. The converse is also of interest: namely, the careful observation of behaviour to detect possible ictal events during known, and apparently subclinical, EEG discharges. The results may be surprising: for instance, in a study of patients who were thought to have been seizure-free for more than 3 years, monitoring showed that in more than 10% there were EEG discharges accompanied by brief seizures, which had not been noticed (Overweg et al 1987). Sometimes the difficulty in detecting seizures arises from their brevity and the lack of subjective events detected or remembered by the patient. If the clinical ictal manifestations fall within the patient's normal behavioural repertoire they are unlikely to be identified except by simultaneous EEG registration. For instance, a momentary hesitation in speech, a blink, a glance to one side, or a brief smile without obvious cause may all pass as normal behaviour, until it is shown that these events are consistently accompanied by an epileptiform discharge. For addressing this problem, the importance of synchronizing the EEG with the video recording of behaviour will be appreciated and split-screen video recording will generally be the most appropriate technology.

Where no spontaneous ictal behaviour is seen during monitoring, it may nevertheless be possible to detect effects of subclinical discharges on the performance of a continuous task. The discovery of 3/s spike-wave activity in absences was rapidly followed by the realization that these discharges could occur without an evident seizure (Gibbs et al 1936). However, it was then soon found that continuous psychological testing might reveal brief episodes of impaired functioning, during apparently subclinical discharges (Schwab 1939). Some 50 subsequent published studies have, with only two exceptions (Milstein & Stevens 1961, Prechtl et al 1961), succeeded in confirming the occurrence of transitory cognitive impairment during subclinical generalized EEG discharges (for a review, see Binnie 1980). The findings are similar even in patients with epileptiform activity who had not been considered previously to suffer from epilepsy (Ishihara & Yoshii 1967).

On several aspects there is general agreement. The probability of demonstrating transitory cognitive impairment (TCI), is dependent on task difficulty (Tizard & Margerison 1963a, Mirsky & Van Buren 1965): simple, repetitious motor acts such as tapping or following a pursuit rotor

(Browne et al 1974b) are relatively insensitive to the effects of subclinical discharges, whereas more complex tasks, particularly those involving signal detection, language or memory, are much more likely to be disrupted (Shimazano et al 1953, Tizard & Margerison, 1963a, Mirsky & Van Buren 1965, Geller & Geller 1970, Hutt et al 1976, Hutt & Gilbert 1980). Generalized, symmetrical, regular discharges, particularly 3/s spike-wave activity, are most likely to produce demonstrable TCI. The effects gradually increase in the course of the discharge and then diminish towards the end (the so-called 'trough of consciousness') and discharges of 3 seconds duration or longer are more likely to produce apparent effects than are shorter episodes. Despite differences in the patient populations studied and in the sensitivity of the tasks employed, most authors were able to demonstrate TCI in approximately half of the patients investigated.

Until recently, TCI appears to have been regarded chiefly as a research topic rather than as a matter of practical clinical importance. One reason may be the difficulty of investigating TCI routinely as a clinical service. To demonstrate convincingly that TCI occurs during subclinical discharges, they must occur with sufficient frequency to allow a substantial number to be captured within a period acceptable for psychological testing. The tests used in research have generally been so tedious that patients could not reasonably be required to perform them for more than a few minutes and, moreover, attending to the task often suppressed the discharges. Research studies were therefore restricted to selected subjects with very large amounts of epileptiform activity. To test patients with subclinical discharges for TCI as a routine service, it is necessary to devise tasks which can acceptably be used over long periods and which are sufficiently sensitive, yet do not demand such concentration that the discharges are suppressed. Aarts et al (1984) presented a short-term memory task as an entertaining video game, which appeared to meet these requirements. They showed that TCI was demonstrable not only during generalized epileptiform activity but also when very brief focal spikes occurred. Moreover, it was found that left-sided discharges selectively impaired performance of a task using verbal stimuli, whereas right-sided discharges had a greater effect when the material to be recalled was topographic. Lateralized effects are also shown by an increase in reaction times when stimuli are presented in the visual field contralateral to the focus or responses made with the contralateral hand (Shewmon & Erwin 1988).

The phenomenon of TCI itself calls into question the definition of an epileptic seizure, and it may be considered that an EEG discharge accompanied by cognitive changes cannot properly be called 'subclinical'. Whether or not one accepts the view of Tizard & Margerison (1963b) that TCI 'should be considered evidence of a seizure', the phenomenon is of practical importance for some patients whose everyday psychosocial function is demonstrably affected by episodes of impaired cognition related to EEG discharges. Without endorsing the all too widespread practice of treating the EEG rather than the patient, it can be argued that where an adverse psychosocial effect of TCI can be demonstrated, therapeutic intervention is required. The most obvious approach is to attempt to suppress the discharges by means of antiepileptic drugs, and indeed some people have undoubtedly been helped by this means (Aarts et al 1984, Rugland 1990). However, the drugs themselves produce cognitive side effects, and, moreover, are rarely effective in suppressing EEG discharges. The indications and most appropriate methods for treating TCI are at the present time unclear. In any event, monitoring of EEG and behaviour, preferably under the constraints of psychological testing, can play an important part in assessing the problems of a particular patient, by determining whether the epileptiform activity has clinical consequences.

Precipitating factors

In many patients, seizures may be precipitated by environmental, biological or psychological factors. These range from the general (stress, sleep or lack of it, biorhythms) to the highly particular as in reflex epilepsies triggered by specific cognitive activities (Forster 1977). Estimates vary concerning the importance of such factors but, in any event, one easily recognized group, patients with visually precipitated seizures, make up 3% of all people with epilepsy. Recognition of precipitating factors may be of importance in the management of the individual patient who may be helped more by avoiding the trigger than by medication. Where the alleged precipitant is not a simple sensory stimulus, such as flicker or pattern, which can be investigated during a routine EEG investigation, monitoring may be required. Seizures precipitated, for instance, by reading, playing chess or playing music may occur only after the activity in question has been practised for an hour or more; here, particularly if some physical activity is involved, monitoring is the appropriate technology for investigating the problem. It should also be noted that some patients deliberately induce seizures or EEG discharges in themselves, most often making use of photosensitivity for the purpose. This problem may be recognized only during monitoring in a natural environment, and it is suggested that monitoring is for this reason probably indicated in all photosensitive subjects, 25% of whom self-induce (see below).

Evaluation studies

Epilepsy monitoring has proved a useful research tool and has brought valuable new insights into the phenomenology of epileptic seizures. It is, therefore, perhaps not surprising that this development has been accepted with general, but often uncritical, enthusiasm. Data collection by telemetry with simultaneous video monitoring is extremely labour intensive, as is the subsequent analysis of the results; particularly when this involves visual searching of cassettes obtained by ambulatory monitoring for events the precise timing of which is unknown.

The cost-effectiveness of monitoring as a routine clinical procedure has been considered by few authors. Several (Table 9.3) have listed indications for monitoring but the earliest valuation study appears to be that of Stålberg (1976). He found that telemetry and video monitoring, undertaken for about half a day at a time, chiefly for purposes of differential diagnosis or determining seizure frequency, yielded useful information in some 65% of instances. Penry, Porter and colleagues (Penry & Porter 1977, Porter et al 1977) stressed the benefits of comprehensive reassessment of epilepsy in a unit which offered a wide range of facilities including monitoring. Sutula et al (1981) suggested that reclassification of the seizures in 43% of patients represented a major contribution of monitoring to the patients' overall clinical improvement. Little objective evidence has been published in support of such claims but one group (Binnie et al 1981, Binnie 1983b) assessed the results of monitoring in terms of practical consequences. At the simplest level of answering the questions of the referring physicians, the success rate increased from 67% over the period 1979–1980 to over 80% by 1981–1982. The clinicians were required to commit themselves to a diagnosis and management plan prior to monitoring and to decide how far these had to be changed in the light of new evidence. The findings were considered to have influenced management in 56% of the original referrals. At long-term follow up, management decisions based on monitoring appeared to have benefited 23% of the original series of over 324 patients. This result appears modest, but compares favourably with the use of other diagnostic aids in neurology (Derouesne et al 1979). It does perhaps serve to emphasize that this costly method of investigation must be employed selectively and for appropriate indications.

Case histories

Two case histories will be given. This first illustrates the use of monitoring to establish the diagnosis of epilepsy in a patient thought to have pseudoseizures only, and to plan successful surgical removal of a focus which could not have been located without monitoring.

A 22-year-old woman with many personal problems had undergone repeated admissions to mental hospitals since the age of 10, on account of attacks which occurred up to 10 times daily. These were characterized by screaming, dropping to the floor without injuring herself, and assuming a classical arc-de-cercle posture, often with rhythmic pelvic thrusting. Numerous interictal EEGs had been normal and other investigations were negative. She attracted some interest as the seizures resembled those of classical 'hystero-epilepsy' as described by Charcot (1887), rarely seen in modern epileptological practice. During video and EEG monitoring by cable telemetry 10 seizures were registered which followed the pattern described above. At seizure onset the EEG was generally obscured by muscle and movement artifact, however on three occasions a run of spikes was recorded at the right superior frontal electrode at the start of the seizure. This finding led to a revision of the provisional diagnosis and it appeared that the patient's attacks were epileptic and arising from a frontal epileptic focus. Magnetic resonance imaging (MRI) showed a localized abnormality in the wall of a sulcus in the right frontal region directly underlying the superior frontal electrode. On the strength of these findings, subdural electrodes were inserted, together with an intracerebral bundle passing through the site of the MRI abnormality. Further monitoring captured another 10 seizures, all of which were characterized by onset with high frequency spikes in the right frontal cortex (Fig. 9.15). The affected area was resected and the patient is now seizure-free. Histological examination of the tissue removed showed patchy gliosis.

The second case illustrates the detection of unsuspected but socially disabling TCI which was then successfully treated.

A 28-year-old man complained of difficulty in concentration at work. This problem had caused him to abandon his studies of law at university, after which he had become a librarian. However, he was greatly hampered in his work by difficulty in concentration when cataloguing. This was attributed by various psychiatrists and psychologists to his obsessional personality and perfectionism. However, he had occasion to write a letter to an ENT surgeon who, noting very astutely that his writing intermittently trailed away, suggested that he might have epilepsy. Routine electroencephalography including sleep recording and 5 hours' monitoring in a relaxing environment was negative; however, when the patient was required to perform a continuous psychological task, repeated generalized spike-wave discharges occurred and these were associated with marked impairment of performance. No other ictal symptoms were detected. The patient was put on sodium valproate, the discharges seen on monitoring during an intellectually demanding task were greatly reduced, and he no longer has any difficulty at work.

PHOTOSENSITIVE EPILEPSY

As indicated in previous sections, intermittent photic stimulation (IPS) can elicit, besides photic following, a wide range of atypical responses, which various authors loosely describe as 'photosensitivity', causing some terminological confusion (Newmark & Penry 1979). Many of these variants are genetically determined, occur most

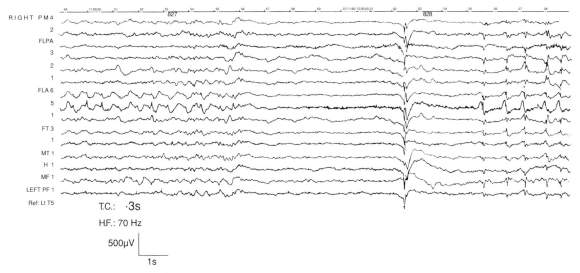

Fig. 9.15 Ictal recording with depth and subdural electrodes from patient with bizarre attacks supposed to be pseudoseizures. Onset of seizure with high-frequency discharge in right frontolateral electrode bundle, FLA 5).

frequently in children and adolescents, and are more common in females than males (Doose et al 1969). Interestingly, similar phenomena are found in other primates. Atypical photic responses are often found in normal subjects, although some types have a weak statistical association with epilepsy. However, the photoconvulsive response (PCR) as described by Bickford et al (1952) is of much greater clinical significance.

The PCR consists of generalized spike-and-wave activity or multiple spikes with a frontal maximum (Fig. 9.16). Arguably, another important feature is that it continues for at least 100 ms after stimulation has ceased (Reilly & Peters 1973). As a self-sustaining response it is more strongly associated with epilepsy. This claim is questioned by Jayakar & Chiappa (1990). However, as examples of self-limited responses, they show two discharges which arguably do outlast the stimulus. They also show an example of a patient exhibiting different types of response at different flash rates; this agrees with the author's experience that application of the criteria of Reilly & Peters (1973) depends on the details of the stimulation technique employed. In practice, amongst patients undergoing clinical EEG examination, a PCR having the characteristics described above is rarely seen in a person who does not have a personal or family history of epilepsy (Reilly & Peters

1973), whereas less typical responses are of less diagnostic significance. For the present purpose the term 'photosensitivity' will be used to describe a liability to produce a PCR in this narrow sense. Regarding asymptomatic photosensitive subjects, it may be added that whenever the author has investigated supposedly unaffected siblings of patients with photosensitive epilepsy, those who exhibited a PCR have themselves invariably had a history of visually induced clinical ictal phenomena which had not been recognized as such.

G. F. A. Harding (cited by Jeavons 1982) estimates the prevalence of photosensitivity in a population aged 5–24 years to be slightly less than 1 in 4000. As the prevalence of active epilepsy is of the order of 0.5% (Pond et al 1960, Gudmundsson 1966, Hauser & Kurland 1975, Goodridge & Shorvon 1983), this figure agrees closely with the finding that some 5% of people with epilepsy are photosensitive, provided most photosensitive subjects also have epilepsy. However, to determine the specificity of the PCR would be very difficult; if only 50% of photosensitive subjects had epilepsy it would be necessary to investigate a population of 4000 to have an even chance of finding one non-epileptic person with a PCR. The 5% prevalence among persons with epilepsy is a general finding in Caucasians and Japanese (Seino, M., personal communication) in

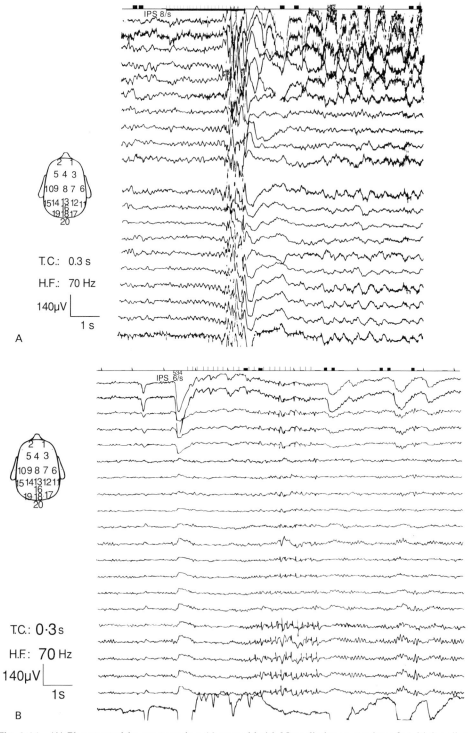

Fig. 9.16 (A) Photoconvulsive response in a 10-year-old girl. Note discharge consists of multiple spikes and slow-waves; although arguably of posterior onset it rapidly becomes generalized with a frontal maximum; the spikes are not phase-locked to the flashes; discharge continues after stimulation has ceased. (B) Occipital spikes; high-amplitude at the back of the head and phase-locked to the stimulus. This is not a photoconvulsive response and is only weakly associated with epilepsy.

Table 9.4 Incidence of photosensitivity in 6500 referrals for EEG investigation of epilepsy (Instituut voor Epilepsiebestrijding, Netherlands 1978–1983)

Idiopathic generalized epilepsy	21.2%
Symptomatic generalized epilepsy	5.1%
Partial	2.8%
Unclassified	2.9%
Overall	5.5%

epileptological practice. A lower incidence is found in Nigerians (Danesi & Oni 1983) and in black, but not white, South Africans (De Graaf et al 1980). Danesi (1985) found a reduced incidence of photosensitivity in the summer in London and concluded that the low incidence in Nigeria was attributable to climatic factors. This observation is, however contrary to the findings of Scott et al (1985) in London and of the author (in the Netherlands): both found a slightly increased prevalence in patients tested during the summer. Danesi's hypothesis also fails to explain De Graaf's observation of differences between whites and blacks in the same country, supporting a genetic basis.

Two-thirds of photosensitive subjects are female and the peak prevalence reported is in early adolescence. Photosensitivity is rare, but not unknown, in infants and the elderly, but is chiefly found between the ages of 4 and 20 years. Age of onset is difficult to determine. The diagnosis is typically made at about the age of 12, but this largely reflects a delay in referral for EEG. Some photosensitive subjects are observed from infancy to have been attracted by bright lights. Being to a considerable extent genetically determined, photosensitivity is most common in the idiopathic generalized form of epilepsy, where the prevalence may be of the order of 25% (Table 9.4). Jeavons (personal communication) finds that on long-term follow up there is not the expected reduction of photosensitivity with increasing age. Possibly the apparent age-dependent prevalence is an artifact, due to the fact that photosensitivity is associated with types of epilepsy which present and are investigated in childhood and adolescence. Adult referrals to an EEG laboratory will be weighted with resistant or late onset epilepsies, both of which are negatively associated with photosensitivity.

In 70% of photosensitive patients with epilepsy,

there is a history of seizures precipitated by environmental stimuli and, indeed, photic stimulation may also trigger seizures in the EEG laboratory. Numerous environmental stimuli may be implicated—including the sun seen through trees or reflected on moving water, discotheque lighting and arcade games—but in western Europe, television is most often the precipitant (in some 50% of patients, Table 9.5). Some patients report seizures on entering a brightly lit environment, even in the absence of flicker. In about 50% of photosensitive subjects no spontaneous seizures occur, all the attacks being apparently triggered by visual stimuli (Jeavons & Harding 1975).

Jeavons & Harding (1975) classify photosensitive subjects into three types:

1. Those with 'pure photosensitive epilepsy', i.e. with visually induced seizures only (40%)
2. Epileptic patients with photosensitivity and spontaneous seizures, with or without known visually induced seizures (the majority)
3. Photosensitive people without epilepsy (rare).

This last group appears (when a strict definition of EEG photosensitivity is used) to be very small and was later discarded (Jeavons 1982).

Table 9.5 Clinical features of 358 photosensitive patients with epilepsy

Sex ratio F/M	2.5
Age (mean)	19 years
Type of epilepsy	
Idiopathic generalized	43%
Symptomatic generalized	23%
Partial	29%
Unclassified	5%
Specific sensitivities	
Sensitive to static pattern	45%
*Sensitive to moving pattern	60%
Sensitive to TV	45%
†Photogenic seizures	
TV induced	46%
Disco-induced	34%
Pattern-induced	18%
All types	61%
†Patient reported symptoms during IPS	42%
‡Visually-induced ocular discomfort	39%
Self-induction	26%

* Not always tested.
† A subsequent study using closer observation and direct questioning suggested an incidence over 75% (Kasteleijn-Nolst Trenité et al 1987a).
‡ Smaller sample (n=250) personally interviewed by the author or by Dr D. C. A. Kasteleinj-Nolst-Trenité.

Most visually-induced seizures reported by patients are tonic-clonic convulsions. However, the PCR elicited in the EEG laboratory is usually accompanied by myoclonus or by strange subjective feelings (Kastelijn-Nolst Trenité et al 1987a). On direct questioning, patients admit to similar sensations when exposed to epileptogenic environmental stimuli; these experiences too should probably be regarded as seizures. Absences, usually with myoclonus, are rarely reported, but are often observed during IPS or in patients with self-induced attacks (see below).

Photic stimulation

Demonstration of photosensitivity in the EEG laboratory depends on adequate apparatus and technique. There is also a risk of inducing a convulsive seizure unless proper precautions are followed. For detailed recommendations see Jeavons (1969), Jeavons & Harding (1975) and Binnie et al (1982). The stimulus intensity should if possible be at least 100 nit-s/flash. The stroboscope lamp must be centrally fixated; if the patient looks at the edge of the lamp housing, a PCR will rarely be obtained. The probability of eliciting a PCR is probably greater if the flash stimulus is patterned (Jeavons et al 1972), although some authors could not confirm this (Engel 1974, Kirstein & Nilsson 1977). Some lamps are patterned, having wire grids in or behind the glass, for reasons of electrical screening or safety; if the glass is clear, pattern can be introduced by inserting a plastic sheet bearing a grid or grating with a spatial frequency of about 2 cycles per degree (i.e. black and white stripes each 1.2 mm wide if the pattern is to be viewed at 30 cm). This measure can increase the likelihood of finding a PCR on routine examination by as much as 50% (assuming that the lamp intensity is adjusted to compensate for light absorption by the pattern). Such a stimulus may be less suitable for use in a research context, as it confounds the effects of flicker with those of pattern.

Red light is reputed to be more epileptogenic than other colours or white. Early studies on which this claim was based failed to consider whether the eyes were open or closed during stimulation (the closed eyelids will selectively transmit red light) or to use adequate photometric calibration of the stimuli used (Walter & Walter 1949, Livingston 1952, Carterette & Symmes 1952, Marshall et al 1953, Pantelakis et al 1962, Brausch & Ferguson 1965, Capron 1966). Harding et al (1975), taking account of these factors, found no effect of the colour of illumination. By contrast, Takahashi, in a series of meticulous experiments (Takahashi et al 1980, 1981), demonstrated red light to be most effective, and to produce a PCR at extremely low levels of intensity (25 candella/m^2 or less). Binnie et al (1984a) confirmed the findings of Takahashi but demonstrated that this effect was obtainable only with monochromatic, deep-red light at the extreme limit of the visible spectrum, probably because this avoided the inhibitory interactions which occur between systems subserving different colours when light is used which is capable of stimulating populations of cones with different spectral sensitivities. Although highly epileptogenic, monochromatic long wavelength flicker is difficult to generate from conventional light sources using filters etc., and should not present an environmental hazard unless novel sources appear, such as laser shows, or instrumentation using deep-red photo-diodes.

Photic stimulation is often performed in darkness in the reasonable expectation that the flashes should appear relatively brighter and therefore be more effective. However, Van Egmond et al (1980) found no consistent effect of environmental lighting on photosensitivity and suggested that photic stimulation should be performed under conditions of normal or subdued room lighting so that the technician could observe the patient, controlling ocular fixation and noting any clinical ictal manifestations. These latter can be identified by close observation and subsequent questioning of the patient, during routine photic stimulation in over 70% of photosensitive subjects (Kastelijn-Nolst Trenité et al 1987a).

Eye opening and closure have a marked effect on photosensitivity, most patients are more sensitive with the eyes open than closed, but the majority exhibit the greatest sensitivity if stimulation commences at the moment of eye closure. The flash rate is important in determining the occurrence of a PCR. A patient is sensitive over a continuous range between upper and lower threshold frequencies, but outside these limits exhibits normal photic following or often an atypical response not meeting the criteria for a PCR. The 'photosensitivity range' may be used as a measure of the severity of sensitivity and is reduced by effective medication (Jeavons & Harding 1975, Binnie et al 1986a). The flash rate most likely to elicit a PCR is of the order of 15–18/s; only 10% of photosensitive patients respond at 6/s or at 60/s (Fig. 9.17).

Once it is established that a patient is photosensitive, the photosensitivity range can be determined by approaching the lower frequency threshold from below and the upper threshold from above. There should thus be no need to employ stimuli at frequencies between these limits, which may induce a convulsive seizure. If a given stimulus frequency is effective in a particular patient, a PCR will develop rapidly, usually within 2 seconds and almost always within 4 seconds. No useful purpose is therefore served by prolonged IPS. Monocular stimulation is usually much less epileptogenic than binocular. During routine examination of a photosensitive patient, it is worth checking the effect of covering one eye with the hand, as, if effective, this manoeuvre may be recommended to protect against environmental epileptogenic stimuli.

As indicated above, subtle ictal events, myoclonus or a subjective sensation of jerking may be observed by the technician or recognized by the patient. Convulsive seizures should, however, be entirely avoidable. The train of stimuli should be terminated as soon as a PCR appears. For this reason the use of preprogrammed photic stimulators is questionable, and the on/off control should be spring-loaded, so that stimulation stops immediately if the technician's hand is withdrawn. It is acceptable to repeat a set of stimulus conditions which has elicited a PCR for purposes of confirmation, but there can rarely be any justification for using a more potently epileptogenic stimulus (e.g. testing at 18 flashes/s when 10/s has already elicited a response). Sleep deprivation markedly increases photosensitivity, and photic stimulation should not in general be performed after prolonged sleeplessness in a known photosensitive subject.

Pattern sensitivity

Viewing static linear patterns elicits epileptiform discharges in over 30% of photosensitive subjects (Stefannson et al 1977, Porter 1985) but, if the pattern oscillates in a direction orthogonal to the line orientation, 70% of patients exhibit discharges. A history of seizures induced by pattern is volunteered by only a small proportion of these subjects (Table 9.5), probably because the causal relationship is not recognized as readily as in the case of environmental flicker. However, close questioning reveals that attacks may be precipitated by stimuli as varied as Venetian blinds, railings, stainless steel escalator treads, striped domestic furnishings and clothing (nurses' uniforms!), and ironing striped shirts.

Pattern sensitive epilepsy was first described by Bickford et al (1953) and was occasionally reported as an interesting rarity up to the mid-1970s (Bickford & Klass 1962, 1969, Gastaut & Tassinari 1966, Chatrian et al 1970a,b). A study by Wilkins et al (1975) showed that the physical characteristics of the pattern were crucial in determining its epileptogenicity and that checker-

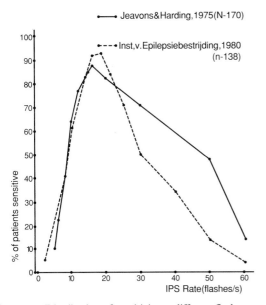

Fig. 9.17 Distribution of sensitivity to different flash-rates in two studies of photosensitivity. The difference in incidence of sensitivity to higher frequencies probably reflects the fact that sodium valproate was not available in the United Kingdom during most of the period covered by the study of Jeavons & Harding (1975).

boards, widely used for eliciting evoked responses, were particularly ineffective. Thus Stefannson et al (1977), using stimuli more appropriate than those employed by previous investigators, were able to demonstrate pattern sensitivity in a majority of photosensitive subjects. This finding in turn encouraged more detailed enquiry after possible pattern-induced seizures.

Pattern stimuli lend themselves to physiological studies of photosensitivity (Wilkins et al 1979a) as much is already known from experimental work about pattern vision and the influence of the physical characteristics of the stimulus on events in neurones within the visual system. To be epileptogenic, a pattern requires a high contrast (usually at least 0.4) and an illumination generally greater than 50 lux. Gratings (stripes) are most effective, whereas grids and checkerboards are not so epileptogenic. The optimal spatial frequency is 2–4 cycles/degree (i.e. each pair of stripes should subtend an angle of 15–30 min of arc). The orientation of the grating is usually unimportant (unless the patient is astigmatic). Binocular stimuli are more effective than monocular but, under conditions of binocular rivalry, e.g. gratings of different orientations exposed to each eye, the patterns become much less epileptogenic. The probability of eliciting a discharge is related to the size of the stimulus or, more precisely, to the area of visual cortex stimulated having regard to the site of the retinal image and the cortical magnification factor. Thus, a small central stimulus is as effective as a much larger one in peripheral vision. The effects of discrete patterned areas are additive if they fall in the same visual field (i.e. project to the same hemisphere) but there is no spatial summation between right and left fields. From these detailed findings, which are reviewed more fully by Wilkins et al (1980) various physiological conclusions follow.

Physiology of photosensitivity

Patterns which are optimally epileptogenic are closely similar in their physical characteristics to those which produce the maximum discharge rate in visual cortical neurones in experimental animals, and also to those which are experienced by normal subjects as being most disagreeable to look at. This may amount to the somewhat trivial statement that physiologically potent stimuli are most effective in inducing seizures and inducing peculiar sensations. However, the physiological data on pattern sensitivity also show that epileptogenicity is abolished by presentation of images with different spatial orientations in the two eyes.

Binocularly innervated orientation selective units are not, apparently, found lower in the visual pathway than the complex cells of the visual cortex. This finding therefore implies a central role for the visual cortex in the triggering of EEG discharges by pattern. Presentation of pattern stimuli within the right or left visual field in pattern-sensitive subjects elicits focal discharges over the contralateral posterior temporal occipital region (Soso et al 1980, Wilkins et al 1981). This finding implies not only that the visual or pre-visual cortex is involved in the triggering of the epileptiform discharge, but also that epileptiform activity arises at this site. Flicker stimulation provides less evidence concerning physiological mechanisms but it is of interest to note that, as the generalized photoconvulsive response is suppressed by effective medication, the discharges may become confined to the posterior regions (Binnie et al 1980a) and eventually the only residual abnormality may be the presence of occipital spikes (Harding et al 1978). Together, these observations suggest that photosensitivity, although seen most often in patients with idiopathic generalized epilepsy, is a model of partial epilepsy with secondary generalization; epileptogenesis thus appears to commence in the occipital regions, giving rise to secondarily generalized discharges, which can be suppressed by drugs such as sodium valproate.

A striking characteristic of flicker stimulation is its temporal rhythmicity, which is not obviously shared by pattern stimuli, and the question arises to what extent entrainment of cortical discharges by the rhythmic stimulus gives rise to synchronous, discharges and how far this is important to the triggering of epileptiform activity. Binnie et al (1985a) report an experiment comparing three types of pattern stimulation: drifting gratings, oscillating gratings and static gratings. It was argued that the contours of drifting gratings should enter and leave the receptive field of different cortical units asynchronously, producing no synchronization of cortical activity. Oscillating gratings, by contrast, should elicit synchronous activity alternately in populations of neurones sensitive to movement in one direction or the other. Static gratings might give rise to some synchronization because of oscillation of the retinal image secondary to ocular tremor. The hypothesis that synchronization by the stimulus contributed to epileptogenesis therefore led to the prediction that the oscillating gratings should be most epileptogenic, the static gratings less so and the drifting gratings virtually without effect. This prediction proved correct.

In conclusion, it appears that triggering of EEG discharges by visual stimuli, particularly pattern, takes place in striate or prestriate cortex; depends on the efficacy of the stimulus in eliciting action potentials in cortical neurones and the size of the neuronal population activated within one hemisphere; and is promoted by synchronizing effects of the stimulus itself. It may be noted that the mechanisms involved in photosensitivity in some other species, notably the Senegalese baboon, are almost certainly different: discharges arise in the frontal cortex under the influence of diffuse subcortical projections, corticocortical pathways from other areas including the visual cortex, and proprioceptive inputs to the frontal eye fields (Menini 1976).

Television epilepsy

As many people spend hours daily watching television, it is not surprising that seizures often occur in front of the television set. However, where a causal relationship to television viewing is demonstrable, the patient can almost invariably be shown to be photosensitive. Early reports stressed the role of malfunction of the television set (Lange 1961, Mawdsley 1961, Charlton & Hoefer 1964), but the crucial factor may in fact be that the patient had approached the set to adjust it or to change channels. Many patients undoubtedly have seizures induced by a normally functioning television (Pantelakis et al 1962) and Stefansson et al (1977) demonstrated that a normal television induced EEG discharges in 70% of photosensitive

patients, although curiously Gastaut et al (1960a) could not. Black and white television is said to be more likely to induce seizures (Connell et al 1975). This may reflect the greater clarity of the raster pattern of a black and white set (see below). However, the difference in epileptogenicity is not great (Wilkins et al 1979b) and the use of a colour set offers no protection against television epilepsy.

The television screen flickers at mains frequency, i.e. 50 Hz in Western Europe, 60 Hz in North America. In Europe, almost 90% of patients with 'pure photosensitive epilepsy' have suffered television-induced seizures. Television epilepsy was recognized later in the USA (Charlton & Hoefer 1964) than in Europe (Klapatek 1959, Richter 1960, Lange 1961, Dumermuth 1961) and is reported less often, possibly because of the higher mains frequency. However, the majority of patients with television epilepsy are not photosensitive at frequencies even as high as 50 Hz and some alternative explanation must be found for the triggering of their seizures. Wilkins et al (1979b) showed two mechanisms to be involved. Patients who are photosensitive at 50 Hz often exhibit EEG discharges whilst viewing at several metres from the television screen. Patients with television epilepsy who are not sensitive to 50 Hz flicker are pattern sensitive and discharges can be elicited only when the viewing distance is so small that the raster pattern of the screen can be resolved. Television pictures are presented at half mains frequency (25 frames/s in Europe) but are actually scanned as two half frames, the odd and even-numbered lines being traced alternately. Thus at several metres distance the only epileptogenic stimulus is the mains frequency flicker of the whole screen, but close up the patient is confronted by a grating pattern, apparently oscillating (actually alternating) at 25 Hz. The distinction between these two different mechanisms is of some practical importance. Those 50-Hz sensitive patients who respond at distances of several metres from the screen are less sensitive when viewing in a well-lit environment. By contrast, the pattern-sensitive subjects responding only at close viewing become more sensitive when the background is brightly lit (Binnie et al 1980b).

The first group of patients may be protected from adverse effects of television by viewing in a well-lit room whilst the second group must adopt other measures; they should avoid close proximity to the screen, for instance by using a remote control unit, should cover one eye if it is necessary to approach the television, or should obtain a set so small (e.g. less than 30 cm diagonally) that the spatial frequency of the raster, even at the near point of vision, is too high to be epileptogenic. A more elaborate way of avoiding binocular television stimulation is to cover the screen with a polarizing sheet and for the patient to wear spectacles, one lens of which is polarized in an axis orthogonal to that of the screen (Wilkins et al 1977, Wilkins & Lindsay 1985). The patient can thus see the television with only one eye, but vision for the rest of the environment is binocular. This method is effective but acceptable to only a minority of patients, because of eye strain or cosmetic considerations.

In view of the undoubted epileptogenicity of television for many photosensitive patients, it has been suggested that visual display units (VDUs) could represent a hazard to people with epilepsy. However, the physical characteristics of a VDU differ from those of a domestic television in ways that, on theoretical grounds, make them unlikely to be epileptogenic. EEG recording from photosensitive subjects whilst viewing VDUs of various types with both static and scrolling displays fails to demonstrate any activating effect (Binnie et al 1985b). A similar procedure elicits discharges in 40% of photosensitive subjects if a black and white television is used. There is no evidence, theoretical, experimental or clinical, that computer displays of text on a professional VDU represent a hazard to photosensitive patients. A possible explanation is the use of slow phosphors on VDUs which flicker less than TV tubes. However, a domestic television set employed as a computer display device may prove even more epileptogenic than when it is used for watching programmes, as the viewing distance will be less. Arcade games often use flashing effects which are themselves epileptogenic, whatever the method of display.

Treatment of photosensitive epilepsy

As indicated in the previous section in the context of television epilepsy, simple practical measures to avoid epileptogenic stimulation may provide protection against visually induced seizures and, in patients with no spontaneous attacks, medication may not be necessary. Other practical measures include the use of dark glasses when exposed to potentially epileptogenic stimuli out of doors. To provide effective protection, these must absorb some 90% of the incident light, which means that the lenses should be very dark, as those worn for winter sports, and may be cosmetically unacceptable. The belief that Polaroid glasses confer particular benefit appears to have no basis except where there is a source of plane polarized flicker (at sea or when the ground is snow-covered). Patients should not be encouraged to obtain expensive photochromatic lenses, as these generally respond too slowly to prevent seizures that may be induced, for instance, on suddenly entering a brightly lit environment. Every patient with photosensitive epilepsy should be taught to cover one eye as an emergency measure, when suddenly confronted with an epileptogenic stimulus. Complete occlusion with the palm is required, not just shading the eye with the radial side of the hand against the forehead.

Where medication is necessary, sodium valproate, ethosuximide and the benzodiazepines are most effective, but tolerance usually develops to the latter. Dosage should be adjusted to abolish photosensitivity if possible. This can be achieved with sodium valproate in a little over 50% of patients (Harding et al 1978) and nearly 80% show a substantial reduction. If it is decided after some years of freedom from seizures to withdraw this drug, at least 6 months follow-up is required, as the suppressant effect on photosensitivity continues for weeks or months after valproate is withdrawn. Various methods of deconditioning have been attempted (Forster et al 1964, Braham 1967, Jeavons & Harding 1975) but with little success.

On acute administration, representatives of all major groups of antiepileptic drugs (AEDs) suppress photosensitivity. This response is not predictive of their chronic effects in photosensitive epilepsy, but may provide a useful means of assessing efficacy of new experimental AEDs (Binnie et al 1986a).

Self-induced seizures

The first descriptions of photosensitive epilepsy date from before the clinical use of EEG and concern patients who induced attacks in themselves by staring at the sun and waving the outspread fingers of one hand in front of the eyes to produce flicker (Radovici et al 1932). Patients displaying this behaviour are often mentally subnormal (Andermann et al 1962). More recently, however, it has been realized that many more photosensitive subjects employ a manoeuvre involving extreme upward deviation of the eyes with slow eyelid closure to induce seizures or epileptiform discharges in themselves (Green 1966). The eye movements may themselves be misinterpreted as an ictal phenomenon, eyelid myoclonia, and indeed some authors have regarded the hand waving in the same way (Ames 1971, 1974, Livingston & Torres 1964). There is, however, compelling evidence that when placed in a poorly-lit environment patients continue to exhibit the slow eye closures, at least for some minutes, but no discharges occur.

The oculographic artifacts accompanying the inducing movements show them to be different from those seen on normal blinking, eye closure to command, or during spontaneous absence seizures. The syndrome of visual self-induction can indeed be recognized from clinical observation alone: since drawing the attention of colleagues to the phenomenon the writer has received referrals of self-inducing patients who were correctly identified on clinical grounds before an EEG had been recorded and before photosensitivity was suspected.

Despite a reluctance to discuss the subject, some patients admit to deliberately practising self induction and describe the sensations produced. Some report using other methods in addition to eye closure and hand waving, viewing patterns or television for instance.

Many other photosensitive patients who do not habitually self-induce have discovered the slow eye closure manoeuvre and can describe the subjective effects.

Some patients learn a technique of initiating a discharge by eye closure and prolonging or enhancing it by hand waving. This is well illustrated in the series of cine stills published by Ames (1974). Some photosensitive patients exhibit epileptiform discharges, either generalized or at the back of the head, on normal eye closure. This appears to be a phenomenon different from self-induction: the oculographic artifact is normal and no pleasurable experience is reported; but obviously the mechanism involved could be related to that used in self-induction. Studies employing telemetric monitoring of photosensitive subjects suggest that some 25% of susceptible patients indulge in self-induction, if not of seizures at least of discharges (Darby et al 1980b, Binnie et al 1980c). Patients are usually embarrassed to discuss this habit but may admit to experiencing a pleasurable sensation or a relief of tension when self-inducing. The rate of self-induction usually increases under stress and frequencies of 100 episodes per hour are not unusual. The self-induced seizures range from pleasurable subjective experiences, through sexual arousal including orgasm, and absence seizures, to tonic-clonic convulsions.

Some patients with television epilepsy are compulsively attracted to the screen. Most are children, with a small preponderance of males. Some of these patients, particularly the adults, admit to using television as a method of self-induction (Harley et al 1967, Andermann 1971). One freely admitted to inducing tonic-clonic seizures with television as a 'do it yourself' convulsive therapy, which relieved the severe bouts of depression from which she suffered. Others insist that the compulsion is distressing to them but irresistible, and it is uncertain whether or not some instances of compulsive attraction to television are to be regarded as self-inducing behaviour or as ictal phenomena. Wilkins & Lindsay (1985) argue from the rapid abolition of compulsive attraction when polarized glasses are worn (see above) that the behaviour is usually not learned but is ictal. However, these patients may be attracted to a television in a shop window from distances at which no epileptogenic effect is demonstrable.

Self-induced epilepsy is notoriously resistant to therapy (Andermann et al 1962, Hutchinson et al 1958, Rabending et al 1969, Rail 1973, Ames & Enderstein 1976). This may in part be due to reluctance to take medication, but even compliant patients appear refractory to AEDs. A few patients have responded to psychotherapy (Libo et al 1971) or can be persuaded to wear dark glasses. Overweg & Binnie (1980) noted an analogy between this behaviour and electrical self-stimulation of the brain in experimental animals, a phenomenon which is suppressed by dopamine antagonists. They therefore attempted therapy with chlorpromazine or haloperidol and reported an improvement in six out of seven patients. Kasteleijn-Nolst Trenité et al (1983) also obtained a reduced incidence of self-stimulation in a controlled trial of pimozide.

Reading epilepsy

Photosensitive epilepsy is by far the most common of the reflex epilepsies. Patients with seizures induced by other stimuli than flicker or pattern, such as eating, are often also photosensitive. One of the less rare forms of reflex epilepsy is characterized by seizures induced by prolonged reading. If a patient with reading epilepsy is also photosensitive, the question arises of whether or not the seizures are induced by sensitivity to the pattern formed by the lines of text (Mayersdorf & Marshall 1970). If this mechanism is ever involved, it is probably rare: very few pattern sensitive patients have reading epilepsy or exhibit EEG discharges on viewing text. Content and context are usually important determinants of epileptogenicity in reading epilepsy. Perhaps the most striking difference between reading epilepsy and visual sensitivity is that reading induces EEG discharges or seizures only after many minutes, whereas photic or pattern sensitivity is demonstrable within seconds of exposure.

Conclusion

Photosensitive epilepsy is of special interest to the electroencephalographer as, even though careful enquiry will usually establish a history of visually induced seizures, in practice the diagnosis is usually made after finding a PCR in the EEG laboratory. Although photosensitive subjects represent only 5% of patients with epilepsy, the condition is of some considerable interest representing, apart from ECT, the only human experimental model of epilepsy, and can be used both to investigate physiological mechanisms of epi-

leptogenesis and for preliminary assessment of antiepileptic drugs. Moreover, the finding of photosensitivity is important to those patients whose seizures are all visually precipitated, as they may often be effectively treated by simple practical measures to avoid visual triggers and may not need medication. Finally, it is important to identify the 25% of photosensitive subjects who practise self-induction. If the problem is not recognized, they may be regarded simply as having therapy-resistant epilepsy and treated unsuccessfully to the point of intoxication with antiepileptic drugs.

APPENDIX: TECHNIQUES OF VISUAL STIMULATION IN THE EEG LABORATORY

Standardized method for photic stimulation (Jeavons & Harding 1975)

1. The procedure is explained to the patient.
2. The same photostimulator is used in all repeat tests as was used initially.
3. Illumination of the room is standardized by drawing blinds and using artificial light.
4. The lowest intensity light is used initially, increased if there is no abnormality and standardized in subsequent tests.
5. A pattern of small squares with narrow black lines (0.3 mm), with spacing of 2×2 mm, or a pattern of parallel lines (1 mm) spaced 1.5 mm apart, is placed behind the glass of the lamp (dry print transfers are cheap and easily available).
6. A circle of 3 cm diameter is drawn in the centre of the glass and the patient looks at this circle.
7. The lamp is placed at 30 cm from the eyes.
8. Testing is carried out with eyes kept open or kept closed, and only if no PCR is evoked is the effect of eye closure tested.
9. 16 Hz can be used as an initial test frequency to identify the photosensitive patient. If no PCR is elicited, testing starts at 1 Hz and rates up to 25 Hz are used, followed by 30, 40, 50 Hz.
10. In the photosensitive patient the duration of the stimulus should not usually exceed 2 seconds.
11. In the photosensitive patient, testing starts at

1 Hz and increases in steps of 1 Hz until a PCR is evoked. The upper limit is then established by starting at 60 Hz and reducing in steps of 10 Hz.

12. The sensitivity limit is defined as the lowest or highest flash rate which consistently evokes a PCR. The sensitivity range is obtained by subtracting the lower from the upper limit.

Some further comments or suggestions may be added (Binnie et al 1986a)

13. In a known photosensitive patient, it is necessary only to find the upper and lower frequency thresholds for producing a PCR in order to determine the photosensitivity range. No useful purpose will be served by performing IPS at frequencies between these limits, and this carries, moreover, the risk of inducing a convulsive seizure.

14. As the probability of eliciting a discharge increases by only 6%/Hz over the range of flash rates 1–18/s, it is inefficient to increase the stimulus frequency in steps of only 1 Hz. The standard frequencies—18, 6, 8, 10, 15, 20, 30, 40, 50, 60—are recommended, corresponding to the optimum for eliciting a PCR (18/s) and those above and below this, to which 10, 20, 40, 60 or 80% of photosensitive subjects respond.

15. Also, in the interests of saving time, if the stimulator is turned on for 8 seconds as the eyes are closed and the patient is asked to open the eyes 4 seconds later, all three eye conditions, closure, closed and open, can be tested at a single stimulus presentation. If a PCR occurs the stimulus train should immediately be terminated, to avoid a possible seizure and to determine whether the discharges are self-sustaining.

16. Many commercially available photic stimulators are unsatisfactory. The maximum flash rate available should be at least 50 Hz (60 Hz in North America) for assessing patients with television epilepsy. The maximum flash intensity (which is rarely specified in photometric units by the manufacturer) should be at least 100 nit-s/flash.

Summary of method of testing pattern sensitivity (Darby et al 1980a)

1. The pattern is circular, diameter 48 cm with stripes of 2.5 mm.
2. The black and white stripes should be parallel and of equal size.
3. The optimal width is 2 cycles/degree of visual angle (15 min of arc) subtending more than 16 degrees.
4. The contrast should be high and brightness above 200 cycles/m^2
5. The patient stares at a spot in the centre of the pattern.
6. Viewing is at arm's length (57 cm) and unless the pattern is itself luminous (e.g. a video display) it should be illuminated by a spotlight behind the patient. (At this viewing distance 1 cm subtends 1°, so the spatial frequency of the pattern described is 2 cycles/degree.)
7. The pattern is held steady for 30 seconds and is oscillated orthogonal to the line orientation if no paroxysmal activity is evoked.
8. The optimal frequency of oscillation is about 20 Hz, this can be achieved by special stimulators, but a hand held card cannot be oscillated at more than 10 Hz.

MISCELLANEOUS DIAGNOSTIC PROBLEMS

Febrile convulsions

As the incidence of febrile convulsions is about 3% (Lennox-Buchtal 1973), the electroencephalographer is often asked to investigate a child who has recently suffered a seizure while pyrexial. Questions which may be asked concern: possible acute cerebral disease underlying both the fever and the seizure, the risk of recurrence of febrile convulsions, and the prognosis for developing epilepsy. Within 24 hours following a febrile convulsion, nearly 90% of children will show an abnormal EEG (Laplane & Salbreux 1963) and after 3–5 days about one-third still have abnormal records (Frantzen et al 1968). Slowing of background rhythms is generally seen, which may be symmetrical or asymmetrical; the latter particularly if the seizure itself was asymmetrical or unilateral.

The more severe abnormalities may be difficult to distinguish from the effects of acute encephalopathy and serial EEG recording may be required to resolve this issue. Reviewing several previous series, Lennox-Buchtal (1973) found that extreme or focal slowing of the EEG was significantly associated with severity of the convulsion, duration and degree of fever, and past history of brain injury. There was a nonsignificant association with a subsequent liability to afebrile convulsions. However, as under 10% of children with extreme or focal slowing subsequently developed epilepsy, this finding was of little predictive value in any individual. Epileptiform discharges in the immediate postictal phase are of little significance in relation to subsequent epilepsy but, particularly if focal, may reflect acute underlying pathology. Gastaut et al (1960b) described a syndrome of a severe unilateral febrile convulsion and an EEG showing contralateral reduction in amplitude of background activity with focal abnormalities, slow waves, spikes or spike-wave complexes, in children who subsequently developed hemiconvulsions, hemiplegia and epilepsy. In the absence of cerebral pathology, the initial EEG does not usually contain epileptiform activity except in the older children and its presence is in any event of no prognostic significance (Frantzen et al 1968).

At follow-up, generalized spike-wave activity shows an association with a family history of convulsions (Frantzen et al 1970) but does not increase the likelihood of further seizures. Serial studies show development of epileptiform EEG discharges in those children who develop epilepsy. However, the first EEG record containing epileptiform activity may follow the first afebrile seizure (Laplane & Salbreux 1963). In summary, the EEG offers less evidence than might be hoped concerning prognosis following febrile convulsions, and its chief value in the first few days after the seizure is for detecting acute underlying cerebral disease.

Psychiatric problems in epilepsy

There is a recognized association between epilepsy, particularly with partial seizures of temporal lobe origin, and psychosis. Most authors find this chiefly in patients with focal discharges over the dominant hemisphere (Slater et al 1963, Flor-Henry 1969, 1972, 1976, Taylor 1977). Kristensen & Sindrup (1978), by contrast, found bilateral spike foci to be most strongly associated with psychosis. Lateralization of the discharges also appears to influence the nature of the psychotic syndrome. Thus Flor-Henry (1969) found schizophreniform features in patients with left-sided or bilateral foci, and manic-depressive symptoms with right-sided discharges. The effects of laterality are complex, however: a schizophreniform picture is associated with left-handedness in subjects with either left-sided (Sherwin 1981), or right-sided foci (Trimble & Perez 1981).

There appears to be an inverse relationship between seizure occurrence and liability to psychosis. Thus Flor-Henry (1972, 1976) and Kristensen & Sindrup (1978) found a reduced incidence of complex partial seizures when patients became psychotic. Similarly, following successful operative treatment of temporal lobe epilepsy, psychosis may develop (Jensen & Larsen 1979, Taylor 1972, Stevens 1966) or deteriorate (Sherwin 1981). These changes are often accompanied by the disappearance of EEG abnormalities, leading to the hypothesis that 'forced normalization' of the EEG by medication precipitates psychosis (Landolt 1958). A speculative neurochemical basis for this relationship is offered by the observation that dopamine antagonists, effective in schizophrenia, are epileptogenic and that conversely some antiepileptic drugs have a secondary dopaminergic action (Trimble 1977).

In children too a relationship exists between lateralization of focal EEG discharges and psychosocial dysfunction. Thus Stores (1978) found that left-temporal discharges in boys, but not in girls, were associated with educational and behavioural problems. Surprisingly perhaps, generalised epileptiform activity, which might have been expected to cause inattention, was less likely to be associated with school difficulties.

Epilepsy, aggression and crime

Despite a widespread belief in the liability of persons with complex partial seizures to display aggressive and/or criminal behaviour during their attacks, convincing evidence of ictal aggression is exceedingly difficult to find. In this context, it is important to distinguish directed ictal aggression from the random, confused, resistive behaviour seen sometimes during seizures and more often in the postictal state. Delgado-Escueta et al (1981) attempted to collect reports documented by telemetric ictal EEG studies of patients who became aggressive during seizures, but found no convincing evidence of directed aggression against persons.

The question of ictal aggression is, however, confused by other electrophysiological evidence. Spiking has been recorded from the mesial part of the amygdala during spontaneous aggressive behaviour in monkeys and in humans (Heath 1954, 1972, 1975, Heath & Mickle 1960). Both psychotic and epileptic patients exhibited 12–18/s spindles in the hippocampus and amygdala during episodes of dyscontrol but, in those with epilepsy, these were intermixed with spike-wave activity. Stevens (1977a,b) suggests that neural spiking, so far from being only a pathological phenomenon, is a means of transmitting information of imperative biological importance and can be found in various species, including humans during aggression, suckling and orgasm (Heath, 1975). Current views of the ethics of human experimentation preclude further systematic investigation of these phenomena in humans but observations incidental to preoperative assessment of people with epilepsy confirm the finding of deep spike discharges, not detectable in the scalp EEG, during aggressive behaviour in humans (Wieser 1983b). If, however, deep temporal discharges can be a correlate of normal, adaptive, aggressive behaviour, it could be argued that all aggression is ictal; in any event, these observations beg the question of what is epilepsy, and make it almost impossible to claim with certainty that an otherwise inexplicable aggressive act did not have an epileptic basis.

There is, however, no evidence to support the proposition that EEG abnormalities in a person without epilepsy reflect an 'epileptic tendency' which can cause criminal behaviour when activated by alcohol. Unfortunately this claim has been established as a precedent in English case law (Regina v. Coster 1959) and persons without epilepsy charged with violent criminal acts (particularly under the influence of alcohol) are regularly referred for EEG investigation in the hope that some anomaly can be found and used as a basis for a plea of insanity or of diminished responsibility. The scope for constructing a dubious medical defence is widened by the existence of the rare syndrome of 'pathological intoxication'. Some individuals who display violent behaviour following consumption of small quantities of alcohol exhibit epileptiform activity when the EEG is activated with alcohol. The effect appears to be specific, and discharges are not elicited with other sedatives (as routinely used for diagnostic investigation of epilepsy) (Chesterman et al 1989). Unfortunately, there is no substantial literature concerning the effects of alcohol, in relevant dosage, on the incidence of epileptiform activity in persons with epilepsy, nor in normal controls. There is an increased incidence of sociopathy, criminality and cerebral disease, including epilepsy, amongst socially disadvantaged groups, and a raised incidence of epilepsy amongst convicted criminals (Gunn & Fenton 1971). There is, moreover, an association between criminality in general and aggressive crimes in particular, and non-epileptiform EEG anomalies (Williams 1969). However, no association exists between violence and epileptiform EEG disturbances (Driver et al 1974).

In summary, psychoses, behavioural disorders and social dysfunction in people with epilepsy are not only of practical importance but also of theoretical interest, and in this latter context EEG findings are highly relevant. However, diagnostic EEG investigation of a psychiatrically disturbed or socially malfunctioning person, with the intention of detecting previously unidentified epilepsy, is rarely useful and often indeed simply misleading. Schizophrenics receiving neuroleptics will often exhibit bitemporal sharp waves, which may either be misinterpreted as evidence of epilepsy or at least lead to a series of further fruitless investigations, including sleep records or repeat EEGs after withdrawal of medication. Aggressive criminals and psychopaths are often victims as well as instigators of violence, and may have suffered multiple head injuries in fights and road traffic accidents by the time they undergo EEG investigation. In the absence of known epilepsy, the clinical or forensic significance of minor EEG abnormalities under such circumstances is uncertain.

EEG and driving licences

Most societies refuse people with epilepsy the right to drive a motor vehicle; however, there is considerable variation in the regulations governing the restoration of a driving licence to a person who has become seizure-free. In some countries, such as the Netherlands, regular neurological follow-up of people who have regained their licence after remission of epilepsy is mandatory, and includes an EEG recording. The use to be made of the EEG information is not further specified. It would appear unreasonable to refuse anyone a driving licence on the basis of interictal EEG anomalies alone. It is, however, established that seemingly subclinical discharges may be accompanied by transitory cognitive impairment (TCI). EEG telemetry during prolonged driving of a suitably instrumented dual-control vehicle has indeed shown that such impairment may include a disruption of driving skills (Kasteleijn-Nolst Trenité et al 1987b). However, to give balance to the last statement, it should be mentioned that the degree of impairment found was equivalent to that produced in the same experimental setting by 10 mg of diazepam in naive subjects, and the drug-induced impairment was continuous whereas that due to TCI was present for only a few seconds in every hour. It would seem a reasonable policy to attempt to demonstrate by simultaneous video recording, and preferably psychological testing, whether or not subclinical EEG discharges are accompanied by demonstrable cognitive impairment and to withhold a driving licence only where this is the case.

MAGNETOENCEPHALOGRAPHY

The electrical activity of the brain produces weak magnetic fields, of the order of 10^{-13} Tesla. (The Tesla is a unit of magnetic field strength and is equal to the force exerted between two infinite parallel wires each carrying a current of 1 amp and separated by a distance of 1 m). The fields from the brain are very small compared with background noise (that of the Earth is about 5×10^{-5} T, and the typical urban magnetic noise, some 5×10^{-7} T$\sqrt{\text{Hz}}$), and recording them presents a technological challenge comparable to that of the EEG in the 1920s. The magnetoencephalogram (MEG) over the surface of the head is not attenuated and distorted by transmission through tissue, as is the EEG. Moreover, MEG is non-invasive and, if it proves capable of locating deep sources which cannot be detected by potential measurements without insertion of intracranial electrodes, this will represent a considerable advantage over EEG.

The activity of a neuronal aggregate produces a 'primary current' between the source and sink within the generator, and in the surrounding medium a 'volume current', producing both potential gradients and a magnetic field. Assuming that such a single, idealized dipole is present, the problem for both EEG and MEG is to locate it from the pattern of electrical potential or magnetic field at or outside the surface of the scalp.

The scalp EEG is produced entirely by volume current flow and its spatial pattern and frequency composition are modified by the low conductivity of the skull and the inhomogeneous impedance of the brain. By contrast, in a spherical conductor the radial magnetic field is determined solely by the primary current, the sum of the contributions of the volume currents being zero. This statement remains true even if the sphere is composed, as is the head, of layers with differing conductivities.

In an idealized homogeneous spherical head, an elemental current generator produces a simple magnetic field, which enters and leaves the head at two points or extrema (Fig. 9.18). The underlying generator lies at the bisector of the line joining the extrema, its direction is perpendicular to this line, and its depth linearly related to the distance between the extrema. The lack of distortion of the MEG offers at least the possibility of localizing cerebral electrical generators.

However, attempting to deduce the underlying current distribution, from either MEG or EEG, belongs to the wider class of 'inverse problems' (Sarvas 1987), which in general have no unique mathematical solution, and are insoluble except when there is known to be only one, spatially restricted generator. On the other hand, the constraints of anatomy and a priori knowledge, often enable the use of plausibility arguments to decide between mathematically equivalent descriptions of the data. EEG and MEG are complimentary,

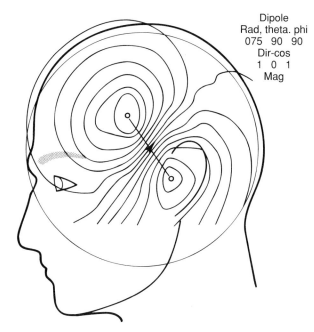

Dipole
Rad, theta. phi
075 90 90
Dir-cos
1   0   1
Mag

Fig. 9.18 A contour plot of the normal component of the external magnetic field produced by a model source (current dipole) embedded in a spherical head of radius 9 cm, at a depth of 1.5 cm beneath the arrow shown in the figure. The plot shows a maximum and a minimum separated by a distance which is linearly related to the depth of the source below the skull.

rather than alternative methods of investigation. Sources which are directed radially make a major contribution to the EEG, but produce no normal component of magnetic field and are silent in the MEG, which is preferentially sensitive to generators lying in the sulci, including much of the primary sensory projection areas. Combined EEG and MEG studies therefore offer a good possibility of localizing generators, in spite of the theoretical difficulties associated with the inverse problem.

MEG performs well in localizing focal epileptogenic generators in comparison with topographic EEG techniques, and invasive ECoG measurements (Barth et al 1982, 1984, Rose et al 1987, Ricci et al 1987). EEG and MEG recordings of the same interictal event often show totally different waveforms, with a variable temporal relationship (Rose et al 1987, Guy et al 1989), evidently reflecting different physiological processes or different, if related, generators. This last feature of variable time relationships appears to have

been overlooked by many investigators who have used EEG spikes as reference events, and taken the average of the associated MEG signals. Modena et al (1982) reported single channel MEG measurements in benign childhood epilepsy, in which the MEG revealed pathological signals absent from both interlictal and ictal EEG records.

Magnetic recording has been hailed as the ideal method of studying the electrophysiological activity of both superfical and deep structures in the brain, and particularly of investigating its topography in three dimensions. If it were to fulfil these expectations, the role of electrical potential recording would be greatly diminished. However, for the foreseeable future it appears more likely that, even when affordable solutions have been found to present technical problems, magnetic techniques will serve rather to complement present methods of potential recording.

THE USES AND LIMITATIONS OF ELECTROENCEPHALOGRAPHY IN EPILEPSY

Misconceptions

It should be apparent from this and previous chapters that EEG findings are fundamental to present concepts concerning both the nature of epilepsy and the classification of its various manifestations. This has led to expectations concerning the value of the EEG for clinical investigation of epilepsy which are either false or subject to important qualifications:

1. That the ictal EEG invariably exhibits epileptiform discharges and the absence of such phenomena during a seizure excludes an epileptic basis for the attack
2. That the interictal EEG can be used to establish or refute the diagnosis of epilepsy
3. That the degree of EEG abnormality, and especially the frequency of epileptiform discharge, closely reflects the severity of epilepsy, particularly the seizure frequency, and is reduced by effective antiepileptic medication
4. That the interictal EEG is predictive of prognosis in epilepsy and specifically that

patients with interictal discharges are less likely to become, or to remain, seizure-free than those with normal EEGs.

Non-fulfilment of these apparently reasonable expectations has led some authors to question the clinical value of electroencephalography in epilepsy, or indeed for any other purpose (Matthews 1964, Hopkins & Scambler 1977).

The negative ictal EEG

As indicated above, an epileptic seizure is by definition accompanied by a cerebral electrophysiological disturbance. With appropriately placed intracranial electrodes, this must always be detectable. Ictal changes in the scalp EEG are not necessarily present, however. Some seizure types, it would appear, are invariably associated with

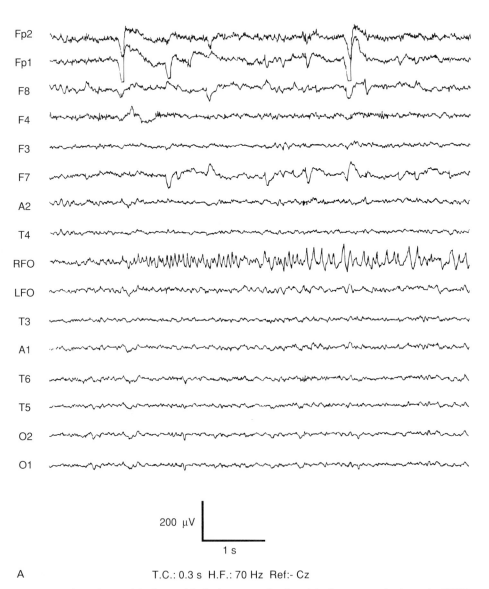

200 µV

1 s

A   T.C.: 0.3 s H.F.: 70 Hz Ref:- Cz

Fig. 9.19 Complex partial seizure with discharges confined to right foramen ovale electrode (RFO). (A), (B), and (C) from beginning, middle and end of seizure. Patient was inaccessible despite active attempts to attract his attention, stared and exhibited chewing movements.

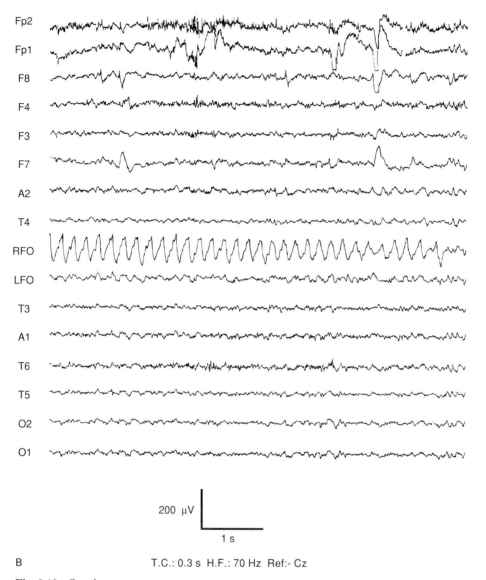

Fp2
Fp1
F8
F4
F3
F7
A2
T4
RFO
LFO
T3
A1
T6
T5
O2
O1

200 μV

1 s

B   T.C.: 0.3 s H.F.: 70 Hz Ref:- Cz

Fig. 9.19 Contd.

ictal EEG change: a convulsive attack without spikes in the EEG (assuming, of course, a technically acceptable tracing has been obtained) is not epileptic; nor probably is an episode of unconsciousness resembling an absence seizure, but without epileptiform EEG activity. Other seizure types sometimes produce ictal EEG changes and sometimes do not, notably simple partial seizures with motor symptomatology. Some kinds of seizures never or rarely produce ictal change in the scalp EEG, particularly simple partial seizures with psychic symptomatology or consisting only of viscerosensory hallucinosis. Complex partial seizures without evident EEG changes are rare but do occur (Fig. 9.19).

Further, it must be recognized that ictal EEG change does not necessarily consist of spikes or spike-and-wave complexes and subtle alterations may be undetectable in the presence of muscle and movement artifact, or if the technical specification of the recording system used is not adequate (see section on monitoring). An electro-

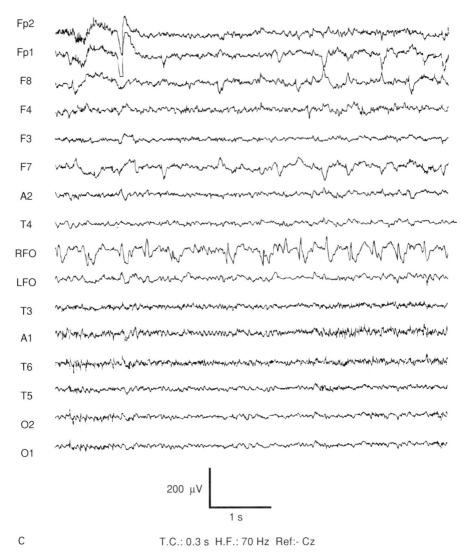

Fp2
Fp1
F8
F4
F3
F7
A2
T4
RFO
LFO
T3
A1
T6
T5
O2
O1

200 µV

1 s

C

T.C.: 0.3 s H.F.: 70 Hz Ref:- Cz

Fig. 9.19   Contd.

decremental event may readily be overlooked, especially when it accompanies an atonic seizure with artifact as the patient falls. If seen, it may be taken to be an effect of increased arousal, possibly accompanying a pseudoseizure. Particular difficulties are presented by the brief anterior slow wave discharge which may be the only EEG manifestation of some complex partial seizures of frontal origin. This activity is readily misinterpreted as oculographic artifact, or as a phenomenon due to awakening, if the seizure occurs from sleep, as is often the case. As the bizarre symptomatology of such attacks often leads to a

suspicion of pseudoseizures, there is a considerable risk of misdiagnosis based on a supposedly negative ictal EEG.

Proof and disproof of epilepsy

The request for an EEG 'to exclude epilepsy' may be only an abbreviated way for the referring physician to indicate his wishes for diagnostic assessment, but is commonplace in most laboratories, and often reflects a serious misconception. As indicated previously, a single interictal waking EEG will fail to detect epileptiform activity in

50% of people with epilepsy. It is difficult to justify, on economic or any other grounds, referring a patient with suspected epilepsy for a waking EEG and then declining the offer of a sleep recording if this first investigation is negative. Even if a full diagnostic series is performed as suggested earlier, almost 10% of patients will consistently fail to exhibit interictal epileptiform discharges. In this event, the only possibility of obtaining electrophysiological evidence in favour of, or against, the diagnosis of epilepsy is by an ictal recording, probably during monitoring.

The confusion concerning the incidence of epileptiform activity in persons without seizure disorders was noted earlier. Where there is a differential diagnosis between epilepsy and, for instance, syncope, or panic attacks (and assuming the patient is not already taking psychotropic drugs), the presence of interictal epileptiform discharges must greatly increase the statistical probability of epilepsy. By contrast, where there is already evidence of cerebral disease, for instance after severe head injury or in the presence of a cerebral tumour or mental subnormality, the presence of interictal epileptiform activity may contribute little to the clinical decision of whether or not a patient's attacks are epileptic.

If only to discourage misguided treatment of abnormal EEGs rather than patients, it must be clearly stated that epilepsy is a clinical diagnosis and that epileptiform EEG discharges without seizures do not constitute epilepsy. However, in interpreting this incontrovertible proposition, it must be also noted that clinical ictal manifestations include subtle cognitive changes which may not be recognized either by the patient or other observers without the help of video monitoring or possibly some form of psychological testing. The incidence and clinical importance of such unrecognized transitory cognitive impairment in patients with subclinical discharges is, at the present time, unknown.

Severity of epilepsy and effects of antiepileptic drugs (AEDs)

The reasonable assumption that the frequency of EEG discharges should relate to seizure incidence does hold good in the case of patients with ab-

sence seizures. In this particular instance, however, it could be argued that all the discharges are in fact ictal and that there is therefore inevitably a one-to-one relationship between generalized spike-wave activity and absences. Certainly it is the case that drugs effective in absence seizures dramatically reduce the incidence of generalized 3/s spike-wave activity and that patients who appear to have become seizure-free show a 95–100% reduction of their discharges. At the other extreme, in symptomatic generalized epilepsy there may be a complete dissociation between seizure frequency and EEG abnormality so that the record may be dominated by generalized discharges, even in a patient who appears to be seizure-free.

In routine epileptological EEG practice covering a wide spectrum of types of epilepsy, Binnie (1986) found a positive association between changes in discharge rate in serial EEGs and changes in seizure frequency (Table 9.6), but the association, although statistically significant, was extremely weak.

Gotman & Marciani (1985) found no clear relationship in more detailed serial EEG investigations and seizure frequency in patients with partial epilepsy. In general, the spiking rate did not change before seizures but increased, sometimes for several days, after them (Gotman & Marciani 1985). In a small series of patients with partial or symptomatic generalized epilepsy, studied with twice-weekly standardized EEGs over many months (Binnie 1983a), the subjects fell into two distinct groups: those who showed a strong, highly significant association between seizure frequency and spike counts, and others who showed no such relationship. There were no other apparent clinical differences between the groups. A tendency to a higher discharge rate following

Table 9.6 Weak association of change in discharge rate in 'routine' EEG with reported seizure frequency

Change in epileptiform activity	Reported change in seizure frequency	
	Increase	Decrease
Increase	75	84
No change	441	507
Decrease	40	97

seizures as reported by Gotman & Marciani (1985) was not found.

In EEGs obtained prior to a reduction of medication in patients on multiple drugs, Duncan et al (1989) found a dominant frequency below the alpha range to be predictive of increased seizure frequency, whereas the amount of epileptiform activity was not. Following drug reduction, an increase in bursts of epileptiform activity was seen in a majority of those patients who deteriorated, but rarely in those who did not.

Gram et al (1982) noted that the majority of controlled trials of AEDs included EEG studies, but that in over a half the findings were apparently of so little interest that the authors had not considered them worth analysing or reporting. Excluding studies of absence seizures, only a handful of controlled trials show that the preferred drug treatment was accompanied by a reduction in EEG discharges (Wilkus & Green 1974, Kellaway et al 1978, Binnie et al 1986b, Ben-Menachem & Treiman 1989). Carbamazepine in particular produces an increase in EEG abnormalities, notably disturbances in background activity. Van Wieringen et al (1987) comparing the findings of six AED trials, found that only one drug (Lamotrigine) produced both clinical improvement and reduction in EEG discharges. In one other case (an experimental benzodiazepine prodrug), the EEG findings could be considered relevant, in that withdrawal gave rise both to an exacerbation of seizures and to an increase in EEG abnormality.

Short-term fluctuation in levels of AEDs in patients with partial epilepsy on chronic therapy have little or no effect on the rate of EEG or depth discharges in telemetric records over 24–48 hours (Martins da Silva et al 1984, Gotman & Marciani 1985).

The failure to find a strong association between seizure frequency and drug effects on the one hand and EEG discharge rate on the other may arise from two sources: first, the statistical sampling problem created by the inherent variability of EEG discharge rate; and, secondly, a possible lack of the expected relationship between discharges and seizures. Spontaneous interictal discharges change systematically with waking and sleep and under the influence of various circadian, ultradian, or infradian biorhythms (Stevens et al

1971, Martins da Silva et al 1984, Binnie et al 1984b, Broughton et al 1985). They also fluctuate in association with uncontrolled and generally undocumented factors as attention, vigilance and cognitive activity (Guey et al 1969). Finally, there are many unexplained fluctuations which, for all practical purposes, must be regarded as random. A typical half-hour 'routine' waking EEG therefore generally represents a statistically unreliable sample of a changing process.

More reliable estimates of discharge rate may be obtained by recording for long periods, by telemetry or otherwise, or by short periods of registration under standardized conditions of vigilance, psychological tasks etc. Where these measures are adopted it may be possible to show a relationship between seizure frequency and discharge rate (Binnie 1983a) or drug effects (Milligan & Richens 1981, 1982, Milligan et al 1982, 1983, Binnie 1986). For purposes of quantitative studies of epileptiform activity in long-term recordings, Burr & Stefan (1987) have proposed a transformation which gives a more nearly Gaussian distribution of the data, and suggest methods of calculating confidence limits.

The theoretical basis of the presumed relationship of interictal discharge rate to seizure liability merits critical examination. The genesis of a clinical seizure involves a hierarchy of events, from the virtually continuous dysfunction of individual neurones, manifest, for instance, in paroxysmal depolarization shifts, through the intermittent synchronous discharges in neuronal populations giving rise to spikes which may be detected with depth or even scalp electrodes, to the occasional recruitment of larger, or specific, populations of neurones required for the clinical expression of a seizure. Rodin (1968) distinguishes 'seizure threshold', a liability to abnormal neuronal discharge, and 'seizure propensity', the tendency for such discharges to find clinical expression. These speculations are underpinned by some physiological evidence. At the core of an experimental epileptic focus are 'Group 1' neurones, which display continuous autonomous abnormal activity uninfluenced by afferent stimuli. Surrounding neurones ('Group 2') also have an abnormal tendency to fire in bursts, but remain under normal afferent control (Wyler et al, 1973, 1974). Recruitment of Group 2 neurones produces a partial seizure (Lockard 1981). Because Group 2 neurones are subject to normal afferent influences, their liability to recruitment (i.e. seizure propensity) depends on such various extrinsic factors as attention, wake and sleep, stress etc. An interictal discharge is, by definition, one which fails to give rise to a seizure. Thus a heightened seizure propensity should result in a smaller proportion of discharges being interictal, and hence a reduced interictal discharge rate.

An effective antiepileptic drug could work at the level of primary neuronal dysfunction, increasing seizure threshold and reducing both epileptiform discharges and seizures. Another agent might act rather at the level of ictal propagation, reducing seizure propensity and thus producing a dissociation between frequency of seizures and discharges. Further investigation of these relationships should provide valuable insights both into the physiology of epilepsy and into the different modes of action of various antiepileptic drugs.

The clinical interpretation of the interictal EEG in epilepsy, appears to be based on the assumption that ictal and interictal discharges represent essentially the same epileptogenic process. Yet apart from 3/s generalised spike-wave activity (which arguably is always ictal) the morphology of interictal epileptiform activity is generally different from that seen during seizures, particularly at the onset of the attack. Seizure onset is usually heralded by attenuation of continuing interictal discharges, possibly an electrodecremental event involving all activities, often a high frequency multi-unit discharge in depth recordings, and then the appearance in depth and on the scalp of regular activity 'rhythmic ictal transformation' (Geiger & Harner 1978). In a patient whose seizures are characterized by an electrodecremental event, rhythmic theta activity or high frequency multi-unit activity, it is perhaps naive to expect any close relationship of the attacks to interictal slow spike-wave complexes or sharp waves. Interictal discharges often resemble the phenomena seen in the later stages of a seizure and possibly are related to inhibitory mechanisms which limit or prevent seizures. Thus a case exists for regarding interictal spikes, not as abortive seizures, but rather as homeostatic phenomena related to seizure preven-

tion. Such an interpretation would explain many of the paradoxes of the EEG in epilepsy.

In addition to showing effects, or sometimes a singular lack of effect, on spontaneous epileptiform discharges, AEDs may also change background activity. The effects range from minimal or absent in the case of sodium valproate (Benninger et al 1985), to marked with carbamazepine, which produces a deterioration of background activity, typically an increase in the slower components. Most other antiepileptic drugs in routine use give an increase in beta and theta activity. The beta activity is most prominent and usually fairly fast (20/s and above) in the case of the barbiturates; whereas benzodiazepines produce a large amount of slower beta activity, often taking the form of a fast alpha variant. The appearance of a slowed EEG with an excess of fast activity in a drowsy patient with epilepsy will generally give rise to a suspicion of AED intoxication, provided the record is not postictal. Similarly, EEG investigation may make a useful contribution in patients with such symptoms as apathy, which could be due either to medication or to depression, and with levels of (usually several) antiepileptic drugs, which are in the upper 'therapeutic range', but not individually toxic. Here the finding of a slowed EEG with an excess of beta activity will suggest that a reduction of the dosage or of the number of drugs is desirable.

Prognosis

In studies based on severely handicapped or institutional populations, gross EEG abnormality is reported as indicating a poor prognosis for becoming seizure-free (Rodin 1968, Rowan et al 1980). However, background abnormalities are as important in this respect as epileptiform activity, and probably reflect the severity of the underlying cerebral pathology, which is itself the main determinant of prognosis in this group of patients. By contrast, two specific and strikingly abnormal EEG patterns, 3/s spike-wave activity with absence seizures and Rolandic spikes, both support the diagnosis of particular epilepsy syndromes which have a good prognosis for seizure control on medication and for terminal remission.

After a single non-febrile seizure, focal epileptiform discharge is reported to be predictive of recurrence in children, the recurrence rate being 68% with focal discharge against 22% without (Camfield et al 1985). This finding is surprising as the authors did not apparently exclude patients with Rolandic spikes from the analysis as a special category. In adults, by contrast, generalized spike-wave activity is associated with recurrence after a first seizure (Hauser et al 1982).

In patients who have remained seizure-free on medication for two years or more, the possibility arises of withdrawing antiepileptic drugs. However, a substantial proportion of patients, as high as 60% in some series, relapse when this is attempted. It is generally regarded as self-evident that the continued presence of epileptiform EEG activity or its recurrence when AEDs are reduced is predictive of relapse. Indeed, many investigators considering it ethically unacceptable to put this proposition to the test, have excluded from studies of AED termination any patients exhibiting epileptiform discharges, and have resumed medication if discharges reappeared during withdrawal (Zenker et al 1957, Juul-Jensen 1964, Van Heycop ten Ham 1980, Holowach et al 1972, Rodin & John 1980). The claim that epileptiform EEG activity is predictive of relapse on drug withdrawal has therefore become a self-fulfilling prophecy.

The few studies of the use of EEG in predicting outcome of AED withdrawal have confirmed that this is indeed the case in children (Emerson et al 1981, Todt 1981, 1984, Shinnar et al 1985, Le Pestre et al 1985, Matricardi et al 1989). Only three investigations appear to have addressed this question in adults (Overweg 1985, Overweg et al 1987, Wallis 1985, Chadwick, personal communication) and none found that the presence of epileptiform discharges was of value for predicting relapse. Overweg, indeed, found a significant positive association between the presence of sharp waves and continued remission. Chadwick did find a weak association between epileptiform activity and relapse on univariate analysis, but this effect was entirely attributable to the relationship of EEG findings to epilepsy syndromes with differing prognoses, and the EEG did not appear as a significant factor in a multivariate analysis including clinical variables.

These findings too can be explained by the concepts put forward in the previous section. Terminal remission may not necessarily indicate a disappearance of the original underlying neuronal dysfunction reflected in the presence of spikes and sharp waves, but rather a reduced seizure propensity, so that the patient's discharges are now self-limiting and no longer give rise to clinical manifestations. The decision whether or not to withdraw AEDs in a patient who is seizure-free is again clearly a matter which should be determined by clinical considerations, without misguided concern for the cosmetic appearance of the EEG.

APPLICATIONS OF THE EEG IN EPILEPSY

The previous section has described at length the limitations of electroencephalography in epilepsy, because the many useful applications of the EEG tend to be obscured by its conspicuous lack of utility, when misused. Where the clinical diagnosis of epilepsy is in doubt and the patient is not suffering from other obvious cerebral disease, the finding of interictal epileptiform activity, either in a single routine EEG or in the course of a full diagnostic series, must importantly reinforce that diagnosis. Negative findings will be of less diagnostic value, although a normal resting EEG and sleep with a normal response to adequate hyperventilation can exclude certain specific epilepsy syndromes. Where clinical assessment and interictal EEGs have not permitted a confident diagnosis, an ictal recording should be obtained, assuming that the attacks occur sufficiently frequently, so that there is a reasonable chance of capturing a seizure during an acceptable period of registration. Where necessary, medication, if already instituted, can be reduced in the hope of increasing the seizure frequency. Usually, the appropriate technology will be telemetric monitoring with simultaneous video registration. Ambulatory monitoring provides an alternative but its limitations for this application have been noted above. Ictal EEG change during a seizure proves its epileptic nature, provided a cardiac cause is excluded by simultaneous ECG registration. The interpretation of negative ictal EEG findings depends on the seizure pattern.

Establishing the diagnosis of epilepsy on clinical

grounds may be less difficult than determining the classification. Here both interictal and ictal EEGs make an important contribution. Where there is an inadequate history of episodes of impaired consciousness, the finding of generalized spike-and-wave activity on the one hand or of a focal abnormality on the other may be crucial to distinguishing idiopathic generalized epilepsy with absence seizures from partial epilepsy with complex partial seizures. In a patient with partial seizures where the possibility of surgical treatment is being considered, the finding of an EEG picture typical of symptomatic generalized epilepsy will cause this programme to be reconsidered. In the recognition of various epileptic syndromes, the role of the EEG ranges from supportive (as in the Lennox–Gastaut and West syndromes) to virtually diagnostic (benign childhood epilepsy, photosensitive epilepsy).

In following the progress of persons with epilepsy and in predicting prognosis, the role of the EEG is limited and often overvalued. In patients with frequent, brief seizures which are difficult to recognize, notably absences, both conventional recordings and ambulatory monitoring can be valuable for following progress. A follow-up EEG to assess progress is clearly of value in absence seizures which are, moreover, often reported unreliably by patients and relatives. In other forms of epilepsy it is of marginal clinical value, except possibly in postoperative assessment where a successful outcome is usually associated with marked EEG improvement (Falconer & Serafetinides 1963) and relapse is often heralded by the return of interictal discharges. 'Routine' EEG follow-up

may occasionally provide unexpected and relevant information, for instance, by detecting unrecognized minor seizures or identifying possible episodes of transitory cognitive impairment. However, an audit of follow-up EEGs which did not address any specific question suggested that only 3% produced information which influenced management (Binnie 1992).

In status epilepticus, particularly in refractory cases where the patient is anaesthetized and artificially ventilated, the EEG may provide the only means of monitoring response to treatment.

The surgery of epilepsy is a specialized field which concerns few clinicians and offers help to only a small proportion of people with epilepsy. Nevertheless, both for the preoperative assessment and during operation, detailed, complex electrophysiological assessment is indispensable.

CONCLUSION

As a functional disorder, epilepsy would appear an ideal application of electroencephalography. Certainly the use of the EEG in investigation of persons with epilepsy is illustrative of various general principles of electroencephalography. Perhaps the most important of these, which this chapter demonstrates, is that the recording of 'routine' EEGs for no clear indication is a misuse of resources which can better be applied to detailed and, if necessary prolonged, investigation of the specific problems of individuals, an activity which can prove valuable to patients and rewarding to the Clinical Neurophysiologist.

REFERENCES

Aarts J H P, Binnie C D, Smit A M, Wilkins A J 1984 Selective cognitive impairment during focal and generalised epileptiform EEG activity. Brain 107: 293–308

Aird R B, Masland R L, Woodbury D M 1989 Hypothesis: the classification of seizures according to systems of the CNS. Epilepsy Research 3: 77–81

Ajmone Marsan C, Abraham K 1960 A seizure atlas. Electroencephalography and Clinical Neurophysiology Suppl 15

Ajmone Marsan C, Zivin L S 1970 Factors related to the occurrence of typical paroxysmal abnormalities in the EEG records of epileptic patients. Epilepsia 11: 361–381

Ames F R 1971 'Self-induction' in photosensitive epilepsy. Brain 94: 781–798

Ames F R 1974 Cinefilm and EEG recording during 'handwaving' attacks of an epileptic, photosensitive child. Electroencephalography and Clinical Neurophysiology 37: 301–304

Ames F R, Enderstein O 1976 Clinical and EEG response to clonazepam in four patients with self-induced photosensitive epilepsy. South African Medical Journal 50: 1423

Andermann F 1971 Self-induced television epilepsy. Epilepsia 12: 269–275

Andermann F, Oguni H 1990 Do epileptic foci in children migrate? The cons. Electroencephalography and Clinical Neurophysiology 76: 96–99

Andermann K, Berman S, Cooke P M et al 1962 Self-induced epilepsy. A collection of self-induced epilepsy cases compared with some other photoconvulsive cases. Archives of Neurology 6: 49–65

Angelieri F 1974 Partial epilepsies and nocturnal sleep. In: Levin P, Koella W P (eds) Sleep. Karger, Basel, p 156–203

Angelieri F, Bergonzi P, Ferroni A 1967 Le fasi ed i cidi del sonno notturno negli epilettici. Rivista di Patalogia Nervosa e Mentale 88: 107–148

Babb T L, Crandall P H 1976 Epileptogenesis of human limbic neurons in psychomotor epileptics. Electroencephalography and Clinical Neurophysiology 40: 225–243

Baldy-Moulinier M 1982 Temporal lobe epilepsy and sleep organization. In: Sterman M B, Passouant P (eds) Sleep and epilepsy. Academic Press, New York, p 347–359

Bancaud J 1972 Mechanisms of cortical discharges in 'generalized' epilepsies in man. In: Petsche H, Brazier M A B (eds) Synchronisation of EEG activity in epilepsies. Springer Verlag, New York, p 368–380

Bancaud J, Talairach J, Waltregny A, Bresson M, Morel P 1968 L'activation par le mégimide dans le diagnostic topographique des épilepsies corticales focales (étude clinique et EEG et SEEG). Revue Neurologique (Paris) 119: 320–325

Bancaud J, Talairach J, Morel P et al 1974 'Generalised' epileptic seizures elicited by electrical stimulation of the frontal lobe in man. Electroencephalography and Clinical Neurophysiology 37: 275–282

Barth D S, Sutherling W, Broffman J 1982 Neuromagnetic localisation of epileptiform spike activity in the human brain. Science 218: 891–894

Barth D S, Sutherling W, Engel J 1984 Neuromagnetic evidence of spatially distributed sources underlying epileptiform spikes in the human brain. Science 223: 293–296

Batini C, Fressy J, Naquet R, Orfanos A, Saint-Laurent J 1963 Etude du sommeil nocturne chez 20 sujets présentant des décharges imitatives focalisées. Revue Neurologique (Paris) 108: 172–173

Bengzon A R A, Rasmussen T, Gloor P, Dussault J, Stephens M 1968 Prognostic factors in the surgical treatment of temporal lobe epileptics. Neurology 18: 717–731

Ben-Menachem E, Treiman D M 1989 Effect of gamma-vinyl GABA on interictal spikes and sharp waves in patients with intractable complex partial seizures. Epilepsia 30: 79–83

Bennett F E 1953 Intracarotid and intravertebral Metrazol in petit mal epilepsy. Neurology 3: 668–673

Bennett D R 1962 Sleep deprivation and major motor convulsions. Neurology 13: 953–958

Bennett D R, Ziter F A, Liske E A 1969 Electroencephalographic study of sleep deprivation in flying personnel. Neurology 19: 375–377

Benninger C, Matthis P, Scheffner D 1985 Spectral analysis of the EEG in children during the introduction of antiepileptic therapy with valproic acid. Neuropsychobiology 13: 93–96

Besset A 1982 Influence of generalized seizures on sleep organisation. In: Sterman M B, Shouse M N, Passouant P (eds) Sleep and epilepsy. Academic Press, New York, p 339–346

Berkovic S F, Andermann F, Andermann E, Gloor P 1987 Concepts of absence epilepsies: discrete syndromes or biological continuum? Neurology (NY) 37: 993–1000

Bickford R G, Klass D W 1962 Stimulus factors in the mechanism of television-induced seizures. Transactions of the American Neurological Association 87: 176–178

Bickford R C, Klass D W 1969 Sensory precipitation and reflex mechanisms. In: Jasper H H, Ward A A, Pope A (eds) Basic mechanisms of the epilepsies. Little Brown, Boston p 543–564

Bickford R G, Sem-Jacobsen C W, White P T, Daly D 1952 Some observations on the mechanism of photic and photometrazol activation. Electroencephalography and Clinical Neurophysiology 4: 275–282

Bickford R G, Daly D, Keith H M 1953 Convulsive effects of light stimulation in children. American Journal of Diseases in Children 86: 170–183

Billiard M 1982 Epilepsies and the sleep-wake cycle. In: Sterman M B, Shouse M N, Passouant P (eds) Sleep and epilepsy. Academic Press, New York, p 269–286

Binnie C D 1980 Detection of transitory cognitive impairment during epileptiform EEC discharges: problems in clinical practice. In: Kulig B M, Meinardi H, Stores G (eds) Epilepsy and behavior 1979. Swets and Zeitlinger, Lisse, p 91–97

Binnie C D 1983a EEG and blood levels of antiepileptic drugs. In: Buser P, Cobb W A, Okuma T (eds) Proceedings 10th International Congress of Electroencephalography and Clinical Neurophysiology, Kyoto. Electroencephalography and Clinical Neurophysiology 36 (suppl): 504–512

Binnie C D 1983b Telemetric EEG monitoring in epilepsy. In: Pedley T A, Meldrum B S (eds) Recent advances in epilepsy 1. Churchill Livingstone, Edinburgh, p 155–178

Binnie C D 1986 The interictal EEG. In: Trimble M R, Reynolds E H (eds) What is epilepsy? Churchill Livingstone, Edinburgh, p 6–125

Binnie C D 1987 Ambulatory diagnostic monitoring of seizures in the adult. In: Gumnit R J (ed) Advances in neurology: International Conference on Neurodiagnostic Monitoring. Raven Press, New York, p 99–107

Binnie C D 1990 Long-term monitoring. In Dam M, Gram L (eds) Comprehensive Epileptology. Raven Press, New York, p 339–349

Binnie C D 1992 EEG audit: increasing cost-efficiency of EEG investigations in epilepsy. Electroencephalography and Clinical Neurophysiology, in press

Binnie C D, Van der Wens P 1986 Diagnostic re-evaluation by intensive monitoring of intractible absence seizures. In: Schmidt D, Morselli P (eds) Intractable epilepsy: experimental and clinical aspects. Raven Press, New York, 99–107

Binnie C D, Coles P A, Margerison J H 1969 The influence of end-tidal carbon dioxide tension on EEG changes during routine hyperventilation in different age groups. Electroencephalography and Clinical Neurophysiology 27: 304–306

Binnie C D, Batchelor B G, Bowring P A et al 1978 Computer-assisted interpretation of clinical EEGs. Electroencephalograpy and Clinical Neurophysiology 44: 575–585

Binnie C D, De Korte J W A, Meijer A J, Rowan A J, Warfield C 1980a Acute effects of sodium valproate on the photoconvulsive response in man. Journal of the Royal Society of Medicine International Congress Series 30: 103–113

Binnie C D, Darby C E, De Korte R A, Veldhuizen R, Wilkins A J 1980b EEG sensitivity to television: effects of ambient lighting. Electroencephalography and Clinical Neurophysiology 50: 329–331

Binnie C D, Darby C E, De Korte R A, Wilkins A J 1980c Self-induction of epileptic seizures by eyeclosure: incidence and recognition. Journal of Neurology, Neurosurgery and Psychiatry 43: 386–389

Binnie C D, Rowan A J, Overweg J et al 1981 Telemetric EEG and video monitoring in epilepsy. Neurology 31: 298–303

Binnie C D, Rowan A J, Gutter T 1982 A Manual of EEG technology. Cambridge University Press, Cambridge

Binnie C D, Estevez O, Kasteleijn-Nolst Trenité D G A, Peters A 1984a Colour and photosensitive epilepsy. Electroencephalography and Clinical Neurophysiology 58: 387–391

Binnie C D, Aarts J H P, Houtkooper M A et al 1984b Temporal characteristics of seizures and epileptiform discharges. Electroencephalography and Clinical Neurophysiology 58: 498–505

Binnie C D, Findlay J, Wilkins A J 1985a Mechanisms of epileptogenesis in photosensitive epilepsy implied by the effects of moving patterns. Electroencephalography and Clinical Neurophysiology 61: 1–6

Binnie C D, Kasteleijn-Nolst Trenité D G A, De Korte R, Wilkins A 1985b Visual display units and risk of seizures. Lancet 1: 1991

Binnie C D, van Emde Boas W, Wauquier A 1985c Geniculate spikes during epileptic seizures induced in dogs by pentylenetetrazol and bicuculline. Electroencephalography and Clinical Neurophysiology 61: 40–49

Binnie C D, Kasteleijn-Nolst Trenité D G A, De Korte R 1986a Photosensitivity as a model for acute antiepileptic drug studies. Electroencephalography and Clinical Neurophysiology 63: 35–41

Binnie C D, Van Emde Boas W, Kasteleijn-Nolst Trenité D G A et al 1986b Acute effects of lamotrigine (BW430C) in persons with epilepsy. Epilepsia 27: 248–254

Binnie C D, Marston D, Polkey C E, Amin D 1989a Distribution of temporal spikes in relation to the sphenoidal electrode. Electroencephalography and Clinical Neurophysiology 73: 403–409

Binnie C D, Polkey C E, Spencer S 1989b Positive spikes over a cortical laceration. Electroencephalography and Clinical Neurophysiology 72: 106P

Binnie C D, Polkey C E, Volans A 1990 Consistency of lateralisation in intracranial recordings of seizures of temporal lobe origin. Acta Neurologica Scandinavica 133 (Suppl): 20

Blume W T 1990 Do epileptic foci in children migrate? The cons. Electroencephalography and Clinical Neurophysiology 76: 100–105

Bordas-Ferrer M, Talairach J, Bancaud J 1966 Incidence des accès sur l'organisation du sommeil de nuit des épileptiques. Revue Neurologique 115: 556–561

Bowden A N, Fitch P, Gilliat R W, Willison R G 1975 The place of EEG telemetry and close-circuit television in the diagnosis and management of epileptic patients. Proceedings of the Royal Society of Medicine 68: 246–248

Braham J 1967 An unsuccessful attempt at the extinction of photogenic epilepsy. Electroencephalography and Clinical Neurophysiology 23: 558P

Brausch C C, Ferguson J H 1965 Color as factor in light sensitive epilepsy. Neurology 15: 154–164

Breakell C C, Parker C S, Christopherson F 1949 Radio transmission of the human electroencephalogram and other electrophysiological data. Electroencephalography and Clinical Neurophysiology 1: 243–144

Bridgers S L 1987 Epileptiform abnormalities discovered on electroencephalographic screening of psychiatric patients. Archives of Neurology 44: 312–316

Bridgers S, Ebersole J S, Purdy P 1987 Supervision of ambulatory cassette EEG screening: a strategy based on the temporal distribution of epileptiform abnormalities. Electroencephalography and Clinical Neurophysiology 66: 219–224

Broughton R, Stampi C, Romano S, Cirignolta F, Barizzi A, Lugarci E 1985 Do waking ultradian rhythms exist for petit mal absences? A case report. In: Martins da Silva A, Binnie C D, Meinardi H (eds) Biorhythms and epilepsy. New York, Raven Press, p 95–105

Browne T R, Penry J K, Porter R J, Dreifuss F E 1974a A comparison of clinical estimates of absence seizure frequency with estimates based on prolonged telemetered EEGs. Neurology 24: 381–382

Browne T R, Penry J K, Porter R J, Dreifuss F E 1974b Responsiveness before, during and after spike-wave paroxysms. Neurology 24: 659–665

Bruens J H, Knijff W 1980 Ambulatory EEG monitoring with a 24 hour cassette recorder in epileptic patients. In: Epilepsy: a clinical and experimental research. Monographs in Neural Science 5: 295–297

Burr W, Stefan H 1987 Day by day variations of the amount of spike-wave activity in 24 hour cassette recordings. Electroencephalography and Clinical Neurophysiology 67: 40–41.

Camfield P R, Camfield C S, Dooley J M, Tibbles J A R, Fung T, Garner B 1985 Epilepsy after a first unprovoked seizure in childhood. Neurology 35: 1657–1660

Capron E 1966 Etude de divers types de sensibilité électroencéphalographique à la stimulation lumineuse intermittente et leur signification. Thesis, Foulon, Paris

Carterette E C, Symmes D 1952 Color as an experimental variant in photic stimulation. Electroencephalography and Clinical Neurophysiology 4: 289–296

Charcot J M 1887 Leçons sur les maladies du système nerveux tome III. Delahaye & Lecrosnier, Paris

Charlton M H, Hoefer P F 1964 Television and epilepsy? Archives of Neurology 2: 239–247

Chatrian G E, Lettich E, Miller L H, Green J R 1970a Pattern-sensitive epilepsy, part 1. An electrographic study of its mechanisms. Epilepsia 11: 125–149

Chatrian G E, Lettich E, Miller L H, Green J R, Kupfer C 1970b Pattern-sensitive epilepsy, part 2. Clinical changes, tests of responsiveness and motor output, alterations of evoked potentials and therapeutic measures. Epilepsia 11: 151

Chatrian G E, Bergamini L, Dondey M, Klass D W, Lennox-Buchthal M, Pettersen I 1974 A glossary of terms most commonly used by clinical electroencephalographers. Electroencephalograpy and Clinical Neurophysiology 37: 538–548

Chemburkar J, Desai A D, Pabini R 1976 The sleeping pattern and incidence of seizure discharges during whole night sleep in grand mal epileptics. Neurology India 24: 141–147

Christodoulou G 1967 Sphenoidal electrodes. Acta Neurologica Scandinavica 43: 587–593

Chesterman P, Binnie C D, Fenwick P B C 1989 Can drink kill? Two cases of pathological intoxication.

Electroencephalography and Clinical Neurophysiology 73: 65

Clemens B, Oláh R 1987 Sleep studies in benign epilepsy of childhood with Rolandic spikes: I sleep pathology. Epilepsia 28: 20–23

Commission on Classification and Terminology of the International League Against Epilepsy 1985 Proposal for classification of epilepsies and epileptic syndromes. Epilepsia 26: 268–278

Commission on Classification and Terminology of the International League Against Epilepsy 1989 Proposal for revised classification of epilepsies and epileptic syndromes. Epilepsia 30: 389–399

Connell B, Jolley D J, Lockwood P, Mercer S 1975 Activation of photosensitive epileptics whilst watching television: observations on line frequency, colour and picture content. Journal of Electrophysiological Technology 1: 281–287

Cooper R, Winter A L, Crow H J et al 1965 Comparison of subcortical, cortical and scalp activity using chronically indwelling electrodes in man. Electroencephalography and Clinical Neurophysiology 18: 217–228

Creutzfeldt O D, Watanabe S, Lux H D 1966 Relations between EEC phenomena and potentials of single cortical cells. II. Spontaneous and convulsoid activity. Electroencephalography and Clinical Neurophysiology 20: 19–37

Danesi M A 1985 Geographical and seasonal variations in the incidence of epileptic photosensitivity. Electroencephalography and Clinical Neurophysiology 61: S216

Danesi M A, Oni K 1983 Photosensitive epilepsy and photoconvulsive responses to photic stimulation in Africans. Epilepsia 24: 455–458

Darby C E, Wilkins A J, Binnie C D, De Korte R A 1980a Routine testing for pattern sensitivity. Journal of Electrophysiological Technology 6: 202–210

Darby C E, De Korte R A, Binnie C D, Wilkins A J 1980b The self-induction of epileptic seizures by eye closure. Epilepsia 21: 31–42

Daskalov D S 1975 Influence of the stages of nocturnal sleep on the activity of a temporal epileptogenic focus. Soviet Neurology and Psychiatry 8: 37–45

De Graaf A S, Van Wyk Kotze T J, Claassen D A 1980 Photoparoxysmal responses in the electroencephalograms of some ethnic groups of the Cape Peninsula. Electroencephalography and Clinical Neurophysiology 50: 275–281

Delange M, Castan Ph, Cadilhac J, Passouant P 1962 Study of night sleep during centrencephalic and temporal epilepsies. Electroencephalography and Clinical Neurophysiology 14: 777

Delgado-Escueta A V 1979 Epileptogenic paroxysms: modern approaches and clinical correlations. Neurology 29: 1014–1022

Delgado-Escueta A V, Mattson R H, King L et al 1981 The nature of aggression during epileptic seizures. New England Journal of Medicine 305: 711–716

Dement W, Kleitmann N 1957 Cyclic variations in EEG during sleep and their relation to eye movements, body mobility and dreaming. Electroencephalography and Clinical Neurophysiology 9: 673–690

Derouesne C, Golmard J L, Bilbeau H, Asselain B, Salamon 1979 Evaluation of the usual supplementary tests in neurological diagnosis. In: Alperovitch A, De Dombal F T,

Gremy F (eds) Evaluation of efficacy of medical action. North Holland, Amsterdam, p179–183

Dimitrakoudi M, Harding G F A, Jeavons P M 1973 The inter-relation of the P2 component of the V.E.R. with occipital spikes produced by patterned intermittent photic stimulation. Electroencephalography and Clinical Neurophysiology 35: 416

Dondey M 1983 Transverse topographical analysis of petit mal discharges: diagnostical and pathogenic implications. Electroencephalography and Clinical Neurophysiology 55: 361–371

Doose H, Gerken H 1973 On the genetics of EEC-anomalies in childhood. IV. Photoconvulsive reaction. Neuropaediatrie 4: 162–171

Doose H, Gerken H, Hein-Volpel K F, Volzke E 1969 Genetics of photosensitive epilepsy. Neuropadiatrie 1: 56–73

Dreifuss F E (Chairman Commission on Classification and Terminology of the International League Against Epilepsy) 1981 Proposal for revised clinical and electroencephalographic classification of epileptic seizures. Epilepsia 22: 489–501

Dreifuss F E, Penry J K, Rose S W et al 1975 Serum clonazepam concentrations in children with absence seizures. Neurology 25: 255–258

Dreyer R, Wehmeyer W 1978 Laughing in complex partial seizure epilepsy: a video tape analysis of 32 patients with laughing as symptom of an attack. Fortschritte der Neurologie, Psychiatrie und ihre Grenzgebiete 46: 61–75

Driver M V, West L R, Faulk M 1974 Clinical and EEG studies of prisoners charged with murder. British Journal of Psychiatry 125: 583–587

Dumermuth G 1961 Photosensible Epilepsie und Television. Schweizerische Medizinische Wochenschrift 91: S1633–S1636

Duncan J S, Smith S J, Forster A, Shorvon S D, Trimble M R 1989 Effects of removal of phenytoin, carbamazepine, and valproate on the electroencephalogram. Epilepsia 30: 590–596

Ebersole J S 1987 Telemetered and ambulatory cassette: Review of current systems and techniques. In: Gumnit R J (ed) International conference on intensive neurodiagnostic monitoring. Raven Press, New York, p 139–155

Egli M, Mothersill I, O'Kane M, O'Kane F 1985 The axial spasm—the predominant type of drop seizure in patients with secondary generalized epilepsy. Epilepsia 26: 401–415

Emerson R, D'Souza B J, Vining E P, Holden K R, Mellits E D, Freeman J M 1981 Stopping medication in children with epilepsy: predictors of outcome. New England Journal of Medicine 304: 1125–1129

Engel J 1974 Selective photoconvulsive responses to intermittent diffuse and patterned photic stimulation. Electroencephalography and Clinical Neurophysiology 37: 283–292

Engel 1989 Seizures and epilepsy. Davis, Philadelphia

Engel J, Driver M V, Falconer M A 1975 Electrophysiological correlates of pathology and surgical results in temporal lobe epilepsy. Brain 98: 129–156

Epstein A W, Hill W 1966 Ictal phenomena during REM sleep of a temporal lobe epileptic. Archives of Neurology 15: 367–375

Falconer M, Kennedy W A 1961 Epilepsy due to small focal temporal lesions with bilateral spike discharging foci: a study of seven cases relieved by operation. Journal of Neurology, Neurosurgery and Psychiatry 24: 205–212

Falconer M A, Serafetinides E A 1963 A follow-up study of surgery in temporal lobe epilepsy. Journal of Neurology, Neurosurgery and Psychiatry 26: 154–165

Fisher R S, Prince D A 1977 Spike-wave rhythms in cat cortex induced by parenteral penicillin. l. Electrographic features. Electroencephalography and Clinical Neurophysiology 47: 592–596

Flor-Henry P 1969 Psychosis and temporal lobe epilepsy. Epilepsia 10: 363–395

Flor-Henry P 1972 Ictal and interictal psychiatric manifestations of epilepsy. Specific or non-specific? Epilepsia 13: 773–783

Flor-Henry P 1976 Epilepsy and psychopathology. In: Granville-Grossman (ed) Recent advances in clinical psychiatry. Churchill Livingstone, Edinburgh

Forster F M 1977 Reflex epilepsy; behavioural therapy and conditional reflexes. Thomas, Springfield

Forster F M, Ptacek L J, Peterson W G, Chun R W M, Bengzon A R A, Campos G B 1964 Stroboscopic induced seizure discharges. Modification by extinction techniques. Archives of Neurology 11: 603–608

Frantzen E, Lennox-Buchthal M, Nygaard A 1968 A longitudinal EEG and clinical study of children with febrile convulsions. Electroencephalography and Clinical Neurophysiology 24: 197–212

Frantzen E, Lennox-Buchthal M, Nygaard A, Stene J 1970 A genetic study of febrile convulsions. Neurology 20: 909–917

Gale K 1985 Mechanisms of seizure control mediated gamma-aminobutyric acid: role of the substantia nigra. Federal Proceedings 44: 2414–2424

Gastaut H 1950 Combined photic and metrazol activation of the brain. Electroencephalography and Clinical Neurophysiology 2: 249–261

Gastaut H 1982 A new type of epilepsy: benign partial epilepsy of childhood with occipital spike-waves. In: Akimoto H, Kazamatsuri H, Seino M, Ward A (eds) Advances in epileptology (XIIIth International Symposium). Raven Press, New York, p 19–24

Gastaut H, Tassinari C A 1966 Triggering mechanisms in epilepsy. The electroclinical point of view. Epilepsia 7: 85–138

Gastaut H, Regis H, Bostem F, Beaussart M 1960a Etude electroencephalographique de 35 sujets ayant présenté des crises au cours d'un spectacle télévisé. Revue Neurologique 102: 533–534

Gastaut H, Poirier F, Payan H, Salamon G, Toga M, Vigouroux M H 1960b H E Syndrome: Hemiconvulsions, hemiplegia epilepsy. Epilepsia 1: 418–447

Gastaut H, Batini C, Fressy J, Broughton R, Tassinari C A, Vitini F 1965 Etude électroencéphalographique des phénomènes épisodiques au cours du sommeil. In: Fishgold H (ed) Sommeil de nuit normal et pathologique. Masson, Paris, p 239–254

Geiger L R, Harner R N 1978 EEG patterns at the time of focal seizure onset. Archives of Neurology 35: 276–286

Geller M R, Geller A 1970 Brief amnestic effects of spikewave discharges. Neurology 20: 380–381

Gibbs F A, Gibbs E L 1953 Atlas of Electroencephalography vol 2: Epilepsy. Addison-Wesley, Cambridge, Mass

Gibbs F A Lennox, W G, Gibbs E L 1936 The electroencephalogram in diagnosis and in localization of epileptic seizures. Archives of Neurology and Psychiatry 36: 1225–1235

Gibbs F A, Gibbs E L, Lennox W G 1937 Epilepsy: a paroxysmal cerebral dysrhyrhmia. Brain 60: 377–388

Gibbs E L, Gillen H W, Gibbs F A 1954 Disappearance and migration of epileptic foci in children. American Journal of Diseases of Childhood 88: 596–603

Gloor P 1968 Generalized corticoreticular epilepsies. Some considerations on the pathophysiology of generalized bilaterally synchronous spike and wave discharge. Epilepsia 9: 249–263

Gloor P 1972 Generalized spike and wave discharge: a consideration of cortical and subcortical mechanisms of their genesis and synchronization. In: Petsche H, Brazier M A B (eds) Synchronization of EEG activity in epilepsies. Springer Verlag, New York, p 382–406

Gloor P 1975 Contributions of electroencephalography and electrocorticography to the neurosurgical treatment of the epilepsies. In: Purpura D P, Penry J K, Walter R D (eds) Advances in neurology, vol 8. Raven Press, New York, p 59–105

Gloor P, Tsai C, Haddad F, Jasper H H 1957 The lack of necessity for sleep in the EEG or ECG diagnosis of temporal seizures. Electroencephalography and Clinical Neurophysiology 9: 379–380

Gloor P, Quesney L F, Zumstein H 1977 Pathophysiology of generalized penicillin epilepsy in the cat: The role of cortical and subcortical structures. II. Topical application of penicillin to the cerebral cortex and to subcortical structures. Electroencephalography and Clinical Neurophysiology 43: 79–94

Gloor P, Pellegrini A, Kostopoulos G K 1979 Effects of changes in cortical excitability upon the epileptic bursts in generalized penicillin epilepsy in the cat. Electroencephalography and Clinical Neurophysiology 46: 274–289

Goldensohn E S 1984 The relevance of secondary epileptogenesis to the treatment of epilepsy: kindling and mirror focus. Epilepsia 25(suppl 2): S156–S168

Goodridge D M C, Shorvon S D 1983 Epileptic seizures in a population of 6000: I. Demography, diagnosis and classification, and role of the hospital services. British Medical Journal 287: 641–647

Gotman J 1981 Automatic recognition of epileptic seizures in the EEG. Electroencephalography and Clinical Neurophysiology 54: 530–540

Gotman J 1982 A computer system to assist in the evaluation of the EEGs of epileptic patients. Behavioural Research Methods 13: 525–531

Gotman J 1990 Automatic seizure detection: improvements and evaluation. Electroencephalography and Clinical Neurophysiology 76: 317–324

Gotman J, Marciani M C 1985 Electroencephalographic spiking activity, drug levels and seizure occurrence in epileptic patients. Annals of Neurology 17: 597–603

Gotman J, Ives J R, Gloor P 1979 Automatic recognition of interictal epileptic activity in prolonged EEG recordings. Electroencephalography and Clinical Neurophysiology 46: 510–520

Gotman J, Gloor P, Quesney L F, Olivier A 1982 Correlations between EEG changes induced by diazepam and the localization of epileptic spikes and seizures. Electroencephalography and Clinical Neurophysiology 54: 614–621

Gotman J, Ives J R, Gloor P 1985 Long-term monitoring in epilepsy. Electroencephalography and Clinical Neurophysiology Suppl 37

Gram L, Drachmann Bentsen K, Parnas J, Flachs H 1982

Controlled trials in epilepsy: a review. Epilepsia 23: 491–519

Green J B 1966 Self-induced seizures: clinical and electroencephalographic studies. Archives of Neurology 15: 579–586

Gross M 1983 Pseudoepilepsy. Heath, Lexington, Mass

Gudmundsson G 1966 Epilepsy in Iceland: a clinical and epidemiological investigation. Acta Neurologica Scandinavica 25 (Suppl): 4–124

Guerrero-Figueroa R, Barros A, de Balbian Verster F, Heath R G 1963 Experimental 'Petit Mal' in kittens. Archives of Neurology 9: 297–306

Guey J, Bureau M, Dravet C, Roger J 1969 A study of the rhythm of petit mal absences in children in relation to prevailing situations: the use of EEG telemetry during psychological examinations, school exercises and periods of inactivity. Epilepsia 10: 441–451

Gunn J C, Fenton G W 1971 Epilepsy, automatism and crime. Lancet 1: 1173–1176

Gutrecht J A 1989 Clinical implications of benign epileptiform transients of sleep. Electroencephalography and Clinical Neurophysiology 72: 486–490

Guy C N, Binnie C D, Cayllesi A et al 1989 Preliminary results of simultaneous MEG, EEG and foramen ovale recordings in epileptic patients. Abstracts 7th International Conference on Biomagnetism, New York

Halasz P 1982 Generalized epilepsy with spike-wave pattern (GESW) and intermediate states of sleep. In: Sterman M B, Shouse M N, Passouant P (eds) Sleep and epilepsy. Academic Press, New York, p 219–239

Halasz P, Devenyi E 1974 Petit mal absences in night sleep with special reference to transitional sleep and REM periods. Acta Medica Academiae Scientiarum Hungariae 31: 31–45

Harding G F A, Pearce K, Dimitrakoudi M, Jeavons P M 1975 The effect of coloured intermittent photic stimulation (IPS) on the photoconvulsive response (PCR). Electroencephalography and Clinical Neurophysiology 39: 428

Harding G F A, Herrick C E, Jeavons P M 1978 A controlled study of the effect of sodium valproate on photosensitive epilepsy and its prognosis. Epilepsia 19: 555–565

Harley R D, Baird H W, Freeman R D 1967 Self-induced photogenic epilepsy. Report of four cases. Archives of Ophthalmology 78: 730

Harris R 1972 EEG aspects of unclassifed mental retardation in the brain. In: Cavanagh J B (ed) Unclassified mental retardation Churchill Livingstone, Edinburgh

Harrison-Covello A, De Barros-Ferreira M 1975 Techniques et premiers résultats de l'enregistrement en telemetrie d'enfants présentant des éléments paroxystiques (1). Revue d'Electroencéphalographie et Neurophysiologie Clinique 5: 427–438

Hauser W A, Kurland L T 1975 The epidemiology of epilepsy in Rochester, Minnesota, 1935 through 1967. Epilepsia 16: 1–66

Hauser W A, Anderson E, Loewenson R B, McRoberts S M 1982 Seizure recurrence after a first unprovoked seizure. New England Journal of Medicine 307: 522–528

Heath R G 1954 Studies in schizophrenia. Harvard University Press, Cambridge, Mass

Heath R G 1972 Pleasure and brain activity in man: deep and surface electroencephalograms during orgasm. Journal of Nervous and Mental Disease 154: 3–18

Heath R G 1975 Brain function and behaviour: emotion and sensory phenomena in psychotic patients and in experimental animals. Journal of Nervous and Mental Disease 160: 159–175

Heath R G, Mickle W A 1960 Evaluation of seven years experience with depth electrode studies in human patients. In: Ramey E R, O'Doherty D S (eds) Electrical studies on the unanaesthetized brain. Hoeber, New York, p 214–247

Hendricksen O 1986 Absence seizures: multiple and reduction of multiple drug therapy In: Schmidt D, Morselli P (eds) Intractable epilepsy: experimental and clinical aspects. Raven Press, New York, p187–193

Heppenstall M E 1944 The relation between the effects of blood-sugar levels and hyperventilation on the electroencephalogram. Journal of Neurology, Neurosurgery and Psychiatry 7: 112–118

Hogan T, Sundaram M 1989 Rhythmic auditory stimulation in generalized epilepsy. Electroencephalography and Clinical Neurophysiology 72: 455–458

Holmes G L 1982 Prolonged EEG and videotape monitoring in children. American Journal of Diseases of Children 136: 608–611

Holowach J, Thurston D L, O'Leary J 1972 Prognosis in childhood epilepsy: follow-up study of 148 cases in which therapy had been suspended after prolonged anticonvulsant control. New England Journal of Medicine 286: 169–174

Homan R W, Jones M C, Rawat S 1988 Anterior temporal electrodes in complex partial seizures. Electroencephalography and Clinical Neurophysiology 70: 105–109

Hopkins A, Scambler G 1977 How doctors deal with epilepsy. Lancet 1: 183–186

Huck F R, Radvany J, Avila J O et al 1980 Anterior callosotomy in epileptics with multiform seizures and bilateral synchronous spike and wave EEG pattern. Acta Neurochirurgica 30 (Suppl): 127–135

Hughes J R 1985 Long-term clinical and EEG changes in patients with epilepsy. Archives of Neurology 42: 213–223

Hughes J R, Cayaffa J J 1973 Is the 'psychomotor variant' 'rhythmic mid-temporal discharge' an ictal pattern? Clinical Electroencephalography 4: 42–49

Hughes J R, Grunener G 1984 Small sharp spikes revisited: further data on this controversial pattern. Clinical Electroencephalography 15: 208–213

Hunter J, Jasper H H 1949a Effects of thalamic stimulation in unanesthetized animals. Electroencephalography and Clinical Neurophysiology 1: 437–445

Hunter J, Jasper H H 1949b A method of analysis of seizure patterns. Electroencephalography and Clinical Neurophysiology 1: 113–114

Hutchinson J H, Stone F H, Davidson J R 1958 Photogenic epilepsy induced by the patient. Lancet 1: 243–245

Hutt S J, Gilbert S 1980 Effects of evoked spike-wave discharges upon short-term memory in patients with epilepsy. Cortex 16: 445–457

Hutt S J, Denner S, Newton J 1976 Auditory thresholds during evoked spike-wave activity in epileptic patients. Cortex 12: 249–257

Ishihara T and Yoshii N 1967 The interaction between paroxysmal EEG activities and continuous addition work of Uchida-Kraeplin psychodiagnostic test. Medical Journal of Osaka University 18: 75–78

Ives J R 1982a A completely ambulatory 16-channel cassette recording system. In: Stefan H, Burr W (eds) Mobile long-term EEG monitoring (Proceedings of the MLE Symposium, Bonn, 1982). Fischer, Stuttgart, p 205–217

Ives J R 1982b Long-term EEG cassette recordings: advantages, limitations and future. In: Stott F D, Raftery E B, Clement D L, Wright S L (eds) Fourth International Symposium on Ambulatory Monitoring. Academic Press, London, p189–194

Ives J R 1982c What time is it? Electroencephalography and Clinical Neurophysiology 54: 37P

Ives J R, Woods J F 1975 4-channel 24 hour cassete recorder for long-term EEG monitoring of ambulatory patients. Electroencephalography and Clinical Neurophysiology 39: 88–92

Ives J R, Woods J F 1980 A study of 100 patients with focal epilepsy using a four channel ambulatory cassette recorder. In: Stott F D, Raftery E B, Goulding L (eds) ISAM 1979: Proceedings of the Third International Symposium on Ambulatory Monitoring. Academic Press, London, p 383–392

Ives J R, Thompson C J, Gloor P 1976 Seizure monitoring: a new tool in electroencephalography. Electroencephalography and Clinical Neurophysiology 41: 422–427

Jackson J H 1873 On the anatomical, physiological and pathological investigation of epilepsies. West Riding Lunatic Asylum Medical Reports 3: 315. Reprinted in: Taylor J (ed) Selected writings of John Hughlings Jackson. Hodder & Stoughton, London, p 90–111

Janz D 1962 The grand mal epilepsies and the sleep-waking cycle. Epilepsia 3: 69–109

Jasper H H, Kershman J 1941 Electroencephalographic classification of the epilepsies. Archives of Neurology and Psychiatry 45: 903–943

Jasper H H, Droogleever-Fortuyn J 1947 Experimental studies on the functional anatomy of petit mal epilepsy. Research Publications of the Association for Research in Nervous and Mental Disorders 16: 271–298

Jayakar P, Chiappa K H 1990 Clinical correlations of photoparoxysmal responses. Electroencephalography and Clinical Neurophysiology 75: 251–254

Jeavons P M 1969 The use of photic stimulation in clinical electroencephalography. Proceedings of the Electrophysiological Technologists Association 16: 225–240

Jeavons P M 1982 Photosensitive epilepsy. In: Laidlaw J, Richens A (eds) A textbook of epilepsy, 2nd edn. Churchill Livingstone, Edinburgh, p 195–211

Jeavons P M, Bower B D 1964 Infantile spasms. Clinics in developmental medicine, no 15. Heinemann, London

Jeavons P M, Harding G F A 1975 Photosensitive epilepsy. Heinemann, London

Jeavons P M, Harding G F A, Panayiotopoulos C P, Drasdo N 1972 The effect of geometric patterns combined with intermittent photic stimulation in photosensitive epilepsy. Electroencephalography and Clinical Neurophysiology 33: 221–224

Jensen I, Larsen J K 1979 Mental aspects of temporal lobe epilepsy. Follow-up of 74 patients after resection of a temporal lobe. Journal of Neurology, Neurosurgery and Psychiatry 42: 256–265

Jovaniovc U J 1967 Das Schlafverhalten der Epileptiker: I Schlafdauer, Schlaftiefe und Besonderheiten der Schperiodik Deutsche Zeitschrift fur Nervenheilk 190: 159–198

Juul-Jensen P 1964 Frequency of recurrence after discontinuance of anti-convulsant therapy in patients with epileptic seizures. Epilepsia 5: 352–363

Kaibara M, Blume W T 1988 The postictal electroencephalogram. Electroencephalography and Clinical Neurophysiology 70: 99–104

Kaiser E 1976 Telemetry and video recording on magnetic tape cassettes in long-term EEG. In: Kellaway P, Petersen I (eds) Quantitative analytic studies in epilepsy. Raven Press, New York, p 279–288

Kamp A 1963 Eight-channel EEG telemetering. Electroencephalography and Clinical Neurophysiology 15: 164

Kamp A, Mars N J I, Wisman T 1979 Longterm monitoring of the electroencephalogram in epileptic patients. In: Amlaner C J, Macdonald D W (eds) A handbook on biotelemetry and radio tracking. Pergamon Press, Oxford, p 499–503

Kasteleijn-Nolst-Trenité D C A, Binnie C D, Overweg J, de Korte R A 1983 Abstracts of XVth Epilepsy International Congress, Washington DC, p 412

Kasteleijn-Nolst Trenité D G A, Binnie C D, Meinardi H 1987a Photosensitive patients: symptoms and signs during intermittent photic stimulation and their relation to seizures in daily life. Journal of Neurology, Neurosurgery and Psychiatry 50: 1546–1549

Kasteleijn-Nolst Trenitè D G A, Riemersma J B J, Binnie C D, Smit A M, Meinardi H 1987b The influence of subclinical EEG discharges on driving behaviour. Electroencephalography and Clinical Neurophysiology 67: 167–170

Kaufman I C, Marshall C, Walker A E 1947 Activated electroencephalography. Archives of Neurology and Psychiatry 58: 533–549

Kazamatsuri H, Kikuchi S, Jujimori M, Tokuda Y 1970 An electroencephalographic study of nocturnal sleep in the epileptic patients. Folia Psychiatrica et Neurologica Japonica 24: 1–22

Kellaway P, Frost J D 1983 Biorhythmic modulation of epileptic events. In: Pedley T A, Meldrum B S (eds) Recent advances in epilepsy. Churchill Livingstone, Edinburgh, p 139–154

Kellaway P, Frost J D, Hrachovy R A 1978 Relationship between clinical state, ictal and interictal EEG discharges and serum drug levels: phenobarbital. Annals of Neurology 4: 197

Kirstein L, Nilsson B Y 1977 Provokation von Spitzen im EEG mittels diffusem Licht und Lichtmustern bei epileptischen und nichtepileptischen Kranken. Zeitschrift fur Elektroenzephalographie und Verwandte Cebiete 8: 155–161

Klapetek J 1959 Photogenic epileptic seizures provoked by television. Electroencephalography and Clinical Neurophysiology 11: 809

Kooi K A, Thomas M H, Mortensen F N 1960 Photoconvulsive and photomyoclinic responses in adults. Neurology 10: 1051–1058

Kostopoulos G, Gloor P 1982 A mechanism for spikewave discharge in feline penicillin epilepsy and its relationship to spindle generation. In: Sterman M B, Shouse M N, Passouant P (eds) Sleep and epilepsy. Academic Press, New York, p 11–27

Kristensen O, Sindrup E H 1978 Psychomotor epilepsy and psychosis. Acta Neurologica Scandinavica 57: 361–377

Landolt A 1958 Serial EEG investigations during psychotic episodes in epileptic patients and during schizophrenic attacks. In: Lorenz de Haas A M (ed) Lectures on epilepsy. Elsevier, Amsterdam, p 91–133

Lange L S 1961 Television epilepsy. Electroenphalography and Clinical Neurophysiology 13: 490–491

Laplane R, Salbreux R 1963 Les convulsions hyperpyrètiques. Revue du Praticien 13: 753–761

Lennox-Buchthal M A 1973 Febrile convulsions: a reappraisal. Electroencephalography and Clinical Neurophysiology Suppl 32

Le Pestre M, Loiseau P, Larrieu E, Cohadons 1985 Stopping medication in adolescent epileptic patients (Abstracts of 16th Epilepsy International Symposium). Ciba-Geigy, Basel

Libo S S, Palmer C, Archibald D 1971 Family group therapy for children with self-induced seizures. American Journal of Orthopsychiatry 41: 506–508

Lieb J P, Woods S C, Siccardi A, Crandall P H, Walter D O, Leake B 1978 Quantitative analysis of depth spiking in relation to seizure foci in patients with temporal lobe epilepsy. Electroencephalography and Clinical Neurophysiology 44: 641–663

Lipman I J, Hughes J R 1969 Rhythmic mid-temporal discharges. An electro-clinical study. Electroencephalography and Clinical Neurophysiology 27: 43–47

Livingston S 1952 Comments on a study of light-induced epilepsy in children. American Journal of Diseases of Children 83: 409

Livingston S, Torres I C 1964 Photic epilepsy: report of an unusual case and review of the literature. Clinical Pediatrics 3: 304–307

Lockard J S 1981 A primate model of clinical epilepsy: mechanisms of action through quantification of therapeutic effects. In: Lockard J S, Ward A A Epilepsy: a window to brain mechanisms. Raven Press, New York, p 11–49

Lombroso C T, Erba G 1970 Primary and secondary bilateral synchrony in epilepsy. A clinical electroencephalographic study. Archives of Neurology 22: 321–334

Ludwig B I, Ajmone Marsan C 1975 EEG changes after withdrawal of medication in epileptic patients. Electroencephalography and Clinical Neurophysiology 39: 173–181

Maheshwari M C, Jeavons P M 1975 The clinical significance of occipital spikes as a sole response to intermittent photic stimulation. Electroencephalography and Clinical Neurophysiology 39: 93–95

Manni R, Galimberti C A, Zucca C, Parietti L, Tartara A 1990 Sleep patterns in patients with late onset partial epilepsy receiving chronic carbamazepine (CBZ) therapy. Epilepsy Research 7: 72–76.

Manson G 1974 EEG radio telemetry. Electroencephalography and Clinical Neurophysiology 37: 411–413

Marcus E M, Watson C W 1966 Bilateral synchronous spike and wave electroencephalographic pattern in the cat. Interaction of bilateral cortical foci in the intact, the bilateral corticocallosal and adiencephalic preparation. Archives of Neurology 14: 601–610

Marcus E M, Watson C W, Simon S A 1968 An experimental model of some varieties of petit mal epilepsy. Electrical-behavioural correlations of acute bilateral epileptogenic foci in cerebral cortex. Epilepsia 9: 233–248

Marshall C, Walker A E, Livingston S 1953 Photogenic epilepsy: parameters of activation. Archives of Neurology and Psychiatry 69: 760–765

Martins da Silva A, Aarts J H P, Binnie C D et al 1984 The circadian distribution of interictal epileptiform EEG activity. Electroencephalography and Clinical Neurophysiology 58: 1–13

Matricardi M, Brinciotti M, Benedetti P 1989 Outcome after discontinuation of antiepileptic drug therapy in children with epilepsy. Epilepsia 30: 582–589

Matthews W B 1964 The use and abuse of electroencephalography. Lancet 2: 577–579

Matsuo F, Knott J R 1977 Focal positive spikes in electroencephalography. Electroencephalography and Clinical Neurophysiology 42: 15–25

Mawdsley C 1961 Epilepsy and television. Lancet 1: 190–191

Mayersdorf A, Marshall C 1970 Pattern activation in reading epilepsy: a case report. Epilepsia 11: 423–426

Mayersdorf A, Wilder B J 1974 Focal epileptic discharges during all night sleep studies. Clinical Electroencephalography 5: 73–87

Menini C 1976 Rôle du cortex frontal dans l'épilepsie photosensible du singe Papio papio. Journal de Physiologie 72: 5–44

Merlis J K 1970 Proposal for an international classification of epilepsies. Epilepsia 11: 114–119

Milligan N, Richens A 1981 Methods of assessment of antiepileptic drugs. British Journal of Clinical Pharmacology 11: 443–456

Milligan N, Richens A 1982 Ambulatory monitoring of the EEG in the assessment of antiepileptic drugs. In: Stott F D, Raftery E B, Clement D L, Wright S L (eds) Proceedings of the 4th International Symposium on Ambulatory Monitoring, Gent, 1981. Academic Press, London, p 224–233

Milligan N, Dhillon S, Oxley J, Richens A 1982 Absorption of diazepam from the rectum and its effect on interictal spikes in the EEG. Epilepsia 23: 323–331

Milligan N, Oxley J, Richens A 1983 Acute effects of intravenous phenytoin on the frequency of interictal spikes in man. British Journal of Clinical Pharmacology 16: 285–289

Milstein V, Stevens J R 1961 Verbal and conditioned avoidance learning during abnormal EEG discharge. Journal of Nervous and Mental Disease 132: 50–60

Mirsky A F, Van Buren J M 1965 On the nature of the 'absence' in centrencephalic epilepsy: a study of some behavioural, electroencephalographic and autonomic factors. Electroencephalography and Clinical Neurophysiology 18: 334–348

Morrell F 1960 Secondary epileptogenic lesions. Epilepsia 1: 538–560

Modena I, Ricci G B, Barbanera S, Leoni R, Romani G L, Carelli P 1982 Biomagnetic measurements of spontaneous brain activity in epileptic patients. Electroencephalography and Clinical Neurophysiology 54: 622

Molaie M, Cruz A 1988 The effect of sleep deprivation on the rate of focal interictal epileptiform discharges. Electroencephalography and Clinical Neurophysiology 70: 288–292

Morimoto K, Goddard G V 1987 The substantia nigra is an important site for the containment of seizure generalization in the kindling model of epilepsy. Epilepsia 28: 1–10

Morrell F, Whisler W W 1980 Secondary epileptogenic lesions in man: prediction of the results of surgical excision of the primary focus. In: Canger R, Angelieri F, Penry J K (eds) Advances in epileptology (XIth Epilepsy International Symposium). Raven Press, New York, p 123–128

Naquet R 1983 The clinical significance of EEG in epilepsy. In: Nistico G, De Perri R, Meinardi H (eds) Epilepsy: an update on research and therapy. Alan R Liss, New York, p 147–164

Naquet R, Louard C, Rhodes J, Vigouroux M 1961 A propos de certaines décharges paroxystiques. Leur activation par l'hypoxie. Revue Neurologique 105: 203–207

Newmark M E, Penry J K 1979 Photosensitivity and epilepsy: a review. Raven Press, New York

Niedermeyer E, Lopes da Silva F 1987 Electroencephalography. Urban & Schwarzenberg, Baltimore,

O'Kane M, O'Kane F, Mothersill I 1982 On the telemetric monitoring of ictal events. In: Stefan H, Burr W (eds) Mobile long-term EEG monitoring (Proceedings of the MLE Symposium, Bonn, 1982). Fischer, Stuttgart, p 137–147

Overweg J 1985 Antiepileptic drug withdrawal in seizure-free patients. Thesis, University of Amsterdam

Overweg J, Binnie C D 1980 Pharmacotherapy of self-induced seizures. Acta Neurologica Scandinavica 79 (suppl): 98

Overweg J, Binnie C D, Oosting J, Rowan A J 1987 Clinical and EEG prediction of seizure recurrence following antiepileptic drug withdrawal. Epilepsy Research 1: 272–283

Pampiglione G 1956 Some anatomical considerations upon electrode placement in routine EEG. Proceedings of the Electrophysiological Technologists Association 7(1): 20–30

Panayiotopoulos C P, Jeavons P M, Harding G F A 1970 Relation of occipital spikes evoked by intermittent photic stimulation to visual evoked responses in photosensitive epilepsy. Nature 228: 566–567

Panayiotopoulos C P, Jeavons P M, Harding G F A 1972 Occipital spikes and their relation to visual evoked responses in epilepsy, with particular reference to photosensitive epilepsy. Electroencephalography and Clinical Neurophysiology 32: 179–190

Pantelakis S N, Bower B D, Jones H D 1962 Convulsions and television viewing. British Medical Journal 2: 633–638

Passouant P 1967 Epilepsie temporale et sommeil. Revue Roumaine de Neurologie 4: 151–163

Passouant P, Cadillac J, Delange M 1965 Indications apportées par l'étude du sommeil de nuit sur la physiopathologie des épilepsies. International Journal of Neurology 5: 207–216

Pedley T A 1983 Differential diagnosis of episodic symptoms. Epilepsia 24: S31–S44

Penfield W, Jasper H 1954 Epilepsy and the functional anatomy of the human brain. Churchill, London

Penin H 1968 Neuartige Diagnostik und Forschungsanlagen in der Universitats-Nervenklinik Bonn. Acta Medizinische Technologie 16: 76–78

Penry J K, Porter R J 1977 Intensive monitoring of patients with intractable seizures. In: Penry J K (ed) Epilepsy: The Eighth International Symposium. Raven Press, New York, p 95–101

Penry J K, Porter R J, Dreifuss F E 1971 Quantification of paroxysmal abnormal discharge in the EEGs of patients with absence (petit mal) seizures for evaluation of antiepileptic drugs. Epilepsia 12: 278–279

Penry J K, Porter R J, Dreifuss F E 1975 Simultaneous recording of absence seizures with video tape and electroencephalography. A study of 374 seizures in 48 patients. Brain 98: 427–440

Perria L, Rosadini G, Rossi G F, Gentilomo A 1966 Neurosurgical aspects of epilepsy: physiological sleep as a means for focalizing EEG epileptic discharges. Acta Neurochirurgica (Wien) 14: 1–9

Pollen D A, Perot P, Reid K H 1963 Experimental bilateral wave and spike from thalamic stimulation in relation to level of arousal. Electroencephalography and Clinical Neurophysiology 15: 1017–1028

Pond D A, Bidwell B H, Stein L 1960 A survey of epilepsy in fourteen general practices: 1. demographic and medical data. Psychiatrie, Neurologie und Neurochirurgie 63: 217–236

Porter A C 1985 Pattern sensitivity testing in routine EEG. Journal of Electrophysiological Technology 11: 153–155

Porter R J, Wolf A A, Penry J K 1971 Human electroencephalographic telemetry. American Journal of EEG Technology 11: 145–159

Porter R J, Penry J K, Lacy J R 1977 Diagnostic and therapeutic re-evaluation of patients with intractable epilepsy. Neurology 27: 1006–1011

Prechtl H F R, Boeke P E and Schut T 1961 The electroencephalogram and performance in epileptic patients. Neurology 11: 296–302

Prince D A, Farrell D 1969 'Centrencephalic' spike and wave discharges following parenteral penicillin injection in the cat. Neurology 19: 309–310

Principe J C, Guedes de Oliveira P, Vaz F, Tome A 1985 Automated event detection and characterization in EEG monitoring. Part II: Signal processing. In: Martins da Silva A, Binnie C D, Meinardi H (eds) Biorhythms and epilepsy. Raven Press, New York, p 177–193

Prior P F, Maynard D E 1976 Recording epileptic seizures. In: Janz D (ed) Epileptology: Proceedings of the Seventh International Symposium on Epilepsy. Thieme, Stuttgart, p 325–328

Quesney L F, Gloor P, Kratzenberg E, Zumstein H 1977 Pathophysiology of generalised penicillin epilepsy in the cat: The role of cortical and subcortical structures. I. Systemic application of penicillin. Electroencephalography and Clinical Neurophysiology 42: 640–655

Quy R J, Fitch P, Willison R G 1980 High-speed automatic analysis of EEG spike and wave activity using an analogue detection and microcomputer plotting system. Electroencephalography and Clinical Neurophysiology 49: 187–189

Rabending G, Klepel H, Krell D, Rehbein D 1969 Selbstreizung bei photogener Epilepsie. Psychiatrie, Neurologie und Medizinische Psychologie 11: 427–434

Radovici A, Misirliou V, Gluckman M 1932 Epilepsie réflexe provoquée par excitations des rayons solaires. Revue Neurologique 1: 1305–1308

Rail L R 1973 The treatment of self-induced photic epilepsy. Proceedings of the Australian Association of Neurologists 9: 121–123

Ralston B L 1958 The mechanism of transition of interictal spiking foci into ictal seizure discharges. Electroencephalography and Clinical Neurophysiology 10: 217–232

Ralston B L, Papatheodorou C A 1960 The mechanism of transition of interictal spiking foci into ictal seizure discharges Part II: Observations in man. Electroencephalography and Clinical Neurophysiology 12: 297–304

Ramsay R E 1982 Clinical usefulness of ambulatory EEG monitoring of the neurological patient. In: Stott F D, Raftery E B, Clement D L, Wright S L (eds) ISAMGENT 1981: Proceedings of the Fourth International Symposium on Ambulatory Monitoring and Second Gent Workshop on Blood Pressure Variability. Academic Press, London, p 234–243

Regina versus Coster 1959 Law Reports, The Times, 3 and 4 December

Reilly E L, Peters J F 1973 Relationship of some varieties of electroencephalographic photosensitivity to clinical convulsive disorders. Neurology 13: 1050–1057

Ricci G B, Romani G L, Salustri C et al 1987 Study of focal epilepsy by multichannel neuromagnetic measurements. Electroencephalography and Clinical Neurophysiology 66: 358–368

Richter R 1960 Télévision et épilepsie. Revue Neurologique 103: 283–286

Riley T L 1983 Normal variants in EEG that are mistaken as epileptic patterns. In: Gross M (ed) Pseudoepilepsy. Heath, Lexington, p 25–27

Riley T L, Roy A (eds) 1982 Pseudoseizures. Williams and Wilkins, Baltimore

Robin J J, Tolan G D, Arnold J W 1978 Ten-year experience with abnormal EEGs in asymptomatic adult males. Aviation, Space and Environmental Medicine 49: 732–736

Robin A, Binnie C D, Copas J B 1985 A within patients comparison of electrophysiological and hormonal responses to three types of electroconvulsive therapy. British Journal of Psychiatry 147: 707–712

Röder-Wanner U U, Wolf P, Danninger T 1985 Are sleep patterns in epileptic patients correlated with their type of epilepsy? In: Martins da Silva A, Binnie C D, Meinardi H (eds) Biorhythms and epilepsy. Raven Press, New York, p 109–121

Rodin E A 1968 The prognosis of patients with epilepsy. Thomas, Springfield

Rodin E A, John G 1980 Withdrawal of anticonvulsant medications in successfully treated patients with epilepsy. In: Wada J A, Penry J K (eds) Advances in epileptology (The Xth Epilepsy International Symposium). Raven Press, New York, p 183–186

Rodin E, Onuma T, Wasson J, Prozak J, Rodin M 1971 Neurophysiological mechanisms involved in grand mal seizures induced by metrazol and megimide. Electroencephalography and Clinical Neurophysiology 30: 62–72

Rodin E, Kitano H, Wasson S, Rodin M 1975 The convulsant effects of bicuculline compared with metrazol. Electroencephalography and Clinical Neurophysiology 38: 106–107

Rodin E, Kitano H, Nagao B, Rodin M 1977 The results of penicillin C administration on chronic unrestrained cats. Electrographic and behavioural observations. Electroencephalography and Clinical Neurophysiology 42: 518–527

Rose D F, Sato S, Smith P D, Porter R J, Theodore W H, Friauf W, Bonner R, Jabbari B 1987 Localisation of magnetic interictal discharges in temporal lobe epilepsy. Annals of Neurology 22: 348–354

Ross J J, Johnson L C, Walter R D 1966 Spike and wave discharges during stages of sleep. Archives of Neurology 14: 544–551

Roubicek J, Volavka J, Matousek M 1967 Elektroencefalogram u normalni populace. Ceskoslovenska Psychiatrie 63: 14–19

Rowan A J, Binnie C D, De Beer-Pawlikowsky N K B et al 1979 Sodium Valproate: serial monitoring of EEG and serum levels. Neurology 19: 1450–1459

Rowan A J, Overweg J, Sadikoglu S, Binnie C D, Nagelkerke N J D, Huenteler E 1980 Seizure prognosis in long-stay mentally subnormal epileptic patients: inter-rater EEG and clinical studies. Epilepsia 21: 219–225

Roy A 1977 Hysterical fits, previously diagnosed as epilepsy. Pschological Medicine 7: 217–273

Rugland A-L 1990 'Subclinical' epileptogenic activity. In: Sillanpää M, Johannessen S I, Blennow G, Dam M (eds) Paediatric epilepsy. Wrightson Biomedical Publishing, Washington, p 217–224

Sarvas J 1987 Basic mathematical and electromagnetic concepts of the biomagnetic inverse problem. Physics in Medicine and Biology 32: 11–22

Sato S, Dreifuss F, Penry J K 1973 The effect of sleep on spike-wave discharges in absence seizures. Neurology 23: 1335–1345

Schwab R S 1939 A method of measuring consciousness in petit mal epilepsy. Journal of Nervous and Mental Disease 89: 690–691

Schwab R S, Schwab M W, Withec D, Cock Y C 1954 Synchronized moving pictures of patients and EEG. Electroencephalography and Clinical Neurophysiology 6: 684–686

Scott D F, Furlong P F, Moffett A M, Harding G F A 1985 Is sunshine protective in photosensitive epilepsy? Electroencephalography and Clinical Neurophysiology 61: S216–S217

Sherwin I 1981 The effect of the location of an epileptogenic lesion on the occurrence of psychosis in epilepsy. In: Koella W P, Trimble M R (eds) Temporal lobe epilepsy, mania, and schizophrenia and the limbic system. Advances in biological psychiatry, 8. Karger, Basel, p 81–97

Shewmon D A, Erwin R J 1988 The effect of focal interictal spikes on perception and reaction time. II Neuroanatomic specificity. Electroencephalography and Clinical Neurophysiology 69: 338–352

Shimazono Y, Hirai T, Okuma T, Fukuda T, Yamamasu E 1953 Disturbance of consciousness in petit mal epilepsy. Epilepsia 2: 49–55

Shinnar S, Vining E P C, Mellits E D et al 1985 Discontinuing antiepileptic medication in children with epilepsy after two years without seizures. A prospective study. New England Journal of Medicine 313: 976–980

Sindrup E 1980 Technical contributions to the differential diagnosis in epilepsy. Acta Neurologica Scandinavica 79 (suppl): 47–48

Slater F, Beard A W, Glithero E 1963 The schizophrenia-like psychoses of epilepsy. British Journal of Psychiatry 109: 95–150

Smith E B O 1982 The value of prolonged EEG monitoring to the clinician in a psychiatric liaison service. In: Stott F D, Raftery E B, Clement D L, Wright S L (eds) ISAMGENT 1981: Proceedings of the Fourth International Symposium on Ambulatory Monitoring and Second Gent Workshop on Blood Pressure Variability. Academic Press, London, p 162–170

So E L, Penry J K 1981 Epilepsy in adults. Annals of Neurology 9: 3–16

Soso M J, Lettich E, Belgium J H 1980 Case report: responses to stripe width changes and to complex gratings of a patient with pattern-sensitive epilepsy. Electroencephalography and Clinical Neurophysiology 48: 98–101

Stålberg E 1976 Experiences with long-term telemetry in routine diagnostic work. In: Kellaway P, Petersen I (eds)

Quantitative analytic studies in epilepsy. Raven Press, New York, p 269–278

Stefan H, Burr W 1986 Absence signs: long term therapeutic monitoring. In: Schmidt D, Morselli P (eds) Intractable epilepsy: experimental and clinical aspects. Raven Press, New York, p 187–193

Stefan H, Froscher W, Burr W, Hubschmann R, Penin H 1980 Diagnostik und mobile 24-Stunden Langzeituberwachung von Absencen unter Carbamazepinetherapie. Nervenarzt 51: 623–629

Stefan H, Burr W, Hildenbrand K, Penin H 1981 Computer-supported documentation in the video analysis of absences: preictal-ictal phenomena: polygraphic findings. In: Dam M, Gram L, Penry J K (eds) Advances in epileptology (XIIth Epilepsy International Symposium). Raven Press, New York, p 365–373

Stefansson D B, Darby C E, Wilkins A J et al 1977 Television epilepsy and pattern sensitivity. British Medical Journal 2: 88–90

Stevens J R 1966 Psychiatric implications of psychomotor epilepsy. Archives of General Psychiatry 14: 461–472

Stevens J R 1977a The EEG spike: signal of information transmission? A hypothesis. Annals of Neurology 1: 309–314

Stevens J R 1977b All that spikes is not fits. In: Shagass C, Gershon S, Friedhofff A J (eds) Psychopathology and brain dysfunction. Raven Press, New York, p 183–198

Stevens J R, Kodama H, Lonsbury B, Mills L 1971 Ultradian characteristics of spontaneous seizure discharges recorded by radio telemetry in man. Electroencephalography and Clinical Neurophysiology 31: 313–325

Stores G 1978 School-children with epilepsy at risk for learning and behaviour problems. Developmental Medicine and Child Neurology 20: 502–508

Sundaram M, Hogan T, Hiscock M, Pillay N 1990 Factors affecting interictal spike discharges in adults with epilepsy. Electroencephalography and Clinical Neurophysiology 75: 358–360

Sutula T P, Sackellares J C, Miller J Q, Dreifuss F E 1981 Intensive monitoring in refractory epilepsy. Neurology 31: 243–247

Takahashi T, Tsukahara Y, Kaneda S 1980 EEG activation by use of stroboscope and visual stimulator SLS-5100. Tohoku Journal of Experimental Medicine 130: 403–409

Takahashi T, Tsukahara Y, Kaneda S 1981 Influence of pattern and red color on the photoconvulsive response and the photic driving. Tohoku Journal of Experimental Medicine 133: 129–137

Tassinari C A, Bureau M, Dravet C, Roger J, Daniele-Natale O 1982 Electrical status epilepticus during sleep in children (ESES). In: Sterman M B, Shouse M N, Passouant P (eds) Sleep and epilepsy. Academic Press, London, p 465–479

Taylor D C 1972 Mental state and temporal lobe epilepsy. A correlative account of 100 patients treated surgically. Epilepsia 13: 727–765

Taylor D C 1977 Epileptic experience, schizophrenia and the temporal lobe. Mclean Hospital Journal Special Issue: 21

Tizard B, Margerison J H 1963a The relationship between generalized paroxysmal EEG discharges and various test situations in two epileptic patients. Journal of Neurology, Neurosurgery and Psychiatry 26: 308–313

Tizard B, Margerison J H 1963b Psychological functions during wave-spike discharge. British Journal of Social and Clinical Psychology 3: 6–15

Todt H 1981 Zur Spatprognose kindlicher Epilepsien:

Ergbnisse einer prospektiven Langsschnittstudie. Deutsches Gesundheitswesen 30: 2012–2016

Todt H 1984 The late prognosis of epilepsy in childhood: results of a prospective follow-up study. Epilepsia 25: 137–144

Treiman D M, Walton N Y, Kendrick C 1990 A progressive sequence of electroencephalographic changes during generalized convulsive status epilepticus. Epilepsy Research 5: 49–60

Trimble M R 1977 The relationship between epilepsy and schizophrenia. Biological Psychiatry 121: 1460

Trimble M R, Perez M 1981 The phenomenology of the chronic psychoses of epilepsy. In: Koella W P, Trimble M R (eds) Temporal lobe epilepsy, mania, and schizophrenia and the limbic system: Advances in Biological Psychiatry, 8. Karger, Basel, p 98–105

Tukel K, Jasper H 1952 The electroencephalogram in parasagittal lesions. Electroencephalography and Clinical Neurophysiology 4: 481–494

Turski L, Cavalheiro E A, Turski W A, Meldrum B S 1986 Excitatory neurotransmission within substantia nigra pons reticulata regulares threshold for seizures produced by pilocarpine in rats. Neuroscience 18: 61–77

Van Egmond P, Binnie C D, Veldhuizen R 1980 The effect of background illumination on sensitivity to intermittent photic stimulation. Electroencephalography and Clinical Neurophysiology 48: 599–601

Van Heycop ten Ham M W 1980 Complete recovery from epilepsy? Discontinuation of antiepileptics after five or more seizure-free years. Huisarts en Wetenschap 23: 309–311

Van Wieringen A, Binnie C D, De Boer P T E, Van Emde Boas W, Overweg J, De Vries J (1987) Electroencephalographic findings in six antiepileptic drug trials. Epilepsy Research 1: 3–15

Veldhuizen R, Binnie C D, Beintema D J 1983 The effect of sleep deprivation on the EEG in epilepsy. Electroencephalography and Clinical Neurophysiology 55: 505–512

Vidart L, Geier S 1967 Enregistrements télééncephalographiques chez des sulets épileptiques pendant le travail. Revue Neurologique 117: 475–480

Vignaendra V, Walsh J, Burrows S 1979 The application of prolonged EEG telemetry and videotape recording to the study of seizures and related disorders. Clinical and Experimental Neurology 16: 81–94

Wada J, Engel J 1987 Appendix III: Potential relevance of kindling and secondary epileptogenesis to the consideration of surgical treatment of epilepsy. In: Engel J (ed) Surgical treatment of the epilepsies. Raven Press, New York, p 701–707

Wallis W E 1985 Withdrawal of anticonvulsant drugs—a prospective study. Journal of Neurology 232 (suppl): 260

Walter V J, Walter W G 1949 The central effects of rhythmic sensory stimulation. Electroencephalography and Clinical Neurophysiology 1: 57–86

Weir B 1964 Spikes-wave from stimulation of reticular core. Archives of Neurology 11: 209–218

Westmoreland B F, Klass D W 1981 A distinctive rhythmic EEG discharge of adults. Electroencephalography and Clinical Neurophysiology 51: 186–191

Westmoreland B F, Reiher J, Klass D W 1979 Recording small sharp spikes with depth electroencephalography. Epilepsia 20: 599–606

White J C Langston J W, Pedley T A 1977 77 Benign

epileptiform transients of sleep: clarification of the small sharp spike controversy. Neurology 27: 1061–1068

Wieser H G 1979 "Psychische Anfalle" und deren stereoelektroenzephalographisches Korrelat. Zeitschrift fur EEG und EMG 10: 197–206

Wieser H G 1983a Electroclinical features of the psychomotor seizure. Fischer, Stuttgart

Wieser H G 1983b Depth recorded limbic seizures and psychopathology. Neuroscience & Behavioural Reviews 7: 427–440

Wieser H G, Bancaud J, Talairach J, Bonis A, Szikla G 1979 Comparative value of spontaneous and chemically and electrically induced seizures in establishing the lateralization of temporal lobe seizures. Epilepsia 20: 47–59

Wilkins A J, Lindsay J 1985 Common forms of reflex epilepsy: physiological mechanisms and techniques for treatment. In: Pedley T A, Meldrum B (eds) Recent advances in epilepsy, 2. Churchill Livingstone, Edinburgh, p 239–271

Wilkins A J, Andermann F, Ives J 1975 Stripes, complex cells and seizures—an attempt to determine the locus and nature of the trigger mechanism in pattern-sensitive epilepsy. Brain 98: 365–380

Wilkins A J, Darby C E, Binnie C D 1977 Optical treatment of photosensitive epilepsy. Electroencephalography and Clinical Neurophysiology 43: 577

Wilkins A J, Darby C E, Binnie C D 1979a Neurophysiological aspects of pattern-sensitive epilepsy. Brain 102: 1–25

Wilkins A J, Darby C E, Binnie C D, Stefansson S B, Jeavons P M, Harding G F A 1979b Television epilepsy: the role of pattern. Electroencephalography and Clinical Neurophysiology 47: 163–171

Wilkins A J, Binnie C D, Darby C E 1980 Visually-induced seizures. Progress in Neurobiology 15: 85–117

Wilkins A J, Binnie C D, Darby C E 1981 Interhemispheric differences in photosensitive epilepsy: I. pattern sensitivity thresholds. Electroencephalography and Clinical Neurophysiology 52: 461–468

Wilkus R J, Green J R 1974 Electroencephalographic investigations during evaluation of the antiepileptic agent sulthiame. Epilepsia 15: 13–25

Williams D 1953 A study of thalamic and cortical rhythms in Petit Mal. Brain 76: 50–69

Williams D 1969 Neural Factors related to habitual aggression. Brain 92: 503–520

Wolf P, Röder-Wanner U U, Brede M, Noachtar S, Sengoku A 1985 Influences of antiepileptic drugs on sleep. In: Martins da Silva A, Binnie C D, Meinardi H (eds) Biorhythms and epilepsy. Raven Press, New York, p 137–153

Wong P K H 1985 Comparison of spike topography in typical and atypical benign rolandic epilepsy of childhood. Electroencephalography and Clinical Neurophysiology 61: S47

Wyler A R, Fetz, E E, Ward A A 1973 Spontaneous firing patterns of epileptic neurones in the monkey motor cortex. Experimental Neurology 40: 567–585

Wyler A R, Fetz E E, Ward A A 1974 Antidromic and orthdromic activitation of epileptic neurones. Experimental Neurology 43: 59–74

Zenker C, Groh C, Roth G 1957 Probleme und Erfahrungen beim Absetzen antikonvulsiver Therapie. Neue Osterreichische Zeitschrift fur Kinderheilkunde 2: 152–163

Zetterlund B 1982 Quantification of spike-and-wave episodes in 24-h tape recordings of EEG. In: Stefan H, Burr W (eds) Mobile long-term EEG monitoring (Proceeding of the MLE Symposium Bonn 1982). Fisher, Stuttgart, p 237–244

Zivin L, Ajmone Marsan C 1968 Incidence and prognostic significance of 'epileptiform' activity in the EEG of non-epileptic subjects. Brain 91: 751–778

10. Neuroradiology

B. Kendall

INTRODUCTION

The logical application of neuroradiological procedures to the study of epilepsy depends on a clear understanding of the advantages, limitations and potential morbidity of the various tests. The clinical features which influence the probability of demonstrating a causative lesion and its likely nature have been discussed in Chapter 5, and the significance of an underlying structural lesion in management and in assessment of prognosis has been stressed.

Some patients with epilepsy require no radiological study. Included in these are patients with clinically and electroencephalographically typical primary generalized seizures, in which neuropathological studies show no demonstrable underlying structural changes; and those in which clinical study resolves the nature of the lesion and decides its treatment, as, for example, most cases of uncomplicated tuberous sclerosis and disseminated known systemic neoplasm. Ideally, all other patients should have only the radiological study or selection of studies relevant to their particular treatment, preferring always the safest test if there are real alternatives.

Neuroradiological procedures fall naturally into two groups: first, those which cause no significant discomfort to the patient, carry no risk of morbidity and do not require admission to hospital; and, secondly, those which involve injections into blood vessels or previously rarely into the cerebrospinal fluid, which are unpleasant and, even in ideal conditions, carry a small risk of permanent morbidity. In the first group, computer tomography (CT), magnetic resonance imaging (MRI) skull and chest X-ray, and occasionally isotope encephalography may be relevant to the study of epilepsy. There is no positive contra-indication to the use of any or all of these procedures and the extent of their application is primarily a matter of the finance to procure the equipment and to employ a sufficient number of trained personnel to ensure an adequate service.

All neuroradiological studies need skilled radiography; the detection of slight abnormalities and the assessment of borderline normal findings is dependent on excellent technique. Good results can only be achieved when the head is completely immobile, which requires co-operating or adequately sedated patients; the clinician should ensure that the patients referred are in a suitable condition for the examination to be performed.

PLAIN RADIOGRAPHS

Plain skull radiographs (SXR) are completely negative in over 85% of intracranial tumours (Hillemacher 1982) and in the presence of other significant pathology. Even abnormal appearances are frequently nonspecific and rarely adequate for management. Plain skull radiographs are not a useful screening test. The use of CT increased positive findings up to 63% in patients with partial and 61% with generalized symptomatic epilepsy and the number of tumours detected from 5% up to 10% of cases investigated when compared with all other studies, except MRI (Gastaut & Gastaut 1976). Lesions were also found in 10% of patients previously considered to have generalized idiopathic epilepsy and CT is therefore the best widely available screening test.

Nevertheless, SXR may have been made prior to referral: significant abnormalities requiring

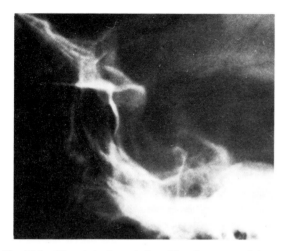

Fig. 10.1 Chronic hydrocephalus with enlargement of the third ventricle; such appearances are often due to aqueduct stenosis. Lateral radiograph of sella turcica. The dorsum sellae is short. The anterior wall of the sella is elongated.

elucidation by CT or MRI should be distinguished from physiological variations and artifacts. Many features to be noted will be equally well or better appreciated on CT. Skull radiographs are useful after CT or MRI for detailed study of bone in vault fractures, osteomyelitis and occasionally for distinction between meningioma and other superficial intrinsic tumours.

Raised intracranial pressure

Raised intracranial pressure causes erosion of the cortex of the sella turcica visible on a good quality lateral film most frequently at the junction of the posterior wall and floor. Erosion was present in 44% of intracranial tumours remote from the sella studied by Mahmoud (1958) and about 20% of patients with erosion have no clinical evidence of raised intracranial pressure.

Aqueduct stenosis may present with fits; it is the commonest cause of a sella deformity characteristic of chronic hydrocephalus with enlargement of the third ventricle in which shortening of the dorsum is combined with elongation of the anterior wall of the sella and often with enlargement of the anterior clinoid processes (Fig. 10.1).

When intracranial hypertension has commenced before the age of 10 years the sutures may be wider than 2 mm or have elongated interdigitations.

Physiological calcification and artefacts

The typical shape and position of the calcification facilitates recognition and distinction from significant lesions. Calcification in the pineal body and/or habenular commissure is visible on SXR in about 60% of European adults; it is much less frequent in African and Asiatic races and in children. Deviation of more than 2.5 mm from the midline is usually due to displacement by a contralateral mass and rarely to ipsilateral atrophy.

Calcification in the choroid plexus of the lateral ventricles is visible in about 10% of normal adults. It occurs usually in the trigone region, but can be elsewhere and is not infrequently unilateral or asymmetrical.

Plaques of ossification commonly occur in the dura lining the vault, in the falx and the tentorium. Curvilinear or circular calcified opacities are frequent in the walls of the carotid vertebral and basilar arteries in elderly patients. A dense artifact may be caused by substances such as EEG paste or lacquer on the scalp and may be recognized if it is outside the line of the vault on any projection.

Pathological calcification

This occurs in many conditions which may cause epilepsy. Frequently, calcification is not specific, but its appearance in a particular position may be diagnostic or it may be associated with other abnormalities making a diagnostic combination.

Tumours

Calcification is visible on SXR in 10–15% of meningiomas, sometimes outlining a considerable part of the tumour. The appearance of the calcification, and the position, if close to the dura, suggests the diagnosis (Fig. 10.2), and hyperostosis at the tumour attachment or enlarged meningeal grooves leading to it (Gold et al 1969) are confirmatory.

Calcification is visible on SXR in only 5.5% of gliomas (Kalan & Borrows 1962), being more frequent in the relatively benign tumours. The extent varies from one or two to an irregular

NEURORADIOLOGY 351

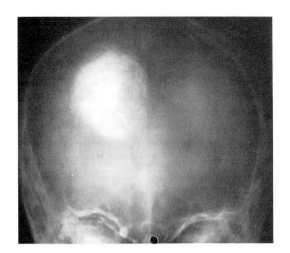

Fig. 10.2 Meningioma. SXR anteroposterior, projection. A well-defined cloud of calcification is present in the right parafalcine region typical of a meningioma with calcification in psammoma bodies.

conglomeration of nodules or an amorphous aggregate. The most typical appearance (Fig. 10.3), which occurs in both astrocytomas and the less common oligodendrogliomas, is of curvilinear streaks, suggesting gyri. Hamartomas, which are most common in the temporal lobe, may show nonspecific calcification indistinguishable from a glioma. The features of the calcification will be reflected in the CT appearances and the location

and extent of the tumour are elucidated by CT and/or MRI.

Tuberous sclerosis

A family history, typical skin manifestations or associated mental retardation usually suggest the diagnosis. Imaging is not necessary as a routine in typical tuberous sclerosis, but CT or MRI should be performed if a tumour is suspected. However, typical clinical features are sometimes absent (Kingsley et al 1986) and the disease may present with predominant manifestations in other systems. Mesodermal dysplasia may occur in bones, especially those of the hands and feet which may show subperiosteal cysts or nodular cortical thickening and sclerotic areas. In a small number of patients the lungs are infiltrated by smooth muscle, which causes a honeycomb appearance; spontaneous pneumothorax is a not infrequent complication. Multiple renal hamartomas, which are usually bilateral, may be shown by ultrasound, intravenous pyelography or CT. Intestinal polyps also are a described feature.

The dysplastic brain lesions of tuberous sclerosis often progressively calcify in older children, causing nodular and curvilinear densities. These are most frequent adjacent to the ventricular system and in the basal ganglia, though they

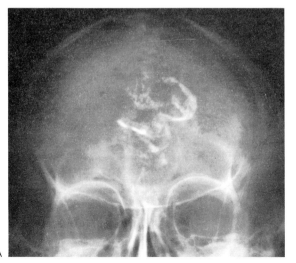

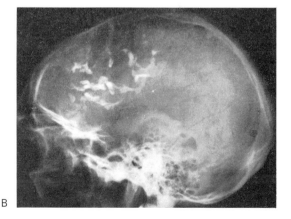

Fig. 10.3 Oligodendroglioma. Skull radiographs: (A) anteroposterior, (B) lateral projections. Gyriform curvilinear calcification is shown in the medial frontal region on both sides of the midline but extending further to the left. The appearances are typical of a glioma. This was an oligodendroglioma but an astrocytoma can cause similar findings.

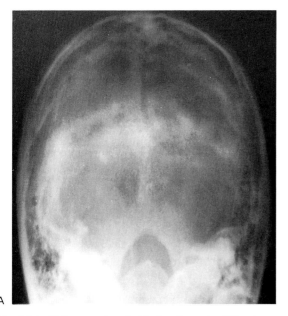

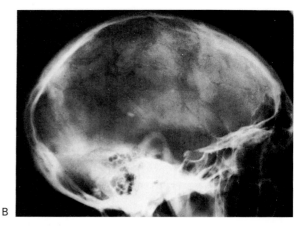

B

A

Fig. 10.4   Tuberous sclerosis. Skull radiographs: (A) anteroposterior, (B) lateral projections. Nodular calcification is present in the region of the basal ganglia on the right side and near the inferior surface of the right cerebellar hemisphere. Several sclerotic areas are present in the bones of the vault.

may occur elsewhere (Fig. 10.4). Tubers rarely obstruct the ventricular system and hydrocephalus is more often caused by a complicating glioma, usually a giant cell astrocytoma encroaching on an intraventricular foramen.

Inflammatory disease

Non-specific calcification occurs occasionally in necrotic tissues, such as old pyogenic abscesses and empyemas. Tuberculomas, which are the most common intracranial masses presenting in India, may also show non-specific nodular calcification.

Combined linear cortical and curvilinear basal ganglia calcifications occur in about 40% of cases of congenital toxoplasmosis and are diagnostic in the clinical context (Fig. 10.5). Hydrocephalus, due to occlusion of the aqueduct or outlets of the fourth ventricle, or microcephaly secondary to destruction of brain substance, occur in about 50% of these patients.

Calcified cysticerci may be shown in skeletal muscles. These are typically about 3 mm in diameter and 12–15 mm in length and lie parallel to the axis of the muscle fibres. They may be observed on films of the skull and chest, but are more frequent in the thighs (Fig. 10.6). Calcification is much less frequent in cerebral cysts and is then usually confined to the scolices, which show as nodules about 3 mm in diameter which are often multiple.

A rare but typical calcification, usually in the parietal regions, occurs in the walls of cysts in the cerebral form of paragonamiasis. The disease is endemic in the Far East particularly in Korea, China and Formosa.

Vascular lesions

Fine calcification is visible in about 15% of intracranial arteriovenous malformations (Fig. 10.7). It is usually curvilinear in the walls of abnormal veins, but it can also be deposited as nodules within old haemorrhages. Meningeal arteries may contribute to the increased blood flow and enlargement of foramina and vascular grooves and channels transmitting these vessels support the diagnosis. Confirmation is best achieved by MRI which may give evidence of blood flow in abnormal vessels or of haemoglobin derivatives in haematoma or thrombosed lesions.

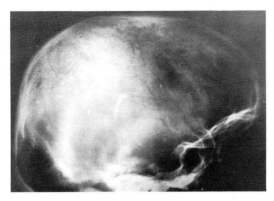

Fig. 10.5 Toxoplasmosis. Lateral radiograph skull. There are multiple nodular calcified lesions. Curvilinear calcification is present in one of the basal ganglia. The dorsum sellae is shortened due to erosion by an enlarged third ventricle, secondary to aqueduct obstruction caused by the disease.

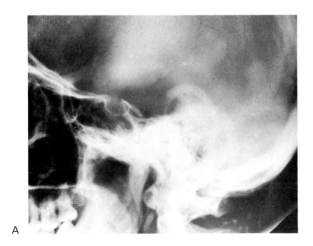

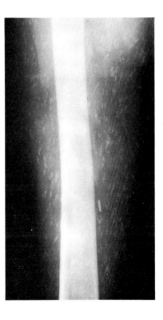

Fig. 10.6 Cysticercosis. (A) Lateral radiograph skull. Fusiform nodular shadows of calcified cysticerci are present in the neck and facial muscles. Nodular calcification is also present in the frontal and parietal lobes in the scolices of intracerebral cysticerci. (B) Right thigh. Large number of fusiform calcified lesions due to cysticerci in the muscles.

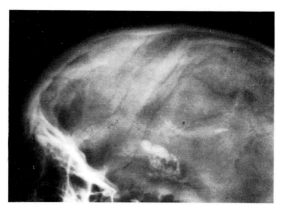

Fig. 10.7   Angiomatous malformation. Lateral radiograph skull. Aggregates of nodular calcification are shown in the inferior frontal region, confirmed by angiography to be in an angiomatous malformation.

In the Sturge–Weber syndrome, characteristic sinuous double lines of calcification are laid down in superficial layers of the atrophic cortex underlying the meningeal angioma, which is usually in the occipital and posterior parietal regions (Fig. 10.8). Calcification is visible on radiographs in only 50–60% of cases; it may be evident by 18 months of age but tends to increase in density up to adult life. The calcification is shown more frequently and at an earlier age on CT (see Fig. 10.32). Imaging is indicated for diagnosis only in clinically atypical cases and to show the extent and location of the disease process if surgery is contemplated.

New bone formation

The bone changes to be described are often better shown on CT than on SXR. Localized thickening of the inner table of the skull is commonly present at the site of attachment of a meningioma. It is sometimes associated with sclerosis of the adjacent diploe and less frequently with bone formation on the outer table of the skull. Enlarged and tortuous meningeal vascular channels extending to the hyperostosis and pits in the bone where small branches from the meningeal and scalp arteries perforate the vault to supply a tumour are useful confirmatory signs (Fig. 10.9). Bone reaction to solitary metastases from carcinoma of the prostate or breast may simulate a meningioma; extension of sclerosis into the facial skeleton and evidence of metastases elsewhere may aid differential diagnosis.

Meningioma-en-plaque (Fig. 10.10) typically produces a more diffuse and extensive sclerosis of bone, usually at the base, which could be confused with fibrous dysplasia. The latter is not a cause of epilepsy but may present as an incidental finding (Fig. 10.11). In its sclerotic form the bone is thickened and has a more homogenous chalky density without trabecular structure. In all tumours, the soft tissue components are elucidated by MRI and/or CT. Absence of any intracranial soft tissue mass or of meningeal enhancement distinguishes fibrous dysplasia from tumour.

Bone erosion

Meningioma may cause isolated erosion much less frequently than sclerosis and hyperostosis. The erosion is typically ill defined, more extensive on the inner aspect of the vault and is usually accompanied by enlarged meningeal channels, a combination strongly suggesting the diagnosis (Fig. 10.12), which is confirmed by CT and/or MRI.

Metastases, the rare primary tumours of bone and haematogenous osteomyelitis (Fig. 10.13) commence within and tend to more extensively destroy the diploe; they are an unusual cause of fits.

Pressure from any subadjacent mass, such as a superficial glioma, a meningioma or a por-

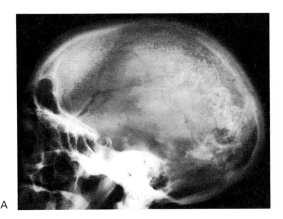

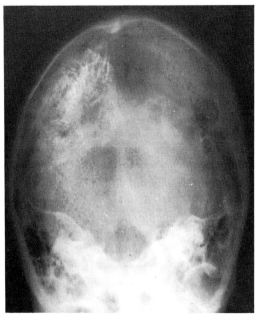

Fig. 10.8 Sturge–Weber syndrome. Skull radiographs: (A) lateral, (B) anteroposterior. Typical gyriform calcification is shown in the right posterior parietal and occipital regions. The right side of the vault is considerably smaller than the left due to associated hemiatrophy.

encephalic or arachnoid cyst, may cause smooth corticated erosion of the inner table or localized expansion of the vault. These lesions are distinguished by CT and/or MRI.

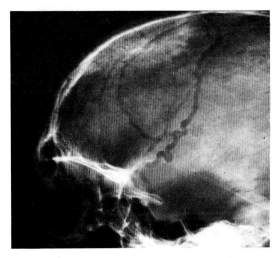

Fig. 10.9 Frontal convexity meningioma. Lateral radiograph skull. Localized sclerosis is evident in the superior frontal region. The groove of the middle meningeal artery is enlarged and tortuous and branches of the vessel extend to the abnormal bone. Large diploic vascular shadows are also shown.

Cerebral hypoplasia or atrophy

Because growth of the skull is secondary to that of the brain, which takes place mainly in the first 2 years of life, radiological findings are most marked when a lesion occurs early in this period. Lesser changes may be seen with severe damage occurring up to puberty.

With predominantly unilateral involvement, the capacity of the skull over the smaller hemisphere or lobe is less than that of the corresponding normal region. This may be recognized by flattening of the curve of the vault, elevation of the base with enlargement of the air cavities in the sinuses or mastoids and deviation of the falx or superior sagittal sinus towards the affected side. The skull overlying the atrophic lobe is usually thickened, but it may be thinned and smooth if there is a wide fluid-filled space between the atrophic brain and the vault. The SXR is diagnostic and further imaging is unnecessary for confirmation.

Post-traumatic epilepsy

Linear fractures, especially in young patients, usually heal without trace. In depressed fractures, deformity remains and occasionally bone fragments may be shown projecting medially from the

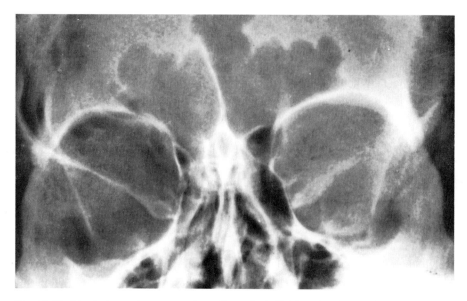

Fig. 10.10 Meningioma. Anteroposterior radiograph skull. There is sclerosis of the left lesser and greater wings of the sphenoid.

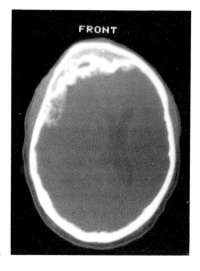

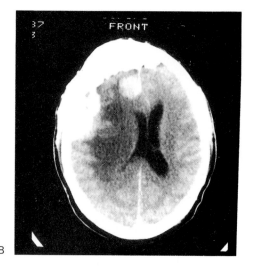

A

B

Fig. 10.11 Fibrous dysplasia plus meningiomas. (A) CT section imaged with wide window to show bone. There is thickening of the frontal bone, mainly on the right side, but extending across the midline. The thickening involves all tables, but the inner table is both thickened and irregular and a partly ossified mass extends into the cranial cavity from the posterior frontal convexity. (B) Same level after intravenous contrast medium. The mass enhances and a further well circumscribed tumour enhances adjacent to the right side of the falx. There is vasogenic oedema in the white matter of the right hemisphere and there is moderate mass effect. Histology confirmed tumours to be meningiomas and thickening of diploe due to fibrous dysplasia.

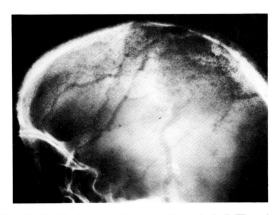

Fig. 10.12 Meningioma. Lateral radiograph skull. There is a large area of erosion high in the right parietal and frontoparietal regions. Enlarged meningeal vascular channels extend towards the abnormal region, large diploic venous channels drain away from it. The changes are diagnostic of a meningioma, but bone lysis is much less common than sclerosis in these tumours.

edge and are commonly associated with scarring in the adjacent brain. When the dura is torn the fracture line may widen (Fig. 10.14). In adults, this is associated with leptomeningeal cyst formation, which may cause bevelled thinning of the inner table beyond the limits of the fracture. In children, such erosion may be due to herniated brain, often damaged with cystic change, as well as extracerebral cyst in direct contact with the bone. The cyst may herniate through the fracture line and expand under the scalp, eroding the outer table. Widening fractures, especially in children, are usually associated with underlying brain damage which should be defined with CT or MRI.

A meningocerebral cicatrix may result in expansion of the ventricle or formation of an arachnoid cyst; even in the absence of fracture, trauma may cause contusion and haemorrhage sufficient to induce formation of an intracerebral cyst. Any of these conditions may incite thinning or lateral bulging of the adjacent inner table; in all of them the pathology is elucidated by CT or MRI.

CHEST RADIOGRAPHS

A chest radiograph is indicated in every patient with an intracranial mass. Bronchial carcinoma is by far the most common tumour metastasizing to the brain. Cerebral metastases from other neoplasms are frequently associated with pulmonary metastases. Occasionally, unsuspected cardiac lesions or chronic lung disease is first revealed on chest films.

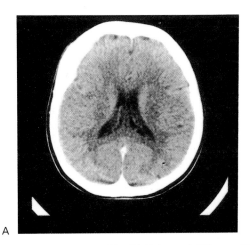

A

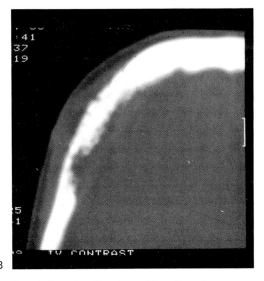

B

Fig. 10.13 Osteomyelitis. (A) Enhanced CT scan. (B) Same section windowed to show bone. There is erosion involving all tables of the skull with adjacent enhancing extradural and subgaleal inflammatory tissue.

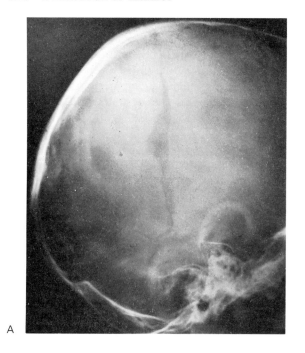

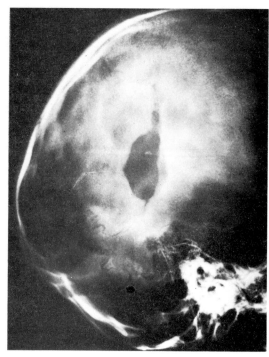

A

B

Fig. 10.14   Post-traumatic leptomeningeal cyst. Lateral radiographs skull. History of trauma 3 months previously. (A) A linear cleft, wider than a fresh fracture, is shown extending vertically in one of the parietal bones. (B) Seven months later; the fracture is considerably wider. At surgery a tear in the dura and arachnoid was associated with the leptomeningeal cyst.

COMPUTED TOMOGRAPHY (CT)

On radiographs it is only possible to recognize such marked differences in density as distinguish bone or calcification, soft tissue or water, fat and air. CT (Hounsfield 1973) gives quantitative readings of tissue density sufficiently sensitive to discriminate between the various intracranial tissues and to distinguish white and grey matter.

The method requires that the patient lies immobile for periods of between a few seconds and a minute, varying with the type of machine, while a series of contiguous sections of the head are scanned through their edges from a large number of directions by a finely collimated beam of X-rays with a thickness of 1–10 mm. The intensity of the beam is measured before and after transmission through the head, and many such readings are taken in each direction from multiple angles. A computer assembles the data from each section and, using a mathematical method, reconstructs it as a matrix of cells (pixels) between 0.75 mm^2 and 1.5 mm^2 A digital value approximating to

within 0.5% of the average radiation absorption within the tissues contained in the cell volume (voxel) represented by each particular pixel is calculated, resulting in a format simulating the structure and shape of the original section. An image with corresponding points of variation of light intensity is displayed simultaneously on a cathode ray tube and can be recorded on film.

The most radio-opaque tissue encountered normally in the skull is compact bone and the least is air; these have been made the extremes of a scale of absorption, in which water was assigned zero value, and they have been arbitrarily designated +1000 and −1000 Hounsfield units (HU) respectively. Most of the normal intracranial soft tissues fall into the narrow range of 0 to +60 HU. The grey matter of the cortex, basal ganglia and thalami has a value of +36 to +56 HU and can be distinguished (see Fig. 10.15) from white matter, which ranges between +20 and +38 HU with an average value of +24 HU. The pineal gland is always evident and the glomeri of the choroid plexuses are usually outlined by calcium (Ca): each mg Ca/ml increases absorption by 2 HU at 120 kV and can be appreciated when insufficient to be shown on the skull radiographs, which requires a density equivalent of 80 HU. Cerebrospinal fluid, with an absorption value of between 0 and +10 HU is shown and gives a close approximation to the configuration of the ventricles and intracranial subarachnoid spaces (Synek et al 1979); because of their small height, the normal temporal horns may be averaged out by brain tissue in thicker sections and 4–5 mm sections should be used to image the temporal lobes.

Intravenous contrast media do not cross the blood–brain barrier, so that the attenuation of the normal brain is only increased by a relatively small amount (up to 5 HU) by contrast medium which is retained within the blood stream. Repeat scanning following intravenous injection of contrast medium causes an increase in the attenuation of some lesions. This is sometimes related to vascularity (see Fig. 10.21) but more commonly to interstitial extravasation of contrast medium within the lesion or to abnormalities induced in the blood–brain barrier by neoplasm, inflammation or tumour; it may also occur transiently in the cerebral cortex following prolonged status epilepticus in the absence of any other factor. Enhancement is particularly valuable for defining pathologies which are of similar attenuation to adjacent normal or oedematous brain, but it may be useful in other cases also, to obtain the maximum information about the morphology of an abnormality. Cystic or necrotic regions, which do not increase in attenuation, are more evident when surrounding tumour tissue (see Fig. 10.23) or an abscess capsule is enhanced.

Apart from being more generally available, CT has a few advantages over magnetic resonance imaging; these include:

1. The machine is more open and less frightening and the procedure is much less noisy than MRI; fewer patients find CT intolerable and fewer children need sedation or anaesthesia
2. No limitation in the presence of critically situated magnetic materials, such as clips on aneurysms, or equipment influenced by radio waves, such as cardiac pacemakers

3. Demonstration of detail in cortical bone and of calcified lesions.

Pathological findings

The incidence of CT scan abnormalities is markedly influenced by clinical selection. It is increased particularly by the presence of interictal focal signs and/or focal EEG abnormalities with slowing and spikes. A coarse approximation of the incidence of CT abnormalities may be gained from analysis of the series in which the cases were either unselected (McGahan et al 1979, Dellaportas et al 1982, Weisberg et al 1984) or only partly selected on clearly defined criteria (Bogdanoff et al 1975, Langenstein et al 1979, Yang et al 1979). Normal examinations or varying degrees of diffuse atrophy will be found in between 65% and 86% and focal atrophy, hemiatrophy or porencephaly in between 4% and 16%. In most series, neoplasm and infarct have an incidence of just under 5%, and angiomatous malformation or aneurysm about 1.5%. In general, surgically amenable lesions are rarely detected by CT in patients without neurological symptoms or signs after more than 5 years' duration of seizures (Jabbari et al 1979, Gilsanz et al 1979).

Though primary generalized epilepsy was associated with CT abnormality in 10% of cases in two series (Gastaut & Gastaut 1976, Langenstein et al 1979), other series, which fit in with the more general experience differ from matched controls in only two respects. Firstly, patients who had suffered episodes of status had a higher incidence of cerebral atrophy; and, secondly, prolonged therapy with phenytoin was not uncommonly associated with cerebellar cortical atrophy (Weisberg et al 1984).

In secondary generalized epilepsy atrophic changes are shown in CT in almost two-thirds of cases (Gastaut & Gastaut 1976) and an incidence of over 90% has been recorded (Langenstein et al 1979). The incidence of CT abnormalities is high in simple partial seizures, ranging in different series between 52% and 68%, with tumours between 4% and 38%. It is also high in complex partial seizures, ranging between 40% and 70%. Mesial temporal sclerosis is the most common abnormality; it is caused by anoxia selectively

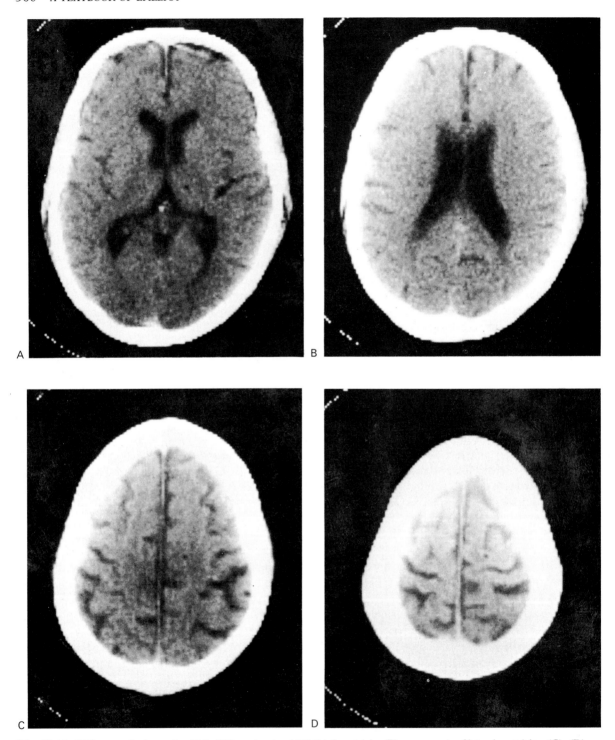

Fig. 10.15 Diffuse cerebral atrophy. Plain CT, section level (A) third ventricle, (B) upper parts of lateral ventricles, (C), (D) near vertex. The cerebrospinal fluid in the ventricular system and cerebral subarachnoid spaces is of lowest attenuation (0–6 H) and outlines the enlarged lateral ventricles, upper part of the third ventricle and the Sylvian and interhemispheric fissures. The hemispheric and capsular white matter (20–38 H) can be distinguished from the grey matter (36–56 N) in the basal ganglia and thalami.

affecting the H1 and H3 sectors of the hippocampus which may be precipitated by prolonged seizures and is usually manifested as temporal lobe atrophy with dilatation of the temporal horn (see Fig. 10.39). Jabbari et al (1979) reported one case with an arcuate non-enhancing region of calcification on CT. Small focal tumours, including hamartomas, have formed up to 23% of lobectomized series (Falconer & Serafetinides 1963).

The age of onset of the epilepsy considerably influences the incidence and nature of the abnormalities shown; the incidence is highest with onset during the first year of life when it may reach 68%, with a high proportion due to congenital malformations and perinatal brain damage (Yang et al 1979). Focal seizures after the first year and under 15 years of age are uncommonly due to tumour (Holowach et al 1958); CT infrequently reveals an abnormality of therapeutic significance (Bachman et al 1976), though, occasionally, low density changes in white matter or symmetrical calcification may suggest an unsuspected metabolic disturbance. When epilepsy arises in adult life, the incidence of abnormality increases with the age of onset (Bogdanoff et al 1975, Collard et al 1976, Scollo-Lavizzari et al 1977). Under the age of 35, head injury and neoplasm predominate; between 35 and 60 cerebral ischaemia and neoplasm are dominant, with an increasing proportion of metastases; and after 55, ischaemia (Shorvon et al 1984) and degenerative disorders are most likely.

Epilepsy follows in over 12% of severe head injuries but it is rare after more minor injuries. If CT does not reveal a focal lesion soon after injury, epilepsy is unlikely; with intracerebral haemorrhage the incidence is about one in six; if both intra- and extracerebral haemorrhage are present there is about a 75% incidence of epilepsy.

Atrophy and hydrocephalus

Generalized atrophy (Fig. 10.15), hemiatrophy (Fig. 10.16), focal atrophy, cortical and cerebellar atrophy (Fig. 10.17), hydrocephalus (Fig. 10.18) and cystic expansion of the ventricles or

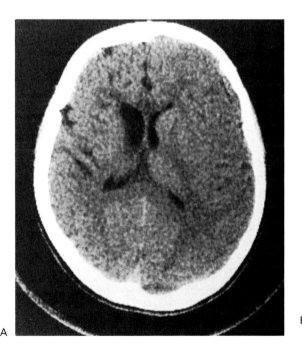
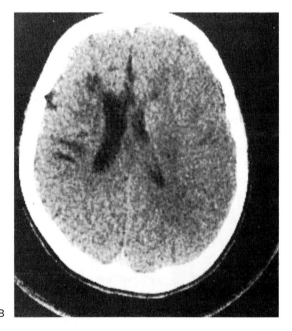

A

B

Fig. 10.16 Right hemiatrophy. (A), (B) Plain CT scan. The right hemicranium is relatively small and the vault is thickened on this side. The right lateral ventricle, the Sylvian fissure and some sulci over the frontal lobe are enlarged. There is a small region of low density in the deep frontal white matter suggesting focal accentuation of the brain damage associated with the hemiatrophy.

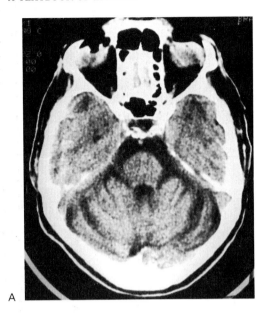 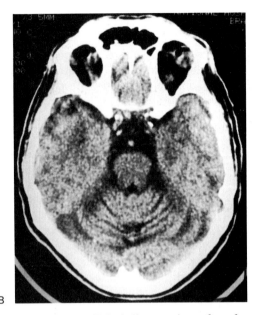

Fig. 10.17 Cerebellar atrophy. Plain CT sections: (A) level of fourth ventricle, (B) including superior surface of cerebellar hemisphere. The fourth ventricle is prominent. The basal cisterns around the brainstem are enlarged and the curvilinear dilated superior cerebellar sulci are evident.

subarachnoid space are all clearly shown. The more minor degrees of temporal atrophy associated with temporal sclerosis may be difficult to recognize, even with high resolution scanners. They are better shown with MRI, as are most midline stenosing lesions causing hydrocephalus (Fig. 10.18, and see Fig. 10.44).

Vascular lesions

A typical infarct (Fig. 10.19) shows a low attenuation region involving both the white and cortical grey matter, sometimes wedge-shaped when in the distribution of a cortical artery and without displacement of adjacent structures. In a recent infarct, however, oedema may cause the lesion to appear ill-defined and may produce swelling sufficient to suggest the possibility of a tumour. Repeat study may distinguish by showing a tendency of the infarct to resolve towards more typical appearances within a few days. The blood–brain barrier is damaged by infarction and enhancement may occur until recovery has taken place, which is usually less than 1 month after the stroke but can be up to 3 months.

Sometimes infarction is patchy and shows as multiple regions of decreased attenuation in the distribution of the occluded vessel. An old infarct may eventually form a cyst, which causes a sharply defined region of low attenuation, or a scar, associated with focal atrophy (Fig. 10.20). Small vessel disease commonly causes patchy ill-defined low density in the deep white matter of the cerebral hemispheres, sometimes associated with lacunar infarcts in the white matter and/or corpus striatum.

The attenuation of clotted blood (+56 to +80 HU), which increases as serum is expressed from the contracting clot, is characteristic of a recent haematoma (Fig. 10.21). Angiography is necessary if details of a causative lesion need to be defined, but large aneurysms and angiomas can be identified by re-examination by CT after intravenous injection of contrast medium (Fig. 10.22). As a clot is absorbed, its density diminishes and eventually a cyst or scar, indistinguishable from an old infarct, may remain.

Tumours

Neoplasms cause mass effect of very variable degree, resulting in displacement and deformity of normal structures due to compression and/or invasion. The attenuation of tumour tissue varies

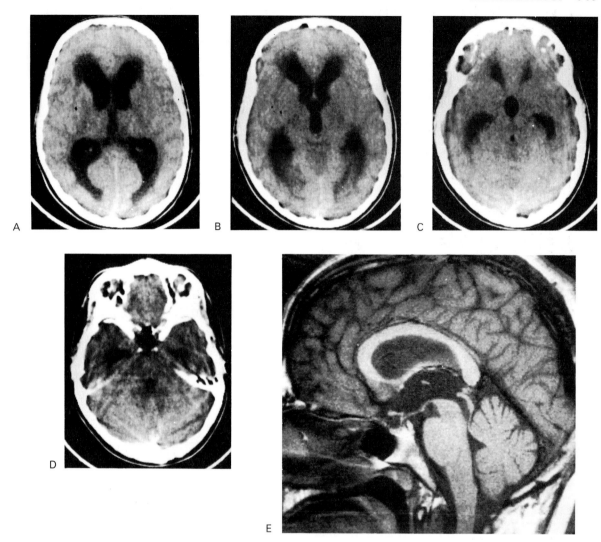

Fig. 10.18 Hydrocephalus due to stenosis of lower end of the aqueduct. (A)–(D) Plain CT scan. The dilated lateral (A)–(C) and third (B), (C) ventricles and aqueduct (C) are evident. The fourth ventricle (D), basal cisterns and cortical sulci are not dilated. There is periventricular lucency around the frontal horns due to transependymal passage of CSF. Aqueduct stenosis (different case). (E) MRI, sagittal section, spin echo sequence. Note the distension of the third ventricle and of the aqueduct, which tapers to stenosis at its lower end. The fourth ventricle and the basal cisterns are normal.

markedly: it may be higher, similar to or less dense than the adjacent brain but it tends to be higher in tumours with more compact cell structure. Calcified, haemorrhagic, cystic, necrotic and oedematous regions in or adjacent to tumours may cause superadded focal variations of the basic attenuation due to the tumour tissue. Grade I and II gliomas (Fig. 10.23) are mainly of diminished attenuation, apart from calcified foci, which are often evident when they are not visible on radio-graphs. Higher grade gliomas (Fig. 10.24) tend to be heterogeneous, usually of diminished attenuation but with areas of similar or greater attenuation than the normal white matter, and over 90% enhance with intravenous contrast medium. Fluid in cystic and necrotic parts is common in malignant tumours; it may be suspected if there are low density non-enhancing regions, but can only be diagnosed definitely when there are fluid levels. The edges of gliomas are commonly poorly

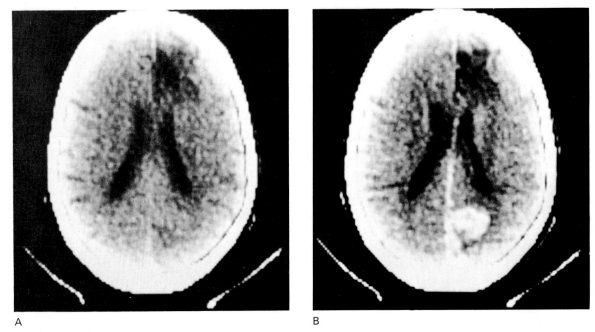

Fig. 10.19 Cerebral infarcts right frontal and parieto-occipital regions. (A) Plain scan. Low attenuation lesions with no mass effect. (B) After intravenous contrast medium. There is enhancement of the low attenuation parieto-occipital region and of the surrounding brain indicating injury to the blood–brain barrier and that the infarct is recent. There is no enhancement in the frontal infarct which is probably mature.

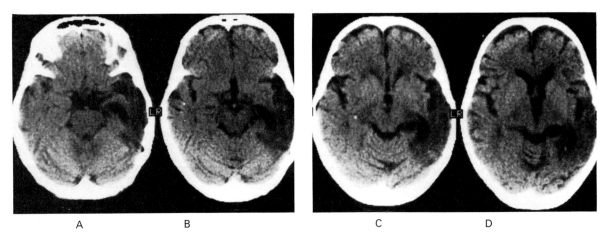

Fig. 10.20 Temporal lobe epilepsy associated with mature infarction of left temporal lobe. Plain CT scan, (A)–(D) contiguous sections. There is low density involving most of the left temporal lobe. The left temporal horn is dilated. There is also more diffuse atrophy, with enlargement of cortical sulci and of the wings of the ambient cistern.

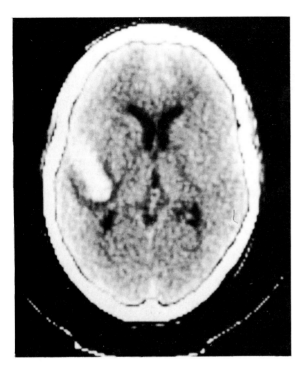

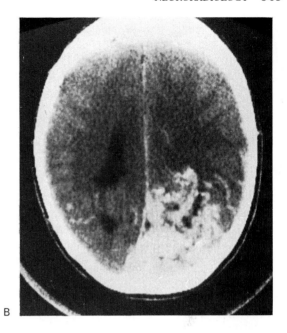

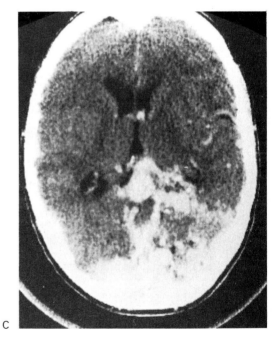

Fig. 10.21 Intracerebral haematoma. Plain CT. There is a region of homogeneously increased attenuation in the posterior part of the left temporal lobe, with well-demarcated, surrounding low attenuation blood clot from a recent haemorrhage. There is also subarachnoid blood, which accounts for the increased attenuation around the interhemispheric fissure anteriorly.

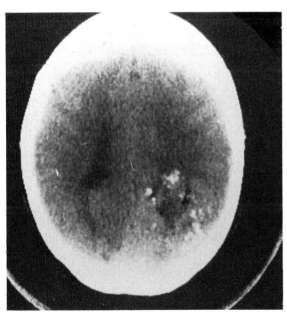

A

B

C

Fig. 10.22 Angiomatous malformation. (A) Plain scan. There is high density lesion containing nodular calcification in the left parieto-occipital lobes. (B) Scan at similar level after intravenous contrast medium. There is marked enhancement throughout the high density region, with a suggestion of curvilinear structures in the anterior part of the enhancement. (C) At a lower level after enhancement. The rounded and curvilinear structures, due to enlarged arteries supplying veins draining the angiomatous malformation, are evident.

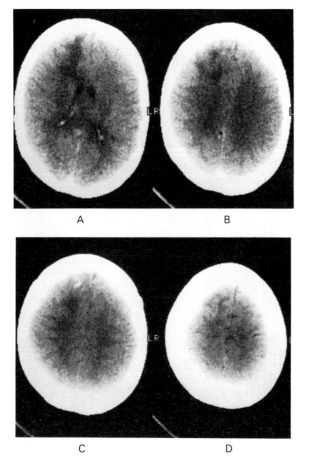

A   B

C   D

Fig. 10.23 Low grade oligodendroglioma. (A)–(D) Plain scan, contiguous sections. There is extensive low density in the right frontal white matter with a little calcification peripherally near the anterior convexity. The sulci over the right hemisphere are not visible but there is no other evidence of mass effect.

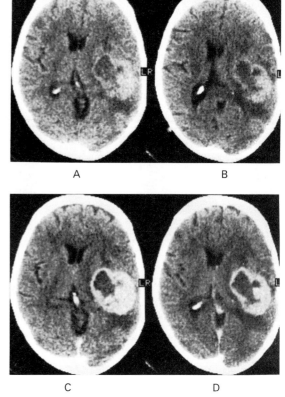

A   B

C   D

Fig. 10.24 Astrocytoma grade IV left temporal and parietal lobes. Plain scan. Mass attenuation enclosing a low attenuation region which is compressing the anterior horn and trigone of the left lateral ventricle. (B)–(D) After intravenous contrast medium, irregular ring enhancement around the low attenuation region, which was necrotic. There is also low attenuation due to oedema posterior to the mass.

demarcated although, occasionally, they may be well defined.

Metastases (Fig. 10.25) usually show relatively well-defined masses which may vary in density from less to greater than normal brain. Not uncommonly there is irregular central necrosis and there may be extensive oedema of the adjacent white matter. If a solitary lesion is revealed, re-examination after intravenous contrast injection or by MRI may show further metastases and is especially important if surgery is contemplated.

Meningiomas (Fig. 10.26) show as peripheral well-defined enhancing masses of greater attenuation in most instances, but sometimes isodense with brain. Associated cerebral oedema is not un-

common and, if the section does not pass through a small meningioma, the oedema may be mistaken for a primary intrinsic pathology.

Developmental abnormalities

Dermoids, which may be recognized from the presence of fat which is less dense than water, rarely present with epilepsy; but epidermoids more frequently do so when they encroach on the surfaces of the cerebral hemispheres. They are usually low density masses, without surrounding oedema. There may be some calcification and occasionally enhancement in the capsule (Fig. 10.27).

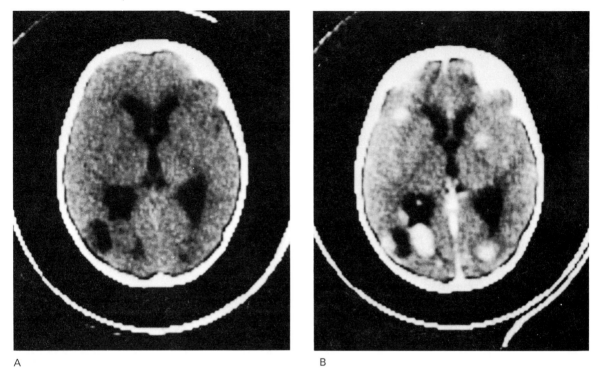

A   B

Fig. 10.25 Multiple metastases. (A) Plain scan. (B) Same section after intravenous contrast medium. There are masses of both low and brain attenuation most of which enhance. One in the left occipital region remains of low attenuation centrally and could be cystic. There is low attenuation due to oedema around some of the lesions, but this is rather less than is usual with metastases. There is moderate hydrocephalus, which was caused by further metastases in the posterior fossa partially obstructing the fourth ventricle.

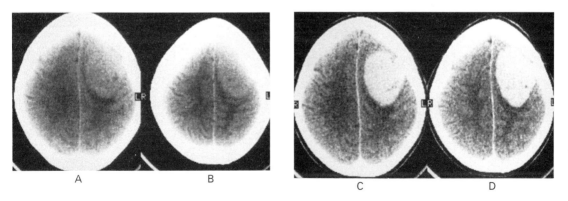

Fig. 10.26 Meningioma. (A), (B) CT above level of lateral ventricles. There is a peripheral area of increased density in the left frontal region due to a meningioma, with diminished density due to intracerebral oedema posterior to it. (C), (D) Following intravenous contrast medium, there is marked uniform enhancement of the meningioma.

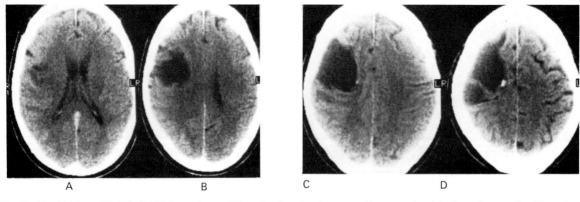

Fig. 10.27 Epidermoid. (A)–(D) Enhanced scan. There is a low density mass adjacent to the right frontal convexity. There is a small nodule of calcification in its medial margin and there is a little enhancement along the medial margin of the mass, possibly in the adjacent cortex. There is no oedema. The sulci over the right hemisphere are occluded and the roof of the lateral ventricle is depressed.

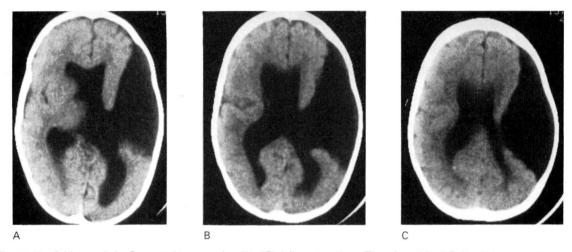

Fig. 10.28 Schizencephaly. Computed tomography. (A)–(C) Adjacent sections. There is a wide cleft, lined by grey matter, extending through the right cerebral hemisphere and linking the body of the ventricle with the subarachnoid space. The septum pellucidum is absent and parts of the margins of the dilated lateral ventricles are slightly irregular, suggesting heterotopia.

The more gross brain malformations, in which the ventricles show characteristic anatomical deformities (Fig. 10.28), are evident on both CT and MRI imaging. Neuronal migration and proliferation abnormalities arising at a later time in development, in which the brain substance itself may be mainly affected, are more exactly depicted by MRI but may be diagnosed by CT. They include heterotopia, in which nodules of grey matter may deform the lateral ventricular outlines, expand within the white matter or thicken the cortex (Fig. 10.29) causing refractory seizures, and sometimes microcephaly. In pachygyria, in which the gyri are wide and diminished in number, and agyria or lissencephaly (Fig. 10.30), which is characterized by absence of sulcation over part (Fig. 10.31) or all of the cerebral hemispheres so that the cortex appears smooth, epilepsy is generally combined with retardation and microcephaly. In agyria the ventricles are large, the subarachnoid space generally wide and the Sylvian fissures shallow and wide. Recessively inherited microcephaly shows no abnormality on CT or MRI.

The dysplastic lesions of tuberous sclerosis are usually evident by the second year of life and are

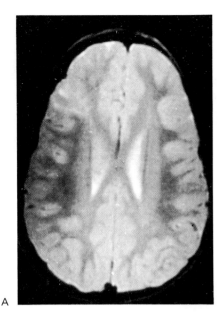

A

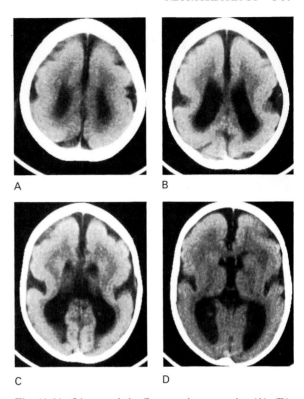

A   B

C   D

Fig. 10.30 Lissencephaly. Computed tomography. (A)–(D) Adjacent sections. The subarachnoid space is wide and outlines the abnormally smooth cortex and the shallow Sylvian fissures. The lateral and third ventricles are dilated. The septum pellucidum is absent.

commonly associated with infantile spasms. Most frequent are the typical subependymal, partly calcified tubers, which do not enhance on CT (Fig. 10.32). Recently, however, some tubers in the region of the interventricular foramina have been shown to enhance after intravenous gadolinium on MRI (Martin et al 1990). Parenchymal and subcortical lesons may also be calcified, of low attenuation or less well defined. When these are solitary manifestations (Fig. 10.33) a definite CT diagnosis may not be possible, but should be recognized as being consistent in the presence of clinical signs of tuberous sclerosis (Kingsley et al 1986). Nodules enhancing on CT are usually due to giant cell astrocytomas or occasionally to other types of glial tumours. The former are most commonly found in the region of the foramina of Monro and tend to cause obstructive hydrocephalus (Fig. 10.34).

In Sturge–Weber the subcortical calcification is

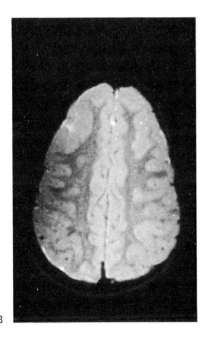

B

Fig. 10.29 Localized cortical dysplasia. Spin echo sequence TR 2000 TE 90: (A) at and (B) above the upper border of the lateral ventricles. There is localized thickening of right frontal convexity cortex with widening of the overlying sulci and reduction in thickness of the sub-adjacent white matter.

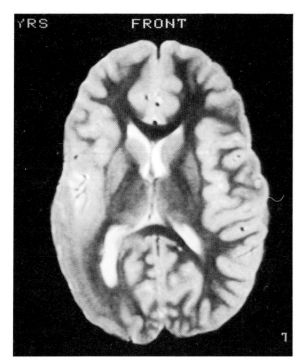

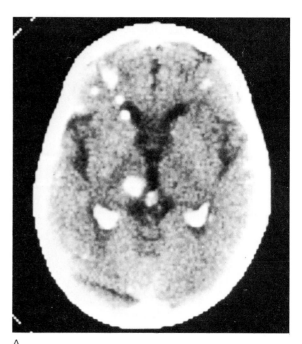

A

Fig. 10.31 Localized agyria or pachygyria. Spin echo TR 2000, TE 90. There is abnormal cortex and thinning of white matter involving the right temporal and lateral half of the right occipital lobe. Within the thickened cortex there is a low signal band which in some cases has been shown to correspond histologically to a cell sparse zone of migration arrest. The tissue between this band and the white matter contains the incompletely migrated heterotopic neurones.

shown earlier and is usually much more extensive than on skull radiographs. Abnormal enhancement occurs in affected cortex and atrophy causes enlargement of the adjacent subarchnoid space and/or ventricle (Fig. 10.35).

Inflammatory disease

Abscess is an unusual cause of isolated epilepsy. It is a clinical diagnosis, confirmed on CT by the presence of a relatively thin and even, approximately isodense enhancing ring with a low density centre and surrounding oedema. However, about one-third of abscesses are atypical. These are often due to low grade organisms, sometimes in an immune deficient patient. They tend to cause irregular, uneven ring or nodular enhancement on CT, with little or no central low density and relatively less oedema.

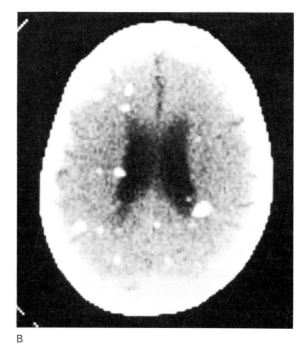

B

Fig. 10.32 Tuberous sclerosis. Plain CT, sections at the level of (A) third ventricle, (B) upper parts of bodies of lateral ventricles. There are multiple calcified paraventricular and intraparenchymal tubers. There is also physiological calcification in the pineal gland and the choroid plexuses of the lateral ventricles.

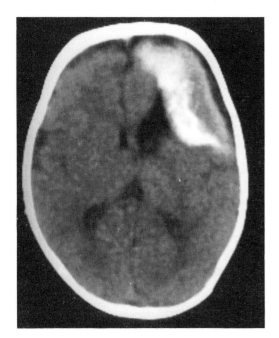

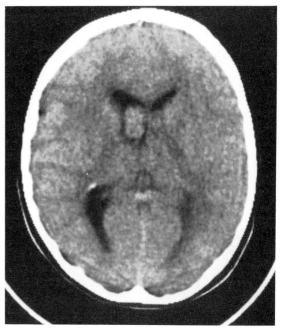

Fig. 10.33   Tuberous sclerosis. There is a large, partly calcified tuber occupying the anterior half of the left frontal lobe and associated with ventricular dilatation and dilatation of the subarachnoid space overlying it.

B

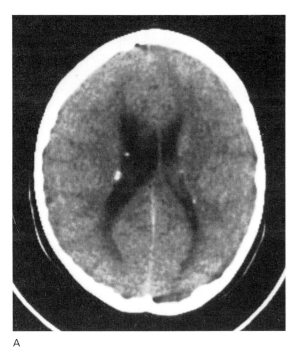

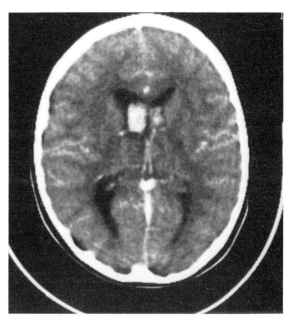

A

C

Fig. 10.34   Tuberous sclerosis, with giant cell astrocytoma. (A), (B) Plain scan. There are calcified tubers around the lateral ventricles. There are isodense masses impinging on the anterior horns of the lateral ventricles from the regions of the heads of the caudate nuclei. There is minimal dilatation of the right lateral ventricle. (C) Similar level to (B) after intravenous contrast medium. There is homogeneous enhancement of the tumours.

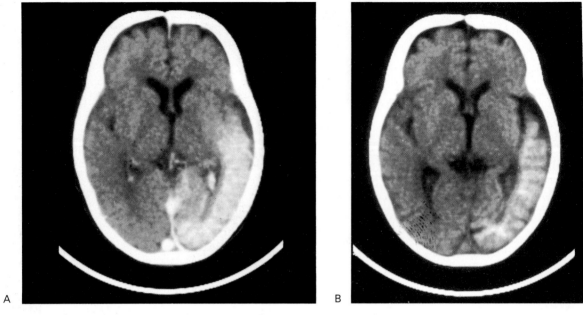

A   B

Fig. 10.35 Sturge–Weber syndrome. (A) Plain scan. (B) Similar section after intravenous contrast medium. In the left temporal and occipital lobes, there is extensive subcortical calcification, which was not visible on SXR. There is left hemiatrophy. Abnormal enhancement is present throughout the temporal and occipital lobes, extending beyond the calcified region and also involving the choroid plexus.

Tuberculomas and other granulomas are usually isodense with brain, but may be of lower density. About 40% show some calcification. There is homogeneous or irregular ring enhancement in the lesions and a variable amount of surrounding oedema, but generally less than with acute inflammatory lesions (Fig. 10.36).

Convulsions are commonly precipitated by cysticerci within the brain parenchyma at the stage when they have died and provoked granuloma formation (Fig. 10.37). Convulsions may continue at a later stage also, when the larva has undergone fibrosis and calcification (see Fig. 10.6). Single enhancing ring or hyperdense lesions with or without surrounding oedema shown within 2 weeks of a seizure and with substantial resolution occurring spontaneously within 8–12 weeks on repeat CT have been described from India. Many of these lesions have proved to be cysticerci (Ahuja et al 1989).

Hydatid cysts commonly present as slow-growing mass lesions, but convulsions occur in about 50% of cases. The CT findings are typical: a large unilocular, well-defined mass of water density, without contrast enhancement or adjacent oedema unless the cyst has ruptured.

Herpes encephalitis causes low density and brain swelling with predilection for the temporal lobes, which is usually evident on CT by the end of the first week of the illness and at an earlier stage on MRI. Focal haemorrhagic changes are not infrequent and patchy enhancement is usual. Early treatment may avoid the extensive brain damage which was frequently associated with considerable and rapidly progressive atrophy. In most other encephalitic illnesses, MRI is the imaging modality of choice; CT may show swelling and/or low brain density but often remains normal throughout the illness (see Fig. 10.38).

Antenatal infection, with toxoplasma, cytomegalic inclusion virus, rubella or herpes simplex, causes necrosis of brain tissue, which may calcify (see Fig. 10.40), and atrophy leading to microcephaly, retardation and epilepsy. Cytomegalic inclusion and, less frequently, rubella cause linear calcification around the margins of the dilated ventricles. In toxoplasmosis similar changes may occur but more often there is nodular and

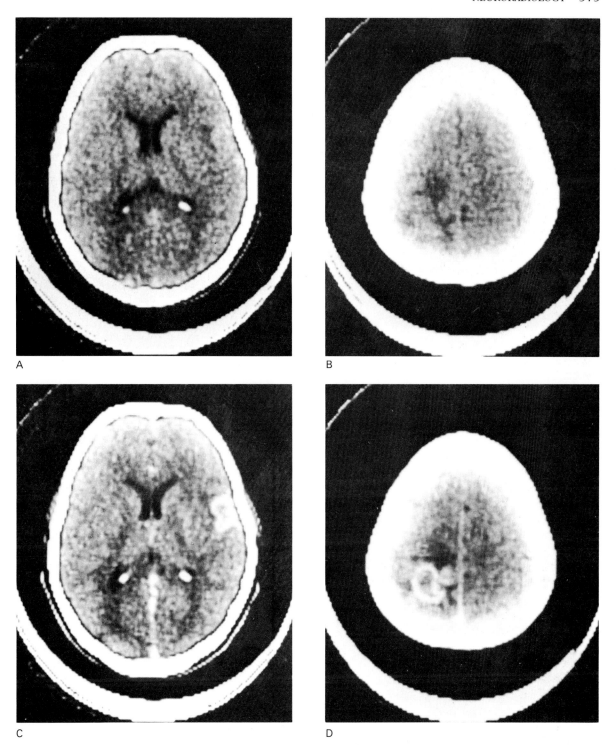

A

B

C

D

Fig. 10.36 Tuberculomas. Plain CT sections, at levels of (A) frontal horns, (B) at the vertex. (C), (D) Same sections after intravenous contrast medium. There are multiple lesions in the right frontotemporal and left parietal regions. Some are isodense with brain and others of slightly higher attenuation; all show enhancement, mostly peripheral, homogeneous in the medial right parietal region. The patient is an Asian with pulmonary tuberculosis and the lesions responded to antituberculous chemotherapy.

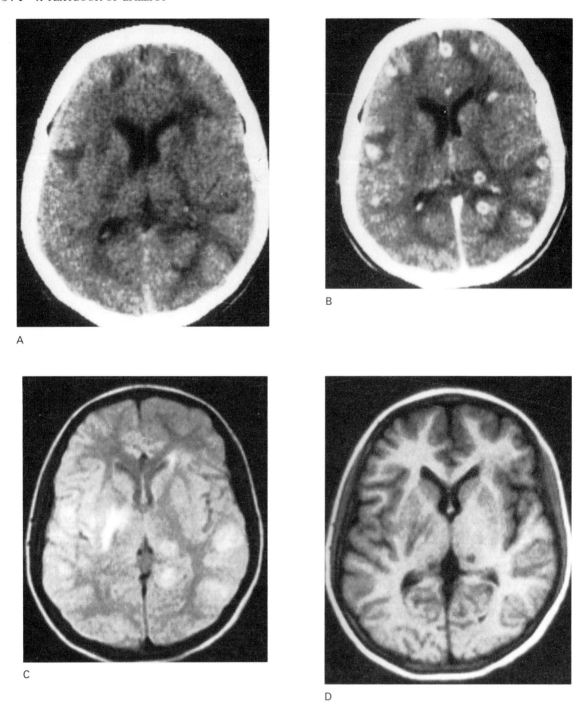

Fig. 10.37 Cysticercosis. CT scan, (A) plain and (B) postcontrast at similar levels. There are multiple low density regions of white matter oedema, and within or impinging on these are isodense nodules in both white and grey matter showing small ring or, occasionally, homogeneous enhancement due to granuloma formation. Some of the isodense nodules contain a high density dot representing the scolex in a cysticercus. MRI, (C) spin echo (TR 1600, TE 60) and (D) inversion recovery (TR 1000, T 1500) sequences. The oedematous regions give high signal in (C) and some of the cysticerci give discrete low signal regions in (D). Rather unusually, the abnormalities on MRI are less extensive than those shown on CT.

curvilinear calcification in brain substance. Necrosis involving the aqueduct may cause hydrocephalus and surface lesions may be associated with subdural effusions resulting in macrocrania.

Carefully performed CT will detect some abnormality in about 98% of supratentorial tumours, infarcts and intracerebral haemorrhages and in most atrophic lesions. In most cases, the nature of the lesion can be suggested and in a considerable proportion its exact pathology can be predicted. In a recent analysis, 6.5% of cases diagnosed as glioma on CT were proven to be benign (Kendall et al 1979); so that whenever CT findings suggest malignancy their compatibility with a benign lesion should always be considered.

MAGNETIC RESONANCE IMAGING

In magnetic resonance, image production is by fourier transformation of spatially encoded signals produced by sensitive nucleons, which have been induced to resonate by the application of radiofrequency pulses.

Certain nucleons, by virtue of their structure, possess a magnetic moment and will therefore gyrate around the axis of a strong external magnetic field with a frequency specific for each type of nucleon. Each gyrating nucleon produces an oscillatory magnetic field and therefore induces a radio signal. If the gyrating nucleons are brought into phase, by absorption of energy induced by the application of a short external radio signal at the specific frequency of the gyrating nucleons, they will produce a recordable evanescent radio signal as they: 1. lose the energy in realigning with the magnetic field and 2. dephase because of variations in the molecular environments of the individual nucleons. The time taken for each of these processes has considerable influence on signal strength. They are referred to as relaxation times and designated T_1 and T_2 respectively.

Signal strength is also particularly influenced by the concentration of sensitive nucleons, movement including bulk flow perfusion and diffusion of the nucleons within or through the magnetic field and strength of the field.

MRI has some major advantages over computer tomography:

1. Ionizing radiation is not involved and, with field strengths of under 2 Tesla, the method appears to lack biological hazard. Ferromagnetic implants or foreign bodies which could move in the high magnetic field, and certain types of pacemaker which are activated in the radiofrequency field, are contraindications. Otherwise MRI can be performed whenever indicated and repeated as often as necessary on clinical criteria alone.

2. Each of the several parameters which influence signal intensity in magnetic resonance can be made the dominant factor, reflected in the contrasting tissues shown in a particular image. Variations of pulse sequence produce a series of images in which differential contrast between normal brain and different pathological processes can be accentuated. Certain lesions commonly isodense with brain on CT and, in a proportion of which CT has been completely normal, can be demonstrated by MRI; amongst these are demyelinating diseases, encephalitis (Fig. 10.38), including both direct infection, as in subacute sclerosing panencephalitis, and postinfective demyelination, ischaemic lesions, low-grade gliomas (Brant Zawadski et al, 1983) and late temporal lobe damage following radiation therapy (Lee et al 1990). In one study (Laster et al 1985) of 34 patients with complex partial seizures of more than 5 years duration, in which pre- and post-infusion CT scans were negative, MRI revealed focal structural temporal lobe lesions of potential surgical therapeutic significance in four cases (11.7%); a cryptic arteriovenous malformation and a glioma were excised from two of these. The not uncommon declaration of a progressive organic lesion on a follow-up CT scan in patients with previously CT negative focal epilepsy (Young et al 1982) clearly implied an indication for MRI in such cases and has been rewarded by the detection of mesial temporal sclerosis (Fig. 10.39), occult tumours and cryptic angiomas (Brooks et al 1990, Jackson et al 1990). In partial epilepsy of childhood MRI not only demonstrates the lesions shown by CT but also abnormalities in more than one-third of cases which are not visible on CT. These include more or less symmetrical high signal areas on T_2 weighted sequences in the peritrigonal white matter; the significance of these abnormalities is uncertain (Peretti et al 1989).

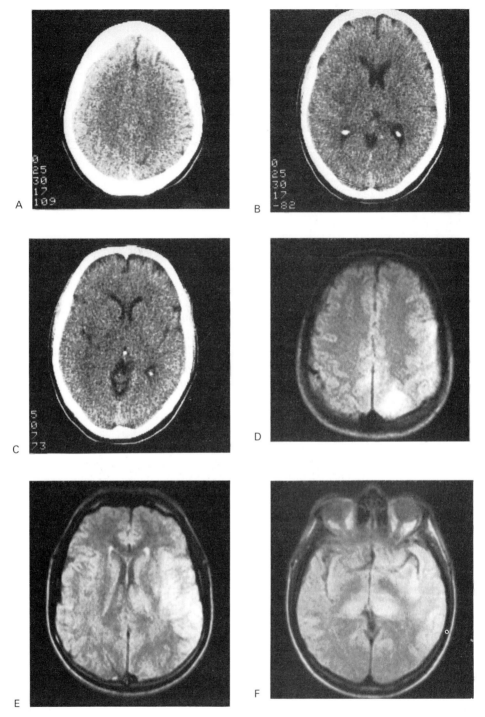

Fig. 10.38 Encephalitis. CT scan. (A)–(C) Serial sections. There is a minor degree of swelling of the left cerebral hemisphere (reader's left) with compression of the left lateral ventricle and cortical sulci. No focal abnormality. There was no abnormal enhancement. MRI. (D)–(F) similar sections; spin echo sequence. The left hemisphere (reader's right) swelling is evident and there is increased signal from the left thalamus, occipital lobe and left temporal and parietal cortex.

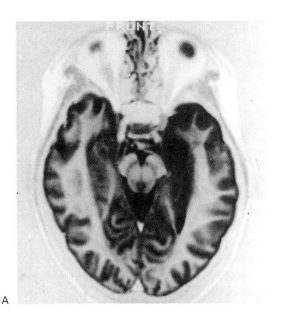

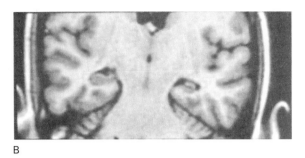

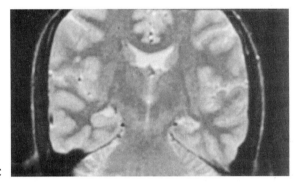

Fig. 10.39 Left mesial temporal sclerosis. (A) Axial. (B) Coronal. (T_1 weighted) sequences. There is atrophy of the left hippocampal formation with some dilatation of the left temporal horn. (C) Coronal T_2 weighted sequence. High signal return from left hippocampus.

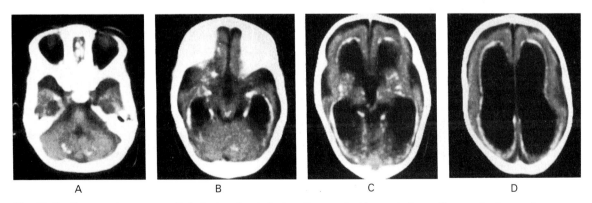

Fig. 10.40 Intra-uterine cytomegalic inclusion virus infection. Presented with retardation, epilepsy and microcrania. (A)–(D) Plain CT scan sections. There is irregular calcification, mainly around the dilated lateral and third ventricles but also within the brain substance. The cerebral mantle is narrow, the subarachnoid space is wide and the vault is thick due to atrophy.

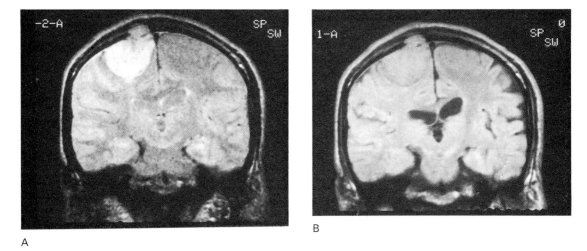

Fig. 10.41 Parasagittal meningioma. Coronal spin echo sequence. (A) TR 2000, TE 27. (B) TN 2000 TE 70. The extra-axial parasagittal mass is of similar intensity to grey matter on the short echo sequence but hyperintense in the long echo sequence on which a thin rim of cortex can be seen depressed under the tumour. The tumour erodes into the skull vault. Its medial edge lies against the falx and the sagittal sinus. However there is no evidence of invasion of the sinus which is outlined by the low signal of flowing blood.

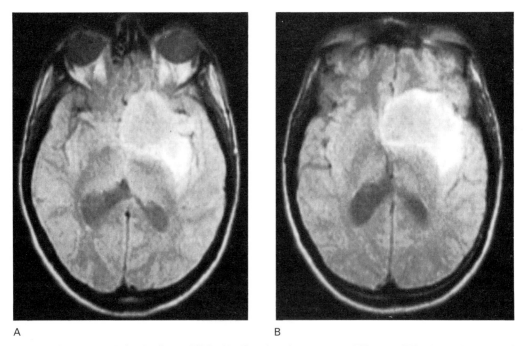

Fig. 10.42 Deep frontal-hypothalamic glioma. MRI, (A)–(C) spin echo sequences (TR 1500, TE 60), contiguous sections. The tumour gives rise to a high signal. Involvement of the deep frontal region and hypothalamus is evident and the tumour extends across the midline. Precise relationship to the Sylvian fissure is difficult to assess in these sections. (D)–(F) Inversion recovery sequence (TR 2100, T 1500), contiguous coronal sections. The upper border of the tumour extends up to the frontal horn and the lower margin extends across the Sylvian fissure, to involve the superior temporal white matter and hippocampal gyrus.

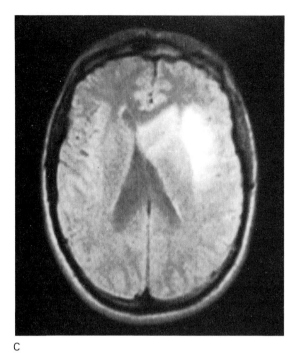

C

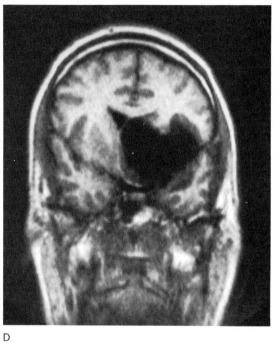

D

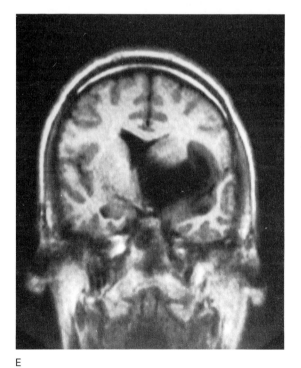

E

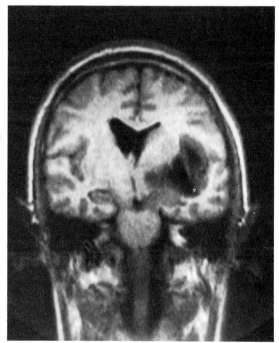

F

Fig. 10.42 (contd)

Magnetic resonance imaging generally shows the pathological processes revealed by CT to be more extensive (Fig. 10.40) and significant differences in internal structure of lesions may be more clearly defined on some of the MRI sequences.

3. The image plane in MRI, being determined electronically, is unrestricted by the mechanical constraints which influence computed tomography. For practical purposes, sagittal images can only be produced on CT by computer reformatting of multiple thin sections made in an accessible plane, a process which is accompanied by some loss of resolution and is also distorted by any patient movement; vertical plane images are particularly valuable in assessing the brainstem, high convexity (Fig. 10.41) and parasagittal regions, relationship of abnormalities to the Sylvian fissure (Fig. 10.42) and transcallosal extension of tumour. Imaging along and perpendicular to the axis of the temporal horn in the coronal plane, using an anatomy-sensitive heavily T_1 weighted sequence, has proved effective in detection of hippocampal atrophy which is the cardinal feature of medial temporal sclerosis (MTS) (Jackson et al 1990), though high signal return from the damaged grey matter on T_2 W sequences provides confirmatory evidence. Volume acquisition is even more useful for more exact volumetric assessment (Jack et al 1990): from the data thus acquired very thin sections (1.0–1.5 mm), can be formed in any plane and very exact estimates of the volume of grey matter in the hippocampus (or any other structure which can be defined anatomically) can be achieved.

4. Bone-induced artifacts limit the value of CT, especially for the diagnosis of small lesions adjacent to the skull base.

Complex partial seizures are the most common adult form of epilepsy. In two-thirds of these patients the focus of origin is in the temporal lobe and it is often small. The mode of acquisition of MRI and the lack of signal from cortical bone has made it particularly valuable for detection of such lesions adjacent to the floor of the middle

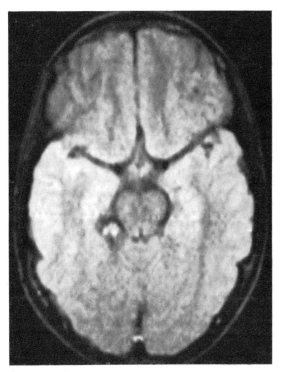

A

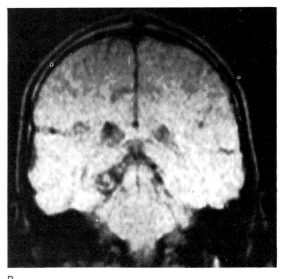

B

Fig. 10.43 Hamartoma. MRI. (A) Axial; spin echo sequence. High signal mass protruding from medial surface of right temporal lobe. (B) Coronal; inversion recovery sequence. The relation of hamartoma to medial surface of temporal lobe and upper border of tentorium is shown.

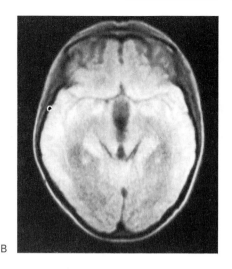

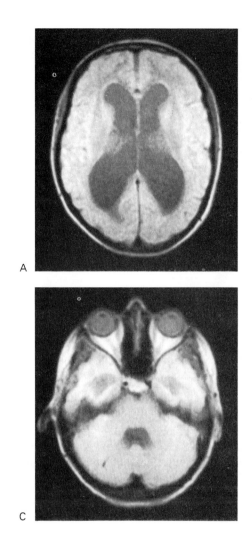

Fig. 10.44 Hydrocephalus. MRI. (A)–(C) Axial sections, spin echo sequence. Communicating hydrocephalus. There is enlargement of the whole ventricular system and of the basal cisterns. There is slightly increased signal around the ventricles due to transependymal passage of fluid into the adjacent brain substance.

fossa (Fig. 10.43) (Young et al 1983). Most other complex partial seizures arise from the frontal lobes. Here the causative lesions detected tend to be larger but even so, atrophy, dysplastic cortex (see Fig. 10.29) and gliosis are generally more effectively demonstrated by MRI than by CT. The detail of the cortical ribbon which can be achieved with modern MRT rivals that of anatomical sections. Subtle abnormalities may be revealed which have potential significance but may be difficult or impossible to detect by visual inspection. The cortical white matter interface of the frontal lobes are well suited to fractal analysis (Lancet anonymous editorial, 1991), and this method has been shown to have considerable diagnostic significance, particularly in frontal lobe

seizures due to cortical dysplasia and migrational abnormalities (Cooke et al).

The very long T_1 of normal cerebrospinal fluid (CSF) can be used to delineate clearly the margins of the subarachnoid space and ventricles. The higher water content of the grey matter is associated with prolongation of T_1 relative to that of white matter; grey matter therefore gives a relatively lower signal when a short pulse repetition time is used and the intensity increases and eventually exceeds that from white matter as the repetition time is increased. The clear delineation of the cerebrospinal spaces (Fig. 10.44) and of the white and grey matter facilitates localization of intra-axial, extra-axial (see Fig. 10.41) and intraventricular masses. The change in signal

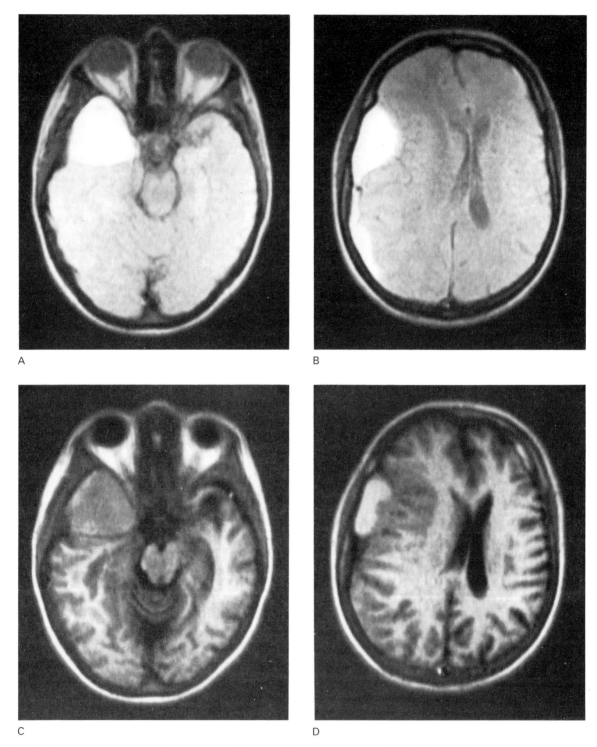

Fig. 10.45 Arachnoid cyst, with haemorrhage. MRI. (A), (B) Spin echo sequence (TR 1000, TE 60) axial sections, and (C), (D) inversion recovery sequence (TR 2000, TE 1500) similar sections. The high signal from the fluid over the convexity in (D) and the slightly higher signal than cerebrospinal fluid (C) is due to the short T_1 relaxation induced by break down products of blood in this distribution.

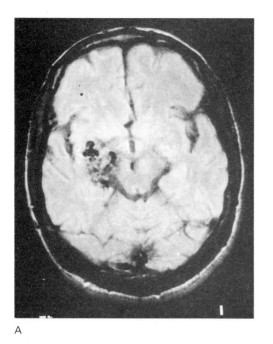

A

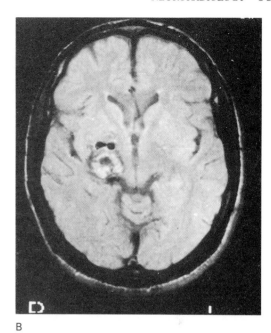

B

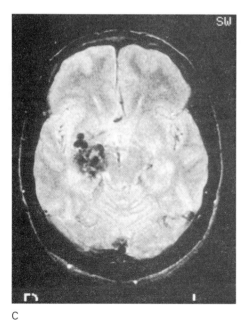

C

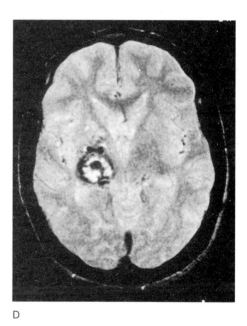

D

Fig. 10.46   Angiomatous malformation. MRI axial sections, spin echo sequences: (A) and (B) TR 2000, TE 27, (C) and (D) corresponding levels, TR 2000, TE 70. Note absence of signal from flowing blood outlining the large abnormal vessels. This is evident on all images but more prominent in the short echo sequence. An old haemorrhage from the posterior part of the lesion has resulted in peripheral haemosiderin deposition which is causing low signal on the long echo sequence, best shown in (D). Inside this there is a thicker ring of high signal due to methaemoglobin from more recent blood clot.

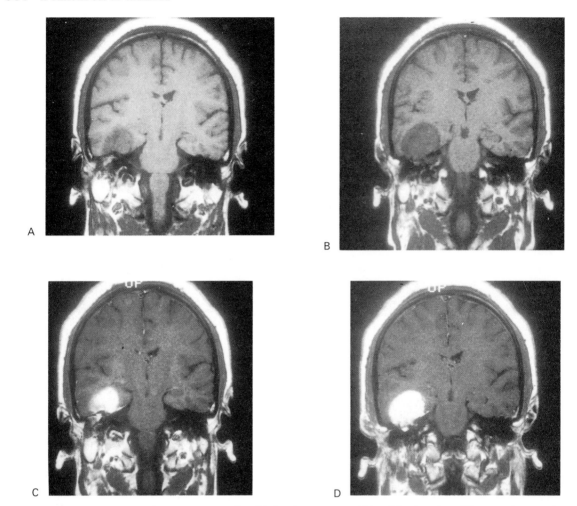

Fig. 10.47   Seventh cranial nerve neuroma. (A), (B) Contiguous coronal T_1 weighted sections. There is a low signal mass involving the right temporal lobe and eroding the floor of the middle fossa. (C), (D) Similar sections after intravenous GdDTPA. The mass is now of high signal due to marked enhancement. Part of the tumour is within the petrous bone and the enhancement of this component corresponds to a thickened genu of the VIIth nerve.

induced by blood flow allows flow-dependent sequences to be formulated for visualization of the major blood vessels. This is a further facility in aiding localization of intra- and extra-axial masses and defining relationships of critical structures.

In general, the most significant information from MRI has been the precise anatomical distribution of pathology. Tissue specific characterization is much less common, as might be expected, since increase in water content in general causes prolongation of the T_1 and T_2 relaxation time regardless of whether it is caused by oedema, infarction, encephalitis or demyelination. The paramagnetic effects of extracellular iron in methaemoglobin from lysed red blood cells in subacute and chronic haematomas (Figs 10.45 and 10.46), and of melanin in melanoma metastases, are manifested in short T_1 relaxation; and triglyceride fat in lipomas and teratomas, as well as in subcutaneous and intermuscular fat planes, is also characterized by a very short T_1 relaxation time. Low signal on T_2 weighted images results from local shortening of the T_2 relaxation time caused by paramagnetic products of haemoglobin retained within cells. Such products include deoxyhaemoglobin, ferritin and haemosiderin (Fig. 10.46). The lack of signal from rapidly flowing blood and increasing signal with turbulence

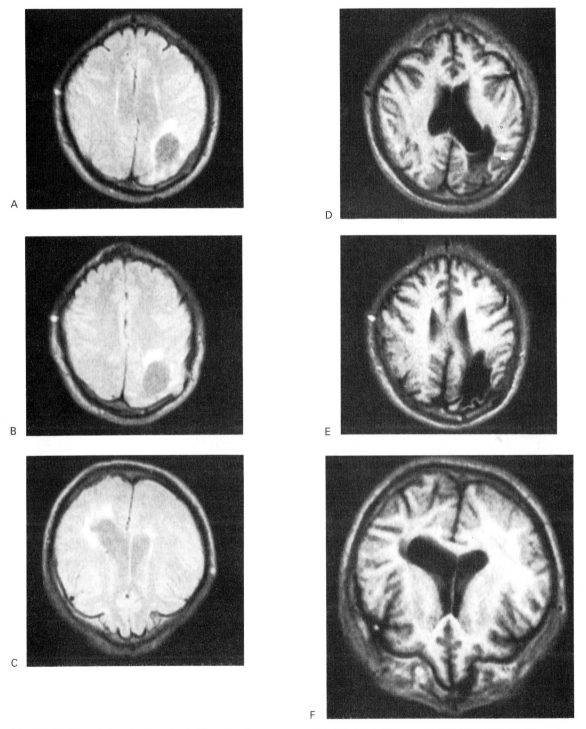

Fig. 10.48 Encephalomalacic cavity. MRI, spin echo sequences. (A), (B) Axial, (C) coronal (TR 1500, TE 60). There is a region of diminished signal intensity, similar to that of the cerebrospinal fluid, within the left parietal lobe, with some surrounding high signal from damaged brain substance. (D)–(F) Inversion recovery sequence (TR 2100, TE 500) similar sections. The myelomalacic cavity, with the dilated trigone extending towards it, is well defined on this sequence and, again, gives a similar signal to the ventricular cerebrospinal fluid.

and slow flow clearly delineates and specifically characterizes aneurysms and angiomatous mal-formations and their connecting vessels when flow-dependent sequences are used (Fig. 10.46).

The lack of clear demarcation between some tumour margins and adjacent brain or surround-ing oedema has proved to be a limitation of MRI. This has been a feature of some metastases, infiltrating malignant gliomas, haemangioblastomas and meningiomas. Certain paramagnetic ions, of which gadolinium (Gd) is currently the most suitable, can be administered in biocompatible compounds such as DTPA, which render them among the safest of contrast media, anaphylactic reactions occurring at the rate of less than 1/100 000 injections. These are, for practical con-siderations, retained within the normal blood–brain barrier but they penetrate the disrupted barrier in damaged brain tissue and through the permeable capillaries of tumours and granulation tissue, in a very similar fashion to iodide contrast media used in CT and technetium DTPA used in radionucleide studies (Carr et al 1984). The para-magnetic agents shorten T_1 relaxation time and thus enhance contrast on T_1 weighted sequences (Fig. 10.47); not only is the tumour demarcated but details of its structure tend to be better defined.

Loculated CSF, as within arachnoid cysts or porencephaly (Fig. 10.48), is distinguished by signal intensities close to those of the rest of the cerebrospinal fluid. The T_1 relaxation time shortens when protein concentration is increased (Brant Zawadski et al 1985), as within cystic or necrotic regions of tumours, though it is still generally longer than that of the solid tissues. Haemorrhagic changes may be suggested by re-latively short T_1 or T_2 relaxation times (see Figs 10.45 and 10.46) causing high or low signal on T_1 and T_2 weighted sequences respectively.

Heavy calcification gives no signal on MRI and may be suspected for this very reason on a combi-nation of T_1 and T_2 weighted images. However, calcification, hyperostosis and bone erosion are, in general, better revealed by CT, at least in the supratentorial compartment.

If no abnormality is shown on computed tomography or magnetic resonance imaging, it is unlikely that other investigations will show a significant lesion in patients suffering from well-controlled epilepsy and no other symptoms.

POSITRON EMISSION TOMOGRAPHY (PET)

This is a high-cost technique currently requiring a specialist operated cyclotron for the production of the so-called physiological radionucleides, in-cluding $O_2 15$ (2.1 min half-life), N13 (10 min half-life), C11 (20.1 min half-life) and F18 (110 min half-life). PET measures tomographically the uptake and distribution of these tracers in vivo and thus allows investigation of some of the biochemical processes essential to life, utilizing chemical amounts small enough not to perturb the phenomena being studied. The response within the tomograms is quantitative, reflecting absolute units of tracer concentration, enabling the method to be used for the absolute measurement of re-gional cerebral blood flow, oxygen and glucose utilization, amino acid synthesis, amine neuro-transmitter metabolism and blood volume estima-tion. Such measurements have been used in the study of focal pathophysiology in epilepsy, psy-chosis, glioma and cerebrovascular disease amongst other pathologies.

Metabolic studies in epileptic patients have been mainly performed using fluorodeoxyglucose. These have shown diminished glucose metabo-lism in the region of a discrete focus, which gener-ally includes, but tends to be more extensive than, any structural changes shown by histopathological examination of resected tissue (Engel et al 1982a). Sperling et al (1986) reported hypometabolism on PET studies in 18 cases of histologically proven mesial temporal sclerosis with normal MRI and in another small recent study involving 15 cases subjected to temporal lobectomy (Heinz et al 1990b) PET was significantly more accurate (74%) than MRI (48%) in detecting temporal lobe epileptic foci. These were mainly caused by mesial temporal sclerosis and it should be noted that the detection rate of MRI was unusually low in this series.

Multifocal and diffuse EEG changes are asso-ciated with a corresponding distribution of hypo-metabolism (Engel et al 1982b). In a few patients, diminished regional cerebral blood flow and cerebral metabolic rate for oxygen has been demonstrated on the side of the focus, mainly in the temporal lobes and basal ganglia (Kuhl et al 1980). Similarly reduction of 99mTc HMPAO uptake (Smith et al 1989) and changes in blood flow using 133-Xenon (Chiron et al 1989) have been shown using SPECT scanning. The focus also demonstrates diminution in the stimulus-induced metabolic response to glucose metabolism. During an ictus hypermetabolism and hyperfusion in combination with EEG abnormalities may provide useful identification of the site of the focus for surgical excision.

PET has demonstrated very variable levels of blood flow and glucose metabolic rate in middle grade and malignant gliomas, but the mean lies close to that of the corresponding contralateral brain substance: in high grade gliomas, because of the anaerobic pattern of metabolism of glucose by these tumours, there is consistent, marked reduction in oxygen extraction (Ito et al 1982, Rhodes et al 1983). This feature may be useful in cases in which distinction between intrinsic tumour and acute infarction is required immediately and where more simple tests have failed to elucidate. In the acute ischaemic lesion, blood flow may be reduced but oxygen extraction is increased up to 90% (normal 40–50%) per passage, indicating survival, by utilization of the normal reserve in oxygen carriage, of some cerebral tissue within the infarct. After about a week, this uncoupling of flow and metabolism may be reversed as perfusion is re-established: the reduced oxygen extraction is accompanied by increased glucose utilization related to glycolytic activity of infiltrating white cells (Wise et al 1984). After about a month, blood flow and metabolic rate of oxygen are reduced but coupling is restored (Lenzi et al 1982). In some patients with clinically transient cerebral ischaemia, cerebral vasodilatation, as shown by increase in cerebral blood volume relative to flow or focally reduced blood flow associated with increased oxygen extraction, is observed (Gibbs et al 1984) indicating chronic ischaemia.

In low grade astrocytomas glucose consumption is usually decreased, but 11C-L-methionine uptake is increased in both low and high-grade gliomas and distinguishes the tumour tissue from oedema (Bergstrom et al 1983).

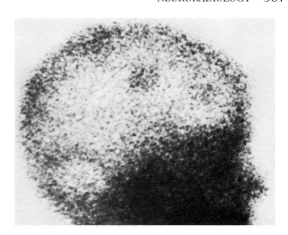

Fig. 10.49 Metastases. Gamma encephalogram. Right lateral.

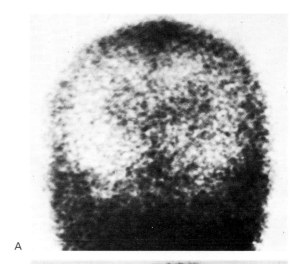

A

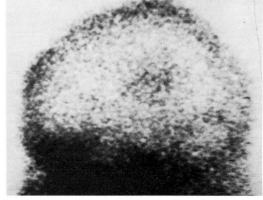

B

Fig. 10.50 Glioma of the corpus callosum. Gamma encephalogram. (A) Anteroposterior, (B) lateral views. There is bilateral parietal uptake, more extensive on the left, joined across the midline.

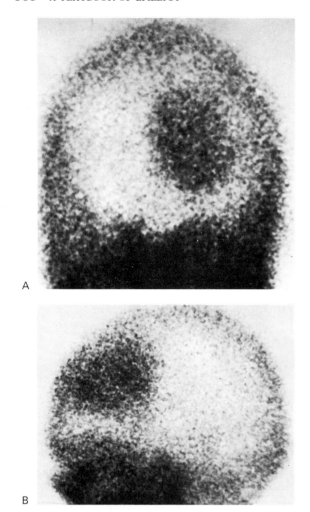

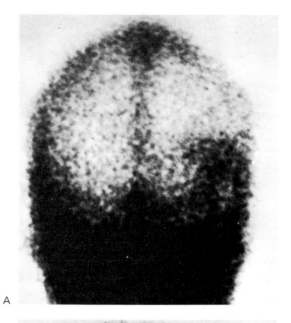

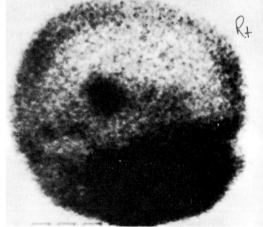

Fig. 10.51 Meningioma. Gamma encephalogram.
(A) Anterior, (B) left lateral views. There is a peripheral area
of dense increased uptake in the frontal region.

Fig. 10.52 Angiomatous malformation. Gamma
encephalogram. (A) anterior view, (B) right lateral view,
taken immediately after injection of isotope. There is marked
increased density in the angiomatous malformation; increased
uptake is shown extending from it in the draining veins.

Radiation necrosis and recurrent high grade glioma may give markedly similar appearances on both MRI and CT scanning. However, high grade glioma is hypermetabolic for glucose and postirradiation necrosis is hypometabolic; PET scanning has proved useful in distinguishing between the two conditions in a number of cases.

ISOTOPE ENCEPHALOGRAPHY

Computed tomography or MRI give more exact localization and more specific information in a much wider range of conditions than does isotope encephalography. Also, CT is a simpler routine

procedure than detailed gamma encephalography performed over a period of hours. Consequently the latter has been replaced, and only when CT and MRI are not available is isotope encephalography ever used as a screening test for those important conditions in which isotope uptake is usually increased.

Most departments use a simple technique, employing a modern gamma camera and the isotope 99mTc, which has the advantages of easy standardization and availability with a half-life of 6 hours, in combination with DTPA (TcDTPA) so that it is retained within the normal blood–brain barrier. Both lateral, anterior and posterior views are necessary to obtain images in both planes of all regions of the brain, and for scanning purposes these are commonly taken at about 30 minutes after intravenous injection of the isotope. Abnormal uptake occurs in lesions lacking a normal blood–brain barrier and is recognized in virtually all abscesses, in over 90% of meningiomas and malignant gliomas, 85% of metastases and about 30% of benign gliomas. Abnormal uptake is not usually detected until lesions reach a critical size of about 2 cm and they may be obscured by superimposition of the normal uptake in large venous sinuses, mucous membrane and the large muscles attached to the skull base.

In most cases the appearance of the uptake is non-specific but consideration of intensity, size, shape and position can be suggestive of a particular pathology. Multiple areas of uptake in patients with a known primary neoplasm are virtually diagnostic of metastases (Fig. 10.49), although abscesses and infarcts can also be multiple. The butterfly distribution of a corpus callosum glioma (Fig. 10.50) and diffuse peripheral uptake in a subdural haematoma are suggestive of these diagnoses. High intensity, well-demarcated uptake in a peripheral site is usual in meningiomas (Fig. 10.51); the diagnosis may be confirmed by plain film changes.

Rapid serial filming immediately after injection of TcDTPA may give further information about the nature of the lesions. Angiomatous malformations show very early (Fig. 10.52) and fade quickly as the isotope is rapidly carried into the veins. Sometimes an irregular serpiginous shape, giving a vague outline of the vascular pattern of the malformation, is evident. Very vascular tumours, such as some meningiomas, also show early uptake, but this increases and is retained as the circulation clears. Malignant gliomas and some metastases have a slower build-up of uptake through the capillary and venous stages of transit, which then persists. Most metastases are not shown until 40–70 seconds after the injection and then progressively retain more of the isotope.

In gliomas and metastases the ratio of uptake between abnormal and normal tissues increases up to about 4 hours after injection.

Isotope accumulates in infarcts and haemorrhages when cellular reaction is occurring about 7–10 days from their onset and it persists for several weeks or even months, gradually diminishing.

It should be noted that occasionally abnormal uptake is found after repeated focal seizures in the absence of any demonstrable pathology. It is presumably due to alteration in the blood–brain barrier since it returns to normal on subsequent examinations.

Though a positive gamma encephalogram alone, or considered with plain film studies, may give sufficient information for management, in most cases, other studies are necessary to decide the diagnosis or confirm that biopsy is necessary. A negative gamma encephalogram is of no value since many of the more benign gliomas and virtually all the atrophic processes will not be revealed.

CONTRAST STUDIES

Pneumoencephalography is now obsolete. It was an uncomfortable and potentially harmful procedure: in general, the information gained was limited and based on indirect or secondary effects on the CSF spaces. A more specific indication of the nature of a mass was evident only when it was situated within or encroached upon one or more CSF spaces (Fig. 10.53): this is in contrast with CT or MRI, by which most lesions are themselves revealed. Atrophy, both focal and general, was apparent on pneumoencephalograms and sufficient information for clinical management was frequently achieved. This applied, for example, in mesial temporal sclerosis, (Sumie et al, 1978), even though the structure of the hippocampus itself was not shown as it is using MRI. The use of cerebral angiography has diminished; as noninvasive studies are more accurate in the diagnosis and exclusion of structural lesions associated with epilepsy, angiography is inappropriate for this purpose, particularly if CT or MRI is negative.

With modern facilities and skilled technique selective angiography still carries a risk of inducing permanent neurological deficit of about 0.2%. If

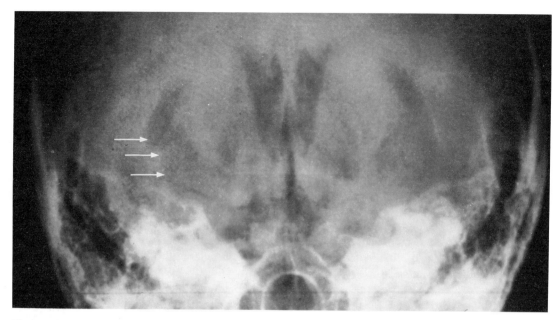

Fig. 10.53   Astrocytoma. Air encephalogram, brow-up Towne's projection. The tip of the right temporal horn is dilated and there is an irregular filling defect in its lateral part (arrows). The anterior half of the right temporal lobe was resected and contained a Grade II astrocytoma.

the information required concerns the detection of atheroma in the large cervical arteries or of major cerebral venous or sinus occlusive disease, this can be obtained by MRI using flow sensitive sequences or, without risk of arterial catheterization and at reduced cost, by using good quality intravenous digital subtraction angiography (Takahashi et al 1983).

Cerebral angiography and vascular imaging

The localization of an intracranial mass may be evident from the stretching and splaying of cerebral vessels around the periphery of the swelling (Fig. 10.54). The gyral pattern may be distorted and the circulation locally delayed in the region of the mass. Intracerebral masses which compress the surface vessels towards the skull may be distinguished from extra-axial masses which displace the vessels away from it.

The nature of a lesion may be suspected from changes in vessel structure evident on the angiogram. The vascular bed of a tumour may show an abnormal pattern. This tends to be more florid in malignant tumours (Fig. 10.55), in which some vessels are sinusoids lined by tumour cells,

through which arteriovenous shunting occurs; irregular dilatations may be formed in regions of tumour necrosis. This pattern is most usual in anaplastic primary brain tumours, occurring in about half of malignant gliomas, but is also present in some metastases. Less often, malignant tumours have fine, irregular vessels or a capillary blush which tends to be patchy in gliomas and more homogeneous in metastases; necrotic and cystic parts of tumours are avascular and residual vascularized tissue may form an irregular ring around them.

The vasculature of benign tumours tends to have a radiating or reticular basis with distal tapering, like that of normal tissues. When vascularity is increased, as is typical of most meningiomas, the capillary circulation may show as a prolonged blush. In about half the malignant and a greater proportion of more benign intracerebral tumours, vascular changes are absent or minor and non-specific.

Extracerebral tumours, especially meningiomas (Fig. 10.56), usually obtain a blood supply from meningeal arteries which often become enlarged and tortuous. This is not a pathognomonic feature, since intracerebral masses which invade or

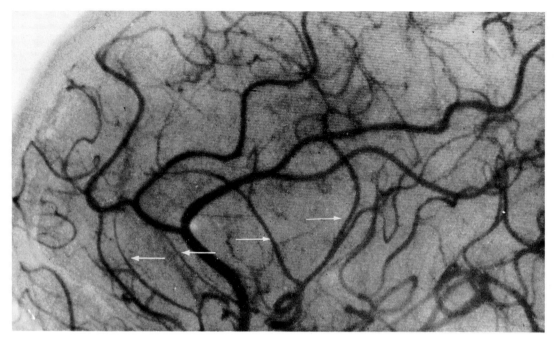

Fig. 10.54 Astrocytoma. Left internal carotid angiogram, lateral projection. Ascending frontal branches of the middle cerebral artery (arrows) are splayed apart due to a sub-adjacent swelling, without positive angiographic evidence of its nature. It proved at surgery to be a solid astrocytoma.

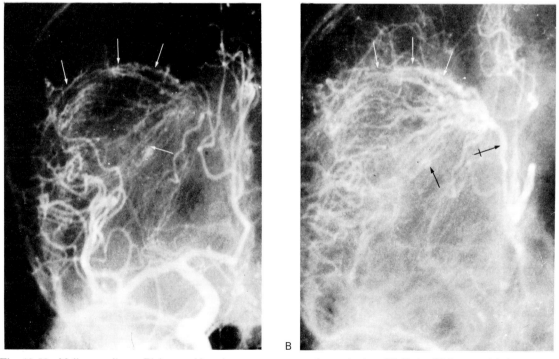

A   B

Fig. 10.55 Malignant glioma. Right carotid angiogram, anteroposterior projection. (A) Early, (B) late arterial phases. There is displacement of the anterior cerebral artery and of the internal cerebral vein to the left. Pathological vessels (arrow) are shown extending from the cortical branches of the middle cerebral artery medially through the white matter to drain into the thalamostriate vein (crossed arrow). The appearances are typical of a malignant glioma.

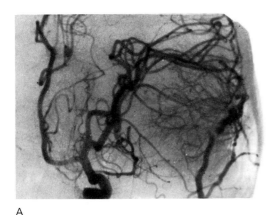

A

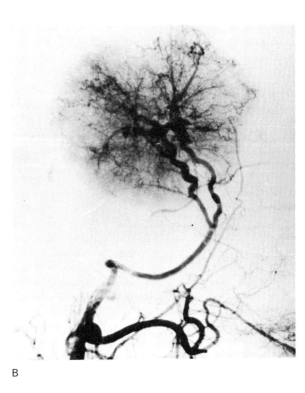

Fig. 10.56 Meningioma. (A) Left common carotid angiogram, anteroposterior projection. The trunk of the middle cerebral artery is elevated. Its branches over the insula are displaced medially and those in the lateral ramus of the Sylvian fissure are elevated and splayed apart by an extracerebral mass which is supplied with a rich abnormal circulation from the middle meningeal artery. (B) Left external carotid angiogram, lateral projection. The middle meningeal artery is enlarged. It gives a large number of small branches radiating from the point of attachment to supply and delineate the meningioma with a capillary blush.

B

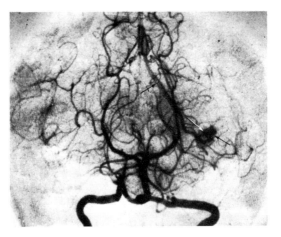

Fig. 10.57 Angiomatous malformation. Vertebral angiogram, arterial phase, anteroposterior projection. Small angiomatous malformation lying medially in the anterior part of the left temporal lobe (arrows), with early drainage to the basal vein (crossed arrow).

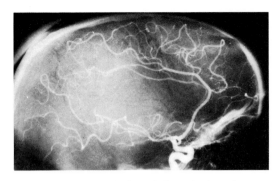

Fig. 10.58   Middle cerebral cortical arteries branch occlusion. Female, aged 55, who presented with left-sided focal fits of recent onset. Right carotid angiogram, arterial phase, lateral projection. There is marked delay of filling of the ascending frontal and anterior parietal branches of the middle cerebral artery.

adhere to the dura may acquire a meningeal supply, though it is usually less pronounced than in meningiomas. Such intracerebral lesions may be recognized with certainty when they receive blood from penetrating arteries or drain to subependymal veins.

The capsule of an intracerebral abscess contains small vessels which may be seen as a ring-like blush. As in any system lacking normal arteriolar resistance, arteriovenous shunting may occur in the capsule.

Arteriovenous malformations (Fig. 10.57) and occlusions of moderate-sized vessels (Fig. 10.58), which are not infrequent causes of focal epilepsy, are shown directly.

It has been emphasized that CT or MRI frequently give sufficient information for management or even suggest a specific diagnosis. Virtually all tumours, infarcts and haemorrhages, and most inflammatory lesions, are recognized; and, in some cases, where swelling is slight or absent, a lesion is obvious when angiography reveals either minimal non-specific changes or is normal. The nature of avascular masses with no evidence of the type of the pathology on angiography may also be resolved by CT or MRI. Ambiguous findings on CT or MRI are sometimes resolved by angiography but, overall, it provides positive evidence of the nature of the pathological process in only about 30% of the unusual cases in which

an equivocal or inaccurate diagnosis of glioma is suggested from CT appearances.

Some information considered helpful for planning surgery could until recently be obtained by no other method than angiography. MRI is now capable of fulfilling this role. For example, the relationship of major blood vessels to a lesion, including the presence or absence of tumour cuffing, or of invasion of the venous sinuses by meningioma may be shown by either modality. When CT reveals a small infarct or focal atrophy, especially in a middle-aged or elderly patient with sudden onset of seizures, digital angiography or flow sensitive sequences on MRI of the appropriate neck vessels may reveal a significant ulcerating or stenosing atheromatous plaque. Focal atrophy may also be caused by an arteriovenous malformation: even if small, this will almost always produce a diagnostic abnormality on the non-invasive studies but may require elucidation by angiography.

When CT and MRI are not available, the role of angiography is extended. Abnormal uptake shown on isotope encephalography is often non-specific and angiography of the appropriate vessel may be helpful in deciding the nature of the pathological process or underlying lesion. When isotope encephalography is negative and there are unexplained focal features, appropriate angiograms should be performed. Unexplained raised intracranial pressure may be elucidated by non-dominant carotid angiography—vessel displacement may indicate a supratentorial mass: the subependymal veins outline the size of the lateral ventricles and deformity of the deep veins may provide a useful indicator of the cause of hydrocephalus. Venous occlusion may be recognized, either directly or by slowing of venous flow towards the obstructed region and filling of collateral veins.

Following focal status epilepticus, capillary dilatation may temporarily occur in the affected region of the brain. Rarely, this may be shown as a blush or be associated with early venous filling on angiography: failure to consider this possibility may lead to an erroneous diagnosis of significant pathology.

REFERENCES

Ahuja G K, Behari M, Prasad K, Goulatia R K, Jailkhani Bansi 1989 Disappearing CT lesions in epilepsy: is tuberculosis or cysticercosis the cause? Journal of Neurology, Neurosurgery and Psychiatry 52: 915–916

Anonymous 1991 Fractals and medicine (Editorial) Lancet 338: 1425–1426

Bachman D S, Hodges F H, Freeman J M 1976 Computerised axial tomography in chronic seizure disorders of childhood. Pediatrics 58: 828–832

Bergstrom M, Collins V P, Ehrin E et al 1983 Discrepancies in brain tumour extent as shown by computed tomography and positron emission tomography using 68Ga-EDTA, 11C-glucose and 11C-methionine. Case report. Journal of Computer Assisted Tomography 7: 1062–1066

Bogdanoff B M, Stafford C R, Green L, Gonzalez C F 1975 Computerized axial tomography in the evaluation of patients with epilepsy. Neurology 25: 1013–1017

Brant Zawadski M B, Davis P L, Crooks L E et al 1983 NMR demonstration of cerebral abnormalities: Comparison with CT. American Journal of Neuroradiology 4: 117–124

Brant Zawadski M, Kelly W, Kjos B et al 1985 Magnetic resonance imaging and characterisation of normal and abnormal intracranial cerebrospinal fluid (CSF) spaces. Neuroradiology 27: 3–8

Brooks B S, King D W, El Gammal T et al 1990 MR Imaging in patients with intractable complex partial seizures. American Journal of Neuroradiology 11: 93–99

Carr D H, Brown J, Bydder G M et al 1984 Intravenous chelated gadolinium as a contrast agent in NMR imaging of cerebral tumours. Lancet i: 484–486

Chiron C, Raynaud C, Dulac O, Tzvurio N, Plouin P, Tran-Dinh S 1989 Study of cerebral blood flow in partial epilepsy of childhood using the Spect method. Journal of Neuroradiology 16: 317–324

Collard M, Dupont H, Noel G 1976 Summary: computerized transverse axial tomography in epilepsy. Epilepsia 17: 339–340

Cook M, Free S, Manford M et al 1992 Fractal description of normal and abnormal cerebral cortex abstracts of proceedings of the Society of Magnetic Resonance in Medicine, Berlin

Dellaportas G I, Dawson J M, Reynolds E H 1982 Computerised tomography in new referrals with epilepsy. British Journal of Clinical Practice Suppl 18: 201–203

Engel J Jr, Brown W J, Kuhl D E, Phelps M E, Mazziotta J C, Crandall P H 1982a Pathological findings underlying focal temporal lobe hypometabolism in partial epilepsy. Annals of Neurology 12: 518–528

Engel J Jr, Kuhl D E, Phelps M E, Mazziotta J C 1982b Interictal cerebral glucose metabolism in partial epilepsy and its relation to EEG changes. Annals of Neurology 12: 510–517

Falconer M A, Serafetinides E A 1963 A follow up study in temporal lobe epilepsy. Journal of Neurology, Neurosurgery and Psychiatry 26: 154

Gastaut H, Gastaut J L 1976 Computerised transverse axial tomography in epilepsy. Epilepsia 17: 325–336

Gibbs J M, Wise R J S, Leonders K L, Jones T 1984 Evaluation of cerebral perfusion reserve in patients with carotid artery occlusion. Lancet i: 310–314

Gilsanz V, Strand R, Barnes P, Nealis J 1979 Results of presumed cryptogenic epilepsy in childhood by CT scanning. Annals of Radiology 22: 184–187

Gold L H A, Kieffer S A, Petersonn H O 1969 Intracranial meningiomas. A retrospective analysis of the diagnostic value of plain skull films. Neurology 19: 873–878

Heinz E R, Crain B S, Radtke R A et al 1990a MR imaging in patients with temporal lobe seizures. American Journal of Neuroradiology 11: 827–832

Heinz E R, Radtke R, Hoffman J, Henson M, Protger W 1990b Comparison of MR and PET imaging in temporal lobe epilepsy. Symposium Neuroradiologicum Abstract Proceedings

Hillemacher A 1982 Der wert amnetischer und klinischer Daten sowie apparativer Intersuchungsbefunde bei der Diagnose von Hirntumoren. Fortschritte der Neurologie Psychiatrie 50: 93–112

Holowach J, Thurston D L, O'Leavy J 1958 Jacksonian seizures in infancy and childhood. British Journal of Paediatrics 52: 670–686

Hounsfield G N 1973 Computerised transverse axial scanning (tomography). Part I, description of system. British Journal of Radiology 46: 1016–1022

Ito M, Lammertsma A A, Wise R J S et al 1982 Measurement of regional cerebral blood flow and oxygen utilisation in patients with cerebral tumours using 15O and positron emission, tomography: analytical techniques and preliminary results. Neuroradiology 46: 1016–1022

Jabbari B, DiChiro G, McCarthy J P 1979 Medial temporal sclerosis detected by computed tomography. Journal of Computer Assisted Tomography 3: 527–529

Jack C R, Sharborough F W, Twomey C K et al 1990 Temporal lobe seizures: evaluation with MR volume measurements of the hippocampal formations. Radiology 175: 423–429

Jackson G D, Berkovic S F, Tress B M et al 1990 Hippocampal sclerosis can be reliably detected by MRI. Neurology 40: 1869–1875

Kalan C, Burrows E H 1962 Calcification in intracranial gliomata. British Journal of Radiology 35: 589–602

Kendall B E, Jakubowski J, Pullicino P, Symon L 1979 Difficulties in diagnosis of supratentorial gliomas by CAT scan. Journal of Neurology, Neurosurgery and Psychiatry 42: 485–492

Kingsley D P E, Kendall B E, Fitz C R 1986 Tuberous sclerosis; A clinico-radiological evaluation of 110 cases with particular reference to atypical presentation. Neuroradiology 28: 38–46

Kuhl D E, Engel J Jr, Phelps M E, Selin C 1980 Epileptic patterns of local cerebral metabolism and perfusion in humans determined by emission computed tomography of 18FDG and 13NH. Annals of Neurology 8: 348–360

Langenstein D K, Sternowsky H J, Rothe M 1979 Computerized cranial transverse axial tomography (CTAT) in 145 patients with primary and secondary generalized epilepsies. I. Neuropaediatrie 10: 15–28

Laster D W, Perry J K, Moody D M, Ball M R, Witcofski R L, Riela A T 1985 Chronic seizure disorders: Contribution of MR imaging when CT is normal. American Journal of Neuroradiology 6: 177–180

Lee A W M, Chang Lol, Ng Sh, Tse V K C, Au Skogkh, Poon V F 1990 MRI in the clinical diagnosis of late temporal lobe necrosis following radiotherapy for nasopharyngeal carcinoma. Clinical Radiology 42: 24–31

Lenzi G L, Frackowiak R S J, Jones T 1982 Cerebral oxygen metabolism and blood flow in human cerebral ischaemic infarction. Journal of Cerebral Blood Flow and Metabolism 2: 321–335

Mahmoud M el S 1958 The sella in health and disease: Value of the radiographic study of the sella turcica in morbid anatomical and topographic diagnosis of intracranial tumours. British Journal of Radiology Suppl. 8

Martin N, Debussche C, DeBroucker T, Mompoint D, Marsault C, Nahum H 1990 Gadolinium-DTPA enhanced MR imaging in tuberous sclerosis. Neuroradiology 31: 492–497

McGahan J, Dublin A B, Hill R P 1979 The evaluation of seizure disorders by computerized tomography. Journal of Neurosurgery 50: 328–332

Peretti P, Raybaud Ch, Dravet Ch, Mancini J, Pinsard N 1989 Magnetic resonance imaging in partial epilepsy of childhood. Journal of Neuroradiology 16: 308–316

Rhodes C G, Wise R J S, Gibbs J M et al 1983 In vivo disturbance of the oxidative metabolism of glucose in human cerebral gliomas. Annals of Neurology 14: 614–626

Scollo-Lavizzari G, Eichhorn K, Wuthrich R 1977 Computerized transverse axial tomography in the diagnosis of epilepsy. European Neurology 15: 5–8

Shorvon S D, Gilliatt R W, Cox T C S, Yu Y L 1984 Evidence of vascular disease from CT scanning in late onset epilepsy. Journal of Neurology, Neurosurgery and Psychiatry 47: 225–230

Smith D F, Smith F W, Knight R S G, Roberts R C, Gemmel H G 1989 99TcHMPAO single photon emission computed tomography in partial epilepsy. British Journal of Radiology 62: 970–973

Sperling M R, Wilson G, Engel J, Babb T L, Phelps M, Bradley W 1986 MRI in intractable partial epilepsy. Annals of Neurology 20: 57–62

Sumie H, Kuru Y, Kurokawa S, Kondo R 1978 Ammon's horn sclerosis on pneumoencephalotomography. Neuroradiology 16: 335–336

Synek V, Reuben J R, Gawler J, du Boulay G H 1979 Comparison of the measurement of the cerebral ventricles obtained by CT scanning and pneumoencephalography. Neuroradiology 17: 149–151

Takahashi M, Hirota Y, Bussaka W et al 1983 Evaluation of prototype equipment for digital subtraction angiography in diagnosing intracranial lesions. American Journal of Neuroradiology 4: 259–262

Wiesberg L A, Nice C, Katz M 1984 Cerebral computed tomography, 2nd edn. Saunders, Philadelphia

Wise R J S, Rhodes C G, Gibbs J M et al 1984 Disturbance of oxidative metabolism of glucose in recent human cerebral infarcts. Annals of Neurology 14: 627–637

Yang P J, Berger P E, Cohen M E, Duffner P K 1979 Computed tomography and childhood seizure disorders. Neurology 29: 1084–1088

Young A C, Costanzi J B, Mohr P D, St Clair Forbes W 1982 Is routine computerised axial tomography in epilepsy worthwhile? Lancet ii: 1446–1447

11. Neuropsychiatry

T. A. Betts

INTRODUCTION

Epilepsy originates in the brain; so do our thoughts, our feelings and our behaviour. Epilepsy results from changes in chemical activity at transmitter sites and in cell membranes in the brain; so does how we comprehend the world and how we react to it. Epilepsy, therefore, can change the way we think, feel and behave; but, equally, thought, emotion and behaviour can change epilepsy.

Epilepsy is, therefore, important to the psychiatrist, and the psychiatrist is important to epilepsy. Epilepsy lies in the borderland between what is understood conventionally as a province of psychiatry and a province of neurology. Epilepsy and its associated phenomena cannot be understood without a firm grounding in both brain and behavioural sciences.

An understanding of epilepsy requires the co-operation of several disciplines. It requires more than that, however: each discipline must have some understanding of the role of the others. The treatment of epilepsy is not the prerogative of any one speciality, but can be a job for any doctor, whether neurologist, psychiatrist, paediatrician or general physician, providing he or she has a particular interest in epilepsy and is prepared to learn something of the skills and attitudes of other branches of the profession so that total care can be offered to the patient.

This chapter is an attempt to describe the various aspects of epilepsy with which a psychiatrist is particularly concerned, and for which his or her skills have something to offer.

THE ROLE OF THE PSYCHIATRIST

There are three main ways in which the psychia-trist has a unique contribution to make to the management of people with epilepsy.

It is probable that psychiatric disturbance of all kinds is more common in people with epilepsy than in the general population; although this bold statement needs qualification. Most psychiatric disturbance in people with epilepsy can be seen as no more than a reaction to the stress of being epileptic. The skills of psychiatrists and their colleagues in nursing, clinical psychology, occupational therapy and social work are very pertinent here.

Some people with epilepsy, because of concomitant brain damage or the effect that having epilepsy has had on their emotional development, grow up with persistent disturbances of behaviour or in their relationships to other people which classify them as having a personality disorder. This is one of the most contentious areas of the psychiatry of epilepsy. Again, the skills that a psychiatrist and his or her colleagues possess may have a lot to offer such people. Even more important, perhaps, if we can study these problems carefully enough, we may be in a position eventually to offer some kind of preventative treatment. A few people with epilepsy have such gross disorders of feeling, behaviour, thinking, or in the way they relate to the external world and other people, that they have to be described as mentally ill; here, of course, the psychiatrist's help is essential.

The second way in which the psychiatrist has a contribution to make is in helping to diagnose attack disorder. Often the diagnosis of epilepsy is easy but sometimes it is not: particularly with complex partial seizures, it may be difficult to distinguish between a phenomenon relating to epilepsy and a phenomenon relating to psychiatric disturbance. The differential diagnosis of attacks may need psychiatric experience.

Thirdly, new and developing methods of treatment in psychiatry, particularly those based on learning theory, may have a great deal to offer people with epilepsy in terms of the actual treatment of their seizures. Although still largely experimental, behavioural treatments may become a powerful adjunct to more conventional forms of therapy.

Since this is a medical textbook, a medical model has tended to be followed in describing psychological reactions to epilepsy. There are, however other equally appropriate models that could have been used, which help to explain why people with epilepsy behave in the way they do. Although it says very little about epilepsy directly, Goffman's book, on stigma and spoilt identity (Goffman 1963) is well worth reading by those who wish to pursue this idea further. Wing (1974) presents a model of handicap, which although related to schizophrenia, is also extremely applicable to epilepsy:

1. *Primary handicaps*, which are the result of chronic impairment of physiological or psychological function (e.g. loss of a limb, obsessions, or seizures).
2. *Secondary handicaps*, extra handicaps which would not be present had the primary handicap not also been present (e.g. seizures leading to hospitalization which leads to institutionalization or seizures leading to fear which leads to an increased number of seizures).
3. *Extrinsic handicaps*, which are pre-existing handicaps which are independent of the main one but which influence it—like poor social circumstances or a lack of social or cognitive skills which are relevant to treatment planning.

PSYCHOLOGICAL EFFECTS OF HAVING EPILEPSY

To have epilepsy is to be stressed. Stress itself can influence the frequency of seizures, and it is possible sometimes for this to become a self-reinforcing phenomenon. If patients can come to

terms or deal with the stress that epilepsy induces, their lives will be made much more comfortable and their seizure frequency may diminish. It is, therefore, important for any doctor who is helping people with epilepsy to know something about the effects of stress, the factors that influence the way an individual reacts to stress and the means available to help people to cope with stress. It is also important for doctors to know when reactions to stress should be classified as abnormal.

The word 'stress' itself is ill-defined in the literature: sometimes it is applied to that which causes reactive and unpleasant symptoms in individuals; and sometimes it is applied to the actual symptoms themselves. In this chapter the word 'stress' implies the impact that becoming epileptic has on the patient and also the chronic effects that having epilepsy has on the individual and his or her relationships with others. In terms of its effects on the individual, help given should really be considered under two headings: firstly, helping him to come to terms with the diagnosis of epilepsy and secondly trying to minimize the effects that epilepsy will have on his or her life, i.e. on social life, interpersonal relationships and on his or her job.

In looking at how somebody is reacting to a particular stress, it should be remembered that stress reactions in themselves can often be considered as normal, are usually self-limiting and are part of the normal biological mechanisms of adaptation to new situations. In considering whether a particular reaction is abnormal or not, one should pay particular attention to whether the reaction is helping that person to deal with the situation, and also whether the reaction is becoming self-reinforcing (i.e. that the person is, for instance, becoming afraid of being afraid).

The term 'normal mental health' certainly does not imply an absence of stress symptoms or emotional conflicts. At any one time, the majority of the population are under some kind of stress, and so may be experiencing appropriate feelings or showing evidence of this stress in their behaviour. Indeed, if the criteria are set wide enough, almost every normal person will be classified as having emotional symptoms. For instance, an epidemiological study which used such broad criteria, the Manhatten Midtown Study (Srole et al 1962), found an estimated 87% of the normal population in the survey to have some emotional disturbance. In any population of supposedly ill patients, a careful distinction must, therefore, be made between normal and abnormal reactions to stress.

The way a particular individual reacts to stress depends on certain factors; some of them independent and some of them interdependent. There is the significance of the stress to the individual involved. It has been shown, for instance, that the psychological effects of head injury are dependent partly on the relative meaning of the injury to the individual. Dysphasia in a school-master, for instance, is of much more importance in terms of his emotional response to it than dysphasia in a farm labourer. The support which a person receives from family and friends and society will also affect his or her ability to cope with a particular stress. Someone recently bereaved, for instance, is much less able to meet the impact of physical illness.

It has also been shown (Slater & Shields 1969) that the genetic constitution of an individual and the responsiveness of his or her autonomic nervous system to stress, may play an important part in shaping the particular way the stress responses are presented. Lacey et al (1953) propose the concept of *response specificity*: that people respond to stress in a relatively stereotyped way through their autonomic system.

Stress responses are also influenced by a person's educational and cultural background. The West Indian response to stress, for instance is different from the British; it is easy to misinterpret the behaviour of people not of our own culture and 'medicalize' normal expression of grief and stress. Stress is not an isolated event and a person's response to it is influenced by coincident problems and difficulties affecting him or her at the time. In other words, stress is easier to cope with if one is not already overburdened. Stress reactions are learned as part and parcel of growing up: children are influenced greatly in terms of the way they learn to respond to stress by the example set by their parents and by the social values of their family.

Various extra influences which fall on people with epilepsy are perhaps particularly pertinent to the way they respond to stress. There is a growing body of evidence to suggest that social learning, particularly in childhood (which will include learning about how to cope with common stresses and difficulties), is impaired by epilepsy acquired in early childhood; and it is possible that some of the chronic personality difficulties that adults with epilepsy may show are related to mal-learning in childhood.

There is no doubt as well that brain damage, particularly perhaps in the temporal lobes, impairs the ability of a person to respond in a normal way to a stressful situation: minor neurotic symptoms and hysterical reactions are probably more common in people who are brain damaged.

There is also some evidence to suggest that the antiepileptic drugs needed by a person with epilepsy may also impair learning and interfere with normal responses to stress. A person with epilepsy then, not only has to suffer the normal stresses that any chronic illness would impose, but also may be handicapped in terms of responding to those stresses by the illness itself and by its necessary treatment. In some ways, then, epilepsy is a unique illness compared to other chronic handicaps.

COMING TO TERMS WITH EPILEPSY

The first problem for the patient newly diagnosed as having epilepsy is to come to terms with it. It is easy for doctors in the confines of outpatients (where patients' behaviour is usually subservient and controlled) to believe that this is easy. The patient who nods and smiles when told the diagnosis and says 'thank you doctor, at least it's nothing more serious', is very pleasing; but one should not imagine that he or she is necessarily going to behave the same way at home and, even if that is the case, friends, parents, spouse or children may not react similarly.

What the patient has to come to terms with is not just epilepsy as it actually is, but the misinformation, myths and fears about epilepsy that exist in his own mind, in his family and in his culture. This is why it is so important when telling people that they have epilepsy to find out first what they think epilepsy is and to begin the educational process at once. But there is only a limited amount of information that patients can absorb at any one time in a medical consultation; and even that small amount is drastically reduced if the information given to the patient has an emotional import, so that information will need to be repeated.

Some doctors conceal the truth from their patients about the diagnosis of epilepsy and merely use vague terms like 'blackouts'. I believe most firmly that all patients with epilepsy should know their diagnosis, but one should remember that in addition to the diagnosis the patient will require a whole range of information about lifestyle, treatment, risks and his or her responsibilities to others. If one tries to give this information at the same time as giving the patient the diagnosis it will often fall on deaf ears, and the education of the patient about all the implications of epilepsy may take several months of painstaking effort, particularly as one is often overcoming the patient's own prejudice and ignorance about the disorder.

In many chronic illnesses, including epilepsy, the use of printed handouts for the patient and his family (and the use of videotape material) to further explain the illness is necessary. I think it important that people with epilepsy actually see seizures presented to them on videotape or film: they may need support as this is done, but they will at least know, and be able to come to terms with, what happens to them. Many patients, as they come to terms with the diagnosis, will benefit from the support of other people with epilepsy. Most countries are now developing, or have developed, such patient support groups.

As people come to terms with any emotionally significant or life threatening physical disability, they commonly show a range of mental mechanisms to deal with the anxieties and stress that the situation has caused. Most of these mental mechanisms are quite normal, and help to maintain emotional equilibrium under stress and preserve self-respect. The work of Bowlby (1960) and Hinton (1967) on children deprived of maternal care, and people facing unpleasant situations such as dying, shows that a common initial reaction to such situations is one of *denial*, followed by a period of *struggle* in which the individual consciously tries to assimilate the new knowledge into his self-concept and image. This period of struggle and denial may be particularly painful, and may also, of course, occur in relatives. It is during this period of denial and struggle that one may see the phenomenon of the patient dragged from one useless consultation to another (often of an esoteric or fringe medicine type) because the devastating truth cannot be accepted. The consultant, flattered by being asked to provide a second opinion, should remember that the reasons for this may have much more to do with the emotional struggle that the patient is going through than with the consultant's own particular prowess.

Many patients (adolescents in particular) will often deny their epilepsy by erratic (or non-existent) taking of medication. Adolescents will often test our their need to take medication by stopping it to see what happens—it is important for doctors to remember that this is *normal* adolescent behaviour.

The period of denial is often followed by a period of *depression* as the person begins to assimilate the unpleasant situation. This depression, providing it does not go on for too long and can be worked through, should be regarded as normal. It usually gives way eventually to a period of acceptance and resignation. These reactions need support rather than treatment, except in unusual circumstances. People passing through these emotional reactions may have transient periods of the most profound depression which, unless they become prolonged and therefore pathological, should not be treated, since there is evidence that the successful working through of grief is necessary for later emotional stability.

During this struggle to assimilate the diagnosis, both patients and their relatives may show profound feelings of *guilt* and particularly *anger* in addition to depression. This is particularly likely to happen, of course, if there is some known reason for the epilepsy, such as a head injury or a febrile convulsion. It should be remembered that patients often invent their own mythology to explain the cause of their epilepsy, something the doctor should be aware of when discussing possible causes for a patient's epilepsy.

Anger can be destructive, negative and self-defeating but can also be positive. If the patient turns his anger at acquiring epilepsy on himself, his family or his particular God or sense of fate he will achieve misery: but if he allows his anger to fuel his drive to rehabilitation and to defeat his epilepsy he will achieve much.

Although not all patients pass through a period of emotional distress on learning of the diagnosis (some may actually be relieved, having feared far worse, i.e. that they were going mad), it should be assumed that most patients will. It is important as patients go through this period of turmoil that one does not interpret it as anything else than it is and not to 'medicalize' it.

Case History 1

This patient was a language student at university. At the age of 19 she began to have complex partial seizures. These became frequent and, since they were rather prolonged consisting of absences in which occasionally frightened behaviour would occur, were socially disabling. Despite the concern of her friends, she initially denied there was anything wrong with her and referred to her attacks as her 'little faints'. She developed a blasé, flippant attitude to them, so much so that at one time her apparent unconcern made one doctor suspect that she had the 'belle indifférence' of hysteria (but if one talked to her for long enough, her underlying anxiety became apparent). Later, as she accepted both the diagnosis and its implications (of lifelong taking of antiepileptic drugs and restrictions on her future career) she passed through a fairly profound period of depression, but later was able to accept the illness for no more or no less than it actually is, and has found comfort in being able to help others in a worse predicament. Her emotional reaction was never treated as an illness but merely supported and interpreted, and she was given the opportunity of working through it.

THE SOCIAL EFFECTS OF HAVING EPILEPSY

To have epilepsy means to be exposed to the fear of having attacks; it means being somebody who frightens and disturbs others; it means being at a disadvantage in terms of work and personal relationships; it means being open to prejudice (which exists both in the lay public and in the medical and nursing professions); and it means sometimes to suffer disturbing symptoms not always directly connected with the epilepsy.

Among the many problems with which a person with epilepsy has to deal are the unpredictability of attacks, and the reactions that other people have to them. This description given by one patient is typical: 'to awaken in a street which, for a moment, I cannot recognize, lying in a filthy gutter, wet and messy because I soiled myself, my thoughts confused, surrounded by strangers who are half curious, half disgusted, this is the nightmare with which I have to live'. Many people with epilepsy will recognize those feelings. Through most of his or her life the person with epilepsy does not appear disabled, but well. Unpredictably he or she thrusts the disability unexpectedly on unprepared and uninformed strangers.

There is widespread prejudice against epilepsy in almost all cultures. Among many primitive people, people with epilepsy are regarded with hostility and denied access to whatever medical and social care may be available. A person with epilepsy may become an outcast from his society; exposed to social and religious taboos; sometimes denied the right to procreate; seen as different and threatening to the stability of society; and often the victim of cruel and useless medical treatment.

It is easy to be complacent, to say that such things do not happen in our own society, and that the reaction of rejection of epilepsy is essentially primitive. However, we must remember that, until very recently, similar attitudes and practices occurred in our own societies, and to some extent still exist. In some western countries, laws forbidding people with epilepsy to marry were repealed only very recently. Officially, there is little overt prejudice against people with epilepsy. However, there is still important and significant latent or covert prejudice even amongst those highly educated and with a tradition of liberalism and compassion—the medical, nursing and teaching professions, and the churches.

Intensive educational efforts to change public attitudes towards epilepsy have been made particularly in the United States, and, as has been shown (Caveness et al 1969), these have had considerable success. As might be expected, the most favourable changes have been found amongst the better educated and younger people living in large towns in the United States. The greatest remaining prejudice against epilepsy was found in the southern states where there seems to be a relationship between it and racial prejudice. People with epilepsy tend to be viewed with the same hostility as the racial minorities (Bagley 1971). In Western societies, both the coloured person and the person with epilepsy are feared for their supposed primitiveness and violence, and for their unpredictability.

In the UK 30 years ago only 57% of the population surveyed felt that people with epilepsy should be employed and 32% said that they would object to their child playing with a child with epilepsy (Office of Health Economics 1971). Have these entrenched attitudes changed?

That they may be changing in this country is illustrated by a 1979 Gallup survey (Epilepsy News 1979) which showed that 78% of respondents then felt that people with epilepsy should be employed and 88% were happy for their children to associate with an epileptic child. Of course, what people say they will do and what they will actually do are not necessarily the same. How much this poll reflected specific attitude changes to epilepsy or how much it merely related to a general liberalization of attitudes in the British people is hard to say. A disquieting feature of the survey was that prejudice is still common in adolescents and young adults reflecting the need for better education about epilepsy in schools. Recognizing this fact, the British Epilepsy Association has recently developed a schools pack of information about epilepsy for both teachers and pupils designed both to give unbiased information about epilepsy and to help school children to examine their attitudes towards epilepsy and those who have it. The effectiveness of this approach is high (Corbidge & Bullock 1986).

However, a recent survey of its members by the British Epilepsy Association has shown that nearly two-thirds encounter difficulty in living with epilepsy, particularly in the areas of transport and work: a substantial minority also experience difficulties in communication with the medical profession. This has lead the Association to develop a charter for people with epilepsy, related to fair practice in employment and education.

In purely material terms, money spent on social education about epilepsy in the UK would be a way in which preventative medicine might save, not only many people much unhappiness, but also an immense amount of time for psychiatrists and their colleagues in trying to relieve personality and behavioural reactions to faulty social attitudes.

It is important to emphasize that the medical and related professions themselves are not free from prejudice and may still entertain irrational attitudes about people with epilepsy. The British Medical Association Working Party on Immigration as recently as 1965 recommended that people with epilepsy should not be allowed to enter this country 'for social and economic reasons'. It is difficult for people even with well-controlled epilepsy to enter the medical, nursing or teaching professions (Betts 1986), although this is slowly improving.

Doctors, nurses and school teachers (and their colleagues) are an important source of unbiased education for the public, and removal of prejudice in these groups is therefore very important. The teacher, whether medical, nursing or lay, has a vital role in educating others about epilepsy. In the classroom the teacher, by his or her acceptance of the child with epilepsy and calmness and unconcern if a child has a seizure, by example helps to dispel fear and prejudice in the rest of the class. It is easy for busy doctors immersed in their clinical work to forget the importance that such preventative work may have, and the effect that it may have even on their own practice.

A large number of problems with family relationships can be averted by the understanding, sympathy and common sense of the family doctor. Those problems which are more severe or which have been allowed to develop unnoticed need the special experience of the psychiatrist, and his or her psychologist, nursing and social work colleagues to put them right. Reactions of rejection or hostility against the child with epilepsy by parents may occur and, as previously mentioned, are often associated with feelings of guilt. However, a more common reaction is over concern or overprotection. Occasionally this is a reaction to the guilt that parents feel about their hostile feelings towards their child with epilepsy. Much more often overprotection is a reaction to the anxiety that parents feel about their child's seizures.

Overprotection is extremely damaging, particularly as its effects, being meant kindly, are the more difficult to resist and can be reinforced by society and yet can totally destroy an individual. It is the worst handicap that people with epilepsy can acquire and its recognition and prevention (and the treatment of parental anxiety) is vital to the health, welfare and happiness of the child with epilepsy.

Case History 2

John was 40 and was 'severely handicapped'; he had never been out on his own, never been on a bus on his own, never swum, never ridden a bike, never climbed a tree, never been to the pictures, never eaten out, never so much as kissed a girl, never got drunk, never been in a fight. All his life he had been looked after by his devoted parents (held up as a shining example of caring by the congregation of the church to which John and his parents belonged). Yet John had but two seizures a month, could read and write and has an unrivalled knowledge of Great Western Railway rolling stock. His life long epilepsy had led his parents to put him in cotton wool and prevent him from joining in anything that might be dangerous or embarrassing if a seizure should occur and he had been thoroughly taught to be afraid of his seizures. At 40 he showed signs of mild rebellion and was taken to the doctor by his worried parents who interpreted his protests as a sign of mental illness. When he came to the clinic, supported on each arm by his devoted family, this man of 40 entered the consultation room with both parents. When asked how he was, a parental voice answered 'not too bad, thank you' for him. Two years later John is living apart from his parents and now feels responsible for *them*. He is working and has a steady relationship and is beginning to enjoy his sexuality; he has also learnt to swim. He has not had a seizure for a year despite (or because of?) a drastic reduction in his antiepileptic medication.

This is perhaps an extreme example of over-protection (but not, sadly, an unusual one). The management and prevention of overprotection is one of the most important elements in the treatment of people with epilepsy and yet has been little researched or written about: much unnecessary overprotection is unfortunately taken for granted and never looked at critically and often reinforced by the medical and nursing professions. Our first prescription for epilepsy is often a list of negative prohibitions rather than a positive affirmation that the patient can still live a normal life. Often the patient, rather like Samson pulling the temple down about his ears, will, in his misery, invent his own prohibitions and voluntarily give up much that he finds enjoyable, or parents, still suffering from the emotional shock of seeing their child have his first seizure will, as a treatment for their own distress and anxiety, make similar prohibitions.

It is important to do two things in a first consultation. The first is to acknowledge and confront the distress that parents (and the patient) will have felt ('that must have been very disturbing—how did you feel, what did you think was happening?') and the second is, when relatives or the patient ask about 'what can't he do?', to be *positive* and say 'Rather, lets talk about what he *can* do'. Apart from the legal proscription against driving and certain high risk occupations, there is nothing that a person with epilepsy cannot do that he was not doing before his seizures started. If precautions have to be taken they must not be blanket prohibitions, but relate to the actual circumstances and seizures of the individual patient.

The prevention of overprotection depends upon our willingness and ability to prevent it: to treat parental and patient anxiety, to prevent and treat fear of seizures, and to recognize that a full and enjoyable life is the right and true goal for people with epilepsy and that this entails helping patients to be prepared either to take risks, or otherwise to face a life of boredom and underachievement. Those of us who also counsel people with cancer recognize the need to help the patient develop a 'fighting spirit': such an attitude is also needed in epilepsy.

Case History 3

At the age of 8, this girl sustained a cerebrovascular accident of unknown aetiology in the territory of the right middle cerebral artery. After investigation in a neurosurgical unit, she recovered quite well although she was left with residual hemiplegia. This, however, did not interfere with her school performance and she eventually obtained a job in the Civil Service and married. She was the youngest of her family, and, particularly after her stroke, was babied by the rest of the family, so that she grew up with a rather histrionic and attention-seeking personality. About a year after her marriage she began to develop brief absences accompanied by bilateral twitching in the arms. The attacks worsened rapidly. There had always been a definite startle component to them, but now, instead of lasting a few seconds and being followed by instant recovery, they started to last up to half an hour. She would respond to unexpected sounds in her environment by a brief akinetic absence plus a few bilateral jerks of the arms. This was followed by weeping, kicking, screaming and rolling about. She would frequently cry out 'get off' and appeared to be struggling with an imaginary, evil and presumably lecherous assailant. (This change in her attack pattern had followed her visit to hospital for a brain scan which involved an intravenous injection—which she hated—and also a visit to a film called *The Exorcist*).

The family's reaction to these very noisy attacks was interesting in that, when she had them, they would rush to her and start rubbing her legs, patting her on the face, and mopping her brow with a damp cloth. At the same time the mother and the husband would have a bitter quarrel over the struggling body of the young woman, the mother accusing the husband of being the cause of the attacks, saying: 'She wasn't like this until she married you', whilst the husband would be hurling similar accusations back at the mother. Eventually the mother took the girl back into her own home to live with her. The frequency of the attacks increased until she was admitted to hospital, having up to half a dozen in a single day, exhausting both herself and her family. She was rapidly transferred from a general medical ward to a psychiatric unit where the attacks were treated simply by ignoring them and they disappeared fairly rapidly. The startle seizures were controlled with clonazepam. When she went home on weekend leave, the postictal elaboration returned and it became apparent that they were the woman's reaction to pre-existing family stresses which had been intensified by the development of her genuine attacks. A family conference was held in which a common policy for dealing with the attacks was thrashed out, and they declined in frequency at home. Over the next few years the elaborated attacks reappeared at times of family stress, and occasionally at such times she also had other brief hysterical symptoms such as aphonia.

She developed a good therapeutic relationship with her social worker who encouraged her to develop independence and self-reliance, which was particularly needed after the birth of her child. As she became more mature in her relationships and more self-assertive, family attitudes to her changed and eventually her husband left home taking the child with him; she was then rejected by her mother, so that she is now having to make her own way in the world. It seems that neither the family nor the husband were able to accept the girl when she was no longer in a relationship emotionally dependent on them. It is interesting that, as she has developed a more mature personality, she has ceased having even her genuine attacks and she has recently been withdrawn from medication.

Overprotection during childhood may well lead to the kind of battle which I have just described, with mother and husband competing to give unnecessary succour to the daughter or wife. It is often as difficult and painful for the victims of such family battles to break away as it is for the family to let them go: but full independence will not be achieved until such a break has been made.

Case History 4
This 30-year-old woman, born of a prolonged and difficult labour and who later had several febrile convulsions, developed complex partial seizures originating in the left temporal lobe at the age of 11. The seizures consisted of an absence lasting a couple of minutes, during which the girl felt intense jamais vu and had micropsia: occasionally, seizures would continue for a great deal longer. They were frequent and showed little response to medication and were most likely to occur in the early morning.

This family's reaction to them was pathological. Mother and father denied themselves the opportunity of having other children and devoted themselves to the care of their child. The mother gave up work, the child was kept in a school near home: due to frequent seizures, school attendance was poor. She was never allowed to play with other children or go out on her own, but had to be accompanied everywhere by her mother. She eventually left school and tried to obtain employment. Her mother was so anxious that the young woman might possibly have an attack whilst on her own, that her anxieties were communicated to the daughter. She, in turn, became so tense and anxious at the prospect of new employment, that she had many seizures whenever she started a new job, and therefore was unable to keep the job. Consequently, she spent a very restricted life at home merely helping her mother with domestic tasks. Occasionally, she would go to a youth club, but, again, was always accompanied by her mother. At the club she met and fell in love with a young man with whom she had a prolonged courtship, marrying 6 years after they first met. They moved into a house only a few doors away from her parents' house. The woman now finds herself in a very difficult situation. A combination of intensive behavioural treatment and new chemotherapy has made her far more independent and has taught her to deal with her anxieties better, and has reduced significantly the number of her attacks, but she is still trapped in a dependent situation with both her mother, who interprets independence as ingratitude and her husband, who is the kind of man who wanted a dependent domesticated woman to look after him. When she had a child her mother took over its care. For a long time the girl, although now having very few seizures, and despite having an automatic 'dead mans handle' brake on the pram, was not allowed to take the child out on her own. When the clinic staff supported the girl against her mother in her desire for freedom the mother apparently acquiesced: but a couple of weeks later was discovered by one of the community staff 'shadowing' the girl on her way to and from the shops like an actress in a third rate spy film: the girl's father would follow the girl in the family car when her mother could not manage a spying expedition and the parents would often try to meet her 'accidentally' in the shopping centre. When the clinic staff confronted this behaviour and tried to treat the parents' anxiety the mother removed her daughters care to another doctor.

Several studies (Pond & Bidwell 1959, Bagley 1971) have shown that the earlier the age of the onset of epilepsy, the more likely it is that the child will have behavioural problems during childhood and also in later life. Pathophysiological factors are obviously important, but psychological ones even more so, particularly the debilitating effects of overprotection.

STRESS DISORDERS

Many stress responses are normal. They become abnormal either when they are very severe, so that they interfere significantly with the person's life or with the life of others; when they become prolonged and continue to exist long after the stress itself has resolved; when they are maladaptive (in other words they inhibit a person's correct response to a particular stress so that it cannot be resolved); or when they become self-reinforcing so that the stress symptoms themselves become the stressor.

Reinforcement can also occur because of the effect that the patient's symptoms have on other people, or because the patient's symptoms do, in an unhealthy way, solve the problem. Psychiatrists talk about 'primary gain' which the patient may obtain from his or her symptoms; and 'secondary gain', which is the reinforcement or encouragement that other people may unwittingly give to the patient's symptoms. As we have seen, some parents have a need for a child to be totally dependent on them, and may, as the child comes to adolescence, encourage such dependency needs. The patient whose symptoms are cutting him or her off from a stressful situation (like the development of paraplegia in a teenager who is in conflict about whether or not to leave home) may find that there is a kind of collusion between himself or herself and other people so that the symptoms are unintentionally reinforced by other people who cheerfully push the paralysed teenager around in a wheelchair and help the person to adapt to the life of somebody who is paralysed.

Just as we cannot consider epilepsy in isolation (epilepsy is certainly not just about having seizures), so we cannot consider psychiatric symptoms in isolation—we have to take into account not only the patient's reaction to them but also the reaction of other people, and the situation in which they are occurring.

The particular stress disorder which occurs in an individual is the sum of many forces and influences acting on him or her and is partly determined by constitution and by previous experience. Stress disorders tend to be fairly consistent, although modified by the factors we have already considered, and they can also be modified by treatment.

The most common stress disorder is probably anxiety, which may be seen as a 'flight or fight' reaction which has become distorted by the requirements of civilization. Some people under stress develop disabling depressive symptoms; some may show maladaptive ritualistic or obsessional behaviour, others (although this is now rare), 'cut off' from their stress and develop hysterical conditions. Occasionally, people under stress may break down into acute psychotic states. Stress is, of course, also a most important causative factor in some physical illnesses and a significant adjunct to many others. The role of stress in the precipitation of epilepsy itself will be considered later on in this chapter. The types of maladaptive responses to stress which have been described are not necessarily exclusive: many people who are anxious, for instance, can also feel depressed and vice versa.

By and large, stress disorders should not be seen as illnesses. There is no doubt that psychiatric illnesses in the true sense do occur in people with epilepsy and these will be considered later in this chapter. Except perhaps in rare situations, it is not useful to see anxiety, mild depression or hysteria as an illness, particularly as this tends to imply that there is a 'medical' treatment.

Do stress disorders occur more commonly in people with epilepsy than in the general population? The answer is that they probably do, and that epilepsy, in some ways, is unique in causing stress disorders. Life experiences may either be pathogenic to a disorder (in other words they may actually *cause* the disturbance) or they may be pathoplastic (in that they alter the form that the disturbance takes in the particular individual).

Studies of the epidemiology of stress disorders and psychiatric illness in people with epilepsy have been made, but there are many difficulties in carrying out an accurate epidemiological survey of the psychological difficulties of people with a chronic relapsing disorder like epilepsy. It is known, for instance, that in the UK only about half the people with epilepsy in the community treated by their general practitioners will be seen at a hospital clinic. Those that are seen are often referred, not because of the severity of their epilepsy as such, but because of other handicaps, both physical and psychological, or because of co-existent personality and stress disorders. Some kinds of epilepsy are also more difficult to treat (like partial seizures). If they are associated with psychiatric disturbance (as they probably are) then, since the more difficult to treat patients will tend to accumulate in hospital clinics, psychiatric illness will be over represented in studies confined to hospital clinic populations. Any studies that concentrate on a hospital population of people will, therefore, be biased by the selected population being studied.

Although general practitioners frequently know a great deal about their patient's social problems, emotional disorders and psychological difficulties, such information may not be recorded or assessed accurately. It is also true that there are, in the general population, some people with epilepsy (and certainly many people with mental disorders) who do not seek help from their general practioners. The sickest people often may be those least likely to seek help. Again, therefore, it is likely that those who do not seek help from their general practioner will be a biased sample. Some people with epilepsy may not themselves realize that they have it, or their families may accept it without asking for help. In one study (Betts 1974) of people with epilepsy admitted to psychiatric hospitals, it was found that 28% of the sample (who had proven epilepsy) had never consulted their general practitioners about their attack disorder, and were not receiving medication.

Therefore, to determine accurately the relationship between epilepsy, stress disorders and mental illness, field studies should be carried out in which a total population of a particular town or district is sampled by specially trained personnel who can carry out a formal examination of all people with a particular disorder. Even a study such as this will miss those people in the population who have been removed to an institution.

The results, therefore, of studies carried out in the past few years should be interpreted cautiously. There does seem to be general agreement, however, that stress disorders (neurotic disorders) are more common in people with epilepsy that in the general population (Gudmundsson 1966).

A survey of all handicapped children on the Isle of Wight (Graham & Rutter 1968) suggested that about one-third of children with epilepsy had significant psychiatric disturbance. This proportion rose in those cases that had associated neurological symptoms, and was particularly high in those who were also mentally handicapped. The survey showed that the prevalence of psychiatric disorder was twice as frequent in children with epilepsy compared with children who had other chronic disabilities, e.g. asthma, and was about four times the expected rate in the general child population. Pond & Bidwell (1959) demonstrated in a pioneer survey in General Practice that psychiatric illness was common in people with epilepsy particularly those with temporal lobe epilepsy. The survey had methodological flaws related both to the ascertainment of psychiatric illness and to the determination of the type of epilepsy the patient was experiencing. However, a recent General Practice survey (Edeh & Toone 1987) using an accurate measure of psychiatric disorder and a detailed examination of the type of epilepsy that patients had, has also shown that psychiatric morbidity (especially anxiety and non-psychotic depression) occurs more commonly in people with epilepsy than would be expected by chance and is particularly common in patients with focal epilepsy as opposed to primary generalized epilepsy.

It may be that one other unique factor in the burden that epilepsy imposes on people (apart from the fear of the attacks themselves and the limitations on day-to-day living) is the fear of loss of control which epilepsy engenders. In this regard a comparison can be made between people with epilepsy and sufferers from Menière's syndrome, some of whom may also be toppled to the ground by their vertigo. Patients with this disease may also feel very keenly the ignominy of their disability, which they are also helpless to control, and it has been shown that they too are particularly liable to develop anxiety and depression (Pratt & Mackenzie 1958).

ANXIETY

A widely used classification of anxiety is:

A. Generalized anxiety disorder
B. Phobic disorder
   1. agoraphobia
   2. social phobia
   3. simple phobia
C. Panic disorder
D. Obsessive compulsive disorder
E. Post-traumatic stress disorder.

As has already been said, anxiety is part of normal experience; it becomes pathological when it becomes overwhelming or self-reinforcing, or when it prevents the individual from dealing with the problem which is causing the anxiety. Anxiety has a psychological component—a feeling of morbid dread or fear, which is subjectively most unpleasant—and a somatic component, which consists of symptoms referrable to stimulation of the sympathetic and the parasympathetic autonomic nervous systems (palpitation, nausea, diarrhoea, muscle aching, shaking etc). In some patients the psychological component is more prominent and in some the somatic component. Since anxiety often presents with somatic symptoms, it can easily be mistaken for physical illness, and the corollary is also true. In epilepsy, it is particularly important to distinguish between querulousness, irritability and agitation found in organic brain disease and anxiety itself. Likewise, anxiety is often a component of depression and, in somebody who is agitated, it is important to look for a possible underlying depressive illness.

Anxiety may be generalized and, therefore, despite some fluctuation, be with the person all the time (so called 'free-floating anxiety') or it may be situational, occurring in response to certain definite identifiable stimuli to which the patient is exposed ('phobic anxiety') occurring only when the patient is travelling, going into shops or encountering, say, cats or moths. A variety of severe phobic anxiety is 'agoraphobia'; the patient is crippled by intense anxiety when stepping over the threshold of home, and may, in fact, become totally housebound. In somebody who has anxiety sympoms, it is important to distinguish any phobic element, as this may alter management.

As will be seen later, patients who become acutely anxious often have so-called 'panic attacks' and these can be sometimes difficult to distinguish from epilepsy itself (Spitz, 1991). Panic attacks (sudden intense anxiety feelings both psychological and somatic), often occur in their own right with hyperventilation which may give rise to somatic symptoms and collapse resembling epilepsy (see section on non-epileptic attack disorder). Many anxiety symptoms (like depersonalization and derealization) also resemble epileptic symptoms. In my experience, phobic anxiety and agoraphobia seem particularly common in people with epilepsy and relate clearly to the patient's fear of having a seizure in a crowded place or in the street. Often, as we shall see later, the patient's anxiety increases the likelihood of having seizures so that, as the seizure anxiety increases so does the frequency of seizures, with each reinforcing the other. Indeed, the relationship between anxiety and epilepsy is extremely complex: an understanding of the nature of anxiety, its role in exacerbating and complicating epilepsy and its management is necessary for anyone who cares for people with epilepsy. It is particularly important to distinguish between 'state' and 'trait' anxiety—between anxiety as a response to a situation and anxiety as a permanent part of a persons personality.

I have suggested (Betts 1981a) a classification of the relationship between anxiety and epilepsy, which I have subsequently modified slightly as follows:

1. Anxiety reaction to acquiring epilepsy, which may become a chronic post-traumatic disorder
2. Generalized anxiety related to the fear of having a seizure
3. Anxiety reaction to the social and family stigmatization of epilepsy
4. Prodromal anxiety
5. Anxiety as an aura
6. Ictal anxiety
7. Anxiety (agitation) occurring in an epileptic psychosis
8. 'Organic anxiety'
9. True phobic anxiety related to seizures
10. Anxiety which precipitates a seizure
11. Panic disorder or other anxiety phenomena mistaken for epilepsy

12. Anxiety occurring as part of complex partial, simple partial or non-convulsive generalized status epilepticus.

Anxiety, as already indicated, is a common reaction to the stress of the discovery that one has epilepsy or to family, friend's or society's reaction to it or as a chronic post-traumatic disorder. Anxiety can also occur as a prodromal symptom of epilepsy—in other words, often for several days before an attack, a definite increase in a person's anxiety levels is apparent, culminating in a seizure (usually tonic-clonic) and usually with relief of the anxiety afterwards.

Case History 5
This simple man of 40, despite taking phenobarbitone in adequate dosage, had had tonic-clonic seizures about once a month ever since a closed head injury 20 years before. Both he and his family noticed that about one week before his seizure he became irritable, restless and agitated, sweated more, his pulse rate rose and he became hypochondriacal and preoccupied with bodily sensations. About 2 days before his attack he developed an urticarial rash on his trunk and arms, his sleep became disturbed and he developed a feeling of anxious expectation. At this time his sensorium was intact, physical examination normal and an EEG normal. Within 2 days of the rash developing he would have a tonic-clonic seizure, usually in his sleep. When he woke, he was his usual calm, sunny self.

On one occasion full control of his seizures was obtained with phenytoin and for nearly a year he had no attacks; but his distraught relatives approached his doctor requesting that he be allowed to have the ocasional seizure as without them he had become anxious and irritable all the time, and the phenytoin was withdrawn. Later it was found that if he took clobazam 30 mg daily for 10 days from the onset of his anxiety he had neither the anxiety nor the rash nor the seizure; and he has now been successfully maintained on this regimen (plus his usual phenobarbitone) for 2 years.

The mechanism of prodromal anxiety is uncertain although it is unlikely to be directly related to epileptic activity itself. Occasionally, anxiety is experienced as part of the ictal experience, either as an aura or as the ictus itself.

Case History 6
This 15-year-old girl was referred, when she grew too old for the paediatric service, with a diagnosis of probable pseudoseizures. Her attacks consisted of shouting, screaming, and rolling on the floor with kicking and jerking. She was a very reserved girl, difficult to get to know and the despair of a harassed and divorced mother who was finding her daughter's behaviour more and more difficult to cope with.

Ambulatory EEG monitoring showed that there was no discernible paroxysmal activity during the convulsive struggling, but that these episodes were always preceded by a 30 second spike discharge from the right temporal lobe. Observation of the girl's attacks showed that they started with the girl looking frightened; her eyes would glaze and she would rub her lower abdomen with her left hand; she would then given a sudden start, throw herself on the floor and begin to scream and kick. She eventually revealed that her attacks started with an intense feeling of fear 'as though the end of the world was coming'. This fear was felt in the pit of her stomach which tightened and tightened and the feeling would then rise up into her throat; she felt that when it reached her throat she would die. It was to escape from these feelings that she would scream and struggle. She found it difficult to tell others of these terrifying experiences lest she be judged mad.

Subsequently, these attacks lessened in frequency as the result of new medication. She no longer reacts to them with her previous dramatic behaviour, because she has been taught an effective anxiety management technique, so that she no longer fears the feeling, nor feels out of control: latterly intense anxiety management using a cue controlled technique (Boden et al 1990) has abolished the attacks altogether.

Case History 7
This 20-year-old girl was referred with a diagnosis of panic attacks. From the age of 3 she had suffered from brief episodes of anxiety. From 3 until 12 she had sudden feelings of anticipatory anxiety ('like going to the circus'). These would come on suddenly, last a few seconds and go as quickly as they came. She found them mildly pleasant: 'like something nice was going to happen' could not relate them to any particular event or circumstance and held them of no consequence.

When she was about 12 the attacks continued but the nature of the feeling changed. Now the anxiety was unpleasant 'like going to the dentist', and tended to last longer and she became visibly upset. She became afraid that others might notice the attacks and laugh and stopped going out or mixing with people as a result. At the time of change in the emotional tone of the attacks there was a great deal of family turmoil.

By the time she was seen she had had a year of psychiatric treatment to no avail (including interpretive psychotherapy and behaviour therapy) and was housebound, as she was having several attacks a day. Observation in hospital showed that she would suddenly go quiet; consciousness would be clouded; there would be some swallowing followed after about 10–20 seconds by brief tachypnea; sometimes she would rub her nose. Ambulatory EEG monitoring showed at these times that there was a clear-cut spike discharge in the right posterior temporal region.

Treatment with carbamazepine has reduced both the frequency and duration of these attacks, but they still occur, and tend to increase during times of stress. The girl needed a great deal of counselling to enable her to accept her epilepsy and admit its existence to others.

Case History 8
This woman believed herself to be a witch, as did many of the inhabitants of the small Herefordshire village where she lived. She had been able to predict many natural disasters and had become an object of fear and veneration in her village. She eventually became greatly distressed by her prophecies and by the effect they were having on others; she had several episodes of depression and was referred for further investigation. A careful history showed that she was not predicting natural disasters in a direct way, but would merely develop sudden brief intense feelings of apprehension of impending disaster. These forebodings did not occur every time there was a natural disaster, and it was clear that selective forgetting of occasions when she did not predict correctly and retrospective falsification of memory were responsible for her reputation. Careful observation revealed that she was having a brief attack disorder in which she would suddenly slump forward for a few seconds, breathing stertorously with a vacant glazed expression. During the attacks she could not be roused, and would wake up suddenly, although she was dazed for a few seconds afterwards; she was quite unaware of having had an attack although she remembered the premonitory feeling before it. The relationship between her attacks and the premonitory experiences became clear when it was found that there was EEG evidence of a right temporal lobe epileptic focus. The attacks ceased with medication.

Case History 9
This woman had had an undiagnosed attack disorder thought to be psychogenic for 8 years before she was referred for a second opinion. Her turns started the day after the delivery of her third child. Although she had had them for 8 years, only her husband had ever witnessed one. She could only describe them vaguely, although she knew that in them she was very badly frightened. She described feeling hot and very anxious for no apparent reason and thought the attacks lasted for about 15 minutes. At first they might come on at any time, but for some time they had occurred invariably on a particular day of her menstrual cycle. In addition to these symptoms, she was undoubtedly prone to depression and anxiety and had a markedly obsessional personality. She had a very unhappy childhood, with a complete disruption of normal family relationships. Over the 8 years she had had frequent EEG examinations, all of which revealed no abnormality, and had taken a large amount of psychotropic medication, including tranquillisers and anti-depressants, all of which had failed to relieve her

symptoms. Most doctors who had seen her over this 8-year period thought she was suffering from anxiety attacks.

For some reason it was 8 years before anyone got a description from her husband, the only witness of the attacks. What he had observed was very different from his wife's account. He said the attacks were very brief, seldom lasting more than 30 seconds; he appreciated when she was having one since she became vacant and clouded and he was not able to reassure her. After the attacks, she was intensely anxious and frightened. She was admitted to a specialized unit for observation at the phase of her menstrual cycle when an attack might be expected. The attacks began, as anticipated, and were as her husband had described. They began quite suddenly: for 20–30 seconds she was dazed and unrousable and was observed to flush violently over the face and upper arms and she chewed and smacked her lips. She came to suddenly, although she appeared somewhat dazed and confused for some seconds afterwards, and was also intensely frightened (it was this part of the attack she remembered).

During the day of the attacks themselves, but at no other time, her EEG showed evidence of strong epileptic activity in her left temporal lobe. She is an example of how, during a temporal lobe attack, time sense may become distorted so that the patient gives an inaccurate estimate of how long the attack lasts. The attacks have diminished over the years, but have not really responded to medication, and paradoxically, have continued into the menopause, still in their cyclical fashion.

Williams (1956) in his classic paper on ictal emotion felt ictal anxiety to be the most common of the ictal feelings and to be confined to the anterior part of the temporal lobes, either the left side or bilateral. My experience, as shown above, is different. Ictal anxiety can be accompanied by autonomic manifestations of anxiety like sweating, belching, vomiting, piloerection, tachycardia or, as in one patient, even micturition. Automatism related to the anxiety may occur, and visual hallucinations of a frightening nature may be observed. Williams felt that the fear often has an unnatural quality like fear of the supernatural, rather than being reality based.

True epilepsy may start in some patients at a time of stress in their life. The stress triggers off an epileptic response in an individual with a low convulsive threshold and the epilepsy then becomes self-perpetuating, often assisted by the continuing stress of the original problem and the added stress of having epilepsy. Such epilepsy is likely to increase in frequency at times of other life stresses and often will have an anxiety component contained within it. Ictal fear or anxiety may powerfully reinforce a patient's own anxiety about his seizures which will increase seizure frequency— and may, although ictally based, respond to behavourial manipulation (see later in this chapter). Patients with ictal fear may especially learn to associate their seizures with particular stimuli (such as music). Often this is no more than seizures occurring by chance in a particular situation, and associated with that situation by the patient who now associates the particular stimulation with an expectation and fear that a seizure will occur, making that occurrence more likely as a result. Rarely a true conditioned response will develop (see later in this chapter).

It is clear from the above case histories that ictal anxiety may not be recognized and may carry a psychiatric label. Occasionally, the converse is true and anxiety attacks may be mistaken for an ictus.

Case History 10

This woman, aged 38, had a long history of psychiatric illness. For some years before admission to a psychiatric hospital she had become agoraphobic, being unable to pass over the threshold of her front door without experiencing symptoms of anxiety. She became particularly anxious when entering shops and, shortly before her admission to hospital, began to experience peculiar attacks of depersonalization in this situation, eventually falling to the floor if she entered a supermarket. She was aware of a rising tide of anxiety before these phenomena happened; suddenly, the anxiety would seem to leave her, and was replaced by intense depersonalization. She became aware of a feeling of lightheadedness, tingling in her hands and feet, followed by tetany of the hands and feet, and she would then pass into a brief period of apparent unconsciousness. When one of these attacks was witnessed, she was put into an ambulance and initially taken to a nearby general hospital, but from there transferred to the local psychiatric hospital. During the course of her investigations there, an EEG was performed which showed some dysrhythmia in the right temporal lobe (a not uncommon finding in people with phobic anxiety— Harper & Roth 1962). On the basis of this abnormal EEG she was diagnosed as having temporal lobe epilepsy and was referred for neurosurgical advice. She was seen at the request of the neurosurgeon before surgery was contemplated; admitted to a general hospital psychiatric unit; treated with intensive behaviour therapy; and, eventually, made a full recovery from the attacks which were clearly not epilepsy, but panic attacks. The phenomena

of light-headedness, which were considered as epileptic, are of course symptoms and signs of hyperventilation which, rarely, even may cause a major convulsion.

Case History 11

This man of 36 was referred from another consultant with a diagnosis of intractable temporal lobe epilepsy which large doses of antiepileptic drugs had failed to control. Two years previously, following a road accident, he had begun to develop attacks which were described as starting with 'an aura of fear' and which were accompanied by stereotyped behaviour described as an automatism. This was sometimes followed by a tonic-clonic seizure. The attacks were occurring many times a week and had totally disrupted his life and the life of his family — he had also been dismissed from a couple of jobs because of his epilepsy.

On admission to hospital, he was noted to be intoxicated with the various antiepileptic drugs he was taking and the usual policy of withdrawing them gradually was pursued. He became very apprehensive as they were withdrawn, and warned that he would have many seizures as a result. It was interesting that, as so often happens both with people with epilepsy and also those with pseudoseizures, he did not have an attack for about 10 days after his admission to hospital. He had several attacks on his first weekend visit home, however, being returned to hospital in an ambulance accompanied by various worried relatives. He then began to have many attacks whilst in hospital and most of them followed the same curious stereotyped form. Nurses would notice that he had become somewhat distant and vague; he would then suddenly jump to his feet, run to the nearest water tap which he would turn on (it was always the cold tap), and then allow a stream of cold water to flow over his head whilst holding his nose and groaning incoherently. His attacks would usually terminate after this and he would lie on his bed for about half an hour recovering, declaring himself to have a headache and to feel sleepy. On two or three occasions, however, whilst kneeling with the cold water pouring over his head, he would have an undoubted tonic-clonic seizure.

If he was arrested in his dramatic flight down the ward to find the nearest cold tap, however, it was possible to hold a rational if somewhat fraught conversation with him, and there was no evidence of a diminution in or clouding of consciousness and he would express himself at these times as feeling intensely anxious and frightened and said that the sensation of cold water, plus the act of holding his nose, seemed to prevent the anxiety from becoming more intense. It was also noted that at these times he was hyperventilating and it seemed that his nose holding was a way of slowing his breathing.

EEGs before and after such a seizure failed to reveal any significant abnormality: during one of his EEGs hyperventilation precipitated one of his seizures up to nose holding with no concomitant EEG change. There was no doubt, however, that occasionally, what came to be regarded as acute panic attacks were followed by genuine tonic-clonic seizures. As he came to be better known (when detoxified he became a somewhat amiable rogue) the connection between his anxiety attacks and his road accident became more clear. The car he had been driving was stolen, he was uninsured, he did not have a driving licence and he was also drunk. He had been terrified ever since that the police might investigate the accident and charge him with the various offences that he had committed. However, in the accident itself he had suffered a head injury with slight concussion afterwards and it was interesting that air encephalography of the brain revealed a discrete area of cortical atrophy in the right parietal area consistent with the previous head injury.

He was treated by an intensive regimen of behaviour therapy aimed at anxiety reduction and whilst on the ward he stopped completely having his anxiety attacks and after this no spontaneous tonic-clonic seizures were seen. It was concluded that he was suffering primarily from anxiety attacks, which occasionally were severe enough to precipitate a tonic-clonic seizure from hyperventilation, due perhaps to a low convulsive threshold induced by his head injury. He was eventually discharged and attended an employment rehabilitation unit.

Unfortunately, with the stresses of work and family life, he began to have panic attacks again and eventually had another tonic-clonic seizure and persuaded his general practitioner to put him back on antiepileptic drugs. The reason that he was keen to go back on drugs was to gain respectability in the eyes of his family who, when told that his attacks were primarily anxiety attacks, rejected him and told him to 'pull himself together'. When he had a further tonic-clonic seizure at home following rehabilitation they became very angry with the hospital, insisted that he change consultants and complained to their Member of Parliament who instituted enquiries into the 'gross incompetence' of the hospital. It was difficult to convince the MP that one could have an epileptic attack without necessarily being 'an epileptic'.

In my experience anxiety attacks (or panic attacks) can be a trap for the unwary and can be confused with epilepsy. In a personal series of patients with pseudoseizures, panic attacks account for about 30% of the total. Their recognition and management will be dealt with further in this chapter.

Sometimes anxiety or agitation may accompany a psychosis associated with epilepsy. A particular kind of agitation can also be seen in the brain-damaged, often accompanied by obsessionality (or 'organic orderliness'). Sometimes, in both, the agitation can be so prominent that the underlying cause goes unrecognized.

Complex partial and simple partial status and sub-convulsive generalized status may also present as an apparent generalized anxiety disorder: but clouding or constriction of consciousness will usually be apparent—see later in this chapter.

The management of anxiety involves careful investigation of the patient and his or her symptoms, with a physical history and examination followed by detailed analysis of the patient's emotional symptoms and life situation. Some patients with anxiety need counselling to help them to discover the best way of dealing with the situation that is making them anxious. Some, whose anxiety relates to interpersonal conflict, may need formal psychotherapy (a therapeutic relationship with a professional therapist who uses interpersonal skills and the emotional relationship that develops between therapist and patient to lead to an understanding of the emotional or interpersonal conflict causing the anxiety). Formal psychotherapy is a skilled undertaking with a large investment in terms of time and resources and, although sometimes extremely useful, need not be applied routinely in every patient who is anxious.

Behavioural methods of treatment, i,e. treatment aimed at helping the patient to overcome symptoms or to control them without worrying too much about the antecedents of the anxiety, are gaining popularity. They were originally used successfully in patients with phobic anxiety, but are now also being used in those with free-floating anxiety. There are various available methods of teaching a patient to control his or her anxiety involving types of relaxation training which will be described in the section on the self-control of seizures. The advantages of behavioural methods is that they teach the patient self-reliance and self-control, and also teach *discrimination*, so that the patient can recognize anxiety symptoms at an earlier stage in their development and learn how to control them before they become too overwhelming. Cognitive therapy techniques which aim to help the patient recognize and control the negative thinking which accompanies anxiety and which may reinforce or even precipitate it, are also very useful.

The use of psychotropic medication in those who are anxious should be kept to an absolute minimum. Far too many people in this country are given minor tranquillisers or hypnotic drugs to deal with anxiety symptoms which can be much better dealt with by other methods. Once started, tranquillisers are difficult to stop: they lead to dependence, they are a potent source of overdoses, and they teach the patient nothing about self-reliance. This applies particularly to patients with epilepsy, as most minor tranquillisers of the benzodiazepine group have antiepileptic properties and it may be even more difficult to take a patient with epilepsy off diazepam or chlordiazepoxide than somebody who does not have epilepsy. Occasionally, other medication may be useful temporarily in treating anxiety, particularly beta-blocking drugs if the anxiety has a large somatic component (Tyrer 1974). If tranquillizers are used, they should be given in short diminishing courses of 2–3 weeks duration only, during which time the patient must be encouraged to deal with the situation which is causing the anxiety.

MOOD DISORDER (AFFECTIVE DISORDER)—DEPRESSION AND MANIA

Depression is a term much used but often little defined. As a symptom of reaction to stress it is probably less common than anxiety, but can be much more disabling. It is also common as an illness in its own right. Mania, pathological excitement, is much rarer. The classification of affective disorder is contentious, but a commonly used and practical clinical classification of mood disorder is as follows:

1. a. *episode severity* (mild moderate or severe)
   b. *type* (depressive, manic or mixed)
   c. *associated symptoms*
      i. neurotic
      ii. psychotic
      iii. agitated
      iv. retarded
2. *Course*—unipolar, bipolar
3. *Aetiology*—predominately reactive, predominately endogenous.

Depression, like anxiety, has both psychological and somatic components. It is a feeling of pathological sadness or lowness of spirits (which may pass beyond ordinary human understanding), often accompanied by feelings of guilt, unworthiness and self-blame.

In severe depression, delusions and hallucinations of a gloomy nature may occur. These psychological symptoms are accompanied by biological symptoms of a change in sleep pattern, loss of weight, loss of appetite and loss of libido. In milder forms of depression, the appetite and sleep changes sometimes go in the reverse direction and there is oversleeping and overeating, with a consequent weight gain.

Classically, two forms of depression are described, reactive and endogenous (or neurotic and psychotic), implying that in some people depressive symptoms are a clear result of life stress or interpersonal difficulty; in other patients no such relationship can be seen, and it is assumed that the depression is an illness sui generis. This is sometimes a useful concept, although it is probable that in the majority of patients with a depressive illness no completely clear separation between the two can be made. Both reactive and endogenous depressive illnesses do seem to be more common in people with epilepsy, as will be described later, although depression itself is anyway very common. The relationship between depression and epilepsy is basically similar to that between anxiety and epilepsy (modified from Betts 1981a).

1. Depressive reactions to acquiring epilepsy ('grief')
2. Depressive reaction to the social and family stigmatization of epilepsy
3. Prodromal depression
4. Depression as an aura
5. Ictal depression
6. Depression (or mania) occurring as part of an epileptic psychosis
7. Depressive (or manic) psychosis occurring in people with epilepsy, possibly related to a change in seizure frequency
8. Depressive symptoms (rarely mania) occurring in organic brain disease related to epilepsy
9. Depression (or mania) occurring as part of a complex or simple partial status or non-convulsive generalized status.

As already indicated, depression is a natural component of the grief reaction, although it can be suppressed or denied. Likewise, it can be the product of a person's reaction to family or social stress caused by the epilepsy.

Prodromal depressive symptoms have been described (I have one current case), although, like ictal depression, they are much rarer than prodromal anxiety. Depression as part of an aura is likewise less common. In a personally observed series of 2000 patients with epilepsy Williams (1956) knew of 100 who felt emotion as part of the attack: the majority felt frightened (61), 21 experienced depression and the rest had some other feeling.

Since both anxiety and sadness is so much part of our life it may be difficult to distinguish normal sadness from ictal sadness, but the sadness often has a bizarre quality and is so out of context that it is usually easy to recognize. Almost invariably, if looked for, something else recognizable as part of a partial seizure will be present.

Case History 12

This 63-year-old man tumbled off a ladder in a seizure whilst painting his house. One of his lumbar vertebrae was shattered. Whilst lying in an orthopaedic ward, alone in the early hours of the morning, he cut his throat with a razor blade, and his life was barely saved. On admission to the psychiatric ward he was in profound depressive stupor: he had had lifelong poorly controlled epilepsy and was still having several major seizures a week, despite heroic attempts to control them with antiepileptic drugs. He had had several previous psychiatric admissions for depressive illnesses. Because of his precarious physical condition, his depression was not treated for a few days. In that time it was noted that he was passing very rapidly from the depth of profound despair and depression to near normality and back again. In the middle of a sentence he might slump forward into an intense stupor, the picture of unhappiness, responding painfully and slowly to all questions, and was full of suicidal ideas, only suddenly, some minutes or an hour or so later, to lift in mood back to an almost normal state. His EEG showed generalized spike and wave discharge. He was treated with clonazepam. A relatively small dose of this drug rendered him attack free and within a few days of starting it his depressive mood changes disappeared and have not returned.

Peri-ictal depression will sometimes persist, after the ictus is over, for a variable length of time. Although persistent depression more usually comes on as attack frequency is declining (Flor-Henry 1969, Betts 1974), occasionally it is found as part of an increase in attack frequency and I have rarely seen it as a kind of 'depressive delerium' (Betts 1981a). Williams (1956) likewise describes depression as being sometimes associated with 'a bad phase in the epilepsy'.

Case History 13

At the age of 14, this girl developed brief complex partial seizures supposedly from a closed head injury at the age of 7. At 16, tonic-clonic seizures developed and tended to run in clusters a few months apart. They continued despite treatment with phenytoin and phenobarbitone and , when she was 22, she began to develop severe but short-lived depressive illnesses that came on when there was an exacerbation of her epilepsy, and in which several determined attempts at suicide occurred. Antidepressant medication had little effect but both the seizures and the depression would paradoxically disappear quickly if electroconvulsive therapy was used. In these depressive episodes she was not confused or disorientated, but developed profound guilt feelings, woke early, was retarded, lost weight and heard hallucinatory voices in the second person telling her she was unworthy and should kill herself. Eventually, episodes of frequent seizures and depression occurred several times a year. Depot flupenthixol was tried and since its use, despite having occasional clusters of major seizures, there has been no recurrence of the depression.

Depression and possibly mania can be part of what otherwise would be seen as a schizophrenic illness occurring in relation to epilepsy. Indeed, careful studies of the phenomenology of epileptic psychosis (Perez & Trimble 1980) suggest that an affective component to these states is common, and will be considered again in the section on psychotic illness.

The management of depression involves a detailed history and examination of the patient, both physically and mentally, and an enquiry into life circumstances. Some depressions can be supported and worked through using techniques of counselling or psychotherapy. In contrast to anxiety, however, some patients will need chemical support as well; the indications for using these drugs, even in reactive depression, are much stronger than in anxiety. The tricyclic antidepressants should be considered first, although their convulsant action needs to be remembered.

The drug treatment of the depressions of epilepsy has recently been reviewed (Robertson 1985).

Theoretically a non-convulsant antidepressant might be more appropriate because of the risk of induced seizures but, in practice, Robertson found that neither amitriptyline nor nomifensine (which has subsequently been withdrawn because of untoward side-effects) were particularly effective in the depressive states of epilepsy, the depressions often spontaneously remitting. Neither drug significantly increased seizure frequency in the patients with epilepsy who were already taking antiepileptic drugs (but may cause seizures in patients with low convulsive thresholds who are not taking antiepileptic medication). Occasionally electroconvulsive therapy (ECT) is needed.

Case History 14
This 23-year-old girl developed complex partial seizures at the age of 16. There was a previous history of febrile convulsions as a child. The attacks were initially frequent and responded poorly to antiepileptic drugs. Physical examination showed no abnormality although an EEG showed some right posterior spike-and-wave activity. A year before her admission to hospital, her seizures spontaneously declined in frequency and she had not had one for 3 months. Shortly after her attacks stopped, she quite suddenly became profoundly depressed with early morning waking, loss of weight, and appetite, loss of sexual interest and marked diurnal variation in mood. she developed profound ideas of guilt related to childhood masturbatory episodes, and was admitted to hospital following a determined attempt at suicide with her antiepileptic drugs. Treatment with amitriptyline in hospital failed to resolve the depression (although there was a concomitant return of her seizures and, in addition, she had two tonic-clonic attacks which she had never had before). Amitriptyline was, therefore, stopped. Because of the severity of her depression and her continuing suicidal feelings, she was treated with a course of electroconvulsive therapy. After six applications of ECT, her depression had largely resolved and she was able to go home. It is interesting that the electrically-induced seizures produced a remission in her depression which the spontaneous tonic-clonic seizures had not (this is not always the case). Over the subsequent year she had two further shortlived episodes of depression which did not require hospitalization or treatment as they resolved fairly rapidly, and since then she has been both depression and seizure free.

Apart from possible drug treatment, patients with depression need the support of somebody who understands how disabling depression can be. As a person's depression starts to improve, so he or she will need careful rehabilitation, because, like anxiety, there is no doubt that depression can be self-reinforcing, The loss of confidence in one's abilities which depression can engender may eventually be more disabling than the depression itself, and can persist long after the depression is over.

In the management of depression the risk of suicide must always be kept in mind. Those with epilepsy have a readily available source of dangerous antiepileptic drugs with which to overdose. It is probable that suicide attempts (Mackay 1979) as well as completed suicide (Barraclough 1981) are more common in people with epilepsy than in the general population. A patient with epilepsy is also more likely to repeat previous overdoses. Part of the explanation for the increased incidence of repeated overdoses in people with epilepsy may, of course, lie in the chronic nature of the epileptic patients problems which are not resolved by the overdose attempt.

In a busy general hospital, I see many people with epilepsy who have taken overdoses of their antiepileptic drugs. One particular phenomenon which is not well described in the textbooks is worth reporting: following recovery of consciousness in patients who have taken large overdoses of such drugs as phenytoin, phenobarbitone, primidone or the benzodiazepines, there may be an interval of several days of unruly acting-out behaviour which may be mistaken for the patients' normal state. (This may occur after generalized status epilepticus, particularly if intravenous benzodiazepines are used to control it.)

Case History 15
A 17-year-old girl with poorly controlled epilepsy (probably due to her reluctance to take antiepileptic drugs because of their side-effects) discovered herself to be pregnant and immediately swallowed a large quantity of the phenobarbitone and phenytoin she was supposed to take. She was admitted to hospital unconscious, and recovered consciousness 24 hours later. Shortly after regaining consciousness she was found on a window ledge of the general hospital to which she had been admitted, threatening to jump. When taken back to bed and restrained, she bit, fought and scratched the nursing staff, broke two thermometers on her bedside locker and attempted to swallow them and later broke a cup and attempted to cut her wrists. Unless constantly watched, she would get out of bed and dash around the wards, screaming and shouting and attempting to leave the hospital. She was, therefore, transferred to a psychiatric unit (where

this kind of behaviour after antiepileptic drug overdosage was well known) and the behaviour was merely contained, as it has been found that sedating such disturbed patients merely makes them worse.

An EEG at this time showed changes compatible with drug intoxication, but there was no evidence of subictal epileptic activity (which might also have been a cause of her mental state). Three days after her admission to the psychiatric unit her behaviour settled rapidly and a pleasant and co-operative, if somewhat troubled, teenager emerged from underneath it. Her antiepileptic medication was changed to carbamazepine; her compliance with treatment improved, and she was counselled about her pregnancy, which she decided to keep.

In patients with epilepsy, threats of suicide should always be taken seriously and carefully assessed. Any patient who is depressed should be asked specifically about whether or not he or she has had any thought or plans of self-harm. (Many patients are relieved to be asked this question.) It has been shown that most people who succeed in killing themselves have given clear warning to somebody of their intention beforehand. Patients who are considered likely to make active attempts at suicide (whether their depression is reactive or endogenous) should be admitted to hospital for treatment of their depression and, if necessary, they should be compelled to come into hospital.

Even if initial assessment suggests that the patient is not potentially suicidal, it is important to keep in close touch with him or her until the depression has clearly resolved. It should also be remembered that somebody with intractable epilepsy, which has not responded to treatment, may attempt to take his or her life, not because of depression but because it is felt to be a rational solution to an intolerable situation.

A high-seizure frequency may make effective treatment of the depression more difficult and concomitant with the treatment of depression every effort should be made to bring the patients seizures under as good control as possible, short of intoxication. (It should be remembered that the symptoms of depression can resemble those of drug intoxication and vice versa.) It cannot be emphasized too strongly that, if a family doctor or neurologist has any doubts about the suicidal intent of a depressed patient whom he or she is treating, it is important that the patient be referred urgently for a psychiatric opinion.

Symptomatic alcoholism is common in depression and may also occur in people with epilepsy; although one survey has suggested that drinking problems are less common in people with epilepsy than in the general population (Mackay 1979). If alcoholism does occur in somebody with epilepsy, it complicates considerably the management of the epilepsy. Excessive alcohol intake may cause seizures in the predisposed (as may alcohol withdrawal), although it can be debated whether such 'rum fits' constitute established epilepsy. However, alcohol affects the metabolism of antiepileptic drugs, and it is difficult to control serum levels if they are liable to be influenced by excessive and erratic alcohol intake. Patients who drink excessively are usually unreliable in the taking of prescribed drugs. The relationship between alcohol and epilepsy has been recently well reviewed by Hauser et al (1988).

Moderate drinking is quite acceptable in people with epilepsy, although in view of the potential epileptogenic effects of overhydration, an excessive fluid intake should be avoided. A very few people with epilepsy are very sensitive to the effect of alcohol and regularly have attacks induced by even a very small amount. I know of two patients who *only* have attacks if they drink alcohol, and have been able to abolish their attacks (and the need to take antiepileptic drugs) by avoiding it. It should also be remembered that those who are brain damaged are probably more sensitive to the effects of alcohol: occasionally, a small amount of alcohol in such people may produce 'mania a potu', an excited, aggressive state, induced by what would otherwise have been a non-intoxicating amount of alcohol, and resembling to some extent epileptic furore.

Those patients with anxiety and depression who are faced with a loss of employment or severe social disadvantage (like the break-up of a marriage), will need further measures to help them. Antidepressants will not be enough and skilled help from a counsellor and a theraputic relationship can be of tremendous importance to such patients. Despair which has evoked a call for psychiatric help will often be associated with an increased frequency of seizures, and this in its turn exacerbates the psychiatric problems which then exacerbate the difficulties in controlling the epilepsy. Inpatient care, which provides a constant refuge with careful observation of seizures, good medical management, adjustment of antiepileptic drugs, and a controlled programme of work rehabilitation is essential. Even specialized neurological units with good psychiatric support may not be able to look after such patients long enough or provide adequate work programmes, and specialized psychiatric units, which in some ways are more suitable, may not have all the necessary medical facilities. For the patients just described with multiple handicaps the Special Centres for Epilepsy, where there are complementary hospital and residential units, may be particularly useful but may not be able to take the very disturbed.

Effective treatment and management of the patient depends not on the skills of one particular discipline but rather on the understanding by each specialist discipline of the skills of the others and on their constructive co-operation. A member of any discipline who treats people with epilepsy must have a good working knowledge of the skills of the other disciplines which are necessary for the total care of a patient with epilepsy, and must know when to call in other specialized help. Any psychiatrist who sets out to treat the psychological complications of epilepsy must know a lot about epilepsy itself.

The psychological opposite to depression is mania or hypomania in which there is elevated mood, sleeplessness, overactivity, often grandiose delusions, flights of ideas, irritability and weight loss. The condition is in itself much rarer than depression. It is probably more common in people with epilepsy than could be expected by chance. It can be difficult to distinguish between an excited schizophrenic state and hypomania; affective symptoms are certainly common in the psychoses of epilepsy (Perez & Trimble 1980).

It is certainly my experience that brief hypomanic episodes (often miscalled schizophrenia) do occur in people with epilepsy (Barzak et al 1988, Gillig et al 1988, Johnson & Campbell 1990) and that the condition is not rare as usually stated. My own experience is that the disorder is usually brief, usually follows sudden exacerbation of seizures and tends to occur in patients with right hemisphere spike-wave discharge. Controlling the seizures often seems to control the psychosis,

which usually responds well to tranquillizers like haloperidol. Other patients are described who have a vulnerability to emotional change (Blumer 1991) in which the emotional change is usually depression or irritability, but occasionally can be a mild and brief euphoria.

Barzak et al (1988) reported three cases of undoubted hypomania (using DSM III criteria) which occurred in patients with right temporal discharge following exacerbation of seizure frequency. The paper contains full details of their case histories. Since that time other patients have been seen with similar short episodes of hypomania, an example of which is given below.

Case History 16

A 37-year-old man had recurrent episodes of hypomania from the age of 20 and complex partial seizures from the age of 16. He was an intelligent man and earned his living as a musician. On first presentation at the neuropsychiatry service a study of his previous hospital notes revealed that there was a close association between exacerbations of his complex partial seizures and of his mood disorder. His mood disorder was a florid hypomania with delusions of grandeur, pressure of speech, overactivity and warm and friendly auditory hallucinations of the voice of God. These were always preceded by a sudden increase in seizure frequency and on several occasions he was admitted to hospital with complex partial status. The acute excited state would usually develop 2 or 3 days after the seizures began to increase (they were usually treated in hospital with diazepam, given intravenously). His psychosis could be severe enough to be a management problem in a general hospital and he had many mental hospital admissions transferred from the district general hospital. On two or three occasions he became mute and unresponsive, although this was not thought to be typical catatonic stupor, but more in the nature of a manic stupor. On occasions he could be aggressive and violent in his psychotic state.

Although his hallucinations were warm and friendly, occasionally he could have command hallucinations inciting him to violent acts but he had no first rank symptoms of schizophrenia. The psychosis would usually respond to intravenous and then oral haloperidol and would settle quickly and he would be discharged rapidly from hospital. He was an erratic taker of his antiepileptic medication and refused to take antipsychotic therapy, but would always return to a normal intercurrent mental state until his next episode of complex partial seizures, which usually occurred because of poor compliance with antiepileptic medication. When he did comply with the medication he would still have occasional isolated complex partial seizures. For the last 2 years he has been taking lamotrigine and his seizure frequency is now low. He has had no further mood changes and is now in full-time employment.

I now have a personal series of eight patients with these brief hypomanic episodes in association with complex partial seizures, seven of whom have definite right-sided focus for the epilepsy and only one of whom had a left-sided seizure focus. The religious nature of the delusions and hallucinations and the rare occurrence of the psychosis apart from during exacerbations of the epilepsy seem characteristic. Discussion with colleagues suggests that these psychoses are probably quite common but they are often called a postictal psychosis. Other studies of postictal psychoses in fact suggest that many of them do have an affective element (Logsdail & Toone 1980). Some antiepileptic drugs have anti-manic properties (e.g carbamazapine, sodium valproate) and it is my impression that the new antiepileptic drug lamotrigine also has similar mood stabilizing properties and may be a useful treatment in such cases. Some patients of course have epilepsy complicated by a manic depressive or bipolar psychosis and in these patients too it has been suggested that often there is a right-sided seizure discharge (Flor-Henry 1969).

OTHER STRESS DISORDERS

Some people under stress develop compulsive ritualized behaviours (such as compulsive hand washing, checking or thinking) which can be seen as an attempt to ward off the anxiety induced by the particular stress. Compulsive disorders are particularly likely to become self-reinforcing and are subjectively most unpleasant. There is little evidence that they are more common in people with epilepsy than in the general population. They seem to respond best to behavioural methods of treatment. (They should be distinguished from the 'obsessional personality' which is a rigid pedantic personality structure not uncommon in those who are brain damaged.)

Some people under stress, in order to escape an intolerable situation, develop hysterical symptoms. There is no word in psychiatry which has been more abused and misunderstood than hysteria. To a psychiatrist, hysteria means the uncon-

scious adoption of conversion symptoms of an organic nature (often of a pseudoneurological character) which resolve the conflict or stress for the patient often in a symbolic way (e.g the paralysis of the writing hand which prevents a student from writing his or her final examination papers). Most psychiatrists would agree that the symptoms or signs presented are adopted unconsciously in hysteria, although the borderline between conscious simulation of a disorder and conscious malingering is difficult to define. Hysteria nowadays in Britain is rare, and usually easy to recognize, particularly as it usually results from an acute traumatic situation for the patient.

Problems in recognition arise with chronic symptoms which may be hysterical. It is certainly true that acute hysterical symptoms, unless rapidly treated, may become chronic; particularly as they are easily reinforced by the reaction of other people to them. However, it cannot be emphasized enough that, in a patient with chronic neurological symptoms for which no adequate cause can be found, the diagnosis of hysteria must only be made on positive diagnostic criteria for hysteria and not just be a diagnosis of exclusion. Many patients with a definite organic lesion may over-elaborate their symptoms in order to draw the attention of an often doubting medical profession to them. Cases of firmly diagnosed hysteria often turn out later to have either organic or other psychiatric pathology to account for them (Slater 1965).

A syndrome of multiple somatic complaints without a pathological foundation (Briquets syndrome or somatization disorder) is often confused with hysteria although it is not the same thing at all. The patient has a history of many physical complaints (or a belief that he or she is sickly) which persists for several years and begins before the age of 30. The patient must have at least 13 symptoms from a checklist of 31 (or 35 if female) not related to organic pathology and seek frequent medical advice. Pseudo-neurological symptoms, including faints, collapses and apparent seizures or convulsions, are common. Patients tend to resist psychiatric help and present themselves repeatedly for physical examinations often to a multitude of doctors. There is probably a multiple aetiology. Some suffer somatic symptoms related to tension and anxiety. It is possible that others have been taught to present distress and unhappiness in a somatic form. Treatment of this condition is difficult. If a satisfactory therapeutic relationship can be established and maintained with the patients their behaviour may gradually change over time.

Hysteria has usually been treated by some form of psychotherapy but there is a growing interest in treating hysteria along behavioural lines (Bird 1979). A full account of the management of hysteria will be found in Mersky (1979). The condition will be considered further in this chapter in the section on simulated seizures and non-epileptic attacks.

Occasionally, people under stress break down into what appears to be an acute psychotic illness of either an undifferentiated or schizophrenic type. In some patients who break down like this under acute stress, there is no doubt that it is an unconsciously simulated psychotic disorder (like the Ganser syndrome), which can be seen as a variant of hysteria, often with a clear message from the patient to the outside world, 'look how mad you have made me', but occasionally a true acute schizophrenic illness can be precipitated by stress. Such illnesses have a good prognosis if the stress can be removed: in people with epilepsy they need to be distinguished from those psychotic illnesses of a schizophrenic type which are found in association with epilepsy itself, or from partial status.

PSYCHOSIS AND EPILEPSY

The relationship between psychotic illness and epilepsy has held interest and fascination for centuries; unfortunately the whole subject is confused both by conflicting information, by conflicting theories and interpretation of what information there is and by semantic and terminological muddle. It is an area of particular controversy at the moment and there are several excellent recent reviews (Trimble 1991a,b, Stevens 1991), which particularly highlight differing views on the subject between British and American workers. There is a European view as well (Bruens 1974).

The term 'psychosis' implies the presence of a constellation of symptoms which are characteristic of a particular condition and which are so severe, or which alter the patients thinking or behaviour

or feeling so profoundly, as to have no basis in reality (as opposed to so called 'neurotic' symptoms in which although the patients suffering or experience may be extreme there is a basis within common human experience). Major mental disorders such as severe affective illness, schizophrenia and the paranoid illnesses are usually regarded as psychotic illnesses. In them there is profound behavioural, cognitive and emotional change occurring in the setting of clear consciousness. Some descriptions and classifications of psychotic illness occurring in the context of epilepsy also include mental states which are clearly related to continuing ictal activity within the brain (partial status and sub-convulsive status), and also organic mental illnesses such as delirium. These are conditions not occurring in clear consciousness and are considered later on in this chapter. The discussion in this section of the chapter therefore will be confined to schizophrenia and to chronic paranoid illnesses, as affective illness has already been considered.

SCHIZOPHRENIA AND EPILEPSY

Schizophrenia is a mental disorder characterized by persistent disturbance in the perception and evaluation of reality which leads to characteristic changes in the way the patient behaves, thinks, perceives his environment and responds emotionally to it. Like epilepsy schizophrenia is a common condition although its precise classification and diagnostic criteria are still open to discussion and differences of opinion. In this country particular weight is given to possession by the patient in clear consciousness of certain 'first rank symptoms' (Mellor 1970), particularly if they occur in clear consciousness without evidence of primary mood change and are not fleeting. They are characteristic auditory hallucinatory experiences (such as hearing one's own thoughts spoken out loud, voices talking about the patient in the third person or voices keeping up a running commentary on the patient's behaviour) or certain delusional experiences such as thought insertion or withdrawal, delusional perceptions, thought broadcasting, or feelings, impulses or actions which the patient feels are imposed upon him by outside agencies.

Although in British descriptions of the disease

these first rank symptoms are seen as important and most British literature on schizophrenia is based on first rank symptoms of psychiatric illness, this is not so in American literature, and in the main American classification, DSM III R. This is gaining in acceptance, particularly because DSM III R pays some attention to the duration of symptoms and is also an operational and multiaxial description. Diagnostic confusion is also made worse by the common error of diagnosing an excited, hallucinated and deluded patient as having schizophrenia when he is, in fact, suffering from a manic illness. There is some evidence that American psychiatrists are much more likely to make this mistake than British psychiatrists, but, as has been pointed out (Stevens 1991), British psychiatrists preoccupied with first rank symptoms, (which are largely verbal and auditory and therefore much more likely to relate to left hemisphere dysfunction), may be led into the trap of over emphasizing the left temporal lobe in the genesis of the schizophrenia-like syndromes of epilepsy.

It is also becoming recognized that schizophrenia is not a single disease entity. Not only are there common patterns of presentation which vary according to the age of the patient, but also if one takes a longitudinal view of schizophrenia it is possible to recognize a Type 1 and Type 2 schizophrenia. Type 1 schizophrenia is said to have an acute onset with mainly positive symptoms (active hallucinations and delusions, thought disorder and disturbed emotional response), has a good prognosis and has a good response to treatment. Type 2 schizophrenia is characterized by a chronic state with mainly negative symptoms (poverty of speech, apathy, loss of drive, slowed thinking and movement and affective flattening) and a poor response to treatment. An enlarged ventricular system is detectable on CT scanning in Type 2, but not in Type 1.

Some patients, although they have chronic (usually persecutory) delusions and hallucinatory experiences do not have the other diagnostic characteristics of schizophrenia, particularly because affective contact and emotional responsiveness is maintained. Such psychoses are termed paranoid psychoses: they are common in middle and old age, carry a different prognosis to schizophrenia

and usually are regarded as being separate from it. Patients with paranoid psychoses are often able to conceal them for long periods of time and may be able to maintain their position better in society than patients with the more florid and more personality destroying schizophrenias.

If the literature describing the relationship between psychotic illness, particularly schizophrenia and paranoid psychosis, and epilepsy is reviewed (Trimble 1991b) it will be seen that interest in possible links between the two has been maintained for many years. Unfortunately descriptions in the early literature were often referring to patients with partial status, to patients with delirium resulting from frequent seizures or to patients with affective illness. In the older literature many patients who were described as having psychotic illnesses may have had schizophrenia, but, because at that time the actual classification and recognition of schizophrenia was different, and the symptoms and signs to which we now pay attention were ignored as being irrelevant (Betts 1981b) it is impossible to tell. Thus the very early work on the connection between psychosis and epilepsy, interesting as it is, may not be very helpful to our present understanding of the relationship, if there is one, between the two conditions.

By the 1930s it was possible to find in the literature (Betts 1981b) two totally differing views, one that there was a biological antagonism between epilepsy and schizophrenia (a view which still finds echoes today—Stevens et al 1979), the other that there was a positive biological relationship between the two. The fact that both views could be held sincerely and backed with evidence was because whether or not a writer was seeing fewer or more patients with epilepsy who also had schizophrenia than would be expected by chance depended entirely on where he worked. In chronic mental hospitals patients with epilepsy and schizophrenia tend to accumulate because of the difficulty of rehabilitating patients with this double disability (Betts 1974, Betts and Skarrott 1979, Betts & Kenwood 1988), whereas in academic and university institutions chronically ill patients were often not admitted. In the 1930s convulsive therapy, initially with camphor injections, latterly with electrical stimulation, was introduced as a treatment for schizophrenia (it is largely useless for the condition, but much more effective in affective illness) because of the belief that there was a biological antagonism between the two conditions. It is also possible that, since both epilepsy and schizophrenia are common conditions, they must occur occasionally together purely by chance.

By the 1970s in the UK the view was firmly established that there was a positive biological relationship between epilepsy and schizophrenia, particularly influenced by the work of Slater et al (1963). This highly influential paper, which reviewed numerous cases of patients with both epilepsy and schizophrenia, came to the conclusion that there was a positive relationship between the two conditions, and that the schizophrenia tended to come on some years after the onset of the epilepsy (often when the epilepsy itself was beginning to decline). It was also noted that although the psychoses the patients suffered were indistinguishable from those of schizophrenia, there seemed to be a better preservation of personality and affective contact than is usual in schizophrenia. Since most of the patients described had epilepsy originating in the temporal lobe, it was postulated that the schizophrenia was the result of the disorderly activity in the temporal lobe which had originally caused the epilepsy. The number of patients with combined epilepsy and psychosis that the authors had seen was far higher than would be expected by chance within the catchment area of the two hospitals which were involved in the study, but it is likely that selective referral of patients with epilepsy and psychosis accounted for much, if not all, of the preponderance of the two conditions occurring together. The authors presented evidence concerning the time relationship between the onset of the psychosis and the onset of the epilepsy which is also now open to doubt (Slater & Moran 1969). A survey of a mental hospital population of patients with epilepsy and schizophrenia (Betts & Skarrott 1979) suggested that almost as many patients started their schizophrenia before their epilepsy as those who started the epilepsy before their schizophrenia.

In the United Kingdom in the 70s and 80s the idea that there was a special biological relationship between epilepsy and schizophrenia was developed and elaborated. It was assumed that the two conditions existed together more commonly than would be expected by chance and also occurred quite frequently. Retrospective studies of the patient populations of neuropsychiatric units with a particular interest in epilepsy such as those at The National Hospital or the Maudsley Hospital all seemed to find many examples of the two conditions existing side by side and such populations became extensively studied (see Trimble 1991a,b for a review). The consensus of such studies appear to be that these are interictal psychoses not directly related to ictal events— Logsdail & Toone (1988) have shown that postictal psychoses are different. If the patient possessed nuclear schizophrenic symptoms then the left hemisphere, particularly the left temporal lobe, was more likely to be involved: as Slater et al (1963) had already suggested personality and affective response seemed to be better preserved than is usual in schizophrenia. The partial epilepsies (whether or not they are secondary generalized) were much more likely to give rise to psychosis: there was often a definite affective element to the psychosis as well as the schizophrenic symptoms.

This particular interest in the partial epilepsies which are associated with psychosis probably relates to a general interest in brain localization and the belief in the importance of the left hemisphere as opposed to the right which exists in neuropsychiatry. Latterly the possible links between the transmitter chemistry of epilepsy and the transmitter chemistry of schizophrenia (and also affective disorder) is gaining attention. Recently (Sander et al 1991) interest has focused on the apparently relatively frequent incidence of psychosis in patients treated with vigabatrin. Perhaps 5% of patients treated with vigabatrin for their intractable complex partial seizures, with or without secondary generalization, develop a psychosis. In my own experience (Kenwood & Betts 1992) such vigabatrin psychoses only seem to occur if the patient's epilepsy comes under sudden control and will usually resolve eventually, even if the vigabatrin is continued, if appropriate psychotropic medication is used. They are usually affective in nature, either depressive or manic, with a psychotic colouring and resemble, as Trimble (1991b) has pointed out, the rare psychoses that occur with ethosuximide. Such psychoses in my experience can often be avoided by starting the patient with a very small dose of vigabatrin and building the dose up slowly. They do seem to occur in those patients whose seizures stop suddenly or where there is a preceding history of psychotic illness.

As Stevens 1991 has argued, the British preoccupation with psychoses related to epilepsy, particularly if they have a schizophrenic nature, may be possibly an artifact of the British preoccupation with the first rank symptoms of schizophrenia and also may be an artifact of the collection of such patients in neuropsychiatry centres that have a particular interest in psychosis and epilepsy. Patients with the double disability of psychosis and epilepsy may be particularly difficult to rehabilitate and therefore may accumulate in psychiatric institutions so that the relationship appears to be more common than it actually is. There is little evidence that the two conditions are commonly associated in patients with epilepsy in the community (Edeh & Toone 1987). In a survey of acute admissions of people with epilepsy to all the psychiatric institutions within a single city over a calendar year (Betts 1974) there were relatively few patients admitted with epilepsy and psychosis. The majority of the patients with epilepsy who were admitted for psychiatric care were admitted for depressive illness, acute situational reactions, or acute organic states related to the epilepsy. Only 3% of the patients surveyed were actually admitted with a psychotic illness resembling schizophrenia. However over 50% of the patients in the same hospitals who had been in the hospitals for at least 2 years (and often of course for much longer) did have a psychotic illness in addition to their epilepsy, suggesting that factors of accumulation were very important.

When a combination of psychosis and epilepsy does occur it is likely that the two conditions in some way exist together because of the changes in transmitter chemistry occurring in the parts of the brain that are responsible both for the psychosis and for the epilepsy itself. However other views on aetiology do exist. It is still possible that some cases are no more than the coincidence of two common conditions occurring together. There is also the view that sometimes the alienating experience of epilepsy itself may eventually change into the alienation of schizophrenia, although such experiences may be pathoplastic rather than pathogenic for the psychosis. The patient described below in case history 20 illustrates this. Many patients with schizophrenia are known to have low convulsive thresholds (Hill 1957). This low convulsive threshold means that patients with schizophrenia are particularly likely to have epileptic seizures if given psychotropic medication: one of the problems in managing psychoses in patients with epilepsy is that although the psychosis may be controlled the epilepsy is often exacerbated (see case history 21).

The treatment of the psychoses of epilepsy is well reviewed by Trimble (1991b). In my own experience these psychoses seem to respond well to non-sedating neuroleptic medication such as haloperidol, pimozide or sulpiride, although control of the psychosis is often accompanied by an increase in seizures: in some patients the decision has to be made with the patient and the patient's relatives as to whether they can cope better with the psychosis or the seizures (see case history 21). A European concept of the relationship between epilepsy and psychoses is that which is termed in English 'forced normalization' (Landolt 1958). However this phrase 'forced normalization', although a literal translation from the German, is not an accurate one as Landolt was merely implying that during the psychotic episodes that he was observing the EEG of the patients with epilepsy became temporarily normal: he was not implying an active process (Trimble 1991b). It is possible that although the epileptic activity has shifted from the surface electrodes it is still continuing deep in the cortex.

In conclusion, many patients during the time they have epilepsy (and sometimes before it and sometimes after the epilepsy itself has disappeared) will develop psychotic episodes. Many of these patients clearly have an affective psychosis, or are passing through a period of delirium or have partial or sub-convulsive status. Some patients however will be having a schizophrenic or a paranoid psychosis, which occasionally will be postictal, but will usually be interictal. Such patients, if both the epilepsy and the psychosis continue and do not respond to treatment, may be difficult to rehabilitate and therefore may accumulate in institutions. Such patients are also of particular interest to psychiatrists and neuro-psychiatrists seeking a link between schizophrenia and epilepsy. They may therefore assume an importance disproportionate to the actual frequency of the condition, although it is possible that the two conditions do exist together slightly more commonly than would be expected by chance and may pose some problems in management. It is interesting that the affective psychoses of epilepsy, which are certainly more common, do not excite the same interest and have been curiously little studied, although they have been clearly recognized in people with epilepsy since ancient times.

Case History 17
This woman of 53 developed epilepsy at the age of 40, following the removal of a left temporal turberculoma. Her attacks had usually been generalized without any evidence of a partial focus although EEG evidence showed clearly that they were left temporal in origin. She had had relatively few attacks which were controlled with a mixture of phenobarbitone and phenytoin. Three years before her first psychiatric admission she developed status epilepticus and was unconscious for some time after the status was controlled. She was left with a gross dysmnesic state which slowly cleared over the following year. As this improved so she began to develop paranoid symptoms, becoming hostile towards her neighbours and entertaining delusional ideas about them. She finally developed a complex delusional system involving Jehovah's Witnesses and the Post Office whom she felt were tampering with her mind and had inserted an electronic listening device into her brain so that her thoughts were broadcast to other people. She began to develop auditory hallucinations and her behaviour became so disturbed at home that she needed admission to hospital. She was treated with small doses of haloperidol and within a fortnight the delusional ideas encapsulated and then disappeared and she was no longer troubled by auditory hallucinations. She remained well on a small dose of haloperidol for 2 years but then had to be re-admitted with a further exacerbation of her psychosis which followed self-withdrawal from her medication. She recovered, was maintained on haloperidol for some 3 years, which was then slowly withdrawn and she has continued well since and there has been no return of the psychosis. Her last seizure occurred just before the onset of her original psychotic illness and she has had no seizures since.

Case History 18
This woman of 30 with poorly controlled left temporal epilepsy began to develop religious ideas which gradually became so obtrusive and insistent that she would read her Bible loudly and continually all day long, both at work, on the bus going to and from work, and at home. Her readings became more angry and voiciferous and eventually she began to express religious delusions that she had had a visitation from The Almighty and had been sent with a special purpose to cleanse the world of sin. She always denied having auditory hallucinations although it was felt that her loud Bible reading was an attempt to drown out hallucinations, and other aspects of her behaviour suggested that she did actually have auditory hallucinations. Her epilepsy continued (she had both complex partial and secondary generalized seizures) although there was a clear relationship between the intensity of her psychotic symptoms and the temporary absence of seizures. On several occasions, after spontaneous attacks of serial epilepsy, lasting 2 or 3 days, her psychotic symptoms would clear temporarily. Investigations showed marked atrophy of the left temporal lobe and also a colloid cyst of the third ventricle. She was treated with large doses of haloperidol and on this regimen her psychotic symptoms gradually disappeared and she was able to return to sheltered employment. Her psychotic symptoms did not return and she had only the occasional epileptic seizure since her original admission. She was found dead in bed one day following a nocturnal seizure.

Case History 19
This woman was admitted to a mental hospital at the age of 27 with a history of the insidious onset of a schizophrenic illness. On admission she displayed delusions of passivity and influence, ideas of reference, somatic illusions and auditory hallucinations which failed to respond to treatment. At the age of 32 she began to have tonic-clonic seizures, often at night, which were not very frequent but which were described as very severe when they did occur as she would remain unconscious for several hours afterwards. Both the epilepsy and the psychosis continued but the psychotic symptoms disappeared after she was given haloperidol at the age of 46. For the next 10 years of her life her mental state remained normal although she continued to have two or three major tonic-clonic seizures a year despite treatment with phenobarbitone and phenytoin. About once or twice a year she would have episodes of acute excitement, lasting 2 or 3 hours, in which she would become quite aggressive and destructive. These were unpredictable, swiftly resolved and she seemed to have little memory of them. Shortly before her death at the age of 57 she began to have more tonic-clonic seizures than usual although her mental state remained unchanged and there was no evidence of dementia or organic brain impairment. She was found dead one morning: there was no post-mortem examination. EEG examination at the age of 46 had shown a right temporal slow-wave focus.

Case History 20

This man of 30 had developed simple partial seizures at the age of 16 which gradually evolved into complex partial seizures (there was evidence of a right temporal lobe focus on EEG). There was a history of previous febrile convulsions. His seizures initially consisted of an epigastric sensation which he found hard to describe, but which would occur in his stomach, gradually rise into his throat, again in a way that he could not describe, but which was associated with the colour blue so that he described the experience as a blue bubble developing in his stomach and rising up into his throat during which he seemed to have some mystically erotic feeling so that he quite welcomed the experience. After 2 or 3 years of merely experiencing this as a simple partial seizure and retaining full consciousness he began to lose consciousness as the experience rose into his throat. He would become unconscious and uncommunicative for some 2 minutes, and would stand or sit without moving, smacking his lips and swallowing repeatedly until suddenly recovering consciousness but being a little confused after waking. He became preoccupied with the meaning of the experience, kept many notebooks full of his descriptions of his ictal experience and his interpretation of it, and gradually his preoccupation with and his description and interpretation of the experience became all pervading and bizarre, leading him to develop the idea that the 'blue bubbles' were inserted into his abdomen by an X-ray device operated by his neighbours and triggered off by passing cars sounding their horns outside his house. He became reclusive and if he did go out believed himself to be being followed and spied upon and that car radio aerials were communicating with each other about his movements (on his first visit to the clinic he presented me with 57 car aerials that he had snapped off and removed between the railway station and the hospital). Because of his intense preoccupation with the colour blue and the bizarre description of the epigastric experience it was not realized immediately that he was actually describing a simple partial seizure so that he was treated initially with haloperidol which removed the preoccupation but not the experience. The epileptic nature of the experience was eventually realized partly by observation of him during an attack and partly by the observation that, as his preoccupation with the experience faded so it was clear that he was having paroxysmal and episodic experiences of the phenomena. His seizures responded to carbamazepine and he has been psychosis and seizure free for many years.

Case History 21

This 32-year -old woman with limited intelligence had had generalized seizures (with a primary generalized pattern on EEG) since the age of 6. By the age of 32 her seizures, which had previously been so severe and frequent that she could only take sheltered employment, had become rare and she was only having two or three a year. She gradually become reclusive in her room, developed obsessional behaviour related to the way that pictures were hung on her wall and the way that her patterned bed quilt was arranged and, to use her mother's phrase, 'Talked of nothing but colours'. She developed an elaborate hierarchy of colours, their meanings and their relationships to people and began to develop auditory hallucinations which commented on her actions in the third person but gave her direct advice in the second person about changing the colour of her room. Treatment with various antipsychotic drugs including trifluoperazine, haloperidol, pimozide and sulpiride always resulted in a swift resolution of the psychosis but on each occasion caused a sudden exacerbation of her seizures so that she would have two or three a week despite an increase in her antiepileptic medication. A family conference was eventually held where it was realized that her epilepsy was easy for the family to manage and did not mean that she could no longer go to her sheltered workshop but that the psychosis was difficult for the family to cope with and had led to her exclusion from sheltered employment. She is therefore being maintained on antipsychotic medication and the resulting increased seizure frequency has been tolerated: it is gradually falling.

NON-EPILEPTIC ATTACK DISORDER (PSEUDOSEIZURES)

In the last 20 years or so it has become increasingly recognized that many patients, who have often carried the label of being a 'known epileptic' for many years, do not actually have the condition at all. The term pseudoseizure has been coined to describe such patients. Pseudoseizure however is a pejorative term and is also technically incorrect. It is pejorative because it is blaming the patient for something which is almost certainly not the patient's fault. The error in diagnosis is the doctor's and not, except very rarely, due to the patient's deliberate deception. The term is also technically wrong because pseudoseizures, although not epileptic, are as real as epileptic seizures but just have a different cause. I much prefer the term non-epileptic attack disorder (NEAD—Betts 1990). I think the term pseudoseizure needs to be abandoned partly for the reasons given above and also because it prevents us from making a readjustment of our attitudes to attack disorder in general, which it is important to do if we are to understand completely these attacks and their relationship to epilepsy.

Immersed in the work of busy clinics we seldom step back and look at epilepsy with any different perspective, but I think that it is important that we do. We need to look at it both in a biological and a human context. The fact that sudden changes in the chemistry of receptors in the brain produce characteristic changes in the behaviour of an animal is not just an accident. Epilepsy has a biological purpose in the animal kingdom or it would have long since disappeared. It conveys a biological advantage—a swift automatic response to threat and startle which may lead to escape from threat or produce fear in a predator—a tonic-clonic seizure in a mouse is expressed as running behaviour, but is a blind unpredictable dash which a predator cannot follow. A rabbit that convulses when it is picked up by a predator will be dropped.

A convulsion in a human being is seen as threatening and frightening and, until we are used to it, we respond to it with alarm and fear and we have the primitive feeling that the person is out of control. Often when trying to educate patients and their families about epilepsy we have to be reassuring that the person in the seizure can feel nothing and is not distressed because we also have in our language and in our concepts the view that a seizure or a fit is an acceptable or appropriate response to severe emotion ('Surprised? I nearly had a fit'). In mediaeval England and up to the eighteenth century and also nearer our own time physicians talked of 'fits of the mother' a term which, although it had some relationship to convulsions, was also related to sudden changes in behaviour of a paroxysmal nature or, at least, of a quasi-neurological nature but probably with a psychological cause (Williams 1990). Even today we still use terms such as 'blue fit' to indicate that we recognize that paroxysmal changes in behaviour or sudden alterations in mood or feeling may have an emotional basis and an impact on and import for other people.

We often express strong emotions through the idiom or through the action of a seizure. Children enraged or intensely frustrated have a tantrum in which they lie on the floor and kick and scream (so do disadvantaged adults). Sudden overwhelming emotion or circumstances will cause some people to withdraw suddenly and to cut off from the overwhelming emotion by closing their eyes and sinking to the floor or by showing other signs of withdrawal. I sometimes wonder if there is actually much difference between the patient in whom intense anxiety triggers off the chemical events which lead to an epileptic seizure, and the patient in whom intense anxiety triggers off an imitation of the seizure as a way of escaping from an intolerable situation. Both serve the same biological purpose.

The problem is that we have over medicalized convulsive and paroxysmal responses: and because epilepsy is medical, treatable and understandable we tend to label any sudden paroxysm, convulsion or alteration in behaviour as epileptic (because that makes it acceptable and potentially controllable) and become angry with and rejecting of the person whose seizure turns out to be non-epileptic, because of our need to use medicine to understand behaviour. We have forgotten to think about the person who has the seizure and the meaning of seizures (whether they are epileptic or not). Although we tend to regard all seizures as epileptic (and we call non-epileptic seizures 'pseudoseizures') we should really recognize that there is a class of conditions that we should call 'seizure or paroxysmal disorders' of which epilepsy is only one. We have made the mistake of putting epilepsy on a pedestal.

The importance of this is not only that we should be less rejecting and more accepting of patients that have a non-epileptic seizure disorder, but also because non-epileptic seizure disorders do not respond very well to treatment for epilepsy. We would also be better prepared for dealing with uncertainty because, as will be shown, it is becoming increasingly clear that the distinction between an epileptic seizure and a non-epileptic seizure is often difficult to make despite all the technology currently at our disposal. We need to use a non-medical model for understanding seizure disorder much more frequently than we do.

Also, it must not be forgotten that although most non-epileptic seizure disorders are of a psychological origin there are also physical non-epileptic seizure disorders, and that the psychological disorders which lead to a non-epileptic seizure have their own differential diagnosis. Because we are preoccupied with epilepsy, when we discover that the patient does not have epilepsy we fail to look critically at the patient's behaviour which has led to the erroneous diagnosis and label it as a 'pseudoseizure' without recognizing that there are several distinct types of pseudoseizure.

Non-epileptic attack disorder (NEAD) is of some economic importance. It has been defined as 'A sudden disruptive change in a person's behaviour, which is usually time limited, and which resembles, or is mistaken for, epilepsy but which does not have the characteristic electrophysiological changes in the brain detectable by electroencephalography which accompanies a true epileptic seizure' (Betts & Boden 1991). NEAD may occur in up to 20% of patients seen in specialist epilepsy practice, particularly in patients labelled as having intractable epilepsy who undergo intensive monitoring and assessment (Ramani 1986). NEAD may also be important at the very start of diagnosing epilepsy. In a recent study of newly diagnosed epilepsy in general practice (Sander et al 1990) it was shown that some 28% of patients presented to the research team as having suspected epilepsy either did not have it (7%) or the diagnosis could not be substantiated, at least in the short term (21%). It was felt that some of the patients had other physiological causes for seizures resembling epilepsy (e.g. migraine) and some were labelled as having probable 'pseudoseizures'. This term is not further defined but presumably means emotionally based seizure activity. This was a study where very careful diagnostic criteria were laid down for epilepsy and patients were not included in the study as having epilepsy unless there was clear evidence that they did. In ordinary clinical practice many of the 28% of patients not included in the study would probably have been labelled clinically as having epilepsy and would have been treated accordingly. This is often how NEAD becomes labelled as epilepsy. The problem is that once someone has been given the label of epilepsy it becomes very difficult to remove it as the patient becomes a 'known epileptic' and nobody thereafter ever looks critically at what the patient's seizures are like.

There is another side to the coin. Many patients with actual epilepsy presenting as a seizure disorder do not have the epilepsy diagnosed, as other explanations are given for the seizure behaviour, or the patient or family do not actually bring the attention of the medical profession to the seizure disorder because they can cope with it and live with it or have their own private explanation for it. 'Mummy's little turns' are incorporated into family mythology. What people do about seizures, whether epileptic or not, depends very much on the cultural values and expectations of the society in which they live. Certainly there are a number of people with epilepsy who although they have had it for a long time, never have it recognized, investigated or treated (Betts 1974).

NEAD becomes a problem if, having recognized that the patient has a NEAD as opposed to epilepsy, the recognition of the NEAD is seen as the end point of the interaction between patient and doctor. If the doctor can however recognize that there are several distinct types of NEAD and that there is very good management for it, his job will be easier and the patient's lot a bit happier, particularly as making the distinction between NEAD and epilepsy is often difficult, time consuming and uncertain, and both NEAD and epilepsy may be existing side by side in the same patient.

Classification of attack disorders

I am going to be very unorthodox for a moment in terms of this classification, and look at attack disorder as a whole, including epilepsy as well as non-epileptic attack disorder, and consider how these disorders actually present themselves to other people.

1. Convulsive behaviour
2. Collapse but no convulsion—'syncope'
3. Sudden change in external awareness or relationship to the environment (brief or prolonged)
4. Sudden change in internal awareness, thinking or sensation (brief or prolonged)
5. Sudden change in emotion, either felt or expressed, which may be brief or prolonged
6. Sudden change in behaviour or in relationship to others which may be brief or prolonged, may be simple or complex motor activity
7. Sudden change in awareness, behaviour or feelings whilst apparently asleep.

Table 11.1   Types of convulsive behaviour (Collapse and Convulsion)

a. Tonic-clonic seizure (primary or secondary generalized)
b. Tonic-clonic seizure (exogenous cause)
c. Tonic-clonic seizure (endogenous cause)
d. Convulsion—non-epileptic but physically caused (e.g. agonal seizure)
e. Convulsive behaviour emotionally based (e.g. imitation, 'tantrum', 'abreactive')

All such attacks may or may not be accompanied by loss or abrogation of consciousness.

Patients whose attacks are frightening or disturbing, either to themselves or others, are likely to present early and may have had only one or two attacks before they are seen. Other patients may not present until the attacks have been present for some considerable time, either because of denial or because the importance of the attacks is not recognized, or because they are accepted by the patient and his or her family who have a ready explanation for them. Once presented however, particularly if they are disturbing or the question of epilepsy has been raised (with the implications of loss of a driving licence or employment and other social disadvantages), there is usually intense pressure upon the doctor to make a diagnosis and to institute treatment as rapidly as possible, which is why a hasty ill-considered diagnosis is sometimes made, or treatment is started blindly which then makes it impossible to diagnose what kind of attack disorder the patient actually had.

Differential diagnosis of attack disorder

Table 11.1 lists the differential diagnosis of convulsive behaviour which usually consists of a collapse followed by a convulsion. This may occur without warning, or there may be a warning beforehand which the patient comes to recognize as regularly preceding his attacks (it is important to determine as well whether the patient gets the warning at other times without a convulsion following). Often the warning is a true epileptic aura, such as déjà-vu or an olfactory experience, but often its nature is not so clear cut or may eventually point to a different cause of the convulsion (a feeling of anxiety before a convulsion

may mean that the patient is hyperventilating himself into a seizure) or prior feelings of dizziness may mean that there is a cardiovascular cause for the seizure, particularly if it is accompanied by pallor and if quickly sitting or lying down stops it: likewise a paroxysmal headache before the attack or transient weakness in a limb may suggest a cerebrovascular cause.

Tonic-clonic seizures tend to be stereotyped in their nature and are usually brief. Classically there is a sudden loss of consciousness, characteristic stiffening, sometimes a cry as air is forced out of a closed glottis and a fall. Stiffening of the body usually continues for a short while, with a characteristic tonic posture of the limbs followed by clonic jerking. (It is important for doctors who are likely to have to diagnose tonic-clonic seizures to see several on video tape and study their characteristics carefully: it is often useful to show a typical tonic-clonic seizure on video tape to the witness of a convulsion so that they can judge if it was similar.) Tonic-clonic seizures may be due to primary or secondary generalized epilepsy, may be due to an exogenous cause initiating a tonic-clonic seizure in a patient who has a low convulsive threshold, or may be due to some physical condition like hypoglycaemia which triggers off a tonic-clonic seizure, in a patient with a low convulsive threshold. It is important to recognize this because removing the exogenous or endogenous cause will stop the seizures without the patient needing to be labelled as having epilepsy: such symptomatic epilepsies, anyway, are usually resistant to antiepileptic treatment. If the brain is suddenly deprived of oxygen an agonal seizure will occur, which is convulsive but which is not a true epileptic seizure.

Some apparent convulsions with falling, apparent unconsciousness and with vigorous body movement relate to emotional causes. Conscious simulation of epilepsy is rare, but is often quite accomplished when it does occur, as the patient may be imitating a friend or relative with genuine epilepsy. Many patients simulate epilepsy apparently unconsciously without obvious deliberate intent (although it is often very difficult to tell if the patient is aware of what he is doing). Apparently unconscious simulation of epilepsy occurs in hysteria or Briquet's syndrome and is usually an imitation of the lay concept of epilepsy and does not look like a tonic-clonic seizure.

The patient falls but usually not stiffly. There is often a cry but it is usually a gasping intake of breath rather than an exhalation. There may be a tonic phase but the limbs are usually extended rigidly rather than having the tonic posture of a tonic-clonic seizure. Subsequent jerking is not usually rhythmical but is an incoordinate thrashing of the limbs and the body. The patient may transport himself across the room during the seizure. Breathing is not suspended and is often noisy and gasping. External movement of the limbs or body during the seizure or eye opening is resisted, and gentle restraint is often met by redoubled convulsive efforts. Seizure activity may go on for a long time, may stop and restart, there may be biting of the inside of the mouth or the tip of the tongue. There may be repetitive banging of the head on the ground with cuts and bruises: injuries may occur during falling: incontinence may occur and I know of at least one patient who not only urinates but defecates during the attacks. The patient is usually flushed rather than blue, and may be sleepy, exhausted and have a headache after the seizure is over. The patient may appear to be in the grip of some strong emotion. In true hysterical seizures other neurological signs are commonly present, such as hemianaesthesia or hemiplegia either as part of the attack or separately.

I would emphasize that I have been describing up until now patients whose intent, even though it appears to be unconscious, is to imitate actual epilepsy for some primary or secondary gain. Non-epileptic convulsive behaviour can also occur in settings and situations where it is clear that the patient is not attempting to imitate epilepsy but that the behaviour has been labelled as epileptic by the medical profession. These patients, in my experience, are commoner than the patients who are actually imitating epilepsy and who wish to have the behaviour so labelled.

There are two main types: the first is the *tantrum*. Tantrums are sudden collapses with convulsive behaviour. They tend to occur following environmental challenge or demands that the patient cannot cope with. They are usually noisy, and often start with a wild scream. The patient throws him- or herself to the ground kicking, screaming and thrashing about, often with minor injury to the victim or to those who try to restrain the victim. The patient may bite himself or onlookers. The attacks resemble the tantrums of childhood and are usually the result of the patient feeling frustrated and angry and tend to occur in the underprivileged or the brain damaged or patients who have grown into adult life without losing their childhood behaviour. They can be seen as a form of 'acting out behaviour'. Usually anger or frustration is being acted out but sometimes fear or other unpleasant emotions.

Abreactive attacks are also convulsive, are not meant to imitate epilepsy but usually get labelled as epilepsy—they account for over 20% of the patients that I have seen with non-epileptic attacks (Betts & Boden 1991). The attacks often occur at night although the patient is not asleep. There may be initial overbreathing followed by stiffening of the body (the patient will fall if she is on her feet) and there is then breath holding followed by gasping intakes of breath, incoordinate jerking of the body with characteristic back arching and pelvic thrusting. The attack does not look like a tantrum, nor like a convulsive seizure but does resemble sexual intercourse. It may continue for hours (most cases of 'pseudostatus-epilepticus' are this kind of seizure). This kind of seizure very commonly occurs in women who have had previously suffered sexual abuse and in my experience is often a result of unpleasant memories of abuse entering consciousness.

Table 11.2 Types of collapse (but no convulsion)

a.	Generalized epilepsy
b.	Partial epilepsy (temporal lobe and frontal)
c.	Vasovagal attack (syncope)
d.	Basilar migraine
e.	Cataplexy
f.	Menières disease
g.	TIA and 'cerebral grey out'
h.	Aortic stenosis
i.	Atrial myxoma
j.	Mitral valve prolapse
k.	Stokes–Adams attacks
l.	Hypoglycaemia
m.	IIIrd ventricular cyst
n.	Emotional syncope
o.	Hyperventilation (panic attack)
p.	Cutting off behaviour (swoon)

Some patients collapse but do not convulse (Table 11.2) or following a collapse have only slight movement. Primary generalized seizure discharge, usually brief, can lead to a jerk, an absence and a fall. Most patients usually have brief attacks: often no sooner have they landed on the floor than they are awake and able to get up again. Occasionally they may be dazed by striking their head on the floor or they may have an absence, a fall and a tonic seizure (it is always important to check in patients that fall and who then lie still whether they are stiff or flaccid). Some partial seizures can result in a fall followed by unconsciousness. This is usually for a fairly brief period but sometimes can last for longer. Such patients are usually flaccid and may occasionally be aware dimly of what is happening around them but be unable to respond: they are usually confused afterwards. Patients who fall in a frontal lobe seizure may have characteristic head or eye turning and may have peculiar incoordinate bicycling movement of the legs or may behave in a bizarre way, which can often be mistaken for hysterical behaviour.

Non-epileptic collapse is usually caused by syncope which may be frequent (and may have an emotional cause). Usually there are premonitory feelings of faintness and dizziness: there is pallor and a characteristically slow pulse (patients having partial seizures usually have a rapid pulse) and recovery is usually quick. (Some patients who faint may be inadvertently kept propped up in which case unconsciousness may go on for much longer and the patient may be very confused afterwards.) Occasionally a faint is sufficient to trigger off an epileptic seizure: patients in a faint can injure themselves, may twitch and occasionally can be incontinent. There are several cardiovascular causes of sudden unconsciousness with a fall including sudden changes in cardiac rhythm, aortic stenosis, atrial myxoma and possibly mitral valve prolapse.

There are several cerebral causes for sudden loss of consciousness. Transient ischaemic attacks may present in this way. Basilar migraine may present with unconsciousness, cataplexy may present with what looks like attacks of unconsciousness (though of course the patient is actually conscious), as may occasionally Menière's disease (although

there will be other symptoms to suggest the diagnosis such as tinnitus, true vertigo and deafness). A third ventricle cyst may also sometimes present with recurrent abrupt losses of consciousness.

The commonest causes of non-epileptic loss of consciousness are, however, emotional. Emotional syncope (true fainting induced by strong emotion) is common, as is a panic attack leading to hyperventilation and unconsciousness. Characteristically, patients feel a rising sense of anxiety and panic as they overbreathe (they are usually unaware of their hyperventilation or describe it as not being able to get their breath). As the attack continues they get tingling in their extremities (which often increases the panic) and there may be actual tetanic spasm of the hands and feet and, sometimes, the face. If the overbreathing continues the patient will often pass out and lie inert, often not breathing for 2 or 3 minutes and may even go slightly blue in the face until respiration recovers. Characteristically the patient also feels lightheaded and dizzy during the attack and may feel unwell afterwards. Panic attacks are commonly mistaken for epilepsy and it often happens that the two conditions may exist side by side. Diagnostic difficulty also occurs when the panic attack is preceded by other anxiety symptoms which can be mistaken for epilepsy such as derealization or depersonalization.

Some patients faced with an unpleasant reality or a situation with which they cannot cope withdraw from the reality in a 'swoon'. This cutting off behaviour, usually not consciously motivated, is common. Often the patient closes his eyes and sinks to the floor and then lies flaccidly inert often with peculiar eyelid flickering (rather like children taking surreptitious peeps at their surroundings whilst playing dead). Attacks may be prolonged and the patient may be unrousable even if vigorous stimulation is applied. Some patients feel refreshed after such episodes and most wake up quickly with little confusion.

Drop attacks, particularly with prolonged unconsciousness and flaccidity, can be very difficult to diagnose with certainty. In any series of patients with non-epileptic attack disorder there is a small group of patients, mostly with drop attacks, who remain undiagnosed and in whom the elucidation of whether or not the attack has an epileptic basis

Table 11.3 Types of changes in awareness, cognition, emotion and behaviour—brief or prolonged

---

a. Primary generalized epilepsy
b. Partial seizures
c. Sub-convulsive status
d. Simple partial status
e. Complex partial status
f. Catalepsy
g. Cortical stroke: TIA
h. Hypoglycaemia: phaeochromocytoma: carcinoid
i. Unusual tics: Tourette's syndrome
j. Movement disorders
k. Depressive/anxiety phenomena: fugues
l. Hysteria (cutting off behaviour): fugues
m. Psychotic illness
n. Episodic dyscontrol syndrome

---

may take years to discover. This is partly because EEG ambulatory monitoring shows gross artifact if the patient falls and hits his head, so at the very time one wants to know what is going on in the patient's brain it is impossible to do so. Most patients who swoon are escaping from environmental stress or unpleasant obtrusive thoughts. In a few patients this seems to be a learnt pattern of behaviour or it may be consciously motivated but in most patients it takes a long time to get them to connect their behaviour with whatever is causing it, so it is probably an unconscious mechanism. Not all patients who swoon sink slowly to the floor and some may throw themselves down quite violently.

Table 11.3 illustrates the possible causes for sudden changes in external awareness, in internal awareness, in emotional tone and in behaviour, whether they are brief or prolonged. This is, as one might expect, a rich field for differential diagnosis. Sudden loss of awareness of surroundings can be due both to primary generalized epileptic discharge or a partial seizure: more prolonged states of loss of awareness and loss of contact with surroundings can be due to sub-convulsive status or to complex partial status. Repetitive motor movements (simple or complex) may be due to a partial epilepsy and prolonged motor movements may be due to simple partial status (epileptic movement disorder can sometimes be a tonic motor phenomenon rather than a clonic one and may be followed by temporary loss of function—Todd's paralysis—and may or may not be accompanied by change in sensation).

Other physical phenomenon that may be implicated in changes in awareness, cognition, emotion or behaviour, either brief or prolonged, are catalepsy, cortical stroke, transient ischaemic attacks, transient global amnesia (the aetiology of which is uncertain but is probably vascular), hypoglycaemia (often characteristically preceded by emotional symptoms which may look bizarre and be mistaken for hysteria), phaeochromocytoma and the carcinoid syndrome. Unusual tics (particularly in the Tourette's syndrome) and complex movement disorders may also be mistaken for epilepsy (particularly as in Tourette's syndrome the disorder is often brief and stereotyped).

Paroxysmal changes in feeling or internal awareness are common accompaniments of stress, high arousal, anxiety and depression (Silberman et al 1985) and brief lapses of awareness or contact with reality are also common presenting symptoms in general practice (Morrell et al 1971)—most of these have an unknown aetiology or are related to emotional stress. In patients who are anxious many of the symptoms commonly associated with epilepsy can occur such as déjà-vu, derealization, depersonalization, and may need careful assessment. Paroxysmal disorders such as catalepsy and the episodic dyscontrol syndrome may also be mistaken for epilepsy, particularly if they are recurrent (there does seem to be a need to try to label episodes of aggressive behaviour as epileptic, although they very rarely are). Fugue (a confused wandering away) is usually emotional in origin relating to depression or is a form of cutting off behaviour. It is rarely epileptic but easily may be labelled as such. It should be remembered, however, that frontal seizures in particular may present with such bizarre and odd behaviour as to be labelled psychogenic when they do in fact have an epileptic basis.

Table 11.4 Types of sleep related paroxysmal attack disorder

---

a. Primary generalized epilepsy (usually on waking)
b. Partial seizures (temporal and frontal lobe)
c. Sleep paralysis
d. REM sleep disorder
e. Hypnopompic/hypnogogic phenomena
f. Sleep walking and variants
g. Night terrors
h. Nocturnal anxiety attacks

Table 11.4 outlines the differential diagnosis of paroxysmal disorders which occur in sleep. Between 10% and 20% of epileptic attacks seem only to occur in sleep, so a sudden paroxysmal disorder in sleep may well have an epileptic basis. (Epileptic attacks may occur in sleep without awakening the patient and therefore remain un-detected unless they happen to wake a partner or they are overheard.) In my clinical experience the differential diagnosis of paroxysmal disorders in sleep is a wide one and often difficult to make: many patients are labelled as having nocturnal epilepsy when in fact they have some other sleep phenomenon. It is now recognized that frontal lobe discharge often occurs in sleep and may produce very wild and disturbed behaviour (so called hypnogenic paroxysmal dystonia) which is labelled as a movement disorder or as hysteria (Tinuper et al 1990). REM sleep disorder in which the patient is dreaming but able (because of lack of the usual paralysis during the dream) to physically express his dream has only been recog-nized comparatively recently: since the patient is in a dreamy state it may well be mistaken for epilepsy, as may sleep paralysis. Patients with sleepwalking, particularly if it is severe or leads to injury or to anxiety in parents, may be referred for investigation of possible epilepsy. Night terrors in children are often mistaken for epilepsy. Night terrors also occur in adults although this is not widely known and are often labelled as epilepsy as may be nocturnal anxiety attacks (attacks of sudden panic and intense anxiety which occur either just as the patient is on the point of falling asleep or in stage one or stage two sleep). Since they are sudden, paroxysmal and apparently are occurring in sleep they are often thought to be epileptic in nature.

Diagnosis

It is important to try to distinguish between epi-lepsy and a non-epileptic attack disorder as quickly and as early as possible. Just as one needs to try to determine the type of epilepsy that the patient has (if the patient's attacks are clearly epi-leptic) one also needs to try to determine the type of non-epileptic attack disorder that the patient has, if it is decided that the patient's attacks are

not epileptic. There is an unfortunate trend in the literature and in clinical practice to label a non-epileptic attack as a pseudoseizure without trying to differentiate what type of pseudoseizure it is the patient has. It is important however to distinguish between non-epileptic attacks which have a physical basis from non-epileptic attacks which have an emotional basis.

Unfortunately it can be easy to recognize that the patient's attacks are epileptic in nature: it can be extremely difficult to prove that they are not. There must always remain in many patients an element of doubt and a lack of certainty, and there is a small group of patients (perhaps 5%) in whom it can be impossible to tell if one is dealing with epilepsy or non-epilepsy. In many patients both epileptic and non-epileptic attacks occur side by side (in my own experience about one-third of patients with a non-epileptic attack dis-order, although, depending on the particular circumstances in which the patients are seen, this figure will vary from 10% to 90%).

The diagnosis of epilepsy still depends initially on a clinical history, as epilepsy is still a clinical diagnosis. The problem with the clinical history however is that it is often given by a patient who has a distorted recollection of what occurred or by a witness who was terrified by the attack and was perhaps so busy attempting to restrain the patient that he did not observe clearly what happened and therefore cannot give a very clear account of the event. It is received and analysed by a doctor who may have little knowledge of epi-lepsy and of the bewildering variety of events that can occur as part of an epileptic attack (and even less knowledge of the phenomena of non-epileptic attacks) so that confusion, fear and ignorance are compounded into grave errors of judgement. These sources of error may be increased by the pressures of the need to 'do something' and by the desire to turn the mysterious into the understand-able. There is little doubt, therefore, that clinical descriptions of attacks, although useful, will often lead to the erroneous diagnosis of epilepsy (or the failure to recognize epilepsy when it exists). It is better if witnesses can be trained not to interfere with attacks but to observe them carefully and it is even better if observers can record the attack in some way (say by using a video camera so that the patient's behaviour can be analysed in detail). It is extremely important that doctors, particularly those that are likely to make the diagnosis, are better educated and have had the opportunity of reviewing on videotape the common types of seizure. Certainly, all medical students should see such videotaped material during their training.

It is also useful in taking a history from a witness of an attack to take a little time confronting and diffusing the anxiety and the fear that he felt until a less distorted account of the seizure is obtained. It is likely that in at least 30% of seizures at first presentation there will be an element of diagnostic doubt and it is important not to rush into a diagnosis of epilepsy without being certain that that is what the patient actually has. It may be necessary to admit the patient to hospital for skilled observation and further investigation.

A prolactin level taken 20 minutes to a half an hour after the seizure and compared with a base line prolactin level is often helpful. There is a characteristic rise in prolactin level after a tonic-clonic seizure (although if the patient is having serial seizures this rise is not sustained) and there is a lesser although potentially helpful rise after complex partial seizures (Rao et al 1989).

EEG studies are also essential. Very little reliance can be placed on the results of an interictal EEG because many patients with epilepsy have normal EEG readings between their seizures and some people who do not have epilepsy have spike-wave activity in their EEG, sometimes even of a focal nature. Characteristic changes often take place in a postictal EEG which can be of help (such as postictal slowing or flattening of the record) but these are not invariable and the absence of postictal change, particularly after a partial seizure, does not mean that the patient does not have epilepsy.

Continuous EEG recording during a seizure (preferably several seizures) is more helpful. This can be by ambulatory EEG recording with eight or 16 channels or by telemetered EEG devices. There are however limitations to this technique. Some patients will not be having seizures sufficiently often to be recorded. In such patients it is sometimes acceptable to withhold medication for a while, providing it is certain that, if medication is withheld, the seizures that occur as a result

are similar to the ones in question and not merely withdrawal seizures. The seizure itself needs to be accurately observed as well as recorded on the EEG because the phenomena of the seizure such as movement, head shaking, teeth grinding for example may cause artifactual change in the EEG which may be misinterpreted: movement artifacts may obscure any epileptic change in the EEG. Conventionally, recording is also made on videotape either in a specially constructed room using a system whereby EEG and behaviour are recorded simultaneously for later analysis, or if ambulatory monitoring is done at home (there is some evidence that one is more likely to catch a seizure in the patient's home than in the artificial confines of hospital) the patient's friends or relatives can be given a portable video camera, or a community worker can make the recording.

However even with these methods some diagnostic doubt may remain. If undoubted epileptic activity is recorded during a seizure which starts when the behaviour in question starts and ceases at about the time that the seizure stops then there can be little doubt that one is dealing with epilepsy. If an apparent convulsion occurs without any change in the surface EEG electrodes, particularly if there is no rise in prolactin as well, then again one can be fairly certain clinically that the seizure, whatever it is, is not an epileptic one. But partial seizures may not be detected by surface electrodes even when there is alteration in consciousness. This is particularly true of simple partial seizures and of seizure discharge in the frontal lobes. Special electrode placements may therefore be necessary including sphenoidal leads, foramen ovale recording and, in selected cases, the use of cortical electrodes using subdural strips or other invasive procedures. Such recording will need the co-operation of a neurosurgeon skilled in inserting foramen ovale leads or subdural strips and begins to pose some risk to the patient. It is possible that even such invasive recording may miss very localized seizure discharge and there will remain a very small group of patients where ictal EEG recording even in a specialized centre may still not solve the problem of what the patient's attacks are, and one then has to fall back on a clinical decision. Since invasive EEG recording is not without its risks or may not be obtainable, at some prior point in the patient's management one may have to decide that pursuing investigation further is not justified and again have to make a clinical decision based on the best available evidence. This may include information from other investigations such as MRI or PET scanning.

By and large, the briefer and more stereotyped the attack the more likely it is to be epilepsy and the longer and less stereotyped the attack the more likely it is that some other phenomenon is causing the attack: this general rule has important exceptions. Monitoring patients whose attacks consist of sudden falls is difficult for the reasons stated earlier, and frontal lobe seizures in particular may take a lot of detection and a long time to realize that, although the patient's behaviour is wild and bizarre, it does actually have a stereotyped nature. No reliance can be placed on the fact that the patient, in addition to having an attack disorder, also has a psychiatric disorder. Although affective disorder, personality disorder and somatization disorder including Briquet's syndrome are over represented in patients with non-epileptic attack disorder and a history of overdoses, self mutilation, eating disorder or sexual difficulty is also a pointer to the attack being non-epileptic (Roy 1979, Savard & Andermann 1990). This can be misleading as many patients with epilepsy also have co-existent psychiatric disorder, particularly anxiety and depression.

Correct diagnosis is therefore not easy, may occasionally be impossible and must not be rushed or hurried. Unfortunately all the phenomena that can be seen in an epileptic attack can also be seen in a non-epileptic attack and vice versa. Although I have come to recognize the abreactive attack, referred to earlier, and its characteristic flailing limbs, back arching and gasping, such behaviour may also be part of a frontal seizure. Tables drawn up to help doctors distinguish between epileptic and non-epileptic attacks (e.g Molder 1990) need a great deal of qualification and personally I think they are misleading. Above all if it is decided that a patient's attack disorder is non-epileptic it is important then to ask the question what type of non-epileptic attack is it (being careful to exclude those that are being caused by physical disorder) and what is its aetiology?

Management of the non-epilepic attack disorder cannot be achieved until this has been achieved. It is also important not to be dogmatic: often diagnosis is based on a balance of probabilities and may always be wrong. Diagnosis needs reviewing: time and experience often changes it.

Management

Non-epileptic attacks are as real as epileptic ones and it is very important that the first step in managing a non-epileptic attack disorder is to keep a good relationship with the patient. It is important not to reject the patient (and sending the patient to a psychiatrist can be seen as rejection) but to help the patient understand that his seizures are still as real as they were but do require different management. The diagnosis must be put over in a positive way and if at all possible the patient should remain under the care of the same team that made the original diagnosis. If psychiatric help is required then it should be provided by a psychiatric team that is well versed in managing non-epileptic attacks and there should be good communication between such a team and the unit that referred the patient, particularly because diagnostic certainty is often not obtainable.

It is important to look at the circumstances surrounding the first seizure and its possible symbolic meaning. Chemical or hypnotic abreaction can be helpful to recall the emotions or events that were occurring at about the time the seizure started. Although it is true that epilepsy itself can start at a time of stress, psychological non-epileptic attack disorder is particularly likely to do so. Most studies have suggested that psychological NEAD is more common in women than in men and there is a growing recognition that some kinds of non-epileptic attack disorder—in my experience, particularly swoons and abreactive attacks (Betts & Boden 1991)—are likely to occur in women who have been previously sexually abused. For a full discussion of this see Betts & Boden (1991) and Goodwin (1989). Women who have been sexually abused will often not reveal it at first until they can trust the person they want to tell, or genuinely may not remember it because they have suppressed the painful memories. Direct enquiry, on first meeting the patient, about sexual abuse is therefore often met with a negative reply but information is finally forthcoming as one gets to know the patient better.

It is also important to look at the patient's present circumstances and environment to try to determine what factors are reinforcing the patient's behaviour and what primary or secondary gain is accruing. It should be remembered that epilepsy itself may obtain secondary gain and may be reinforced. Family or medical concern and attention at the time of seizure occurrence will 'reward' seizure activity whether it is epileptic or not. Secondary gain is often more important in keeping seizures going, once they have started, than the original cause itself and it certainly helps to explain why a number of disadvantaged people with epilepsy develop non-epileptic attack disorder. An examination of the patient's feelings or thoughts just before an attack is also useful as many NEADs are anxiety related or occur in response to internal feelings or thoughts or memories that the patient may not recognize immediately as a precipitant. It is sometimes useful to show the patient a video of his or her own seizure, asking him to try to recall his feelings and thoughts just before and during the seizure, analogous in a way to the technique used by Feldman & Paul (1976) for epilepsy.

In addition to exploring the underlying meaning of the NEAD and its possible reinforcers, using exploratory abreactive and psychotherapeutic techniques to understand the patient and the seizure better (which may in itself be very therapeutic), it is important to take a behavioural approach to the NEAD, treating it as an unwanted piece of behaviour that needs to be extinguished. An operant conditioning approach is best: seizure activity is ignored and seizure-free intervals are rewarded praised and reinforced. Ignoring seizure activity can be difficult and needs the co-operation of the family, if the patient is being treated at home, or all ward staff and fellow patients, if the patient is being treated in hospital. However noisy and dramatic the seizure performance the patient is merely stepped over and paid no attention. If this is done, seizure frequency often rises for a while to a crescendo for about 10 days and then will often suddenly extinguish. It is not easy to keep such a behavioural paradigm running in hospital and is much more difficult in the patient's home or school, but it is worth attempting.

Intensive anxiety management and cognitive therapy directed at the point at which anxiety or negative feelings start in the seizure cycle is also very helpful. The patient learns to discriminate between tension and relaxation and learns control skills so that he or she can apply them at the point where a seizure starts to come on. Once the patient has learnt discrimination the prognosis improves considerably. Likewise if a patient can recognize negative thoughts that start a seizure off or reinforce it, learn to stop them and replace them with positive thoughts the prognosis improves.

For some patients, particularly those in which there was a definite traumatic event like incest which started the seizures, formal counselling and psychotherapy may be needed. Abuse counselling is certainly necessary for those patients who have been sexually abused or were victims of incest. This involves initial abreactive work allowing the patient to talk out the experience and begin to discharge and express some of the associated emotions of shame, disgust, anger and build up a trusting relationship with her therapist. Often two therapists are needed, particularly as feelings of anger are eventually directed not so much at the male therapist (who represents, in the initial stages of therapy, the perpetrator) but at the female therapist who comes to represent the mother who so often knew what was happening but did nothing about it. Abuse counselling often takes a couple of years from the initial exploratory and abreactive stage, followed by a confrontation stage within the family (particularly of the perpetrator if possible), followed by a group experience as the victim shares her experience with others who have been similarly traumatized. In my experience NEAD related to abuse will not resolve unless this counselling has been done, and even then may return at times of further stress.

The prognosis of NEAD obviously depends on the cause. A number of patients respond to simple confrontation, discussion and reassurance, particularly if the confrontation is a non-judgemental one. Patients whose attack disorders relate to psychiatric disorder often do well, particularly patients with panic attacks. Patients whose non-epileptic attack disorder relates to previous emotional trauma can do well if they have full counselling. Patients whose non-epileptic attack disorder is being reinforced by secondary gain, particularly if it becomes enmeshed in family psychopathology, are much more difficult to help and intensive family therapy may be necessary. My own experience is that in hospital about two-thirds of patients with non-epileptic attack disorder obtain complete, or a very significant, resolution of their symptoms but on follow-up many have regained the attack disorder because of the difficulty of treating the whole family or in preventing reinforcement of seizures. It is also true that if one can withdraw such patients from antiepileptic medication they are in great danger of being put back on it by general practitioners or by casualty officers and I suspect that overall prognosis is not very good. This does not mean to say that attempts should not be made to help the patient.

As we gain experience with NEAD it is also important to recognize that one can be wrong about the diagnosis. We have all had the experience of treating somebody's epilepsy for years only to discover eventually that it was a NEAD. (There is a natural 'oneupmanship' about discovering that somebody else's patient does not have epilepsy, but we should avoid this feeling particularly because it is likely to be our turn next.) Many of us by now will also have had the experience of having made a confident diagnosis of non-epileptic attack disorder in a patient only to discover eventually, with better monitoring techniques, that in fact the patient has frontal seizures. It is better to be honest with patients and not pretend that there is a certainty in these matters: often it is best to say that this diagnosis is our working hypothesis and that we will try this form of management and see how we get on rather than implying a certainty which is not there. The management of NEAD is helped by the fact that many of the techniques such as anxiety management, operant conditioning and cognitive therapy used in such patients will also be effective and useful in treating epilepsy.

Case History 22

Walter was an engaging and pleasant unmarried man of 43 who lived with his elderly and dominant mother. Walter may have had epilepsy at one time although this is doubtful. For at least the last 15 years he had an attack disorder (having at least one seizure a day) where he would rock backwards and forwards very rapidly going somewhat red in the face as he did so, followed by falling to the floor with rather incoordinate thrashing and jerking of his limbs and noisy gasping, followed by a period of stiffness in which all his limbs were held rigidly out in front of him. This rigidity would then subside and he would lie still for some minutes moaning softly and then apparently wake up. This 'intractable epilepsy' had been treated with a wide variety of antiepileptic drugs and by several different consultants without avail. Walter was very cheerful about his intractable epilepsy which he wore as a badge of pride within the small West Midlands town where he lived (a town, incidentally, which seems to have more than its fair share of patients with non-epileptic attack disorder).

By the time I saw him first he was taking four different antiepileptic drugs. His medication was supervised by his mother and I was somewhat startled on my first consultation with Walter and his mother to have my conversation with Walter interrupted by his mother rapping him firmly on the head with her walking stick and saying in a loud voice, 'Walter, its time for your next pill.' Walter meekly broke off the conversation, found a glass of water and swallowed his pill. I then discovered that, apart from 6 hours in the night, he was taking a different pill at every hour of the day according to a schedule worked out by his mother. It was very clear, on observing his seizures, that seizure activity could be modified by suggestions made during the seizure itself (on one occasion an EEG technician accidently introduced incontinence to Walter's repertoire by idly observing to a student who was assisting in recording an EEG during one of his seizures that 'most patients pass water at this stage of the attack'. Walter had never been incontinent before but about 30 seconds later it became apparent from the pool of water on the floor that he had obliged).

It was difficult at first to see what Walter got from his seizures but after two or three community visits it became clear that these seizures had started shortly after his father had died and seemed to be part of a symbiotic ritual played out between mother and son. Direct reinforcement of the seizures was observed by a community worker who reported that when she saw Walter have a seizure at home his mother banged on the party wall of her house with her stick and a next door neighbour came round and helped the mother to strip Walter naked whilst he was having the seizure and then wash him all over in warm water. The next door neighbour was young and pretty which probably helped to explain the beatific smile that crossed Walter's features towards the end of his attack. Walter's medication was slowly withdrawn. It was explained to him that during his seizure on several occasions no abnormal electrical activity had been observed and he very cheerfully adopted the new diagnostic badge of a pseudoseizure. His seizure frequency did fall gradually and he was encouraged to be more independent of his mother. Sadly the old lady died suddenly of a myocardial infarction and Walter's seizure frequency subsequently increased as he went through a very prolonged mourning period for his mother. He is, at the moment, undergoing rehabilitation and learning independent living skills and his seizure frequency is a great deal less and he is slowly gaining insight into his condition. He has been withdrawn from all antiepileptic medication.

Case History 23

This woman was transferred to a psychiatric unit via a medical ward where she had been admitted at the request of her general practitioner with what was described as 'near-status epilepticus'. She had begun to have epileptic attacks, some 10 years before. At first they were infrequent but in the 2 years before admission she was having three or four major convulsions a day, despite heroic doses of antiepileptic drugs. On admission she was ataxic and dysarthric. This had been ascribed to her uncontrolled epilepsy but in fact was due to intoxication. From the time of her admission to the medical ward she had had numerous seizures in which she would fall, emit a loud cry and then thrash about screaming loudly banging her head on the ground as she did so, often drawing blood, and making a great deal of noise. She was described as having a difficult personality and after she had been rude to a senior member of the consultant staff during one of her attacks (she had also attempted to bite his ankle) she was removed smartly to the psychiatric ward. When she arrived on the psychiatric ward the attacks were discretely observed but no intervention was made. She occasionally had brief episodes of confusion lasting no more than 10 seconds in which she would drop whatever she was carrying, stare fixedly at the wall and would swallow in a dazed way. She would also have attacks which were the major event already described. These latter events would always occur at times of frustration or anger or when she was asked to do something which did not suit her (like helping with the ward chores). At these times she would fling herself violently to the ground, often throwing herself out of a chair to do so and would kick and scream in a manner reminiscent of a 3-year-old in a tantrum. Her antiepileptic drugs were totally withdrawn (she was later placed on monotherapy with phenytoin when the underlying complex partial seizures that she did have were recognized). Ignoring her non-epileptic attacks made them rise to a crescendo. She would go off the ward to have her attacks in the neighbouring lift or in front of visitors, some of whom became quite angry at the 'callous way' she was being treated by the staff on the ward.

However, on a psychiatric ward with a common therapeutic plan formulated after discussion with all members of staff the anxieties that such patients and policies can arouse can be supported and contained. About 10 days after the attacks were studiously ignored they stopped abruptly and then more attention could be paid to the patient's real problems. It was clear that she was using simulated epilepsy for secondary gain in a battle with her husband. The threat of the attacks was sufficient to keep him at home in the evenings and to get him to do the various domestic chores around the house which he had done uncomplainingly for several years. Undoubtedly her control over her behaviour had been made more difficult by drug intoxication. Her rehabilitation was largely concerned with preventing her husband from allowing the same pattern of behaviour to develop when she returned home and encouraging her to talk out her anger, frustration and difficulties rather than resorting to seizure behaviour. This was eventually successful and she has been seizure free for several years.

Case History 24

A student teacher, aged 20, began to have attacks in front of her class which became so frequent and so unpleasant as to force her removal from teaching. She was subsequently admitted to a gynaecological hospital for investigation of continued amenorrhoea. It proved impossible to manage her in this hospital because when any attempt was made to get her out of bed she collapsed on the floor. She became bed-fast and a nurse had to sit with her at all times because she would otherwise fall out of bed and at least three nurses had to escort her to the toilet. She was transferred to a psychiatric unit at which time she was having several attacks a day. She said she had no warning of the attack but would merely find herself on the floor, obviously having fallen but with no memory of having done so. She did not feel sleepy or confused after the attacks in which she would sink gently to the floor without hurting herself and lie as though asleep for several minutes although it was noticed that her eyelids would be flickering. On several occasions she fell out of bed in an attack. At these times she would edge herself carefully towards the side of the bed for several minutes before she would suddenly fling herself out of bed and drop to the floor. No epileptic activity was seen during these attacks on EEG and they were ignored in the usual way. Lack of reinforcement led them to disappear and she then was able to talk out her underlying problems which related to previous sexual abuse.

Case History 25

This 45-year-old man was referred for in-patient treatment of his intractable epilepsy by another physician. His attacks had begun suddenly, a month after his wife's unexpected death. In the attacks he would have a premonitory feeling of unsteadiness or dizziness and would then slump forward lying inert and unrousable for as long as 2 or 3 minutes. These attacks would occur several times a day, had prevented the man from working for some months, and had failed to respond to antiepileptic drugs. On admission he was taking a mixture of phenytoin, phenobarbitone, ethosuximide and troxidone. His EEGs had been consistently normal. After one or two of the attacks were witnessed doubt was felt about whether they were in fact epileptic particularly as during the attack it was noticed that he became very pale, flushed after the attack and that during the attack his pulse rate was extremely slow. ECG 24-hour monitoring showed that he had a marked cardiac dysrhythmia with runs of ventricular abnormalities leading presumably to low cerebral perfusion pressure and a 'cerebral grey out'. His antiepileptic drugs were withdrawn completely (after which he said he felt a great deal better in himself) and he was treated successfully by a cardiologist.

Case History 26
A young woman physician was referred for treatment of 'personality disorder and epilepsy'. For the preceding year she had had periods of irritability and querulousness and her work standard had slipped. She often seemed inexplicably careless and disinhibited and occasionally her behaviour was very bizarre (on one occasion for instance removing all her clothing in the middle of a ward round). On several occasions in the preceding year she had had witnessed tonic-clonic seizures. She was under a great deal of domestic and personal stress related to an unsatisfactory relationship with a married man and doubts about the profession that she had chosen. It was noted during one of her episodes of irritability that she was quite confused: during this time there was no abnormal EEG activity but a blood sugar was extremely low and her plasma insulin high. An insulinoma was diagnosed and successfully removed since which time there have been no further personality changes and her seizures have stopped.

Case History 27
This patient was admitted from the intensive treatment unit of a local general hospital for further assessment of her epilepsy. She had had frequent tonic-clonic seizures since the age of 14 and on several occasions was admitted to hospital with status epilepticus which was difficult to control (and oddly enough seemed to get worse when diazepam was given intravenously). An EEG at the age of 14 had shown bitemporal theta activity which was taken as indicative of epilepsy. She was taking heavy doses of several antiepileptic drugs. Her seizures often seemed to occur when she was asleep although they also would occur occasionally in the day time. They would start with an increase in breathing rate and retching and spitting, followed by stiffening of her body, back arching, pelvic thrusting and then inco-ordinate thrashing of her limbs accompanied by gasping and crying and biting of her

right arm. These attacks would continue for some hours but then would subside eventually. Ambulatory EEG monitoring failed to reveal any epileptic activity during these attacks.

The attacks were video recorded and shown to the patient. She had denied any problems during routine questioning but when looking at the video and asked to describe what her feelings were during the attack she broke down and described sexual abuse by her father and some of his friends over a period of years from 8 until the age of 16. She was one of the very few patients that I have seen where ritualized sexual abuse occurred (including forced fellatio). Abused people with a non-epileptic attack disorder who have had to perform or endure oral sex often do have retching, spitting or vomiting during their attack. Her counselling, because of the amount of abuse and trauma she had undergone, was stormy and difficult but eventually successful and the attacks have ceased. She was able to confront her father with what he had done which seemed to aid her recovery considerably but declined eventually to have him prosecuted. Initially the details she gave of the ritualized abuse were so horrific and bizarre that many people found it difficult to believe her but the facts were eventually confirmed by a younger sister who had witnessed them and her father admitted them. Her seizures began shortly after she had attempted to tell her mother about what was happening and her mother had punished her for telling lies.

Case History 28
John was 12 when he began to have attacks which were almost invariably nocturnal. He would be asleep, or apparently asleep, would then begin to thrash with his legs, extend his right arm and move his head from side to side for about 1 minute. The attack would then subside and he would apparently fall asleep again. Attacks would occur perhaps a dozen to 20 times in the night. Since his vocal ejaculations were somewhat noisy he would wake his parents and his mother eventually moved into his bedroom to sleep with him as she was so distressed by his seizures. The seizures started at a time when the mother and father were ending their marriage rather painfully and were interpreted as possibly a means of trying to keep mother and father together, as both parents felt guilty about the boy's seizures and ascribed them to the break up of their relationship. EEG examination was normal and eight channel ambulatory EEG monitoring during the attacks also showed no epileptic abnormality. It was assumed, therefore, that they were a non-epileptic attack disorder (particularly as the EEG had also shown that the patient was awake when the attacks occurred) and it was also noted that, even in the middle of an attack, if he was firmly told to stop the attack would cease. In hospital attack frequency declined remarkably.

Attempts were made to engage both himself and his

family in counselling and he had some anxiety management. For a while the seizures did improve considerably, but later they returned. Observation of the seizures on videotape suggested that they were stereotyped, always taking the same form and were brief: it was thought that they were possibly frontal epileptic seizures. This was confirmed by invasive EEG monitoring with foramen ovale electrodes which showed that during the attack there was seizure activity in the right frontal lobe. However, despite antiepileptic medication and despite an attempt at surgery, the seizures continue.

PERSONALITY DISORDERS IN PEOPLE WITH EPILEPSY

There is a long-held belief that people with epilepsy are more prone to disorders of personality than people without epilepsy. This question needs to be considered critically, without the prejudices of those who have preconceived ideas, or those who are over-anxious to alleviate the problems that their patients have by refusing to accept that some people with epilepsy may have problems in interpersonal relationships.

A personality disorder is not easy to define. It is true, however, that some people seem to have chronic problems of adjustment to society, with living, or with relating to other people, which appear to be persistent and long-standing (often dating from childhood) producing stress symptoms either in the person concerned or in those who have to live with him or her. Problems arise in the definition and measurement of such apparent personality disorders, as the definition of a personality disorder is very much bound up with the values of the particular society which is defining it. A particular trait may be seen by one society as pathological; in another it may even be the norm. In societies such as ours, which are changing rapidly, definitions become even more difficult.

The diagnosis of a personality disorder must rest on definite reliable criteria and not on the personal prejudices either of the psychiatrist making the diagnosis or of society. Attempts have been made recently to try to clarify and refine the concept of personality disorder, and even to develop rating scales which can be used to define it accurately (Walton & Presly 1973, Tyrer & Alexander 1979, Tyrer et al 1979).

Most of the published observations on the relationship between personality disorder and epilepsy, however, are not based on reliable criteria which have been scientifically evaluated but merely on descriptions of the patient's behaviour. Such descriptions (which classify people as, for example, 'obsessional' or 'hypochondriacal' or 'overdependent') miss 90% of the patient's other behaviours; and it may be better to see patients on a continuum from normality in terms of a particular personality trait and also to see their personalities as multidimensional. As Walton & Presly (1973) point out, any classification of personality disorder should be based on clinical observation of behaviour rather than intuitive hunches. No symptom of neurotic or psychotic illness is required to make the diagnosis, the abnormality is in the personality itself and is based on the clinical history and examination and the observation of behaviour, plus a history from a relative who has known the patient for some time. Deviation from normal behaviour shows itself primarily in the patient's relationship with other people and is a continuing, not an episodic, phenomenon.

American authors rely heavily on measuring personality by using psychological instruments such as the MMPI, but this is not an approach much favoured in this country (see Trimble & Bolwig 1986 for review). Various personality traits have been attributed to people with epilepsy from time to time. The most famous (or infamous) personality type historically related to epilepsy is, of course, the 'epileptic personality' itself.

The balance of evidence suggests that a small number of patients with chronic epilepsy living under conditions of institutionalization or environmental handicap may develop a characteristic pattern of personality change which has attracted many descriptive adjectives in its time; many of them pejorative. Such patients are commonly described as pedantic, circumstantial, meticulous, hyposexual, religiose, egocentric, hypercritical, hypochondriacal, hypergraphic, suspicious and quarrelsome, and possessing a slowness and stickiness of thought which may suggest subnormality or early dementia (see Geschwind 1979 for a persuasive presentation of this concept). Such patients in an institution, even if few in number, are bound to colour opinion and must also represent a continuing problem in management.

The problem in an institution is that if one has ideas about the personality of patients it is extremely easy to find evidence which supports one's hypothesis and, indeed, the hypothesis may even become self-fulfilling. If one is expecting a certain form of behaviour from a patient one may well behave towards him or her in such a way as actually to induce the behaviour. The other problem about having a fixed belief that certain patients have an abnormal personality characteristic, is that one is then not motivated to change them, (although there is some evidence that even organic personality traits can be treated and changed).

However, there is little doubt that the constellation of personality traits described above does occur and is found in people with epilepsy. This apparent association is due to factors of selection in that those with unfavourable personality traits will tend to enter institutions more often than whose personalities enable them to manage much better in the outside world, and, once admitted, they tend to stick there. Referral of patients with epilepsy to general hospital outpatients unconnected with psychiatry is more likely to occur if the patient has psychological problems (Pond et al 1960).

The epileptic temperament, if it exists or when it occurs, is the result of multiple handicap: childhood environmental and physical deprivation; brain damage; and, perhaps, the chronic effects of antiepileptic drugs. Other prolonged disabilities, e.g. rheumatoid arthritis and chronic pain, also cause personality change (Merskey & Tonge, 1974).

Some authors suggest that the 'epileptic personality' may be a brain damage syndrome (Guerrant et al 1962) and there is some evidence that a similar clinical picture may occur in those patients with bi-temporal lobe damage but without epilepsy (Slater et al 1963). It is certainly true that the epileptic personality has lost its importance in the thinking of those psychiatrists with an interest in epilepsy as, indeed, has the interest in trying to substantiate the relationship between epilepsy and other types of personality disorder. The methodological drawbacks and difficulties are well described by Tizard (1962). Another widely believed 'fact' has been that people with epilepsy are overly religious. However, when put to proper enquiry

the opposite appears to be the case (Sensky 1983).

There remains, however, a generally held view in the literature and elsewhere that people with epilepsy are aggressive. Whether aggressiveness is more common in people with epilepsy than in the general population has never been tested formally, except in children where the evidence is conflicting. One study (Mellor et al 1974) suggested that epileptic children are somewhat more miserable than their peers but, if anything, are less aggressive. Bagley (1971) found an increase in aggressiveness in certain types of epilepsy in children. Aggression in someone with epilepsy is usually due to brain impairment (Mungas 1988) or is a symptom of associated mental illness. The evidence has recently been reviewed by Rodin (1982), Fenton (1983), Volavka (1990) and particularly Treiman (1991). This latter review repays careful study by anyone interested in this topic and presents compelling evidence to suggest that when factors of brain impairment, mental illness and personality disorder with low impulse control are taken into account there is no association between epilepsy and aggression. So called ictal aggression (primary ictal aggression) is also extremely rare and most violence occurring in the setting of an ictus is either secondary to disinhibition occurring during the seizure or is a reaction to emotional events in the seizure such as fear. Violent behaviour, 'resistive violence', commonly occurs at the end of a seizure during postictal confusion (equivalent to epileptic furore) or may occur as part of a postictal psychosis. A stereotyped automatism may also accidently result in violence due to the context in which it is occurring. Resistive violence is the commonest type.

Whether or not aggressiveness is more common in adults with epilepsy than in the general population there is no doubt that people with epilepsy are feared for their aggressiveness. In my experience this is an irrational fear which stems from a small group of hospitalized epileptic patients who may show aggressiveness, and from the general fear of epilepsy itself; and, as shown elsewhere (Betts 1981b), from experiences in the asylums at the turn of the century.

The management of those few patients with epilepsy who do show extreme rage, whether it is ictal, peri-ictal or apparently unassociated with ictal events, may be difficult and requires the resources of a secure unit until the aggression can be investigated by video and EEG monitoring, its nature established and then controlled or contained.

Case History 29

I first saw this man in 1967 when he had been in hospital for 11 years having been admitted at age of 35. He had a history of meningitis as a child and also of a forceps delivery. His epilepsy began at the age of 11, and was described as 'grand mal' in type. From the age of 20 he almost invariably suffered from epileptic furore after each fit, and was eventually admitted to a mental hospital because of these furores. Following his admission to hospital he continued to have many epileptic seizures (up to about 20 a month) and for a long time was the terror of the hospital being confined to a locked room on a locked ward; and there was a record of several attacks on staff and patients. Most of the aggressive episodes occurred after a major tonic-clonic seizure but occasionally, in between his major seizures, he would have sudden short lived outbursts of violence. They would start without warning or obvious precipitant and last for 5 to 30 minutes (during which time he was entirely unapproachable). He seemed to have no memory of them afterwards. At the time of his admission he appeared to be suffering also from a paranoid psychosis, in which he was described as having ideas of reference, grandiose delusions and auditory hallucinations. This psychotic state cleared within a few months after his admission without specific treatment.

He had been taking large doses of phenytoin and phenobarbitone since his admission. His epilepsy had not been investigated until 1967 when an EEG showed phase reversal of spike and wave activity in the right anterior and midtemporal region. In addition to his regular antiepileptic drugs, chlordiazapoxide, 25 mg, three times a day was added in 1967. Subsequently he had no further seizures and there were no further aggressive outbursts. His whole personality seemed to change in that he became pleasant and sociable, and within 6 months of starting chlordiazapoxide he was allowed out into the grounds for the first time ever. He eventually started work in the occupational therapy unit. He was seen again in 1979 (Betts & Skarrott 1979). He was still in hospital, although clearly he would have been quite suitable for hostel accommodation if any had been available. He was a pleasant, cheerful man with a wry sense of humour, and a good grasp of current affairs. There was no evidence of a dementing process. The chlordiazapoxide had been withdrawn in 1974; he had had occasional short-lived aggressive episodes since that time (but none for 2 years) and he had had no seizures since originally taking chlordiazapoxide, although he remained on heavy doses of phenobarbitone and phenytoin.

Case History 30

This man had already been in hospital for 29 years when I saw him first in 1967. He was 19 years old on admission. His epilepsy was known to have begun at the age of 13 and was simply described in his notes as 'grand mal' in type. In 1967 he was still having a couple of seizures a month. He was admitted originally 'confused and demented' and elated with auditory hallucinations. This seems to have been an acute organic psychosis of paranoid type, which disappeared quite rapidly after his admission to hospital without any specific treatment. Subsequently, he suffered from many attacks of epileptic furore following his tonic-clonic seizures and occasionally would suffer from acute aggressive outbursts in between his major seizures. These rages occurred without provocation, although it was noted that a specific phrase 'who's got wooden legs' would always precipitate an aggressive outburst.

In 1967 he was taking 240 mg of phenobarbitone a day in divided doses; this dosage has continued until the present day. His medical notes had continued to describe him as suffering from 'epileptic insanity', although no psychotic features had been observed in his mental state for many years and he was also described as suffering from 'epileptic dementia', although in fact he was correctly orientated in space and time and had a reasonable knowledge of current events. On review in 1979 he was found to be pleasant and equable in temperament. He was a somewhat simple man of 60 who showed no evidence of a dementing process and no psychotic features. His last seizure had occurred in 1974, and since then there had been no further episodes either of furore or of aggressive outbursts.

Case History 31

This 30-year-old publican had been in good health and there was no evidence of previous seizure activity. One evening, whilst working with his wife in their public house, he went down into the cellar to change a beer cask and failed to return after a few minutes. His wife, who suspected that he was having an affair with one of the barmaids, crept down to the cellar to see what was going on. When she got into the cellar she saw her husband in the throes of a tonic-clonic seizure. Shortly after the attack ended, her husband rose in a dazed fashion from the floor and kicked in several of the barrels in the cellar. His wife remonstrated with him and was irritably pushed out of the way by her husband, who then ran upstairs into the bar and began to assault his customers. Although he hurt several of them, his violence did not seem to be directed against any one in particular. If people kept out of the way he failed to pursue them, but if they tried to restrain him, he would respond with violence. The police were summoned and he was eventually taken away with some difficulty to a local hospital where, in the casualty department, further attempts were made to restrain him. During the struggle two members of the staff were injured but attempts to inject him with a sedative were fruitless. He was eventually locked in a side room where, left to himself, he quietened down very rapidly and fell asleep. Subsequent investigations revealed a temporal glioma which was ultimately fatal. Similar behaviour occurred following further seizures but without the violence as no further attempts were made to restrain him and he was just confused and irritable. Attempts at conversation with him during such states were fruitless as, although he was clearly awake, he rarely made any reply.

These patients (one of whom may have had primary ictal violence and the rest resistive violence) are representative of the epileptic patients with aggressive outbursts that can be found in mental hospitals. Both seizures and the aggressive outbursts seem to wane at about the same time. They do not resemble at all closely the patients described by Maletzky (1973) with the 'episodic dyscontrol syndrome'—these were men without epilepsy (but many of whom had temporal lobe EEG abnormalities) who were subject to episodes of senseless, unprovoked violence in the setting of severe personality disorder; some improved with phenytoin.

The treatment of such violent aggressive outbursts is difficult and somewhat controversial. Occasionally, patients may respond well to benzodiazepine drugs, whether intravenously or by chronic oral medication; but not all will do so, and it should be remembered that these drugs, like alcohol and barbiturates, may have a disinhibiting action, making the violence worse. Some patients will have their outbursts better controlled by parenteral butyrophenone drugs or chlormethiazole. A particularly useful drug for calming the acutely disturbed is droperidol which can be given safely intravenously. Patients with acute aggressive outbursts are often better left alone and unrestrained, as the outburst is usually self-limiting.

Some patients, then, do have episodes of severe aggression. It is widely reported in the literature, although few controlled studies have been done, that many patient with epilepsy are chronically or episodically irritable and therefore potentially aggressive. It is not certain that this is necessarily more than one would find in an equivalent population of either institutionalized patients or normal people; but if it is accepted for a moment that perhaps some people with epilepsy do show undue irritability (Blumer 1991), is it possible to find any correlation between the aggression and their social and epileptic history? Men with epilepsy may be more aggressive than women: the earlier the onset of the epilepsy, the more likely it is that aggression will develop later, suggesting the importance in the pathogenesis of aggression of early social disadvantage and failure of social learning (Herzberg & Fenwick 1988).

The evidence to date suggests that, although brain mechanisms may be important, the influence of social and learning factors may be paramount in causing chronic aggressiveness in people with epilepsy. This is important because prevention may be possible with better management of children with epilepsy.

One important factor that has come out of studies of aggressiveness in epilepsy (Taylor 1969a) is that, in those patients going forward for temporal lobe surgery, aggressiveness is a good prognostic sign in terms of successful rehabilitation after the operation and cessation of seizures. It is interesting that the other psychiatric disorders that may occur in association with temporal lobe epilepsy are seldom improved by temporal lobectomy, and may even be made worse. It has been suggested that some of the depressive illnesses which occur after otherwise successful temporal lobe surgery (Hill et al 1957) are the result of the 'turning in' of this aggression onto the patient himself. Postoperative depression is certainly common after temporal lobectomy, but may have other causes.

Gunn (1969), in his study of people with epilepsy in prisons, found little evidence of an increased degree of aggressiveness and violence in epileptic prisoners—confirmed by Treiman (1991)—although he recognized that some more difficult patients might have been sent to Special Hospitals. He also found that in those people with epilepsy in prisons who were aggressive there was no particular correlation with any type of epilepsy. Others also have found no evidence that aggressiveness is especially common in temporal lobe epilepsy (Guerrant et al 1962, Small et al 1966). Lishman (1968), in his study of the psychiatric sequelae of brain injury, found that aggressiveness was more common after frontal rather than temporal lobe injuries.

EPILEPSY AND CRIME

If there is uncertainty about a relationship between epilepsy and aggressiveness, what is the relationship between epilepsy and crime itself? It has long been held that there is such a relationship (Lombroso 1889). In a survey of prison and borstal receptions in England and Wales, followed by a study of a representative sample of male epileptic prisoners (Gunn 1969), it was shown that the prevalence of epilepsy in the prison population is well above that to be expected. Many of these epileptic prisoners were also psychiatrically abnormal, but they were no more aggressive than the general population of prisoners, although they had attempted suicide more often. There was no relationship between the kind of crime the prisoners had committed and whether or not they had epilepsy, and no relationship between type of crime and type of epilepsy.

A further study (Gunn & Fenton 1971) of epileptic patients in a special hospital to assess the possible connection between criminal acts and epileptic automatism showed automatism to be an extremely rare explanation for crime in people with epilepsy: crime related to a seizure tends to be postictal rather than ictal. Those people in England and Wales whose crimes were directly related to the ictus or automatism were particularly disadvantaged as until recently English case law (Regina v. Sullivan) defined such a state as insanity, with the likelihood that an offender would be committed to a special hospital. For a full discussion see Fenwick (1985). The legal definition of insane automatism is in the process of being changed.

Many people with epilepsy are socially disadvantaged and deprived, and tend to drift into crime and possibly are caught more easily. Most people with epilepsy in prison are there for thieving, as is the general prison population, and the increased prevalence of people with epilepsy in prison is almost certainly related to social rather than medical factors.

EPILEPSY AND SEXUALITY

The general public tends to fear epilepsy because of an imagined association with hypersexuality, in the same way as they tend to associate it with criminality and violence. How much of this prejudice can be blamed on Lombroso (1889) is uncertain, but the actual facts about sexuality in epilepsy are very different.

There is a relationship between sexuality and temporal lobe epilepsy (Shukla et al 1979). Temporal lobe lesions may produce disturbances of sexual function, usually hyposexuality with lowered sex drive, occasionally total impotence, and, in women, loss of sexual response (Hierons & Saunders 1966). Social and psychological factors may play at least as important a part as biological ones, although accumulating evidence does suggest that there is a neurophysiological factor present.

There is some evidence that successful treatment of the epilepsy, particularly by surgery, may improve sexual performance (Taylor 1969b). It may be that treatment of epilepsy by enzyme-inducing drugs may affect sexual performance, as such drugs lead to the rapid metabolism of testosterone with lowering of free testosterone blood levels. Testosterone has a relationship with sexual arousal and activity, although it is a complex one. It has been suggested that this effect on testosterone metabolism causes the hyposexuality of epilepsy (Toone et al 1980). In a further study (Toone et al 1989) of a community sample of men with epilepsy compared with a normal healthy population there was evidence of lowered sex drive in the men with epilepsy, particularly those with partial epilepsy: testosterone levels were decreased and anterior pituitary hormone levels increased— there was a significant relationship between behavioural measures of hyposexuality and those of luteinizing hormone (LH). Testosterone depot injections have been suggested as a remedy but a formal trial has not been undertaken. Regular testosterone injections are not without their dangers and tend to induce non-specific feelings of well being and increased appetite that may be mistaken for therapeutic improvement.

Free testosterone blood levels are difficult to measure (usually bound and free levels are measured together). Interpretation of the significance of low levels is also difficult (unless they are pathologically low), particularly as infrequent intercourse leads to a low level of testosterone: a high frequency of intercourse tends to increase testosterone levels. Except for patients with hypogonadism, however, there is little evidence that increasing testosterone levels artificially leads to increased intercourse. Leiderman et al (1990) have also shown a strong positive correlation between total plasma testosterone and aggression in a sample of men with partial (limbic) epilepsy.

Most of the work on the relationship between sexuality and epilepsy (as might be expected in a male dominated medical profession!) has been on male sexuality. However, testosterone does have a relationship with female sexual arousal and so changes in its metabolism may affect sexual response in women. However Demerdash et al (1991) have demonstrated an unusual incidence of hyposexuality in women with epilepsy compared with controls. Interestingly it was also shown that women who experienced ictal or preictal sexual feelings were likely to experience sexual problems within relationships. The authors also found that 'sexual exhibitionism' was more common in women with epilepsy than in a control population of women without epilepsy, but this may have been due to the strict culture to which the control population belonged.

My own experience (Betts 1984) suggests that social and psychological factors are important in the causation of sexual difficulty and lack of responsiveness in both men and women with epilepsy. In a review of people with epilepsy attending a psychosexual clinic (Betts 1984) they were shown to have the same kind of problems as the non-epileptic in roughly the same proportion (the over-representation of people with epilepsy within the clinic was probably due to my interest both in epilepsy and in sexual disorder). The recovery rate of the sexual problems of people with epilepsy was also the same as those without epilepsy, using standard behavioural methods of treatment (and without testosterone supplements).

However, two aetiological factors did seem prominent in those with epilepsy who had a sexual problem: lack of practice due to social isolation and, more important, the inhibitory effect of fear of an attack during sexual activity. This fear usually inhibited the person with epilepsy, but occasionally would inhibit the partner. Because of the bonding effect of a happy sex life and its effect on morale and feelings of well-being, help to achieve a satisfactory sexual union, where appropriate, seems to me to be an important part of the rehabilitation of someone with epilepsy. The fear of a seizure during intercourse is common, but may well not be volunteered and must be directly enquired for.

Case History 32
This man of 50 had had tonic-clonic seizures since the age of two. They had not responded well to medication (he was taking a mixture of phenytoin and phenobarbitone). He had grown up friendless and isolated and had shunned the company of women believing that they would 'not want an epileptic like me'. He suppressed his sexual feelings because a doctor had told him when he was young that masturbation led to attacks and he obeyed this injunction rigorously.

In his late forties his attacks began to abate and he was befriended by a woman at work 10 years younger. As the romance developed she indicated that she wanted it to sexualize and he was confronted with his lack of experience and low sexual arousal. He became miserable and, as his feelings for the women deepened, suicidal. He was referred for professional help. He was treated with a behavioural programme (a modified sexual growth programme of LoPiccolo) which included the development and shaping of masturbatory fantasies and developed a strong sexual response which he was able to develop into a fully satisfying sexual relationship with his partner, with the aid of some joint counselling. His self-esteem grew as he was able to allow the warm and tender part of his nature to show itself for the first time. When last seen he was contemplating marriage and had been attack free for nearly a year.

Case History 33
This girl of 24 was referred from a family planning clinic for advice as a case of 'oral contraceptive induced epilepsy'. When she was younger she had had tonic-clonic seizures (probably secondarily generalized) and, although these had stopped when she was 12, she continued to have occasional brief complex partial attacks which passed almost unnoticed (she stopped antiepileptic medication at 16). At the age 18 she became engaged and started taking an oral contraceptive and a month later had a tonic-clonic seizure whilst in bed at night. Her fiancé, who had known nothing of her epilepsy, fled and the relationship ended. Six years later she was engaged again, took the pill, and again a week or two later had a nocturnal tonic-clonic attack. Her present fiancé was made of sterner stuff than the last and stayed with her.

It became clear that the problem had nothing to do

with the pill. Both attacks had occurred when she was attempting intercourse for the first time. She had hated and feared her major attacks and was terrified that during the abandonment and loss of control of sexual activity they would return. This fear was reinforced by the experience of her first attempt, so that she approached a sexual encounter rigid with fear and overbreathing as soon as a direct sexual approach was made. She was treated with a sexual growth programme, which allowed her to develop a sexual relationship with her fiancé with her fear confronted and controlled by anxiety reduction techniques. She has now developed a satisfactory sexual relationship and has had no further tonic-clonic attacks.

There is possibly a slight increase of perverse sexuality in temporal lobe epilepsy, although the evidence for this is slight. It has been reviewed by Hoenig & Kenna (1979), and, again, neurophysiological factors as well as social ones may be playing a part. The temporal lobes, after all, are probably the seat of sexual awareness in humans and it is, therefore, not surprising that aberrations in function in these areas in the brain may give rise to aberrations in sexual behaviour. There is very little evidence that hypersexuality—except of a primitive kind such as excessive masturbation—occurs in epilepsy, although it may do so in very rare cases. Often, of course, hypersexuality is bound up with mental illness or severe brain damage.

Occasionally, sexual functioning may get bound up in the epileptic event itself, as in those patients whose attacks sometimes have a sexual component (Mitchell et al 1954), or in those patients whose major seizures are triggered off by a sexual experience as a form of reflex epilepsy (Hoenig & Hamilton 1960).

Case History 34
This girl of 16 had brief complex partial seizures, often premenstrual. After they had occurred she would become disturbed, tearful and angry, and would sometimes show acting out behaviour, running around the room and screaming. Even when the attacks came under much better control with carbamazepine the acting out continued. Ambulatory EEG monitoring showed that her complex partial seizures were brief and the acting out was not an ictal event.

She eventually made a confiding relationship with her clinic doctor (particularly when her mother was encouraged not to accompany her daughter during every interview) and the cause of her acting out behaviour was revealed. Her partial complex seizure was a brief abrogation of consciousness followed by lip-smacking, of which she was dimly aware. In addition, she revealed this was accompanied by an intense, pleasurable, erotic feeling arising in her vagina and apparently rising upwards towards her throat. She was sexually inexperienced and her mother had given her such strong warnings about sexuality that she was frightened and confused by the feelings and her acting out behaviour was an attempt to escape from their overwhelming presence. She was counselled and educated about sexual feelings, lost her fear of them and the acting out behaviour disappeared.

Case History 35
This 26-year-old woman had a history of abruptly broken relationships (including two engagements). She had a 10 year history of secondary generalized epilepsy partly controlled by phenytoin. Her partial attacks, which were not always followed by a tonic-clonic seizure, were a feeling of warmth in the vagina which rose in intensity until she had an orgasmic feeling (but only on one side of her vagina and pelvis). A tonic-clonic fit might then follow. Unfortunately, when having intercourse she discovered that a sexually-induced orgasm would be followed by a tonic-clonic seizure. Although one of her partners claimed not to notice, she found the event embarrassing and distressing and several of her partners (she enjoyed her sexuality) abruptly broke off the relationship. It had been planned to try some form of behavioural management of her reflex epilepsy (perhaps by habituation therapy) and she was the subject of one of the clinics more unusual requests to the ambulatory monitoring service. A change of medication to carbamazepine led to complete control of her attacks, both reflex and otherwise, and further investigation and treatment was not needed.

There is a recognized relationship between previous incest and the later development of pseudo-seizures (Goodwin 1989). Occasionally, sexual assault or an incestuous sexual relationship may be followed by true epilepsy and I have several patients with undoubted epilepsy whose attacks followed closely upon such a traumatic event. In several of them the automatic behaviour they show during a complex partial seizure has sexual connotations such as brushing the thighs with their hands. Psychotherapy is helpful but may initially lead to an increase in attacks as painful memories are uncovered.

EMOTIONAL AND PSYCHOLOGICAL CONTROL OF SEIZURES

It has been known for a long time that certain physical and emotional stimuli and certain somatic and mental states can influence, either directly or indirectly, the number of attacks which a patient is having (for recent reviews see Fenwick, 1991 and Mattson, 1991). Occasionally, patients may have a measure of control over their seizures. I feel that a great deal more attention should be paid to these phenomena, partly because they may help to explain one of the fundamental problems of epilepsy—why do seizures occur when they do?—and partly because they hold out therapeutic possibilities.

Physical stimuli adequate to precipitate attacks may, on occasion, be replaced by the psychological equivalent of such stimuli, and many of the methods of psychological treatment whose aim is a reduction of anxiety or a lowering of arousal, may have some therapeutic benefit in these forms of epilepsy, and indeed, in epilepsy in general.

Photic epilepsy induced by flickering light, sudden changes in light intensity or complex patterns, is the commonest form of reflex epilepsy. A variation of this is television epilepsy, which is particularly common in young adolescents. Rarely, reading may provoke attacks in which initial twitching of the jaw progresses to a generalized convulsion if the subject does not stop reading at once. There is an excellent review by Wilkins & Lindsay (1985).

Case History 36
This 20-year-old student was referred with a study phobia to a psychiatrist. He gave a history that, in the previous year at university, whenever he attempted to study hard at night, he had a blackout and was either found by his friends wandering in a dazed state outside his room or slumped before his open books. He said that when reading he suddenly became aware of a throbbing in his throat, followed by a twitching in his jaw, and then he remembered no more for up to an hour. This was clearly reading epilepsy which disappeared when he was given antiepileptic drugs.

Photic simulation is the commonest way in which subjects, usually children, physically induce their own seizures; although in my experience this type of directly self-induced epilepsy is rare. Visual self-inducers are characterized by exceptionally high light sensitivity, frequent seizures and subnormal intelligence. Most of these visually induced attacks are of the generalized absence or myoclonic type, and the frequency of attacks depends to a certain extent on the available light intensity. For example, they are more common in Australia than in the UK.

Most children that do this cannot give an adequate explanation of their behaviour, although it would seem from observation that pleasure and escape from stress or boredom are important aetiological factors. Some seem almost compelled to do it, in the same way that children with television epilepsy seem irresistably drawn towards a television set. Whether this urge is an epileptic phenomenon or related to some other phenomena, like counter-phobic behaviour, is not known. Self-induced visual epilepsy is very difficult to treat and, in many cases, it is necessary to help the family rather than the child, and advise them on how the child and his or her symptoms should be handled.

Hyperventilation is a common method of inducing epilepsy in children and adolescents: some people with self-induced epilepsy seem able to produce an attack at will, or on request, but without any realization of how they do it: some unconsciously hyperventilate; others do it by an effort of concentration.

Seizures may be precipitated by other sensory stimuli, such as loud unexpected sounds: an element of startle is essential since a loud sound that the patient is expecting will not induce an attack (Doube 1965).

Musicogenic epilepsy, another rare condition, has aroused considerable interest. In most patients with this type of epilepsy an affective associative response to the music is required to bring on a seizure. In a few cases, however, there is evidence that the musical sound itself is the epileptogenic stimulus, possibly at a subcortical level.

Case History 37
An 18-year-old student had had several complex partial seizures a month since the age of 12. They were definitely epileptic (proven by EEG) but seemed only to occur when she heard or listened to music for more than a few minutes. She would feel uncomfortable, have a mounting feeling of anxiety, an epigastric sensation and a brief abrogation of consciousness. A keen musician, she had had to avoid her musical pursuits and, due to the prevalence of 'muzak' in the environment, had also to avoid much social activity. The seizures had not responded to any antiepileptic drug. It became clear that music had been playing at the time of her first seizure and she had associated the two together in her mind to such an extent that when

she heard music she became anxious and thereby induced a seizure. She was treated by a cue-controlled anxiety reduction technique (using aromatherapy) and is now seizure and medication free (Boden et al 1990).

A number of other stimuli effective in inducing seizures have been described, including voice and language; skin touching or tapping; vibration; eating food or the sight of it; immersion in hot or cold water; taste; sexual stimulation; arithmetical calculation; mental calculation; strategic thinking and card playing (Gastaut & Tassinari 1966, Epstein 1990).

The important emotional and psychological component to most cases of reflex epilepsy is perhaps best illustrated by Goldie & Green's (1959) classic study. They described a man who could produce a reflex seizure by rubbing his face. The psychological stimuli of preparing to rub his face, or thinking about rubbing it, were as effective as actual rubbing in provoking epileptic EEG activity or the attack itself.

The reflex epilepsies are difficult to treat: it may be impossible to shield the patient from the provoking stimulus without great difficulty, or it may be that the patient does not want to be shielded, either because he or she likes the stimulus or because it gives some kind of emotional pleasure. Antiepileptic drugs are often unsatisfactory. Recently attempts have been made, mainly by Forster (1972) to use conditioning or extinction techniques which may have great possibilities in treating reflex epilepsies, although they are at present too time consuming for widespread use. They may also work by a therapeutic shift of the patient's attention away from the triggering stimulus (Mostofsky & Balaschak 1977), or by techniques aimed at altering levels of arousal (Fenton 1991).

Forster (1972) presents the particular triggering stimulus to the patient continually, until the convulsive and EEG responses to the stimulus have extinguished. He may also train the patient to give himself a different stimulus if he encounters the actual triggering stimulus (as for instance when reading) which prevents the usual convulsive response. Forster appears to have had a great deal of success with these techniques and is also engaged in developing portable devices which can continue the patient's treatment at home, as much of the treatment at the moment is laboratory based.

SELF-CONTROL

The phenomenon of the self-control of seizures has been well known since the days of Hughlings Jackson and Gowers but seems to have been studied curiously little and, in many cases, little effort seems to have been made to discover exactly what it is that some patients actually do to stop their attacks. Symonds (1959), Fenwick (1991) and Lubar & Deering (1981) review the evidence that voluntary mental and physical activity could inhibit seizures. It is well known that patients with sensory or motor epilepsy can sometimes inhibit their attacks, once they have started, either by vigorous sensory stimulation of the involved area or by brisk muscular activity.

In my experience, patients who can stop their seizures in this way do not always feel comfortable afterwards and they may feel better if they allow themselves to have an attack at a time and place of their choosing. Symonds was more concerned with those patients who could inhibit seizures by an effort of concentration or an effort of will. This may involve thinking very hard about not having an attack or the repetition of some phrase which has the property of stopping the attacks, or occasionally the induction of an emotional state in which the attack will not occur. Of Symond's patients, 5.3% could stop their attacks in this way, although how they did it was not usually obvious. Patients may not volunteer to their doctors that they have these control mechanisms and they may only be discovered by accident.

Although little is known about how these patients actually stop their seizures, it is known that desynchronizing and other control mechanisms do exist in the brain and quite possibly they could be better utilized. That certain psychological methods of treatment might be used in potentiating such control mechanisms is illustrated by the example of the woman that Efron (1956) described, where a controlling mechanism which the patient herself had noticed and brought to the attention of her doctor was shaped and refined, so that it became easier to use. It will be interesting to see whether patients with other sensory auras could be treated in the same way. Certainly it is worthwhile trying Efron's technique of applying an adversive olfactory stimulus with patients who have an olfactory aura of sufficient duration that they can use the technique. In my own clinic we now use a cue controlled relaxation technique using a pleasant olfactory stimulus to which a relaxation response has been conditioned by using aromatherapy (Boden et al 1990).

It has been held for a long time that emotional states can lead to an increase in the number of patients' attacks, and therefore, one could suppose that altering such states could reduce seizure frequency. Direct induction of seizures by emotional stimuli is probably rare and certainly Gastaut & Tassinari (1966) in their extensive review could find very little evidence that direct induction occurs. However, most doctors experienced in epilepsy are aware that changes in a patient's emotional state often towards higher arousal may lead to an increased number of attacks (Servit et al 1963). In recent years, a fair amount of laboratory evidence has emerged to support these beliefs.

Mattson et al (1970) and Mattson (1991) have carried out detailed and important neurophysiological studies of the effects of psychic stress on the frequency of seizures, although not as a direct stimulus. In other words in a patient under stress more seizures are likely to occur than usual but not as a direct result of the stress itself. A search was made for any measure of an increase in arousal or stress that could be related to the increase in seizure frequency. There was little relationship between any of the usual parameters of arousal (e.g. plasma cortisol levels) and seizure frequency, but it was noted that increase in seizure frequency under stress was related to involuntary hyperventilation, with a resulting fall in carbon dioxide concentration. The aetiological importance of this finding was supported by the observation that such an increased seizure frequency under stress could be prevented if the patient was made to breathe an increased concentration of carbon dioxide. It is suggested that involuntary overbreathing may be an important psycho-physiological precipitant of seizures, as it is in those patients who induce their attacks deliberately by hyperventilation.

Gotze et al (1967) using telemetered EEG recordings, showed that physical exercise tended to normalize the EEGs of patients with epilepsy. After exercise, in patients who were made to hyperventilate, less EEG abnormality was produced than if they had hyperventilated without previous physical exercise. It would seem, therefore, that physical exercise raises the seizure threshold and reduces the likelihood of seizures occurring.

It may be that involuntary hyperventilation was also responsible for the effect that Stevens (1959) noted in her experiment which showed that emotionally stressful interviews had an adverse effect on EEG stability in a large proportion of people with epilepsy. Hyperventilation is often seen in those who are anxious and, of course, is amenable to behavioural manipulation.

The telemetered EEG is a powerful tool in the study of the effects of various kinds of stress and emotional states on both EEG and seizure activity. Two studies in this field (Vidart & Geier 1968, Bureau et al 1968) are of interest. Vidart was concerned with adults, and measured the occurrence of diffuse episodes of spike-and-wave activity in the EEGs of patients with known epilepsy as they went about a normal life. Intellectual work which did not overtax the capacity of the patient to deal with it, such as mental arithmetic, caused a reduction in EEG abnormalities, and presumably, therefore, a reduction in seizure frequency. If the intellectual effort required to solve the problem exceeded a level critical for the patient, the number of abnormalities increased again (Bureau et al 1968). As might be expected, fatigue and tiredness increase the amount of spike-and-wave activity in the EEG. The relationship between a patient's mental state and abnormalities in the EEG was shown to be complex. Changes in mood might either increase or decrease the amount of abnormal epileptic activity.

Stressful events always seemed to increase the amount of abnormal activity occurring; whereas, if interest was shown in the patient, the number of abnormalities would decrease. In adults or children, boredom or inactivity led to the most abnormalities per unit time in the EEG, whereas if their attention were engaged and they were interested in their work, the amount of EEG activity decreased dramatically. It is likely that there is an optimum level of arousal for any person with epilepsy at which seizures are least likely to occur.

Such states as emotional stress, sleep deprivation, fatigue, boredom and prolonged overtaxing intellectual effort and hyperventilation seem, therefore, to be important factors in precipitating seizures. Physical exercise and interesting intellectual work seem to decrease seizures. In this field it is clear that psychological methods may have an important part to play in the management of seizures and that further research is necessary. There is no doubt that psychological methods of treatment along behavioural lines are probably the treatments of choice for people who self-induce their seizures: and it is also a reasonable assumption to make that those seizures which are associated with an increase in anxiety will also be amenable to psychological methods of treatment aimed at reducing anxiety levels.

Scattered reports occur in the literature (Mostofsky & Balaschak 1977) which suggest that anxiety reducing treatment using relaxation or desensitization are effective in treating patients whose anxiety levels are increasing their seizure frequency, and the behavioural treatment results in a reduction in the frequency of seizures or even their disappearance. These are reviewed by Fenton (1991). The problem of assessing the results of behavioural treatment is that like all treatments there are many non-specific factors present in the therapy which may be responsible for the patient's improvement, rather than the specific therapeutic technique itself. Thus, relaxation therapy is common to many behavioural treatments: it may just be this that is producing the improvement. Likewise, many behavioural techniques have an indirect cognitive effect (i.e. change the way an individual thinks about him or herself). Again, cognitive restructuring may actually provide the benefit.

Case History 38

This 28-year-old woman had occasional tonic-clonic seizures between the ages of five and 11, but then remained seizure free until the age of 26 when she suddenly had an attack in the supermarket. At the time this happened she was under a great deal of personal and marital stress and had been feeling anxious for some weeks. She was still taking antiepileptic drugs. She was extremely embarrassed about the spectacle she had made of herself, and although the personal stress resolved itself, she continued to feel anxious whenever she approached the particular supermarket in which the seizure had occurred. On several occasions her anxiety levels were so high that further seizures occurred there. As a result, she became generally more anxious and attacks began to occur in other places, at home or on the street, and she eventually became so frightened of going out that she became totally housebound. Her antiepileptic drugs were increased but had no apparent effect on her seizure frequency: there was no doubt that her seizures were epileptic in nature.

She was admitted to hospital for behavioural treatment of her agoraphobia. This consisted of intensive relaxation training so that she could have some control over her anxiety feelings, followed by gradual exposure to the outside world, with encouragement and verbal reward as she was able to progress outside the hospital. As a result her anxiety symptoms diminished markedly but she was still afraid of having a seizure in a supermarket or public place. Accordingly, Standage's (1972) method of getting the patient whilst relaxed to imagine herself having a seizure (desensitization in imagination) was used. As a result, she lost her fear of attacks and from that time she has not had another one despite being able now to go anywhere. Her drugs were subsequently withdrawn.

Case History 39

This 24-year-old man had developed secondarily generalized complex partial seizures from a right anterior temporal lobe focus 6 years before. Despite medication with carbamazepine and sodium valproate, his attacks occurred on a daily basis. Ambulatory EEG monitoring confirmed their epileptic nature and he was referred for a second opinion as to his suitability for surgery. Observation during his hospital stay showed that he had no attacks in hospital but invariably had half a dozen on his return home for the weekend. This was initially thought to be due to family stresses but he eventually revealed that he almost invariably had a seizure when walking past a particular lamp-post at the end of his street. Since he lived at the bottom of a cul-de-sac there was little he could do to avoid it. The cause of this reflex epilepsy was initially obscure, but eventually he recalled that it was the spot where he had had his first attack and he now approached this lamp-post feeling that he was bound to have another one. He was taught a relaxation method that involved breathing control which he could apply when he approached the lamp-post; he also had some desensitization in imagination before attempting this and was also taught to think positive thoughts about not having an attack as he passed the lamp-post. This combination of relaxation, desensitization and cognitive therapy certainly worked, in that he lost his lamp-post attacks (and had so few spontaneous attacks afterwards that he declined surgery), but which of these techniques was the effective one?

Case History 40

This 16-year-old boy had complex partial seizures involving an automatism and a lapse of consciousness (occasionally becoming secondarily generalized) from a left temporal focus. The seizures had not responded to medication: they often occurred at times when he was relaxing from stress (e.g. after school examinations or after he had been playing his musical instrument in an orchestra for some time and had lost his performance anxiety and begun to relax and enjoy himself). Using a cue controlled anxiety reducing technique to try to reduce his seizures actually led to an increase in seizure frequency. However, when cue control was used to increase arousal there was almost complete resolution of the seizures. Using an autohypnotic technique he now uses the cue (the aroma of lemon grass oil) to induce swiftly the state of mind needed to practise a perfect golf swing, something he enjoys but which needs high arousal. Although he still occasionally needs to smell his bottle of oil, recollecting the aroma of the oil is now usually enough to stop a seizure.

Sometimes, a technique may be effective for reasons other than those the therapist thinks are the effective ones. For instance, an interesting variant of desensitization was described by Feldman & Paul (1976), in which video tape recordings of their seizures were played back to five patients. The authors believed that the videotapes provided a means by which the patients could acquire otherwise unrecognized or forgotten information and thereby identify specific emotional triggers which precipitated their seizures. The video tapes were therefore used as a specific adjunct to classical psychotherapy. Another way of seeing the procedure, however, would be as a desensitization to the patient's fear of their own seizures and this may be the more likely explanation. Many of my patients find it helpful to see their own seizure (or something resembling it) on video-tape whether or not it is part of an anxiety management programme.

Certainly where the epilepsy is made worse by anxiety, behavioural methods of treatment have now an established place in management. The question arises as to whether behavioural methods of treatment, or indeed psychotherapy itself, has a part to play in the management of epileptic seizures when neither self-inducement, anxiety, or high arousal appear to be playing a precipitating part. This matter is still controversial and has not been subjected to vigorous experimental proof, but there are indications (Mostofsky & Balaschak 1977, Fenwick 1991) that, even in patients where there does not appear to be an emotional precipitant, behavioural methods aimed at extinguishing seizure behaviour may be beneficial.

These behavioural methods include relaxation; cue controlled changes in arousal; operant conditioning (rewarding non-seizure behaviour and 'punishing' seizure activity); desensitization; psychotherapy; extinction and habituation techniques and biofeedback. Biofeedback has not been widely used but is still successful in skilled hands, particularly as it may be possible to predict, by psychological testing, those patients most likely to respond to it (Lantz & Sterman, 1988). In individual cases, the techniques work well, though few studies have controlled for placebo effects (placebo effects are, of course, also psychological in nature) or for non-specific effects of treatment.

Because behavioural treatment is time consuming it tends only to be applied when obvious seizure-related anxiety is present, or when the patient's attacks are unusual or have a marked behavioural component. This means that some of the case reports in the literature are probably accounts of the treatment of non-epileptic attacks (whose treatment is obviously psychological). What is needed is a formal trial of these techniques in epilepsy uncomplicated by anxiety or other special features. The brain has its own mechanisms for preventing or aborting seizure activity; behavioural treatment should be directed at enhancing or reinforcing these mechanisms and thus become a truly holistic technique.

ORGANIC MENTAL ILLNESS AND EPILEPSY

Brain damage and impairment of brain function is often found in epilepsy. It may be responsible for, or a factor in, mental illness occurring in people with epilepsy.

In a person with epilepsy who is of limited or impaired intelligence, almost invariably both the epilepsy and the impairment are related to a single aetiological cause. In general terms epilepsy itself does not cause a reduction in intelligence, and studies which have suggested that it does have usually looked at highly selected populations. However, there is now good evidence that both ictal activity (Jus & Jus 1962) and subictal activity (Goode et al 1970) may interfere with registration of information and also occasionally cause a brief retrograde amnesia. Epileptic activity occurring in specific brain areas, particularly the left temporal lobe, may also interfere with intellectual functioning and learning in children, and can therefore lead to behaviour problems (Stores 1978). There is also growing evidence that antiepileptic drugs may play a part in learning difficulty in children with epilepsy (Stores 1978), and these effects, occurring at an early age, may account partly for the observation that patients with temporal lobe epilepsy have a lower intelligence the earlier the onset of their epilepsy (Taylor & Falconer 1968). It has been shown that actual mental retardation in children with epilepsy is restricted to those who have suffered acute cerebral insults in the form of perinatal damage, head injury or infection, or who have had status epilepticus at an early age (Ounsted 1966).

Up until recently, discussion about the effects of brain damage and epileptic activity, whether ictal or subictal, and medication on intelligence and learning, was difficult to quantify due to the relative crudity of tests of intelligence, intellect and cortical functioning. However, recent advances in the neuropsychology of epilepsy (Dodrill 1978) have led to more discriminatory tests of intellectual and cognitive function. Also being developed are reliable tests of vigilance, attention, performance and learning in a laboratory setting (Hutt & Fairweather 1971, Hutt 1979). There is little doubt from these studies that specific, cognitive learning and performance difficulties do occur in people with epilepsy and, that, for some children with epilepsy, special teaching methods and skills are necessary to obtain optimum learning performance.

Many people with epilepsy complain of memory difficulty, particularly increased forgetfulness, and sometimes difficulty in retaining new information. This may be a complex interaction between seizure activity, pre-existing structural damage, ongoing transmitter instability and possible drug effects. Ictal amnesia, defined as a 'transient disturbance of memory function which is caused by a seizure (or by its after effect) and which has no other clinical manifestation' (Rowan & Rosenbaum 1991) is rare, and there is a wide differential diagnosis, but cases do occur.

Case History 41
Two years after a closed head injury in a road traffic accident (which led to atrophy of the right temporal lobe) this 20-year-old girl had episodes of amnesia: she would suddenly come to her senses having no recollection of the preceding period of time (from several minutes to several hours), and yet during which she had apparently behaved normally, had carried out rational acts and had spoken normally so that her boyfriend had no idea that anything was wrong—and yet she had no memory of the period. There was a persistent spike-wave focus in the right temporal lobe: the lapses of memory disappeared following treatment with carbamazapine.

EPILEPSY AND DEMENTIA

It used to be accepted without much question that people with epilepsy were liable to dement, and the concept of epileptic dementia was part of older psychiatric teaching. This concept requires critical examination.

Dementia may be described as a syndrome of chronic, irreversible and usually progressive intellectual and memory loss in which both recall and retention of information are affected. Usually, recent memory is more affected than distant memory. An important early sign of dementia is an emotional lability with which may go a 'catastrophic reaction' in which the patient over-reacts emotionally to quite trivial changes in his or her environment.

As the disorder progresses, so there is a deterioration of judgement and critical faculties which may lead to inappropriate behaviour. There may also be a release of previously controlled elements in the patient's personality, revealing themselves for the first time, so that, for instance, antisocial behaviour may be expressed in a previously well-behaved middle-aged man.

Poverty of thought and ideation occurs. Patients show difficulty in shifting from one topic to the next and eventually develop severe perseveration. They lose the ability to think logically or handle symbols and develop 'concrete thinking'. Later they may become disorientated in time and place, but very rarely in person, and they suffer from episodes of confusion; infection and sedatives may make confusion worse. Very often chronic emotional changes occur, usually those of depression and may appear when the patient is aware of his or her failing powers.

The diagnosis of dementia is largely a clinical diagnosis, although assisted by psychological tests and radiological investigation. It should not be a diagnosis that is made lightly and only after the fullest possible investigation. The value of careful investigation of people suspected of having dementia has been shown by Marsden & Harrison (1972), who found that a proportion of patients referred with a diagnosis of dementia did not have the condition at all and that some who were demented had treatable causes of the dementia.

Follow-up studies of patients with dementia (Mann 1973) show that, even in patients diagnosed radiologically as having dementia, some turn out on follow-up not to have the disorder at all. Both clinical, radiological, and also psychological investigations in patients with suspected dementia may therefore give rise to misleading results, particularly in the case of psychological testing which is relatively crude and inaccurate, except in advanced cases.

The inaccuracies in the diagnosis of dementia should be particularly borne in mind in considering the relationship between epilepsy and dementia. Whether epilepsy itself is associated with progressive dementia is uncertain. The term 'epileptic dementia' occurs quite commonly in the psychiatric literature but is often mistaken, either for the chronic changes of psychotic illnesses, for the personality changes that occur in epilepsy, for institutionalization, for depression (which so often occurs in epilepsy), or for chronic drug intoxication. In my experience chronic depression and unrecognized intoxication with phenytoin are easily labelled as dementia in people with epilepsy.

Apart from those children who suffer devastating brain insults as a result of febrile status epilepticus, it is unlikely that even repeated epileptic seizures lead to any degree of dementia. In those people who do have epilepsy and have presenile dementia, almost certainly the two syndromes are the result of a single brain disease of a progressive nature (for an example see Betts et al 1968). Some dementing illnesses are associated with symptomatic epilepsy, especially in the later stages (e.g. Alzheimer's disease and multi-infarct dementia). Occasionally, therefore, epilepsy may be the presenting sign of such a condition (patients with Alzheimer's disease often have partial seizures which, because of the prevailing dementing symptoms, often pass unnoticed), or even, occasionally, of something more exotic like porphyria (Scane et al 1986). It is occasionally speculated that some people with epilepsy are suffering from chronic viral infections or from the punch-drunk syndrome (traumatic encephalopathy). These hypotheses are unproven, apart from occasional case reports.

It should be expected, however, that people with epilepsy who are brain damaged, even if the brain damage is static, will tend to dement earlier than the general population, as they have already lost some of their cortical reserves. It is still generally accepted that considerable neuronal damage may occur without any apparent loss of intellectual function but that, after a critical level of brain tissue has been lost, there will be a rapid and obvious loss of function.

However, it does appear that a small number of patients with severe epilepsy do have progressive intellectual loss, the aetiology of which is obscure (Brown & Vaughan 1988).

In assessing a patient with suspected dementia associated with epilepsy, full investigation should be undertaken, both neurological and psychiatric, because there is a wide differential diagnosis (Shorvon 1988). Psychological testing should be employed by using relevant tests (Dodrill 1978). Psychiatric illness, drug intoxication, and apathy and inertia due to chronic illness should be excluded rigorously. Computer-assisted tomography (CT) of the brain should also be carried out; although it should be noted that the procedure is not as helpful in the diagnosis of dementia as was thought originally (reviewed by Ashworth 1986) and, when fully evaluated, investigative procedures such as magnetic resonance imaging (MRI) may well be more valuable. Occasionally, cerebral biopsy may be necessary to elucidate the cause of a particular dementing syndrome (Sim et al 1966), although use of this particular form of investigation had become rare. AIDS now enters into the differential diagnosis of epilepsy and dementia and hence cerebral biopsy may be more widely used.

THE CONFUSIONAL STATES OF EPILEPSY

Various organic mental states occur in people with epilepsy either with a time relationship to a clinical seizure or occurring at the same time as subictal seizure activity in the EEG. They are becoming increasingly recognized and have both psychiatric and forensic importance. Their classification has been confused and arbitrary and they have gone under a bewildering variety of names.

Postictal twilight states

These may occur after any type of seizure; any attempt to restrain the confused patient may lead to outbursts of aggression. The EEG shows profuse irregular slow activity. Hughlings Jackson thought that such states might be due to the exhaustion of cerebral neurones, but it is possible that they may represent a continuing ictal event. It is also possible that the now very rare epileptic furore is related to these states. Some patients, however, after their seizures are not aggressive but remain in a prolonged confused dreamlike state which seems to occur regularly after their attacks (twilight state).

Generalized absence status

This is a mental state directly related to generalized epileptic discharges. Originally termed petit mal status, it has been described by several authors under different names. I use a term coined by Roger et al (1974), that of generalized status epilepticus expressed as a confusional state. This describes a clinical picture and avoids using terms like absence and petit mal because not all patients who develop absence status have either a previous history of convulsions or of absences (Roger et al 1974, Ellis & Lee 1978). Indeed these states do sometimes seem to start de novo in middle age without a previous epileptic history. They are characterized by a confusional state which varies in intensity and presentation from patient to patient and also varies within the same patient from time to time. There may be only a slight degree of confusion, often then accompanied by apparent histrionic or neurotic behaviour, but with clear-cut evidence of an organic deficit on formal psychological testing. There may be episodes of severe confusion, often with a patchy loss of intellectual function (i.e. the patient may remember one thing but forget others during the attack, or may have transient signs of parietal lobe disturbance). There may be the most profound stupor. Those confusional states, which are related to previous epilepsy of a generalized nature, usually respond well to intravenous diazepam or clonazepam but this treatment may make them worse particularly if the patient had atypical absences: lamotrigine seems particularly useful in preventing such atypical absence status, which often respond poorly to other antiepileptic drugs. The ictal confusional states of middle age seem to respond well to conventional drugs, once the underlying epileptic diathesis is identified.

Occasionally, during the ictal period, in addition to the confusion previously described, frank psychotic symptoms may appear. These can often be seen as the patient's attempt to explain puzzling internal feelings which cannot be understood. This phenomenon is more common in the acute prolonged confusional states of later life (Ellis & Lee 1978).

Case History 42
This 13-year-old girl, who had recurrent generalized absences and tonic-clonic seizures since the age of 3, poorly controlled with conventional medication, was admitted from a neurological ward to a psychiatric unit with the diagnosis of schizophrenia. On admission she was fatuous and giggling, appeared to have visual hallucinations, and described herself as married to a well-known pop singer. In addition, to this, however, she was vague and distant, appeared to be disorientated and had little memory of recent events. She had been admitted to the neurological unit in this state some days previously. EEG examination on her admission to the psychiatric unit showed generalized 3 per second spike-and-wave activity. Oral nitrazepam was given and, within a day, the EEG abnormality had stopped and a somewhat bewildered but now normal 13-year-old girl emerged from underneath the apparent psychotic behaviour. On reviewing her history it would seem that, in the preceding few years, she had had many attacks like this lasting up to a day which had greatly interfered with her school work. Under a small dose of nitrazepam these attacks no longer occurred although she continued to have the occasional tonic-clonic seizure. Her school work improved markedly.

Simple partial status

Previously called epilepsia partialis continua this, after tonic-clonic convulsive status, is the most common form of status epilepticus and is repeated clonic twitching and jerking of a limb, usually the arm and usually on one side of the body (sometimes of just a few muscle groups). Although clonic movements are the most common rarely there is tonic spasm. The condition may be very persistent and difficult to treat.

Complex partial status

This involves a prolonged alteration in mental state resulting from epileptic discharge in the cortex, usually in the temporal lobes. This has not been described extensively in the British literature and is said to be rare (Fenton 1983) but in my experience it is more common than is generally thought. Five case histories have been appended to illustrate the clinical features. Some twilight states which resemble complex partial status but which are chronologically related to seizures, appear to occur in other types of epilepsy. These are the ones particularly described by Landolt (1958) who maintains that such twilight states can result from overdosage of antiepileptic drugs—a statement with which I would agree.

Case History 43

This 40-year-old man had never sought help for the brief seizures which he had had for 20 years, and which were of a brief muddled feeling accompanied by a déjà vu experience. He had had one of his usual attacks on the bus on his way to work; after the attack he walked away from his regular bus stop in a dazed state, removing his clothing as he did so. Completely naked, he wandered up and down a shopping precinct muttering incoherently. He was arrested, struggling violently, and covered in the regulation blanket, removed to a police station. When questioned he did not make coherent replies except occasionally to mutter 'protest'. He remained in this state for 12 hours and then suddenly recovered his senses, and demanded to know where he was and who had removed his clothing. He has not shown similar behaviour since, but passed through a transient period of depression on knowing what he had done. Subsequent investigation showed a right temporal epileptic focus on EEG examination.

Case History 44

A man of 23 was found wandering in a dazed fashion in the middle of a large city. He had given no coherent reply to questions by the police, and search of his clothing revealed no identifying mark or documents. He was accordingly admitted to a psychiatric hospital where he was observed to spend most of his time in a catatonic-like stupor, crouched in a chair. Occasionally he was thought to be visually hallucinating as he seemed to be watching some insect or bird flying round his room. Rarely he would become violently aggressive, when he would dash up out of his chair and fly around the ward overturning tables and chairs and smashing windows for a few minutes before returning to his previous still posture. He was thought to have catatonic schizophrenia and was treated with psychotropic drugs but with little effect. A week after admission whilst asleep in bed he was observed to have a tonic-clonic seizure. On awakening the next morning he was lucid and rational, knew his name and where he came from, and was surprised to find himself in hospital. Over the next few hours, the previous psychotic state returned; an EEG at this time showed continuous spike-and-wave discharge from the left temporal lobe. He was given intravenous diazepam and his mental state returned to normal, at the same time as the abnormal EEG discharges stopped. He made a complete recovery with regular antiepileptic drugs.

Case History 45

A woman with left temporal lobe epilepsy stopped her antiepileptic drugs suddenly. A day later she passed into a peculiar clouded mental state in which she was irritable and tearful and had obvious memory difficulty. Definite organic impairment was confirmed on formal mental state testing. She would not eat, lost weight rapidly and complained of bone pain. She would wander distracted round the house in a confused state and was incapable of looking after her children. An EEG showed continual epileptic activity in the left temporal area, which previously had only been present during her actual attacks. Ten days after this episode started she awoke one morning in a normal frame of mind; on that day the EEG abnormality had disappeared and has not returned.

Case History 46

A girl of 18 had had complex partial seizures originating in the right temporal lobe since the age of 7: their aetiology was obscure. She had occasional tonic-clonic attacks as well. Her attacks became more frequent, despite increasing dosages of carbamazepine. It had been intended to try sodium valproate but publicity about the side-effects of this drug in the national press made the patient request the use of another drug. Clobazam was tried and the girl rapidly passed into a peculiar mental state of perplexity and irritability, and left to herself would sit listlessly all day avoiding her usual pursuits. If questioned, she would appear orientated in time and place but was very slow to respond and would not co-operate in psychological testing. An EEG (and ambulatory EEG monitoring) showed dense spike-and-wave activity originating in the posterior part of the right temporal lobe. Clobazam was withdrawn and within a few days the original bright vivacious teenager returned. Subsequently she has been taking sodium valproate and her attack frequency has declined markedly and she has returned to college.

Case History 47
This 15-year-old girl is one of identical twins, both of whom have generalized epilepsy although their attacks are infrequent. They had been treated by their general practitioner with phenobarbitone. This girl suddenly developed an acute mental illness where she became mute and immobile; except occasionally to ejaculate the words 'British Constitution' and wander about. She was sleepless and incontinent. An EEG showed a continual spike focus in the left temporal area. Intravenous clonazepam temporarily altered her mental state but it would return a few hours later. Oral carbamazepine was ineffectual, as was oral clonazepam. After a week she was given one treatment with electroconvulsive therapy under brietal anaesthesia (brietal anaesthesia on its own was ineffective) and the mental state cleared and has not returned; the left temporal focus on EEG has also not returned and she has had no further attacks whilst taking carbamazepine. A year after this her twin sister developed a rather similar mental state but this was not accompanied by EEG changes and was found to be a deliberate imitation of her sister's attacks for purposes of gaining more attention. Firm persuasion abolished it.

These cases illustrate the wide variety of phenomena which may be seen in association with continual epileptic activity occurring in one temporal lobe though, if looked for, confusion and evidence of organic impairment can always be found. Pseudoneurotic behaviour may also be prominent. Sometimes, automatisms are the main feature to be seen in the patient's mental state and, occasionally, the patient may wander away in the twilight state in a kind of fugue. Twilight states may be prolonged and last for several days. Both non-convulsive generalized and complex partial status should be considered in the differential diagnosis of any case of stupor or confusion, particularly if there is a history of epilepsy, but even if there is not. The EEG is needed to make the diagnosis and will usually make a distinction between general and partial non-convulsive status— but not invariably, and it may be difficult to diag-

nose the condition in patients who always have prominent epileptic activity in their EEGs.

Confusion and delirium

Profound confusional states can also occur in epilepsy in the absence of subconvulsive status, and some people with epilepsy develop a frank delirium although not apparently as an ictal experience. Epileptic delirium was frequently described in the older literature on epilepsy and in fact is still encountered (Betts 1981b). The usual characteristics of delirium are present: psychomotor overactivity; perceptual distortions; hallucinatory experiences, usually of a visual nature; confusion; disorientation in time and place; and a degree of clouding of consciousness. Delusional ideas may also be present, usually persecutory, although I have seen the occasional patient with a depressive element to his delirium.

Landolt (1958) associates these delirious states with suppressed seizures and the forced normalization of the EEG. However I would agree with Bruens (1974) that forced normalization does not occur in states in which there is also clouding of consciousness. It has been my experience that these delirious conditions are relatively common, often associated with the patient's admission to hospital, and usually seem to be associated with a sudden increase in attack frequency and carry a relatively good prognosis (Betts 1974). It has usually not been possible to do an EEG at the time of the patient's admission (so that subconvulsive status cannot be completely excluded), but it has been my clinical impression that one is seeing a confused state related to frequent seizures rather than to ictal activity itself.

Case History 48
This man of 60 had about four tonic-clonic attacks a year from the age of 30 which had never been investigated, although he had been taking phenobarbitone for years. Just before his sixtieth birthday he had eight attacks within a week, possibly connected with a reduction in his antiepileptic drugs. During this period he became suspicious, truculent and hostile, and later became physically aggressive and overactive and developed florid paranoid ideas; imagining that he was being spied upon, that his neighbours were pumping gas under his doors; he appeared to have auditory hallucinations and began to see visions of the devil. Finally he attacked his

son-in-law with an axe, mistaking him for the devil himself. On removal to hospital he was noted to have the classic symptoms of delirium, and was markedly confused with severe disorientation and a poor retentive memory. His antiepileptic drugs were increased and within a few days the excited delirious state had disappeared pari passu with cessation of his seizures, and has not returned.

The patient seems to have been left with no residual organic deficit although in my mental hospital experience some patients who develop a delirious state related to epilepsy seem afterwards to have a permanent organic defect state, although it can be difficult to say whether or not they had it before (Betts 1974).

REFERENCES

Ashworth B 1986 Who needs a CT brain scan? British Medical Journal 292: 845–846

Bagley C 1971 The social psychology of the child with epilepsy. Routledge & Kegan Paul, London

Barraclough B 1981 Suicide and epilepsy. In: Reynolds E, Trimble M (eds) Epilepsy and psychiatry. Churchill Livingstone, Edinburgh, p 72–76

Barzak P, Edmunds E, Betts T 1988 Hypomania following complex partial seizures. British Journal of Psychiatry 152: 137–139

Betts T 1974 A follow-up study of a cohort of patients with epilepsy admitted to psychiatric care in an English city. In: Harris P, Mawdsley C (eds) Epilepsy: proceedings of the Hans Berger Centenary Symposium. Churchill Livingstone, Edinburgh, p 326–336

Betts T 1981a Depression, anxiety and epilepsy. In: Reynolds E, Trimble M (eds) Epilepsy and psychiatry. Churchill Livingstone, Edinburgh, p 60–71

Betts T 1981b Epilepsy and the mental hospital. In: Reynolds E, Trimble M (eds) Epilepsy and psychiatry. Churchill Livingstone, Edinburgh, p 175–184

Betts T 1984 Sexual problems in people with epilepsy. Paper presented at British–Danish–Dutch Epilepsy Symposium, Elsinor, October 1984

Betts T 1986 Employment of people with epilepsy within the National Health Service. In: Edwards F, Espir, M, Oxley J (eds) Epilepsy and employment. RSM Services No 88. Oxford University Press, Oxford, p 59–66

Betts T 1990 Pseudoseizures: Seizures that are not epilepsy. Lancet 336: 163–164

Betts T Kenwood C 1988 A 20 year follow-up study of a group of patients with epilepsy and psychosis. Paper presented at the British–Danish–Dutch epilepsy conference Meer-en-Bosch, Sept 1988

Betts T, Skarott P 1979 The mental hospital and epilepsy. Research and Clinical Forums. 2(2): 129–137

Betts T, Boden S 1991 Pseudoseizures (non epileptic attack disorder). In: Trimble M (ed) Women and epilepsy. John Wiley, Chichester, p 237–252

Betts T, Smith W T, Kelly R E 1968 Adult metachromatic leucodystrophy (sulphatide lipidosis) simulating acute schizophrenia. Neurology 18: 1140–1142

Bird J 1979 The behavioural treatment of hysteria. British Journal of Psychiatry 134: 129–137

Blumer D 1991 Epilepsy and disorders of mood . In: Smith D, Treiman D, Trimble M (eds) Advances in neurology, vol. 55. Raven Press, New York, p 185–195

Boden S, Betts T, Clouston T 1990 Use of olfactory stimuli (aromatherapy) to successfully control epileptic seizures. Acta Neurologica Scandinavica 82 (suppl. 133): 54

Bowlby J 1960 Grief and mourning in infancy and early childhood. Psychoanalytic Study of the Child 15: 9–17

Brown S, Vaughan M 1988 Dementia in epileptic patients. In: Trimble M, Reynolds E (eds) Epilepsy, behaviour and cognitive function. John Wiley, Chichester, p 177–188

Bruens J H 1974 Psychoses in epilepsy. In: Vinken P L, Bruyn L W (eds) Handbook of clinical neurology 15. North Holland, Amsterdam, p 593–610

Bureau M, Guey J, Dravet C, Roger J 1968 A study of distribution of petit mal absences in the child in relation to his activities. Electroencephalography and Clinical Neurophysiology 25: 513

Caveness W, Merritt H, Gallup G 1969 A survey of public attitudes towards epilepsy in 1969. US Dept of Health Education and Welfare, Public Health Service, Washington DC

Corbidge P, Bullock K 1986 Production of a teaching package about epilepsy—an analysis. Paper presented at Northern European Epilepsy Meeting, York, September 1986

Demerdash A, Shaalan M, Midani A, Kamel F, Bahri M 1991 Sexual behaviour of a sample of females with epilepsy. Epilepsia 32(1): 82–85

Dodrill C 1978 A neuropsychological battery for epilepsy. Epilepsia 19: 611–623

Doube J R 1965 Sensory precipitated seizures—a review. Journal of Nervous and Mental Disease 141: 524–539

Edeh J, Toone B 1987 Relationship between interictal psychopathology and the type of epilepsy. Results of a survey in General Practice. British Journal of Psychiatry 151: 95–101

Efron R 1956 The effect of olfactory stimuli in arresting uncinate fits. Brain 79: 267–281

Ellis J M, Lee S I 1978 Acute prolonged confusion in late life as an ictal state. Epilepsia 19: 119–128

Epilepsy News 1979 12, British Epilepsy Assoc. Leeds.

Epstein A 1991 What the reflex epilepsies reveal about the physiology of ideation. Journal of Neuropsychiatry 2(1): 69–71

Feldman R G, Paul N L 1976 Identity of emotional triggers in epilepsy. Journal of Nervous and Mental Disease 162: 345–353

Fenton G 1983 Epilepsy, personality and behaviour. In: Rose F (ed) Research progress in epilepsy. Pitman, London, p 188–209

Fenwick P 1985 Regina v Sullivan; the trial and judgement. In: Fenwick P, Fenwick E (eds) Epilepsy and the law. Royal Society of Medicine, London, p 3–8

Fenwick P 1991 Evocation and inhibition of seizures. Behavioural treatment. In Smith D, Treiman D, Trimble M (eds) Advances in neurology, vol. 55. Raven Press, New York, p 163–183

Flor-Henry P 1969 Psychosis and temporal lobe epilepsy. Epilepsia 10: 363–395

Forster F M 1972 The classification and conditioning treatment of the reflex epilepsies. International Journal of Neurology 9: 73–86

Gastaut H, Tassinari C A 1966 Triggering mechanisms in epilepsy. Epilepsia 7: 85–138

Geschwind N 1979 Behaviour changes in temporal lobe epilepsy. Psychological Medicine 9: 217–219

Gillig P, Sackellares J, Greenberg H 1988 Right hemisphere partial complex seizures: mania, hallucinations, and speech disturbances during ictal events. Epilepsia 29(1): 26–29

Goffman E 1963 Stigma. Notes on the management of spoiled identity. Prentice Hall, New Jersey

Goldie L, Green J M 1959 A study of the psychological factors in a case of sensory reflex epilepsy. Brain 82: 505–524

Goode D J, Penry J K, Dreifuss F E 1970 Effects of paroxysmal spike wave on continuous visual motor performance. Epilepsia 11: 241–254

Goodwin J 1989 Sexual abuse : incest victims and their families, 2nd edn. Mosby, Chicago

Gotze W, Kupicki S T, Munter F , Teichman J 1967 Effect of exercise on seizure threshold. Diseases of the nervous system 28: 664–667

Graham P, Rutter M 1986 Organic brain dysfunction and child psychiatric disorder. British Medical Journal 3: 695–700

Gudmundsson D 1967 Epilepsy in Iceland. Acta Neurologica Scandinavia 43 (suppl 25): 1–124

Guerrant J, Anderson W W, Fisher A, Weinstein M R, Jaros R M, Deskins A 1962 Personality in epilepsy. Thomas, Springfield

Gunn J C 1969 Epileptics in prison. MD Thesis, University of Birmingham, England

Gunn J C, Fenton G 1971 Epilepsy, automatism and crime. Lancet 1: 1173–1176

Harper M, Roth M 1962 Temporal lobe epilepsy and the phobic anxiety–depersonalisation syndrome. Part 1: a comparative study. Psychiatry 3: 129–151

Hauser W, Ng S, Brust J 1988 Alcohol, seizures and epilepsy. Epilepsia 29(suppl 2): 566–578

Herzberg J, Fenwick P 1988 The aetiology of aggression in temporal lobe epilepsy. British Journal of Psychiatry 153: 50–55

Hierons R, Saunders M 1966 Impotence in patients with temporal lobe lesions. Lancet 2: 761–763

Hill D 1957 The electroencephalogram in schizophrenia. In: Richter D (ed) Schizophrenia, somatic aspects. Pergamon Press, Oxford

Hill D, Pond D A, Mitchell W, Falconer M A 1957 Personality changes following temporal lobectomy for epilepsy. Journal of Mental Science 103: 18–27

Hinton J 1967 Dying. Penguin, Harmondsworth

Hoenig J, Hamilton C M 1960 Epilepsy and sexual orgasm. Acta Psychiatrica Scandinavia 35: 448–456

Hoening J, Kenna J C 1979 EEG abnormalities and transexualism. British Journal of Psychiatry 134: 293–300

Hutt S J 1979 Cognitive processes and EEG activity in patients with epilepsy. Paper presented at the International Conference on Psychology and Medicine. University College of Swansea, Wales.

Hutt S J, Fairweather H 1971 Some effects of performance variables upon generalized spike wave activity. Brain 94: 321–326

Johnson B, Campbell L 1991 Mood disorder, 'pre-ictal' psychosis and temporal lobe damage. British Journal of Psychiatry 157: 441–444

Jus A, Jus K 1962 Retrograde amnesia in petit mal. Archives of General Psychiatry 6: 163–167

Kenwood C, Betts T 1992 Psychoses occurring in patients taking vigabatrin. Seizure 1 (4)

Lacey J T, Bateman D E, Van Lehn R 1953 Autonomic response specificity. Psychosomatic Medicine 15: 8–21

Landolt H 1958 Serial electroencephalographic investigations during psychotic episodes in epileptic patients & during schizophrenic attacks. In: Lorentz de Haas A M (ed) Lectures in epilepsy. Elsevier, Amsterdam, p 91–133

Lantz D, Sterman M 1988 Neuropsychological assessment of subjects with uncontrolled epilepsy : effects of EEG feedback training. Epilepsia 29(2): 163–171

Leiderman D, Csernansky J, Moses J 1990 Neuroendocrinology and limbic epilepsy: relationships to psychopathology, seizure variables, and neuropsychological function. Epilepsia 31(3): 270–274

Lishman W A 1968 Brain damage in relation to psychiatric disability and head injury. British Journal of Psychiatry 114: 373–410

Logsdail S, Toone B 1988 Post ictal psychoses: a clinical and phenomenological description. British Journal of Psychiatry 152: 246–252

Lombroso C 1889 L'uomo delinquente. Bocca, Turin

Lubar J, Deering W 1981 Behavioural approaches to neurology. Academic Press, New York

Mackay A 1979 Self-poisoning—a complication of epilepsy. British Journal of Psychiatry 134: 277–282

Maletzky B M 1973 The episodic dyscontrol syndrome. Diseases of the Nervous System 34: 178–185

Mann A H 1973 Cortical atrophy and air encephalography: a clinical and radiological study. Psychological Medicine 3: 374–378

Marsden C D, Harrison M J 1972 Outcome of investigation of patients with presenile dementia. British Medical Journal 2: 249–252

Mattson R 1991 Emotional effects on seizure occurrence. In: Smith D, Treiman D, Trimble M (eds) Advances in neurology, vol. 55. Raven Press, New York, p 453–460

Mattson R H, Heninger G R, Gallagher B B, Glaser G H 1970 Psychophysiologic precipitants of seizures in epileptics. Neurology 20:407

Mellor C 1970 The first rank symptoms of schizophrenia. British Journal of Psychiatry 117: 15–21

Mellor D H, Lowitt I, Hall D J 1974 Are epileptic children behaviourally different from other children ? In: Harris P, Mawdsley C (eds) Epilepsy: proceedings of the Hans Berger Centenary Symposium. Churchill Livingstone, Edinburg, p 313–316

Merksey H 1979 The analysis of hysteria. Bailliere Tindall, London

Merksey H, Tonge W L 1974 Psychiatric illness, 7th edn. Bailliere Tindall, London

Mitchell W, Falconer M A, Hill D 1954 Epilepsy with fetishism relieved by temporal lobectomy. Lancet ii: 626–630

Molder O 1990 Management of pseudoepileptic seizures. In: Dam M, Gram L (eds) Comprehensive epileptology. Raven Press, New York, p 495–504

Morrell D, Gage H, Robinson N 1971 Symptoms in general practice. Journal of the Royal College of General Practitioners 21: 32–43

Mostofsky D I, Balaschak B A 1977 Psychobiological control of seizures. Psychological Bulletin 84 (4): 732–759

Mungas D 1988 Psychometric correlates of episodic violent behaviour : a multidimensional neuropsychological approach. British Journal of Psychiatry 152: 180–187

Office of Health Economics 1971 Epilepsy in Society. London

Ounsted C, Lindsay J, Norman R 1966 Biological factors in temporal lobe epilepsy. Heinemann, London

Perez M, Trimble M 1980 Epileptic psychosis—diagnostic comparison with process schizophrenia. British Journal of Psychiatry 137: 245–249

Pond D A, Bidwell B H 1959 A survey of epilepsy in 14 general practices. II. Social and psychological aspects. Epilepsia I: 285–299

Pond D A, Bidwell B H, Stein L 1960 A survey of epilepsy in 14 general practices I. Demographic and medical data. Acta Psychiatrica Neurologica Neurochirugia 63: 217–236

Pratt R T C, Mackenzie W 1958 Anxiety states following vestibular disorders. Lancet 2: 347–349

Ramani V 1986 Intensive monitoring of psychogenic seizures aggression and dyscontrol syndromes. In: Gunit R (ed) Advances in neurology, vol. 46, intensive neurodiagnostic monitoring. Raven Press, New York, p 203–217

Rao M, Stephan H, Bauer J 1989 Epileptic but not psychogenic seizures are accompanied by simultaneous elevation of serum pituitary hormones and cortisol levels. Neuroendocrinology 49: 33–39

Robertson M 1985 Depression in patients with epilepsy: an overview and clinical study. In: Trimble M (ed) The psychopharmacology of epilepsy. John Wiley, Chichester, p 65–82

Rodin E 1982 Aggression and epilepsy. In: Riley T L, Roy A (eds) Pseudoseizures. Williams and Wilkins, Baltimore, London, p 185–212

Roger J, Lob H, Tassinari C A 1974 Generalized status epilepticus expressed as a confusional state (petit mal status or absence status epilepticus). In: Vinken P L, Bruyn G W (eds) Handbook of clinical neurology 15. North Holland Publishing, Amsterdam, p 145–188

Rowan A, Rosenbaum D 1991 Ictal amnesia and fugue states. In Smith D, Treiman D, Trimble M (eds) Advances in neurology, vol. 55. Raven Press, New York, p 357–367

Roy A 1979 Hysterical fits previously diagnosed as epilepsy. Psychological Medicine 7: 271–273

Sander J, Hart Y, Johnson A, Shorvon S 1990 National general practice study of epilepsy : newly diagnosed epileptic seizures in a general population. Lancet 336: 1267–1271

Sander J, Hart Y, Trimble M, Shorvon S 1991 Vigabatrin and psychosis. Journal of Neurology, Neurosurgery & Psychiatry 54: 435–439

Savard G, Anderman G 1990 Convulsive pseudoseizures: a review of current concepts. Behavioural Neurology 3: 133–141

Scane A, Wight J, Godwin-Austin R 1986 Acute intermittent porphyria presenting as epilepsy. British Medical Journal 292: 946

Sensky T 1983 Religiosity, mystical experience and epilepsy. In: Rose F (ed) Research progress in epilepsy. Pitman, London, p 214–220

Serafetinides E 1965 Aggressiveness in temporal lobe epileptics and its relation to cerebral dysfunction and enviromental factors. Epilepsia 6: 33–42

Servit Z, Machek J, Stercova A, Kristof M, Servenkova V A,

Dudas B 1963 Reflex influences in the pathogenesis of epilepsy in the light of clinical statistics. In Servit Z (ed) Reflex mechanisms in the genesis of epilepsy. Elsevier, Amsterdam

Shorvon S 1988 Late onset seizures and dementia: a review of epidemiology and aetiology. In: Trimble M, Reynolds E (eds) Epilepsy behaviour and cognitive functions. John Wiley, Chichester, p 189–198

Shukla G D, Srivastava O N, Katiyar B C 1979 Sexual disturbances in temporal lobe epilepsy—a controlled study. British Journal of Psychiatry 134: 288–292

Silberman E, Post R, Nurnberger J, Theodore W, Boulenger J 1985 Transient sensory, cognitive and affective phenomena in affective illness: a comparison with complex partial epilepsy. British Journal of Psychiatry 146: 81–89

Sim M, Turner E, Smith WT 1966 Cerebral biopsy in the investigation of presenile dementia. British Journal of Psychiatry 112: 119–133

Slater E 1965 The diagnosis of hysteria. British Medical Journal 1: 1395–1399

Slater E, Moran E 1969 Schizophrenia like psychoses of epilepsy : relation between ages of onset. British Journal of Psychiatry 115: 599–603

Slater E, Shields J 1969 Genetical aspects of anxiety. In: Lader M H (ed) Studies in anxiety. Headley brothers, Ashford

Slater E, Beard A W, Glithero E 1963 The schizophrenia-like psychoses of epilepsy. British Journal of Psychiatry 109: 95–150

Small J, Hayden M, Small I 1966 Further psychiatric investigations of patients with temporal and non-temporal lobe epilepsy. American Journal of Psychiatry 123: 303–310

Spitz M 1991 Panic disorder in seizure patients: a diagnostic pitfall. Epilepsia 32(I): 33–38

Srole L, Langner T S, Micheal S T, Opler M K, Rennie T A C 1962 Medical health in the metropolis, the Mid-town Manhattan study. McGraw Hill, New York

Standage K F 1972 Treatment of epilepsy by reciprocal inhibition of anxiety. Guys Hospital Reports 121: 217–219

Stevens J R 1959 Emotional activation of the electro-encephalogram in patients with convulsive disorder. Journal of Nervous and Mental Disease 128: 339–351

Stevens J 1991 Psychosis and the temporal lobe. In: Smith D, Treiman D, Trimble M (eds) Advances in neurology, vol. 55. Raven Press, New York, p 79–96

Stevens J, Bigelow L, Denney D et al 1979 Telemetered EEG-EOG during psychotic behaviours of schizophrenia. Archives of General Psychiatry 36: 251–262

Stores G 1978 School children with epilepsy at risk for learning and behavioural problems. Developmental Medicine and Child Neurology 20: 502–508

Symonds C 1959 Excitation and inhibition in epilepsy. Brain 82: 133–146

Taylor D C 1969 Aggression and epilepsy. Journal of Psychosomatic Research 13: 229–236

Taylor D C, Falconer M A 1968 Clinical socio-economic and psychological changes after temporal lobectomy. British Journal of Psychiatry 114: 1247–1261

Tinuper P, Cerullo A, Cirignotta F, Curtelli M, Lugaresi E, Montagna P 1990 Nocturnal paroxysmal dystonia with short lasting attacks : three cases with evidence for an epileptic frontal lobe origin of seizures. Epilepsia 31: 549–556

Tizard B 1962 The personality of epileptics. Psychological Bulletin 59: 196–210

Toone B, Wheeler M, Fenwick P 1980 Sex hormone changes in male epileptics. Clinical Endocrinology 12: 391–395

Toone B, Edeh J, Nanjee M, Wheeler M 1989 Hyposexuality and epilepsy : a community survey of hormonal and behavioural changes in male epileptics. Psychological Medicine 19: 937–943

Treiman D 1991 Psychobiology of ictal aggression. In: Smith D, Treiman D, Trimble M (eds) Advances in neurology, vol. 55. Raven Press, New York, p 341–356

Trimble M 1991a Interictal psychoses of epilepsy. In: Smith D, Treiman D, Trimble M (eds) Advances in neurology, vol. 55. Raven Press, New York, p 143–152

Trimble M 1991b The psychoses of epilepsy. Raven Press, New York

Trimble M, Bolwig T 1986 Aspects of epilepsy and psychiatry. John Wiley, Chichester.

Tyrer P 1974 The role of bodily feelings in anxiety. Oxford University Press, Oxford

Tyrer P, Alexander J 1979 Classification of personality disorder. British Journal of Psychiatry 135: 163–167

Tyrer P, Alexander J, Cicchetti D, Cohen M, Remington M 1979 Reliability of a schedule for rating personality disorder. British Journal of Psychiatry 135: 168–174

Vidart L, Geier S 1968 Work, fatigue and the psychic state in epileptic patients: a telemetric EEG study. Electroencephalography and Clinical Neurophysiology 25: 511

Volavka J 1990 Aggression, electroencephalography and evoked potentials: a critical review. Neuropsychiatry, Neuropsychology and Behavioural Neurology 3(4): 249–259

Walton H J, Presly A S 1973 Use of category system in the diagnosis of abnormal personality. British Journal of Psychiatry 122: 259–268

Wilkins A, Lindsay J 1985 Common forms of reflex epilepsy: physiological mechanisms and techniques for treatment. In: Pedley A, Meldrum B (eds) Recent advances in epilepsy 2. Churchill Livingstone, Edinburgh, p 239–271

Williams D 1956 The structure of emotions reflected in epileptic experiences. Brain 79: 29–67

Williams D 1981 The emotions and epilepsy. In: Reynolds E, Trimble M (eds) Epilepsy and psychiatry. Churchill Livingstone, Edinburgh, p 49–59

Williams K 1990 Hysteria in seventeenth century case records and unpublished manuscripts. History of Psychiatry 1: 383–401

Wing J 1974 Paper 5. In: People with handicaps need better trained counsellors. Central Council for Education and Training of Social Workers, London

12. Neuropsychology

C. B. Dodrill

INTRODUCTION

Neuropsychology is the discipline which deals with the relationship between the brain and behaviour. As applied to human beings, neuropsychology is especially concerned with pathological conditions of the brain and their effects upon abilities, behaviour, and ultimately the total adjustment of the person.

The important role of neuropsychological assessment in epilepsy is evident from an examination of the nature of this disorder. In epilepsy, the brain is known to be dysfunctional, at least during the epileptic attacks. While this is beyond dispute, it is less well appreciated that brain dysfunction continues to exist between attacks in most people with epilepsy. The EEG demonstration of this fact is the observation that interictal EEG tracings often show both epileptiform and nonepileptiform changes. Were this not the case, the EEG would be of little value except during periods where epileptic attacks were recorded. Because the brain constitutes the basis for mental abilities and behaviour, it is only reasonable to expect that alterations in these areas would be found even between attacks in many persons with epilepsy. This has been shown to be the case when a comprehensive battery of tests has been used (Dodrill 1978), and while exceptions to the rule clearly exist, this should not distract us from focusing upon the more typical circumstance. Because of both the frequency of brain dysfunction and the importance of brain functions for daily life adjustment in the patient with epilepsy, it is suggested that a neuropsychological study of the underlying brain problem is of equal importance as is a medical study of the symptoms (epileptic attacks) of the same underlying neurological difficulty.

In this chapter, the basic areas of neuropsychological assessment in epilepsy will be discussed. This includes: 1. approaches to neuropsychological assessment in epilepsy, 2. seizure history variables, 3. effects of antiepileptic drugs upon performance, and 4. surgery for epilepsy.

NEUROPSYCHOLOGICAL ASSESSMENT IN EPILEPSY

The brain is a complex organ with many functions, and because of this, the extent to which there may be impairment in these functions cannot be assessed adequately without evaluating a number of them. Inevitably, this calls for the use of a battery of tests rather than one or two measures. Furthermore, epilepsy is typically found accompanied by various matters of neuropsychological importance such as underlying brain disturbance, both epileptiform and nonepileptiform EEG discharges, immediate and long-term effects of the attacks themselves, and the chronic effects of antiepileptic drugs. These issues and others argue for a systematic and comprehensive neuropsychological assessment of people with epilepsy, and especially is this true for persons with this disorder who are evidencing various difficulties in adjustment. With the administration of a battery of tests which are sensitive to the particular types of difficulties frequently found in epilepsy, there is hope of describing the problems for each case and also in devising courses of remedial treatment tailored to the limitations found.

Although the rationale for neuropsychological assessment of people with epilepsy just presented appears reasonable, it is the exception rather than the rule that they receive any type of systematic neuropsychological testing. When evaluation is provided, it is typically brief with an emphasis upon standard areas of functioning such as 'intelligence' and with no systematic effort to evaluate brain functions. While the argument of limited manpower and the costs of this evaluation is often raised, a closer inspection shows that the value of such an assessment is not always appreciated relative to its limited cost. Most people with epilepsy who are institutionalized or maintained on disability incomes for years at great expense have never had such an assessment and an adequate description of their brain-related limitations has never been made. It is little wonder then that satisfactory remedies to their problems have not been forthcoming. While an adequate resolution of problems is certainly not guaranteed by a neuropsychological evaluation, a directed assessment of abilities in combination with specialized guidance has led to improved quality of life for persons with epilepsy (Fraser et al 1986).

Approaches to neuropsychological testing

Two general approaches to neuropsychological testing of patients with epilepsy have emerged. These approaches are disparate from one another, the assumptions underlying them are dissimilar, and their strengths and weaknesses also vary. Because of these differences, it is important to differentiate between them at the outset. By so doing, needless criticism between proponents of each method is avoided and the way is paved for a more constructive integration of the approaches.

Method 1

The first method of neuropsychological assessment is the best known and it has been available for many years. It consists of the use of a systematically established and validated battery of neuropsychological tests. In the best developed form of this general method (Reitan & Wolfson 1985), in order for a test to be labelled 'neuropsychological' and included in the battery, it must have demonstrated sensitivity to the 'neuro-' part of the term. That is, a test is included in the battery not on the basis of the technology which is available or on the basis of what the test appears to measure, but on the basis of its actually demonstrating its sensitivity to pathological conditions of the brain. The rationale is that unless it is able to make such a basic distinction, changes in scores are of uncertain significance with respect to the functioning of the nervous system.

The tests used in this general method are not automated and they involve an examiner who gives instructions, asks questions, and records answers. Test materials and pieces of equipment are involved routinely. The tests are selected to cover a number of areas of functioning, and in most batteries labelled as 'comprehensive', an effort is made at least to sample the major areas of mental abilities. These include memory, language, visual–spatial function, attention/concentration, perceptual abilities, motor functions, and problem solving.

The mere accumulation of a group of brain-sensitive tests which appear to cover various areas of functioning is not, however, adequate alone to permit the construction of a test battery. It is also important that the tests which comprise a battery be constructed in such a way that they utilize complementary methods of assessing brain functions. These include: 1. level of performance (how well a patient does compared to a normative group), 2. a comparison of the performances of the right and left sides of the body, 3. a search for signs of neurological deficit such as aphasia, and 4. the use of patterns of test scores rather than isolated findings from the individual tests. It is only by the use of such a method that the power of the procedure can be appreciated adequately, and the weaknesses of each of these methods can be supplanted by the strengths of the others. For example, a group of tests relying primarily upon level of performance measures can be affected by a wide variety of factors including general testing conditions, rapport with the examiner, and motivation, whereas the other methods are much less affected by these factors.

The method of neuropsychological assessment being described here appears to be that of traditional neuropsychology, but the method is defined somewhat more exactly than is often done. In recent times, there has been a tendency to use the term 'neuropsychological' quite loosely. Often, psychological tests are devised without attention to establishing the validity of each as brain-sensitive measures, groups of tests are assembled without attention to interrelationships between them, the use of complementary methods of brain assessment such as those indicated in the last paragraph are neglected, and then the term 'neuropsychological' is applied. Such a general procedure often results in unvalidated groups of tests of uncertain value, the vast majority of which depend upon the 'level of performance' method of analysis. Clearly, a more tightly defined method is the one under discussion here.

The first psychologist to develop fully this more precise method of neuropsychological assessment was Ward Halstead of the University of Chicago in the 1930s. The numerous studies done by himself and others using his tests have provided an excellent understanding of the effects of pathological conditions of the brain upon his tests, especially as the method was developed by Reitan (Reitan & Davidson 1974). Utilizing the strengths of this method, an expanded form of the approach has been advanced explicitly for people with epilepsy (Dodrill 1978). In this approach, not only were the basic criteria applied for test selection, but tests were included only if they had previously demonstrated sensitivity to variables of importance in epilepsy including various epileptiform and nonepileptiform EEC parameters (Dodrill & Wilkus 1978, Wilkus & Dodrill 1976), antiepileptic drugs (Dodrill 1975, Dodrill & Troupin 1977), and seizure history variables (Matthews & Klove 1967, Klove & Matthews 1974). In establishing the final battery of 16 neuropsychological variables, 100 test variables were screened for sensitivity to brain dysfunction found in epilepsy, tested for overlap with one another, and evaluated for ability to cross-validate to new samples. A list of the tests used in this battery is given in Table 12.1.

A number of studies have accumulated which have pointed to the value of this battery of tests in epilepsy, only a few of which will be mentioned here. Its utility has now been shown in a number of contexts in addition to those identified above. These include biographical and seizure history variables (Batzel & Dodrill 1984), performance in life (Batzel et al 1980, Dodrill & Clemmons 1984), psychogenic seizures (Wilkus et al 1984),

Table 12.1 Tests constituting the Neuropsychological Battery for Epilepsy

Category Test	Reitan–Klove Perceptual Exam
Tactual Performance Test	Name Writing Procedure
Seashore Rhythm Test	Seashore Tonal Memory Test
Finger Tapping Test	Stroop Test
Trail Making Test	Aphasia Screening Test
Wechsler Memory Scale (Form I, selected portions)	

surgery for epilepsy (Dodrill et al 1986, Ojemann & Dodrill 1987), effects of seizures (Dodrill 1986), speech lateralization (Woods et al 1988), and psychosocial variables (Dodrill 1983). Thus, it appears to be a reasonably useful tool in dealing with a number of topics of interest in epilepsy.

While the advantages of this method of neuropsychological assessment for epilepsy have now been demonstrated, its disadvantages must also be enumerated. Among the most important of these is the length of time required for evaluation which is approximately 4 hours for the 16 test measures. Also, examiners must be trained extensively but despite this training, some variability in the presentation of test materials is certain to ensue. In addition, while minimized by extensive cross-checking, errors in recording of information are certain to occur. While everyone seems to agree that these are disadvantages of the method, how critical they are is less well established, particularly in view of the demonstrated value of the method. For example, while the stimuli are presented in a somewhat variable manner, the difference may be of little consequence. Likewise, while examiner errors undoubtedly exist in the recording of responses and scoring, their significance in the typical case is unclear.

Two other general types of criticisms have been levelled at this approach, but the points in question are actually seen as assets by proponents of the system. These points include the selection of tests on an empirical basis rather than on a theoretical basis and the fact that the original development of the tests was in part for purposes of localizing brain lesions. Persons preferring other neuropsychological methods see both of these points as restrictive. Proponents of the system, on the other hand, point to the fact that an adequate theoretical model of brain functioning does not exist, that tests identified to measure certain constructs often do not do so as clearly as would be hoped, and that the long history of the use of the tests in neurological populations has resulted in knowledge which is of great advantage in understanding what changes in test scores mean both with respect to the nervous system and in relation to performance in everyday life.

Method 2

The second general method of neuropsychological assessment is one which utilizes computer-assisted tests either primarily or solely. It has achieved great popularity in recent years, especially in Europe and in the United Kingdom. This method appears to have been utilized first in the United States (Dekaban & Lehman 1975), but it was popularized by Trimble and Thompson (Thompson 1981, Thompson & Trimble 1982) and others (Tomlinson et al 1982, Aldenkamp et al 1987). Recently, it has been presented in perhaps its best developed form by Alpherts and associates (Alpherts 1987).

This method is characterized by the use of computers for the presentation of test material and the recording of resulting data. One of the most detailed descriptions of a battery of available tests has been presented by Moerland et al (1986). It is evident that a considerable amount of time has been spent on the technical aspects of the system with the hardware and software which is required. Once operational, however, a variety of tests can be given with this equipment. The tests which are administered seem to fall into two categories, namely, those which represent automated forms of well known neuropsychological tests and those which represent new procedures. Well known procedures adapted to this system include Digit Span, Finger Tapping, Block Tapping, Seashore Rhythm, and the 15 Word Test (variant of Rey Auditory Verbal Learning). The system is especially well adapted to all measures of reaction time and in fact to most procedures where precise timing is required.

An examination of the strengths and weaknesses of this system reveals that they complement very well those of the first basic method of neuropsychological assessment. Advantages include greater precision in the presentation of

stimuli and more accurate recording of responses. In addition, the use of computers may itself be interesting to the patients taking the test and may help to stimulate cooperation and attention. Other advantages include the automatic recording of information in a form amenable to analysis, the more precise pursuit of hypotheses pertaining to the ways in which the brain functions, and the possibility of performing shorter and more economical evaluations. Also, proponents of this system point to the value of utilizing theory from cognitive psychology as a basis for test development.

There are several disadvantages of this second method of neuropsychological assessment which must be mentioned. To date, it has been applied primarily to the evaluation of the effects of anti-epileptic drugs, the results of which will be discussed in a subsequent section. It has not yet been systematically related to a variety of variables including seizure-related information (seizure type, age at onset of seizures, duration of seizures, etc.) EEG abnormalities (both epileptiform and nonepileptiform), ability to perform in everyday life, and to a variety of abnormal brain conditions. The tests are not normed, and interpretation of scores is therefore difficult. There is still little information dealing with technical problems such as practice effects and test–retest reliability. The adaptation of existing tests to computerized administration is difficult in some cases and impossible in others (Alpherts 1987). The equipment is clearly more expensive and more difficult to maintain than that used in standard neuropsychological testing. Software development is also not within the capability of most users, and therefore widespread use of the procedures may have to await general availability of both software and hardware. These constitute the primary disadvantages of this approach at the present time.

Evaluation of the neuropsychological approaches

The two methods of neuropsychological assessment have advantages and disadvantages which are largely complementary. Some combination of the approaches would therefore appear to be most desirable, but there has been almost no effort to combine the two areas effectively. An exception to this has been the work of one group of investigators (Aldenkamp et al 1987, Alpherts 1987). Nevertheless, no one has yet presented even nominal information concerning the degree to which tests arising from the two areas statistically intercorrelate.

Since little information is available on the interrelationships between computerized and standardized neuropsychological tests, the results of a preliminary study by the author are reported here. Forty adults with epilepsy averaging 33.14 years of age (SD = 10.60) and 12.26 years of education (SD = 3.02) were administered a full standard neuropsychological battery (Dodrill 1978) as well as measures of simple visual reaction time (patients pressed a button as quickly as a light appeared on a screen), choice reaction time (patients determined if people were or were not obviously present in pictures), and decision making which requires basic colour and animate vs inanimate discriminations (adapted from Thompson 1981). In Table 12.2, correlations are presented between these three computerized procedures and five groups of standard neuropsychological tests. As expected, simple reaction time was not related to the vast majority of standard neuropsychological tests. However, choice reaction time was related to several of the cognitive areas and especially to tasks emphasizing motor performance. The decision making task showed significant relationships with all cognitive areas and not just with problem solving, where one might expect to find the strongest relationships.

Several implications arise from the material presented in Table 12.2. First, tasks thought to measure various constructs (such as 'decision

Table 12.2 Correlations of three computerized tests with standard neuropsychological tests

Standard neuropsychological test	Computerized test		
	Simple reaction time	Choice reaction time	Decision making, total latency
Problem solving			
Category Test	0.14	0.37*	0.61**
Tactual Performance, Time	0.14	0.35	0.47*
Trail Making, Part B	0.15	0.64**	0.56**
Intelligence			
WAIS-R Verbal IQ	−0.16	−0.33	−0.43*
WAIS-R Performance IQ	−0.10	−0.47*	−0.56**
WAIS-R Full Scale IQ	−0.15	−0.41*	−0.52**
Memory			
WMS, Logical Memory	−0.14	0.20	−0.23
WMS, Visual Reproduction	−0.13	−0.33	−0.48**
WAIS-R Digit Span	−0.40*	−0.40*	−0.62**
Attention			
Stroop, high interference	0.33	0.61**	0.72**
Seashore Rhythm	−0.27	−0.55**	−0.49**
Seashore Tonal Memory	−0.16	−0.34	−0.37*
Motor			
Name writing, total	0.10	−0.61**	−0.53**
Finger Tapping, total	−0.12	−0.64**	−0.57**
Marching, Total Time	0.31	0.66**	0.74**
Dynamometer, total	−0.08	−0.48**	−0.40*
Computer tests			
Simple Reaction Time	—	0.24	0.40*
Choice Reaction Time	0.24	—	0.68**
Decision Making	0.40*	0.68**	—

* $P < 0.01$
** $P < 0.001$

Note: WMS Logical Memory is Wechsler Memory Scale (Form I), Logical Memory, immediate recall; WMS Visual Reproduction is Wechsler Memory Scale (Form I), Visual Reproduction, immediate recall. WAIS-R = Wechsler Adult Intelligence Scale—Revised.

making') may not always measure these as simply as might be hoped. Second, taken together, the two tasks which measured anything more complex than simple reaction time were more related to motor functions (and especially to motor speed) than to any area which requires thinking or cognition. Thus, it is clear that these tasks have a very strong motor speed component. Finally, from the bottom portion of Table 12.2, it is also clear that the more complex tasks are highly related to each other and much more so than standard neuropsychological tests (Dodrill 1978). Thus, there is danger that a battery of computerized tests may be substantially overlapping with each other, significantly influenced by motor speed, and othervise diffusely related to a variety of cognitive areas.

As one evaluates the basic neuropsychological approaches, one must bear in mind that the computerized testing method has only been available in the last decade. Thus, the strengths and weaknesses of this general approach have yet to be fully explored. However, the present author has now used this approach for several years and has been pleased with its precision and accuracy. It is hoped that with time some of the limitations can be overcome at least in part. The best approach is to explore it further without abandoning the established value of the other primary approach. Ultimately we should look towards a method which utilizes the strengths of both methods while side-stepping the weaknesses in so far as this is possible.

NEUROPSYCHOLOGICAL CORRELATES OF SEIZURE HISTORY VARIABLES

There has long been an interest in investigating the relationship between aspects of the seizure history and abilities, especially intelligence. The literature relevant to this will be briefly summarized here. As will be seen, in most cases the relationship of these variables with mental abilities is fairly limited. Because of this, the findings are difficult to apply in individual cases.

Aetiology

One of the better established findings in the area

is the relationship between intelligence and whether or not the aetiology of the seizure disorder is known. Most studies have shown that when aetiology is known, intelligence and neuropsychological abilities are mildly diminished in comparison to cases where it is unknown. A series of studies in the area summarized years ago showed that the difference was approximately 5–10 IQ points (Tarter 1972). The likely reason for this difference is that when a specific cause is known, detectable damage to the brain is more probable. Decreased mental abilities may reflect both this underlying impairment and the epilepsy itself.

Klove & Matthews (1966) performed one of the most detailed studies in this area. Using the Halstead-Reitan Neuropsychological Battery, they matched their subject groups for age and education and appeared successful in achieving good control for non-relevant variables across their groups. Results show that the groups with known aetiology did indeed perform just a little more poorly, but that only on a portion of the variables did the differences achieve statistical significance. Their results support the general contention advanced that while there is a relationship with aetiology, it is limited in both scope and magnitude.

Age at onset of epilepsy

There is a definite trend in the literature to suggest that the earlier in life epilepsy appears, the lower the mental abilities. Again, the studies supporting this date back many years. In one of the largest patient series reported, Lennox & Lennox (1960) presented data indicating that the differences were most prominent when persons were considered who had generalized tonic-clonic rather than partial seizures. The trend to find poorer abilities with earlier age at onset has been found using both ratings of mental abilities and standardized tests of intelligence.

Because the major studies in the area are significantly dated now, the present author compiled data from his own file to update the information which is available. A total of 510 adults aged 21 and over (263 males, 247 females) with confirmed epilepsy were found who averaged 31.73 years of age (SD = 9.43) and 12.05 years of education (SD

= 2.73). The group was heterogeneous with respect to principal presenting seizure type (57 simple partial, 274 complex partial, 33 absence, 15 atonic/myoclonic/tonic/clonic, 86 tonic-clonic, 45 others/unclassified) and also with respect to other variables such as age at onset, aetiology, etc. The group represented the majority of people who had been given a neuropsychological evaluation at a specialized epilepsy centre over a 12-year period. Age at onset ranges were as follows: 0–1 (n = 37); 2–5 (n = 72); 6–10 (n = 77); 11–15 (n = 107); 16–20 (n = 88); 21–63 (n = 129). Application of one-way analysis of variance across these age at onset groups for the WAIS Full Scale IQ resulted in highly statistically significant differences (F = 14.62, P< 0.0001) with higher intellectual levels associated with progressively later age at onset. The results are shown in Figure 12.1. The youngest age at onset group averaged a WAIS FSIQ score of 83 while the oldest group averaged 102. This is one of the greatest differences reported in the literature for this variable. The Pearson correlation between age at onset and intelligence was 0.31 (P<0.001).

Interpretation of the data just presented and the literature on the topic must recognize that there is an interplay of potentially contaminating factors with the variable of interest. For example, earlier age at onset is associated with a larger number of seizures at any particular point in later life, and there is now some evidence (Dodrill 1986) that the total lifetime number of tonic clonic seizures may be as important as age at onset or possibly more so. Also, earlier age at onset routinely means that medications have been taken for more years and also that other psychosocial and emotional factors have been operative for longer periods. Thus, although data such as that presented in Figure 12.1 are helpful, they need to be interpreted with due caution.

Duration of disorder

Not unexpectedly, longer duration of disorder has often been associated with diminished mental skills. This variable is weaker than many others no doubt partly due to the degree of seizure control which fluctuates substantially from one person to the next. For example, in the 510 persons described in the last section, the Pearson correlation between duration and intelligence was only –0.18 (P<0.001).

In an effort to strengthen the duration of seizure disorder variable, Farwell and associates (Farwell et al 1985) modified it to include only those years in which seizures had been experienced. They found that this modified variable was more potently related to mental abilities than the traditional duration measure of number of years since first attack. In effect, these investigators combined duration and seizure frequency factors and thereby obtained a stronger measure. That this works when applied to the entirely new sample described in the last section is demonstrated by a correlation of –0.28 (P<0.001) between number of years in which seizures were experienced and WAIS Full Scale IQ.

Seizure frequency, temporal pattern of seizures, and seizure type

These variables are considered together because of their interrelationships with each other. While it is reasonable to postulate that the more frequent the seizure the lower the mental abilities, there are at least two reasons why this has not been well demonstrated in most investigations. In the first place, nearly all investigations have considered only recent seizure history such as the last several months. This is probably not long enough to appreciate losses in abilities which may accumulate over time. Secondly, it is almost certainly true that different seizure types have substantially different impacts upon abilities. Convulsive seizures of most types are likely to have many more effects

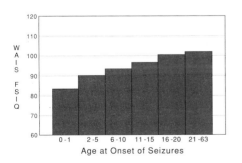

Fig. 12.1 Average Wechsler Adult Full Scale IQ score for 510 patients grouped by age at onset of seizures.

upon cognitive abilities than absence attacks or focal seizures which do not secondarily generalize (Matthews & Klove 1967, Farwell et al 1985). Furthermore, the mere presence of more than one type of seizure is likely to be associated with decreased functioning (Rodin et al 1976) with no necessary reference to seizure frequency at all.

The greatest correlations of seizure frequency with abilities have been reported when generalized convulsive seizures have been studied over the lifetime of patients with attention paid not only to total number of attacks but also to the temporal sequencing of the episodes. In one study (Dodrill 1986) it was shown that diminished mental abilities accompanied typically either a history of status epilepticus (30 or more minutes of repetitive or continuous attacks without the regaining of consciousness) or when more than 100 convulsions had occurred in a person's lifetime. Interestingly, persons with typically only one episode of status performed a little more poorly on tests of abilities than persons with greater than 100 lifetime attacks, but emotional and psychosocial adjustment was decidedly worse with more than 100 attacks than with status epilepticus. Thus, it is not merely the number of seizures but also the type of attack and the temporal sequencing which is important.

ANTIEPILEPTIC DRUGS AND PERFORMANCE

In recent years, there has been an awareness that the medications used to control epileptic attacks may have adverse effects upon mental abilities. The result is that probably more research has recently been done in this area than in any other aspect of the neuropsychology of epilepsy. Significant reviews of the area now appear in many places including some recent publications (Dodrill 1990, Trimble 1987a, Vining 1987). The general findings for the various antiepileptic drugs are summarized below. However, it should be noted that there are a number of methodological problems which exist in the area which have generally resulted in attributing to medications adverse effects which are probably due to other factors. Thus, the general conclusions often reached may ultimately require modification, and a section on these methodological problems is included.

Phenytoin

The most consistent report of adverse changes associated with this drug is with respect to speed of response. This is seen most clearly with very high serum levels. A number of other effects have been reported in the literature including decreased memory, psychomotor performance, and attention. However, more recent literature suggests that such findings were on tasks which typically had speed of response (and especially motor speed) as a common factor (Duncan et al 1990). When speed of response is factored out, the drug effect shown on these tests also tends to disappear (Dodrill & Temkin 1989). This is an important recent finding which awaits additional confirmatory research at the present time. Should such research become forthcoming, this could alter significantly current views of the cognitive effects of this very commonly used medication.

Carbamazepine

In general, few adverse cognitive effects have been associated with this drug, and at one point it was thought that it might even have some positive effects upon abilities. Such a positive effect is now generally disbelieved in the area of abilities, although it should be pointed out that it does have favourable effects upon affective disorders (Trimble 1987b). In terms of adverse effects upon abilities, it is thought that they are fairly minimal despite recent suggestions of adverse effects upon motor speed and occasionally upon cognitive tasks as well (Duncan et al 1990, MacPhee et al 1986).

Barbiturates

The medications which most commonly fall within this group include phenobarbitone and primidone. The adverse cognitive effects of these drugs are more clearly established than for any other. They often include decreased performance in visual–motor functions, ability to attend to the task, memory, problem solving, and motor speed. Recent studies continue to show these negative impacts in both children (Farwell et al 1990) and adults (Meador et al 1990). Studies comparing the effects of primidone with those of phenobarbitone are lacking, but since primidone breaks down into primidone and phenobarbitone, it is unlikely to have fewer effects.

Sodium valproate

This medication has been on the market for a relatively limited period and to date, relatively few adverse cognitive or behavioural effects have been found in connection with its use. It may be found ultimately to have a slight adverse impact upon motor speed (Duncan et al 1990) and various cognitive tasks (Brodie et al 1987), but it is not clear that substantial adverse effects will be found.

Ethosuximide

Relatively few studies have been done with respect to the neuropsychological effects of this drug, even though it has been used for many years. Occasional favourable (Browne et al 1975) and unfavourable (Guey et al 1967) papers have appeared, but there is no compelling evidence for substantial adverse neuropsychological effects of this drug.

Other medications

All other antiepileptic medications have been investigated with only occasional neuropsychological studies, and it is therefore not possible to develop profiles of adverse effects for them.

Methodological problems

In any rapidly developing area, methodological problems are commonly found, and the assessment of the neuropsychological effects of antiepileptic drugs is no exception. In general, these problems have tended to result in attributing cognitive difficulties to the drugs which are more appropriately related to other factors. While at least six of these factors exist (Dodrill 1988), only the three most important of these will be briefly discussed below.

Selection factors

The neuropsychological effects of antiepileptic drugs are often studied with subject groups whose drug regimens have been established or altered solely for clinical reasons. In the typical case, patients are matched on the variables of age, sex, education, seizure type, aetiology, and age at onset of seizures, and it is concluded that any differences in neuropsychological performances across the groups must be due to differences in drug regimens. This thinking is flawed, however, since drugs are not prescribed in a random manner by physicians. When two drugs are equally efficacious in stopping a certain type of seizure but one is prescribed by a particular physician for one patient and the other for another patient, there are probably intrinsic differences between the patients which are unrelated to such variables as age, sex, and seizure type. A few of such factors are ability to deal with complex drug regimens, general intelligence, financial status of the patient, various emotional factors, and distance from the clinic (with curtailed ability to do serial laboratory tests). The result may be that despite superficial resemblance of the groups, important intrinsic differences exist between them which account for the findings on tests of abilities.

The importance of this error can be illustrated with data from the author's own laboratory. Intending to study the neuropsychological effects of sodium valproate, 28 adults on that medication were administered the Neuropsychological Battery for Epilepsy (Dodrill 1978) and they were matched with the next 28 cases in the file who were not on valproate but who had been tested in the same manner. The groups were not statistically different on a host of variables including age, years of education, sex, age at onset of seizures, aetiology of seizures, seizure type, seizure frequency, and total years in which antiepileptic medications had been taken. However, the valproate group had decidedly lower abilities on a variety of tests of abilities. For example, the average WAIS Full Scale IQ for the valproate group was 87.29 and the score for the group not on valproate was 99.00 (t = −2.47; P<0.02). It is improper to conclude that sodium valproate decreases intelligence, however, since all of these people were tested 5 years previously when valproate was not yet available. At that time, the group which was ultimately placed on valproate had an average Full Scale IQ score of 85.36 while the controls averaged 96.69 (t = −2.67; P<0.02). It is clear that our physicians had given valproate to duller (and more difficult to manage) patients who were not controlled on other drugs.

From the above, it is clear that selection factors are of enormous importance. When it is not possible to have random assignment of drug conditions in clinical investigations, selection factors should be suspected and guarded against.

Statistical factors

Statistical problems are often found in these studies. An all too common problem pertains to over-interpretation of a few statistically significant findings when a large number of statistical tests have been run. It is typical that only a few differences between drug groups are noted in these papers, but they are discussed at great length in the report while a host of tests not producing statistically significant findings are scarcely mentioned. Frequently also, variables which are associated with statistical findings are highly overlapping (i.e. tapping with preferred hand, tapping with nonpreferred hand, tapping with both hands). While this statistical problem of few independent findings is elementary in nature, it appears repeatedly in these studies.

Another frequent statistical error is the inappropriate choice of statistical tests in situations where the homogeneity of variance assumption is violated. Suppose, for example, that seizure frequencies under two drug regimens are being compared to be sure that seizure frequency is not responsible for some of the differences noted between the drugs on the neuropsychological tests. If one drug is clearly better than the other in stopping the attacks as shown by obvious differences in the average seizure frequencies, but if there is even a single patient with a seizure frequency far higher than all others, the Student t statistic or analysis of variance may fail erroneously to report such a difference. This is due to a substantially increased standard deviation and the consequent inability of the statistic to be confident of the difference between means. The result will be that the investigator will conclude there is no difference in seizure frequency and that therefore the differences on the neuropsychological tests are due to differences in the drugs. Use of non-parametric statistics obviates this important but subtle problem and would raise the possibility that seizure rather than drug effects are responsible for the differences on the neuropsychological tests.

Type of psychological test given

The likelihood of finding a drug effect is directly related to the type of test given. In particular, the more highly timed the test the greater the probability of a statistically significant finding. In one major review of the literature (Dodrill 1988), for example, across 40 studies of the neuropsychological effects of drugs with patients with epilepsy it was found that there was an 85% chance of finding a drug effect with tests such as reaction time measures which are recorded in milliseconds of latency, a 79% chance if tests were timed in whole seconds, a 59% chance for tests of intelligence which are usually partially timed, and a 43% chance of finding a drug effect with untimed tests.

In view of the above, to find small drug effects one should use the more highly timed measures. Computerized testing may make a helpful contribution at this point. However, attention is drawn to two points. Firstly, as was documented in a previous section, many computerized tests have a strong element of speed and are significantly overlapping with one another. Thus, it is important not to accept uncritically the contention that these tests measure various psychological constructs such as *memory* or *attention* without empirical support for these assertions. In fact, all may be measuring one aspect or another of speed. Secondly, attention is drawn to the fact that the practical importance has yet to be established of differences between drugs which are reported in milliseconds. Statistical significance does not imply practical significance.

SURGERY FOR EPILEPSY

The vast majority of the surgery done for people

with epilepsy in the world today is cortical resection surgery. Because only a few neuropsychological studies have been reported with respect to other types of surgery, only those changes after cortical resection surgery will be reviewed here. Neuropsychological evaluation prior to surgery serves to identify areas of brain-related deficit for correlation with EEG and other data in evaluation of the patient with respect to suitability for surgery. It also serves as a baseline for the evaluation of the effects of surgery after it is completed. Postsurgical evaluation makes possible the evaluation of changes after surgery for clinical and research purposes.

Presurgical identification of brain-related deficits

Since a comprehensive battery of neuropsychological tests is designed systematically to evaluate brain functions, it is reasonable to presume that it might constitute a way of assessing brain-related problems in epilepsy which would complement the EEG and various neuroradiological procedures. Investigators at the Montreal Neurological Institute were the first to confirm that this in fact is possible (Bengzon et al 1968). In their research, it was demonstrated that surgery was more likely to be successful in stopping seizures when the neuropsychological tests lateralized dysfunction to the cerebral hemisphere where surgery was ultimately performed than when such tests failed to do so. This was very encouraging, not only because a significant portion of persons taken to surgery do not experience seizure relief, but also because predictors of outcome have limited power and are considerably unstable (Dodrill et al 1990).

Encouraged by the results at Montreal, several other investigators have attempted to use psychological and neuropsychological variables to predict the outcome of cortical resection surgery and two summaries of the literature have appeared (Dodrill et al 1986, Rausch 1987). Both of these have provided data pointing to the value of this assessment in terms of determining suitability for surgery.

One of the more comprehensive papers on prediction of surgical outcome using psychological and neuropsychological measures involved 100

patients with refractory complex seizures (Dodrill et al 1986). Other types of predictive variables were simultaneously evaluated including EEG, neuroradiological, and neurological seizure-related variables. A total of 71 predictors were used, 14 of which were intellectual, 20 were neuropsychological, and 14 pertained to emotional factors. The subjects were 100 adults with refractory seizure disorders who had undergone cortical resection surgery for epilepsy in a variety of cortical areas at least 2 years previously. Evaluation of seizure relief was based upon seizure frequency in the second postoperative year with classification as: 1. seizure free (no attacks at all), 2. significantly improved (at least a 75% reduction in seizure frequency), and 3. not significantly improved (less than a 75% improvement). The first two groups were considered to have been helped by the surgery and the last group not to have been helped. Subjects were randomly assigned to predictive (n = 75) and cross-validation (n = 25) groups.

While this study failed to identify any seizure history or radiological variable as a consistent predictor of surgical success, four psychological and neuropsychological variables were found. These, with their ranges of favourable prediction in terms of being helped by the surgery, are as follows:

1. WAIS Digit Symbol (scaled score of nine or greater or a raw score of 47 or greater on the WAIS-R)
2. Marching Test (time of 20 s or quicker with the preferred hand)
3. MMPI Hysteria scale (T score of 75 or less)
4. MMPI Paranoid scale (T score of 80 or less).

Four reliable EEG predictors were also found:

1. Single focus
2. Discharges from the anterior mid-temporal area
3. Discharges only from side of surgery
4. Discharges from surgical area no more frequent than one per minute on average.

A general result from this study was that no one of either the EEG or the neuropsychological variables was successful in predicting consistently in more than about two out of three cases whether

Table 12.3 Surgical outcomes with patients grouped by number of favourable preoperative prognostic indicators (n = 100)

Number of favourable prognostic indicators	Outcome		
	Seizure-free	Significantly improved	Not significantly improved
0–3	0%	0%	100%
4	9%	9%	82%
5	37%	20%	43%
6	27%	53%	20%
7	64%	32%	4%
8	75%	25%	0%

or not a patient would be helped. However, when the predictive variables were added together by finding the number which fell within a favourable prognostic range, it was possible to predict whether or not a person would be helped in four out of five cases. Both EEG and neuropsychological variables were required to bring the prediction up to this improved (though imperfect) level. It was also found to be possible to provide a prognostic statement of outcome for individual patients based upon the number of favourable indicators. Table 12.3 summarizes this information; it can be used to give patients a predictive statement more directed to their individual case and it appears to be better than giving all patients the same general prognostic figures.

Overall, it appears that neuropsychological tests have a role in the prediction of seizure relief from cortical resection surgery which is not duplicated by variables arising from other specialties.

Establishment of baseline presurgical functioning

Because there are risks involved in the surgical procedure and because not all patients profit from it, the decision to undertake surgery is one which should be made with great care. While there is little risk of mortality, there is a low risk of losses in mental abilities (especially memory and language-related), particularly when surgery is on the speech-related side. The importance for the individual patient of estimating these losses in advance has been stressed (Ivnik et al 1988). Presurgical neuropsychological assessment not only helps to predict surgical outcome as was

shown in the previous section, but it may also help to presage losses which may occur. For example, it has been shown that persons with very good memories are at greater risk for memory loss after surgery than persons who have only limited memory skills prior to surgery (Ojemann & Dodrill 1987). In addition, pre-operative neuropsychological assessment provides a baseline which is useful in many contexts. An example of how a comprehensive neuropsychological battery can help in the full evaluation of a surgical candidate is given below.

Case History
K.B. was an 18-year-old girl who had just completed high school when she was hospitalized for her presurgical workup. She had experienced generalized tonic-clonic seizures beginning at the age of 18 months during an episode of high fever. Although she had been taking antiepileptic medication constantly since her first attack, she soon began to experience other types of seizures. Complex partial seizures began at 6 years and by 18 years were the only type of attack reported. They occurred on average 10 times per month and were poorly controlled by a wide variety of drug regimens. EEG studies including closed circuit television/long-term monitoring recorded eight seizures, all of which arose from the left sphenoidal area. The interictal tracings also demonstrated occasional diffuse atypical spike-wave patterns as well as moderate to marked generalized abnormalities. Her cerebral angiogram was normal, but a CT scan revealed herniation of the left mesial temporal structures. The intracarotid sodium amytal procedure (Wada test) showed speech to be associated with the left hemisphere only in this strongly right-handed person. The study also demonstrated a substantial loss in short-term memory when the left hemisphere was perfused and thereby suggested that the left hemisphere did perform important memory functions. The neuropsychological testing showed her to be of

above average intelligence both in the verbal and visual–spatial areas. This encouraged us since it was clear that she had good potential for rehabilitation. Likewise, although 16 neuropsychological test measures were given, only three were performed outside normal limits. This meant that her performances across a broad range of perceptual, motor, and cognitive tasks were normal. It was noted, however, that memory for verbal materials as evaluated by the Wechsler Memory Scale was definitely below her visual–spatial memory which was normal. Also, her right hand was relatively deficient on the Finger Tapping Test. This agrees with and explicitly confirms the EEG focus.

A review of the eight predictors of surgical outcome revealed that because of occasional generalized EEG discharges and because discharges in the surgical area were very frequent, only one of the four EEG indicators was positive. All four neuropsychological indicators were positive, however, so that the overall outlook was moderately positive (37% chance of being seizure free, 20% chance of at least a 75% reduction in seizure frequency although not seizure free, and a 43% chance of not being significantly improved). She was taken to surgery where a markedly gliotic left temporal lobe was noted along with 4–5 mm of uncal herniation over the incisura. A left temporal lobectomy was performed which was guided by corticography and language testing. At the conclusion of surgery, the resection was noted to extend 7 cm posteriorly at the level of the inferior temporal gyrus and about 3.5 cm posteriorly at the level of the superior temporal gyrus. The resection included the uncus, the amygdala and the anterior hippocampus.

Postsurgical neuropsychological evaluation

Patients such as K.B. are clearly at risk for additional losses in short-term verbal memory, especially because the intracarotid amytal test indicated that important memory functions were associated with the left hemisphere. Because of this risk, special procedures (Ojemann & Dodrill 1987) were used to map cognitive functions at the time of surgery. A postsurgical evaluation was required to determine if losses had occurred.

Case History
Thirteen months after surgery, K.B. received a repeat neuropsychological assessment, and the findings are compared with those obtained preoperatively. Intelligence was essentially at the same level as seen preoperatively, and the neuropsychological tests overall were performed also at the same level (two of 16 tests were outside normal limits). However, in the area of verbal memory there was a definite improvement with 21 correct recollections instead of 14 for immediate

recall and 18 instead of 12 with 30 minute delayed recall conditions. There were also several other slight improvements on the neuropsychological tests of lesser consequence. The MMPI demonstrated no adverse change in emotional adjustment. At the point of this evaluation, it was discovered that she had not had a seizure since surgery. Additional follow-up 2 years after surgery revealed that she was seizure free, off medication, and was making an excellent psychosocial adjustment.

The improvement in verbal memory which this patient noted was an unexpected result from her surgery. It illustrates the fact that using local anaesthesia and cortical mapping, an extensive re-section on the hemisphere associated with speech can be done with excellent clinical results and without losses in mental abilities. While the results are not always as positive as this, they are frequently encouraging and by no means do we shy away from performing surgery on the side associated with speech.

There have now been several reports of improvement in memory following surgery for epilepsy, especially if the surgery is successful in stopping the attacks, and if it is on the side associated with speech (Novelly et al 1984, Rausch & Crandall 1982). The present case is in accord with these findings, but it is important to stress that the tailor-made procedure guided by mapping at the time of surgery was a vital part of the procedure. Had a smaller standardized resection been undertaken under general anaesthesia, control of seizures may have been incomplete with the possibility of a less favourable finding in the cognitive area.

CONCLUSIONS

The objective of this chapter has been to cover several current areas of interest in the neuropsychology of epilepsy. It has been stressed that a neuropsychological evaluation of patients with epilepsy is of great importance. This remains true even though there are differences in the approaches to this type of assessment and even though there are important questions which are yet to be answered. Research currently in progress in many places around the world should help to bring answers to the most important of these questions in the years to come.

ACKNOWLEDGMENTS

The preparation of this chapter and a portion of the research reported therein was supported by grants NS 24823 and NS 17111 awarded by the National Institute of Neurological Disorders and Stroke, PHS/DHHS, USA.

REFERENCES

Aldenkamp A P, Alpherts W C J, Moerland M C, Ottevanger N, Van Parys J A P 1987 Controlled release carbamazepine: cognitive side effects in patients with epilepsy. Epilepsia 28: 507–514

Alpherts W C J 1987 Computers as a technique for neuropsychological assessment in epilepsy. In: Aldenkamp A P, Alpherts W C J, Meinardi H, Stores G (eds) Education and epilepsy: proceedings of an international workshop on education and epilepsy. Swets & Zeitlinger, Amsterdam, p 101–109

Batzel L W, Dodrill C B, Fraser R T 1980 Further validation of the WPSI Vocational Scale: comparisons with other correlates of employment in epilepsy. Epilepsia 2l: 235–242

Batzel L W, Dodrill C B 1984 Neuropsychological and emotional correlates of marital status and ability to live independently with epilepsy. Epilepsia 25: 594–598

Bengzon A R A, Rasmussen T, Gloor P, Dussault J, Stephens M 1968 Prognostic factors in the surgical treatment of temporal lobe epileptics. Neurology 18: 717–731

Brodie M J, McPhail E, Macphee G J A, Larkin J G, Gray J M B 1987 Psychomotor impairment and anticonvulsant therapy in adult epileptic patients. European Journal of Pharmacology 31: 655–660

Browne T R, Dreifuss F E, Dyken P R, et al 1975 Ethosuximide in the treatment of absence (petit mal) seizures. Neurology 25: 515–524

Dekaban A S, Lehman E J B 1975 Effects of different dosages of anticonvulsant drugs on mental performance in patients with chronic epilepsy. Acta Neurologica Scandinavica 52: 319–330

Dodrill C B 1975 Diphenylhydantoin serum levels, toxicity, and neuropsychological performance in patients with epilepsy. Epilepsia l6: 593–600

Dodrill C B 1978 A neuropsychological battery for epilepsy. Epilepsia 19: 611–623

Dodrill C B 1983 Development of intelligence and neuropsychological impairment scales for the Washington Psychosocial Seizure Inventory. Epilepsia 24: l–10

Dodrill C B 1986 Correlates of generalized tonic-clonic seizures with intellectual, neuropsychological, emotional and social function in patients with epilepsy. Epilepsia 27: 399–411

Dodrill C B 1988 Cognitive effects of antiepileptic drugs. Journal of Clinical Psychiatry 49 (suppl): 31–34

Dodrill C B 1990 Neuropsychology. In: Dam M, Gram L (eds) Comprehensive epileptology. Raven Press, New York, p 473–484

Dodrill C B, Clemmons D 1984 Use of neuropsychological tests to identify high school students with epilepsy who later demonstrate inadequate performances in life. Journal of Consulting and Clinical Psychology 52: 520–527

Dodrill C B, Temkin N R 1989 Motor speed is a contaminating variable in the measurement of the 'cognitive' effects of phenytoin. Epilepsia 30: 453–457

Dodrill C B, Troupin A S 1977 Psychotropic effects of carbamazepine in epilepsy: comparison with phenytoin. Neurology 27: 1023–1028

Dodrill C B, Wilkus R J 1978 Neuropsychological correlates of the electroencephalogram in epileptics: III. Generalized nonepileptiform abnormalities. Epilepsia 19: 453–462

Dodrill C B, Wilkus R J, Ojemann G A et al 1986 Multidisciplinary prediction of seizure relief from cortical resection surgery. Annals of Neurology 20: 2–12

Dodrill C B, van Belle G, Wilkus R J 1990 Stability of predictors of outcome of surgical treatment for epilepsy. Journal of Epilepsy 3: 29–35

Duncan J S, Shorvon S D, Trimble M R 1990 Effects of removal of phenytoin, carbamazepine, and valproate on cognitive function. Epilepsia 31: 584–591

Farwell J R, Dodrill C B, Batzel L W 1985 Neuropsychological abilities of children with epilepsy. Epilepsia 26: 395–400

Farwell J R, Lee Y J, Hirtz D G, Sulzbacher S I, Ellenberg J H, Nelson K B 1990 Phenobarbital for febrile seizures—effects on intelligence and on seizure recurrence. New England Journal of Medicine 322: 364–369

Fraser R T, Clemmons D C, Dodrill C B, Trejo W R, Freelove C 1986 The difficult-to-employ in epilepsy rehabilitation: predictions of response to an intensive intervention. Epilepsia 27: 220–224

Guey J, Charles C, Coquery C, Roger J, Soulayrol R 1967 Study of psychological effects of ethosuximide (Zarontin) on 25 children suffering from petit mal epilepsy. Epilepsia 8: 129–141

Ivnik R J, Sharbrough F K, Laws E R 1988 Anterior temporal lobectomy for the control of partial complex seizures: information for counselling patients. Mayo Clinic Proceedings 63: 783–793

Klove H, Matthews C G 1966 Psychometric and adaptive abilities in epilepsy with differential etiology. Epilepsia 7: 330–338

Klove H, Matthews C G 1974 Neuropsychological studies of patients with epilepsy. In: Reitan R M, Davidson L A, (eds) Clinical neuropsychology: current status and applications. V H Winston & Sons, Washington DC, p 237–265

Lennox W G, Lennox M A 1960 Epilepsy and related disorders, 2 vols. Little, Brown, Boston

MacPhee G J A, Goldie C, Roulston D et al 1986 Effect of carbamazepine on psychomotor performance in naive subjects. European Journal of Clinical Pharmacology 30: 37–42

Matthews C G, Klove H 1967 Differential psychological performances in major motor, psychomotor, and mixed seizure classifications of known and unknown etiology. Epilepsia 8: 117–128

Meador K J, Loring D W, Huh K, Gallagher B B, King D W 1990 Comparative cognitive effects of anticonvulsants. Neurology 40: 391–394

Moerland M C, Aldenkamp A P, Alpherts W C J 1986 A neuropsychological test battery for the Apple II-E. International Journal of Man-Machine Studies 25: 453–467

Novelly R A, Augustine E A, Mattson R H et al 1984 SE

Selective memory improvement and impairment in temporal lobectomy for epilepsy. Annals of Neurology 15: 64–67

Ojemann G A, Dodrill C B 1987 Intraoperative techniques for reducing language and memory deficits with left temporal lobectomy. In: Wolf P, Dam M, Janz D, Dreifuss F E (eds) Advances in epileptology: the XVIth Epilepsy International Symposium. Raven Press, New York, p 327–330

Rausch R 1987 Psychological evaluation. In: Engel J (ed) Surgical treatment of the epilepsies. Raven Press, New York, p 181–195

Rausch R, Crandall P H 1982 Psychological status related to surgical control of temporal lobe seizures. Epilepsia 23: 191–202

Reitan R M, Davidson L A (eds) 1974 Clinical neuropsychology: current status and applications. V H Winston & Sons, Washington DC

Reitan R M, Wolfson D 1985 The Halstead-Reitan Neuropsychological Test Battery: theory and clinical interpretation. Neuropsychology Press, Tucson

Rodin E A, Katz M, Lennox K 1976 Differences between patients with temporal lobe seizures and those with other forms of epileptic attacks. Epilepsia 17: 313–320

Tarter R E 1972 Intellectual and adaptive functioning in epilepsy: a review of fifty years of research. Diseases of the Nervous System 33: 763–770

Thompson P 1981 The effects of anticonvulsant drugs on the cognitive functioning of normal volunteers and patients with epilepsy. Doctoral thesis, University of London

Thompson P J, Trimble M R 1982 Anticonvulsant drugs and cognitive functions. Epilepsia 23: 531–544

Tomlinson L, Andrewes D, Merrifield E, Reynolds E H 1982 The effects of antiepileptic drugs on cognitive and motor functions. British Journal of Clinical Practice 18 (Symposium Suppl): 177–183

Trimble M R 1987a Anticonvulsant drugs and cognitive function: a review of the literature. Epilepsia 28 (suppl 2): S37–S45

Trimble M R 1987b Antiepileptic and psychotropic properties of carbamazepine. International Clinical Psychopharmacology 2 (suppl 1): 1–9

Vining E P G 1987 Cognitive dysfunction associated with antiepileptic drug therapy. Epilepsia 28 (suppl 2): S18–S22

Wilkus R J, Dodrill C B 1976 Neuropsychological correlates of the electroencephalogram in epileptics: I. Topographic distribution and average rate of epileptiform activity. Epilepsia 17: 89–100

Wilkus R J, Dodrill C B, Thompson P M 1984 Intensive EEG monitoring and psychological studies of patients with pseudoepileptic seizures. Epilepsia 25: 100–107

Woods R P, Dodrill C B, Ojemann G A 1988 Brain injury, handedness and speech lateralization in a series of amytal studies. Annals of Neurology 23: 510–518

13. Neuropharmacology

J. Davies   A. Richens

INTRODUCTION

The traditional approach to the development of new antiepileptic drugs has involved the screening of all newly synthesized compounds to identify anti-seizure activity by testing them in rodent models of epilepsy. It was by this approach that phenytoin was discovered in 1938. The most widely used initial screening test involves the use of two complementary test models which together will identify the anticonvulsant activity of all the major antiepileptic drugs in clinical use (Krall et al 1978). The maximal electroshock test in mice involves the detection of a modification of the seizure pattern by the test drug and correlates fairly well with the potency of the drug against partial and generalized tonic-clonic seizures in patients. The second test uses a chemical convulsant, pentylenetetrazole, in mice; activity in this test predicts drugs likely to be effective in the suppression of absence seizures. Recently, various genetic models of epilepsy have been described where seizures occur either spontaneously or in response to specific sensory stimulation (e.g. auditory seizures in certain mice) and these models may be more analogous to human epilepsy than the experimental seizures caused by unnatural chemicals and electrical methods (Loscher & Meldrum 1984). Primate models of epilepsy have been developed such as the alumina gel model of focal epilepsy in monkeys (Lockard 1980) and the spontaneously photosensitive Senegalese baboon, *Papio papio* (Naquet & Meldrum 1972). Although the results of drug testing in such primate models are more likely to be predictive of probable efficacy in human epilepsy, they are impractical for initial screening of large numbers of chemicals.

A second approach to the development of new antiepileptic drugs is to modify the chemical structures of existing drugs in order to increase the potency but with fewer undesirable features. After the anticonvulsant potency of phenobarbitone was recognized in 1912, many other barbiturates were synthesized but none had antiepileptic activity superior to phenobarbitone. Similarly, none of the many analogues of phenytoin proved clinically superior to the original drug. More recently, following the discovery of the anticonvulsant activity of the 1,4-benzodiazepines, the possible advantages of the 1,5-benzodiazepines are being explored in an attempt to reduce sedative and psychomotor adverse effects. Oxcarbazepine, an analogue of carbamazepine, also has been developed with the aim of finding a compound with a lower incidence of adverse effects.

NEUROTRANSMITTERS

Neurotransmitters in the central nervous system (CNS) may be divided into two major groups depending on the speed of the transduction process at the postsynaptic membrane. These two groups have been designated: 1. fast, i.e. postsynaptic responses in the millisecond range, and 2. slow, postsynaptic responses in seconds or even minutes. These responses may be mediated either via ionic mechanisms (ionotropic) or through a second messenger system (metabotropic).

The two major fast neurotransmitters used in the CNS are glutamate for excitation and γ-amino butyric acid (GABA) for inhibition. Signalling in a large majority of synapses in the CNS is by one or other of these transmitters. On the other hand, the slow neurotransmitters such as the monoamines and the neuropeptides have a modulatory role and are used by only a small proportion of synapses. While the slow neurotransmitters may have some role to play in epilepsy, in particular to account for the decrease in convulsive thresholds seen following treatment with psychoactive drugs, the major underlying cause of epilepsy is most probably a defect in transmission at those synapses using GABA or glutamate as a neurotransmitter. Historically the defect has been considered to be in GABA-mediated systems solely on the evidence of drug treatment. Of the drugs available for the treatment of this condition many are thought to act by facilitating transmission at GABA-mediated synapses. Direct evidence for the involvement of GABA is, however, not convincing and the loss of neurones seen in brain tissue from epileptic patients could well be a secondary neurotoxic phenomenon either as a consequence of seizure activity or as a result of excitatory amino acid release.

With the recent burgeoning of research into excitatory amino acids producing a greater understanding of the role of glutamate in the CNS (see TIPS 1990), a case may be made for the primary defect in epilepsy being one of excessive glutamate-mediated transmission. This may occur either as increased release of transmitter, possibly as a result of failure of inhibitory mechanisms, or as a consequence of the postsynaptic glutamate receptors becoming hypersensitive. The excitatory amino acids are neurotoxic and this may account for the toxicity seen following prolonged febrile convulsions. There is a loss of neurones in the hippocampus and this damage can act as a focus for the development of complex partial (temporal lobe) seizures. Also there is evidence that cerebral ischaemia during an epileptic seizure, particularly during status epilepticus, can cause neuronal loss.

GABA AS AN INHIBITORY NEUROTRANSMITTER IN THE CNS

GABA is the major inhibitory neurotransmitter in the CNS and is found in all brain regions and it has been estimated to be the transmitter at 30% of all the synapses in the brain. There are two types of inhibitory mechanisms in the CNS, presynaptic

and postsynaptic. In the former GABA acts on a presynaptic terminal of an excitatory neurone to prevent release of transmitter; this form of inhibition is found predominantly in the spinal cord. Postsynaptic inhibition is the main inhibitory mechanism found in the brain, and it is at this site that most of the antiepileptic drugs have their action.

The ubiquitous distribution of GABA in the brain can be accounted for by its utilization as a neurotransmitter in both interneurones and in long-axoned tracts. As an inhibitory transmitter in interneurones it plays a vital part in the functioning of neuronal local-circuits within well-defined brain areas. The interneurones of the cerebral cortex, such as the large and small basket cells and the chandelier cells, are responsible for regulating the output of the cortex and also the activity of the association fibres. The basket cells of both the hippocampus and the cerebellum, likewise, via the release of GABA, regulate the output of these regions. The major long-axoned tracts which use GABA as a neurotransmitter are those from the cortex to the substantia nigra, the striatum to the nigra and those from the hypothalamus to the cortex. However, it is the GABAergic interneurones which are most probably more important in the aetiology of epilepsy.

Gaba receptors and transduction mechanisms

GABA receptors when occupied by the endogenous ligand invariably produce hyperpolarization in the postsynaptic neurone. There are two types of receptor designated $GABA_A$ and $GABA_B$ (Matsumoto 1989). $GABA_A$ receptors are the 'classical' bicuculline-sensitive receptors and it is these which are important in the treatment of epilepsy, while the $GABA_B$ receptors are activated by baclofen (Bowery et al 1989). Both these sub-types of receptor are found pre- and postsynaptically and stimulation of these results in either pre- or postsynaptic inhibition. In addition to these actions, $GABA_B$ receptors are considered to be the autoreceptors situated on terminals of GABA neurones, activation of such receptors leads to a decrease in GABA release (Bormann 1988).

Molecular cloning techniques for the isolation and cloning of GABA$_A$ receptors originally described the GABA$_A$/benzodiazepine receptor complex as consisting of two α and two β subunits with the GABA$_A$ receptor localized on the β subunit and the benzodiazepine receptor being on the α subunit (Levitan et al 1988). However, recent reports indicate that there is a third type of subunit (γ) in the GABA$_A$/benzodiazepine complex in the brain (Olsen & Tobin 1990). Also, multiple forms of the α subunit have been described which, when combined with β and γ subunits, would result in complexes having different sensitivities to GABA and also differing pharmacological properties. This latter point offers undoubted therapeutic potential.

GABA$_A$ and GABA$_B$ receptors have differing postsynaptic transduction mechanisms. Activation of GABA$_A$ receptors (Fig. 13.1) opens the chloride channel in the GABA/benzodiazepine complex and this allows an influx of Cl$^-$ which leads to hyperpolarization of the postsynaptic neurone and consequently an inhibition of firing. As this mechanism involves ionic fluxes it has been termed ionotropic transmission (McGeer et al 1987). GABA$_B$-mediated transmission has been classified as metabotropic in that the transduction mechanism at these sites involves a second messenger and metabolic changes result from activation of these receptors. A linkage of the GABA$_B$ receptors to a G protein(s) is the most probable transduction process (Wojcik et all 1989). Activation of GABA$_B$ receptors leads to a decrease in Ca^{2+} conductance (infux) and/or an increase in K$^+$

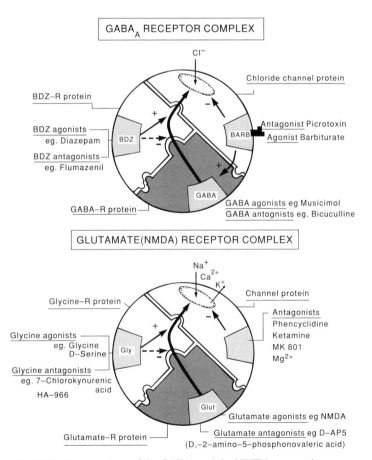

Fig. 13.1 A comparison of the GABA$_A$ and the NMDA-operated channel complexes showing the superficial similarity with both complexes having multiple binding sites providing possibilities for allosteric modulation of neurotransmission.

conductance. The latter, producing an efflux of K$^+$, would lead to hyperpolarization of the neurone. Either of these possibilities would decrease transmitter release.

Gaba synthesis and degradation

GABA is found in high concentrations (μmol/g tissue) in the brain and spinal cord, but it is only present in very low concentrations in peripheral tissue. The major source of GABA in the CNS is most probably glucose entering the tricarboxylic acid (Krebs) cycle via pyruvate and the subsequent production of α-ketoglutarate (Fig. 13.2). The transamination of α-ketoglutarate produces L-glutamic acid (glutamate), the immediate precursor of GABA. Fundamental to GABA synthesis is the so-called 'GABA shunt' which operates entirely within the terminal of the neurone. This is a closed loop which conserves the supply of GABA by producing a molecule of glutamate for every molecule of GABA that is metabolized. GABA is formed by decarboxylation of L-glutamic acid by the enzyme glutamic acid decarboxylase (GAD) which is found only in neurones and this decarboxylation is probably the rate-limiting step in the synthesis of GABA. The next reaction in the shunt is the transamination of GABA to succinic

semialdehyde via GABA-transaminase (GABA-T). However, this can only take place if there is α-ketoglutarate present to accept the amine group that is produced. This ensures that a molecule of glutamate (produced by GABA-T transaminating α-ketoglutarate) is synthesized to take the place of the molecule of GABA destroyed. The succinate semialdehyde formed from GABA is oxidized to succinate and this enters the tricarboxylic acid cycle (Fig. 13.2).

The main inactivating process for GABA which is released from the neurone is by a specific sodium-dependent high-affinity uptake system located in the presynaptic membrane and also in the glial cells. GABA taken up into the neurone can be stored for re-use or some may be metabolized as outlined above. A third mechanism exists where GABA is taken up into glia and converted to glutamate by GABA-T. However, the glutamate formed in glia cannot be used to synthesize GABA as glia do not contain GAD. The glutamate is therefore converted into glutamine by glutamine synthetase and this glutamine can then be transported from glia into neurones whence it can be converted into glutamate by glutaminase, thus conserving the supply of GABA precursor and completing the so-called 'glutamine loop' (Fig. 13.2).

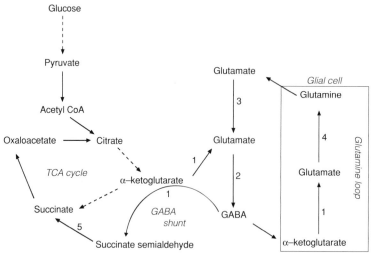

Fig. 13.2 Metabolic pathway for the synthesis and degradation of GABA and glutamate. 1: GABA-transaminase (pyridoxal phosphate required as co-factor); 2: Glutamic acid decarboxylase; 3: Glutaminase; 4: Glutamine synthetase; 5: Succinic semialdehyde dehydrogenase.

Clinical applications

GABA agonists and prodrugs

Because GABA itself does not cross the blood–brain barrier it is not possible to give GABA systemically to patients with epilepsy. Thus various compounds have been synthesized as GABA prodrugs. They contain a lipid-soluble moiety that facilitates brain penetration and subsequently they undergo enzymic conversion within the brain to release GABA itself or a related analogue, e.g. progabide, acetyl GABA. Progabide was found to be effective against seizures in animals (Worms et al 1982, Cepeda et al 1982), but appears less impressive in human epilepsy (Dam et al 1983, Loiseau et al 1983, Van der Linden et al 1981). Another approach has been the design of lipid-soluble agonist molecules which act at the postsynaptic GABA$_A$ recognition site to reproduce the hyperpolarizing action of GABA itself, e.g. 4,5,6,7-tetrahydroisoxazolo (5,4-c)pyridin-3-ol (THIP), muscimol. THIP is an effective anticonvulsant in some animal seizure models, but was ineffective when tried in baboons with photosensitive epilepsy and in patients with epilepsy (Meldrum & Horton 1980, Petersen et al 1983). Why these agonists are ineffective in clinical epilepsy is not clear—possibly they have too diffuse an inhibitory action or perhaps they are not specific for the GABA$_A$ receptor.

GABA-transaminase inhibitors (e.g ethanolamine-O-sulphate, τ-acetylenic GABA)

These compounds are specific enzyme-activated, irreversible (suicide) inhibitors of the enzyme GABA-transaminase and they thus prevent the breakdown of GABA in neurones and glia. The brain concentration of GABA is raised after administration of these compounds to animals and it is thought that the pool of GABA available for synaptic release from nerve terminals is also increased. Most research so far has been done with vigabatrin (Fig. 13.3) which has been shown to be anticonvulsant in animal models of epilepsy, both rodents (Schechter et al 1979) and primates (Meldrum & Horton 1978). These studies predicted efficacy in man, and clinical trials have shown it to be a useful antiepileptic drug in partial and secondarily generalized seizures (see Ch. 15).

GABA uptake inhibitors (e.g. nipecotic acid, 4,5,6,7-tetrahydroisoxazolo (4,5-c) pyridin-3-ol (THIP)

Compounds which inhibit GABA re-uptake will enhance the inhibitory effect of GABA. Those chemicals which are selective inhibitors of glial re-uptake are likely to have the most consistent anticonvulsant action. Many of the available uptake inhibitors do not cross the blood–brain barrier but, when evaluated by intracerebral injection in mice, they have been shown to be anticonvulsant (Schousboe et al 1983). Tiagabine is an experimental compound which has been designed to cross the blood–brain barrier. It consists of nipecotic acid joined by a linker to a lipophilic anchor. Following administration by intraperitoneal injection or gastric lavage it has potent anticonvulsant activity in animals. It is undergoing clinical trials (Pierce et al 1991).

Enhancement of GABA action at the GABA receptors (e.g. benzodiazepines)

Another possible way to augment GABA inhibition is by using drugs which bind to the various sites on the GABA receptor complex and enhance the effect of synaptically released GABA. Theoretically, this type of pharmacological action should preserve the necessary spatial and temporal linkage to suppress abnormal neuronal output but have little effect on normal neuronal function. This is how benzodiazepines and anticonvulsant barbiturates are thought to exert their antiepileptic effect (see below). Thus the development of other compounds which act at the GABA receptor complex is a possible source of new drugs which might lack the limitations of those currently

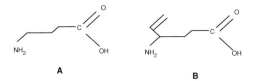

Fig. 13.3 The structure of GABA (A) and vigabatrin (gamma-vinyl GABA) (B).

available, i.e. habituation/dependence, development of tolerance, undue sedation.

GLUTAMATE AS AN EXCITATORY NEUROTRANSMITTER IN THE CNS

Besides being the essential immediate precursor for the synthesis of GABA in the CNS and an important intermediate in neuronal metabolism, glutamate is the predominant excitatory neurotransmitter in the brain and spinal cord. The postsynaptic action of glutamate when applied to neurones is always excitatory, mediated through either an ionotropic or metabotropic action.

The many roles of glutamate in the CNS has made the mapping of neuronal pathways difficult and the evidence for glutamergic axonal tracts is based mainly on changes in neuronal uptake following lesioning. However, immunocytochemical techniques are now available which are overcoming the presence of large amounts of glutamate not involved in neurotransmission. There is good evidence for glutamate being the major transmitter in corticofugal pathways innervating the thalamus, striatum, pontine nuclei and the spinal cord. The output of the hippocampus is also glutamergic, as are the Schaffer colateral interneurones. While in the cerebellum one of the inputs, i.e. the mossy fibres, and the relay neurones, i.e. the granule cell/parallel fibre, use glutamate as a transmitter.

Glutamate receptors and transduction mechanisms

Stimulation of glutamate receptors powerfully depolarizes the postsynaptic neurone with, in most instances, a very fast onset and rapid termination of effect. Four sub-types of postsynaptic glutamate receptor have been described and these have been named after the agonists which preferentially bind to the receptor i.e. N-methyl-D-aspartate (NMDA), kainate, quisqualate and α-amino-3-hydroxy-5-methyl-5-isoxazolepropionic acid (AMPA, for review, see Collingridge & Lester 1989). There is a further receptor which is most probably presynaptic and is stimulated by L-2-amino-4-phosphonobutyrate (L-APB) the function of which is to regulate the release of glutamate from the presynaptic terminal.

Transduction mechanisms mediated by the various sub-types of glutamate receptor are predominantly ionotropic. However, stimulation of at least some populations of quisqualate receptors, notably in the cerebellum, have been shown to be metabotropic via the formation of inositol-1,4,5-trisphosphate (IP_3, Blackstone et al 1989). The ionotropic transduction mechanisms mediated by kainate, quisqualate, AMPA and NMDA receptor occupation open ion channels which allow the passage of Na^+ and K^+, while those activated by NMDA also allow the influx of Ca^{2+}.

Of the various sub-types of glutamate receptors it appears that NMDA receptors are the most likely candidates for a role in epilepsy as antagonists for this receptor have been shown to be effective anti-convulsants in animal models (Meldrum et al 1989). In order to discuss the possible role of NMDA receptor-gated ion channels (NMDA channel) in epilepsy it is necessary to consider the structure of the receptor/channel complex. Superficially there is a marked similarity between the NMDA (Fig. 13.4) and the GABA receptor complexes (Fig. 13.1). Both have multiple binding sites which modulate the affinity of the endogenous ligand for its receptor. The receptor/ionophore complex is most probably made up of membrane spanning sub-units surrounding the cation channel although the complex has not, as yet, been cloned. The NMDA channel allows the influx of Na^+ and Ca^{2+} and the efflux of K^+ and within this channel there is a binding site for Mg^{2+} which at resting potentials blocks the channel. However, depolarization of the postsynaptic neurone by, for example, stimulation of the quisqualate or AMPA receptor removes the Mg^{2+} block on the NMDA channel, the block is thus voltage dependent. The dissociative anaesthetics, phencyclidine and ketamine, have been shown to bind to another site within the channel to produce non-competitive blockade and are anticonvulsant (Aram et al 1989). This has been termed the PCP site. Blockade of the NMDA channel at the PCP site thus offers a mechanism whereby drugs may act and one such compound that has shown potent anticonvulsant activity in animal models is dizocilpine (MK 801, Patel et al 1988). However, any compounds binding to the PCP site and blocking the cation channel show

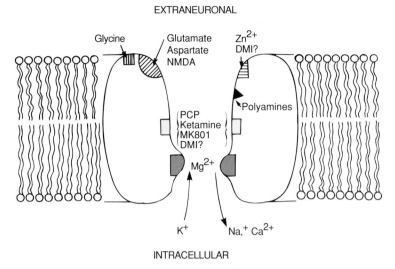

Fig. 13.4 The NMDA receptor-operated ion channel showing the variety of binding sites (DMI: desmethylimipramine; PCP: phencyclidine).

PCP-like psychotomimetic effects and consequently may not be acceptable for use clinically as anticonvulsants. Antagonists acting at this site are also very effective in preventing neuronal degeneration following ischaemia (Iversen et al 1989) and may therefore prove to be of value in protecting against neuronal damage in stroke and other types of cerebral ischaemia in man.

Compounds have been developed which act as competitive antagonists at the NMDA receptor site. While these have exhibited anticonvulsant effects in animal models the majority do not cross the blood–brain barrier. However, orally active compounds are now becoming available and are undergoing toxicity testing and it is most probable that from this group effective antiepileptic drugs will be developed.

There are recognition sites on the receptor complex for the endogenous ligands (glutamate/aspartate) and also for other modulators (Fig. 13.1). A recognition site for glycine, which facilitates NMDA-mediated transmission, has been well documented (Johnson & Ascher 1988) and can be compared with the allosteric modulation seen with benzodiazepines at the GABA receptor/ionophore complex. The modulators in both cases facilitating neurotransmission. The glycine site, adjacent to the NMDA receptor, is not strychnine sensitive and thus antagonists at this site, by de-

creasing NMDA-mediated transmission would have anticonvulsant potential. Thus, glycine at this site on the NMDA complex is excitatory whereas its action at other glycine receptors is inhibitory through activation of Cl⁻ ionophores.

Other binding sites (Fig. 13.4) on the NMDA receptor complex have not been thoroughly investigated, however, spermidine and spermine, acting on a postulated distinct, polyamine site, potentiate NMDA-induced convulsions in animals (Singh et al 1990). The presence of high concentrations of zinc (Zn^{2+}) in the neurones in the CNS, particularly in the mossy fibres of the hippocampus, has been reported. That Zn^{2+} can be released during neuronal activity in a calcium-dependent manner (Assaf & Chung 1984) and subsequently inhibits NMDA-mediated transmission (Westbrook & Mayer 1987) suggests a neuromodulatory or neuroprotective role for this ion. Tricyclic antidepressants, such as desmethylimipramine, are also known to block the effects of NMDA and it is thought that this action is either via the Zn^{2+} recognition site or in the channel at the PCP site.

Clinical applications

Impaired maximal rate of synthesis of excitatory transmitters

This could theoretically have a selective action on

the pool of glutamate and/or aspartate available for neurotransmission. However, the routes of synthesis of the excitatory amino acids are not known with certainty. Sodium valproate has been shown to decrease brain aspartate concentrations but how this is done and the significance of this effect is unknown.

Decreased synaptic release of excitatory transmitters

Decreased release of excitatory amino acid transmitters might be achieved by an effect on autoreceptors on presynaptic terminals or via $GABA_B$ receptors. Lamotrigine, a new drug at an advanced stage of clinical testing, is thought to act in this way (Leach et al 1986).

Decreased postsynaptic action

Analogues of the excitatory amino acids that act as competitive antagonists at the postsynaptic receptors have been evaluated in test animals and are anticonvulsant against audiogenic and various chemically-induced seizures in mice. The most potent specific antagonists are 2-amino-5-phosphonopentanoic acid (AP5) and 2-amino-7-phosphonoheptanoic acid (AP7) which are selective for the NMDA receptor site. AP7 is also effective against photically-induced seizures in baboons. Unfortunately, when these compounds are administered systemically, there is only limited entry into the brain because of poor lipid solubility. However, two experimental compounds, CGP37849 and CGP39551, have been synthesized which are orally active and show promise for clinical development (Schmutz et al 1990).

An alternative approach is by the administration of noncompetitive NMDA antagonists. Dizocilpine (MK801) was tested in pilot clinical trials but showed unacceptable psychotomimetic effects. Remacemide is a novel acetamide compound which weakly blocks NMDA receptors but whose desglycine metabolite is more potent in this respect. It is currently undergoing early Phase II studies in epileptic patients. So far, psychotomimetic effects do not appear to have been prominent.

MODE OF ACTION OF STANDARD ANTIEPILEPTIC DRUGS

Although drugs like phenytoin and carbamazepine have been used for many years their mode of action is still open to debate. The evidence is summarized below. The reader is referred to McDonald & Meldrum (1983) for a further account.

Phenytoin

Phenytoin is a diphenyl substituted hydantoin (Fig. 13.5). A phenyl or another aromatic substituent at position 5 appears to be essential for anticonvulsant activity while alkyl substituents in this position confer sedative properties on the molecule. The mechanism of antiepileptic action of phenytoin is not known but it appears to affect the electrical excitability of the neuronal membrane rather than an action on synaptic transmission. Many effects of the drug have been identified experimentally but the relevance of these to its antiepileptic action is not clear. However, it is the ability of phenytoin to block Na^+ channels which most probably confers its therapeutic action.

Presynaptic actions include reduction of Na^+ conductance through voltage-sensitive channels which is required for the initiation of action potentials; blockade of repetitive firing through use- and frequency-dependent block, i.e. the more frequently the channels open the greater the degree of blockade; by reducing the recovery rate from inactivation of sodium channels; reduction of post-tetanic potentiation possibly via an action on the sodium pump decreasing the excitability of the neuronal membrane following repetitive activity as is seen in epilepsy. Also, presynaptically, phenytoin reduces Ca^{2+} entry into neurones and as a result may decrease neurotransmitter release.

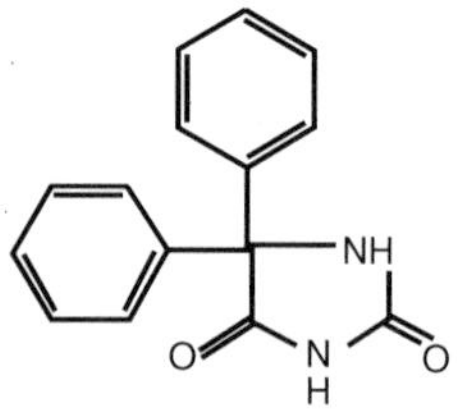

Fig. 13.5   The structure of phenytoin.

Postsynaptic effects include enhancement of GABA-mediated inhibition and subsequent reduction of excitatory transmission possibly via GABA uptake inhibition or the proliferation of postsynaptic GABA$_A$ receptors. At high concentrations the drug inhibits the release of both serotonin and noradrenaline and also inhibits monoamine oxidase.

Many of the actions of phenytoin outlined above only occur with high concentrations of the drug, often far above relevant therapeutic concentrations. The exception to this is its ability, at low concentrations, to decrease the rate of recovery of sodium channels following repetitive firing and this could prove to be its true mechanism of action.

Phenobarbitone

The structure of phenobarbitone is given in Figure 13.6. The structure–activity relationships of the barbiturates has been extensively studied and shows that one of the substituents at the 5

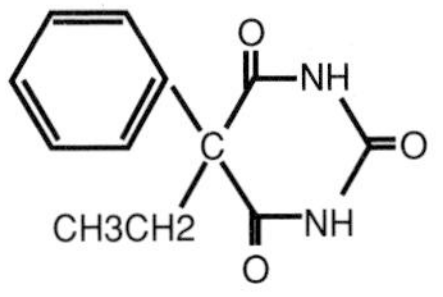

Fig. 13.6 The structure of phenobarbitone.

position must be a phenyl group in order to confer anticonvulsant activity on the molecule. Two phenyl groups at the 5 position give less anticonvulsant activity but also reduce sedative activity. As in the hydantoin group, an alkyl moiety at position 5, as is the case with phenobarbitone, confers sedative properties on the molecule.

The mechanism of action of the barbiturates has been throughly investigated and the ability of some barbiturates to show a specific anticonvulsant action rather than a sedative action suggests that different mechanisms may be involved. The most probable mode of action of phenobarbitone is through an enhancement of GABA-ergic neurotransmission, especially as these

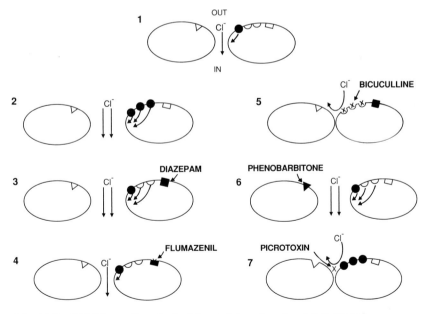

Fig. 13.7 GABA/benzodiazepine/barbiturate interaction. 1 and 2: Increased occupation of postsynaptic GABA$_A$ receptors potentiates the entry of Cl$^-$. 3: Diazepam enhances this effect so that basal levels of GABA open the channel more frequently. 4: The benzodiazepine antagonist, flumazenil, has no effect on transmission. 5: GABA antagonists such as bicuculline inhibit the action of benzodiazepines. 6: The presence of phenobarbitone also enhances entry of Cl$^-$. 7: Picrotoxin, a channel antagonist, blocks Cl$^-$ entry even when GABA receptors are fully occupied.

responses are seen at relatively low concentrations ($<100\,\mu$M). The GABA-receptor complex, on the postsynaptic neuronal membrane, surrounds and controls Cl^- channel opening. This complex has many binding sites. As well as the GABA and benzodiazepine receptor sites, as discussed earlier, there is a third distinct, allosteric site most probably situated adjacent to the Cl^- channel protein, which binds the convulsant, picrotoxinin, it is to this site that barbiturates are known to bind (see Fig. 13.1). Phenobarbitone, by binding to this allosteric site facilitates the GABA-mediated entry of Cl^- into the neurone (Fig. 13.7). Barbiturates have been shown to prolong the open-time of these channels and thus entry of Cl^-, down its concentration gradient, is increased leading to hyperpolarization of the postsynaptic neurone and enhancement of GABA-induced inhibition.

Phenobarbitone has also been shown to antagonize the excitatory effects of glutamate at relatively low concentrations through an inhibitory action at the quisqualate/AMPA receptor, however, whether this is a direct action through reduction of release or a postsynaptic effect is not clear. Either of these effects could well be mediated through inhibition via an action on GABA transmission as described above.

The release of neurotransmitters from synaptosomal preparations has been shown to be decreased with barbiturates, this occurs at very high concentrations and is probably due to blockade of Ca^{2+} entry into the terminal. It is unlikely that this mechanism has any relevance to the anticonvulsant actions of the barbiturates as the concentrations needed would only be attained in heavily sedated or anaesthetized patients.

Primidone

Primidone (2-desoxyphenobarbitone) has been shown to be an effective anticonvulsant. However, it is metabolized to the two active metabolites phenobarbitone and phenylethylmalonamide (PEMA) as shown in Figure 13.8

As a result of the formation of the active metabolites it has proved to be very difficult to determine the mechanism of action of the parent compound due to interference from the metabolites. However, the probability is that an action

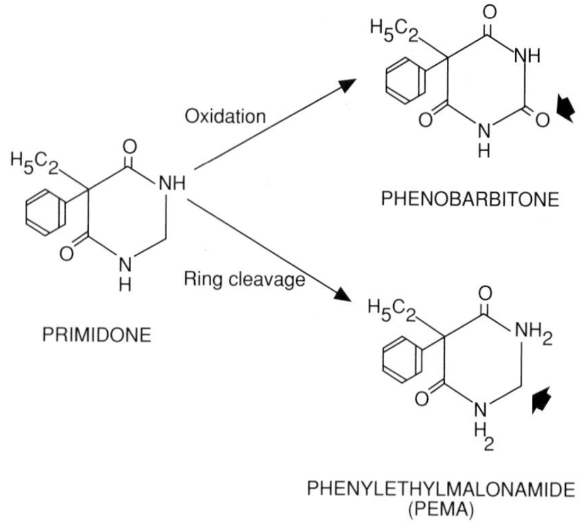

Fig. 13.8   The structure of primidone and its two active metabolites, phenobarbitone and phenylethyl malonamide (PEMA).

similar to that of the barbiturates accounts for the anticonvulsant effects of primidone.

Carbamazepine

Carbamazepine is related chemically to the tricyclic antidepressant imipramine, and is effective in the treatment of bipolar affective disorders and trigeminal neuralgia as well as being anticonvulsant. It is a derivative of iminostilbene with a carbonyl group in position 5 (Fig. 13.9), and it is this moiety which confers the anti-epileptic activity on the molecule. The ureide group occurs in the heterocyclic ring of many anticonvulsants as it is this group which is used in the synthesis of barbituric acid.

Carbamazepine and phenytoin have very similar actions on Na^+ channels in that both are effective in reducing the generation of high-frequency repetitive firing. Thus, carbamazepine-induced blockade of Na^+ channels is use- and frequency-

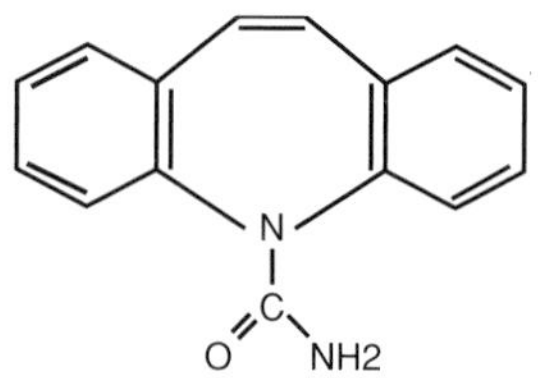

Fig. 13.9   The structure of carbamazepine.

dependent and this action occurs at therapeutic concentrations (2 μg/ml).

A recent report has shown that carbamazepine (50 μM), but not phenytoin, blocks NMDA-activated currents in spinal cord neurones. Under normal conditions the NMDA-activated channel would be blocked by Mg^{2+}, however, this block would be relieved during the excessive activity seen in an epileptic focus. The decrease in Na^+ and Ca^{2+} fluxes through the NMDA-operated channel could account for some of the anti-convulsant activity seen with carbamazepine.

Carbamazepine also blocks the re-uptake of noradrenaline into the presynaptic terminal. It is unlikely that this effect contributes to its anti-convulsant action as the tricyclic antidepressants also block amine reuptake but lower convulsive thresholds. There is no evidence that carbamazepine influences GABA-ergic transmission.

Ethosuximide

Ethosuximide (Fig. 13.10) has very little protective effect against maximal electroshock-induced seizures in experimental animals but is effective against pentylenetetrazol-induced seizures. Substitution with phenyl moieties at position 2 confers activity against electroshock-induced seizures. The mode of action of ethosuximide is not known but it may be postulated that a novel mechanism is involved as this drug does not inhibit Na^+ entry into the neurone terminal and it does not enhance the post-synaptic actions of GABA. Ethosuximide has been shown to specifically block transient (T) calcium-channel activation in neurones and it has been suggested that this accounts for the action of those drugs used in absence seizures (Coulter et al 1989). However, valproate, an effective drug in this condition, does not block T-type channels. These channels are involved in the control of neuronal activity and burst firing

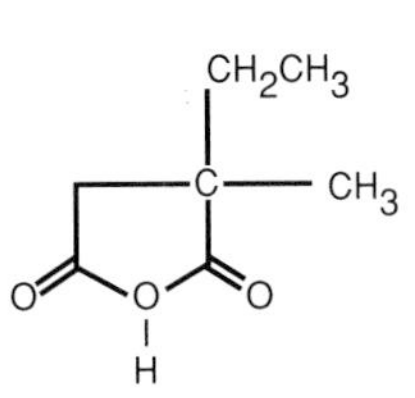

Fig. 13.10   The structure of ethosuximide.

rather than in transmitter release. The former action offers an attractive hypothesis for the action of ethosuximide, especially as it has been shown to reduce the T-type calcium current in thalamic neurones (Coulter et al 1989).

Sodium valproate

Sodium valproate is a simple, branched-chain carboxylic acid (Fig. 13.11). In animal models of epilepsy sodium valproate is effective against pentylenetetrazol-induced convulsions and shows a greater potency than ethosuximide, it also protects against electroshock-induced seizures.

The mechanism of action of sodium valproate is far from clear. It has been shown to inhibit repetitive firing in neurones as do phenytoin and carbamazepine, however, there is no evidence to suggest that this action of valproate is via blockade of sodium channels.

Great interest has been shown in the ability of valproate to affect GABAergic transmission and thus increase CNS inhibitory pathways. Two possibilities have been suggested for this action. One is that valproate inhibits GABA-T, the enzyme responsible for the degradation of GABA, and the other is through a facilitation of GAD, the enzyme responsible for the synthesis of GABA from glutamate (see Fig. 13.2). However, sodium valproate inhibits seizures in animal models at concentrations far lower than those required to block GABA-T or stimulate GAD. It might well be that the increases observed in GABA levels are due to the accumulation of a metabolite of valproate (2-en-valproic acid) which in itself causes the accumulation of GABA in vivo.

At relatively low concentrations sodium valproate has been shown to hyperpolarize neurones although the mechanism through which this occurs is unknown. However, high concentrations of the drug do increase potassium conductance and so the possibility that the hyperpolarization is mediated through the opening of potassium channels in the neuronal membrane cannot be ruled out.

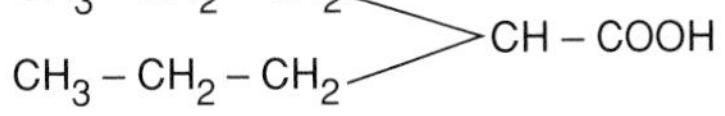

Fig. 13.11   The structure of sodium valproate.

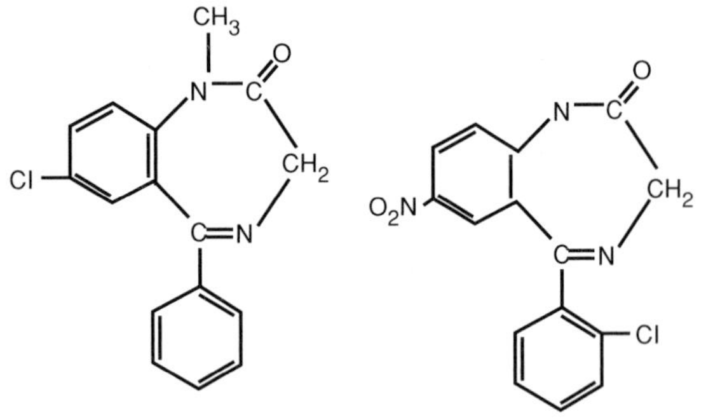

Fig. 13.12   The structure of the two benzodiazepine drugs, diazepam and clonazepam.

Benzodiazepines

All the benzodiazepines have anticonvulsant properties as do the many active metabolites of this large group of sedative/hypnotic drugs. The two most commonly used, whose structures are shown in Figure 13.12, are diazepam and clonazepam.

In animals, the benzodiazepines are much more effective against pentylenetetrazol-induced convulsions than against maximal electroshock-induced seizures, whilst both clonazepam and diazepam suppress convulsions in kindled rats.

The mode of action of the benzodiazepines has been throughly investigated and as discussed earlier in this chapter the mechanism is via facilitation of GABA-mediated neurotransmission (see Fig. 13.1). The $GABA_A/Cl^-$ ionophore complex has binding sites for benzodiazepines and, as discussed earlier, for barbiturates. The benzodizepine sites are located on the α sub-units of the receptor complex and occupation of these allosteric sites facilitate GABA-mediated transmission and consequently increase hyperpolarization of the postsynaptic neurone (Fig. 13.7). Although both the barbiturates and benzodiazepines allosterically modulate GABA transmission they have distinct binding sites on the receptor complex. Also, the facilitation seen with the benzodiazepines leads to an increase in the frequency of opening of Cl^- channels without affecting the channel open time; the barbiturates, on the other hand, prolong the channel open time. The actions of the benzodiazepine outlined above occur at clinically relevant concentrations.

REFERENCES

Aram J A, Martin D, Tomczyk M et al 1989 Neocortical epileptogenesis in vitro: studies with N-methyl-D-aspartate, phencyclidine, sigma and dextromethorphan receptor ligands. Journal of Pharmacology and Experimental Therapeutics 248: 320–328
Assaf S Y, Chung S-H 1984 Release of endogenous Zn^{2+} from brain tissue during activity. Nature 308: 734–736
Blackstone C D, Supattapone S, Synder S H 1989 Inositolphospholipid-linked glutamate receptors mediate cerebellar parallel-fiber-Purkinje-cell synaptic transmission. Proceedings of the National Academy of Sciences USA 86: 4316–4320
Bormann J 1988 Electrophysiology of $GABA_A$ and $GABA_B$ receptor subtypes. Trends in Neurosciences 11: 112–116
Bowery N G, Hill D R, Moratalla R 1989 Neurochemistry and autoradiography of $GABA_B$ receptors in mammalian brain: second-messenger system(s). 1989 In: Barnard E A, Costa E (eds) Allosteric modulation of amino acid receptors. Raven Press, New York, p 159–172
Cepeda C, Worms P, Lloyd K G, Naquet R 1982 Action of progabide in the photosensitive baboon, Papio papio. Epilepsia 23: 463
Collingridge G L, Lester R A J 1989 Excitatory amino acid receptors in the vertebrate central nervous system. Pharmacological Reviews 40: 143–210
Coulter D A, Huguenard J R, Prince D A 1989 Characterization of ethosuximide reduction of low-threshold calcium current in thalamic neurones. Annals of Neurology 25: 482–593

Dam M, Gram L, Philbert A et al 1983 Progabide: a controlled trial in partial epilepsy. Epilepsia 24: 127
Iversen L L, Woodruff G N, Kemp J A et al 1989 Non-competitive NMDA antagonists as drugs. In: Watkins J C, Collingridge G L (eds) The NMDA Receptor. Oxford University Press, Oxford, p 217–226
Johnson J W, Ascher P 1988 The NMDA receptor and its channel. Modulation by magnesium and by glycine. In: Lodge D (ed) Excitatory amino acids in health and Disease. Wiley, Chichester, p 143–164
Krall R L, Penry J K, White B G, Kupferberg H J, Swinyard E A 1978 Antiepileptic drug development. II. Anticonvulsant drug screening. Epilepsia 19: 409
Leach M J, Marden C M, Miller A A 1986 Pharmacological studies on lamotrigine, a novel potential antiepileptic drug. II. Neurochemical studies and mechanism of action. Epilepsia 27: 490
Levitan E S, Schofield P R, Burt D R et al 1988 Structural and functional basis for $GABA_A$ receptor heterogeneity. Nature 335: 76–79
Lockard J S 1980 A primate model of clinical epilepsy: mechanisms of action through quantification of therapeutic effects. In: Lockard J S, Ward A A (eds) Epilepsy. A window to brain mechanisms. Raven Press, New York, p 11
Loiseau P, Bossi L, Guyot M, Orofiamma B, Morselli P L 1983 Double-blind cross-over trial of progabide versus placebo in severe epilepsies. Epilepsia 24: 703
Loscher W, Meldrum B S 1984 Evaluation of anticonvulsant drugs in genetic animal models of epilepsy. Federation Proceedings 43: 276

Macdonald R L, Meldrum B S 1989 Principles of antiepileptic drug action. In: Levy R, Mattson R, Meldrum B, Penry J K, Dreifuss F E (eds) Antiepileptic drugs. Raven Press, New York, p 59–83

Matsumoto R R 1989 GABA receptors: are cellular differences reflected in function? Brain Research Reviews 14: 203–225.

McGeer P L, Eccles J C, McGeer E G 1987 Molecular neurobiology of the brain. Plenum Press, New York, p 151–173

Meldrum B, Horton R 1978 Blockade of epileptic responses in the photosensitive baboon, Papio papio by the two irreversible inhibitors of GABA-transaminase, γ-acetylenic GABA (4-amino-hex-5-ynoic acid) and γ-vinyl GABA (4-amino-hex-5-enoic-acid). Psychopharmacology 59: 47

Meldrum B S, Horton R W 1980 Effects of bicyclic GABA agonist, THIP, on myoclonic and seizure responses in mice and baboons with reflex epilepsy. European Journal of Pharmacology 61: 231

Meldrum B S, Chapman A G, Patel S, Swan J 1989 Competitive NMDA antagonists as drugs. In: Watkins J C, Collingridge G L (eds) The NMDA receptor. Oxford University Press, Oxford, p 207–216

Naquet R, Meldrum B S 1972 In: Purpura D, Penry J K, Tower D B, Woodbury D M, Walter R Q (eds) Experimental models of epilepsy. Raven Press, New York, p 373

Olsen R W, Tobin A J 1990 Molecular biology of GABA_A receptors. FASEB Journal 4: 1469–1480

Patel S, Chapman A G, Millam M H, Meldrum B S 1988 Epilepsy and excitatory amino acid antagonists. In: Lodge D (ed) Excitatory amino acids in health and disease. Wiley, Chichester, p 353–378

Petersen H R, Jensen I, Dam M 1983 THIP: a single blind controlled trial in patients with epilepsy. Acta Neurologica Scandinavica 67: 114

Pierce M W, Suzdak P D, Gustavson L E, Mengel H B, Mckelvy J F, Mant T 1991 Tiagabine. In: Pisani F, Perucca E, Avanzini G, Richens A (eds) New antiepileptic drugs. Elsevier, Amsterdam

Richens A 1989 Vigabatrin. In: Levy R H, Dreifuss F E, Mattson R H, Meldrum B S, Penry J K (eds) Antiepileptic drugs, 3rd edn. Raven Press, New York, p 937–946

Schechter P J, Tranier Y, Grove J 1979 Attempts to correlate alterations in brain GABA metabolism by GABA-T inhibitors with their anticonvulsant effects. In: Mandel P, De Feudis F V (eds) GABA-biochemistry and CNS functions. Plenum, New York, p 43

Schmutz M, Portet Ch, Jeker A et al 1990 The competitive NMDA receptor antagonists CGP37849 and CGP39551 are potent, orally-active anticonvulsants in rodents. Naunyn-Schmiedeberg's Archives of Pharmacology 342: 61–66

Schousboe A, Larsson O M, Wood J D, Krogsgaard-Larson P 1983 Transport and metabolism of τ-amino-butyric acid in neurons and glia: implications for epilepsy. Epilepsia 24: 531

Singh L, Oles R, Woodruff G 1990 In vivo interaction of a polyamine with the NMDA receptor. European Journal of Pharmacology 180: 391–392

Trends in Pharmacological Sciences 1990 11: Nos 1–12. A series of articles on excitatory amino acids.

Van der Linden G J, Meinardi H, Meijer J W A, Bossi L, Gomeni C 1981 A double blind crossover trial with progabide (SL 76002) against placebo in patients with secondary generalized epilepsy. In: Dam M, Gram L, Penry J K (eds) Advances in epileptology. 12th Epilepsy International. Raven Press, New York, p 141

Westbrook G L, Mayer M L 1987 Micromolar concentrations of Zn^{2+} antagonize NMDA and GABA responses of hippocampal neurones. Nature 328: 640–643

Wojcik W J, Paez X, Ulivi M 1989 A transduction mechanism for GABA_B receptors. In: Barnard E A, Costa E (eds) Allosteric modulation of amino acid receptors. Raven Press, New York, p 173–193

Worms P, Depoortere H, Durand A, Morselli P L, Lloyd K G, Bartholini G 1982 Aminobutyric acid (GABA) receptor stimulation. I. Neuropharmacological profiles of progabide (SL 76002) and SL 75102 with emphasis on their anticonvulsant spectra. Journal of Pharmacology and Experimental Therapeutics 220: 660

14. Assessing new drugs for epilepsy

L. Gram   S. Schwabe   P. K. Jensen

THE NEED FOR NEW ANTIEPILEPTIC DRUGS

Since the introduction of phenobarbitone, in 1912, the first effective treatment for epilepsy, a significant number of antiepileptic drugs have been developed. In the majority of countries, between 10 and 20 drugs are currently approved for the treatment of epilepsy. Consequently, one may question if there is still a need for a continued search for new antiepileptic compounds.

Today, despite the significant number of drugs available, at least 20% of all patients with epilepsy are still uncontrolled. In addition, many well controlled patients suffer from adverse effects caused by the antiepileptic drug(s) they are treated with. Consequently, there is a significant need to develop new and even more effective antiepileptic compounds, or to identify drugs that are equally effective but with less pronounced toxicity.

Fortunately, at the moment, a significant number of new substances have reached, or are approaching the stage of clinical testing in man. This has resulted directly from an increasing knowledge of the cellular mechanisms of neuronal excitability and has been supported by the Antiepileptic Drug Development Programme, which was launched in 1975 by the National Institute of Health in USA (Porter et al 1984). As a result, recently updated Guidelines for the clinical testing of antiepileptic drugs were issued by the International League Against Epilepsy (Commission on Antiepileptic Drugs 1989).

STUDIES IN HEALTHY VOLUNTEERS

In the development of new drugs in general, Phase I studies in healthy volunteers pose highly specific ethical and practical problems. It is during this phase that new, potential antiepileptic compounds are administered to man for the first time. Phase I is also the only phase in the clinical development of a new compound in which the subjects obviously derive no benefit from the treatment. The purpose is to obtain the first information with regard to tolerability, pharmacodynamic, and pharmacokinetic properties of a new compound in humans, in order to be able to plan the further clinical development in a rational and safe manner.

Phase I testing of a new potential antiepileptic compound differs from that of many other compounds, in that the pharmacodynamic information that can be obtained on the potential antiepileptic effect is very limited. Investigation of EEGs (including pharmaco-EEG) cannot reliably predict any therapeutic effect of the compound. The prediction of antiepileptic activity by more sophisticated methods, such as MRI or PET scans, still needs to be explored.

The main purpose of Phase I studies is to define a well-tolerated dose range, and to determine the highest tolerated dose in healthy volunteers. Based on the available animal pharmacological and toxicological data, an initial dose expected to be well tolerated in humans must be defined. In the first single-dose study at least three dosages per volunteer should be investigated in a placebo-controlled trial design. A minimum of 16 healthy male volunteers should be included (Commission on Antiepileptic Drugs 1989). Close monitoring of safety, including adverse effects, EEG, and haematological and biochemical parameters, is essential. Also to be included is a pharmacokinetic assessment, comprising at least calculations of half-life, T_{max}, protein binding and dose proportionality, in order to be able to administer the compound in an adequate dosage regimen for the multiple-dose studies.

The multiple-dose studies should include a minimum of 16 healthy volunteers, each being exposed to the compound for at least 28 days (Commission on Antiepileptic Drugs 1989). In order to compare the basic pharmacokinetic parameters a single-dose pharmacokinetic profile should be obtained before the start of the multiple-dose series, in order to allow intraindividual comparison of the pharmacokinetic properties of the compound. As in the case of the single-dose study, close monitoring of the safety parameters is essential. In addition to these, assessment of neurophysiological parameters, including neuropsychometric testing, should be included. Careful monitoring of the pharmacokinetic parameters, including steady-state pharmacokinetics, protein binding, and calculation of half-life after multiple-dose administration is also essential. A placebo-controlled design is mandatory. The compound should be tested using at least three different dose levels, using a rising-dosage regimen.

The information obtained in the above-mentioned trials is essential before proceeding to the clinical testing in patients. The safety profile, including assessment of possible adverse effects, is intended to give the clinician an indication of the nature and severity of the adverse effects to be expected with the new compound. The pharmacokinetic profile obtained in healthy volunteers should be used to establish a rational dosage regimen and to provide a baseline for potential drug interactions to be investigated in patients. This latter profile is especially important for the clinical testing of antiepileptic compounds, as early Phase II trials involve patients on concomitant antiepileptic treatment, and therefore potential drug interactions.

In addition to the trials described in this chapter, further studies in volunteers need to be included in a complete development programme for any new antiepileptic compound. Studies investigating the influence of food on the absorption of the new compound, as well as specific studies in subpopulations, e.g. elderly subjects, and subjects with renal and/or hepatic insufficiency, are also needed. However, such studies are normally not initiated before the start of Phase II, and usually run in parallel to the Phase II programme.

STUDIES IN PATIENTS

The need for controlled clinical studies

Seizure frequency, one of the key endpoints in clinical drug trials, has been shown to be influenced by a number of factors, apart from the drug(s) ingested. This fact may of course give rise to bias, unless adequate control is ensured. An example of a factor which may change seizure frequency despite unchanged treatment is the admission of patients into a hospital. It is well known that in many cases such a procedure alone may cause a dramatic reduction in the number of seizures (Riley et al 1981). Another factor which is much more crucial for clinical drug trials is the so-called placebo effect. Recently, a placebo-controlled double-blind study with a new antiepileptic compound demonstrated that treatment with placebo resulted in a 50% seizure reduction in 23% of the patients (Group for the evaluation of Cinromide in the Lennox–Gastaut syndrome 1989). Consequently, adequate randomisation and blinding is very important. A review of the controlled clinical trials of antiepileptic drugs up to 1981 has appeared (Gram et al 1982).

Trial designs

Two main types of design exist; the parallel design, comparing groups of patients, i.e. *between patient* comparisons; and the cross-over design, undertaking *within patient* evaluations. Parallel investigations represent the more robust design, but have the disadvantage that they require large numbers of patients in order to achieve adequate statistical power. For this and other reasons, cross-over designs are very popular, and extensively used in the clinical testing of antiepileptic drugs. In general, the prerequisite for using cross-over designs is a purely symptomatic treatment of a stable chronic disorder. The main advantage of the cross-over design is that it can be undertaken with fewer patients than the parallel study, but with identical statistical power. This is because in cross-over designs, variation in the statistical analysis is reduced due to the fact that intra-patient comparisons are performed. Scoville et al (1981) have provided estimates suggesting that between 2.7 and 6.4 times as many patients would be needed in a parallel study, compared to a cross-over trial in order to detect a given difference between treatments.

However, a number of problems are linked to the use of cross-over designs:

- carry-over effects
- period effects (e.g. regression towards the mean).

The *carry-over effect* implies that the effect of one treatment may continue into the next treatment period. This may involve pharmacokinetic or pharmacodynamic carry-over effects. If the test drug has a very long half-life, the effect may continue into the subsequent period of placebo treatment. Another possibility for introducing a carry-over effect is where the effect of the investigated drug turns out not to be completely reversible, or if the effect only disappears slowly, e.g. due to receptor binding. The best method of avoiding this type of carry-over effect is to introduce a washout period of sufficient duration between treatments to ensure against this phenomenon.

The occurrence of a *period effect* may be due to test–retest phenomena, spontaneous fluctuations in the disease, or regression towards the mean. It is well known that epilepsy does not exhibit a uniform frequency of seizures (Hopkins et al 1985).

Francis Galton (1885) described a phenomenon which later became known as regression towards the mean. This term refers to the fact that a variable which attains an extreme value during one measurement will tend to approach a mean value at subsequent measurements. This problem is especially relevant in the clinical testing of antiepileptic drugs, due to the selection of patients. It is customary to include patients with a high seizure frequency in order to increase the possibility of demonstrating a difference between treatments. Consequently, regression towards the mean has been demonstrated to occur frequently in controlled trials of antiepileptic drugs, as patients with a high seizure frequency at entrance tend to experience a decrease in seizure frequency independent of the treatment (Spilker & Segreti 1984). The opposite has also been shown to occur in patients with an initially low seizure frequency, who tend to demonstrate an increase over a period of time. Regression towards the mean is difficult to avoid. One possibility would be to recruit patients for clinical trials without taking their current seizure frequency into account. Another possibility would be to include long baseline periods, or to make treatment periods very long or very short compared with the random fluctuations in seizure frequency. However, the time course of temporal fluctuations in seizure frequency is rarely known.

Applying a cross-over design implies that a therapeutic regimen, to which the patient may have responded favourably may later be withdrawn. In order to avoid this problem, the response conditional design (incomplete cross-over) has been developed (White 1979). This method implies that only patients showing an 'insufficient' response to the treatment will be crossed over to the alternate treatment (Fig. 14.1). The response conditional design is especially suited to the comparison of a new antiepileptic compound to a standard drug, or to the comparison of two standard drugs. This design procedure is particularly suitable for the inclusion of patients with newly diagnosed epilepsy, as well as the inclusion of patients for long-term studies since there is no risk of withholding a favourable therapy from the patients. However, the problem is that appropriate statistical methods to deal with this type of design are as yet not available. More sophisticated multiple cross-over designs e.g. N of 1, do not avoid the drawbacks of the classical cross-over design.

Patient selection

There is a general consensus that it is unethical to withhold active treatment from patients with proven epilepsy. As mentioned previously, the vast majority of patients may be controlled on existing antiepileptic drugs. Consequently, the patient group most frequently selected for clinical testing of new antiepileptic compounds are patients with chronic, uncontrolled epilepsies

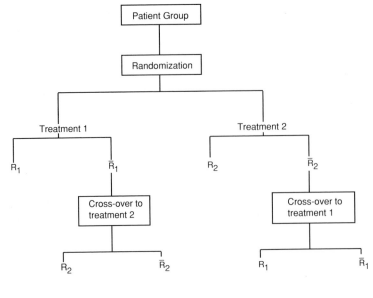

R : Satisfactory response
R̄ : Insufficient response

Fig. 14.1   Response conditional (incomplete cross-over) design.

despite optimal treatment with available drugs. Consequently, the majority of Phase II trials are so-called add-on studies, where the new drug or placebo is added on to the current treatment. This type of patient selection and investigational procedure may cause several problems.

The demonstration of a positive drug-related effect may be more difficult in chronic patients, since it may be assumed that they are particularly resistant to improvement (Gram et al 1982). Highly effective drugs may thus be favoured at the expense of less effective, yet clinically relevant drugs.

It is well known that the majority of antiepileptic drugs have a significant interaction potential. *Consequently, it is very important to keep the plasma concentration of the concomitant treatment constant throughout the trials.* If a significant increase in plasma levels occurs during treatment with the test drug, compared to placebo, the influence of this factor cannot be distinguished from a possible genuine effect of the test drug. During controlled testing of antiepileptic drugs, this problem has frequently invalidated the interpretation of studies. One possibility of eliminating this problem is to introduce a non-blind thera-

peutic monitor, who adjusts the doses of concomitant drugs in order to ensure constant plasma levels throughout the study period (Fig. 14.2).

Effect parameters

The most widely applied parameter of efficacy of new drugs is change in seizure frequency. Generally, this variable is considered to provide 'hard data' for the statistical analysis. However, other measures of efficacy are being explored. Several attempts have been made to develop a 'seizure severity scale', which apart from quantifying the

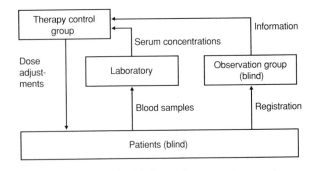

Fig. 14.2   Double-blind design with an open therapeutic control.

severity of the individual seizure, may even take seizure frequency into consideration, thus reflecting changes in the patient's 'quality of life' (Duncan & Sander 1990, Baker et al 1991).

Another possibility would be to measure seizure free intervals, or time to the first, second, or indeed any other number of seizures following entry into the study. Unfortunately, statistical calculations of Monte Carlo simulations of seizure frequency have demonstrated that even measuring the time to the 12th seizure implies a significant decrease in the ability to detect differences between treatments for a fixed sample size (Shofer & Temkin 1986). The number of patients had to be increased several times in order to maintain unaltered statistical power. Consequently, the use of this measurement as an outcome variable may require prohibitively large patient samples.

The recording and quantification of side-effects are as important as measures of efficacy. However, in previous controlled trials, this aspect has been greatly neglected. In the trials published up to 1981, only 25% applied statistical testing with regard to side-effects (Gram et al 1982). This fact was mainly due to unsystematic data collection with an inadequate use of rating scales. However, increasing attention has been focused on this important aspect in recent years.

In daily clinical practice, both efficacy and tolerability determine whether a patient can be successfully treated with any particular compound. One parameter that subsumes both of these factors would therefore be the probability that the patient will remain on the compound within a certain period of time. Survival analysis is a statistical tool that effectively deals with this problem. One of the possible endpoints for this method of analysis could be, for example, the number of patients remaining on a given treatment after 12 months.

Dosing of test drug

Three possibilities exist:

- fixed dose
- fixed plasma level
- dosing according to clinical effect.

All of these possibilities are being used in antiepileptic drug trials, depending on the status of the pharmacokinetics of the new compound. It is important to realize that the majority of antiepileptic drugs exhibit great inter-patient variability with regard to their pharmacokinetics. Consequently, fixed dose trials may imply the testing of a very wide range of plasma concentrations of the experimental drug. However, extrapolating an effective plasma level of the test drug from animal experiments may be very difficult.

Enzyme induction is another confounding factor when attempting to extrapolate the pharmacokinetics from healthy volunteers to patients. The majority of antiepileptic drugs exhibit enzyme induction to a greater or lesser extent. For this reason, the correlation between dose and plasma concentration may be quite different in healthy volunteers and in patients treated in polytherapy. This fact may of course have implications, with regard to both tolerability and efficacy. For this reason, it is usual to start out by performing uncontrolled and preliminary dose-ranging trials in a limited number of patients before embarking on formal controlled clinical studies (Gram et al 1983). At the same time important interactions may be discovered, which may have crucial implications for the planning of future controlled trials (Binnie et al 1986).

Clinical testing in children

Up to now, the general opinion has favoured postponing the testing of new antiepileptic compounds in children until they have been assessed in adults, i.e. Phase III. However, recently, for several reasons, this approach has been questioned. Children cannot simply be regarded as 'small adults'. In fact, from a drug-related point of view in many instances they behave quite differently compared to adults (Morselli et al 1983). In addition, they may suffer from a number of special seizure types or epileptic syndromes which are seldom or never found in adults. One example of this is infantile spasms (West syndrome). Therefore the lack of effect of a presumed antiepileptic compound in adults by no means precludes a potential effect in children. Consequently, there is an increasing realization that the clinical testing of potential antiepileptic compounds should start much earlier in children (Commission on Antiepileptic Drugs 1989). Recently, at an international level, a consensus with regard to this aspect has been reached (Dulac & Gram 1991).

CONCLUSION

The testing of putative antiepileptic compounds causes a number of highly complex theoretical, statistical, and practical clinical problems. This is due, among other things, to the fact that the frequency of epileptic seizures varies greatly both inter- and intraindividually. Further compounding this complexity, the seizure frequency for *each*

different seizure type within the same patient may vary greatly, ranging from seizure clusters to long periods in which the patient may be seizure free. No reliable methods for predicting the fluctuations in the course of the disease exist. In addition, studies in patients with epilepsy often require long observation periods in order to ensure that a sufficient number of seizures will be recorded to make statistical analysis meaningful. For these and other reasons clinical testing of new antiepileptic drugs should be performed only in clinical centres with specific experience in this field.

REFERENCES

Baker G A, Smith D F, Dewey M et al 1991 The development of a seizure severity scale as an outcome measure in epilepsy. Epilepsy Research 8: 245–251
Binnie C D, Emde Boas W, Kasteleijn-Nolste-Trenite D G A et al 1986 Acute effect of lamotrigine (BW 430 C) in persons with epilepsy. Epilepsia 27: 248–254
Commission on Antiepileptic Drugs 1989 Guidelines for clinical evaluation of antiepileptic drugs. Epilepsia 30: 400–406
Dulac O, Gram L 1991 International workshop in antiepileptic drug trials in children. A consensus report. Epilepsia 32:284–285
Duncan J S, Sander J W A S 1990 The Chalfont seizure severity scale. Acta Neurologica Scandinavica 82(Suppl 133): 31
Galton F 1885–6 Regression towards mediocrity in hereditary stature. Journal of Anthropological Institutes of Great Britain and Ireland 15: 246–263
Gram L, Bentsen K D, Parnas J, Flachs H 1982 Controlled trials in epilepsy: A review. Epilepsia 23: 491–519
Gram L, Lyon B B, Dam M 1983 Gamma-vinyl-GABA: A single-blind trial in patients with partial epilepsy. Acta Neurologica Scandinavica 68: 34–39
Group for the evaluation of cinromide in the Lennox–Gastaut syndrome 1989 Double-blind, placebo-controlled

evaluation of cinromide in patients with Lennox–Gastaut syndrome. Epilepsia 30: 422–429
Hopkins A, Daview P, Dobson C 1985 Mathematical model of patterns of seizures. Archives of Neurology 42: 463–467
Morselli P L, Pippenger C E, Penry J K 1983 Antiepileptic drug therapy in pediatrics. Raven Press, New York
Porter R J, Cereghino J J, Gladding G D et al 1984 Antiepileptic drug development program. Cleveland Clinical Journal of Medicine 51: 293–305
Riley T L, Porter J R, White B G, Penry J K 1981 The hospital experience and seizure control. Neurology 31: 912–915
Scoville B, White B, Cereghino J J, Porter R J 1981 Suitability and efficiency of cross-over drug trials in epilepsy. In: Dam M, Gram L, Penry J E (eds) Advances in epileptology: XII Epilepsy International Symposium. Raven Press, New York, p 113–122
Shofer J B, Temkin N R 1986 Comparison of alternative outcome measures for antiepileptic drug trials. Archives of Neurology 43: 877–881
Spilker B, Segreti A 1984 Validation of the phenomenon of regression of seizure frequency in epilepsy. Epilepsia 25: 443–449
White B G 1979 A class of ethical designs for controlled clinical trials. Doctoral dissertation. Johns Hopkins University, Baltimore

15. Clinical pharmacology and medical treatment

A. Richens   E. Perucca

INTRODUCTION

With the currently available drugs, approximately 80% of patients presenting with epilepsy will have their seizures controlled. This leaves a significant number of patients, particularly those with complex partial seizures or symptomatic epilepsy, who will continue to have seizures which will prove refractory to optimal drug therapy. Others will develop unacceptable acute or chronic adverse effects from their antiepileptic medication. Thus there is an urgent need for new antiepileptic drugs with greater efficacy and less toxicity.

Although we are still far from understanding completely the underlying neurochemical mechanisms of epilepsy or the mode of action of most of the antiepileptic drugs in use today, advances have been made in our understanding of central nervous system neurotransmitters and the pathophysiological changes underlying seizures (see Chs 13 and 8). Consequently, a more rational approach to the development of new antiepileptic drugs is evolving and we look forward to a time when the new drugs in use will specifically modify the abnormal mechanisms that cause seizures.

Nevertheless, we have learnt a great deal more about the presently available drugs and how to use them to better effect. Increased knowledge of antiepileptic drug pharmacokinetics has been invaluable and the use of serum drug concentration monitoring can be very useful for selected antiepileptic drugs. Because of our greater awareness of the hazards of polytherapy, in particular the risks of chronic drug toxicity and the dangers of drug interactions, monotherapy has become the general policy. No longer should a newly diagnosed patient presenting for the first time with seizures be immediately assigned to combination therapy.

However, there are still many unanswered questions about the natural history and optimal drug management of epilepsy, many of which are being currently investigated. When should drug treatment be started? How long should drugs be continued after a patient has been rendered seizure free? Does drug treatment really influence the natural history of epilepsy? Can we predict which patients will respond well to drug therapy? Which drugs are best for which seizure types? In time it is hoped that clear and definite guidelines will emerge so that a concensus on the best management of epilepsy will be achieved.

In this chapter we describe the principal drugs currently available to treat epilepsy and outline some general principles of management. In the last section we will describe some of the new drugs currently under assessment.

PART 1

PRINCIPAL DRUGS USED IN THE TREATMENT OF EPILEPSY

SODIUM VALPROATE

Sodium valproate is the sodium salt of valproic acid (dipropylacetic acid, 2-propylpentanoic acid or 2-propylvaleric acid). The acid itself, the magnesium salt and the amide are also marketed as antiepileptic drugs in some countries. It was first used to treat epileptic patients in 1964 and has been licensed for clinical use in the UK since

1973 and the USA since 1978 (limited indications only). Its structure and mode of action are described in Chapter 13.

Pharmacokinetics

These are summarized in Table 15.1. The reader is referred to Pinder et al (1977) and Gugler & von Unruh (1980) for a detailed account of the pharmacokinetics of sodium valproate.

Absorption

Sodium valproate has been shown to be completely absorbed following oral administration, with peak plasma concentrations of valproic acid occurring at 1 to 4 hours after ingestion of the plain tablets or syrup and at 4 to 8 hours after enteric-coated tablets. Absorption may be delayed if the drug is taken after a meal.

Distribution and plasma protein binding

The distribution of valproic acid is largely restricted to the extracellular water. Values for the apparent volume of distribution have been reported as 0.1–0.4 l/kg. Concentrations in brain and cerebrospinal fluid are much lower than plasma levels and appear to be related to the

Table 15.1 Summary of pharmacokinetic data on sodium valproate

Range of daily maintenance dosage	Adult: 500–3000 mg/day Child: 10–40 mg/kg/day
Time to peak serum level	1–4 h (plain tabs) 2–8 h (enteric-coated)
Oral absorption	>95%
Percentage bound to plasma proteins	Approx. 90% (see text)
Apparent volume of distribution	0.1–0.4 l/kg
Elimination half-life (adults)	9–21 h
Time to steady state after starting therapy	4 days
Major metabolites	β, ω and ω-1 oxidation products
Minimum dose frequency	Once daily

free drug concentration in plasma. In humans, the brain concentration has been shown to be 6.8–27.9% of plasma concentrations. At plasma levels within the accepted therapeutic range, valproic acid is highly bound (approximately 90%) to the plasma proteins, mainly albumin, but the binding is concentration dependent and the free fraction increases as total plasma valproate concentrations rise (Gugler et al 1980). This gives rise to a non-linear relationship between dose and serum level and affects the interpretation of total serum valproic acid concentrations during therapeutic drug monitoring (Gram et al 1980). Valproic acid binding is reduced by free fatty acids as well as in patients with hypoalbuminaemia, liver and renal disease (Gugler & Mueller 1978). Because of the drug's low pKa (4.95) it is secreted into saliva in small amounts which do not reflect the free plasma concentration.

Metabolism and excretion

Valproic acid is almost completely metabolized prior to excretion, only 1–3% of the ingested dose being excreted unchanged in the urine. Its metabolism is complex. The major elimination pathway is via conjugation with glucuronic acid (20–70%). The remainder is largely metabolized via oxidative pathways (β, ω and ω-1) particularly ω-oxidation. The 2-en metabolite of valproic acid possesses antiepileptic activity, although less than that of the parent compound. The clinical significance of this is uncertain but it has been calculated that the parent drug itself is responsible for more than 90% of the therapeutic effect.

Plasma half-life

The plasma half-life varies between 9 and 21 hours, with a mean of 12–13 hours. In patients who are taking other antiepileptic drugs, shorter values can be measured and this is the result of the induction of the oxidation of valproic acid. Because of the relatively short half-life, it is generally administered two to three times daily. However, there is evidence from animal and patient studies (Lockard & Levy 1976, Rowan et al 1979) that the antiepileptic effect may come on more slowly than would be predicted from the time to peak plasma concentration following a single dose, and that it may long outlast the presence of drug in the plasma. Thus, once-daily administration appears feasible and patient studies have shown that seizure control was at least as good with once-daily dose as with divided dosage (Covanis & Jeavons 1980).

Concentration–effect relationship

Because sodium valproate appears to have a prolonged pharmacological effect in epilepsy, with delayed onset of action and carry-over of effect, it would not be expected that measurements of plasma drug concentration would correlate closely with antiepileptic effect. A therapeutic range for seizure control of 350–700 μmol/1 (approximately 50–100 μg/ml) was first suggested by Schobben et al (1975) but many subsequent studies have failed to show such a relationship. Some of the toxic effects of valproic acid, such as tremor, appear to be related to plasma concentrations of the drug and are more common with levels greater than 700 μmol/1. Besides interindividual variations in serum valproic acid concentrations when patients are given the same dose there are large intraindividual fluctuations in the concentrations throughout the day depending on the frequency and time of drug administration. Thus, standardization of sampling times is necessary. Furthermore, the extent of protein binding is very variable due to concentration-dependent binding and the displacing effect of plasma free fatty acids, the level of which also varies. As it is the free drug concentration that is responsible for the therapeutic action, it would perhaps be more relevant to attempt to relate free valproate concentration to clinical effect.

Consequently, the value of therapeutic drug monitoring for valproate is doubtful.

Pharmacokinetics in special situations

The half-life of valproic acid is prolonged in neonates (20–67 hours) but falls rapidly in the first few months of life so that in older infants it reaches adult values. Placental transfer of valproate and its metabolites has been demonstrated with reports of higher concentrations in cord than in maternal blood. Small amounts of the drug are secreted into breast milk with levels reported as 0.17–5.4% of maternal plasma concentrations and therefore unlikely to affect the baby adversely (see Ch. 19). Doses of valproate in patients with renal disease should be reduced and valproate should be avoided in patients with liver disease.

Drug interactions

Unlike most of the other antiepileptic drugs in common use, sodium valproate does not induce hepatic metabolism but rather appears to act as a non-specific inhibitor of drug metabolism (Perucca et al 1979, 1980). Below are most of the significant interactions which have been documented so far.

Pharmacokinetic interactions

Effect of valproate on other drugs Serum phenobarbitone concentrations may increase when sodium valproate is introduced concurrently and result in excessive sedation. This interaction is thought to arise because of the inhibition of the metabolism of phenobarbitone by valproic acid resulting in a prolonged elimination half-life. The interaction between phenytoin and valproic acid is more complex. The latter drug displaces phenytoin from its binding site on albumin and also inhibits the metabolism of phenytoin, thus reducing its intrinsic clearance. This results in increased free levels of phenytoin and either decreased or unchanged total levels (Perucca et al 1980). Because of these conflicting effects on phenytoin kinetics, in some circumstances it may be necessary to measure free rather than total phenytoin concentrations in patients on phenytoin–valproate combination therapy. Valproic acid can also inhibit the metabolism of primidone but its effects on carbamazepine and ethosuximide kinetics are less consistent.

Effect of other drugs on valproate Several antiepileptic drugs can reduce serum concentrations of valproic acid by increasing the intrinsic clearance by enzyme induction. Such an interaction is seen with phenytoin, carbamazepine and phenobarbitone. Salicylates have been reported to displace valproic acid from plasma protein binding sites.

Pharmacodynamic interactions

Sodium valproate may enhance the effects of central nervous system depressants including ethanol.

Adverse drug reactions (Turnbull 1983)

The incidence of adverse effects with sodium valproate is difficult to gauge exactly because many patients are on polytherapy and the method of determining side effects varies between studies. Schmidt (1984b) estimated the incidence of adverse reactions based on analysis of 16 trials on a total of 1140 patients as 26%, but in only 2% were problems so severe that discontinuation of valproate therapy was necessary.

Gastrointestinal disorders

Recognized problems include anorexia, nausea, vomiting, dyspepsia, diarrhoea and constipation. The incidence of gastrointestinal adverse reactions is reduced by use of the enteric-coated preparation. They may also be minimized by starting valproate in a low dose and gradually increasing it, and by taking the drug with food and in divided doses. Pancreatitis has occasionally been reported in association with valproate therapy and rare deaths have occurred.

Weight gain

An increase in weight is a recognized problem with sodium valproate; the reason is uncertain.

Skin and hair

Rashes are a rare occurrence with valproate but reversible hair loss occurs quite frequently with a reported incidence between 2.6 and 12% Occasionally the hair regrows curly.

Haematological disorders

Thrombocytopenia and bruising may occur during therapy with valproate. There have also been reports of abnormal platelet function.

Neurological

Tremor is a well-recognized adverse effect of sodium valproate. It is usually of the benign essential type and is probably dose related and reversible. Reports on the effects of sodium valproate on cognitive function conflict, probably due to difficulty in interpretation when patients are on multiple drug therapy and have variable seizure frequency. In normal volunteers, impairment in decision making was found but the adverse effects were much less than with phenytoin.

Hepatotoxicity

Severe hepatotoxicity, occasionally with a fatal outcome is a rare adverse effect of valproate. It appears to be due to an idiosyncratic reaction and usually occurs during the first 6 months of treatment. Most of the reported cases have occurred in children and many had already been noted to have developmental delay or associated neurological disease. Most were taking other enzyme-inducing drugs and in some cases the causative role of sodium valproate was not clear cut. It is possible that the 4-en metabolite of valproic acid is responsible, perhaps interacting with an intrinsic metabolic abnormality in some patients. The incidence of liver toxicity is low, approximately one in 50 000, but the risk increases when treating children with severe epilepsy, progressive neurological disease and taking multiple drug therapy. Asymptomatic elevations of hepatic transaminases are not uncommonly found and usually respond to dose reduction.

Hyperammonaemia

Valproate may cause various metabolic disturbances because it inhibits several enzymes involved in intermediary cell metabolism (Kay et al 1986). Moderate asymptomatic elevations in blood ammonia levels are common during valproate therapy, but in a few cases encephalopathy has resulted, occasionally with fatal outcome.

Teratogenicity

Sodium valproate has been shown to be teratogenic in animals and reports of abnormalities in the offspring of epileptic mothers taking sodium valproate have been published (see Ch. 19). Spina bifida is the most common abnormality and occurs in about 1% of babies born to mothers taking valproate.

Indications for the use of sodium valproate

Sodium valproate has a broad spectrum of antiepileptic effects. It is very effective therapy for absence seizures, with success rates approaching 100% in uncomplicated previously untreated absence seizures. Valproate is comparable with phenytoin and carbamazepine in the control of tonic-clonic seizures and is the drug of choice in patients with photosensitive epilepsy. It may also be beneficial in the treatment of myclonic seizures. Although sodium valproate is less effective for the treatment of partial seizures than it is in primary generalized seizures, it appears to be as effective as phenytoin or carbamazepine. Valproate has also been shown to be effective for the prophylaxis of febrile convulsions. It is unsuitable for use in status epilepticus because its onset of action occurs several hours after administration.

CARBAMAZEPINE

Carbamazepine was developed in the late 1950s and its anticonvulsant properties were demonstrated in animals in 1963. Over the last 20 years it has been used extensively as an antiepileptic drug. It is an iminostilbene derivative and is closely related structurally to the tricyclic antidepressant drug imipramine. Its structure and mode of action are described in Chapter 13.

Pharmacokinetics

These are summarized in Table 15.2. The reader is referred to Pynnönen (1979) for a general review of the pharmacokinetics of carbamazepine.

Absorption

Carbamazepine is absorbed slowly and erratically

Table 15.2 Summary of pharmacokinetic data on carbamazepine

Range of daily maintenance dosage	Adult: 400–1800 mg/day Child: 10–30 mg/kg/day
Time to peak serum level	4–8 h (but may be delayed up to 24 h)
Percentage bound to plasma proteins	75%
Apparent volume of distribution	1.2 l/kg
Elimination half-life	Single doses: 20–55 h After chronic therapy: 10–30 h (adults) 8–20 h (children)
Time to steady state after starting therapy	Up to 10 days (but subsequent fall may occur due to autoinduction)
Major metabolite (active)	10, 11-epoxide
Others:	Dihydrodiol Hydroxy-metabolites Iminostilbene
Minimum dose frequency	Adult: twice daily Child: twice daily

after oral administration. Absorption is inversely dependent on dose and may be enhanced by giving the drug with food (Levy et al 1975). Because of the lack of an intravenous formulation, the absolute bioavailability of carbamazepine in humans is not known precisely, but is probably of the order of 75–85%. Slow-release formulations may have a slightly lower bioavailability than conventional release.

Distribution and plasma protein binding

Carbamazepine is highly lipid soluble and it distributes rapidly to tissues. The apparent volume of distribution has been calculated as 0.8–2.0 l/kg by various workers. The plasma protein binding of carbamazepine is 70–80% and of the epoxide metabolite is 48–53%. The interindividual variation in carbamazepine plasma protein binding is small and is unlikely to be of clinical importance due to the fairly high free fraction under normal conditions. Other antiepileptic drugs do not appear to influence carbamazepine binding. Concentrations of carbamazepine in the brain are similar to those in plasma, as are those of carbamazepine epoxide. Cerebrospinal fluid carbamazepine concentrations are between 17% and 31% of those in plasma. Saliva concentrations of carbamazepine and the epoxide also reflect the free fraction of the drug in plasma and measurement of saliva drug concentrations has been used for monitoring of free plasma concentrations (Chambers et al 1977).

Metabolism and excretion

Carbamazepine is largely metabolized into a stable epoxide metabolite, carbamazepine 10,11-epoxide, which is pharmacologically active (Bertilsson & Tomson 1986). It is further metabolized to hydroxy-derivatives which are excreted in the urine. Only about 2% of the drug is excreted unchanged in the urine.

Carbamazepine exhibits dose-independent kinetics. The plasma half-life may be up to 55 hours after a single dose of carbamazepine but following repeated treatment the half-life decreases to between 5 and 24 hours. This is due to 'auto-induction' of the hepatic microsomal enzyme systems and leads to what is known as 'time-dependent kinetics'. As the clearance of carbamazepine increases during chronic therapy, increases in dose of the drug are required to maintain the same plasma carbamazepine level. It takes 3 to 4 weeks for maximal autoinduction to occur. Autoinduction of carbamazepine metabolism seems to accelerate preferentially the elimination reaction of the epoxide by increasing the production of the dihydroxide. The metabolism of carbamazepine is also induced by other antiepileptic drugs, such as phenytoin. Thus the dose of carbamazepine required by epileptic patients who are already taking enzyme-inducing antiepileptic drugs is higher than in drug naive patients (Cereghino et al 1975). Heteroinduction by other drugs preferentially induces the formation of the epoxide rather than its subsequent oxidative product. Reported plasma half-lives for the carbamazepine 10,11-epoxide range from 3 to 23 hours.

Dose–serum concentration relationship

There is little correlation between dose of carbamazepine and serum concentration when blood samples from different patients are analysed. In addition to the usual variation in the rate of metabolism between individuals, there are two other probable reasons for this: the variable bioavailability of the drug; and autoinduction of metabolism. When carbamazepine is given with other drugs, such as phenytoin, phenobarbitone and primidone, heteroinduction of carbamazepine metabolism complicates the picture further. Levels of the 10,11-epoxide also vary widely between individuals. The serum concentration of the epoxide in adults is reported as between 15 and 55% of the concentration of unchanged drug and may be higher in children (Bertilsson & Tomson 1986). The ratio of epoxide to carbamazepine also varies according to the co-medication, being higher in patients on other enzyme-inducing antiepileptic drugs. There is a cross reaction on enzyme immunoassay testing between carbamazepine itself and the epoxide. This interference is probably not a problem for routine plasma determinations, but immunoassay methods may overestimate carbamazepine concentrations in cerebrospinal fluid or saliva due to a relatively higher proportion of epoxide in these fluids.

Concentration–effect relationship

A relationship between serum concentration and antiepileptic efficacy has been demonstrated for carbamazepine (Sillanpää et al 1979). The commonly quoted therapeutic range is 20–40 μmol/l (approximately 5–10 μg/ml) although patients with mild epilepsy may be controlled with much lower levels. Adverse effects do not usually occur until serum levels reach 40–50 μmol/l (9.5–12 μg/ml). Although the 10,11-epoxide possesses antiepileptic activity in animals equivalent to that of the parent drug itself, its antiepileptic potency in humans is uncertain. However, it probably contributes to the overall pharmacological effects of carbamazepine, particularly when allowance is made for its lower degree of plasma protein binding. In children, its relative concentration in plasma can be much higher and its contribution may therefore be greater. There is, however, insufficient data as yet to justify routine measurement of the epoxide metabolite during therapeutic drug monitoring. In children, measurement of saliva concentrations of carbamazepine may be preferable to serum level monitoring. These correlate closely (Chambers et al 1977).

Dose interval

With half-life values of 10–30 hours after chronic dosing in the adult, twice-daily dosing is appropriate. Johannessen et al (1977) showed that the variation is serum level with twice-daily dosing is about 50% of the mean value. However, with large total daily doses in some patients, adverse effects may occur 2–4 hours after drug administration and it may then be necessary to divide the total daily dose into three or more divided doses to avoid high peak serum concentrations or to give a slow-release formulation.

Pharmacokinetics in special situations

In neonates whose mothers take carbamazepine during pregnancy, placental transfer of carbamazepine occurs, resulting in fetal enzyme induction in utero. Thus, clearance of the drug in such neonates may be similar to adults. In children, carbamazepine metabolism is greater than in adults and the epoxide:carbamazepine ratio is significantly higher (Rane et al 1976). The plasma protein binding of carbamazepine in children may be lower than in adults. In pregnancy, there is evidence of increased metabolism of carbamazepine resulting in lower carbamazepine levels but higher epoxide levels (Battino et al 1985). Although carbamazepine binding may be reduced by liver or renal disease, an increased toxicity of the drug due to this mechanism is unlikely. Severe liver disease may also be associated with reduced metabolism of carbamazepine.

Drug interactions

Most of the documented interactions are pharmacokinetic (Perucca & Richens 1980, 1985).

Effect of carbamazepine on other drugs

Carbamazepine can induce the metabolism of other drugs given concomitantly, including other antiepileptic drugs such as sodium valproate, ethosuximide, phenytoin and clonazepam and other medications, such as warfarin and the oral contraceptive steroids.

Effect of other drugs on carbamazepine

Levels of carbamazepine are significantly lowered when phenytoin, phenobarbitone or primidone are added to carbamazepine therapy, but the ratio of the 10,11-epoxide to parent drug may be increased. Enzyme-inhibiting drugs, such as cimetidine, propoxyphene and verapamil, can elevate carbamazepine levels. Protein binding interactions do not appear to be important for carbamazepine.

Adverse drug reactions with carbamazepine

Adverse effects occur in approximately one-third of patients treated and are more frequent in patients on polytherapy. In 5%, withdrawal of carbamazepine is necessary. Carbamazepine causes various dose-related neuropsychiatric adverse drug reactions including alteration in mental function and impaired co-ordination. The more serious idiosyncratic side-effects, including toxic hepatitis and blood dyscrasias, are exceedingly rare. Experience with carbamazepine over recent years has confirmed its relatively low toxicity.

Neuropsychiatric

The most common dose-related adverse effects of carbamazepine are those that affect co-ordination and they usually consist of a disturbance of eye movements resulting in dizziness, blurred vision and diplopia, or a disturbance of balance causing ataxia. Other more complex eye movement disturbances are seen more rarely. Such dose-related side-effects often occur early on in the course of treatment and are transient. If the starting dose of carbamazepine is small and the dose is increased gradually there are usually fewer problems. It is not unusual for patients to complain of intermittent side effects, often occurring between 2 and 4 hours after a dose and coinciding with peak serum carbamazepine concentrations. This is due to the fluctuations in plasma levels which occur during the dosing intervals, and these fluctuations are greater when other antiepileptic drugs are taken concomitantly. It can be managed by administering the drug in three or four divided doses or administering a slow-release formulation. If very high serum carbamazepine levels occur, for example after acute overdose, enhancement of seizures may occur.

Carbamazepine appears to have relatively less adverse effect on mental functioning than some of the other antiepileptic drugs. The reported incidence of neurotoxicity varies considerably, but there are no published reports of irreversible neurological toxicity. In volunteers, deficits in association with carbamazepine occurred in relation to motor rather than mental speed and in one task measuring processing speed and perceptual registration the administration of carbamazepine was associated with a significant improvement in performance (Thompson et al 1981). In studies of epileptic patients where medication was altered by reducing the number of different antiepileptic drugs prescribed, and in some cases subsituting carbamazepine for the original medication, improvement in the performance of psychological tests was recorded (Thompson & Trimble 1982). Those patients who changed to carbamazepine, either alone or in combination with existing treatment, displayed more widespread improvements in test performance particularly on measures of memory. It was not clear whether these improvements were due to withdrawal of polytherapy, better seizure control or an independent beneficial effect of carbamazepine on psychomotor performance.

Dyskinesias and asterixis have been reported to occur and psychoses can be provoked by carbamazepine. There is no evidence to incriminate carbamazepine in the development of peripheral neuropathy (Shorvon & Reynolds 1982).

Haematological disorders

Adverse haematological reactions to carbamazepine are very rare but are potentially serious (Pisciotta 1982). They include bone marrow depression in the form of leucopenia, anaemia and thrombocytopenia, and more rarely proliferative effects such as eosinophilia and leucocytosis. The incidence of aplastic anaemia has been estimated at 0.5/100 000/year. It has been observed more often in patients being treated with carbamazepine for trigeminal neuralgia than for epilepsy. Haematological disturbances other than agranulocytosis and aplastic anaemia are almost always reversible. Transient leucopenia occurs in about 10% of patients, usually in the first month of therapy. More substantial persistent leucopenia is rare and responds to discontinuation of carbamazepine (Hart & Easton 1981).

Gastrointestinal disturbances

Gastrointestinal disturbances during carbamazepine therapy are mostly found in the first few weeks of treatment. They include anorexia, nausea and vomiting.

Hepatic disturbances

Hepatic toxicity has been reported in association with carbamazepine therapy but is a very rare occurrence: 21 cases reported in the literature during the first 20 years of use. Mostly, symptoms occurred within the first month of therapy, which suggests a hypersensitivity reaction. On withdrawal of the drug most patients recovered.

Skin reactions

The incidence of skin reactions with carbamazepine is at least 3%, although some studies have found a higher rate of skin reactions which may have been related to higher initial dose of the drug (Chadwick et al 1984). Most occur early in the course of treatment. Many of the skin rashes are mild maculopapular, morbilliform, urticarial or vesicular eruptions which do not necessitate cessation of the drug. Less frequently, exfoliative dermatitis may occur and this type of reaction necessitates discontinuation of carbamazepine. Reversible alopecia has also been reported.

Endocrine disturbances

Hyponatraemia and low plasma osmolality may occur in patients receiving carbamazepine

(Perucca et al 1978). The mechanism of this effect is not clear. There is some evidence of increased release of antidiuretic hormone from the posterior pituitary gland, but other investigators have suggested that there is increased renal sensitivity to normal plasma concentrations of antidiuretic hormone. Hyponatraemia may result in weight gain, oedema, irritability and loss of seizure control. Carbamazepine can reduce circulating throxine concentration, probably by a mixture of central and peripheral effects, but clinical hypothyroidism is rare. Carbamazepine therapy has been associated with changes in circulating androgens and exaggerated luteinizing hormone (LH) responses to gonadotrophin-releasing hormone consistent with enhanced sex hormone metabolism due to hepatic enzyme induction (Richens 1984). Induction of hepatic metabolism by carbamazepine leads to reduced levels of exogenous contraceptive hormones and may result in oral contraceptive pill failure (see Ch. 19).

Biochemical features of osteomalacia have been found in patients on carbamazepine but without clinical evidence of bone disease (Hahn 1976).

Teratogenicity

There is little evidence from animal studies to implicate carbamazepine as a teratogen but recent clinical studies have shown a higher incidence of craniofacial defects and spina bifida in the offspring of carbamazepine-treated mothers (Jones et al 1989). The possibility of the epoxide metabolite possessing teratogenic potential has been raised, based on the observation of a high rate of congenital abnormalities after prenatal exposure to certain combinations of antiepileptic drugs which result in accumulation of the epoxide (Lindhout et al 1984).

Indications for the use of carbamazepine

Carbamazepine is an effective drug in the control of partial and tonic-clonic seizures but has no therapeutic effect in absence seizures.

PHENYTOIN

Phenytoin (5,5-diphenylhydantoin) was first iden-tified as an antiepileptic drug in 1938, and since then has been extensively used. Of the various antiepileptic drugs in common use, phenytoin has been studied in greatest depth because it is the most widely used, is relatively easy to measure in serum and has some interesting pharmacokinetic properties which are responsible for the wide variation in response to the drug. The structure and mode of action of phenytoin are described in Chapter 13.

Pharmacokinetics

These are summarized in Table 15.3. The reader is referred to Richens (1979) for a detailed review of the pharmacokinetics of phenytoin.

Absorption

The acid form of phenytoin is poorly soluble in water but the sodium salt is much more soluble. The acid, unless in the microcrystalline form, is poorly and erratically absorbed, whereas the sodium salt which is macrocrystalline in form is reliably absorbed. The excipient in a formulation may influence bioavailability by altering the rate of deaggregation of the particles. In Australasia in 1968, an outbreak of phenytoin intoxication occurred when the manufacturers of Dilantin capsules changed the excipient from hydrated

Table 15.3 Summary of pharmacokinetic data for phenytoin

Range of daily maintenance dose	Adult: 15–600 mg/day Child: 5–15 mg/kg/day
Minimum dose frequency	Adult: once daily Child: twice daily
Time to peak serum level	4–12 h (oral) Many hours (intramuscular)
Percentage bound to plasma proteins	85–90%
Apparent volume of distribution	0.45 l/kg
Elimination half-life in adults	9–140 h (saturation kinetics)
Time to steady state after starting therapy	7–21 days
Major metabolite	5-(p-hydroxyphenyl)-5-phenylhydantoin (inactive)

calcium sulphate to lactose, which resulted in an unexpected increase in bioavailability (Tyrer et al 1970). Elsewhere, similar problems have arisen with inequivalence between the various marketed preparations and this should be borne in mind if substitution of one formulation for another is contemplated. In the UK and USA a chewable microcrystalline tablet formulation for paediatric use (Epanutin Infatabs) appears to be better absorbed than standard tablets (Stewart et al 1975). However, Infatabs contain 50 mg of phenytoin acid, which is equivalent to 54 mg of the sodium salt contained in standard tablets and capsules.

Parenteral preparations of phenytoin should not be given intramuscularly because crystals of drug precipitate and phenytoin is very poorly and unreliably absorbed by this route (Wilensky & Lowden 1973). Also considerable muscle damage may occur (Serrano & Wilder 1974). The serum concentrations produced by intramuscular administration may be inadequate and a change from oral to intramuscular administration to cover, for instance, an abdominal operation, may cause seizures. On the other hand, rebound intoxication may occur on resumption of the oral therapy because considerable quantities of drug remain in the tissues to be absorbed (Wilder & Ramsay 1976). Thus it is more satisfactory to give phenytoin by intravenous infusion (into a saline drip) in a single daily dose when oral administration is not possible for a short period.

Distribution and plasma protein binding

Phenytoin is approximately 90% bound to plasma proteins in adults (Porter & Layzer 1975). The binding is mainly to albumin, but there are also secondary low affinity sites on other proteins. Although there is controversy over the degree of intersubject variation in protein binding, it would appear that in most epileptic patients, who do not have a medical condition known to alter drug protein binding and are not taking concurrent drugs which interfere with phenytoin binding, the amount of variability in protein binding is very small. However, hypoalbuminaemia reduces protein binding as do liver and renal disease (see below). Only the free (unbound) drug is available to produce a pharmacological effect at the site of

action and, therefore, ideally it would be more relevant to measure free drug concentrations in serum as a therapeutic guide. However, the currently available methods for doing this are too time consuming and costly. Thus routine measurement of free serum phenytoin concentrations is not indicated. An alternative approach is to measure saliva phenytoin concentration, which is closely related to free drug concentration in serum. The salivary glands act as a simple dialysis membrane across which free drug molecules are able to diffuse and equilibrate (Paxton et al 1977). There are methodological difficulties to this technique and it is necessary to take precautions to avoid direct contamination of the saliva by the oral formulation.

Phenytoin diffuses rapidly into the tissues including the brain. Following intravenous administration the distribution phase lasts about 2 hours. Brain binding is of the same order of magnitude as protein binding in serum and thus brain concentrations are very similar to serum concentrations (Houghton et al 1975b). Penetration into brain tissue is rapid and this explains the efficacy of phenytoin in the treatment of status epilepticus (Wilder et al 1977). Cerebrospinal fluid concentrations mirror serum free drug concentrations.

Metabolism and excretion

Phenytoin is extensively metabolized by hydroxylase enzymes in the liver and less than 5% appears unchanged in the urine. The rate of hepatic metabolism is under genetic control and varies between individuals (Richens 1979). There is a continuous unimodal distribution of rates of metabolism, with very slow and very fast metabolizers at the extreme ends of the distribution but there is a small subgroup of slow metabolizers in whom a dominant gene may be responsible for their phenotype. Race may also be an important determinant of the rate of metabolism as Negroes metabolize phenytoin more slowly than Caucasians.

The major metabolite of phenytoin is 5-p-hydroxyphenyl-5-phenylhydantoin (p-HPPH) which is pharmacologically inactive. This is conjugated to glucuronide and excreted in the urine. The conversion of phenytoin to this metabolite by liver microsomal enzymes is saturable within the therapeutic range of serum concentrations, i.e. the liver is unable to increase its rate of metabolism proportionately as the drug serum concentration rises (Richens 1979). Instead, it moves towards a situation in which a fixed amount of drug is removed regardless of increases in the serum level (zero order kinetics). The ratio of metabolite to parent drug is influenced both by genetic differences in drug metabolism and by steady state serum concentrations of parent drug. As the latter rises, the hydroxylation mechanism becomes saturated and p-HPPH production fails to rise in proportion, and relatively more parent drug appears in the urine (Houghton & Richens 1974). p-HPPH appears to be actively excreted by the renal tubules as its renal clearance exceeds the glomerular filtration rate.

Plasma half-life and dose interval

The effective plasma half-life of phenytoin gradually lengthens as the steady-state concentration rises as a result of the saturable nature of its metabolism (Richens 1979). On average, the effective half-life at very low serum concentrations is about 13 hours, but this lengthens to 46 hours when the steady-state concentration reaches the top of the therapeutic range. The time to steady state (approximately equal to five half-lives) depends upon the dose and the final concentration reached, and may be as long as 2 weeks or more in a patient given a dose yielding a high therapeutic or toxic concentration. Similarly, the rate of elimination of phenytoin on discontinuing therapy may be much slower than expected, particularly in a patient who started with toxic serum concentrations.

Also, the fluctuations in serum concentrations may be less than expected. The higher the steady-state serum concentration, the smaller (in percentage terms) is the fluctuation in serum concentration. The degree of fluctuation in serum levels throughout 24 hours is quite acceptable for clinical purposes and therefore once-daily dosage in adults is compatible with effective control of seizures. However, in children twice-daily dosing is preferable because the serum half-life of phenytoin is shorter. If a more immediate

therapeutic effect is required a loading dose may be administered (Wilder et al 1973), but such dosing schedules may be associated with a higher incidence of adverse effects. When intravenous administration for the treatment of status epilepticus is needed a dose of 10–15 mg/kg body weight given over 5–10 min will lead to plasma levels of 40–80 μmol/l (10–20 μg/ml).

Dose–serum concentration relationship

As a consequence of the great variability in rate of phenytoin metabolism between individuals, the steady state serum concentrations achieved with a given dose of phenytoin will vary greatly. A dose of 200 mg/day of phenytoin may be enough to produce a therapeutic concentration in one adult patient, while another may require in excess of 500 mg/day. Although age, sex and body weight influence the dose–serum concentration relationship, in adults the relative contribution of each is fairly small (Houghton et al 1975a). Body surface area correlates most strongly with dose requirements in adult patients.

In children, body size becomes a major determinant of dose. The dose/kg of body weight required to produce a given serum concentration increases as body weight falls. Although dosing related to body surface area is the most reliable guide in practice, it is usually satisfactory to dose according to body weight (Table 15.4). However, because there is such a wide interindividual variation in serum levels produced by a given dose of

Table 15.4 Starting doses of phenytoin in children and infants. The doses have been chosen to produce an average serum concentration of 40 μmol/l (10 μg/ml)

Body weight kg	Phenytoin dose mg/kg/day	mg/day*
6–10	10.0	100
11–15	9.0	125
16–20	8.0	150
21–25	7.0	175
26–30	6.5	200
31–35	5.5	200
36–40	5.5	225
41–45	5.5	250
46–50	5.0	250
51–60	5.0	300

* Doses rounded off to suit 25 mg dose units.

phenytoin, the doses suggested will give levels that are too low in some and toxic in a few.

The saturable nature of phenytoin metabolism is of considerable practical importance because it leads to a non-linear relationship between dose and serum level in each patient (Richens & Dunlop 1975). Figure 15.1 illustrates the relationship between phenytoin dose and serum level in five patients in whom steady-state concentrations were measured at several different doses. In patient PH, an increment of only 55 mg would carry the serum level from the lower limit to the upper limit of the therapeutic range. Thus, on a dose of 200 mg daily, the serum level is below the therapeutic range, yet on a daily dose of 300 mg the level is above the range and could be causing symptoms of toxicity. The same pattern is seen in each patient although the dose range yielding a therapeutic level varies considerably, presumably because of genetic differences in the rate of hydroxylation in the liver. The steepness of the dose–serum level relationship within the therapeutic range is important in a number of ways:

1. If phenytoin therapy is regulated by monitoring serum levels, increments in dose should be limited to 50 mg or less once the level comes close to the lower end of the therapeutic range
2. Monitoring serum phenytoin levels is essential if the dose is to be correctly tailored
3. A small increase in the bioavailability of the drug will readily increase a therapeutic level to a toxic one
4. The effects of drug interactions will be exaggerated. Addition of a second drug which either inhibits or induces phenytoin metabolism will produce a disproportionate change in phenytoin level.

These practical problems make phenytoin therapy difficult to manage. In order to assist the prescriber in achieving levels within the therapeutic range, various schemes have been designed to assist dosage adjustment (Flint et al 1985). Each demands at least one measurement of phenytoin serum concentration, from which a prediction can

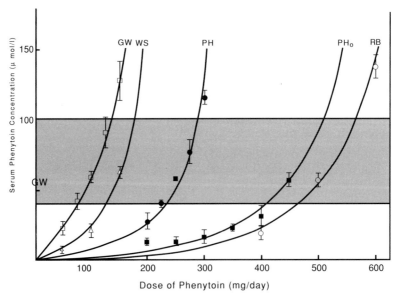

Fig. 15.1 Relationship between phenytoin dose and serum level in five patients whose steady-state concentrations were measured at several different doses. Each point represents the mean ± S D of 3–8 separate estimations of the serum level. The curves were fitted by computer using the Michaelis–Menten equation. The stippled area indicates the 'therapeutic range' of serum levels but is more generous than the usually quoted 40–80 μmol/l (N.B. 4 μmol/l = 1 μg/ml). Reproduced from Richens & Dunlop 1975, by kind permission of the editor.

be made of the increment in dose necessary to increase the level into the therapeutic range. The methods requiring two known doses and plasma concentrations are more accurate than those requiring only one, but no method is sufficiently precise to substitute for confirmatory serum phenytoin concentrations.

Concentration–effect relationship

In view of the great variability between individuals in phenytoin kinetics and the narrow therapeutic ratio of the drug, the case for monitoring serum levels of phenytoin is well established. Buchthal et al (1960) were the first to attempt to define a therapeutic range of serum concentrations of phenytoin. In a prospective study in 12 hospitalized patients with frequent fits, they found no

clinical response until the serum concentration exceeded 40 μmol/l (10 μg/ml). As clinical signs of toxicity were frequently encountered with levels above 80 μmol/l (20 μg/ml) they considered that a therapeutic range of 40–80 μmol/l (10–20 μg/ml) would give optimal control of fits without toxicity. This view was reiterated by Kutt & McDowell (1968) and this range has been widely used in the management of phenytoin therapy. In order to re-examine this point Lund (1974) set up a 3-year prospective study in 32 patients with grand mal seizures. The patients were selected because they had at least one seizure during a 2-month control period. An inverse relationship between seizure frequency and plasma phenytoin was seen (Fig. 15.2). Although the improvement in control was independent of the type of seizures, the optimal phenytoin level for each patient was depend-

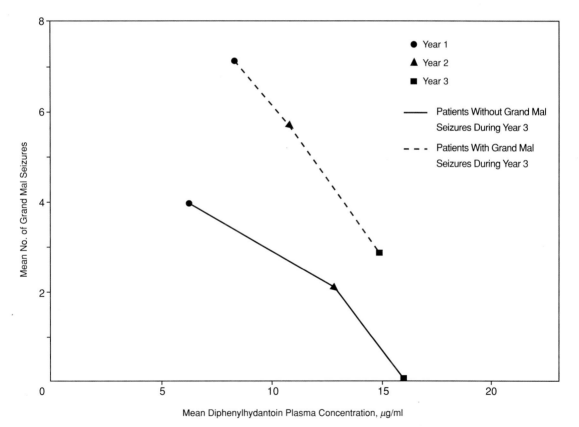

Fig. 15.2 Reduction in mean tonic-clonic (grand mal) seizure frequency in 32 patients studied prospectively by Lund (1974). Phenytoin (diphenylhydantoin) dose was increased over a 3-year period in order to achieve plasma concentrations within the therapeutic range of 10–20 μg/ml (40–80 μmol/l). A dose-related reduction in seizure frequency was seen regardless of whether the patients were seizure free at the end of the study. Reproduced with permission from Lund 1974.

ent on the severity of the epilepsy (Fig. 15.2). This last observation is important because it suggests that many patients with mild epilepsy may be controlled with serum levels below the therapeutic range suggested by Buchthal et al (1960).

Further studies of therapeutic ranges of phenytoin serum concentrations (Gannaway & Mawer 1981, Schmidt & Haenel 1984, Turnbull et al 1984) have emphasized that the efficacy of serum phenytoin concentrations varies not only between patients, but also with the type of seizure within an individual patient. The variation in therapeutic plasma concentration appears to be primarily related to the type and severity of the individual patient's epilepsy. Thus the concept of the lower limit of the therapeutic range of phenytoin concentrations of 40 μmol/l (10 μg/ml) should probably be abandoned. There is general agreement that clinical signs of phenytoin intoxication become more frequent when the serum level rises to between 80 and 120 μmol/l (20–30 μg/ml) but the absolute incidence of toxic effects at a particular concentration varies considerably from one report to another, partly depending on the clinician's criteria for intoxication. However, the rigid use of an upper limit to the therapeutic range is unnecessary and may deny some patients the benefit of extra therapeutic effect without the occurrence of toxicity. The quoted therapeutic range for phenytoin should be used as a guide to dosage adjustment but should not be a substitute for clinical judgement.

Pharmacokinetics in special situations

In neonates who have not been exposed to enzyme-inducing drugs in utero, the metabolism of most drugs will be very slow at birth (Morselli 1977). During the first few months of life, the enzyme systems mature and are capable of metabolizing antiepileptic drugs much faster than in the adult (Blain et al 1981). During childhood the rate of metabolism gradually slows until it reaches adult levels. In neonates who have been exposed to enzyme-inducing drugs such as phenytoin in utero, the half-life of transplacentally transferred phenytoin has been shown to be 6.6 to 34 hours. The plasma protein binding of phenytoin is also lower in neonates. Serum antiepileptic drug levels

tend to fall progressively throughout pregnancy due to an increased metabolic capacity of the maternal liver, the development of drug metabolizing activity in the fetal liver and a reduction in plasma protein binding of drugs (see Ch. 19). Only small quantities of phenytoin are excreted in breast milk. Disease states can alter phenytoin kinetics. Hypoalbuminaemia causes a decrease in the plasma protein binding of phenytoin which can result in drug toxicity appearing at apparently therapeutic serum levels. The plasma protein binding of phenytoin is also reduced in cirrhosis, and hepatocellular diseases can reduce the systemic metabolism (Blaschke 1977). In renal disease the binding of phenytoin to serum albumin is reduced, partly because of hypoalbuminaemia but also more importantly because of the presence of endogenous inhibitors of phenytoin binding (Reidenberg & Drayer 1978).

Drug interactions

Pharmacokinetic

Numerous interactions between phenytoin and other drugs have been described (Perucca & Richens 1980, 1985). Most of these are pharmacokinetic and many occur because of the enzyme-inducing effects of phenytoin.

Effect of phenytoin on other drugs Phenytoin itself is a potent inducer of hepatic microsomal drug metabolizing enzyme activity and this is probably the mechanism responsible for reducing the plasma concentrations or the therapeutic effect of oral anticoagulants, oral contraceptive steroids, carbamazepine, benzodiazepines and other drugs (Perucca 1978).

The effect of other drugs on phenytoin The steep dose–serum concentration relationship and narrow therapeutic ratio of phenytoin makes drug interactions which alter phenytoin serum concentration very important; in particular, those in which phenytoin metabolism is inhibited resulting in elevation of the serum level. Phenytoin is a poor substrate for drug metabolizing enzymes and inhibition of metabolism is relatively common when phenytoin-treated patients are exposed to other drugs, including sulthiame, pheneturide, chloramphenicol, propoxyphene and isoniazid.

Reduction of serum phenytoin concentrations by enzyme induction have been reported with carbamazepine co-medication and chronic ethanol intake. There are, however, conflicting reports on the effect of phenobarbitone on phenytoin metabolism. As phenytoin is highly protein bound, it is also susceptible to displacement from protein binding sites by drugs such as sodium valproate and salicylic acid (Perucca et al 1980). This will result in a fall in protein binding and in a higher free fraction of phenytoin. In the case of valproic acid, which also inhibits the metabolism of phenytoin, the interaction is very complex and results in a higher free phenytoin concentration but a lower total phenytoin concentration than prior to addition of valproate to therapy.

Pharmacodynamic

Interactions between drugs at their site of action in the tissues are termed 'pharmacodynamic interactions'. Combination drug therapy for epilepsy increases the incidence of central nervous system adverse effects, such as drowsiness and inco-ordination.

Adverse drug reactions

The acute dose-dependent adverse effects of phenytoin consist of vertigo, tremor, ataxia, dysarthria, diplopia, nystagmus and headache (Kutt et al 1964). Severe side effects are rare at serum phenytoin levels below 120 μmol/l (30 μg/ml) but great individual variation occurs and some patients experience adverse effects with levels within the therapeutic range while others do not develop toxic reactions with serum levels well above this range.

Peripheral and central nervous system

Several studies in both volunteers and epileptic patients have shown a negative effect of phenytoin on cognitive function although this effect is potentially reversible. In a study by Thompson et al (1981) phenytoin was shown acutely to impair performance of volunteer subjects significantly, compared with placebo, in tests of memory, concentration, mental and motor speed. These neuropsychological impairments seem to be associated with high serum drug levels (Thompson & Trimble 1983). More severe toxic effects of phenytoin on mental function can result in a reversible confused state which has been referred to as encephalopathy, delirium or psychosis. Intellectual deterioration, depression, impairment of drive, initiative and psychomotor slowing are common findings. These changes may develop subacutely or chronically, usually in association with high serum phenytoin concentrations and may be unaccompanied by other signs of phenytoin toxicity, such as nystagmus or ataxia. Occasionally, unusual neurological signs such as dyskinesias have been noted. Such encephalopathy seems more common in children.

Although it is well known that acute toxicity with phenytoin can lead to a reversible cerebellar syndrome, there has been some controversy as to whether permanent pathological or clinical changes can occur (Alcala et al 1978). Seizures themselves can cause loss of Purkinje cells but it appears that the drugs may be responsible in many cases for permanent cerebellar syndromes. Such long-term damage may occur more often in brain-damaged and mentally retarded patients.

There have been several reports of reversible involuntary movement disorders with phenytoin, in particular dyskinesias, similar to those produced by neuroleptics (Chadwick et al 1976). In many cases, the abnormal movements coincided with a period of high serum phenytoin concentrations and again the patients most at risk appeared to be those with pre-existing brain damage.

Peripheral neuropathy, often asymptomatic, is associated with chronic antiepileptic therapy, and the drug most often incriminated is phenytoin. However, there are several difficulties in their interpretation: in many of the studies the patients were taking polytherapy; acute reversible electrophysiological changes were not always distinguished from chronic irreversible abnormalities; and variables, such as length of drug therapy, periods of drug toxicity and folate levels, were not always considered. A study of 51 previously untreated epileptic patients followed prospectively on carefully monitored monotherapy with either carbamazepine or phenytoin for 1–5 years revealed no clinical evidence of neuropathy, although slight abnormalities of sensory conduction were found in 18% of patients on phenytoin, but in none of those on carbamazepine (Shorvon & Reynolds 1982).

Hepatic toxicity

Hepatic toxicity induced by phenytoin is a rare occurrence. It usually develops within 6 weeks of the first phenytoin exposure and appears unrelated to phenytoin dosage or serum levels (Parker & Shearer 1979). The hepatotoxicity is usually accompanied by a rash, fever and lymphadenopathy, and eosinophilia is a common occurrence. These features suggest that the mechanism may be a hypersensitivity reaction. Liver histology shows mixed hepatocellular damage with cholestasis and necrosis.

Long-term therapy with phenytoin may cause asymptomatic biochemical changes such as increased serum alkaline phosphatase and alanine aminotransferase, and enlargement of the liver may also occur (Andreasen et al 1973). These changes are thought to be due to the enzyme-inducing properties of phenytoin and will result in altered metabolism of both endogenous and exogenous substances.

Endocrine and metabolic disorders

A number of different endocrine and metabolic effects have been associated with phenytoin treatment (Bennet 1977). Phenytoin has been shown to accelerate cortisol metabolism due to its effect on hepatic microsomal enzymes. This is compensated for by an increased cortisol secretion rate, presumably due to increased ACTH secretion from the anterior pituitary gland (Werk et al 1964). The increased rate of steroid hormone metabolism may be of clinical importance in epileptic patients who require steroid replacement therapy or steroids for disease suppression, e.g. renal allograft recipients.

Phenytoin also has been shown to have an effect on the secretion of thyroid hormones with reduction in free thyroid hormones and enhanced peripheral conversion of T_4 to T_3 (Finucane & Griffiths 1976). Phenytoin may also have an effect on the pituitary to suppress release of TSH but

this is rarely accompanied by clinical features of thyroid dysfunction.

The role of antiepileptic drug therapy in causing infertility and impotence in epileptic patients is as yet unclear. Phenytoin causes an increase in sex hormone binding globulin and increases the breakdown of oestrogens and androgens (Richens 1984). However, other factors such as an effect on the pituitary or direct toxicity to the germinal tissue are possibly also important.

High serum concentrations of phenytoin have been shown to inhibit insulin release from the pancreas in response to hyperglycaemia.

Long-term antiepileptic drug therapy is associated with a significant incidence of hypocalcaemia and osteomalacia although rarely is the bone disease symptomatic (Richens & Rowe 1970, Bell et al 1978). The biochemical mechanisms involved have not yet been fully elucidated, although phenytoin has been shown to reduce plasma levels of the biologically active vitamin D metabolites.

Haematological toxicity

Phenytoin therapy has been implicated in the development of megaloblastic anaemia, aplastic anaemia, leucopenia and lymphadenopathy. In many patients there is a mild macrocytosis which does not require treatment. Other patients with more severe changes usually respond well to folate therapy without discontinuation of the drug. A transient leucopenia sometimes occurs on starting phenytoin therapy; rarely, phenytoin can cause a pure red cell aplasia or agranulocytosis. Long-term phenytoin treatment can lead to a reversible lymphadenopathy with histology resembling lymphoma and this is thought to be the result of a hypersensitivity reaction (Editorial 1971). Phenytoin has also been shown to cause IgA immunoglobulin deficiency (Meissner et al 1984).

Skin and soft tissue reactions

Skin rashes are a fairly rare adverse reaction to phenytoin therapy, although the incidence appears to be higher if high loading doses of phenytoin are used (Chadwick et al 1984). The rash is usually morbilliform. Rarely, more severe skin disorders such as erythema multiforme may occur. Facial coarsening and thickening of subcutaneous tissue have also been reported as complications of long-term phenytoin treatment. Gum hyperplasia is an adverse effect peculiar to phenytoin. It occurs quite frequently in minor degree and its severity increases with larger drug doses and longer duration of therapy.

Teratogenicity (See also Ch. 19)

There is substantial evidence of an increased incidence of developmental abnormalities in the children of mothers with epilepsy, estimated to be two to three times the usual rate (Janz 1982). The common major abnormalities include cleft lip and palate, congenital heart lesions and malformations of the skeleton, central nervous system and gastrointestinal tract. The increased frequency of malformations has been attributed to the teratogenic effects of the antiepileptic drugs themselves (most are teratogenic in animals), but it is very difficult to differentiate drug effects from the other complicating factors including the seizures and the genetic risk from the maternal epileptic disorder. The occurrence of the so-called 'fetal hydantoin syndrome', including various craniofacial and distal limb anomalies, retarded growth and mental handicap has been disputed. Strickler et al (1985) postulated that a genetic defect in arene oxide detoxification may contribute to susceptibility to phenytoin-induced birth defects.

Indications for the use of phenytoin

Phenytoin has been used extensively over the years although it has been superseded to some extent by the newer drugs such as carbamazepine and valproate, primarily because of its high incidence of adverse effects and difficult pharmacokinetic profile. It is an effective drug in the treatment of tonic-clonic and partial seizures but is ineffective in absence seizures. It also has a role in the emergency treatment of status epilepticus.

Methoin (mephenytoin) and ethotoin

Methoin and ethotoin are hydantoin compounds related to phenytoin (Sjö et al 1975, Troupin et al 1976). Although methoin has been shown to have marked antiepileptic activity and has been used clinically for more than 30 years its use has declined due to excessive risk of serious toxicity, particularly rashes and blood dyscrasias. Ethotoin is rarely used because of its low efficacy, despite its minimal incidence of adverse effects.

VIGABATRIN

Vigabatrin was developed as an inhibitor of the enzyme GABA-transaminase and its ability to increase inhibition in the central nervous system led to its early testing in animal models of epilepsy and subsequently in epileptic patients. At the time of writing, vigabatrin had been marketed in a number of European countries. Its structure and detailed mode of action are given in Chapter 13.

Pharmacokinetics

A summary of the pharmacokinetics of vigabatrin (reviewed by Schechter, 1989 and Perucca & Pisani, 1991) is provided in Table 15.5.

Absorption

The absorption of vigabatrin from the gastrointestinal tract is rapid and almost complete, peak plasma levels being usually attained within 2 hours after a single dose irrespective of whether the drug is taken in the fasting state or after a meal. The peak concentration of the active S(+)-enantiomer is about one-half the concentration of the R(–)-enantiomer in both adults (Haegele et al 1988) and children (Rey et al 1990).

Table 15.5 Summary of pharmacokinetic data of vigabatrin*

Range of daily maintenance dosage (adults)	2.0–4.0 g/day
Time to peak serum level	1–2 h
Percentage bound to plasma proteins	nil
Apparent volume of distribution	0.8 l/kg
Elimination half-life	5–7 h
Time to steady state after starting therapy	2 days
Major metabolite(s)	none
Minimum dose frequency	once daily

* Due to the irreversible mode of action, the time course of pharmacological effect does not parallel the time course of serum drug levels

Distribution and plasma protein binding

Vigabatrin is negligibly bound to plasma proteins and has a volume of distribution of about 0.8 l/kg.

Route of elimination, clearance and half-life

The total plasma clearance of vigabatrin is 1.7 ml/min/kg on average. The drug is excreted primarily by the kidney, the renal clearance of unchanged drug accounting for about 60–70% of the total clearance. Approximately 60% of a single oral dose is excreted in urine within 24 hours. Although the renal clearance of the two enantiomers is similar, the urinary recovery after a single dose is about 50% for the S(+)-enantiomer and 65% for the S(–)-enantiomer.

In adults, the half-life of vigabatrin ranges between 5 and 11 hours and is similar for the two enantiomers. Longer half-life values have been described in elderly patients with age-related impairment of renal function.

Dose–serum concentration relationship

Little information is available on the relationship between vigabatrin dosage and serum drug concentration at steady-state. After single dosing, however, the concentration of vigabatrin is linearly related to dose (at least within the 1 to 3 g range) and there is no reason to anticipate deviation from linearity during chronic administration.

Concentration–effect relationship

Since vigabatrin is an irreversibly acting drug, its pharmacodynamic effects outlast the elimination from the plasma compartment. In other words, the intensity of pharmacological effect does not mirror the profile of the concentration of the drug in plasma and monitoring of plasma drug concentrations is not expected to provide a useful guide for adjusting vigabatrin dosage. Since in animal models the inhibition of GABA transaminase shows similar dose–response and time course profiles in brain and in platelets, it has been suggested that measuring the activity of this enzyme in platelets may provide a non-invasive tool for monitoring vigabatrin therapy (Bolton et al 1989).

Dose interval

Despite the short chemical half-life of the drug, the irreversible nature of GABA-transaminase inhibition results in a relatively long duration of action, as indicated by the fact that the concentration of GABA may remain significantly elevated in human CSF after as long as 120 hours following a single oral dose. For practical purposes, twice or even once daily dosing appears to be adequate. Alternate-day regimens have also been tested, but these seem to achieve less satisfatory therapeutic responses compared with once daily dosing.

Pharmacokinetics in special situations

The pharmacokinetics of vigabatrin in children have been investigated by Rey et al (1990). In six children aged 5 months to 2 years, the half-life of the active S(+) enantiomer was 5.6 + 1.5 h, while that of the S(–) enantiomer was 2.9 + 1.0 h. Corresponding values in another group of six children aged 4 to 14 years were 5.5 + 1.9 h and 5.7 + 2.9 h respectively. In the same study, areas under the plasma concentration curves and drug recovery in urine were found to be considerably lower than those reported in adults, but this difference requires confirmation because a formal control group of adults was not included in the same study. In any case, since renal clearance values in children were similar to those described for adults, the putative differences in plasma and urinary drug concentrations between children and adults could be explained by a lower oral bioavailability in the paediatric age group.

The occurrence of an age-related decrease in renal function provides an explanation for the slower elimination of the drug in elderly patients. In a recent study, Haegele et al (1988) compared the kinetics of vigabatrin enantiomers in elderly and young subjects. The renal clearance of the active S(+) enantiomer fell progressively with increasing age. The reduction in drug clearance in the elderly was found to be non-linearly related with the decrease in creatinine clearance. To compensate for the reduced efficiency of the elimination processes, elderly patients and other patients with impaired renal function should receive lower daily dosages.

Drug interactions

No interactions affecting the pharmacokinetics of vigabatrin have been described to date. By contrast, it has been reported that vigabatrin lowers the serum concentration of concurrently administered phenytoin (Rimmer & Richens 1989). The interaction may occur after a latent period of up to 4 weeks and the decrease in serum phenytoin concentration averages 20 to 30% of the baseline level, though the interindividual variability is considerable. The mechanism of this effect is unknown but it is likely to involve a decrease in phenytoin bioavailability. In most patients, the interaction is of limited practical significance and adjustments in phenytoin dosage are not necessarily required.

The serum levels of concurrently administered carbamazepine and valproic acid are not affected by vigabatrin. A reduction in serum levels of phenobarbitone and primidone has been reported occasionally, but it does not appear to occur consistently and is generally of little or no clinical significance.

Therapeutic efficacy

Following promising results in pilot open studies, the efficacy of vigabatrin (1.5–3 g daily) has been investigated in seven double-blind, placebo controlled trials conducted in a total of 153 patients, mostly with partial seizures refractory to conventional therapy (Mumford & Dam 1989, Mumford & Lewis 1991). All these trials (except one, which was based on a parallel group comparison) followed a randomized cross-over design, according to which vigabatrin or placebo was added to existing antiepileptic therapy for periods of 7 to 12 weeks. The results of these investigations have shown remarkable agreement, approximately 50% of patients in each trial showing a reduction in seizure frequency of more than 50% compared with the placebo period. Partial seizures appeared to respond better to vigabatrin treatment, although a significant decrease in the frequency of generalized tonic-clonic seizures was also seen (Rimmer & Richens 1984).

An overall evaluation of 1400 patients receiving vigabatrin as add-on therapy has confirmed a significant benefit in about half of cases uncontrolled by conventional drugs (Mumford & Lewis 1991). In this evaluation, patients with partial seizures showed generally a better outcome compared to patients with generalized seizures and this seems to be true for both adults and children, although it has been suggested that infantile spasms may be peculiarly responsive (Chiron et al 1990). There are occasional observations suggesting that absence seizures and non-progressive myoclonic epilepsy do not improve and may actually be aggravated by the drug.

In adults, clear-cut therapeutic effects have been observed at daily dosages as low as 2 g/day, but many patients require larger dosages (up to 4 g/day). Clinically, the drug shows a rapid onset of action and the effect is relatively short-lived after withdrawal of therapy. A number of long-term investigations and follow-up studies have indicated that the therapeutic benefit is generally mantained during maintenance treatment and that tolerance to the antiepileptic effect does not develop (Browne et al 1987, Tartara et al 1989).

Adverse effects

Vigabatrin is generally well tolerated and the need to discontinue treatment because of adverse effects is unusual. The side effects most frequently reported during short-term clinical trials are somnolence, fatigue, irritability, dizziness and headache, but only for the first of these symptoms has the incidence during vigabatrin treatment (27%) been significantly higher than that observed during administration of placebo (12%) (Mumford & Dam 1989). Allergic reactions such as skin rashes are virtually unknown. During long-term treatment, weight gain has been reported in an appreciable proportion of patients (Tartara et al 1989). Vigabatrin may cause a decrease in serum transaminases (SGOT and SGPT), an effect probably of no clinical significance which is ascribed to an inhibitory action of the drug on these enzymes.

In certain animal species administration of vigabatrin has been associated with the development of microvacuolization in the white matter, but long-term intensive clinical monitoring has provided no evidence that this effect may also occur in man. To date, perhaps the most serious adverse effect which has been observed clinically is the development of psychotic symptoms. Although this reaction is fortunately rare, there is suggestive evidence that patients with a positive psychiatric history may be predisposed to develop a psychosis. Pending further information, it is probably wise to avoid using the drug in these patients.

Abrupt discontinuation of vigabatrin treatment has resulted in withdrawal seizures. If treatment needs to be terminated, gradual reduction of dosage is recommended, as for other antiepileptic drugs.

PHENOBARBITONE

Phenobarbitone was introduced into the drug treatment of epilepsy in 1912. Phenobarbitone is a substituted barbituric acid and it was the first effective organic epileptic agent. It is much more potent as an anticonvulsant than as a sedative. The structure and mechanism of action of phenobarbitone are described in Chapter 13.

Pharmacokinetics

These are summarized in Table 15.6. The reader is referred to Butler (1978) and Wilensky et al (1982) for a detailed review of the pharmacokinetics of phenobarbitone.

Table 15.6 Summary of pharmacokinetic data on phenobarbitone

Range of daily maintenance dose	Adult: 30–240 mg/day Child: 2–6 mg/kg/day
Minimum dose frequency	Once daily
Time to peak serum levels	1–6 h
Percentage bound to plasma proteins	45%
Apparent volume of distribution	0.5 l/kg
Elimination half-life	Adult: 50–160 h Child: 30–70 h
Time to steady state after starting therapy	Up to 30 days
Major metabolite (inactive)	Para-hydroxyphenobarbitone

Absorption

Absorption of phenobarbitone after oral administration is virtually complete but the rate of absorption is variable. Jalling (1974) found peak serum concentrations 1–6 hours after oral dosing but slower absorption has been described in earlier reports (Sjögren et al 1965). This may be due to differences in pharmaceutical formulation, and the effect of food on absorption may be important. Intramuscular injections of phenobarbitone reach peak serum concentrations in 0.5–6 hours (Wilensky et al 1982) but this is too slow for the emergency treatment of status epilepticus.

Distribution and plasma protein binding

Although the distribution of phenobarbitone to vascular tissues occurs fairly rapidly after absorption, the penetration of the drug into the brain is slow and this is another reason why phenobarbitone is not an ideal drug for the treatment of status epilepticus. The later phases of drug distribution result in almost equal phenobarbitone concentrations in all tissues of the body. The distribution of phenobarbitone is sensitive to variations in the pH of plasma because it has a pKa close to physiological plasma pH. Acidosis causes a shift of the drug from plasma to tissues, and alkalosis results in an increased phenobarbitone concentration in the plasma (Waddell & Butler, 1957).

Phenobarbitone is about 45% bound to plasma proteins. This relatively low degree of protein binding means that the drug is less susceptible to alterations in plasma protein concentrations and is unlikely to be significantly involved in drug interactions in which there is competition for binding sites. Cerebrospinal fluid concentrations of phenobarbitone reflect the free drug concentrations in plasma (Houghton et al 1975b) but the saliva concentrations do not because they are sensitive to pH changes (Schmidt & Kupferberg 1975). It is therefore unwise to use saliva for serum drug level monitoring in the case of phenobarbitone.

Metabolism and excretion

Phenobarbitone is partly metabolized and partly

excreted unchanged in the urine (Butler 1978). Studies in patients have reported between 11 and 55% of the dose is excreted unchanged by the kidneys. The remainder is hydroxylated in the para position to p–hydroxyphenobarbitone, which is then excreted both unchanged and as the glucuronide by the kidneys.

Para-hydroxyphenobarbitone lacks antiepileptic activity. Both the biotransformation and renal clearance of phenobarbitone proceed slowly. The plasma half-life in adults ranges from 50–160 hours (mean 96 h). Thus, once-daily dosing with phenobarbitone is possible. Because of phenobarbitone's pKa of 7.3, the rate of excretion of the parent compound by the kidneys can be altered significantly by changes in urine pH. Alkalinization of the urine increases the renal excretion of unchanged phenobarbitone by reducing the non-ionic back diffusion from the distal renal tubule to the plasma. This property has been exploited in the treatment of phenobarbitone overdose. The renal clearance can be increased from 4–6 ml/min to 30 ml/min by bicarbonate administration.

Dose–serum concentration relationship

Over the therapeutic range of serum concentrations there is a nearly linear relationship between dose and serum level within subjects. Thus phenobarbitone is an easier drug to manage clinically than phenytoin. However, there is considerable variation between subjects in the serum level produced by a given dose. Children metabolize the drug more quickly than adults and therefore require proportionally larger mg/kg doses.

Concentration–effect relationship

Although studies examining the relationship between plasma level of phenobarbitone and seizure control have produced some conflicting results, it would appear that plasma phenobarbitone levels greater than 40 μmol/1 (10 μg/ml) are associated with improved clinical efficacy (Buchthal et al 1968). With plasma levels over 170 μmol/l (40 μg/ml) the additional therapeutic benefits decline and there is a higher incidence of adverse effects (Plaa & Hine 1960). However, it is well recognized that tolerance occurs to the sedative effects of the drug so that a serum level of 20 μmol/l (4.8 μg/ml) produced acutely may have a greater sedative effect than a level of 200 μmol/l (48 μg/ml) which has been maintained chronically. However, it is less certain whether tolerance to the antiepileptic effect occurs in humans. A therapeutic range of 40–170 μmol/l (10–40 μg/ml) has been suggested as a guide to therapy but, because of the phenomenon of tolerance, it could be argued that the value of therapeutic drug monitoring for this drug may be less than previously thought.

Pharmacokinetics in special situations

Phenobarbitone can cross the placental barrier and enter the fetus. The amount in breast milk is fairly small and the dose reaching the breast-fed infant is unlikely to result in side-effects (Kaneko et al 1979). Phenobarbitone's half-life is prolonged in neonates but in children is less than in adults. Because phenobarbitone is cleared partly by renal excretion patients with poor renal function (creatinine clearance < 30 ml/min) may be at risk of phenobarbitone toxicity.

Drug interactions

Most of the reported drug interactions involving phenobarbitone occur in situations where phenobarbitone has altered the kinetics of other drugs (Perucca & Richens 1980, 1985). Alteration in protein binding has not been implicated as an important factor in any reported interactions. However, phenobarbitone is a potent inducer of hepatic mixed function oxidase enzymes and thus can alter the metabolism of numerous drugs, e.g. warfarin and oral contraceptive steroids and various endogenous substances. However, the effect of enzyme induction by phenobarbitone on other drugs in individual patients is largely unpredictable and seems to depend on genetic factors and previous contact with environmental inducing agents. There is no evidence of autoinduction of phenobarbitone metabolism in humans. Inhibition of phenobarbitone's own metabolism by other drugs may also occur, e.g. the valproate-phenobarbitone interaction which can result in phenobarbitone toxicity.

Adverse reactions to phenobarbitone

Phenobarbitone has been widely used for over 70 years and thus experience with the drug has led to the accumulation of considerable information about its toxicity. Serious systemic adverse reactions appear to be very uncommon. The most frequent problems encountered are neuropsychiatric toxicity.

Neuropsychiatric toxicity

Even with serum concentrations of phenobarbitone within the therapeutic range of 40–170 μmol/l (10–40 μg/ml) adverse changes in affect, behaviour and cognitive function are often encountered. High serum concentrations can result in nystagmus, dysarthria and ataxia (Plaa & Hine 1960). The most common adverse reaction in adults is sedation, although marked tolerance to it can develop. In children and the elderly a paradoxical effect may occur resulting in insomnia and hyperkinetic activity. The incidence of behaviour disturbances in children has been reported as over 50% in some studies (Wolf & Forsythe 1978). Those children most at risk are the ones with organic brain disease. Phenobarbitone therapy can cause alteration in mood, particularly depression. Cognitive function may also be disturbed, and the resulting deficits in attention and memory may be subtle and difficult to measure.

Dependence, habituation and withdrawal

Physical dependence on phenobarbitone occurs and abrupt discontinuation after high dosage produces abstinence symptoms, including anxiety, insomnia, tremors, confusion and seizures. If a decision is made to stop phenobarbitone therapy, it must be tapered off very slowly to avoid withdrawal seizures. A neonatal withdrawal syndrome has been described in infants born to epileptic mothers taking phenobarbitone.

Haematological toxicity

Megaloblastic anaemia and macrocytosis have been described during therapy with phenobarbitone alone or more commonly when in combination with other antiepileptic drugs, especially phenytoin. As with phenytoin, folate deficiency occurs, but does not require treatment unless anaemia results.

Coagulation defects can occur in neonates whose epileptic mothers take phenobarbitone during pregnancy (Mountain et al 1970). They are due to a deficiency of vitamin K dependent clotting factors, and vitamin K administration to the baby post partum will prevent this coagulation deficiency.

Bone disorders

Biochemical osteomalacia can occur in epileptic patients treated with phenobarbitone but clinical demineralization of bone is rare (see p. 510).

Hepatic toxicity

There is a low incidence of liver damage resulting from treatment with phenobarbitone.

Endocrine changes

Phenobarbitone stimulates the peripheral metabolism of T_4 which is countered by an increased secretion of T_4 from the thyroid gland so that most patients remain euthyroid.

Skin reactions

Various types of skin rashes have been reported with phenobarbitone. They are usually mild maculopapular or morbilliform eruptions. The incidence of such reactions is low and more serious skin problems, such as exfoliative dermatitis are extremely rare.

Teratogenicity

As previously discussed (see p. 511) there is an increased risk of fetal malformations in the offspring of epileptic mothers, but the role played by the various antiepileptic drugs in their aetiology is far from clear. Evidence for the teratogenic potential of phenobarbitone is much less than for phenytoin.

Other barbiturates

Over the past 30 years other barbiturate derivatives have been developed but none has been shown to be clinically superior to phenobarbitone itself. One such compound, methylphenobarbitone, is less reliably absorbed than phenobarbitone and following absorption it is demethylated to phenobarbitone with a half-life of about 20 hours (Eadie et al 1978). Most of its pharmacological effect resides in its phenobarbitone metabolite. Thus, there is no advantage in giving methylphenobarbitone rather than phenobarbitone itself and the drug has not achieved any widespread popularity.

PRIMIDONE

Primidone is a desoxybarbiturate which was first marketed as an antiepileptic drug in 1952. Its structure and mode of action are given in Chapter 13.

Pharmacokinetics

A summary of the pharmacokinetics of primidone is given in Table 15.7. The reader is referred to Baumel et al (1972) for a detailed review.

Table 15.7 Summary of pharmacokinetic data on primidone

Range of daily maintenance dosage	Adult: 250–1500 mg/day Child: 15–30 mg/kg/day
Minimum dose frequency	Twice daily
Time to peak serum level	2–5 h
Percentage bound to plasma proteins	Less than 20%
Apparent volume of distribution	0.6 l/kg
Major active metabolites	Phenobarbitone Phenylethylmalonamide (PEMA)
Elimination half-life (adults)	Primidone 4–12 h Derived phenobarbitone 50–160 h Derived PEMA 29–36 h
Time to steady state after starting therapy	Up to 30 days for derived phenobarbitone

Absorption

Peak serum concentrations are achieved within 2–5 hours after administration of a single dose but after chronic administration peak levels appear to occur later (Schottelius 1982).

Distribution and plasma protein binding

Studies of the distribution of primidone in humans are not extensive. Reported CSF:serum ratios range from 0.53 to 1.13 and brain concentrations have been shown to correlate well with plasma concentrations with a brain:plasma ratio of 0.87 (Houghton et al 1975b). Saliva:serum ratios are 73–100%. The degree of protein binding of primidone is low, unbound primidone levels being about 80% of the total serum level.

Metabolism and excretion

Primidone is metabolized in the liver to phenobarbitone and phenylethylmalonamide (PEMA) although a relatively high percentage of primidone may be excreted unchanged via the kidneys (Kaufmann et al 1977). On average 20–25% is converted to phenobarbitone but there is extensive interindividual variation in the degree of conversion and this leads to a wide scatter of serum phenobarbitone : primidone concentration ratios. The metabolism to phenobarbitone is very slow after single dose administration but after chronic dosing the conversion occurs more rapidly. Metabolism to PEMA is rapid following a single dose of primidone. Primidone has a half-life of 4–12 hours and therefore considerable fluctuation in serum concentrations occur throughout the day. The derived phenobarbitone has a much longer half-life and therefore the serum concentration of this metabolite exceeds the serum concentration of the parent drug despite the fact that only a relatively small proportion of primidone is metabolized to phenobarbitone. PEMA also accumulates because it is eliminated more slowly than primidone. The ideal dose interval for primidone administration is uncertain because the role played by unchanged primidone and PEMA in the anticonvulsant effect of the drug is uncertain. In animals both primidone and PEMA have antiepileptic activity against experimental seizures (Bourgeois et al 1983) but whether they contribute significantly in the treatment of epileptic patients is not certain. However, Oxley et al (1980) have shown that, in some patients, primidone is a superior antiepileptic drug to phenobarbitone when given in doses which produce similar serum phenobarbitone concentrations. Whether the parent drug itself or the derived PEMA accounts for this additional activity is not known. In view of all the uncertainty it is probably wise to administer primidone in twice-daily divided dosage.

Dose–serum concentration relationship

An approximately linear relationship exists between primidone dose and derived serum phenobarbitone concentrations. The ratio of the primidone: phenobarbitone concentrations at steady state is an average 1:2.5 but there is wide variation between subjects. The co-administration of other enzyme-inducing antiepileptic drugs, e.g. phenytoin, increase the ratio by increasing the rate of metabolism of primidone to phenobarbitone and leading to accumulation of phenobarbitone, and possibly a potentiation of pharmacological effect. Changes in the primidone:phenobarbitone ratio during pregnancy have been reported with a fall during later pregnancy, although the mechanism of this change is not clear and the possibility of non-compliance with medication has not been excluded (Battino et al 1984).

Serum concentration–effect relationship

Correlation of plasma concentrations of primidone with clinical control of seizures is complicated because of its conversion into two active metabolites as well as possibly being active in its own right. Thus for a full assessment it may be necessary to monitor plasma levels of all three compounds. The most practical approach is to monitor derived phenobarbitone. The potential benefit of also measuring unchanged primidone is in detection of non-compliance because those patients who have only started to take the primidone a few days prior to clinic attendance will have a low serum phenobarbitone : primidone ratio. Plasma primidone concentrations in excess of 70 μmol/l (15 μg/ml) are likely to be accompanied by side-effects.

Adverse effects of primidone

Many patients experience side-effects of drowsiness, weakness and dizziness at the initiation of primidone therapy. These symptoms may be severe and last several days. They may occur even when the starting dose is low, and appear to be related to serum concentrations of the parent drug rather than the metabolites. When primidone is added to other enzyme-inducing antiepileptic drug therapy, this initial intolerance is usually less, due to the more rapid conversion of the parent drug to its metabolites. These adverse effects usually subside with time due to functional tolerance to side-effects of primidone (Leppik et al 1984) so that the dose of primidone may be gradually increased. Primidone shares much of the adverse reaction spectrum of phenobarbitone. Only rarely has primidone been implicated in severe haematological or idiosyncratic reactions. There is some evidence that primidone intake during pregnancy may be important in the pathogenesis of minor abnormalities and poor somatic development in the children of epileptic women (Rating et al 1982).

ETHOSUXIMIDE

The clinical effectiveness of ethosuximide against pure absence seizures was first reported in 1958, and it remains an important drug for this indication. The structure and mode of action of ethosuximide are considered in Chapter 13.

Pharmacokinetics

These are summarized in Table 15.8. The reader is referred to Sherwin (1978) for a detailed account.

Absorption

Ethosuximide is rapidly and completely absorbed from the gastrointestinal tract, peak plasma levels occurring after 1–4 hours (Buchanan et al 1973). Absorption is quicker with syrup preparations.

Table 15.8 Summary of pharmacokinetic data on ethosuximide

Range of daily maintenance dosage	Adult: 500–1500 mg/day Child: 10–15 mg/kg/day
Minimum dose frequency	Once daily
Time to peak serum level	1–4 h
Percentage bound to plasma proteins	Negligible
Apparent volume of distribution	0.7 l/kg
Major metabolites (inactive)	2 (1-hydroxyethyl)-2-methylsuccinimide 2-(2-hydroxyethyl)-2-methylsuccinimide 2-acetyl-2-methylsuccinimide
Elimination half-life	Adult: 40–70 h Child: 20–40 h
Time to steady state after starting therapy	Up to 14 days (adult) Up to 7 days (child)

Drug distribution and plasma protein binding

Plasma protein binding of ethosuximide is negligible and therefore the drug is present in saliva and CSF in concentrations which approximate to that of plasma (McAuliffe et al 1977). Ethosuximide appears to be distributed throughout body water, without much selective regional concentration. It crosses the placenta to the fetus rapidly and ethosuximide concentrations in breast milk are about 94% of the plasma levels (Kaneko et al 1979).

Metabolism and urinary excretion

Ethosuximide is extensively metabolized to two hydroxylated metabolites and a ketone derivative. These are largely excreted as glucuronides. Only 10–20% of the drug is excreted unchanged in the urine.

Elimination half-life and dose interval

The elimination half-life is longer in adults than children, but at all ages is long enough for once daily administration to be feasible (Buchanan et al 1976). However, with larger doses, gastro-intestinal adverse effects may make divided dosing preferable.

Dose–serum concentration relationship

Although there is some evidence that the dose–serum concentration relationship may not be linear over the therapeutic range it is not sufficient to have important practical implications for prescribing of ethosuximide. A daily dose of 20 mg/kg yields a serum level of about 450 μmol/l (65 μg/ml) on average (Browne et al 1975).

Concentration–effect relationship

There is good evidence from clinical studies that control of absence seizures is related to the plasma level of the drug and that most patients require a level in the range 200–700 μmol/l (40–100 μg/ml) to achieve optimal control, although some patients may benefit from increased doses to produce levels of 850 μmol/l (120 μg/ml) or more (Sherwin 1982). There does not appear to be a clear relationship between serum levels and adverse effects. Saliva levels of ethosuximide are an alternative way of monitoring ethosuximide therapy in children.

Drug interactions

Because ethosuximide does not bind to plasma proteins and does not induce hepatic microsomal enzymes the number of documented interactions with other drugs is relatively small, and most are of little clinical importance (Perucca & Richens 1980, 1985). Occasionally, addition of valproate to a patient's ethosuximide therapy has caused elevation of plasma ethosuximide levels resulting in toxicity. Also, when enzyme inducing drugs such as carbamazepine are given concurrently, higher doses of ethosuximide may be required to achieve the same plasma ethosuximide levels.

Toxicity

Ethosuximide has a relatively good record regarding incidence of adverse effects. Most problems relate to the acute dose-related side-effects, such as nausea, hiccough, abdominal discomfort, drowsiness, anorexia and headache. Nausea is the most common adverse effect and usually occurs within the first few days of ethosuximide administration. It frequently responds to dose reduction. Ethosuximide has also been reported to cause exacerbation of various types of seizures, particularly tonic-clonic convulsions. However, because tonic-clonic seizures occur at some time during the course of absence seizures in about 25% of patients it is difficult to be sure whether the tonic-clonic seizures were coincidental or causally related to the ethosuximide therapy. Behavioural and cognitive adverse effects have been ascribed to ethosuximide including psychotic episodes, but it is difficult to be sure about how frequently this occurs from the reported studies. They may be a manifestation of drug intoxication.

Skin reactions

Skin rashes have been frequently described with ethosuximide and include erythema multiforme and the Stevens–Johnson syndrome. Systemic lupus erythematosus-like syndromes have been reported in association with ethosuximide administration.

Haematological toxicity

Blood dyscrasias have been reported with ethosuximide but are very rare.

Teratogenicity

There is little information available regarding the risk to the fetus exposed to ethosuximide.

Phensuximide and methsuximide (Porter et al 1977)

Phensuximide is less potent than ethosuximide and its clinical use is declining. Methsuximide's antiepileptic activity rests almost entirely with its metabolite, N-desmethyl-methsuximide. It is used relatively little compared with ethosuximide.

BENZODIAZEPINES

The 1,4-benzodiazepines were first synthesized in 1933. They have antiepileptic activity in addition to tranquillizing and hypnotic effects. They are the most potent agents for the emergency treatment of status epilepticus but their value in the long-term treatment of epilepsy is severely limited by their adverse effects of sedation and psychomotor retardation; the development of tolerance to their antiepileptic effects; and by the problem of withdrawal reactions. There is some evidence that clobazam, a 1,5-benzodiazepine, impairs psychomotor performance less than the 1,4-benzodiazepines, but it suffers from the other drawbacks of this class of drug.

The individual benzodiazepine drugs which are most frequently used in the clinical management of epilepsy will be selected for discussion. Their mode of action is discussed in Chapter 13.

Pharmacokinetics

Tables 15.9, 15.10 and 15.11 summarize the main pharmacokinetic properties of diazepam, clonazepam and clobazam (Mandelli et al 1978, Richens 1983).

Diazepam

When given orally, diazepam is rapidly absorbed with peak plasma concentrations occurring within 30–90 minutes (Gamble et al 1975). Although the presence of food in the stomach delays oral absorption, the extent of absorption may actually increase (Greenblatt et al 1978). Diazepam is very insoluble in water and is prepared for parenteral use in a vehicle which is irritant and often causes local thrombophlebitis on intravenous administration. Preparations in an emulsion form are less irritant. The drug will come out of solution if it is diluted with small amounts of saline but it may be diluted with large amounts for intravenous infusion. However, administration of diazepam by intravenous infusion is not altogether satisfactory because diazepam and its active metabolite, N-desmethyldiazepam accumulate and prolonged coma can result. It also adsorbs on to the intravenous tubing. When given intramuscularly, its absorption is slow and unreliable (Gamble et al 1975, Kanto 1975) and it is therefore inadvisable to administer diazepam by this route for the emergency treatment of status epilepticus where a

Table 15.9   Summary of pharmacokinetic data on diazepam and its N-desmethyl metabolite

	Diazepam	N-Desmethyldiazepam
Range of daily adult maintenance dosage	5–60 mg/day	
Minimum dose frequency	Twice daily	
Time to peak serum level (oral)	0.5–2 h	
Percentage bound to plasma proteins	97%	97%
Apparent volume of distribution	1–2 l/kg	
Major active metabolite	N-desmethyldiazepam Temazepam Oxazepam	Oxazepam
Inactive metabolites	Conjugated derivatives	Conjugated derivatives
Elimination half-life	20–60 h	30–90 h
Time to steady state after starting therapy		Up to 20 days

rapid effect is required. The absorption of diazepam solution from the rectum is rapid and peak serum levels occur within 6–10 minutes in most patients (Milligan et al 1981). Rectal diazepam can be used prophylactically for febrile convulsions but is less satisfactory than intravenous diazepam for the treatment of acute convulsions (Knudsen 1979). Suppositories of diazepam are much more slowly and erratically absorbed and produce lower serum levels.

Following intravenous diazepam, drug distribution to body tissues is rapid. Peak brain concentrations are seen within 1–5 minutes. The apparent volume of distribution is 1–2 l/kg. It is highly bound to plasma proteins (approximately 97%) and CSF and salivary concentrations correspond to the free serum diazepam concentrations.

Diazepam is extensively metabolized by demethylation and hydroxylation. Its major metabolite, N-desmethyldiazepam, is pharmacologically active and accumulates because it has a longer half-life than the parent drug. The hydroxylated derivatives of diazepam and N-desmethyldiazepam are temazepam and oxazepam, which are both pharmacologically active but have short half-lives. All three metabolites are conjugated with glucuronic acid and excreted in the urine. Only traces of the parent drug are eliminated unchanged. The long half-life of diazepam (20–60 h) and N-desmethyldiazepam (30–90 h) allows the

Table 15.10   Summary of pharmacokinetic data on clonazepam

Range of daily adult maintenance dosage	1–10 mg/day
Minimum dose frequency	Once daily
Time to peak serum level (oral)	1–3 h
Percentage bound to plasma proteins	85%
Apparent volume of distribution	2–5 l/kg
Inactive metabolites	7-aminoclonazepam 7-acetaminoclonazepam
Elimination half-life	20–60 h
Time to steady state after starting therapy	Up to 14 days

Table 15.11   Summary of pharmacokinetic data on clobazam

Range of daily adult maintenance dosage	20–60 mg/daily
Minimum dose frequency	Once daily
Time to peak serum level (oral)	1–4 h
Percentage bound to plasma proteins	Approx. 90%
Apparent volume of distribution	?
Elimination half-life	18 h (42 h N-desmethylclobazam)
Active metabolite	N-desmethylclobazam
Time to steady state after starting therapy	Up to 4 weeks for N-desmethyclobazam 1 week for clobazam

drug to be administered once daily. However, when larger doses are given, the sudden rise in serum concentration may cause adverse effects and divided dosage may then be preferable. The half-life is reduced in patients on enzyme-inducing antiepileptic drugs and may be prolonged in the elderly and in patients with liver disease. Diazepam itself does not significantly induce hepatic enzymes.

Clonazepam (Pinder et al 1976)

Clonazepam is fairly rapidly absorbed wih peak serum levels at 1–3 hours. It distributes to body tissues equally rapidly and is approximately 85% bound to plasma proteins. It is extensively metabolized to 7-aminoclonazepam and 7-acetaminoclonazepam, both of which are inactive. The elimination half-life of clonazepam is 20–60 hours in adults so that once daily dosing is possible. Clearance of the drug is more rapid in children. Enzyme-inducing antiepileptic drugs, e.g. phenytoin, can lower serum clonazepam concentrations.

Clobazam (Schmidt 1984a)

In humans, clobazam is virtually completely absorbed after oral administration with peak plasma levels within 1–4 hours. It is 90% protein bound. The terminal half-life of elimination of the parent compound is approximately 18 hours. The major metabolite is N-desmethylclobazam which is active but has considerably less potency than the parent drug. The elimination half-life of the N-desmethyl metabolite is much longer than that of the parent compound (approximately 42 h). The metabolism of clobazam is induced by concomitant antiepileptic medication (Jawad et al 1984).

Serum concentration–effect relationship

Tolerance occurs to the therapeutic effects of the benzodiazepines. Diazepam has been used principally in the emergency treatment of status epilepticus and should not normally be used for the long-term treatment of chronic epilepsy. Thus there is little data on therapeutic serum concentrations in chronic use of diazepam. Clonazepam has been used more extensively in the chronic treatment of epilepsy as well as in the acute therapy of status epilepticus. The correlation between plasma concentrations and therapeutic effect has been found to be somewhat variable although levels greater than >100 nmol/l (0.03 μg/ml) are recommended. In view of the development of receptor tolerance, the value of serum level monitoring is doubtful. Intermittent therapy with benzodiazepines in chronic epilepsy may be valuable and avoid the development of tolerance, e.g. in catamenial epilepsy (Feely et al 1982).

Adverse reactions to benzodiazepines

Adverse reactions such as drowsiness, ataxia, dizziness and behavioural changes occur commonly at the beginning of treatment. Irritability, inattention, sedation and hypotonia are more common in children. These dose-related adverse effects tend to lessen with the duration of treatment because of the development of tolerance. Older patients do appear to be more sensitive to the effects of benzodiazepines. There may be additive effects on the central nervous system when benzodiazepines are administered with other sedating drugs or alcohol. Clobazam may cause less psychomotor impairment than the 1,4-benzodiazepines but otherwise it seems to share all the other adverse features. There is little evidence for haematological, hepatic or renal toxicity of the benzodiazepines. Occasionally, skin rashes occur.

Teratogenicity has been reported with diazepam in particular an increased risk of cleft palate, but the evidence is far from conclusive.

Dependence develops with benzodiazepines and in adults, agitation, anxiety, insomnia, tremor, hallucinosis and tonic-clonic seizures have been seen in relation to diazepam withdrawal. A neonatal withdrawal syndrome has also been reported in newborn babies who have been exposed to long-term benzodiazepine treatment in utero.

When benzodiazepines are given intravenously for the emergency treatment of seizures the most serious adverse effects are respiratory depression, hypotension and cardiac arrest. The incidence of such problems is low, but equipment and personnel prepared for cardiopulmonary resuscitation should be available. Newborns of mothers who have been given a dose of diazepam in the 24 hours preceding delivery may have transient respiratory depression, hypotension and poor feeding.

TROXIDONE

Troxidone (trimethadione) is an oxazolidinedione drug used primarily in the treatment of absence seizures. Over recent years its use has declined because of the greater clinical efficacy of ethosuximide and sodium valproate in absence seizures.

Pharmacokinetics (Withrow 1982)

Troxidone is rapidly and almost completely converted in vivo to dimethadione which because of its very slow excretion rate accumulates in large quantities during chronic troxidone therapy. Dimethadione concentrations in plasma are about 20 times higher than the parent compound.

Although troxidone itself can protect against seizures, it is thought that the dimethadione active metabolite accounts for most of the antiseizure effects of troxidone treatment. Because of the long half-life of dimethadione it could probably be given once daily, although traditionally it is prescribed in divided doses. It may take several weeks for plasma concentrations of dimethadione to reach steady state.

Plasma concentration–seizure control relationship

Retrospective studies indicate that most patients whose absence seizures are controlled by the drug have concentrations of dimethadione, the active metabolite, greater than 5400 μmol/l (700 μg/ml) (Booker 1982). There is often delay in response of 2 weeks or more because it takes such a long time for dimethadione levels to reach steady state.

Toxicity

The known complications of troxidone therapy were summarized by Wells (1957) and little has been added since. Most of the adverse effects on the central nervous system are dose dependent and reversible. Day blindness and photophobia are the most common side-effects. Sedation, lack of concentration, dizziness and ataxia are recognized problems; and insomnia, confusion and psychotic reactions have also been reported. The milder reactions can usually be controlled by dose reduction. Skin reactions are common and include serious eruptions such as erythema multiforme and exfoliative dermatitis. The most serious adverse drug reactions include bone marrow depression, and fatal pancytopenia has been reported. Maternal ingestion of troxidone has been closely linked with an increased incidence of fetal anomalies, sometimes so characteristic that the term 'fetal trimethadione syndrome' has been applied (Feldman et al 1977). The evidence for teratogenicity of trimethadione is stronger than for any other antiepileptic drug and thus its use in pregnancy is absolutely contraindicated.

Indications for use

It would appear from clinical trials that troxidone is a less effective drug for the treatment of absence seizures than ethosuximide and sodium valproate. In view of the serious adverse effects of troxidone its use should seldom be necessary.

PART 2

GENERAL PRINCIPLES IN THE DRUG TREATMENT OF EPILEPSY

WHEN TO START ANTIEPILEPTIC DRUGS?

It is essential that before antiepileptic drug therapy is started a correct diagnosis is made. A clear distinction between epileptic and non-epileptic attacks is of major importance because the attachment of the label of 'epilepsy' to a person has grave medical, therapeutic and social implications that will greatly influence his future life. When diagnostic difficulty persists despite appropriate investigations, it is often the best course to let time make matters clear. Therapeutic trials of antiepileptic drugs in cases of doubt are rarely justified and often only make the management of the patient more difficult. An erroneous diagnosis of epilepsy is a frequent cause of treatment failure.

The variable prognosis of epilepsy makes it difficult to decide when to start drug treatment in the individual patient or indeed when to stop it. The clinical management of epilepsy is based as much on empirical practice as on scientific evidence. There has been debate as to whether early drug therapy improves the prognosis of epilepsy or whether it simply controls seizures (Chadwick & Reynolds 1985). Proponents of the former argue that seizures beget seizures and therefore early control will break a vicious circle and improve the eventual outcome. Others argue that drugs suppress seizure activity while they are being taken, but when they are stopped the tendency to seizures returns to a course determined by the natural history of the disorder. The authors of this chapter find no evidence in support of the first argument.

The decision to start treatment in an individual patient should take into account not only the number of attacks experienced but also, the circumstances in which they occurred, the presence or absence of precipitating factors, the type and severity of the attacks, whether or not there are any accompanying neurological, pyschiatric or social problems, and whether the patient wants treatment.

There are no hard and fast rules but most neurologists in the UK would not recommend treatment after a single tonic-clonic seizure. In the United States, there is a greater tendency to start drug therapy after single seizures, although this may be primarily for medicolegal reasons. The reports on the prognosis of a single untreated seizure are conflicting, and this is probably due to variation in the delay between the occurrence of the first seizure and the time of medical review. In their retrospective general practice study, Goodridge & Shorvon (1983) found that a single seizure was followed by others in 80% of patients. Elwes et al (1985) found a cumulative probability of recurrence of 20% at 1 month, 28% at 2 months, 32% at 3 months, 46% at 6 months, 62% at 1 year and 71% at 3 years. The most recent

prospective study of first seizures in general practice in Britain has shown a 3-year recurrence rate of 78% (Hart et al 1990). In contrast, hospital based studies have shown lower recurrence rates of 38% (Cleland et al 1981) 27% (Hauser et al 1982) and 29% (Hauser et al 1990), probably due to a selection bias. Also, American patients (both studies by Hauser et al) are more likely to receive treatment and this reduces the recurrence rate while it is being administered (Musicco et al 1989).

Although most doctors would not treat an isolated seizure, if two or more tonic-clonic seizures occur within a short time interval, e.g. 1 year, antiepileptic drug treatment is generally considered advisable. With seizures other than tonic-clonic, however, practice is more variable. Nevertheless, there is considerable variation in practice, because no studies exist on the clinical course of untreated epilepsy. The risk of recurrence is greater after two seizures than after one (Hauser et al 1982). Generally, the longer seizures continue during treatment, the less likely are patients to go into remission (Elwes et al 1984). This supports the view of Gowers (1881) that epilepsy tends to escalate and might be interpreted as supporting the idea that seizures should be suppressed by treatment as soon as possible (Reynolds et al 1983). However, as argued above, it may simply be that an individual patient's epilepsy, once it starts, takes a predetermined course; it may be inherently mild or inherently severe. Drug treatment will offer useful symptomatic benefit but it has yet to be proved that it achieves any more than this. If antiepileptic drug treatment does prevent subsequent evolution to chronic epilepsy, then the use of such drugs is imperative. If, however, it is shown that treatment merely suppresses the fits without any fundamental effect on the disease process itself, then in selected patients with less severe epilepsy, the self-limiting nature of the disease would make routine drug treatment unnecessary.

DRUG TREATMENT OF THE EPILEPSIES

In a review of 250 antiepileptic drug trials, Coatsworth (1971) first documented and emphasized the inadequacies of antiepileptic drug trials.

Since then, a considerable number of excellent clinical trials have been performed and we are therefore in a better position to make a rational choice of drug for the various seizure types. Nevertheless, the specificity of antiepileptic drugs is limited and therefore choice is still often influenced by opinion, fashion and marketing pressures. Even with the established drugs, there is insufficient information to make a completely rational choice of initial drug therapy in a newly diagnosed epileptic patient. The sections that follow will therefore take a dogmatic line. They are designed for the non-expert; those with experience in the field may well disagree with some of the points made, particularly those that question current practice.

For the non-expert a simple approach to starting drug therapy is given in Figure 15.3.

When a diagnosis of epilepsy is first made, there may be insufficient information to hand on which to identify clearly the seizure type, and therefore a choice based on the latter is often not possible. For this reason, sodium valproate is recommended as the drug of first choice because this drug has the widest spectrum of activity and is not contraindicated in any type of seizure. Carbamazepine is a more limited drug in that it may be ineffective in, or even worsen, myoclonus and absences and should therefore be avoided in juvenile myoclonic epilepsy. Unfortunately, it is not always possible to exclude this syndrome in an adolescent who presents with only one or two tonic-clonic seizures because absences and myoclonus may appear later, or sometimes on starting carbamazepine therapy.

If it is possible to identify clearly the seizure

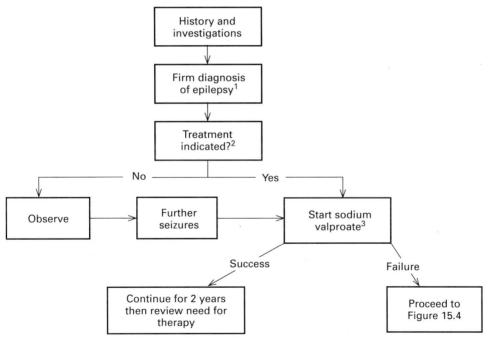

Notes:
1. A diagnosis of epilepsy should not be made until at least two seizures have occurred. This scheme may not be appropriate for very young children.
2. Treatment may not be indicated if only two seizures have occurred with a substantial interval between, if the seizures are mild (e.g. brief complex partial seizures) or if the patient does not wish to receive drug therapy.
3. Adult doses given in Table 15.11. Sodium valproate should not be judged to have failed unless seizures are not controlled by a dose of 3000 mg daily or unacceptable adverse effects occur.

Fig. 15.3 Recommended initial approach to the treatment of epilepsy following diagnosis.

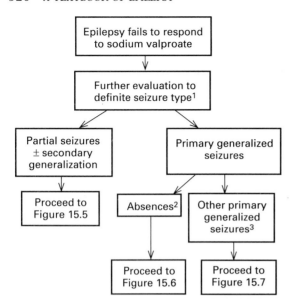

Notes:
1. A detailed description from the patient and eyewitnesses may suffice. Referral to a specialist centre for further investigations may be necessary.
2. Typical (3/second spike and wave) or atypical absences.
3. Tonic-clonic, atonic or myoclonic seizures.

Fig. 15.4 Recommended action if sodium valproate fails as initial therapy (see Fig. 15.3).

type on presentation, the standard teaching in recent years has been to recommend carbamazepine as the drug of first choice for partial seizures with or without secondary generalization although, as argued below, there is little evidence to support this view.

If the strategy in Figure 15.3 is followed and the seizures do not respond to sodium valproate, it is then necessary to focus more clearly on the seizure type in order to develop a further plan of action (Fig. 15.4). It will become apparent that some patients who were thought to have primary generalized tonic-clonic seizures will, in fact, have a focus from which the seizures arise and their seizures will therefore fall into the category of partial seizures with secondary generalization. Sometimes, there may also have been confusion between absences and complex partial seizures in which an alteration of consciousness is the predominant feature. Differentiation is important because the subsequent treatment strategies will be different for these two types of seizure. The accurate definition of seizure type will require a detailed history from the patient, his relatives or any other eye witnesses, particularly concerning the presence or absence of a focal onset (the 'aura'), focal features during or after the seizure. If the history and routine EEGs are unhelpful, 24-hour video-EEG monitoring may be rewarding, especially in patients whose seizures are frequent or occur at times of the day when routine EEGs are not normally done. The reader is referred to Chapters 1 and 9 for further advice.

Drugs effective in tonic-clonic and partial seizures

Tonic-clonic seizures can be primary in origin or can result from secondary generalization of a focal discharge. Drugs effective against tonic-clonic seizures are also active against partial seizures. However, partial seizures and generalized tonic-clonic seizures which start focally tend to show a poorer response to medical treatment.

Recent trials comparing the drugs most commonly used to treat tonic-clonic seizures allow some conclusions about relative efficacy to be made (Mattson et al 1985, Shorvon et al 1978, Callaghan et al 1985, Turnbull et al 1982, 1985). In a comparative trial by Mattson et al (1985) carbamazepine and phenytoin gave the highest overall treatment success, with intermediate success for phenobarbitone and lowest for primidone. Primidone's poor performance was mainly due to a high incidence of intolerable acute adverse effects. Control of tonic-clonic seizures did not differ significantly between the four drugs but carbamazepine provided complete control of partial seizures more frequently than primidone or phenobarbitone. The authors recommended carbamazepine or phenytoin as drugs of first choice for single-drug therapy of adults with partial and/or generalized tonic-clonic seizures. Unfortunately, sodium valproate was not one of the test drugs included in this study because, surprisingly, it is still not licenced for use in these seizure types in the USA.

Turnbull et al (1982, 1985) found no significant difference in efficacy between phenytoin and sodium valproate in a group of newly diagnosed patients with epilepsy. Similar results were obtained by Callaghan et al (1985) in their prospective study of carbamazepine, phenytoin and sodium valproate. Furthermore, monotherapy studies of newly diagnosed epilepsy in adults (E. H. Reynolds, personal communication) have shown no difference between carbamazepine, phenytoin, phenobarbitone and sodium valproate. A similar result occurred in children, although phenobarbitone had to be withdrawn as a trial option because of adverse effects. The success rate for medical treatment of patients with partial seizures seems consistently lower than for those with primary generalized tonic-clonic seizures. However, Chadwick & Turnbull (1985) conclude that, on current evidence, it is not possible to suggest that any individual drug is preferable against the two types of seizure in adult patients.

Despite these conclusions, established practice is to prescribe carbamazepine for partial seizures with or without secondary generalization, and sodium valproate for tonic-clonic seizures which appear to be primary generalized, especially if they are associated with myoclonus, absences or photosensitivity (and therefore fall within one of

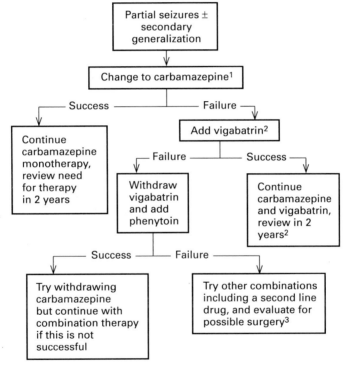

Notes:
1. One of two approaches can be used: a. tail off sodium valproate at the same time as introducing carbamazepine, or b. add carbamazepine until full dose achieved, then withdraw valproate.
2. There is little experience as yet of vigabatrin monotherapy and it is therefore recommended that it is added on to existing therapy.
3. Second-line drugs are given in Table 15.12. Seizures which fail to respond to antiepileptic drug therapy may not be epileptic in origin; a thorough review of the diagnosis is essential if there is doubt. Refer to Chapter 16 for guidance on evaluation for surgery.

Fig. 15.5 Treatment strategy for partial seizures with or without secondary generalization failing to respond to sodium valproate (see Figs 15.3 and 15.4).

the primary generalized syndromes such as juvenile myoclonic epilepsy).

Treatment strategy for partial seizures with or without secondary generalization

If the seizures are clearly partial in nature with or without secondary generalization, the scheme illustrated in Figure 15.5 is recommended. Subdivision of partial seizures into simple and complex has no therapeutic implications, although other aspects of management will be influenced. Carbamazepine is an alternative first line drug to sodium valproate and should therefore be used if sodium valproate has failed to control the seizures adequately. In Table 15.12 the drugs used for partial seizures have been subdivided into three categories according to their position in the therapeutic hierarchy. It is appreciated, however, that the position given to each drug would vary from country to country and centre to centre according to licensing regulations, availability of the drugs, cost and prescribing habit.

Monotherapy is the rule until at least the two first line drugs have been tried. Plasma level monitoring is more helpful in dosage tailoring with carbamazepine than with sodium valproate, although it is far from essential; the dose can simply be increased until seizures are controlled or dose-related adverse effects appear. If vigabatrin is used plasma levels should not be measured because they are unhelpful (p. 539). With phenytoin, however, monitoring plasma levels is essential if the dose is to be tailored correctly (p. 536).

If a combination of two drugs is used, it needs to be borne in mind that the addition of a second drug often fails to achieve improved control of seizures. Indeed, the patient may sometimes have more seizures and is at greater risk of experiencing

Table 15.12 Drugs for partial seizures with or without secondary generalization

First line:	Sodium valproate
	Carbamazepine
Second line:	Vigabatrin
	Phenytoin
Third line:	Phenobarbitone
	Primidone
	Clobazam

adverse drug effects (Shorvon & Reynolds 1979, Schmidt 1982). Studies of monotherapy is previously untreated adolescent or adult epileptic patients with tonic-clonic and/or partial seizures have shown a success rate of about 75% (Shorvon et al 1978).

One of the most common reasons for seizure recurrence is poor compliance with therapy (Elwes et al 1984). Sudden withdrawal of antiepileptic drug treatment may predispose to seizures, particularly with phenobarbitone or benzodiazepine therapy. The management of epilepsy in patients whose seizures do not respond well to the initial drug therapy can be difficult. If the response to full doses of two drugs is inadequate, addition of a third is probably seldom justified. It may be that the drugs are actually making the patient's seizures worse or are causing unacceptable adverse effects in exchange for little therapeutic benefit. Good records of seizure frequency during the period of drug therapy are invaluable and checks on compliance are also necessary. It may be difficult to assess how much benefit the patient is deriving from drug treatment when several years have elapsed since its initiation, especially if many drugs have been tried in a variety of permutations.

Reductions in drug therapy in patients on polytherapy are often justified and will occasionally produce a dramatic improvement in the patient's mental state whilst at the same time not affecting, and sometimes even reducing seizure frequency (Shorvon & Reynolds 1979, Fischbacher 1982, Callaghan et al 1984, Lesser et al 1984). However, such drug reductions are not without hazards and need to be done slowly and carefully to prevent withdrawal seizures during the period of drug reduction. Occasionally, a patient who has been well controlled on combination therapy may relapse when converted to monotherapy and control may not be regained despite return to polytherapy. A message from such experience is that it is more difficult to reduce polytherapy than to avoid it in the first place.

Drugs effective in primary generalized seizures

The treatment of primary generalized seizures is

dependent upon the specific types. The strategies illustrated in Figures 15.6 and 15.7 subdivide the seizures into absences, tonic-clonic seizures, atonic seizures and myoclonic seizures.

Treatment strategy for absence seizures

The two major drugs for the treatment of absence seizures are ethosuximide and sodium valproate. Clinical trials have shown them to be equally effective, with success rates approaching 100% in patients with simple classical absence seizures (Suzuki et al 1972, Callaghan et al 1982, Sato et al

1982). The response is less impressive in patients with atypical absence seizures and the Lennox–Gastaut syndrome. An advantage of sodium valproate over ethosuximide is that it is also effective against tonic-clonic seizures so that in patients with coexisting absences and tonic-clonic seizures sodium valproate would be the initial treatment of choice as in the scheme illustrated in Figures 15.3, 15.4 and 15.6. Troxidone appears less effective than either sodium valproate or ethosuximide and is seldom used. In patients who fail to respond to sodium valproate and ethosuximide given alone, the combination of

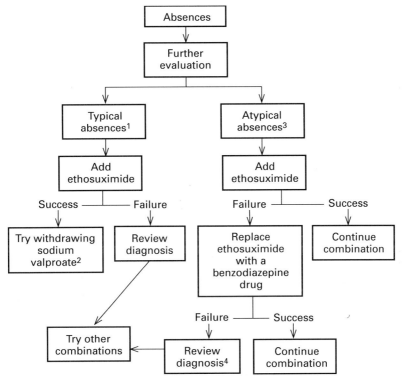

Notes:
1. Typical 3/second spike and wave absences will usually respond to sodium valproate.
2. Ethosuximide has an efficacy similar to sodium valproate in typical absences. If tonic-clonic seizures coexist, sodium valproate or another drug which is active against these seizures will need to be combined with ethosuximide. Resistant absences sometimes respond well to a combination of ethosuximide and sodium valproate.
3. Atypical absences with polyspike and wave or fast spike and wave are less responsive to drug therapy.
4. Resistant slow spike and wave absences may be a feature of Lennox–Gastaut syndrome.

Fig. 15.6 Treatment strategy for absence seizures failing to respond to sodium valproate (see Figs 15.3 and 15.4).

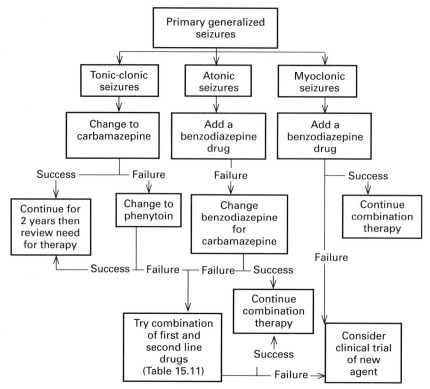

Fig. 15.7 Treatment strategy for primary generalized seizures (other than absences) which have failed to respond to sodium valproate (see Figs 15.3 and 15.4).

the two may prove effective. Long-term benzodiazepine therapy has been used to treat absence seizures but usually in patients whose seizures have not been controlled by other antiepileptic drugs and have had a benzodiazepine added to their other medication. A number of studies report a beneficial effect of benzodiazepines, but there are major deficiences in most of the trials, e.g. lack of uniformity of seizures type in the patients described, small numbers of patients, lack of blind techniques. The major disadvantages of benzodiazepines in the treatment of absence seizures are the marked sedative effects and the development of tolerance to the antiepileptic effect. Thus benzodiazepines are reserve drugs for the treatment of absence seizures.

The EEG can be useful in the assessment of response to treatment in patients with absence seizures. Clinical responce correlates well with the reduction in number of spike-wave paroxysms on the EEG.

Treatment strategy for primary generalized tonic-clonic seizures

Sodium valproate is the drug of first choice in primary generalized tonic-clonic seizures when they are accompanied by absences, myoclonus or photosensitivity. When they occur in isolation there is probably little difference in efficacy between sodium valproate, carbamazepine and phenytoin (Cereghino et al 1974, Troupin et al 1977, Kosteljanetz et al 1979, Turnbull et al 1983, Chadwick & Turnbull 1985, Callaghan et al 1985, E. H. Reynolds, personal communication).

Carbamazepine should therefore be tried if sodium valproate has failed (Fig. 15.7), followed by phenytoin if control has still not been obtained. Combinations of these drugs may be necessary, but the addition of a second or third antiepileptic drug benefits only a minority of patients and carries a greater risk of adverse effects. Vigabatrin does not as yet have an established place in treating primary generalized tonic-clonic seizures.

Phenobarbitone, primidone and benzodiazepine drugs are third-line treatments.

Treatment strategy for atonic seizures

These seizures are generally less amenable to drug therapy. Benzodiazepine drugs play an earlier part in their management (Fig. 15.7) but otherwise they should be treated in a similar manner to tonic-clonic seizures.

Treatment strategy for myoclonic seizures

Myoclonic seizures occur in a variety of syndromes which have different clinical presentations and aetiologies (Jeavons 1977; see also Ch. 4). Some of the severe forms in childhood are difficult to treat and have a poor prognosis.

In infantile spasms, ACTH or corticosteroid therapy has become a conventional form of treatment and there is good evidence that an immediate improvement in the clinical and electro-encephalographic abnormalities occurs (Jeavons & Bower 1974, Hrachovy et al 1979). There seems to be little difference in the efficacy of the two treatments but there is general agreement that the long-term prognosis is not influenced by this treatment and is usually poor (Pollack et al 1979). The Lennox–Gastaut syndrome (myoclonic-astatic epilepsy) is notoriously drug resistant.

Other myoclonic epilepsies, such as myoclonic epilepsy of childhood or adolescence, are more amenable to therapy.

In general, myoclonic phenomena respond best to treatment with sodium valproate or a benzo-diazepine drug. Six large studies reviewed by Browne & Penry (1973) reported a 50% or greater reduction in myoclonic seizure frequency in 36–100% of patients treated with chlordiazepoxide, diazepam or nitrazepam. Studies in which the latter two drugs have been compared indicate that nitrazepam is equal in efficacy or perhaps slightly superior to diazepam.

A number of uncontrolled reports has been published describing the use of clonazepam in myoclonic epilepsies and the results have been uniformly favourable (Pinder et al 1976, Browne 1976).

A satisfactory comparative study of the response of myoclonic epilepsies to clonazepam and to so-dium valproate has not been performed. Sodium valproate, however, appears to be of a similar efficacy to benzodiazepine drugs (Jeavons et al 1977). Patients with myoclonic epilepsy of childhood or adolescence seem to do best; those with Lennox–Gastaut syndrome did less well, although half derived considerable benefit which is worthwhile in such a notoriously drug-resistant condition.

Other drugs such as phenytoin, phenobarbitone and primidone are used in myoclonic and akinetic epilepsies, particularly when other types of seizure co-exist, but no controlled trials of these drugs have been performed. On the whole, the response of myclonic seizures to these drugs is poor.

Treatment of photosensitive epilepsy

Drug treatment is only one aspect of management of photosensitive epilepsy. Sodium valproate would appear to be the drug of first choice in patients with photically induced seizures and the majority of such patients achieve complete seizure control (Harding et al 1978). Clonazepam is also effective but is more sedative (Nanda et al 1977).

Value of the EEG in regulating therapy

The EEG is invaluable as an aid to identify the type of seizures from which a patient is suffering and therefore in enabling a logical choice of drug to be made. As a guide to the subsequent management of therapy, however, it is less useful. It should be remembered that the routine clinical EEG records cerebral activity for a period of only 30 minutes or so during a patient's waking day, and on one occasion the recording may coincide with a period of normal electrical activity and on the next day with an episode of disturbed function. Single records may therefore be unhelpful or even misleading. This has been noted in a number of therapeutic trials, but particularly when carbamazepine has been the drug under study (Cereghino et al 1974). Even prolonged EEG telemetry has failed to show a correlation between the clinical and EEG response to carbamazepine (Rodin et al 1974). When assessing the efficacy of a new drug in an individual patient it is the improvement in seizure control which is important, not changes in EEG activity, which may or may not parallel the changes in the patient's clinical condition.

On the other hand, the improvement in the frequency of absences produced by ethosuximide therapy is accompanied closely by a reduction in the number of spike-wave paroxysms in the EEG (Penry et al 1975). Thus, when treating patients with absence seizures, the EEG can be a very useful monitor of drug therapy.

Hazards of polytherapy

A survey of four European countries by Guelen et al (1975) found that among 11 700 patients from 15 centres, the mean number of drugs per patient was 3.2 of which 84% were antiepileptic. It would seem likely that such figures are representative of the situation in most developed countries. Many factors contribute to the evolution of polytherapy. By its nature, epilepsy is often a chronic disorder and in those patients with chronic drug-resistant epilepsy, the natural response to this is to add more drugs. Traditional approaches to drug treatment often included commencement of a patient on two drugs at presentation and the addition of more drugs when the initial drugs failed.

However, awareness of the hazards of polypharmacy in epilepsy has increased (Shorvon & Reynolds 1979). The points against this type of management are that drug toxicity and interactions become increasingly common as the number of drugs administered increases; the difficulty in identifying the cause of an adverse reaction becomes greater; and errors in drug dosing and deliberate non-compliance become frequent. Although the therapeutic effects of several drugs may be additive, so are the toxic effects.

Thus it is desirable that polypharmacy is avoided and that, wherever possible, one antiepileptic drug should be used alone (Reynolds & Shorvon 1981). However, 20–25% of patients developing epilepsy will not have their seizures adequately controlled by one drug and combinations of two drugs may therefore be necessary, but only rarely should three drugs be used together.

Factors carrying a poor prognosis for successful therapy

There appear to be some patients with epilepsy who prove to be highly resistant to drug treatment (Rodin 1968, Shorvon & Reynolds 1982). However, these patients probably only account for about 20% of all patients presenting with seizures and they are over-represented in specialist epilepsy clinics. Features associated with a poor prognosis include: additional neurological or psychosocial handicap, partial seizure types, mixed seizures, and symptomatic epilepsy. Initial response to treatment may also be determined by the number of seizures prior to the onset of therapy.

Compliance with antiepileptic therapy

It is well recognized that poor compliance is a major reason for drug failure. It may also precipitate status epilepticus and the phenomenon of sudden unexpected death in epilepsy. Peterson et al (1982) identified the following key determinants of patient compliance with antiepileptic drug therapy: concern about health; generalized tonic-clonic seizures; and the absence of barriers to compliance. They have also shown that strategies to improve compliance, such as counselling, special medication containers, self-recording of medication intake and seizures etc, could be effective and lead to a reduction in seizure frequency (Peterson et al 1984). The recent trend towards monotherapy is obviously an aid towards patient compliance. Whenever possible, drugs should be prescribed to be taken once or twice daily rather than three or four times a day. Regular review of patients' treatment is helpful and rationalization of the treatment regime can greatly improve compliance. Serum drug level monitoring can be helpful when poor compliance is suspected.

WITHDRAWING ANTIEPILEPTIC DRUGS

The question of when to withdraw antiepileptic drug therapy is dealt with in Chapter 5. In general, drugs should be withdrawn slowly, especially if they are among those known to cause the development of tolerance such as benzodiazepine and barbiturate drugs.

ANTIEPILEPTIC DRUG PROPHYLAXIS FOLLOWING HEAD INJURY AND NEUROSURGERY

Only a small percentage of patients who sustain a

significant head injury will suffer from fits once they have recovered from the acute stage of the illness. But, because head injuries occur so frequently, there are a considerable number of patients with late post-traumatic epilepsy in the community and fits are a serious cause of long-term morbidity after head injury. The incidence of epilepsy varies according to the nature of the injury. More than 50% of the patients have their first fit within a year of the head injury but the onset of epilepsy may be delayed by several years. Risk factors for the development of late onset epilepsy (i.e. fits occurring after the first week following head injury) have been evaluated (Jennett 1975). Important predictive factors are: the presence of a depressed skull fracture, the development of early epilepsy (within the first week); and the need to evacuate an intracranial haematoma within 2 weeks of the injury. However, the place of prophylactic antiepileptic drug therapy in the management of such patients, especially those at high risk of developing post-traumatic epilepsy, is far from clear. Will the use of drugs early after the cerebral insult prevent the development of an epileptic focus? Which drugs should be used and in what dose? When should they be started and for how long should they be administered?

A study by Young et al (1983a) in which 244 patients were randomly assigned to either phenytoin or placebo within 24 hours after head injury failed to show any significant beneficial effect of phenytoin on the incidence of early post-traumatic seizures. A further paper by these authors, looking at the incidence of late epilepsy in this same group of patients failed to show any effect on late seizures either. However, patient compliance was not good in this second study and the serum phenytoin concentrations were often low (Young et al 1983b). If those patients who develop early fits are excluded from analysis, the incidence of late seizures is relatively low and therefore clinical trials with large numbers of patients (2000) would be necessary in order to prove the efficacy of antiepileptic drug therapy in the prevention of late post-traumatic epilepsy (McQueen et al 1983). Thus the benefit of routine prescription of antiepileptic drugs in severely head-injured patients remains uncertain and any treatment policy for long-term prophylaxis has to consider the likely high level of non-compliance with the drug regime, the risks of adverse drug effects and the uncertain benefit conferred on a group of patients with relatively low risk of developing seizures.

Similar questions arise about the efficacy of prophylactic antiepileptic drug therapy to prevent seizures following neurosurgery. The risk of developing fits following supratentorial procedures for non-traumatic pathology is well recognized and has led to many neurosurgeons giving routine antiepileptic prophylaxis. A retrospective study defined the overall risk of seizures as 17% but it varies according to the condition for which the patient had surgery (Foy et al 1981). Studies of antiepileptic prophylaxis have given mixed results (North et al 1983, Shaw et al 1983) and there is need for larger placebo-controlled studies to determine whether such policies really are of benefit.

PROPHYLAXIS OF FEBRILE CONVULSIONS

Febrile convulsions are discussed in detail in Chapter 4. About 4% of children have a febrile convulsion and in most of them simple febrile convulsions do not lead to epilepsy or produce neurological or learning deficits. There is a small risk that if further febrile convulsions occur, they may be severe or prolonged with the risk of causing structural damage in the temporal lobe leading to chronic epilepsy. Febrile convulsions are, however, a distressing experience for the child and his family. The fits recur in 30–40% of patients. Measures to reduce pyrexia during febrile episodes are essential—increasing fluid intake, removal of clothes and administration of aspirin or paracetamol—but the place of prophylactic treatment with antiepileptic drugs is still under debate (Editorial 1980, 1981). It is clear that certain anticonvulsants, if taken properly, will prevent recurrent febrile convulsions. Well-controlled trials comparing daily phenobarbitone therapy with no treatment or intermittent treatment have established its efficacy in the prevention of recurrent febrile convulsions (Wolf et al 1977) and several studies with continuous sodium valproate medication have shown that it is equally effective (Ngwane & Bower 1980, Wallace & Aldridge-Smith 1980, Lee & Melchior 1981, Herranz et al 1984). However, phenytoin and carbamazepine have been shown to be ineffective (Melchior et al 1971, Bacon et al 1981, Anthony & Hawke 1983). Unfortunately prophylaxis with both phenobarbitone and sodium valproate has drawbacks. There is high incidence of behaviour disorders in children treated with phenobarbitone and it is likely to impair learning ability (Wolf & Forsythe 1978). Consequently, compliance with therapy may be low. Sodium valproate is less frequently associated with adverse effects but there is the rare but very serious problem of hepatotoxicity. Thus neither drug is ideal for treating large numbers of apparently normal children.

An alternative approach is to give intermittent treatment whenever a child who has had a previous febrile convulsion becomes febrile. Phenobarbitone is not a suitable drug for this kind of therapy as effective serum levels are not achieved rapidly enough. Similarly, sodium valproate may have a delayed onset of action. Rectal administration of diazepam solution is satisfactory for such intermittent prophylaxis of febrile convulsions because it is rapidly absorbed and can be administered at home by a parent. Knudsen & Vestermark (1978) showed that prophylactic rectal diazepam at a temperature above 38.5°C is as effective as long-term treatment with phenobarbital. In both groups, 6% of all febrile episodes lead to new convulsions. There were no significant side-effects of such therapy. However, although such treatment strategies can reduce the frequency of subsequent febrile convulsions the risk of subsequent epilepsy does not appear to be altered.

TREATMENT OF EPILEPSY IN DISEASE STATES

Most of the reported pharmacokinetic studies of antiepileptic drugs have been performed in normal volunteers or in patients who were healthy apart from having epilepsy. Sometimes it is necessary to administer these drugs to patients with diseases of other systems and these diseases may alter the way in which they are handled.

Gastrointestinal disease

It is likely that the absorption of drugs can be modified in patients who have undergone gastric or small bowel surgery, or who have small bowel conditions such as coeliac disease. This possibility has been little investigated although one study showed good absorption of phenytoin and ethosuximide in a patient with a jejuno-ileal bypass (Peterson & Zweig 1974).

Hypoalbuminaemia

Changes in plasma albumin concentration can affect the protein binding of some antiepileptic drugs, principally phenytoin and sodium valproate. When the plasma albumin concentration is low, less drug is bound and the total plasma concentration therefore falls. If attempts are made to achieve a total plasma level within the therapeutic range in the presence of a low albumin concentration, drug intoxication can occur because the concentration of unbound drug is higher than normal and it is this which determines the pharmacological effect.

Liver disease (Blashke 1977, Asconape & Penry 1982)

Antiepileptic drug disposition may be altered in several ways by liver disease: 1. bioavailability may be increased because of the development of portal-systemic anastomoses in cirrhosis which may allow drugs to bypass the liver on absorption; 2. systemic metabolism may be reduced by hepatocellular disease; 3. plasma protein binding of drugs may be reduced by hypoalbuminaemia, particularly affecting highly protein-bound drugs such as phenytoin, sodium valproate and diazepam.

Renal disease (Reidenberg & Drayer 1978, Asconape & Penry 1982)

Although renal excretion plays a small part in the elimination of most antiepileptic drugs, renal failure can indirectly alter the distribution of drugs by reducing their binding to plasma proteins. The free fraction may be increased at least two-fold for phenytoin and valproate. The impaired binding may be partly due to a lowered serum albumin concentration but a more important factor is probably a change in the molecular configuration of albumin or the presence of circulating endogenous inhibitors of binding (Reidenberg & Drayer 1978), Thus, when serum levels of phenytoin and sodium valproate are interpreted, allowance must be made for the reduced protein binding of these drugs. Phenobarbitone is cleared partly by urinary excretion, and creatinine clearance values below 30 ml/min may be associated with phenobarbitone toxicity. Vigabatrin is wholly eliminated by renal excretion of the unchanged drug and it may therefore accumulate in renal disease and in the elderly, but this has not been shown to be of any clinical consequence.

Other diseases

It is likely that other disease such as cardiac failure will alter the disposition of antiepileptic drugs but this has not been systematically studied. Acute viral infections may inhibit the metabolism of drugs, and symptoms of drug toxicity may be mistaken for symptoms of intercurrent infection. Drugs given for concomitant diseases may also influence the pharmacokinetics of antiepileptic drugs. The treatment of epilepsy in pregnancy is dealt with in Chapter 19.

TREATMENT OF ACCOMPANYING PSYCHIATRIC DISORDERS

The various types of psychiatric disturbance which can accompany chronic epilepsy are discussed in Chapter 11. Several therapeutic problems can be encountered in treating disorders of this nature in the epileptic patient. Phenytoin, carbamazepine, phenobarbitone and primidone induce the activity of liver enzymes and this effect can result in a much more rapid turnover and excretion of drugs such as the tricyclic antidepressants and phenothiazines. The epileptic patient is likely, therefore to have therapeutically ineffective levels of these psychotropic drugs if standard doses of the latter are used. If failure occurs when treating these patients, there should be no hesitation in increasing the dose beyond the usual limits.

The convulsant activity of tricyclic and related antidepressants and phenothiazines is now well documented and should be borne in mind when prescribing for an epileptic patient (Betts et al 1968, Legg & Swash 1974, Edwards et al 1986). Some tricyclics appear more likely than others to precipitate fits, e.g. maprotiline.

Compliance with antiepileptic drug therapy may also be a problem in those epileptic patients with accompanying psychiatric disorders, and seizures may be precipitated by sudden withdrawal of their antiepileptic medication. Such patients are also at risk of drug overdose which may include their antiepileptic drugs. Drug coma has to be distinguished from the postictal state. Although these are additional problems when treating patients who also have psychiatric disorders, on no account should severe depression or psychosis go untreated.

Antiepileptic drug intoxication can present as a psychotic behaviour disorder and should be borne in mild in the differential diagnosis of this condition in the epileptic patient. Vigabatrin has been shown to precipitate psychosis in some patients, particularly those with a previous history of this condition (Sander et al 1991).

DRUG LEVELS IN THE MANAGEMENT OF EPILEPSY (Richens 1976, Reynolds 1980)

Since the development of spectrophotometric techniques for measuring phenobarbitone and phenytoin in the late 1940s and early 1950s a variety of methods have been described for estimating concentrations of these compounds. The most widely used are gas chromatography, high performance liquid chromatography and immunoassay techniques. Each method his its advantages and drawbacks. Careful attention to quality control within the laboratory is necessary if the clinician is to have confidence in the results and incorrect decisions based on the results are to be avoided (Ayers et al 1980). Several interlaboratory quality control schemes have been set up to assist the analyst to achieve accuracy (Pippenger et al 1978, Griffiths et al 1980). Whether the report is helpful to the clinician, however, depends upon the drug being measured, and the reasons for requesting a drug level.

Not all drugs are suitable for therapeutic drug monitoring. The original criteria were as follows:

1. The action of the drug in question should be reversible
2. No tolerance should occur at receptor sites
3. The drug should have no active metabolites
4. The unbound concentration of the drug in plasma should equate with the unbound drug at the receptor site
5. The therapeutic response should be clearly related to the plasma concentrations of that drug
6. The therapeutic effects of the drug should be measurable with accuracy.

It was expected that most benefit would be obtained with drugs having a narrow therapeutic index. Phenytoin fulfils the above criteria and a therapeutic range of drug in plasma was suggested by Lund (1974) and confirmed clinically (Gannaway & Mawer 1981, Reynolds et al 1981). There is little doubt that the availability of plasma phenytoin assays has greatly improved the clinical use of phenytoin, which can be a difficult drug with which to deal. The same cannot be said for all the other antiepileptic drugs for which plasma concentration assays are available.

There are a number of sound reasons in clinical practice for measuring the serum level of a drug, whether an antiepileptic drug or any other compound. These should be borne in mind whenever a decision to monitor a drug is made:

1. When there is wide interindividual variation in the rate of metabolism of a drug, producing marked differences in steady state levels between patients
2. When saturation kinetics occur, causing a steep relationship between dose and serum level within the therapeutic range
3. When the therapeutic ratio of a drug is low, i.e. when the therapeutic doses are close to toxic doses, most of the available antiepileptic drugs have a low ratio
4. When signs of toxicity are difficult to recognize clinically or where signs of overdosage or underdosage are indistinguishable
5. During pregnancy, or when gastrointestinal,

hepatic or renal disease is present, which is likely to disturb drug absorption, metabolism or excretion
6. When patients are receiving multiple drug therapy with the attendant risk of drug interaction; if a drug is being added which is known to alter the metabolism of an existing drug, it is wise to monitor the level of the latter
7. Where there is doubt about the patient's compliance; up to 50% of epileptic outpatients do not take what is prescribed (Mucklow & Dollery, 1978); serial samples, particularly on admission to hospital may identify these patients
8. During research studies such as controlled therapeutic trials, a correlation between the serum level of a drug and its therapeutic or toxic effect is sound evidence that the effect really is due to the drug.

Obviously for research studies the decision to measure serum levels will be based on different criteria from routine estimations performed to improve the clinical management of the individual patient. Sufficient evidence from prospective studies relating serum levels and effect must be available in order that the results can be interpreted in a way that will lead to improved management. For some drugs there is little to be gained by measuring levels—indeed the clinician may be deluding himself by using an apparently scientific approach to the control of epilepsy and succeed only in treating the serum level and not the patient. Thus it is important to examine each antiepileptic drug in turn and consider the evidence for and against monitoring levels.

Phenytoin

The soundest case can be made out for measuring phenytoin levels. It is a difficult drug to use clinically and therefore most of the reasons given above for monitoring drug levels apply to phenytoin. The rate of metabolism of the drug varies widely from person to person and this is exaggerated by saturation of the enzyme system involved. There is a narrow therapeutic index, so that the therapeutic range of serum levels is close to the toxic range. Sometimes phenytoin intoxication is difficult to recognize when it presents in an unsual way such as with odd psychiatric symptoms, encephalopathy or even as increased fit frequency, and these signs may be misinterpreted as an indication for more intensive antiepileptic drug therapy. These are all compelling reasons why measurement of phenytoin serum levels is worthwhile and aids the clinical management of epilepsy. Perhaps it would be helpful to spell out typical situation in which measuring serum phenytoin levels may be of value:

1. When fits are not controlled by greater than average doses of the drug—the important question here is whether an optimum level of drug has been yet achieved because the patient is a rapid metabolizer or is failing to take his tablets, or whether his epilepsy is resistant to phenytoin
2. If a patient shows clinical signs of phenytoin intoxication, namely coarse nystagmus, ataxia and slurred speech, it is useful to confirm that they are drug-induced by estimating the serum level; sometimes a low or normal level may be found in a patient whose cerebellar signs are caused by cerebellar pathology rather than intoxication
3. If a patient presents with odd neuropsychiatric symptoms or dyskinetic movements; these can result from phenytoin intoxication even in the absence of nystagmus
4. If a previously well-controlled patient has a sudden increase in fit frequency; this can result from a fall in serum level (e.g. because he is failing to take his tablets) or from a rise to toxic levels (e.g. from a change in bio-availability of a formulation)
5. If another drug which might interfere with phenytoin metabolism is added to the patient's treatment
6. In the management of status epilepticus in a patient who has been receiving maintenance doses of phenytoin
7. In the management of childhood epilepsy in which dose adjustment can be more difficult
8. If the epilepsy is complicated by other diseases which might affect phenytoin handling
9. During pregnancy.

The serum concentration–effect relationship is discussed on page 507. The accepted therapeutic range is 40–80 μmol/l (10–20 μg/ml). However, a number of patients with mild epilepsy will be controlled with serum levels which are below this range, and in some patients therapeutic benefit without evidence of toxicity may be achieved with levels above the therapeutic range. Thus it is essential not to stick rigidly to this range but rather to use it as a guide only when evaluating individual patients.

The question of whether we should be monitoring free phenytoin serum concentrations (i.e. unbound drug concentrations) rather than total drug values has been raised. Monitoring of total plasma concentrations assumes lack of variability in plasma protein binding of a drug so that there is a constant relationship between total and free drug concentration. For phenytoin, the degree of variability of protein binding in epileptic patients without evidence of other medical disorders or co-administration of interacting drugs which alter protein binding (e.g. valproate) is probably small (Rimmer et al 1984). The currently available methods for measuring free concentrations are time consuming, expensive and insufficiently robust for routine use; the results therefore may be less reliable than measurement of total levels. In conditions such as hypoalbuminaemia, renal and liver disease and pregnancy, the free fraction of phenytoin may be considerably increased and, under these circumstances, monitoring of free serum phenytoin concentrations may be preferable. Saliva drug concentrations are an alternative, provided precautions are taken during collection to avoid contamination from orally administered drug.

In conclusion, therefore, the object in the management of phenytoin therapy should be to increase the serum concentration until seizure control is achieved, whether this is at 20 μmol/l for a patient with mild epilepsy or 100 μmol/l in severe disease. A knowledge of the serum level makes it possible to achieve this optimal treatment without risk of overdosage. The therapeutic range of 40–80 μmol/l should not be used inflexibly. Serum level monitoring used sensibly and possibly in conjunction with the use of one of the various dosage nomograms available can greatly assist dosage adjustment in many patients.

Carbamazepine

Serum levels of this drug show considerable variation from patient to patient and are markedly influenced by the presence of other enzyme-inducing drugs. However, carbamazepine has an active metabolite, carbamazepine 10,11-epoxide, although its contribution to the overall therapeutic effect of carbamazepine is not certain in humans. Levels of the 10,11-epoxide vary widely between individuals, being relatively high especially in children in whom it may have a substantial therapeutic effect. The ratio of epoxide to parent drug is increased by co-administration of enzyme inducing drugs.

Despite these reservations, a therapeutic range of 20–40 μmol/l (5–10 μg/ml) has been suggested for carbamazepine (Cereghino et al 1974). Adverse effects do not usually occur until serum levels of around 40–50 μmol/l (10–12 μg/ml) are achieved and usually consist of blurring of vision and diplopia. However, there is considerable variability between patients. Although these symptoms are often a good indication of pending toxicity some patients may become hyponatraemic and show impaired water balance before other signs of toxicity develop (Perucca et al 1978). This may be why carbamazepine toxicity can be associated with an increase in fit frequency. As carbamazepine has a relatively short half-life on chronic dosing, standardization of time of blood sampling is preferable.

Sodium valproate

Sodium valproate has a greater therapeutic ratio than some of the other drugs. The therapeutic range of serum concentrations of valproic acid is poorly defined. A range of 350–700 μmol/l (50–100 μg/ml) was first suggested by Schobben et al (1975), and Gram et al (1980) found that serum concentrations greater than 350 μmol/l (50 μg/ml) had a superior clinical effect compared with lower serum concentrations. Other groups have found similar ranges (Henriksen & Johannessen 1980, Klotz & Schweizer 1980) but others have disputed the existence of a therapeutic range (Schobben et al 1980, McQueen et al 1982). Some of the toxic effects of valproate, such as tremor, appear to be related to plasma concentrations of the drug and are more common with levels greater than 700 μmol/l (Turnbull 1983).

Besides interindividual variation in valproic acid levels, there are large intraindividual fluctuations during the day depending on the times of drug administration so that standardization of sampling times is necessary. Also, the extent of protein binding is variable and thus monitoring of total serum concentrations may be less relevant to clinical effect. More importantly, it appears that sodium valproate may have a non-reversible effect (Lockard & Levy 1976, Rowan et al 1979) which, if confirmed, lessens the value of monitoring because fluctuations in the level will not correlate closely with the antiepileptic effect.

In conclusion, because of these reservations, serum concentrations of valproic acid would not be expected to correlate with clinical effect and there is little evidence that measuring levels improves the clinical use of the drug.

Phenobarbitone

Despite the widespread availability and use of phenobarbitone assays, one of the essential criteria for the validity of monitoring is absent in the case of this drug. It is well recognized that tolerance occurs to the sedative effects (Butler 1978), such that a low serum level produced acutely may have a much greater sedative effect than a much higher level which has been maintained chronically. It is less certain whether tolerance occurs to the antiepileptic activity. It is seen in mice (Schmidt et al 1980) but has not been formally studied in humans. Thus the relationship between serum concentration of phenobarbitone and its actions on the central nervous system may not be a constant one and probably depends on the degree of tolerance which has developed. The therapeutic range which was suggested by Buchthal et al (1986) of 40–105 μmol/l is probably too low, and the upper level depends on the degree of tolerance that the patient and the physician have for the sedative effects of the drug. In conclusion, the value of measuring phenobarbitone levels may be much less than previously thought.

Primidone

With primidone, the situation is more complicated because it is converted to two active metabolites, phenobarbitone and PEMA, as well as probably being active in its own right. Thus for a full assessment it may be necessary to measure levels of all three compounds. However, for this to be justified, the relative potencies of the three compounds would need to be known so that the overall antiepileptic drug effect could be assessed. This is not possible on present evidence. The most practical approach is to monitor derived phenobarbitone.

One potential value of measuring unchanged primidone is in detecting non-compliance; for the patient who arrives at the clinic having taken the drug for only a few days beforehand will have a low ratio of phenobarbitone to primidone in his or her serum. Apart from this, primidone estimations for routine purposes are not helpful.

Clonazepam

As with phenobarbitone, tolerance occurs to the effect of clonazepam (and other benzodiazepines) therefore the same limitations apply to the monitoring of the drug. Furthermore, serum levels of clonazepam are much lower than for most of the other antiepileptic drugs and technical difficulties in measurement loom large. In fact, the poor quality of results returned in quality control checks indicate that they may be more misleading than helpful (Griffiths et al 1980). There are no satisfactory studies of the relationship between serum levels and clinical effect, although Morselli (1978) reported that plasma levels over 580–640 nmol/l (180–200 ng/ml) were associated with an increase in seizure frequency, improvement occurring on reduction to 130–180 nmol/l (40–50 ng/ml). Thus, routine monitoring of clonazepam levels is not justified on present evidence.

Vigabatrin

Vigabatrin acts by irreversible inhibition of GABA-transaminase and it therefore has a prolonged duration of action despite its short plasma half-life. There is no correlation between serum levels and its therapeutic or toxic effects, and monitoring levels has no clinical value.

Ethosuximide

As it is used mainly in children, routine monitoring may have a place, although the serum level appears to be fairly predictable for a given dose in mg/kg provided the age of the patient is taken into account (Sherwin 1982). Regular monitoring was found to reduce non-compliance and allowed drug requirements to be individualized, resulting in an improvement of control (Sherwin et al 1973). There is good evidence that control of absence seizures is related to the plasma level of the drug and that most patients require a level of up to 700–850 μmol/l (100–120 μg/ml) to achieve optimum control (Penry et al 1975, Sherwin 1982). A range of 350–700 μmol/l (50–100 μg/ml) has been widely accepted. There does not appear to be a clear correlation between serum levels and adverse effects (Sherwin 1978). The active metabolite of methsuximide (N–desmethylmethsuximide) is responsible for the therapeutic activity of this drug. A therapeutic range of up to 200 μmol/l (40 μg/ml) for the metabolite has been suggested.

Timing of blood sampling

The shorter a drug's elimination half-life the greater the fluctuation in serum levels throughout a 24-hour period. Although the frequency of dosing is adjusted to compensate for this, it is seldom practical to administer a dose during the night, and therefore an early morning trough occurs which, for a drug like sodium valproate may be only about one half of the peak level. With phenobarbitone and phenytoin this fluctuation can usually be ignored and a random sample will give a reasonable estimate of the steady-state level. With carbamazepine, the fluctuation is greater and, therefore, standardization is preferable. Probably a sample taken 6 hours after dosing, using a twice-daily regime, is reasonable. For sodium valproate, a shorter interval of about 4 to 5 hours would be better.

In practice, blood samples will usually coincide with the time of a patient's clinic visit. The advantage to be gained from attempting to achieve the pharmacokinetic ideal is usually too small to be justified.

Abuse of drug monitoring

Table 15.13 summarizes the evidence discussed above and attempts to rank the value of therapeutic drug monitoring for each of the commonly used antiepileptic drugs. Knowledge of plasma concentrations of some of these drugs can be invaluable for the clinical management of the patient, particularly for phenytoin, and less so for ethosuximide and carbamazepine. However, rigidity of interpretation of serum concentrations should be avoided and alterations of drug dosage only made after clinical evaluation.

Monitoring of free drug concentrations

The usefulness of plasma monitoring of drugs rests on the assumption that plasma total drug concentrations reflect free, therapeutically active concentrations and, therefore, depend on protein binding remaining constant. This is especially important for highly bound drugs such as phenytoin and sodium valproate. Situations in which protein binding may be disturbed include pregnancy, old age, liver and renal diseases and when other drugs are prescribed which alter protein binding. However, for most routine measurements it is probably unnecessary to measure free drug concentrations. So far, the methods available for measuring free drug are not completely reliable and are time consuming and expensive and are therefore not applicable for everyday use. Measurement of antiepileptic drugs in saliva samples reflects free serum drug concentrations for phenytoin, primidone and carbamazepine, but is less reliable for phenobarbitone and is unhelpful in the case of sodium valproate. Saliva sampling is less traumatic for the patient than venepuncture, but there are risks of contamination of samples when patients are taking elixirs and uncoated tablets. It is probably of most value in monitoring drug therapy in children (Knott 1983).

Table 15.13 Which drugs should be monitored?

Drug	Therapeutic levels[†] μmol/l (μg/ml)	Value rating[‡]	Comments
Phenytoin	40–80 (10–20)	★★★★★	Monitoring essential for good therapy. Accurate dosing difficult without serum levels, because of saturable metabolism. Low therapeutic ratio, disguised toxicity and frequency of drug interactions add weight to the case for routine monitoring.
Carbamazepine	20–40 (5–10)	★★★	Monitoring useful. Clinical symptoms (especially eye symptoms) are often helpful in determining dose limit, but water intoxication and increase in fit frequency may be caused by high serum level. Standardization of sampling time advisable.
Ethosuximide	350–700 (50–100)	★★★	Monitoring in children is less acceptable, but can be helpful as a guide to correct dose.
Phenobarbitone	70–180 (15–40)	★★	Tolerance develops and therefore therapeutic range difficult to define.
Primidone (unchanged)		★	Phenobarbitone is major metabolite therefore this should be monitored if indicated. Occasional measurement of primidone useful in slow metabolizers.
Valproic acid	350–700 (50–100)	★	Timed specimens essential. Little evidence that management is improved by monitoring. Possibility of 'hit and run' effect.
Clonazepam		★	Sedation is usually dose limiting; serum levels unhelpful because of development of receptor tolerance.

[†] Evidence for these ranges is, in some cases, inadequate.   [‡] The more asterisks, the greater the value of routine monitoring.

PART 3

NEW DRUGS FOR EPILEPSY

FUTURE PERSPECTIVES IN THE DRUG TREATMENT OF EPILEPSY

Although drug therapy is not the only approach to the management of epilepsy, it is likely to retain a central role for the foreseeable future. Presently available drugs are far from ideal. They fail to render all patients fit-free—approximately 20% of patients are drug resistant—and there is also the problem of acute and chronic antiepileptic drug toxicity. Thus there is an urgent need for new drugs which are more potent but less toxic. The ideal antiepileptic drug would have the following features.

1. It should be at least as effective as the currently available drugs with an improved therapeutic ratio
2. It should possess no serious toxicity

3. Tolerance should not develop to it
4. It should be easy to use:
   active orally
   long half-life (24 hours or so)
   simple pharmacokinetic characteristics (i.e. no saturable metabolism or binding)
   no effect on hepatic enzymes.

In recent years, several new drugs have entered pre-clinical and clinical development and a few of these have already reached the marketing stage. Some derive from structural modifications of agents already available, while others result from more innovative experimental approaches which have been made possible by recent progress in the understanding of the basic mechanisms of the epilepsies. Among the latter agents, a prominent place is now held by a new generation of compounds which have been specifically designed to interact, through different mechanisms, with excitatory or inhibitory pathways known to influence the epileptogenic and/or epileptic phenomena in animal models and in humans (see Ch. 13).

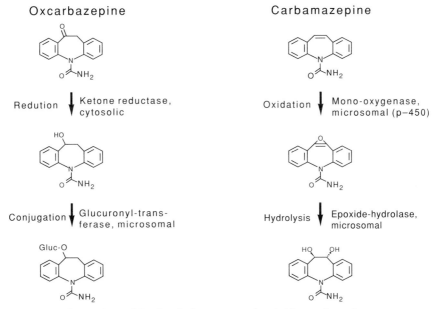

Fig. 15.8 Comparison of the chemical structure and main biotransformation reactions of oxcarbazepine and carbamazepine. The reduction of oxcarbazepine to its 10-hydroxy-derivative (DHC) occurs largely through first-pass metabolism. The latter metabolite is primarily responsible for the pharmacological effects observed after intake of oxcarbazepine.

This section will focus mainly on those drugs which have undergone the most extensive clinical testing, though brief mention will also be made of some agents at an early phase of clinical evaluation. Vigabatrin is considered earlier in this chapter because it is now marketed in many European countries.

OXCARBAZEPINE

Oxcarbazepine is an analogue of carbamazepine which differs from carbamazepine in pharmacokinetic profile, susceptibility to drug interactions and profile of adverse effects. Oxcarbazepine was approved for marketing by the Danish Health Authorities in 1990 and is currently undergoing clinical testing in a number of other European countries.

Structure

Oxcarbazepine is the 10,11-dihydro-10-oxo-derivative of carbamazepine. The structure and metabolic profiles of oxcarbazepine and carbamazepine are shown in Figure 15.8.

Mechanism of action

In animal models, the pharmacological properties of oxcarbazepine resemble those of carbamazepine. There is evidence that the effects of oxcarbazepine are mediated by its 10-monohydroxy metabolite, 10,11-dihydro-10-hydroxy carbazepine (DHC), which shows activity similar to oxcarbazepine and which is present in serum at concentrations much higher than those of the parent drug (Klosterkov Jensen et al 1991).

Pharmacokinetics

The pharmacokinetics of oxcarbazepine have been reviewed by Faigle & Menge (1990) and Perucca & Pisani (1991). Since oxcarbazepine can be considered as a pro-drug for DHC, the parameters summarized in Table 15.14 refer to the latter compound.

Absorption

After oral intake of ^{14}C-labelled oxcarbazepine by normal volunteers, about 95% of the administered radioactivity can be recovered in urine within 6 days, indicating that the absorption of the drug and/or its metabolites from the gastrointestinal tract is virtually complete. Following oral administration of therapeutic doses of oxcarbazepine, however, the serum levels of the parent compound are extremely low and decline rapidly with half-lives of 1.0 to 2.5 hours. A substantial first-pass metabolism occurs, resulting in rapid and extensive conversion to the active metabolite DHC and to other metabolites. In practice, therefore, oxcarbazepine behaves as a pro-drug for DHC. After single oral administration of the parent drug, peak plasma levels of DHC occur at 3 to 8 hours.

Distribution and plasma protein binding

Distribution studies using ^{14}C-labelled oxcarbazepine and DHC indicate that after administration of both compounds the radioactivity penetrates rapidly in all tissues, including the brain. The binding of DHC to serum proteins is estimated to be about 50%.

Metabolism and half-life

Unlike carbamazepine, the metabolic pattern of oxcarbazepine does not involve formation of an epoxide intermediate. The major metabolic pathway involves reduction to the active metabolite DHC, which exists in two enantiomeric forms possessing similar antiepileptic activity in animal models (Schutz et al 1986). Other minor

Table 15.14 Summary of pharmacokinetic data of oxcarbazepine*

Range of daily maintenance dosage (adults)	600–1800 mg/day
Time to peak serum level	3–8 h
Percentage bound to plasma proteins	50%
Apparent volume of distribution	not determined
Elimination half-life	10–13 h
Time to steady state after starting therapy	3 days
Major metabolite(s)*	DHC glucuronide (inactive)
Minimum dose frequency	Twice daily

* Oxcarbazepine is primarily a prodrug for its 10-hydroxy-derivative (DHC). Parameters in this Table refer to DHC.

metabolites, including the O-sulphate and O-glucuronide, have also been identified.

In chronically treated patients, DHC is found in serum at concentrations very much higher than those of the parent drug, in agreement with the concept that this compound is primarily responsible for the pharmacological effect. The elimination of DHC involves primarily conjugation with glucuronic acid, but other metabolic pathways have also been identified. The elimination half-life of DHC is about 10 h and, unlike that of carbamazepine, is the same after single as after multiple dosing.

Dose–serum concentration relationship

The serum concentration of DHC is linearly related to dosage and there is no evidence of dose-dependent kinetics.

Concentration–effect relationship

In patients receiving therapeutic dosages of oxcarbazepine, the serum concentration of DHC has been reported to be generally in the 30–120 μmol/l (8–30 μg/ml) range. Preliminary data suggest that the correlation between serum DHC levels and either therapeutic or adverse effects is poor (Dam et al 1989).

Dose interval

In adults, the recommended dosage of oxcarbazepine is 600–1200 mg/day, though some patients may require higher amounts. The drug has been normally administered in three divided doses, but twice daily dosing may be feasible in some patients. Steady-state conditions are achieved within a few days, as expected on the basis of the relatively short half-life of the active DHC metabolite.

Pharmacokinetics in special situations

Oxcarbazepine and its active DHC metabolite cross the human placenta and are found in neonatal serum at concentrations similar to those found in the mother. In a newborn of an oxcarbazepine-treated mother, the half-life of placentally transferred DHC has been calculated to be about 17 hours, whereas the half-life of parent compound was longer (about 22 hours). It is possible that these values may be artifactually long due to concurrent intake of both compounds with breast milk during the sampling period.

Drug interactions

As compared to carbamazepine, oxcarbazepine is less likely to be involved in pharmacokinetic drug interactions. The serum levels of DHC in monotherapy patients have been reported to be similar to those observed in patients receiving other antiepileptic drugs in combination, suggesting that DHC metabolism may not be susceptible to enzyme induction (Faigle & Menge 1990).

Unlike carbamazepine, oxcarbazepine has little or no hepatic microsomal enzyme inducing properties in man and it does not appear to affect the metabolism of concurrently given drugs (Brodie et al 1989). This may provide a significant advantage in particular subgroups of patients, such as subjects taking oral anticoagulants or women taking the oral contraceptive pill. When oxcarbazepine is substituted for carbamazepine in patients receiving valproic acid or phenytoin, the serum levels of the latter drugs may increase considerably due to the waning of the inducing action of carbamazepine (Houtkooper et al 1987).

Therapeutic efficacy

Up to 1990, about 800 patients with epilepsy had received oxcarbazepine in clinical trials, and 143 of these had been treated for more than 1 year (Klosterkov Jensen et al 1991). Although no placebo-controlled studies have been performed, evidence of therapeutic efficacy has been obtained in a number of clinical investigations in which the drug has been invariably compared with carbamazepine.

In two major double-blind trials, oxcarbazepine and carbamazepine were administered according to a cross-over or parallel group design in addition to other antiepileptic drugs (Bulau et al 1987, Houtkooper et al 1987), while in a third study the two drugs were substituted for phenytoin in patients uncontrolled by phenytoin therapy

(Reinikanen et al 1987). Most of the patients had tonic-clonic and/or partial seizures, and the average daily dosage of oxcarbazepine was 50 to 100% higher than that of carbamazepine. None of these studies showed any significant difference in seizure frequency between the two drugs. Although these data suggest equivalent efficacy, the lack of a placebo control and the fact that, in the cross-over study the concentration of concurrent antiepileptic drugs was higher during the oxcarbazepine period than during the carbamazepine period does not allow unequivocal interpretation of the results.

In a fourth double-blind study, 235 patients with newly diagnosed epilepsy and partial seizures and/or generalized tonic-clonic seizures were randomly allocated to receive either oxcarbazepine or carbamazepine, with an overall follow-up period of about 1 year. In the 194 patients available for final analysis, no significant difference was found in seizure frequency between the two treatments. Complete seizure control was achieved in 43 (52%) of the 83 patients allocated to oxcarbazepine (mean final daily dosage 1040 mg) and in 49 (60%) of the 82 patients allocated to carbamazepine (mean final daily dosage 684 mg).

Overall, available information suggest that oxcarbazepine has similar efficacy to carbamazepine, and that the equivalent effective dose is about 50% higher than that of carbamazepine. Further studies, however, are required to define in more detail the activity of this drug and its indication(s) in specific epileptic syndromes.

Adverse effects

In clinical trials, there has been a trend towards a better tolerability of oxcarbazepine as compared to carbamazepine (Editorial 1989). The most frequently reported side effects, however, are similar to those of carbamazepine and include sedation, headache, dizziness and ataxia. In the largest trial, the overall incidence of side effects in monotherapy patients was 68% during treatment with oxcarbazepine and 74% during treatment with carbamazepine (Dam et al 1989). Although the difference was not statistically significant, side effects requiring discontinuation of therapy

(mostly allergic reactions) were significantly more frequent with carbamazepine than with oxcarbazepine.

Based on available evidence, oxcarbazepine appears to be considerably less likely to cause skin rashes at the onset of treatment, and this is a significant advantage over carbamazepine. In one study 51 patients who developed an allergic skin rash during treatment with carbamazepine were switched to oxcarbazepine: only 27% of them showed evidence of cross allergy (Klosterkov Jensen et al 1991). On the other hand, hyponatraemia seems to be much more common with oxcarbazepine than with carbamazepine. Although this biochemical abnormality is generally asymptomatic, there are reports of confusion and worsening in seizure frequency associated with low sodium levels (Johannessen & Nielsen 1987, Pendlebury et al 1989). Older patients and those on high doses appear to be particularly susceptible to the risk of oxcarbazepine-induced hyponatraemia.

LAMOTRIGINE

Lamotrigine is an antiepileptic drug chemically unrelated to conventional anticonvulsants, which was identified during a search for compounds possessing antifolate activity. Subsequent studies have demonstrated that the action of lamotrigine is mediated by mechanisms other than interference with folic acid metabolism. It has been reviewed by Yuen (1991) and Richens (1991).

Structure

The structure of lamotrigine is shown in Figure 15.9.

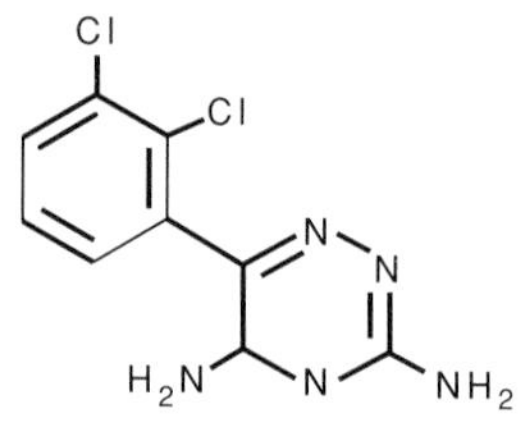

Fig. 15.9 Chemical structure of lamotrigine.

Mechanism of action

It has been proposed that the mode of action of lamotrigine involves blockade of voltage-sensitive sodium channels with consequent inhibition of the release of the excitatory aminoacid glutamate from nerve terminals in the CNS (Leach et al 1986).

Pharmacokinetics

The pharmacokinetics of lamotrigine (Table 15.15) have been reviewed by Perucca & Pisani (1991).

Absorption

Lamotrigine is absorbed rapidly and completely from the gastrointestinal tract, peak serum levels being usually attained within 3 h of drug intake. The first-pass metabolism of the drug is negligible.

Distribution and plasma protein binding

In man, the apparent volume of distribution of lamotrigine is about 1.1 l/kg. The drug is approximately 55% bound to plasma proteins and its concentration in saliva is approximately 45% of the plasma concentration.

Route of elimination, clearance and half-life

The elimination of lamotrigine occurs primarily

Table 15.15 Summary of pharmacokinetic data of lamotrigine

Range of daily maintenance dosage (adults)	50–400 mg/day
Time to peak serum level	2–3 h
Percentage bound to plasma proteins	55%
Apparent volume of distribution	1.1 l/kg
Elimination half-life	
monotherapy	15–50 h
concurrent treatment with enzyme inducers	8–33 h
concurrent treatment with valproic acid	30–90 h
Time to steady state after starting therapy	3–15 days
Major metabolite(s)	Glucuronide (inactive)
Minimum dose frequency	Once or twice daily

through conjugation with glucuronic acid. In subjects not receiving any other drug, the elimination half-life of lamotrigine is about 25 hours (range 14–50 hours) and the plasma clearance is about 0.55 ml/min/kg. The pharmacokinetic parameters determined after multiple dosing are similar to those observed after single dose administration.

As discussed below, the elimination half-life of lamotrigine is shortened by concurrent treatment with enzyme inducing agents (carbamazepine, barbiturates, phenytoin) and prolonged by concurrent intake of valproic acid.

Dose–serum concentration relationship

Serum concentrations of lamotrigine appear to be linearly related to dosage, at least within the 7.5–240 mg single dose range. Due to considerable pharmacokinetic variability, large differences in serum drug levels are observed among patients receiving the same dosage.

Concentration–effect relationship

Insufficient data is available on the relationship between serum drug level and intensity of pharmacological response.

Dose interval

Lamotrigine may be administered normally twice daily or even once daily. More frequent administration (three times daily) may be required in patients receiving concurrent treatment with enzyme-inducing agents which shorten the half-life of lamotrigine.

Pharmacokinetics in special situations

As expected from the route of elimination of the drug (glucuronide conjugation), the half-life of lamotrigine is moderately prolonged in patients with Gilbert's syndrome.

Drug interactions

Lamotrigine lacks enzyme inducing activity and does not affect significantly the kinetics of concurrently administered antiepileptic drugs. By contrast, concomitant antiepileptic therapy has a marked influence on lamotrigine pharmacokinetics. Enzyme–inducing antiepileptics such as phenytoin, phenobarbitone, primidone and carbamazepine markedly accelerate the metabolism of lamotrigine, whereas valproic acid inhibits it. In enzyme-induced patients, the half-life of lamotrigine is on average about 15 hours (range 8–33 hours) whereas in valproate-treated patients the half-life is prolonged to 30–90 hours (mean 60 hours). Patients receiving valproate together with enzyme-inducing drugs exhibit half-lives of about 30 hours, which are similar to those observed in patients not taking other drugs.

Because of these interactions, the recommended dosage of lamotrigine in patients receiving valproate is lower than that recommended for patients taking other anticonvulsants.

Therapeutic efficacy

More than 1600 patients had received lamotrigine in clinical trials at the time of writing.

Four randomized cross-over placebo-controlled trials have been performed in a total of 92 patients refractory to conventional antiepileptics (Binnie et al 1989, Jawad et al 1989, Yuen 1991). Most of these patients had complex partial seizures and the drug (50–400 mg/day) was usually given for 12 weeks in addition to pre-existing medication. The median percent reduction in seizure frequency (as compared to the placebo period) was 60% in one centre (P<0.002) and about 20% in the three remaining centres. Statistical analysis revealed a significant difference in favour of the drug in three out of the four studies. When all data were pooled together, a greater than 50% reduction in seizure frequency was observed in 25 (27%) of the 92 patients. These data clearly show that lamotrigine is effective in reducing seizure frequency. Although in some of these trials the magnitude of response was not dramatic, it should be stressed that the drug was given to patients with severe epilepsy who had already failed on existing therapy. Multicentre placebo-controlled trials in Australia and the USA have confirmed these results.

In these trials, a significant antiepileptic effect could be demonstrated against both partial and generalized tonic-clonic seizures and a similar finding has emerged from open studies in larger populations of patients. In a meta-analysis based on the assessment of the response after 12 weeks of add-on lamotrigine in open studies (Yuen 1991), a >50% reduction in seizure frequency was found in 28% of patients with partial seizures (n = 308), in 52% of patients with tonic-clonic seizures (n = 209) and in 46% of patients with absence seizures (n = 24). The number of patients with other seizure types was too small to allow a meaningful interpretation of data.

Adverse effects

Lamotrigine is generally well tolerated. In controlled studies, the side effects most frequently observed (fatigue, sedation, diplopia and headache) were reported in 12–17% of lamotrigine-treated patients and in 7–13% of patients taking placebo. At the most recent overall evaluation, 123 (8%) out of 1431 patients given lamotrigine were withdrawn because of adverse experiences (Yuen 1991). The most common cause for withdrawal was a skin rash (2.5% of patients treated with the drug). The next common reasons for withdrawal were diplopia and increase in seizure frequency, each of which occurred in less than 1% of treated patients.

GABAPENTIN

Gabapentin is a structural analogue of GABA which was synthesized during systematic studies aimed at developing GABA-mimetic compounds able to cross freely the blood–brain barrier. Although pharmacological studies in animal models confirmed that gabapentin possesses antiepileptic activity, it was surprisingly discovered that the action of the drug probably does not involve an action on GABA receptors or GABA-mediated transmission.

Structure

The structure of gabapentin (Fig 15.10) resembles closely that of GABA. The drug is a stable crystalline substance which does not exist in enantiomeric form.

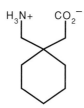

Fig. 15.10 Chemical structure of gabapentin.

Mechanism of action

Despite its structural resemblance to GABA, gabapentin does not bind to GABA receptors, does not affect brain GABA content and does not interfere with GABA metabolism, turnover or uptake. Binding to benzodiazepine, muscarinic and glycine receptors has been excluded. At present, no information is available on the mechanism which mediates the antiepileptic effect of this compound in animal models and in man.

Pharmacokinetics

The pharmacokinetics of gabapentin are summarized in Table 15.16. For more information the reader is referred to Schmidt (1989) and Perucca & Pisani (1991).

Absorption

The absorption of gabapentin from the gastro-intestinal tract is relatively rapid, peak serum levels being usually attained 2–3 hours after an oral dose. No first-pass metabolism occurs and the absolute oral availability is at least 70–80%. The absorption of the drug is not affected by concomitant intake of food.

Table 15.16 Summary of pharmacokinetic data of gabapentin

Range of daily maintenance dosage (adults)	600–1800 mg/day
Time to peak serum level	2–3 h
Percentage bound to plasma proteins	Nil
Apparent volume of distribution	0.7 l/kg
Elimination half-life	5–7 h
Time to steady state after starting therapy	2 days
Major metabolite(s)	None
Minimum dose frequency	Three times daily

Distribution and plasma protein binding

Gabapentin does not bind to plasma proteins. The volume of distribution at steady-state is about 0.7 l/kg.

Route of elimination, clearance and half-life

Gabapentin is not metabolized and is eliminated unchanged in urine. Unchanged drug in urine accounts for 75–81% of an orally-administered dose, the remainder being recovered in the faeces.

In the presence of a normal renal function, the elimination half-life of gabapentin is about 6 hours and the renal clearance is close to the creatinine clearance (120–160 ml/min). The interindividual variation in elimination parameters appears to be relatively small.

Dose–serum concentration relationship

After oral administration of single doses ranging from 100–900 mg, the elimination of gabapentin is independent of dosage whereas the gastro-intestinal absorption appears to be reduced at the highest dose. In patients receiving therapeutic regimens in divided daily administrations the serum concentration of the drug can be considered to be linearly related to dosage. The pharmacokinetics of gabapentin after multiple dosing are similar to those observed after a single dose.

Concentration–effect relationship

Insufficient information is available on the relationship between serum gabapentin levels and therapeutic or adverse effects.

Dose interval

Due to the relatively short half-life, multiple daily doses are recommended. Gabapentin is usually administered three times daily.

Pharmacokinetics in special situations

Since gabapentin is eliminated exclusively by the renal route, a reduction in the clearance of the drug in patients with impaired kidney function can be anticipated.

Drug interactions

The pharmacokinetics of gabapentin are not affected by concomitant administration of other antiepileptic drugs. In a similar way, gabapentin does appear to affect the disposition of other drugs.

Therapeutic efficacy

As of February 1990, about 1800 patients with epilepsy had received gabapentin in clinical trials. Of these, 460 had received the drug for more than 1 year and 119 for more than 2 years.

Evidence of therapeutic activity was first obtained in a double-blind cross-over study in which 25 patients (mostly with partial seizures with or without secondary generalization) received in random order for 8-week periods three different dosages of gabapentin (300, 600 or 900 mg/day) in addition to existing medication. During the 900 mg/day period, seizures were significantly reduced in comparison to both the baseline and the lower dosage periods. Compared to baseline, the median decrease in seizure frequency was 45% at the highest dosage (Crawford et al 1987).

In a subsequent open study in 70 patients with different types of epilepsy, gabapentin was added to pre-existing therapy and its dosage was individually titrated up to a maximum of 1800 mg/day for at least 2 months. As compared to baseline, the median decrease in seizure frequency after gabapentin was 27% for all seizures, 32% for partial seizures, 36% for tonic-clonic seizures and 49% for absence seizures (Bauer et al 1989).

A multicentre, placebo-controlled, double-blind and parallel group trial has been completed in 127 patients with drug resistant partial seizures, of whom 61 were randomized to gabapentin and 66 to placebo (Andrews et al 1990). After a 3-month baseline and a 2-week dose titration period, patients received gabapentin (1200 mg/day) or placebo in addition to existing medication for 3 consecutive months. A reduction of at least 50% in seizure frequency (compared to baseline) was observed in 25% of the patients in the gabapentin group and in 10% of the patients in the placebo group (P < 0.05).

An overall assessment of available data indicates that gabapentin is effective in reducing the frequency of both partial and generalized tonic-clonic seizures (insufficient data is available to assess potential efficacy in other seizure types). As discussed above for lamotrigine, the magnitude of the response has been limited in many cases, but this should be interpreted in the light of the fact that to date the drug has been tried mostly in patients refractory to conventional agents.

Adverse effects

Gabapentin appears to be relatively well tolerated. In the only placebo-controlled study published to date (Andrews et al 1990), side effects were reported in 62% of the patients taking gabapentin and in 41% of those taking placebo. The effects most frequently associated with the drug were drowsiness (15%), fatigue (13%), dizziness (7%) and weight gain (5%). These effects were usually mild and often disappeared during continuation of treatment.

ZONISAMIDE

Zonisamide is a sulphonamide derivative which has been developed in Japan as a result of screening studies on 3-substituted benzisoxazole compounds. In Western countries, its development was discontinued when a relatively high incidence of urolithiasis was observed during clinical trials. This adverse effect does not appear to have been confirmed in Oriental populations and the drug was introduced in the Japanese market in 1989.

Structure

The chemical structure of zonisamide is shown in Figure 15.11.

Mechanism of action

The antiepileptic action of zonisamide has been

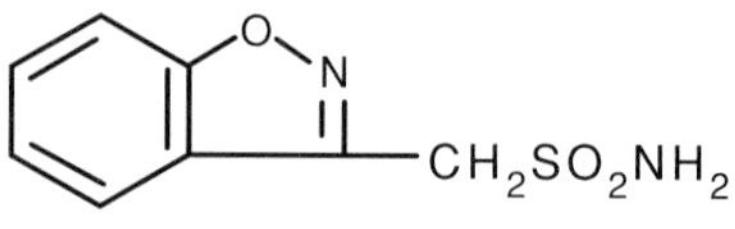

Fig. 15.11   Chemical structure of zonisamide.

related to suppression of epileptic focus activity as well as to blockade of the propagation of seizure discharges. The mode of action at a molecular level is, however, unknown. Zonisamide is a relatively weak inhibitor of carbonic anhydrase but it is unclear to what extent (if any) this property is relevant in mediating the antiepileptic effects of the drug.

Pharmacokinetics

The pharmacokinetics of zonisamide (reviewed by Perucca & Pisani 1991 and Seino et al 1991) are summarized in Table 15.17.

Absorption

Following oral administration, peak plasma zonisamide levels are observed at 2.5–6 hours after dosing.

Distribution and plasma protein binding

Zonisamide is approximately 50% bound to plasma proteins. The degree of plasma protein binding is concentration-dependent and it decreases with increasing drug concentrations within the clinically occurring range.

Zonisamide accumulates extensively in erythrocytes, probably due to binding to red cell carbonic anhydrase.

Route of elimination, clearance and half-life

Zonisamide is partly eliminated unchanged in urine and partly metabolized through glucuronidation, acetylation and other pathways. The proportion excreted unchanged in urine ranges from 8 to 50% of the administered dose. The metabolic pathways of zonisamide may become saturated within the clinically occurring concentration range.

Because of non-linear kinetics, half-life values for zonisamide have been calculated with some approximation. In subjects not taking other drugs, half-lives of 50–68 hours (mean 60 hours) have been reported but in patients treated with carbamazepine or phenytoin, half-life values average 36 and 27 hours respectively.

Dose–serum concentration relationship

Due to the occurrence of saturable metabolism, serum zonisamide concentrations at steady state are higher than predicted from single-dose kinetics. Saturable metabolism may also result in a disproportionately large increase in steady state serum concentration following a given dosage increment, although it has been stated that this phenomenon is of little relevance and that for practical purposes the concentration of the drug can be considered to be linearly related to dose within the therapeutic dose range.

Concentration–effect relationship

A method for the routine monitoring of serum zonisamide levels has been developed in Japan but information on the relationship between serum zonisamide concentration and clinical response is still very limited.

Dose interval

Due to its long half-life, zonisamide may be administered twice daily or even once daily.

Drug interactions

Zonisamide may increase the serum levels of concurrently administered carbamazepine. In patients receiving maintenance therapy with carbamazepine or phenytoin (and probably barbiturates)

Table 15.17   Summary of pharmacokinetic data of zonisamide

Range of daily maintenance dosage (adults)	200–400 mg/day
Time to peak serum level	2.5–6 h
Percentage bound to plasma proteins	50%
Apparent volume of distribution	Not determined
Elimination half-life	50–70 h*
Time to steady state after starting therapy	5–12 days
Major metabolite(s)	Many (probably inactive)
Minimum dose frequency	Twice or once daily

* Half-life is shorter (about 30 h on average) in patients receiving enzyme-inducing drugs such as phenytoin, carbamazepine and barbiturates.

zonisamide half-lives are shorter than those observed in normal subjects, presumably due to induction of metabolism.

Therapeutic efficacy

A large multicentre, double-blind, parallel group, placebo controlled evaluation of zonisamide has been carried out in Europe in 139 patients with refractory partial seizures (with or without secondary generalization). After 12 weeks treatment, the overall improvement rate in seizure frequency was found to be 62% in the zonisamide group as compared to 19% in the placebo group.

A double-blind parallel group trial carried out in Japan compared zonisamide and carbamazepine, each given for 16 weeks at an average daily dose of 330 mg and 600 mg respectively, in 108 patients who were either untreated or treated without good response with one to three conventional drugs (Seino et al 1988). As compared to baseline, the average monthly frequency of partial seizures decreased from 14.9 to 3.4 in the zonisamide group and from 13.3 to 4.4 in the carbamazepine group. The frequency of secondarily generalized tonic-clonic seizures also decreased to about one-third after administration of the two drugs. A similar study in 32 children with convulsive or non-convulsive generalized seizures found zonisamide to be at least as effective as valproic acid (Oguni et al 1988).

A meta-analysis has been performed on data from open studies conducted in a total of 1008 patients treated for an average of 253 days. Of these patients, 712 had partial seizures, 163 had generalized seizures and 132 had mixed seizure types (Seino et al 1991). When zonisamide was used as an add-on drug, improvement rates ranged from a minimum of 29% for myoclonic seizures to a maximum of 73% for atypical absence seizures, with improvement rates of 52% for complex partial seizures and 53% for primarily generalized tonic-clonic seizures. In patients receiving zonisamide monotherapy at the time of the final evaluation, improvement rates were 43% in generalized tonic seizures, 78% in primarily generalized tonic-clonic seizures, 93% in simple and complex partial seizures, and 94% in secondarily generalized tonic-clonic seizures.

Adverse effects

In published clinical trials, most of the reported adverse effects of zonisamide concerned the central nervous system and the gastrointestinal tract. In the meta-analysis performed by Seino et al (1991), adverse effects were found to occur in 517 (51%) out of 1008 patients, of whom 185 (18%) had to discontinue the trial. In polypharmacy patients the most frequently reported effects included drowsiness (24%), ataxia (13%), anorexia (11%), gastrointestinal symptoms (7%), loss or decrease of spontaneity (6%) and slowed mental function (5%). Deterioration of cognitive function has also been described after addition of zonisamide to pre-existing therapy. In monotherapy patients, the most frequently reported side effects were drowsiness (7%), gastrointestinal symptoms (7%), loss or decrease of spontaneity (6%), headache (6%), skin rashes/itching (6%) and weight loss (6%). In 2% of the patients the drug was discontinued because of increased liver enzymes or leukopenia.

As mentioned above, urolithiasis has been observed in some patients participating in clinical trials in Europe and in the United States. In Japan, however, only two out of 1008 patients have been found to suffer from symptomatic calculi during zonisamide treatment, and both of them had a positive family history of uro/nephrolithiasis.

OTHER DRUGS

Many other compounds have been tested for antiepileptic activity in laboratory experiments and in clinical trials during the last few years. These include not only new chemical entities, but also existing drugs which have been initially marketed for indications other than epilepsy and which have been subsequently proposed for investigation as potential antiepileptic drugs on the basis of relevant pharmacological data and/or serependitious clinical observations. Only compounds which have undergone relatively extensive clinical evaluation and which are still being developed at the time of writing will be considered briefly in this chapter. For information about drugs in early development (or compounds of theoretical interest which have been withdrawn from clinical development), the reader is referred to Chapter 13.

Calcium antagonists

Transmembrane calcium currents in cerebral neurones are known to play a significant role in the generation and propagation of epileptic discharges, and many drugs which block calcium channels exert antiepileptic effects in a variety of animal models (De Sarro et al 1988, Meyer et al 1990). In recent years, a large number of case reports or formal trials describing the effects of various calcium antagonists in epilepsy have appeared in the literature (Schmidt & Ried 1989).

Promising results have been obtained initially in some studies with the atypical calcium antagonist flunarizine (Binnie et al 1985), but additional trials have produced less encouraging findings (Alving et al 1990) and this drug is not being developed as an antiepileptic. Verapamil and diltiazem have also been administered to patients with epilepsy, but the assessment of these drugs has been hampered by the occurrence of clinically significant pharmacokinetic interactions with other antiepileptic drugs (particularly an inhibiting effect on carbamazepine metabolism) (Brodie & Macphee 1986).

At present, many investigations are being focused on dihydropyridine compounds, some of which appear to exhibit a relative selectivity for neuronal calcium channels (Meyer et al 1990). In particular nimodipine, one of these compounds, has been found to influence favourably seizure activity in animal models, but available clinical data are as yet insufficient to determine the therapeutic value of this agent (if any). Again, the clinical evaluation of these drugs may be complicated by important pharmacokinetic interactions. It has been shown, for example, that phenytoin and carbamazepine (and presumably also barbiturates) reduce dramatically the oral bioavailability of nifedipine and felodipine by stimulating its first pass metabolism in the liver (Capewell et al l988, Kirch et al 1990). The same drugs were shown also to reduce markedly the serum levels of nimodipine, whereas valproic acid exerts an opposite effect by increasing nimodipine bioavailability about two-fold (Tartara et al 1990).

Eterobarb

Eterobarb is a barbiturate derivative which has been evaluated for efficacy (generally in comparison with phenobarbitone) in a number of controlled trials in the United States and in Italy.

In animal models, eterobarb exhibits a more favourable therapeutic ratio compared with phenobarbitone, despite the fact that it is extensively converted to phenobarbitone itself. In humans, unchanged eterobarb is not detected in blood of patients treated with the drug. Eterobarb is rapidly transformed to its monomethoxymethyl derivative (MMP), which is present in blood at very low concentrations, and to phenobarbitone, which accumulates extensively (Golberg et al 1976).

The results of some clinical studies have suggested that eterobarb retains an efficacy similar to that of phenobarbitone but it is comparatively less prone to produce sedative effects (Mattson et al 1976, Smith et al 1986). To explain this observation, it has been speculated that an additional metabolite of eterobarb (possibly MMP) may counteract the sedative effects of metabolically derived phenobarbitone without interfering adversely with the antiepileptic activity of the latter.

Felbamate

Felbamate is a new compound currently undergoing clinical trials in a number of countries. In animal models, felbamate shows wide-spectrum antiepileptic activity and a lower neurotoxic potential compared with conventional antiepileptic drugs (Leppik & Graves 1989).

In man, felbamate shows rapid absorption from the gastrointestinal tract, low degree of binding to plasma proteins (24–35%) and elimination half-lives of about 10–20 hours. The main route of elimination is metabolic. When added to existing antiepileptic medication, felbamate may cause an increase in serum phenytoin and a decrease in serum carbamazepine concentrations.

Two double blind, cross-over, placebo-controlled add-on studies in patients with partial seizures have been completed in the United States. Only the results of the first of these trials have been analysed to date and demonstrate a significant reduction in seizure frequency during the felbamate period (Leppik et al 1989).

Loreclezole

Loreclezole is a triazole derivative which exhibits broad spectrum antiepileptic activity in animal models (DeBeukelaar & Tritsmans 1991).

In man, the drug is absorbed rapidly from the gastrointestinal tract. Half-lives of 10–34 hours have been described in patients receiving combination therapy with other antiepileptic drugs. The serum levels of loreclezole are known to be reduced by concurrent intake of enzyme-inducing drugs (phenytoin, carbamazepine and barbiturates).

After single dose administration, loreclezole is effective in reducing the photoparoxysmal response in photosensitive patients. A double-blind study has been completed in 62 patients with epilepsy resistant to conventional drugs, who received either loreclezole or placebo for 3 months according to a parallel-group design. In this trial, the loreclezole group showed a reduction in seizure frequency which was significantly better than that observed in the placebo group (DeBeukelaar & Tritsmans 1991).

Stiripentol

Stiripentol is a compound structurally unrelated to existing antiepileptic drugs which also shows a wide spectrum of activity in pharmacological models of epilepsy.

In man, stiripentol is absorbed readily from the gastrointestinal tract, is highly bound to plasma proteins (>90%), and is extensively metabolized.

The biotransformation of the drug is saturable within the clinically used dosage range, resulting in a non-linear relationship between serum concentration and dosage (Levy et al 1984).

The clinical evaluation of stiripentol has been made difficult by the occurrence of a large number of pharmacokinetic drug interactions. Enzyme-inducing antiepileptic drugs stimulate stiripentol metabolism and decrease serum stiripentol levels at steady-state. More importantly, stiripentol inhibits markedly the metabolism of phenytoin and carbamazepine (Levy et al 1984): if the dosage of the latter drug is not reduced after adding stiripentol, serious toxicity may result. Stiripentol has also been shown to inhibit the metabolism of phenobarbitone, primidone and, to a lesser extent, valproic acid. In view of the clinical relevance of most of these interactions, careful monitoring of the serum levels of associated antiepileptic drugs is essential when stiripentol is added to existing therapy.

The efficacy of stiripentol has been evaluated in a number of open trials conducted mostly in France in patients with different seizure types. A reduction in mean seizure frequency after administration of the drug was generally observed, but the non-controlled nature of the observations and the occurrence of pharmacokinetic interactions makes interpretation of the data difficult. In one study in which stiripentol was given as sole therapy to patients with refractory absence seizures, 11 out of 20 patients were found to exhibit a greater than 50% reduction in fit frequency (Loiseau & Tor 1987). These data suggest that stiripentol may be of value in the treatment of seizures of the absence type.

REFERENCES

Alcala H, Lertratanangkoon K, Stenbach W, Kellaway P, Horning M G 1978 The purkinje cell in phenytoin intoxication; ultrastructural and Golgi studies. Pharmacologist 20: 240

Alving J, Krustensen O, Tsiropoulos I, Modrup K 1989 Double-blind placebo-controlled evaluation of flunarizine as adjunct therapy in epilepsy with complex partial seizures. Acta Neurologica Scandinavica 79: 128

Andreason P B, Lyngbye J, Trolle E 1973 Abnormalities in liver function tests during long-term diphenylhydantoin in epileptic out-patients. Acta Medica Scandinavica 194: 261

Andrews J, Chadwick D, Bates D et al 1990 Gabapentin in partial epilepsy. Lancet 1: 466

Anthony J H, Hawke S M B 1983 Phenobarbital compared with carbamazepine in prevention of recurrent febrile convulsions. American Journal of Diseases of Childhood 137: 892

Asconape J J, Penry J K 1982 Use of antiepileptic drugs in the presence of liver and kidney diseases: a review. Epilepsia 23 (Suppl 1): 565

Ayers G, Burnett D, Griffiths A, Richens A 1980 Quality control of drug assays. Clinical Pharmacokinetics 6: 106

Bacon C J, Mucklow J C, Rawlins M D et al 1981 Placebo-controlled study of phenobarbitone and phenytoin in the prophylaxis of febrile convulsions. Lancet ii: 600

Battino D, Binelli S, Bossi L et al 1984 Changes in primidone/phenobarbitone ratio during pregnancy and the puerperium. Clinical Pharmacokinetics 9: 252

Battino D, Binelli S, Bossi L et al 1985 Plasma concentrations of carbamazepine and carbamazepine 10, 11-epoxide during pregnancy and after delivery. Clinical Pharmacokinetics 10: 27

Bauer G, Bechinger D, Castell M et al 1989 Gababentin in the treatment of drug resistant epileptic patients. In: Manelis J, Bental E, Loeber J N, Dreifuss F E (eds), Advances in epileptology, vol 17. Raven Press, New York, p 219

Baumel I P, Gallagher B B, Mattson R H 1972 Phenylethylmalonamide (PEMA). An important metabolite of primidone. Archives of Neurology 27: 34

Bell R D, Pak C Y C, Zerwekh J, Barilla D E, Vasko M 1978 Effect of phenytoin on bone and vitamin D metabolism. Annals of Neurology 5: 374

Bennet E P 1977 Influence of phenytoin and carbamazepine on endocrine function. Epilepsia 18: 294

Bertilsson L, Tomson T 1986 Clinical pharmacokinetics and pharmacological effects of carbamazepine and carbamazepine 10, 11-epoxide: an update. Clinical Pharmacokinetics 11: 177

Betts T A, Kalra P L, Cooper R, Jeavons P M 1968 Epileptic fits as a probable side effect of amitriptyline. Lancet 1: 390

Binnie C D, De Beukelaar F, Meijer J W A et al 1985 Open dose-ranging trial of flunarizine as add-on therapy in epilepsy. Epilepsia 26: 424

Binnie C D, Debets R M C, Engesman M et al 1989 Double-blind crossover trial of lamotrigine (Lamictal) as add on therapy in intractable epilepsy. Epilepsy Research 4: 222

Blain P G, Mucklow J C, Bacon C J, Rawlins M D 1981 Pharmacokinetics of phenytoin in children. British Journal of Clinical Pharmacology 12: 659–661

Blaschke T F 1977 Protein binding and kinetics of drugs in liver disease. Clinical Pharmacokinetics 2: 32

Bolton J B, Rimmer E, Williams J, Richens A 1989 The effect of vigabatrin on brain and platelet GABA-transaminase activities. British Journal of Clinical Pharmacology 27: 35S

Booker H E 1982 Trimethadione. Relation of plasma concentration to seizure control. In: Woodbury D M, Penry J K, Pippenger C E (eds) Antiepileptic drugs. Raven Press, New York, p 697

Bourgeois B F D, Dodson W E, Ferendelli J A 1983 Primidone, phenobarbital and PEMA: seizure protection, neurotoxicity, and therapeutic index of individual compounds in mice. Neurology 33: 283

Brodie M J, McPhee G J A 1986 Carbamazepine neurotoxicity precipitated by diltiazem. British Medical Journal 292: 1170

Brodie M J, Larkin J G, McKee P J et al 1989 Is oxcarbazepine an enzyme inducer in man? 18th International Epilepsy Congress, New Delhi, Abstract 105

Browne T R 1976 Clonazepam. A review of a new anticonvulsant drug. Archives of Neurology 33: 326

Browne T R, Penry J K 1973 Benzodiazepines in the treatment of epilepsy. A review. Epilepsia 14: 277

Browne T R, Dreifuss F E, Dyken P R et al 1975 Ethosuximide in the treatment of absence (petit mal) seizures. Neurology 25: 515

Browne T R, Mattson R H, Penry J K et al 1987 Vigabatrin for refractory complex partial seizures. Multicentre single-blind study and long-term follow-up. Neurology 37: 184

Buchthal F, Svensmark O, Schiller P J 1960 Clinical and electroencephalographic correlations with serum levels of diphenylhydantoin. Archives of Neurology 2: 624

Buchthal F, Svensmark O, Simonsen H 1968 Relation of EEG and seizures to phenobarbital in serum. Archives of Neurology 19: 567

Buchanan R A, Kinkel A W, Smith T C 1973 The absorption and excretion of ethosuximide. International Journal of Clinical Pharmacology and New Drugs 7: 213

Buchanan R A, Kinkel A W, Turner J L, Heffelfinger J C 1976 Ethosuximide dosage regimens. Clinical Pharmacology and Therapeutics 19: 143

Bulau P, Stoll K D, Froscher W 1987 Oxcarbazepine versus carbamazepine. In: Wolff P, Dam M, Janz D, Dreifuss F (eds) Advances in epilepsy, vol 16. Raven Press, New York, p 531

Butler T C 1978 Some quantitative aspects of the pharmacology of phenobarbital. In: Pippenger C E, Penry J K, Kutt H (eds) Antiepileptic drugs: quantitative analysis and interpretation. Raven Press, New York, p 261

Callaghan N, Kenny R A, O'Neil B, Crowley M, Goggin T 1985 A prospective study between carbamazepine, phenytoin and sodium valproate as monotherapy in previously untreated and recently diagnosed patients with epilepsy. Journal of Neurology, Neurosurgery and Psychiatry 48: 639

Callaghan N, O'Dwyer R, Keating J 1984 Unnecessary polypharmacy in patients with frequent seizures. Acta Neurologica Scandinavica 69: 15

Callaghan N, O'Hare J, O'Driscoll D, O'Neill B, Daly M 1982 Comparative study of ethosuximide and sodium valproate in the treatment of typical absence seizures (petit mal). Developmental Medicine and Child Neurology 24: 830

Capewell S, Freestone S, Critchley J A J H, Pottage A, Prescott L F 1988 Reduced felodipine bioavailability in patients taking anticonvulsants. Lancet 2: 480

Cereghino J J, Brock J T, Van Meter J C, Penry J K, Smith L D, White B G 1974 Carbamazepine for epilepsy. A controlled prospective evaluation. Neurology 24: 401

Cereghino J J, Brock J T, van Meter J C, Penry J K, Smith L D, White B G 1975 The efficacy of carbamazepine combinations in epilepsy. Clinical Pharmacology and Therapeutics 18: 733

Chadwick D, Reynolds E H 1985 When do epileptic patients need treatment? Starting and stopping medication. British Medical Journal 290: 1885

Chadwick D, Turnbull D M 1985 The comparative efficacy of antiepileptic drugs for partial and tonic-clonic seizures. Journal of Neurology, Neurosurgery and Psychiatry 48: 1073

Chadwick D, Shaw M D M, Foy P, Rawlins M D, Turnbull D M 1984 Serum anticonvulsant concentrations and the risk of drug induced skin eruptions. Journal of Neurology, Neurosurgery and Psychiatry 47: 642

Chadwick D, Reynolds E H, Marsden C D 1976 Anticonvulsant-induced dyskinesias: a comparison with dyskinesias induced by neuroleptics. Journal of Neurology, Neurosurgery and Psychiatry 39: 1210

Chambers R E, Homeida M, Hunter K R, Teague R H 1977 Salivary carbamazepine concentrations. Lancet i: 656

Chiron C, Dulac O, Luna D et al 1990 Vigabatrin in infantile spasms. Lancet 1: 363

Cleland P G, Mosqvera I, Steward W P, Foster J B 1981 Prognosis of isolated seizures in adult life. British Medical Journal 283: 1364

Coatsworth J J 1971 Studies on the clinical efficacy of marketed antiepileptic drugs. NINDS Monograph No. 12. US Government Printing Office, Washington DC

Covanis A, Jeavons P M 1980 Once-daily sodium valproate in the treatment of epilepsy. Developmental Medicine and Child Neurology 22: 202

Crawford P, Ghadiali E, Lane R, Blumhardt L, Chadwick D 1987 Gabapentin as an antiepileptic drug in man. Journal of Neurology, Neurosurgery and Psychiatry 50: 682

Dam M, Ekberg R, Loyning Y, Waltimo O, Jacobsen K 1989 A double-blind study comparing oxcarbazepine and carbamazepine in patients with newly diagnosed previously untreated epilepsy. Epilepsy Research 3: 70

De Beukelaar F, Tritsmans L 1991 Loreclezole In: Pisani F, Perucca E, Avanzini G, Richens A (eds) New antiepileptic drugs. Amsterdam, Elsevier

De Sarro G B, Meldrum B S, Nistic G 1988 Anticonvulsant effects of some calcium entry blockers in DBA/2 mice. British Journal of Pharmacology 93: 247

Eadie M J, Bochner F, Hooper W D, Tyrer J H 1978 Preliminary observations on the pharmacokinetics of methylphenobarbitone. Clinical and Experimental Neurology 15: 131

Editorial 1971 Is phenytoin carcinogenic? Lancet ii: 1071

Editorial 1980 Febrile convulsions: a suitable case for treatment. Lancet ii: 680

Editorial 1981 Febrile convulsions: long-term treatment. British Medical Journal 282: 673

Editorial 1989 Oxcarbazepine. Lancet 2: 196

Edwards J G, Long S K, Sedgwick E M, Wheal H V 1986 Antidepressants and convulsive seizures: clinical, electroencephalographic, and pharmacological aspects. Clinical Neuropharmacology 9: 329

Elwes R D C, Chesterman P, Reynolds E H 1985 Prognosis after a first untreated tonic-clonic seizure. Lancet ii: 752

Elwes R D C, Johnson A L, Shorvon S D, Reynolds E H 1984 The prognosis for seizure control in newly diagnosed epilepsy. New England Journal of Medicine 311: 944

Faigle J W, Menge G P 1990 Pharmacokinetic and metabolic features of oxcarbazepine and their clinical significance: Comparison with carbamazepine. International Clinical Psychopharmacology 5 (Suppl 1): 73

Feely M, Calvert R, Gibson J 1982 Clobazam in catamenial epilepsy: a model for evaluating anticonvulsants. Lancet ii: 71

Feldman G, Weaver D, Lovrien E 1977 The fetal trimethadione syndrome: report of an additional family and further delineation of their syndrome. American Journal of Diseases of Childhood 131: 1389

Finucane J F, Griffiths R S 1976 Effect of phenytoin therapy on thyroid function. British Journal of Clinical Pharmacology 3: 1041

Fischbacher E 1982 Effect of reduction of anticonvulsants on well being. British Medical Journal 285: 423

Flint N, Lopez L M, Robinson J D, Williams C, Salem R B 1985 Comparison of eight phenytoin dosing methods in institutionalized patients. Therapeutic Drug Monitoring 7: 74

Foy P M, Copeland G P, Shaw M D M 1981 The incidence of postoperative seizures. Acta Neurochirurgica 55: 253

Gamble J A S, Dundee J W, Assaf R A E 1975 Plasma diazepam levels after single oral and intramuscular administration. Anaesthesia 30: 164

Gannaway D J, Mawer G E 1981 Serum phenytoin concentration and clinical response to patients with epilepsy. British Journal of Clinical Pharmacology 12: 833

Goldberg M, Gal J, Cho A K, Henden D J 1976 Metabolism of dimethoxymethylphenobarbital (eterobarb) in patients with epilepsy. Annals of Neurology 5: 121

Goodridge D M G, Shorvon S D 1983 Epileptic seizures in a population of 6000. II. Treatment and prognosis. British Medical Journal 287: 645

Gowers W R 1881 Epilepsy and other chronic convulsive diseases. Churchill, London

Gram L, Flachs H, Wurtz-Jorgensen, A, Parnas J, Andersen B 1980 Sodium valproate, relationship between serum levels and therapeutic effect: a controlled study. In: Johannessen S I et al (eds) Antiepileptic therapy: advances in drug monitoring. Raven Press, New York, p 217

Greenblatt D J, Allen M D, McLaughlin D S, Harmatz J S, Shader R I 1978 Diazepam absorption: effects of antacids and food. Clinical Pharmacology and Therapeutics 24: 600

Griffiths A, Hebdige S, Perucca E, Richens A 1980 Quality control in drug measurement. Therapeutic Drug Monitoring 2: 51

Guelen P J M, Van der Kleijn E, Woudstra U 1975 Statistical analysis of pharmacokinetic parameters in epileptic patients chronically treated with antiepileptic drugs. In: Schneider H, Janz D, Gardner-Thorpe C, Meinardi H, Sherwin A C (eds) Clinical pharmacology of antiepileptic drugs. Springer-Verlag, Berlin, p 2

Gugler R, Mueller G 1978 Plasma protein binding of valproic acid in healthy subjects and in patients with renal disease. British Journal of Clinical Pharmacology 5: 441

Gugler R, von Unruh G E 1980 Clinical pharmacokinetics of valproic acid. Clinical Pharmacokinetics 5: 67

Gugler R, Eichelbaum M, Schell et al 1980 The disposition of valproic acid. In: Johannessen S I et al (eds) Antiepileptic therapy: advances in drug monitoring. Raven Press, New York, p 125

Haegele K, Huebert N D, Ebel M, Tell G, Schechter P J 1988 Pharmacokinetics of vigabatrin: Implications of creatinine clearance. Clinical Pharmacology and Therapeutics 44: 558

Hahn T J 1976 Bone complications of anticonvulsants. Drugs 12: 201

Harding G F A, Herrick C E, Jeavons P M 1978 A controlled study of the effect of sodium valproate on photosensitive epilepsy and its prognosis. Epilepsia 19: 555

Hart R G, Easton J D 1981 Carbamazepine and hematological monitoring. Annals of Neurology 11: 309

Hart Y M, Sander J W A S, Johnson A L, Shorvon S D 1990 For the NGPSE. National General Practice Study of Epilepsy: recurrence after a first seizure. Lancet 336: 1271

Hauser W A, Andersen V E, Loewenson R B, McRoberts S M 1982 Seizure recurrence after a first unprovoked seizure. New England Journal of Medicine 307: 522

Hauser W A, Rich S S, Annegers J F, Anderson V E 1990 Seizure recurrence after a 1st unprovoked seizure: an extended follow-up. Neurology 40: 1163.

Henriksen O, Johannessen 1980 Clinical observations of sodium valproate in children: an evaluation of therapeutic serum levels. In: Johannessen S I et al (eds) Antiepileptic therapy: advances in drug monitoring. Raven Press, New York, p 253

Herranz J L, Armijo J A, Artega R 1984 Effectiveness and toxicity of phenobarbital, primidone and sodium valproate in the prevention of febrile convulsions controlled by plasma levels. Epilepsia 25: 89

Houghton G W, Richens A 1974 Rate of elimination of tracer doses of phenytoin at different steady-state serum phenytoin concentrations in epileptic patients. British Journal of Clinical Pharmacology 1: 155

Houghton G W, Richens A, Leighton M 1975a Effect of age, height, weight and sex on serum phenytoin concentration in epileptic patients. British Journal of Clinical Pharmacology 2: 251

Houghton G W, Richens A, Toseland P A, Davidson S, Falconer M A 1975b Brain concentrations of phenytoin, phenobarbitone and primidone in epileptic patients. European Journal of Clinical Pharmacology 9: 73

Houtkooper M A, Lammertsma A, Meijer J W A et al 1987 Oxcarbazepine (GP 47680): a possible alternative to carbamazepine. Epilepsia 25: 693

Hrachovy R A, Frost J D, Kellaway P, Zion T 1979 A controlled study of prednisone therapy in infantile spasms. Epilepsia 20: 403

Jalling B 1974 Plasma and CSF concentrations of phenobarbital in infants given single doses. Developmental Medicine and Child Neurology 16: 781

Janz D 1982 On major malformations and minor abnormalities in the offspring of parents with epilepsy. In: Janz D, Dam M, Richens A, Bossi L, Helge H, Schmidt D (eds) Epilepsy, pregnancy and the child. Raven Press, New York, p 211

Jawad S, Richens A, Oxley J 1984 Single dose pharmacokinetic study of clobazam in normal volunteers and epileptic patients. British Journal of Clinical Pharmacology 18: 873

Jawad S, Richens A, Goodwin G, Yuen W C 1989 Controlled trial of lamotrigine (Lamictal) for refractory partial seizures. Epilepsia 30: 356

Jeavons P M, Bower B D 1974 Infantile spasms. In: Vinken P J, Bruyn G W (eds) Handbook of clinical neuorology, vol 15: the epilepsies. American Elsevier, New York, p 219

Jeavons P M, Clark J E, Maheshwari M C 1977 Treatment of generalised epilepsies of childhood and adolescence with sodium valproate (Epilim). Developmental Medicine and Child Neurology 19: 9

Jennett W B 1975 Epilepsy after non-missile head injuries, 2nd edn. Heinemann, London

Johannessen A C, Nielsen O A 1987 Hyponatraemia induced by oxcarbazepine. Epilepsy Research 1: 155

Johannessen S I, Barruzzi A, Gomeni R, Strandjord R E, Morselli P L 1977 Further observations on carbamazepine and carbamazepine-10, 11-epoxide kinetics in epileptic patients. In: Gardner-Thorpe C, Janz D, Meinardi H, Pippenger C E (eds) Antiepileptic drug monitoring. Pitman Press, Avon, p 110

Jones I C J, Lacro R V, Johnson K A, Adams J 1989 Pattern of malformations in children of women treated with carbamazepine during pregnancy. New England Journal of Medicine 320: 1661

Kaneko S, Sato T, Suzuki K 1979 The levels of anticonvulsants in breast milk. British Journal of Clinical Pharmacology 7: 624

Kanto J 1975 Plasma concentrations of diazepam and its metabolites after per oral, intramuscular and rectal administration. International Journal of Clinical Pharmacy and Biopharmaceutics 12: 427

Kaufmann R F, Habersang R, Lansky L 1977 Kinetics of primidone metabolism and excretion in children. Clinical Pharmacology and Therapeutics 22: 200

Kay J D S, Hilton-Jones D, Hyman N 1986 Valproate toxicity and ornithine carbamoyltransferase deficiency. Lancet ii: 1283

Kirch W, Kleinbloesem C, Belz G G 1990 Drug interactions with calcium antagonists. Pharmacology and Therapeutics 45: 109

Klosterkov-Jensen P, Gram L, Schmutz M 1991 Oxcarbazepine.In: Pisani F, Perucca E, Avanzini G, Richens A (eds) New antiepileptic drugs. Amsterdam, Elsevier

Klotz U, Schweizer C 1980 Valproic acid in childhood epilepsy: anticonvulsive efficacy in relation to its plasma levels. International Journal of Clinical Pharmacology, Therapy and Toxicology 18: 461

Knott C 1983 Measurement of saliva drug concentrations in the control of antiepileptic medication. In: Pedley T A, Meldrum B S (eds) Recent advances in epilepsy, vol l. Churchill Livingstone, Edinburgh, p 57

Knudsen F U 1979 Rectal administration of diazepam in solution in the acute treatment of convulsions in infants and children. Archives of Diseases in Childhood 54: 855

Knudsen F U, Vestermark S 1978 Prophylactic diazepam or phenobarbital in febrile convulsions: a prospective controlled study. Archives of Diseases of Childhood 53: 600

Kosteljanetz M, Christiansen J, Mouritzen Dam A et al 1979 Carbamazepine vs phenytoin. A controlled clinical trial in focal motor and generalized epilepsy. Archives of Neurology 36: 22

Kutt H, MacDowell F 1968 Management of epilepsy with diphenylhydantoin sodium. Journal of the American Medical Association 203: 969

Kutt H, Winters W, Kokenge R, McDowell F 1964 Diphenylhydantoin metabolism, blood levels, and toxicity. Archives of Neurology 11: 642

Leach M J, Marsden C M, Miller A A 1986 Pharmacological studies on lamotrigine, a novel potential antiepileptic drug. II Neurochemical studies on the mechanism of action. Epilepsia 27: 490

Lee K, Melchior J C 1981 Sodium valproate versus phenobarbital in the prophylactic treatment of febrile convulsions in childhood. European Journal of Paediatrics 137: 151

Legg N J, Swash M 1974 Clinical note: Seizures and EEG activation after trimipramine. Epilepsia 15: 131

Leppik I, Graves N M 1989 Potential antiepileptic drugs: Felbamate. In: Levy R H, Dreifuss F E, Mattson R H, Meldrum B S, Penry J K (eds) Antiepileptic drugs. Raven Press, New York, p 983

Leppik I E, Cloyd J C, Miller K 1984 Development of tolerance to the side effects of primidone. Therapeutic Drug Monitoring 6: 189

Leppik I E, Dreifuss F E, Pledger G W et al 1989 Felbamate in partial seizures: Results of phase II clinical trial. Epilepsia 30: 661

Lesser R P, Pippenger C E, Luders H, Dinner D S 1984 High dose monotherapy in the treatment of intractable seizures. Neurology 34: 707

Levy R H, Pitlick W H, Troupin A S, Green J R, Neal J M 1975 Pharmacokinetics of carbamazepine in normal man. Clinical Pharmacology Therapeutics 17: 657

Levy R H, Loiseau P, Guyot M, Blehaut H, Tor J, Moreland T A 1984 Stiripentol kinetics in epilepsy: non-linearity and interactions. Clinical Pharmacology and Therapeutics 36: 661

Lindhout D, Hoppener R J E A, Meinardi H 1984 Teratogenicity of antiepileptic drug combinations with

special emphasis on expoxidation (of carbamazepine).
Epilepsia 25: 77

Lockard J S, Levy R H 1976 Valproic acid: reversibly acting drug? Epilepsia 17: 477

Loiseau P, Tor J 1987 Stiripentol in absence seizures—an open study. Epilepsia 28: 579

Lund L 1974 Anticonvulsant effect of diphenylhydantoin relative to plasma levels. A prospective three-year study in ambulant patients with generalised epileptic seizures. Archives of Neurology 31: 289

McAuliffe J J, Sherwin A L, Leppik I E, Fayle S E, Pippenger C E 1977 Salivary levels of anticonvulsants: a practical approach to drug monitoring. Neurology 27: 409

McQueen J K, Blackwood D H R, Harris P, Kalbag R M, Johnson A L 1983 Low risk of late post-traumatic seizures following severe head injury: implications for clinical trials of prophylaxis. Journal of Neurology, Neurosurgery and Psychiatry 46: 899

McQueen J K, Blackwood D H R, Minns R A, Brown J K 1982 Plasma levels of sodium valproate in childhood epilepsy. Scottish Medical Journal 27: 312

Mandelli M, Tognoni G, Garatini S 1978 Clinical pharmacokinetics of diazepam. Clinical Pharmacokinetics 3: 72

Mattson R, Williamson P, Hanahan E 1976 Eterobarb (DMMP) therapy in epilepsy. Neurology 26: 1014

Mattson R H, Cramer J A, Collins J F et al 1985 Comparison of carbamazepine, phenobarbital, phenytoin and primidone in partial and secondarily generalized tonic clonic seizures. New England Journal of Medicine 313: 145

Meisser O, Joubert P H, Joubert H F, Van der Merwe C A 1984 The IgA immune system in epileptics on anticonvulsant therapy. European Journal of Clinical Pharmacology 27: 81

Melchior J C, Buchthal R, Lennox-Buchthal M 1971 The ineffectiveness of diphenylhydantoin in preventing febrile convulsions in the age of greater risk, under 3 years. Epilepsia 12: 55

Meyer F B, Anderson R E, Sundt T M Jr 1990 Anticonvulsant effects of dihydropyridine Ca^{2+} antagonists in electrocortical shock seizures. Epilepsia 31: 68

Milligan N, Dhillon S, Richens A, Oxley J 1981 Rectal diazepam in the treatment of absence status: a pharmacodynamic study. Journal of Neurology, Neurosurgery and Psychiatry 47: 914–917

Morselli P L 1977 Antiepileptic drugs. In: Morselli P L (ed.) Drug disposition during development. Spectrum, New York, p 311

Morselli P L 1978 Clinical significance of monitoring plasma levels of benzodiazepine tranquillisers and antiepileptic drugs. In: Deniker P, Radouco-Thomas C, Villeneuve A (eds) Neuropsychopharmacology. Pergamon Press, Oxford, p 877

Mountain K R Hirsch J, Gallus A S 1970 Neonatal coagulation defect due to anticonvulsant drug treatment in pregnancy. Lancet 1: 265

Mucklow J C, Dollery C T 1978 Compliance with anticonvulsant therapy in a hospital clinic and in the community. British Journal of Clinical Pharmacology 6: 75

Mumford J P, Dam M 1989 Meta-analysis of European placebo controlled studies of vigabatrin in drug resistant epilepsy. British Journal of Clinical Pharmacology 27: 101S

Mumford J P, Lewis P J 1991 Vigabatrin. In: Pisani F, Perucca E, Avanzini G, Richens A (eds). New antiepileptic drugs. Amsterdam, Elsevier

Musicco M, Beghi E, Bordo B, Viani F 1989 The effect of drug treatment on the risk of recurrence after a first unprovoked tonic-clonic seizure: an Italian multicentre randomized trial. Neurology 39 (suppl 1): 148

Nanda R N, Johnson R H, Keogh H J, Lambie D G, Melville I D 1977 Treatment of epilepsy with clonazepam and its effect on other anticonvulsants. Journal of Neurology, Neurosurgery and Psychiatry 40: 538

Ngwane E, Bower B 1980 Continuous sodium valproate or phenobarbitone in the prevention of 'simple' febrile convulsions. Archives of Diseases of Childhood 55: 171

North J B, Penhall R K, Hanieh A, Frenwin D B, Taylor W B 1983 Phenytoin and post-operative epilepsy, a double blind study. Journal of Neurosurgery 58: 672

Oguni H, Hayashi K, Fukuyama Y et al 1988 Phase III study of a new antiepileptic AD-810, zonisamide, in childhood epilepsy. Japanese Journal of Pediatrics 41: 439 (in Japanese)

Oxley J, Hebdige S, Laidlaw J, Wadsworth J, Richens A 1980 A comparative study of phenobarbitone and primidone in the treatment of epilepsy. In: Johannessen S I et al (eds) Antiepileptic therapy: advances in drug monitoring. Raven Press, New York, p 237

Parker W A, Shearer C A 1979 Phenytoin hepatotoxicity :a case report and review. Neurology 29: 175

Paxton J W, Whiting B, Stephen K W 1977 Phenytoin concentrations in mixed parotid and submandibular saliva and serum measured by radioimmunoassay. British Journal of Clinical Pharmacology 4: 185

Pendlebury S C, Moses D K, Eadie M J 1989 Hyponatraemia during oxacarbazepine therapy. Human Toxicology 8: 337

Penry J K, Porter R J, Dreifuss F E 1975 Simultaneous recording of absence seizures with video tape and electroencephalography: a study of 374 seizures in 48 patients. Brain 98: 427

Perucca E 1978 Clinical consequences of microsomal enzyme induction by antiepileptic drugs. Pharmacology and Therapeutics 2: 285

Perucca E, Garratt S, Hebdige S, Richens A 1978 Water intoxication in epileptic patients receiving carbamazepine. Journal of Neurology, Neurosurgery and Psychiatry 42: 713

Perucca E, Hebdige S, Gatti G, Lecchini S, Frigo G M, Crema A 1980 Interaction between phenytoin and valproic acid: plasma protein binding and metabolic effects. Clinical Pharmacology and Therapeutics 28: 779

Perucca E, Hedges A, Makki K, Hebdige S, Wadsworth J, Richens A 1979 The comparative enzyme-inducing properties of antiepileptic drugs. British Journal of Clinical Pharmacology 7: 414

Perucca E, Pisani F 1991 Pharmacokinetics and interactions of the new antiepileptic drugs. In: Pisani F, Perucca E, Avanzini G, Richens A (eds) New antiepileptic drugs. Amsterdam, Elsevier

Perucca E, Richens A 1980 Antiepileptic drug interactions. In: Tyrer J (ed) The treatment of epilepsy. MTP Press, Lancaster

Perucca E, Richens A 1985 Antiepileptic drug interactions. In: Frey H-H, Janz D (eds) Handbook of experimental pharmacology, vol 74: antiepileptic drugs. Springer-Verlag, Berlin, p 831

Peterson D I, Zweig R W 1974 Absorption of anticonvulsants after jejuno-ileal bypass. Bulletin Los Angeles Neurological Society 39: 51

Peterson G M, McLean S, Millingen K S 1982 Determinants of patient compliance with anticonvulsant therapy. Epilepsia 23: 607

Peterson G M, McLean S, Millingen K S 1984 Randomized trial of strategies to improve patient compliance with anticonvulsant therapy. Epilepsia 25: 412

Pinder R M, Brogden R N, Speight T M, Avery G S 1976 Clonazepam: a review of its pharmacological properties and therapeutic efficacy in epilepsy. Drugs 12: 321

Pinder R M, Brogden R N, Speight T M, Avery G S 1977 Sodium valproate: a review of its pharmacological properties and therapeutic efficacy in epilepsy. Drugs 13: 81

Pippenger C E, Penry J K, Kutt H (eds) 1978 Antiepileptic drugs: quantitative analysis and interpretation. Raven Press, New York

Pisciotta A V 1982 Carbamazepine. Haematological toxicity. In: Woodbury D M, Penry J K, Pippenger C E (eds) Antiepileptic drugs. Raven Press, New York, p 533

Plaa G L, Hine C H 1960 Hydantoin and barbiturate blood levels observed in epileptics. Archives internationales de pharmacodynamie (et de therapie) 128: 375

Pollack M A, Zion T E, Kellaway P 1979 Long-term prognosis of patients with infantile spasms following ACTH therapy. Epilepsia 20: 225

Porter R J, Layzer R B 1975 Plasma albumin concentration and diphenylhydantoin binding in man. Archives of Neurology 32: 298

Porter R J, Penry J K, Lacy J R, Newmark M E, Kupferberg H J 1977 The clinical efficacy and pharmacokinetics of phensuximide and methsuximide. Neurology 27: 375

Pynnönen S 1979 Pharmacokinetics of carbamazepine in man: a review. Therapeutic Drug Monitoring 1: 409

Rane A, Höjer B, Wilson J T 1976 Kinetics of carbamazepine and its 10,11-epoxide metabolite in children. Clinical Pharmacology and Therapeutics 19: 276

Rating D, Nau H, Joauager-Roman E et al 1982 Teratogenic and pharmacokinetic studies of primidone during pregnancy and in the offspring of epileptic women. Acta Paediatrica Scandinavica 71: 301

Reidenberg M M, Drayer D E 1978 Effects of renal disease upon drug disposition. Drug Metabolism Review 8: 293

Reinikainen K J, Keranen T, Halonen T, Komulainen K, Riekkinen P J 1987 Comparison of oxcarbazepine and carbamazepine: a double-blind study. Epilepsy Research 1: 284

Rey E, Pons G, Richard M O, Vauzelle F et al 1990 Pharmacokinetics of the individual enantiomers of vigabatrin (gamma-vinyl-GABA) in epileptic children. British Journal of Clinical Pharmacology 30: 253

Reynolds E H 1980 Serum levels of anticonvulsant drugs. Interpretation and clinical value. Pharmacology and Therapeutics 8: 217

Reynolds E H, Shorvon S D 1981 Monotherapy or polytherapy for epilepsy. Epilepsia 22: 1

Reynolds E H, Elwes R D C, Shorvon S D 1983 Why does epilepsy become intractable? Prevention of chronic epilepsy. Lancet ii: 952

Reynolds E H, Shorvon S D, Galbraith A W, Chadwick D, Dellaportas C I, Vydelingom L 1981 Phenytoin monotherapy for epilepsy: a long-term prospective study, assisted by serum level monitoring, in previously untreated patients. Epilepsia 22: 475

Richens A 1976 Drug treatment of epilepsy. Henry Kimpton, London

Richens A 1979 Clinical pharmacokinetics of phenytoin. Clinical Pharmacokinetics 4: 153

Richens A 1983 Clinical pharmacokinetics of benzodiazepines. In:Trimble M R (ed) Benzodiazepines divided. John Wiley, Chichester, p 187

Richens A 1984 Enzyme induction and sex hormones. In: Porter et al (eds) Advances is epileptology: XVth Epilepsy International Symposium. Raven Press, New York

Richens A 1991 Lamotrigine. In: Pedley T A, Meldrum B S (eds) Recent advances in epilepsy. Churchill Livingstone, Edinburgh, p 197

Richens A, Rowe D J F 1970 Calcium metabolism in patients with epilepsy. British Medical Journal 4: 803

Richens A, Dunlop A 1975 Serum phenytoin levels in the management of epilepsy. Lancet ii: 247

Rimmer E M, Buss D C, Routledge P A, Richens A 1984 Should we routinely measure free plasma phenytoin concentration? British Journal of Clinical Pharmacology 17: 99

Rimmer E M, Richens A 1984 Double-blind study of gamma-vinyl-GABA in patients with refractory epilepsy. Lancet 1: 189

Rimmer E M, Richens A 1989 Interaction between vigabatrin and phenytoin. British Journal of Clinical Pharmacology 27: 27S

Rodin E A 1968 The prognosis of patients with epilepsy. Thomas, Springfield

Rodin E A, Rim C S, Rennick P M 1974 The effects of carbamazepine on patients with psychomotor epilepsy: results of a double-blind study. Epilepsia 15: 547

Rowan A J, Binnie C D, Warfield L A, Meijer J W A 1979 Epilepsia 20: 61

Sander J W A S, Hart Y M, Trimble M R, Shorvon S D 1991 Vigabatrin and psychosis. Journal of Neurology, Neurosurgery and Psychiatry 54: 435–439

Sato S, White B G, Penry J K et al 1982 Valproic acid versus ethosuximide in the treatment of absence seizures. Neurology 32: 157

Schechter P J 1989 Clinical pharmacology of vigabatrin. British Journal of Clinical Pharmacology 27: 19S

Schmidt B 1989 Potential antiepileptic drugs: Gabapentin. In: Levy R H Dreifuss F E, Mattson R H, Meldrum B S, Penry J K (eds) Antiepileptic drugs. Raven Press, New York, p 925

Schmidt D 1982 Two antiepileptic drugs for intractable epilepsy with complex partial seizure. Journal of Neourology, Neourosurgery and Psychiatry 45: 1119

Schmidt D 1984a Benzodiazepines—an update. In: Pedley J A, Meldrum B S (eds) Recent advances in epilepsy, vol 1. Churchill Livingstone, Edinburgh, p 125

Schmidt D 1984b Adverse effects of valproate. Epilepsia 25 (Suppl.1): S44

Schmidt D, Kupferberg H J 1975 Diphenylhydantoin, phenobarbital and primidone in saliva, plasma and cerebrospinal fluid. Epilepsia 16: 735

Schmidt D, Haenel F 1984 Therapeutic plasma levels of phenytoin, phenobarbital, and carbamazepine: individual variation in relation to seizure frequency and type. Neurology 34: 1252

Schmidt D, Kupferberg H J, Yonekawa W, Penry J K 1980 The development of tolerance to the anticonvulsant effect of phenobarbital in mice. Epilepsia 21: 141

Schmidt D, Ried S 1989 Clinical relevance of calcium antagonists in the treatment of epilepsy. Arzneimittel Forschung 39: 156

Schobben F, Van der Kleijn E, Gabreels F J M 1975
Pharmacokinetics of di-n-propylacetate in epileptic
patients. European Journal of Clinical Pharmacology 8: 97

Schobben F, Van der Kleijn E, Vree T B 1980 Therapeutic
drug monitoring of valproic acid. Therapeutic Drug
Monitoring 2: 61

Schottelius D D 1982 Primidone. Biotransformation. In:
Woodbury D M, Penry J K, Pippenger C E (eds)
Antiepileptic drugs. Raven Press, New York, p 415

Schutz H, Feldmann K F, Faigle J W, Kriemler H P, Winkler
T 1986 The metabolism of 14c-oxcarbazepine in man.
Xenobiotica 16: 769–778

Seino M, Ohkuma T, Miyasaka M et al 1988 Efficacy
evaluation of AD-810 (zonisamide). Double-blind study
comparing with carbamazepine. Journal of Clinical and
Experimental Medicine 144: 275 (in Japanese)

Seino M, Miyazaki H, Ito T 1991 Zonisamide. In: Pisani F,
Perucca E, Avanzini G, Richens A (eds) New antiepileptic
drugs. Amsterdam, Elsevier

Serrano E E, Wilder B J 1974 Intramuscular administration
of diphenylhydantoin. Histologic follow-up. Archives of
Neurology 31: 276

Shaw M D M, Foy P, Chadwick D 1983 Effectiveness of
prophylactic anticonvulsants following neurosurgery. Acta
Neurochirugica 69: 253

Sherwin A L 1978 Clinical pharmacology of ethosuximide.
In: Pippenger C E, Penry J K, Kutt H P (eds) Antiepileptic
drugs: quantitative analysis and interpretation. Raven
Press, New York, p 283

Sherwin A L 1982 Ethosuximide. Relation to plasma
concentration of seizure control. In: Woodbury D M,
Penry J K, Pippenger C E (eds) Antiepileptic drugs. Raven
Press, New York, p 637

Sherwin A L, Robb J P, Lechter M 1973 Improved control of
epilepsy by monitoring plasma ethosuximide. Archives of
Neurology 28: 178

Shorvon S D, Reynolds E 1979 Reduction of polypharmacy
for epilepsy. British Medical Journal ii: 1023

Shorvon S D, Reynolds E H 1982 Early prognosis of epilepsy.
British Medical Journal 285: 1699

Shorvon S D, Chadwick D, Galbraith A W, Reynolds E H
1978 One drug for epilepsy. British Medical Journal 1: 474

Shorvon S D, Espir M L E, Stever T J, Dellaportas C I,
Clifford Rose F 1985 For debate: is there a place for
placebo controlled trials of antiepileptic drugs? British
Medical Journal 291: 132

Sillanpäa M, Pynnönen S, Laippala P, Säklauo E 1979
Carbamazepine in the treatment of partial epileptic seizures
in infants and young children :a preliminary study.
Epilepsia 20: 563

Sjö O, Hvidberg E F, Larsen N E, Lund M, Naestoft J 1975
Dose dependent kinetics of ethotoin in man. Clinical and
Experimental Pharmacology and Physiology 2: 185

Sjögren J, Solvell L, Karlsson I 1965 Studies on the
absorption rate of barbiturates in man. Acta Medica
Scandinavica 178: 553

Smith D B, Goldstein S G, Roomet A 1986 A comparison of
the toxicity effects of the anticonvulsant
eterobarb)(Antilon, DMMP) and phenobarbital in normal
human volunteers. Epilepsia 27: 149

Stewart M J, Ballinger B R, Devlin E, Miller A, Ramsay A C
1975 Bioavailability of phenytoin—a comparison of two
preparations. European Journal of Clinical Pharmacology
9: 209

Strickler S M, Dansky L, Miller M A, Seni M-H, Andermann

E, Spielberg S P 1985 Genetics predisposition to
phenytoin-induced birth defects. Lancet ii: 746

Suzuki M, Maruyama H, Ishibashi Y et al 1972 A double-
blind comparative trial of sodium dipropylacetate and
ethosuximide in epilepsy in children, with special emphasis
on pure petit mal seizures. Medical Progress 82: 470

Tartara A, Manni R, Galimberti C A, Mumford J P, Iudice
A, Perucca E 1989 Vigabatrin in the treatment of epilepsy:
A long-term follow-up study. Journal of Neurology,
Neurosurgery and Psychiatry 52: 467

Tartara A, Galimberti C A, Manni R et al 1991 Differential
effects of enzyme inducing anticonvulsants and valproic
acid on nimodipine bioavailability in epileptic patients.
British Journal of Clinical Pharmacology 32: 335–340

Thompson P, Huppert F A, Trimble M R 1981 Phenytoin
and cognitive function: effects on normal volunteers and
implications for epilepsy. British Journal of Clinical
Psychology 20: 155

Thompson P J, Trimble M R 1982 Anticonvulsant drugs and
cognitive functions. Epilepsia 23: 531

Thompson P J, Trimble M R 1983 The effect of
anticonvulsant drugs on cognitive function: relation to
serum levels. Journal of Neurology, Neurosurgery and
Psychiatry 46: 227

Troupin A S, Ojemann L M, Dodrill C B 1976 Mephenytoin:
a reappraisal. Epilepsia 17: 403

Troupin A S, Ojeman L M, Halpern L 1977 Carbamazepine.
A double blind comparison with phenytoin. Neurology
27: 511

Turnbull D M 1983 Adverse effects of valproate. Adverse
Drug Reactions and Acute Poisonings Review 2: 191

Turnbull D M, Rawlins M D, Weightman D, Chadwick D W
1982 A comparison of phenytoin and valproate in
previously untreated adult epileptic patients. Journal of
Neurology, Neurosurgery and Psychiatry 45: 55

Turnbull D M, Rawlins M D, Weightman D, Chadwick D W
1983 Long-term comparative study of phenytoin and
valproate in adult onset epilepsy. British Journal of Clinical
Practice 27: 3

Turnbull D M, Rawlins M D, Weightman D, Chadwick D W
1984 'Therapeutic' serum concentrations of phenytoin: the
influence of seizure type. Journal of Neurology,
Neurosurgery and Psychiatry 47: 231

Turnbull D M, Howel D, Rawlins M D, Chadwick D W
1985 Which drug for this adult epileptic patient: phenytoin
or valproate? British Medical Journal 290: 815

Tyrer J H, Eadie M J, Sutherland J M, Hooper W D 1970
Outbreak of anticonvulsant intoxication in an Australian
city. British Medical Journal 3: 271

Waddell W J, Butler T C 1957 The distribution and excretion
of phenobarbital. Journal of Clinical Investigation
36: 1217–1226

Wallace S J, Aldridge-Smith J 1980 Successful prophylaxis
against febrile convulsions with valproic acid or
phenobarbitone. British Medical Journal 280: 353

Wells C 1957 Trimethadione: its dosage and toxicity.
Archives Neurology and Psychiatry 77: 140

Werk E E, McGee J, Scholiton L J 1964 Effect of
diphenylhydantoin on cortisol metabolism in man. Journal
of Clinical Investigation 43: 1284

Wilder B J, Ramsey R E 1976 Oral and intramuscular
phenytoin. Clinical Pharmacology and Therapeutics 19: 30

Wilder B J, Serrano E E, Ramsay E 1973 Plasma
diphenylhydantoin levels after loading and maintenance
doses. Clinical Pharmacology and Therapeutics 14: 797

Wilder B J, Ramsay E, Willmore L J et al 1977 Efficacy of intravenous phenytoin in the treatment of status epilepticus; kinetics of central nervous system penetration. Annals of Neurology 1: 511

Wilensky A J, Lowden J A 1973 Inadequate serum levels after intramuscular administration of diphenylhydantoin. Neurology 23: 318

Wilensky H J, Priel P N, Levy R H, Comfort C P, Kaluzny S P 1982 Kinetics of phenobarbital in normal subjects and epileptic patients. European Journal of Clinical Pharmacology 23: 87

Withrow C D 1982 Trimethadione: biotransformation. In: Woodbury D M, Penry J K, Pippenger C E (eds) Antiepileptic drugs. Raven Press, New York, p 689

Wolf S M, Forsythe A 1978 Behaviour disturbance, phenobarbitone and febrile seizures. Paediatrics 61: 728

Wolf S M, Carra A, Davis D C et al 1977 The value of phenobarbital in the child who has had a single febrile seizure: a controlled prospective study. Paediatrics 59: 378

Yuen W C 1991 Lamotrigine. In: Pisani F, Perucca E, Avanzini G, Richens A (eds) New antiepileptic drugs. Amsterdam, Elsevier

Young B, Rapp R P, Norton J A, Hack D, Tibbs P A, Bean J R 1983a Failure of prophylactically administered phenytoin to prevent early post-traumatic seizures. Journal of Neurosurgery 58: 231

Young B, Rapp R P, Norton J A, Hack D, Tibbs P A, Bean J R 1983b Failure of prophylactically administered phenytoin to prevent late post-traumatic seizures. Journal of Neurosurgery 58: 236

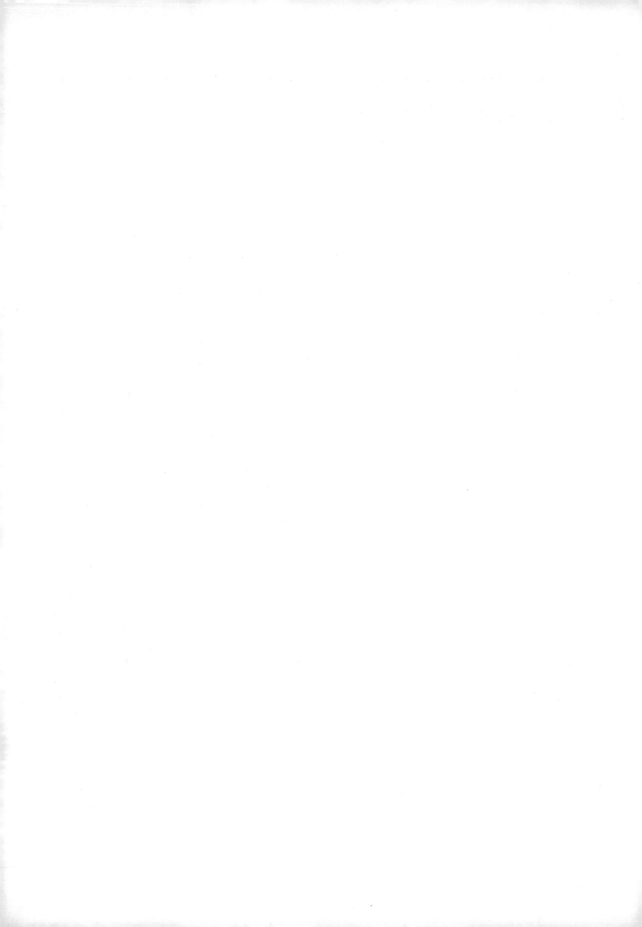

16. Neurosurgical treatment of epilepsy

C. E. Polkey   C. D. Binnie

INTRODUCTION

Epileptic seizures are common in general neuro-surgical practice as a symptom of the underlying disease, or sometimes as a consequence of neuro-surgical interference. However, they present a special and different problem when they are the main symptom, and the underlying pathology is initially obscure. It is with the neurosurgical solution to that problem that the present chapter is concerned.

In many patients with symptomatic epilepsy it is possible to identify an interaction between a cerebral disease process and the individual brain: the apparently identical disease process in the same location in different patients will not necessarily give rise to the same severity of epilepsy, or may not even manifest itself in epilepsy at all. Because of this 'seed and soil' relationship it is not possible to predict with certainty the result of surgical intervention, and therefore the realistic aim of surgical treatment must be the control of seizures rather than their absolute eradication. Although the long follow-up periods now available for the classical resective procedures indicate that in many cases this control is almost perfect, nevertheless it is possible for patients, even many years after a successful operation, to suffer further epileptic attacks.

The physician who wishes to decide whether a patient with chronic drug-resistant epilepsy would benefit from surgery is faced with a multitude of techniques used to assess such patients and a number of different operative procedures apparently available to treat the same condition. The purpose of this chapter is to resolve some of this confusion, and to attempt a rational account of the scope of surgery in epilepsy.

Operations have been used in the treatment of epilepsy since neurosurgery first became practicable and the impressive work of the early pioneers is well described in a review by Talairach et al (1974). The first scientific approach came from the Montreal Neurological Institute where Penfield, expanding the ideas he had worked upon with Foerster, began to try to show that epileptogenic areas of cerebral cortex, identified by stimulation at operation, could be resected with benefit to the patient. The addition of electrical recording from the surface of the brain, and later from the deep structures, together with careful observational and surgical techniques, enabled this group to build up an unrivalled experience of resective surgery, described in their numerous publications, and continuing to the present day.

However, as the Montreal group were developing this approach it became clear also that this technique of local cortical resection was not suitable for all patients with chronic epilepsy, and so in other centres different philosophies and means of treatment were developed. Growth in basic neurophysiological knowledge, outlined below, led to attempts to modify the spread of epileptic discharges within the brain. This was assisted by the application of the techniques of stereotactic localization, originally developed as a tool for the experimental neurophysiologist but subsequently used for clinical purposes. It has played an important part both in the investigation of these patients and to a lesser degree in their treatment.

Although the number of centres carrying out surgical treatment for epilepsy is increasing they remain few, and the number of patients treated in each centre may also be small. There is therefore a tendency for each centre to rely on a few techniques of which there is local experience; consequently, similar patients may be offered a resective operation in one centre and a functional operation in another. Further confusion has been introduced by the fact that when some patients, especially those with temporal lobe epilepsy, undergo stereotactic procedures which alleviate their epilepsy, their accompanying psychiatric disorders are improved because the seizures are controlled. The same procedures are then used, usually with lesser effect, in patients with the personality disorder but no seizures. Finally, as was noted above there is a liability for seizures to recur although operative treatment at first seems successful and therefore to judge the results of any particular procedure prolonged follow-up is necessary. In this review therefore, preference will be given to reports of 5 years follow-up with a minimum of 2 years.

BASIS OF EPILEPSY SURGERY

There are difficulties in relating the experimental data about the pathophysiology of epilepsy with the experience of clinical neurophysiology The vast literature of experimental work in the pathophysiology of epilepsy describes a number of mechanisms such as secondary epileptogenesis and kindling which have been dealt with in detail in other chapters. The part that these mechanisms play in the surgical treatment of epilepsy is largely obscure because of species differences and the uncontrolled nature of the 'experiment' in human epilepsy.

Clinical evidence for the role of these mechanisms is sparse. Patients with bilateral temporal EEG foci tend to have a longer duration of their epilepsy than those with unilateral foci (Hughes & Schlagenhauff 1961, Gupta et al 1973). There is anecdotal evidence from patients subjected to hemispherectomy and those with bilateral EEG changes from unilateral temporal lesions, that EEG abnormalities contralateral to a structural lesion can regress after operation (Falconer & Kennedy 1961, Wieser & Yasargil 1982). Convincing evidence for human secondary epileptogenesis has been presented by Morrell (Morrell et al 1987). Among patients undergoing temporal lobe surgery at the Montreal Neurological Insti-

tute he found a small number who had clinical and electrographic evidence of bilateral foci. The majority, but not all of the secondary foci, regressed after surgical resection of the primary focus. In those patients where the foci persisted the appropriately lateralized seizures also persisted.

Surgery for drug-resistant epilepsy may be effective for each of three reasons which are summarised in Diagram 1. Firstly because it removes pathology, including the primary focus (see page 588); secondly because it disconnects the primary focus from the rest of the brain when complete removal is impossible; lastly because it reduces the mass of neurones which behave abnormally. Functional operations tend to achieve only one or two of these aims whereas resective operations are hybrid in nature and encompass all three. Chronic epilepsy is a dynamic process, which has a continuing influence in some brains. Therefore the length of time for which this adverse influence operates may be important in determining the outcome of the surgery.

It has already been noted that the use of surgical operations for epilepsy has grown up in an idiosyncratic and empirical way, yet it is possible to separate them into two groups, namely those operations which depend upon the resection of a known local pathology and surrounding tissue from the brain, which we will call resective operations, and those operations which aim to alter brain function, and which we will call functional operations. The terms causative and palliative used by Wieser (1986) and other authors make a similar distinction. Lesional surgery is a difficult term to evaluate but it is coming into use for operations in which the resection is restricted, usually without corticographic control, to the

---

STRATEGIES OF EPILEPSY SURGERY

1. Removal of a focus or discrete lesion
   e.g. Removal of frontal scar and surrounding cortex

2. Division of pathways of propagation
   e.g. Callosotomy

3. Gross removal of malfunctioning brain
   e.g. Hemispherectomy

Diagram 1

Table 16.1 Summary of operations undertaken in the Neurosurgical Unit of the Maudsley Hospital since 1986

Procedure	Total	
Temporal resection	194	
Amygdalo-hippocampectomy		34
Lobectomy		160
Other resections	62	
Hemispherectomy	23	
Functional operations	18	
Intracranial electrodes		44
Subdural and depth electrodes		28
Subdural mat electrodes		16
Total resective operations	279	
Total	341	

structural lesion itself. Such lesions are usually some form of hamartoma or benign intrinsic cerebral tumour. Table 16.1 gives a summary of operations undertaken in the Neurosurgical Unit of the Maudsley Hospital since 1976 and illustrates the amount and variety of surgical work which is required to provide a comprehensive programme for the surgical treatment of epilepsy. Table 16.1 is also a useful summary of the main categories of operation. In the temporal lobe the size of the resection varies from a full temporal lobectomy to resection of the medial temporal structures alone, known as selective amygdalo-hippocampectomy. Other resections include cerebral cortical resections which vary from small discrete areas to formal lobectomies. Functional operations include not only callosotomy but also the new procedure of multiple subpial resection in which blocks of eloquent cortex are isolated horizontally but not disconnected vertically (Morrell et al 1989). Resective or causative operations, which of course includes lesional surgery, are commoner and more successful, and therefore will be dealt with first and in greater detail.

PRINCIPLES OF SELECTION OF PATIENTS FOR RESECTIVE SURGERY

In all cases it must be established that the patient is suffering from true epileptic seizures and that this epilepsy is both chronic and drug-resistant and therefore, except in rare cases, the patient's record of drug compliance is important. Occasionally one meets a patient in whom drugs have

made virtually no impact upon their seizures and they have therefore abandoned them. If such patients have genuinely been shown to be totally refractory to drugs and are resolved in their avoidance of drugs, then if operative treatment has a reasonable chance of success it is justified. The frequency of fits which is regarded as disabling will vary from patient to patient and from centre to centre. Unfortunately patients do not usually have attacks at regular intervals but an average of one seizure per week would seem to be the minimum for operation in most cases, bearing in mind that the patient's psychosocial situation has to be considered. Furthermore it should be established that relieving the epileptic seizures would be of some measurable benefit to the patient, and those who care for the patient, and that there is only a minimal possibility of producing a side-effect from the operation which would be more disabling than the original disease. A careful and complete psychiatric history should be taken and particular care should be taken to distinguish between those psychiatric complaints which are known to be associated with chronic epilepsy, and those of independent conditions. The patient, and their relatives, must have the physical and mental resources to cope with the programme of preoperative investigation and the possibility that this may show that no operation is indicated. Finally, what the surgeon hopes to achieve in terms of seizure relief, together with the possible hazard, should be conveyed realistically to the patients, the relatives, and the referring physician.

It is generally agreed that successful resective surgery depends upon demonstrating that the fits originate in one part of the brain, particularly in association with a structural lesion of that part of the brain. Secondary to these considerations is the need to show that the remainder of the cerebral hemispheres is normal and that resecting the affected part, large or small, will not produce an unacceptable neurological, intellectual or personality change.

The evidence that seizures originate in one part of the brain, in which there may be either a structural or a functional abnormality, or both, and which can be safely resected, is obtained from four sources: the clinical details, the results of neurophysiological studies, the results of cognitive

---

PREOPERATIVE ASSESSMENT PROGRAMME

GENERAL CRITERIA FOR ADMISSION

1. Reliable diagnosis of intractable epilepsy:
   Attacks are epileptic, no pseudoseizures
   Failure of appropriate medication
   Patient is compliant

2. Seizures of such a frequency and nature that
   they are disabling, having regard to the
   patient's life style

3. No other contraindication, for example a
   coagulation defect

Diagram 2

PREOPERATIVE ASSESSMENT PROGRAMME

CRITERIA FOR INVESTIGATION FOR RESECTIVE
SURGERY

1. Partial seizures, whether or not secondarily
   generalized

2. Full scale IQ not less than 70 points

3. Age not more than 55 years

4. Patient has the emotional resources to with-
   stand the procedures, including the possibility
   of being found inoperable

Note:
a. a single EEG focus is *not* a requirement
b. psychiatric or behavioural disorder are *not*
   automatic exclusion criteria

Diagram 3

assessment of the patient, and the results of brain imaging studies. In centres dealing with substantial numbers of these patients it is usual to have a scheme of investigation and management which allows patients to progress from simple, non-invasive tests to complex invasive investigations with an opportunity to make decisions about the patient's suitability for surgery at each stage. The scheme used in the Maudsley Hospital is shown in Fig. 16.1 and how it works will become clear as the details of selection are described. The various phases of the investigation referred to in Fig. 16.1 involve associated neurophysiological and neuropsychological tests as well as brain imaging and will be referred to in detail in the section on neurophysiological assessment.

Clinical details

History

This needs to be taken with perseverance and care for detail, and independent corroboration should be obtained both from friends or relatives and from previous hospital case notes. Two objectives should be pursued in such history taking: the first is to try to establish that all the patient's attacks have a common source; the second is to seek evidence of, or a reason for, a structural abnormality in the appropriate part of the patient's brain.

In the first case a careful history of the type of attack which the patient suffers must be obtained. In trying to locate the origin of a fit from clinical details, attention should be paid to the initial events sometimes described as the aura, to any focal or lateralizing features in the attack, as well as its nature, and to any postictal phenomena such as a Todd's palsy. The features of temporal lobe attacks and those originating from the

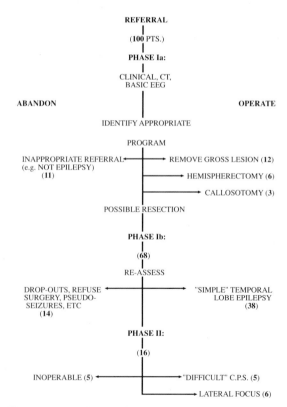

Fig. 16.1   Investigative phases and decision nodes in 100 consecutive patients referred for preoperative assessment. Reprinted with permission from Binnie 1989.

primary motor or sensory areas are well known. There are excellent descriptions of the localizing features of various epileptic phenomena in Penfield & Jasper (1954); Williamson and colleagues (Williamson et al 1985a) have described the variety of seizures which can arise focally in the frontal lobes and there are also now good descriptions of seizures from the supplementary motor cortex (Morris et al 1988). Difficulty may be experienced with the interpretation of speech disturbances for two reasons. Firstly it may be difficult to establish speech dominance and secondly certain phenomena such as automatic speech during an attack may arise in the non-dominant hemisphere as described by Falconer (1967).

It is essential to get a good description of the fit in lay person's terms, not accepting such expressions as 'petit mal' or 'minor' seizure at face value. Witnesses, especially relatives, may display a kind of mirror description in which they attribute the patient's lateralizing features to the opposite side of their own body, but this can usually be clarified by careful questioning. For purposes of postoperative assessment and follow-up the preoperative frequency of fits should be established. Since such attacks are seldom regular we have made a practice of working out from a seizure calendar, or by asking the patient and their relatives to estimate the figures, the average frequency of fits in the year prior to consultation together with the greatest number in one day and the longest fit-free interval, and to note any obvious clustering.

The second point to be established is whether there is any possible pointer to a lesion in the brain. In an elegant monograph Ounstead and his colleagues (1966) showed that in 66 out of 100 children with psychomotor epilepsy there was a history of birth injury or infantile febrile convulsions; in many of the remaining children, where the age of onset of chronic epilepsy was later than in the first two groups, miscellaneous lesions such as small tumours were found. In a similar vein, Falconer (1974) clearly demonstrated that in patients whose temporal lobectomy specimens showed mesial temporal sclerosis there was a high incidence of febrile convulsions, whereas patients with other lesions did not show this.

Such history taking may require some time and considerable background enquiry but will amply repay the time spent.

Physical examination

Except in patients with previous gross brain injury or expanding lesions, physical signs in the interictal period tend to be subtle. Examination in the immediate postictal state should be carried out whenever possible, and special weight placed on any lateralizing or localizing signs found.

Investigations

Neurophysiological studies—I

There is probably no other clinical decision in which the EEG plays such a pivotal role as in the selection of patients for surgical treatment of epilepsy. Electrophysiological investigation is, however, only one aspect of a preoperative assessment which depends on collating evidence from several disciplines, and cannot be considered adequately in isolation. Of the various operative strategies considered above, resection of an epileptogenic focus relies most heavily on electrophysiological data. The role of the EEG in selection of patients for hemispherectomy or callosotomy is not clearly established, and the following section is concerned almost exclusively with those procedures which require focus localization, namely local resection and multiple subpial transection.

Some confusion surrounds the use of the term 'focus' in this context. The success of resective surgery for epilepsy depends on identifying and removing a region of structurally and functionally abnormal brain from which seizures arise. Excising cerebral cortex which is the site of a focus of interictal discharges rarely relieves epilepsy if the tissue is normal. Conversely, removal of a lesion which is not associated with epileptiform activity is not often successful. The theoretical concept of the 'epileptogenic zone' has therefore been introduced to signify that region of brain from which seizures arise. Unfortunately, this term appears to have various meanings to different authors, some of whom use it to signify the area of normal cortex into which interictal discharges spread intermittently from a more discrete and active focus. In the present text the term 'focus' will be used to describe only discrete areas of interictal discharge. 'Primary focus' signifies both the site of electrographic seizure onset and any corresponding interictal focus. 'Epileptogenic zone' is used in its wider sense to indicate a larger region of interictal discharge containing the primary focus.

The best evidence of the location of the primary focus is obtained by repeated, consistent demonstration of the onset of ictal discharge by direct recording with suitably placed intracranial electrodes. However, adequate inferential evidence is provided by the presence of a single, or predominant, focus of interictal discharges, with concordant, localizing findings from neuroradiology, neuropsychology and ictal symptomatology. Electrophysiological focus localization is approached by phased investigations of increasing complexity.

Phase Ia: non-invasive studies. Routine diagnostic EEG investigations, carried out long before any question arose of neurosurgical referral, rarely will have specifically or adequately addressed the issue of localization. A minimum requirement is recording of the EEG both in waking and in sleep in order to demonstrate and locate accurately any focus, or foci, of interictal epileptiform activity. Additional electrodes may be required, either non-standard scalp placements, particularly for recording from the anterior temporal regions, or various special electrodes inserted at the base of the skull. Investigations with basal electrodes will usually include sleep registrations and possibly the intravenous thiopentone test of Lombroso & Erba (1970) (see section on 'Sleep induction' in Ch. 293).

To some extent, the need for additional electrodes arises from the deficiencies of the widely used International 10/20 System of Electrode Placement (Jasper 1958). However commendable the striving after an international convention, the standard 10/20 placements fail to cover one-third of the temporal convexity, including the entire anterior temporal region. Systems providing better coverage without the need for additional electrodes have been described (Pampiglione 1956, Margerison et al 1970) but are not widely used except in the UK. The anterior temporal placement of Silverman (1960) has been more generally accepted and has proved useful. A more comprehensive approach is that of Lüders et al (1982). Using an array of additional electrodes between and below the standard 10/20 sites, they showed that, in scalp recordings from patients with complex partial seizures, the spike focus was most often maximal immediately superficial to the temporal pole (Morris et al 1983). However, they considered it important to use an extensive array to locate the focus, not merely a single anterior temporal electrode to capture spikes.

Basal placements include nasopharyngeal electrodes (Gastaut 1948, Maclean 1949) inserted through the nostrils. They are susceptible to artifact and rarely provide information not obtainable from an anterior temporal placement (Binnie et al 1982). A naso-ethmoid electrode (Lehtinen & Bergstrom 1970) is less widely used, but Quesney et al (1981) found it useful for recording from inferomesial frontal foci. Morris & Lüders (1985) confirm this, but report that very similar results are obtained with electrodes on the side of the bridge of the nose or below the eye. Sphenoidal electrodes (Jones 1951, Pampiglione & Kerridge 1956, Rovit et al 1960) are flexible wires inserted with a needle to lie under the foramen ovale. They certainly provide information not obtainable with the standard 10/20 placements (Christodoulou 1967), but the yield of new data is less if they are compared with anterior temporal placements, and their usefulness has recently been questioned. Wilkus & Thompson (1984) demonstrated that spontaneous or deliberate displacement of the sphenoidal electrode from below the foramen ovale to a more superficial position had no apparent effect on the activity recorded. Similarly, Laxer (1984) claimed that a 'mini-sphenoidal'

PHASE IA—INVESTIGATION

1. Interictal EEG: awake, asleep, barbiturate activation, with sphenoidal or other electrodes
2. Appropriate and available brain imaging
3. Neuropsychological and possibly neuropsychiatric assessment

---

Diagram 4

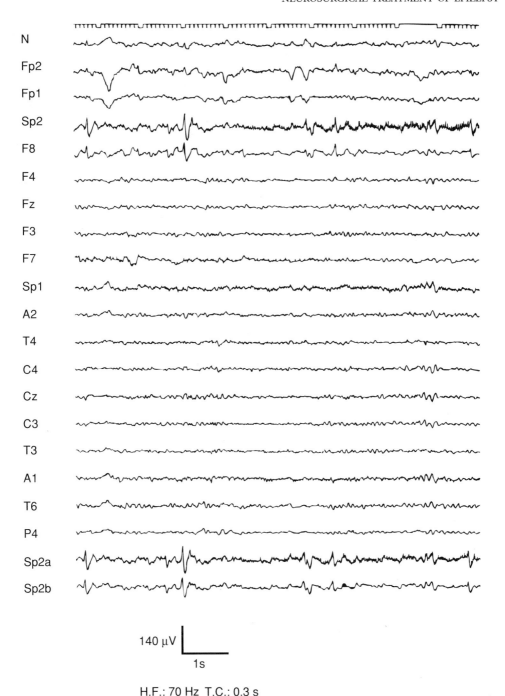

140 µV

1s

H.F.: 70 Hz T.C.: 0.3 s

Fig. 16.2 Multipolar sphenoidal recording in patient with complex partial seizures due to right mesial temporal sclerosis. Common average reference derivation with right sphenoidal contacts at approximate depths of 40 mm (standard location Sp2), 25 mm (Sp2a) and 10 mm (Sp2b). Note shallow potential gradient from deepest to most superficial contact, which is virtually equipotential with anterior temporal scalp electrode (F8). Reproduced with permission from Binnie et al 1989.

needle inserted just under the skin was no less adequate than the standard placement. Such observations must call in question the utility of inserting sphenoidal electrodes at all, and Homan et al (1988) found indeed that they offered little gain of information compared with anterior temporal placements. Binnie et al (1989) found in a large series of temporal foci that spikes demonstrated by sphenoidal recording could in all instances be unequivocally identified at suitably placed scalp electrodes (Fig. 16.2). They concluded that interictal sphenoidal recording served no useful purpose for detecting temporal foci, although the relative amplitudes at sphenoidal and surface contacts did appear to distinguish mesial from lateral temporal lesions. It was argued that sphenoidal recording had been overvalued, due to the inadequate use of surface placements, of pharmacological activation procedures, and of recording montages which emphasized focal events at the sphenoidal electrodes relative to those at adjacent scalp contacts.

Confidence in EEG localization will be increased if other abnormalities, such as focal slow activity and reduction in amplitude of barbiturate-induced fast activity, are found at the same site as the spike focus. The lateralizing value of decreased fast activity was questioned by Margerison & Corsellis (1966), but their study concerned severely handicapped patients with extensive brain damage. In the type of patients considered for surgery, reduction of barbiturate-induced fast activity appears to be a reliable lateralizing sign (Kennedy & Hill 1958, Engel et al 1975).

On conclusion of Phase Ia, various patterns emerge, which determine the next step to be taken:

1. Conventional awake and asleep EEG recording with, as necessary, the use of additional or special electrode placements, may have demonstrated a single, stable temporal focus of epileptiform discharges, together possibly with a local abnormality of background activity, at a site amenable to surgery, and concordant with clinical, neuroradiological and neuropsychological evidence concerning the origin of the seizures. Some teams adopting a traditional, conservative approach would at this point be prepared to proceed with temporal lobectomy (Bloom et al 1959, Polkey 1981). If, however, the available surgical options include amygdalo-hippocampectomy, it may be considered that further studies are required to obtain evidence whether seizure onset is mesial or lateral temporal (see below).

2. Some patients do not fulfil the criteria above, but have obvious non-atrophic lesions demonstrable by neuroradiology, and may proceed directly to surgery at this point, if other findings are consistent. The presence, for instance, of a tumour does not necessarily indicate that the lesion is the source of the patient's seizures, and the decision whether to operate or to obtain ictal EEG recordings will depend on whether the total available evidence supports or casts doubt on such an hypothesis.

3. In very few patients Phase Ia studies will lead to the conclusion that they are not suitable candidates for surgery. Local resection of an established primary focus is rarely successful in patients with numerous, irregular secondarily generalized interictal discharges (Lieb et al 1981a) (a picture which is generally also associated with multiple foci and a diagnosis of symptomatic generalized epilepsy). This finding should usually lead to the conclusion that resective surgery is inappropriate. It should, however, be noted that regular, bisynchronous, generalized 3/second spike-wave activity accompanying a single temporal focus is not an adverse sign (Sadler & Blume 1989, Blume personal communication), nor, in our experience, are irregular generalized discharges in the presence of a discrete mass lesion. Secondary generalization is not a contraindication for other procedures such as callosotomy and hemispherectomy, which may be applicable in some patients unsuitable for localized resection.

4. There is a widespread, and mistaken, belief that, if interictal recordings show either no focus or multiple foci of epileptiform activity, surgery is out of the question. Indeed, many patients are apparently denied referral for preoperative assessment for this reason. However, such findings, confirmed in Phase Ia, signify only that further, more protracted and probably invasive, electrophysiological investigations will be required.

5. In yet other patients, the localization of a focus in the scalp EEG is considered to cast doubt

on the practicability of surgery (for instance, posterior temporal involvement), or EEG localization may be non-concordant with clinical, radiological or neuropsychological findings. In these subjects, together with all those with non-temporal interictal foci (except with clear lesions as considered above), ictal studies are required to determine the precise localization of the primary focus.

Phase Ib: ictal EEG studies. Ictal EEG studies are generally carried out with the help of telemetry (see p. 305). Scalp electrodes may be used alone, or in combination with flexible sphenoidal wires (Ives & Gloor 1977), or foramen ovale electrodes (see below). Recordings of high technical quality are required, with a minimum

---

PHASE IA—DECISION

1. Is there a discrete radiologically demonstrated cerebral lesion

   CONCORDANT WITH:

   Seizure pattern
   Site of interictal EEG discharges
   Abnormalities of background EEG
   Neuropsychological findings?

   YES then OPERATE

2. Is there a clear unilateral temporal focus, in a temporal lobe which probably does not support memory?

   YES then confirm with Wada test and proceed to 'en bloc' resection

3. Do secondarily generalized interictal discharges predominate?
   YES then ABANDON
   or consider callosotomy

   OTHERWISE GO TO PHASE IB

Diagram 5

PHASE IB—INVESTIGATION

1. EEG Telemetry to obtain an ictal EEG record, with foramen ovale electrodes, unless the focus is clearly outside the temporal lobe, and with reduction of antiepileptic drugs

2. Carotid amytal (Wada) test:
   To lateralize cognitive function
   To predict postoperative deficits
   To investigate secondary generalization

Diagram 6

---

of 16 channels to ensure reliable localization and with careful video documentation of the relationship between EEG and clinical events. It is essential to determine whether the site of onset of electrical ictal change is constant: therefore recordings of upwards of five seizures are desirable and some workers prefer to obtain 20 or more (Olivier et al 1983).

Patients referred for preoperative assessment typically have about one seizure a week and to capture five or more attacks would require an unacceptably long period of registration. Seizure frequency may be increased by antiepileptic drug (AED) reduction or withdrawal, or use may be made of any observed pattern in the patient's seizure liability, for instance, a tendency for the attacks to occur in clusters. As seizures provoked by chemical means often differ both clinically and electrographically from the patient's habitual pattern (see p. 294), it may be questioned whether attacks provoked by a drop in blood AED levels may not also exhibit misleading localization. Exceptionally this may be the case (Engel & Crandall 1983, Binnie 1989) but, in general, seizures released by AED reduction appear to conform to the patient's habitual pattern (Spencer et al 1981). Anomalous localization of onset may be observed when a seizure closely follows within the period of gross postictal physiological disturbance produced by a preceding attack. Discordant findings in this situation are apparently of little consequence; they do not indicate that the patient's habitual seizures are likely to arise from multiple foci. Seizures provoked by acute AED withdrawal show an increased tendency to secondary generalization, whereas those occurring more than four half-lives after the most recent drug reduction are likely to be non-generalized (Marciani et al 1985). The occurrence of generalization may cause concern that the attacks are atypical, but this should not be considered to detract from the localizing significance of the initial events.

In selecting the drug to be withdrawn first in a patient on polypharmacy, reduction of carbamazepine appears most effective in producing withdrawal seizures, probably because of the combination of efficacy in partial epilepsy and a short half-life (in patients with enzyme induction).

Valproate withdrawal is unlikely to be useful, as this drug's duration of action appears to be much more sustained than its short half-life would suggest. As a cluster of seizures develops, judgment is required to decide when to restore the medication to avoid status epilepticus. Patients having frequent seizures after drug withdrawal sometimes develop a confusional state with psychotic features, which may persist for several days after seizures are again controlled.

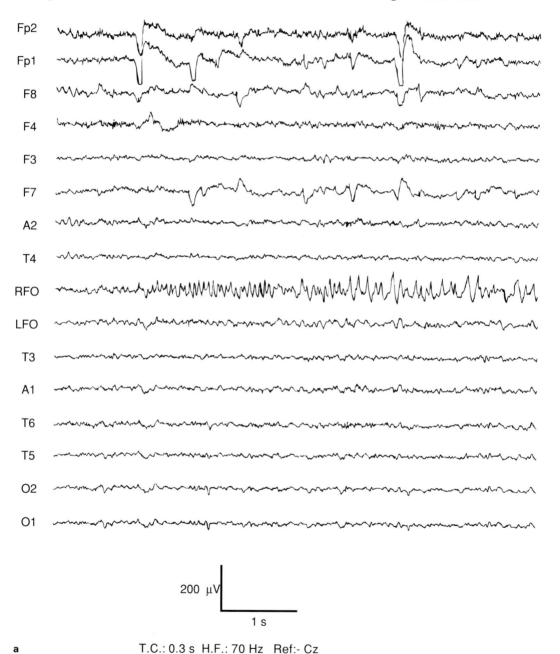

a   T.C.: 0.3 s H.F.: 70 Hz   Ref:- Cz

Fig. 16.3 Ictal record with foramen ovale electrodes. Note discharges confined to RFO (right foramen ovale) at onset (**a**), midpoint (**b**) and towards end (**c**) of complex partial seizure. Patient showed oro-alimentary automatisms, stared ahead and to the right and was unresponsive.

The limitations of ictal scalp EEG recordings can now be overcome to some extent without recourse to conventional implantation of depth or subdural electrodes by the use of foramen ovale electrodes (Wieser et al 1985a). In patients with bitemporal interictal foci the site of origin of the seizures can usually be lateralized by this method and, to meet the criteria for amygdalo-hippocampectomy, a mesial temporal origin of partial seizures can usually be identified reliably by ictal recordings with a combination of scalp and foramen ovale electrodes (Fig. 16.3a–c).

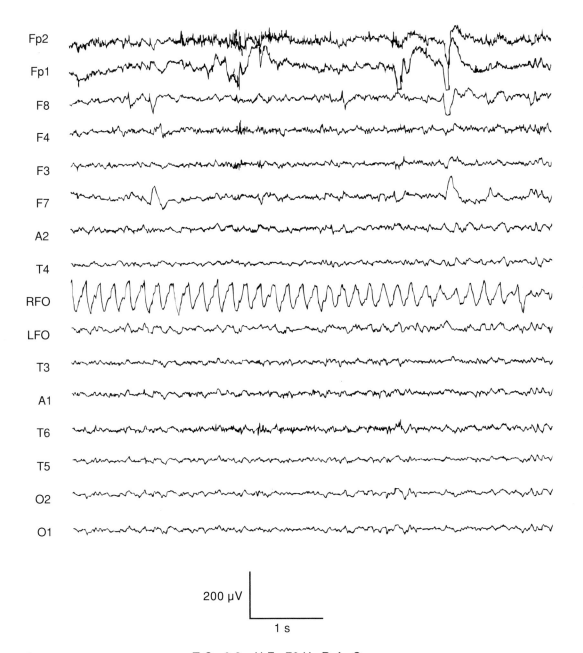

200 μV

1 s

b

T.C.: 0.3 s H.F.: 70 Hz Ref:- Cz

Fig. 16.3 Contd.

The importance of behavioural monitoring in assessing ictal discharges (whether from scalp, foramen ovale or depth electrodes) should be emphasized. If clinical events precede the first apparent or focal electrographic change, it must be concluded that the site of seizure onset has not been detected. In the case of foramen ovale recordings, this does not exclude the possibility of a mesial temporal onset, as early ictal discharges, confined for instance to the amygdala, may not be detected with these placements.

Even where a mesial temporal origin is not found, and possibly not expected, monitoring with scalp and foramen ovale electrodes may nevertheless provide evidence to help decide on further action. For instance, the appearance of epilepti-

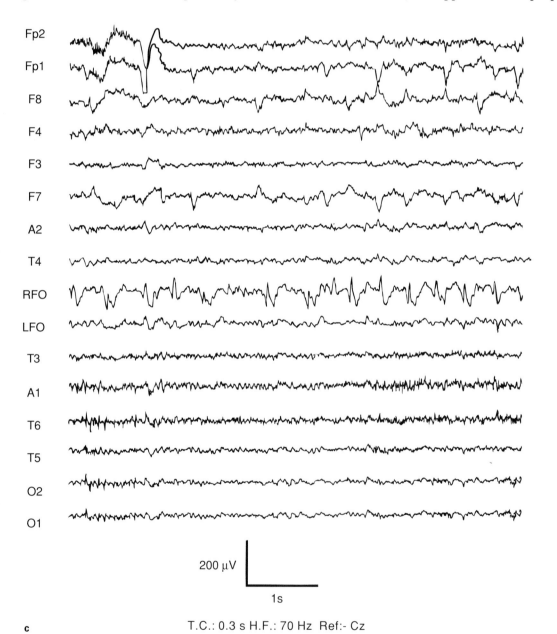

Fp2

Fp1

F8

F4

F3

F7

A2

T4

RFO

LFO

T3

A1

T6

T5

O2

O1

200 µV

1s

c

T.C.: 0.3 s H.F.: 70 Hz Ref:- Cz

Fig. 16.3 Contd.

form discharges at one foramen ovale contact some seconds after the onset of clinical ictal symptoms provides both a guide to lateralization and evidence that the attacks probably (but not necessarily) arise outside the temporal lobes. This information may be of value in selecting sites for placement of depth or subdural electrodes. Conversely, generalized spike-wave activity at seizure onset may indicate that, even if a primary focus can be demonstrated by depth recording, a successful outcome of surgical treatment is unlikely and preoperative assessment should probably be abandoned.

Our view that sphenoidal electrodes provide little information not obtainable by scalp placements applies equally to ictal recording. The most proximal contact of our multipolar foramen ovale electrodes is located approximately at the same site as the standard sphenoidal placement. It records essentially the same activity as is obtained at an overlying surface electrode, and manifestly fails to detect early mesial temporal events demonstrated by deeper foramen ovale contacts (Binnie 1989) (Fig. 16.3).

Reassessment after ictal recordings with scalp and possibly foramen ovale electrodes may show that a consistent focal onset has now been demonstrated corresponding with the site of maximum interictal discharge, attenuation of fast activity and interictal slow wave abnormalities (if any), and that the findings are concordant with clinical, neuroradiological and neuropsychological evidence. On this basis, it should now be possible to proceed to operation, in most patients with an established temporal seizure origin, and in many with a primary focus over the convexity. It may be considered that all patients with a presumed, but radiologically negative, frontal seizure origin require more invasive investigation, unless the focus is clearly in the immediate precentral region.

However, there remain patients in whom ictal scalp recordings will have shown no epileptiform activity, or will have demonstrated an unstable or ill-defined localization. This will usually be the case if only brief simple partial seizures have been recorded, particularly with psychic, viscerosensory or very localized motor phenomena. With fully developed complex partial seizures, 50% or more of scalp EEG recordings may show either no epileptiform activity or, more commonly, bilateral discharges only (Lieb et al 1976).

Few authors (e.g. Spencer et al 1985) have commented on the difficulty of interpreting ictal scalp EEGs. Inter-rater agreement even on lateralization is less than 75% (Spencer et al 1985). Estimates of reliability of scalp EEG against depth recording (which may be taken as the 'gold standard') must depend on how conservatively the findings are interpreted. Thus, Lieb et al (1976) found no instance of incorrect lateralization, but could not lateralize at all in 50% of the patients that they studied. Spencer et al (1985) predicted laterality in two-thirds of cases, but agreement with depth recordings was little better than chance. When unclassified records were excluded, lateralization of temporal foci was about 80% reliable, but that of frontal foci remained random. A detailed study by Delgado-Escueta et al (1982) compared surface EEG, including sphenoidal or nasopharyngeal electrode placements, with clinical events documented by video recording, with similar conclusions. Over half the patients showed non-lateralizing ictal EEG changes. However, those attacks commencing with a motionless stare, which the authors considered on clinical grounds to be of temporal lobe origin, were accompanied in 70% of instances by focal or lateralizing EEG signs, whereas other seizure types, presumed to arise outside the temporal lobes, produced symmetrical or diffuse EEG changes. It was suggested that depth recording would be required only in the patients without staring and a lateralized EEG seizure onset. However, depth studies in such patients also failed in most cases to offer clear evidence of localization and surgical outcome was poor (Delgado-Escueta & Walsh 1983). Thus, a possible conclusion to be drawn from their findings is that patients with complex partial seizures, with no clear ictal focus in the scalp EEG nor staring at seizure onset, should be regarded as unsuitable for surgery.

Occasionally, the EEG localization may seem to conflict with other evidence. False lateralization, in both interictal and ictal EEGs, may result from damage so severe on the affected side that surface discharges can be recorded only from the intact contralateral temporal lobe. However, in patients selected for depth implantation, it is in any case common for ictal discharges, once propagating beyond the deep primary focus, to appear on the convexity predominantly contralateral to the side of onset. Conflict between EEG and other localizing evidence should lead to this possibility being considered (Engel et al 1980) .

A pragmatic approach to interpreting ictal records may permit an early decision as to whether more invasive studies are required. The occurrence of only one seizure in which the electrographic onset follows the first clinical event, is clearly non-localized, or is discordant with observations in other seizures, or with findings from other disciplines (clinical, radiological, etc.) must generally lead to a conclusion either that further implantation is required or that assessment should be abandoned. Less stringent criteria may, however, apply where there is good evidence of an extratemporal site of seizure onset over the convexity. Thus, in simple partial seizures with exclusively motor or somatosensory symptoms, possibly epilepsia partialis continua, or a superficial frontal or parieto-occipital lesion, it may be reasonable to proceed to an exploratory operation with electrocorticography. A consideration here will be whether functional mapping by electrical stimulation is considered necessary, and whether this can be done under local anaesthesia or requires subacute electrode placement (see also p. 582) .

The carotid amytal test requires some explanation at this point as it involves matters of neurophysiological recording and interpretation. The test is described in detail later in relation to neuropsychological assessment but it involves cannulation of one or other internal carotid artery in order to inject sodium amytal into the circulation to one cerebral hemisphere. The chief role of the EEG is to determine the onset and duration of anaesthesia and to establish that the effects are, in fact, unilateral. Typically, high voltage beta activity appears on the affected side within some 20 seconds, rapidly followed by the onset of delta activity. As the effects wear off, the delta activity becomes intermittent and, for a brief period, is intermixed with a returning alpha rhythm. Spontaneous epileptiform discharges are usually suppressed. Occurrence of substantial change over the contralateral hemisphere (with the exception of suppression of bilateral epileptiform discharges) indicates significant cross-flow of amytal.

In most patients, the amytal test is performed chiefly for purposes of neuropsychological evaluation, but it may also contribute to electrophysiological assessment. It may, for instance, help to establish the side of origin of secondarily generalized discharges; these will be abolished bilaterally when the side of the underlying focus is anaesthetized, but only unilaterally when the opposite side is injected. For obvious reasons, well-controlled data to support this claim do not appear to be available and, given current views on the corticocortical mechanisms of generation of generalized discharges (see Ch. 9) the fact that secondary bilateral synchrony is often of mesial frontal origin and that cross-flow often occurs into the contralateral anterior communicating artery, the findings should probably be interpreted with caution. Moreover, as surgical outcome in patients with bilateral discharges is generally poor (Lieb et al 1981a, Spencer et al 1982), little may be gained by locating the underlying focus. Similarly, care is necessary in interpreting effects of intracarotid metrazol, which was formerly administered in conjunction with the amytal test, as a means of determining seizure threshold on the two sides and hence possibly deciding which of two foci is the source of the patient's seizures (Garretson et al 1966). Gloor (1975), whilst advocating both carotid amytal and metrazol tests for identification of secondary bilateral synchrony, concedes that they often fail to give an unequivocal result and suggests this may be due to diffuse or multifocal brain disease.

Activation of foci is not commonly seen in the scalp EEG with the doses of amytal (100–150 mg) commonly used, and detailed EEG assessment may in any event be hampered by the artifacts which occur during psychological testing. However, this last problem is avoided in patients with intracranial electrodes and, using bolus injections of 200 mg of amytal, Hufnagel et al (1990) have reported a characteristic 'spike-burst-suppression pattern' of irregular sporadic spikes against a low amplitude background at the primary focus. In nearly half their patients, the primary focus was also activated by the contralateral injection; this never occurred with a latency of less than 35 seconds and was probably due to recirculation of amytal.

PHASE IB—DECISION

1. Is there is a single temporal ictal EEG focus

   CONCORDANT WITH:

   Seizure pattern
   Site of EEG discharges
   Background EEG activity
   Brain imaging findings
   Neuropsychological findings

   NO then go to PHASE II

   YES If:

   a. Seizure onset is mesial temporal and
   b. Affected temporal lobe supports memory and
   c. No lateral temporal lobe lesion is present:

   THEN perform AMYGDALO-HIPPOCAMPECTOMY

   Otherwise perform EN-BLOC LOBECTOMY

Diagram 7

ABANDON ASSESSMENT FOR SURGERY IF:

1. There are multiple sites of electrographic seizure onset

2. There is generalized epileptiform discharge at seizure onset

3. The probable site of seizure onset cannot be resected without unacceptable complications

Diagram 8

Phase II: subacute intracranial recording.

Subdural and/or depth recording may be acute, lasting up to 12 hours, or subacute, continuing from a few days to several weeks. Subacute intracranial recording may use epidural, subdural or depth electrodes, or a combination of both superficial and deep placements.

Extracerebral electrodes include:

1. small plastic strips bearing 4–8 contacts inserted through multiple burr holes (Ajmone Marsan & Van Buren 1958, Wyler et al 1984)

2. long flexible monopolar electrodes (Broseta et al 1980) or multipolar bundles (Storm van Leeuwen 1982, Van Veelen et al 1990) manipulated under fluoroscopy through the subdural space from bilateral central trephine holes

PHASE II—INVESTIGATION

1. Subacute invasive intracranial recording
   Choice of technique depends upon site of suspected focus
   Temporal or frontal sites may need a combination of subdural and depth electrodes

   If the focus is suspected to be on the superficial (convexity) cortex then some form of subdural mat or strip electrode may be required

2. Functional mapping may be indicated using either electrode system, to record evoked potentials, determine after-discharge and seizure threshold

3. Assess interictal discharges

4. Assess subclinical seizure's spike frequency at different sites, autonomy during sleep or thiopentone activation

Diagram 9

3. large subdural or epidural electrode matrices on plastic sheets introduced through an extensive craniotomy (Goldring 1978, Lesser et al 1984).

Electrodes mounted on mats or plastic strips can cover much of the convexity but cannot readily be placed below the mesial parts of the temporal lobes. Flexible bundles provide considerably more extensive cover and can be manipulated through a central burr hole to reach the entire convexity and to orbital and frontal and subtemporal sites, but have not been widely used (Storm van Leeuwen 1982, Van Veelen et al 1990).

The technique of stereotactic placement of multiple depth electrodes, developed by Bancaud & Talairach (Bancaud et al 1965), has been exploited in particular by Wieser (1983) who has studied clinical and electrographic ictal patterns, documenting meticulously the onset and spread of the ictal discharge and the concomitant clinical manifestations. For the more pragmatic purpose of, for instance, determining which of two known mesial temporal foci is the primary focus, simpler methods may suffice, with the insertion of one or two bundles into the mesial temporal structures of both sides from bilateral central burr holes.

The appropriate electrode technology will be determined by the clinical picture and likely site of the primary focus. Thus in patients with simple partial seizures with motor or somatosensory symptoms, and a presumed peri-Rolandic focus, subdural mats are suitable. This will permit mapping of the ictal discharges and also localization of sensory and motor function by evoked potentials and/or electrical stimulation.

More extensive exploration will be required in patients with seizures of possible temporal, or medial or orbital frontal origin. There do not appear to have been any substantial comparative studies of the diagnostic reliability of depth and subdural electrodes for this purpose. Subdural electrodes may appear simpler to insert and perhaps less invasive, but one may question their reliability for locating the site of seizures arising in deep structures. It is, for instance, possible that discharges spreading from deep structures may first appear at surface contacts over neocortex contralateral to the site of origin, and be wrongly lateralized if only subdural contacts are used. Spencer et al (1987a), using a combination of depth and subdural electrodes in 11 patients, reported that this did not occur. However, in a series of 20 patients studied by the authors the first ictal neocortical discharges were contralateral to the epileptogenic zone in one-third of patients (Binnie et al 1990) (Fig. 16.4). This discrepancy may reflect methods of patient selection—our subjects underwent implantation specifically because of non-congruent findings between foramen ovale telemetry, clinical features and other data. Similarly, Sperling et al (1988) found subdural electrodes detected only late seizure propagation some 35 seconds after onset at deep contacts, and sometimes failed to localize the epileptogenic zone.

Conversely, it is also difficult to sample efficiently the electrical activity of cortical grey matter with radially inserted multipolar depth electrodes. Many contacts may be located uselessly in white matter or may be so positioned that they fail to register any activity from nearby cortical electrical dipoles (Gloor 1987). This difficulty can be overcome to some extent by the use of depth electrodes with large cylindrical contacts (Maxwell et al 1983), but to obtain an adequate picture of the onset and evolution of the seizure with depth electrodes alone, a large number of insertion tracks will generally be needed.

Complications of inserting depth electrodes, haemorrhage and infection, are rare but have been fatal (Ajmone Marsan 1980, Spencer 1981), and Rasmussen (1976) has also questioned whether inserting electrodes into the healthy parts of a brain which has demonstrated an abnormal tendency to generate seizures, could itself cause epileptogenic lesions. Viral infections such as Jakob–Creutzfeldt disease can be transmitted by intracranial electrodes (Bernoulli et al 1977) and some workers would not therefore be prepared to reuse electrodes, despite their considerable cost (Wyler et al 1984).

The above considerations have led an increasing number of workers, including the present authors, to use the combination of as few depth electrodes as is necessary to monitor any suspected deep sites of ictal onset, supplemented by subdural electrode strips or bundles. There are practical difficulties in combining the usual lateral approach for inserting depth electrodes with the use of subdural strips or mats. One solution is to insert the depth contacts through the occipital regions (Spencer et al 1987a), but this carries a risk of cortical blindness if bleeding occurs on an electrode track. According to the method of Van Veelen et al (1990) all electrodes, both subdural and depth, are inserted through two bilateral central trephine holes, radiating from these so that their paths do not cross.

Although the main purpose of subacute intracranial recording is to obtain ictal records, it might be expected that the interictal activity would contain some relevant information. Some authors report that, if multiple foci are present, the rate of spiking will be greater and the variability of interspike intervals less at the primary focus (Lieb et al 1978.) In the probably more highly selected patients whom we implant, bilateral independent foci are almost always present and the seizures do not necessarily arise from the most active focus. The primary focus is, however, less likely to show changes in discharge rate with different sleep stages and yet is more readily activated with thiopentone (Engel et al 1981). Various writers have developed methods of demonstrating the time relations and patterns of spread between functionally interdependent foci (Brazier 1973, Rossi 1973, Mars & Lopez da Silva 1983, Lange

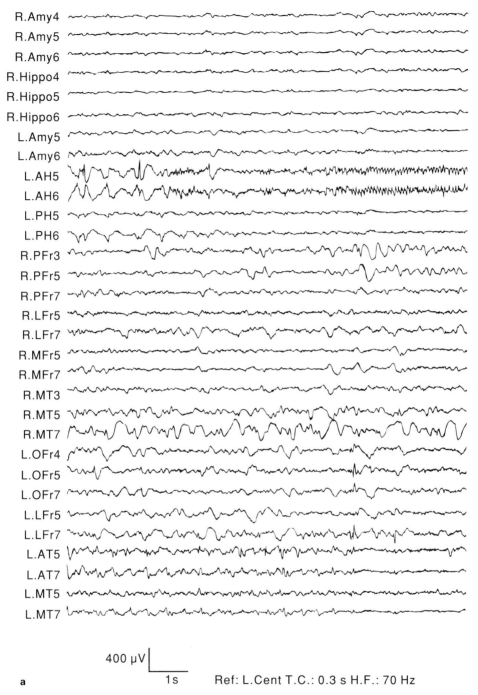

400 µV

a   1 s   Ref: L.Cent T.C.: 0.3 s H.F.: 70 Hz

Fig. 16.4   Propagation of ictal discharges in patient with left mesial temporal sclerosis. At onset
(**a**) interictal spike-wave activity in left anterior hippocampus (L. AH5, 6) gives way to fast
rhythmic activity. This remains sharply localized for 20 seconds (through **b**), and then (**c**)
propagates to the left posterior hippocampus (L. PH5, 6), right mid-hippocampus (R. Hippo6)
and right temporal neocortex (R. MT5, 7). The first ictal changes at subdural electrodes are thus
contralateral to the primary focus.

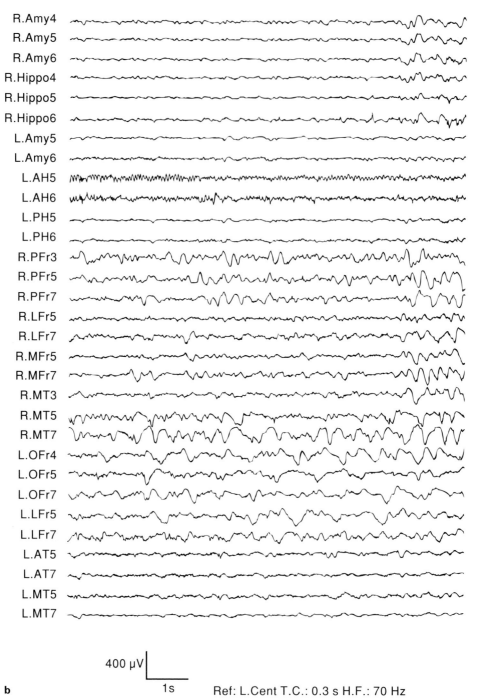

400 μV

1s

b

Ref: L.Cent T.C.: 0.3 s H.F.: 70 Hz

Fig. 16.4   Contd.

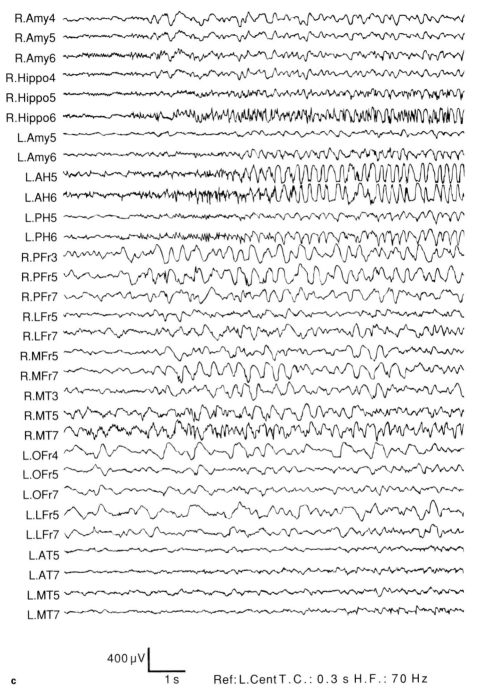

Fig. 16.4 Contd.

et al 1983). It is hoped this may provide a means of identifying the site of origin of seizures on the basis of interictal records.

In those patients who prove amenable to surgery, the electrographic pattern at seizure onset is usually very stereotyped, far more so than in the scalp EEG. In addition to episodes recognized as the patient's habitual attacks, electrographic seizures occur, with minimal or no overt clinical change. These will generally have the same location and morphology as the initial electrographic events of the typical overt seizures, and are therefore of similar localizing value. In the type of patient being considered for surgery, it is usually possible to capture 10 or more overt seizures within a few days, with reduction of medication if necessary, and in the same period dozens of electrographic seizures may be seen.

A recurring problem in evaluating methods of preoperative assessment is the marked difference in the patient populations seen in different centres. This may largely explain apparently irreconcilable differences in practice between different groups, for instance in respect of the use of intracranial recording. It is clearly possible to operate successfully without invasive recording in patients with temporal epileptogenic lesions demonstrable by neuroimaging, and concordant clinical, neuropsychological and interictal surface EEG findings. Even in the radiologically negative subjects, skillful clinical selection (notably of patients with mesial temporal sclerosis) identifies a group operable without invasive recording. Both surgical outcome (Polkey 1983) and confirmation by intracranial recording of the location of the primary focus in such patients (Spencer et al 1987a) confirm the validity of this approach. However, in some centres such a large proportion of patients have extratemporal lesions and/or discordant or negative findings from non-invasive assessment, that intracranial recording is justifiably regarded as routine.

It is also important to recognize that in many centres the only patients who undergo invasive studies are selected by virtue of discrepancies between clinical, imaging, neuropsychological and electrophysiological evidence, and as such are atypical. Reports of findings on depth recording contrary to those of the scalp EEG, do not therefore justify the conclusion that conventional methods of EEG examination are in general unreliable. The selection process was illustrated by the flow chart in Fig. 16.1 which shows the pattern of investigation at the Maudsley Hospital, London, a centre which has a mixed caseload of both complex and relatively simple problems, and where foramen ovale telemetry is used in most patients but full depth or subdural implantation in only 25%.

Spencer (1981) estimated that the use of depth recording increased by 36% the population of patients amenable to surgical treatment of epilepsy, whilst preventing unsuccessful operations in another 18% of patients who prove to have multiple foci. The procedure could thus alter the decision whether or not to operate in half the patients. Olivier et al (1983) interestingly report the experience of increasing the use of routine depth recording in a unit with a vast experience of selecting patients for surgery on conservative criteria using only interictal or ictal scalp EEGs. Their conclusions were similar to those of Spencer.

Discussions of interictal versus ictal recording, or of EEG versus depth registration, generally appear to consider these as alternatives, with the ictal depth recorded data representing the 'correct' findings. Lieb and colleagues (Lieb et al 1981a,b), stress rather that the purpose of electrophysiological assessment is prediction of outcome or identification of operable epileptogenic lesions. By these criteria, ictal, interictal, surface and depth findings contain non-redundant information, and all were used by a non-linear pattern-recognition algorithm for predicting outcome. Specifically, the following were predictive of a poor outcome and negative pathology: interictal bilaterally synchronous surface spikes; interictal independent surface spikes on the side selected for operation; ictal onset with bilateral or unilateral surface involvement (with or without deep spikes); multiple onset sites, and suppression at onset. The outcomes considered above related to removal of abnormal tissue and seizure relief. However, some of the adverse findings listed, notably bilaterally synchronous ictal onset and interictal discharges, were also predictive of postoperative psychological deterioration (Lieb et al 1982a,b).

The proportion of patients considered amenable to surgery after depth recording must depend on the selection criteria for performing this investigation. Half the patients of Spencer et al (1982) exhibited multiple or unlocalizable sites of ictal onset in depth recording and, if the most active focus was excised, results were poor. Unlocalized depth recordings were obtained in 80% of patients with non-localizing ictal scalp recordings. From the studies of Lieb and Spencer and their colleagues it seems that depth recording may often be required to confirm the finding of a focal onset in the scalp EEG but, where the EEG is non-localizing, depth recording is unlikely to offer a basis for successful surgery. The findings of Delgado-Escueta and colleagues (Delgado-Escueta et al 1982, Delgado-Escueta & Walsh 1983) may be considered to lead to the same conclusion, although this is not the view of the authors themselves. In our material (Binnie et al 1990), where invasive recording was employed in only 25% of patients, the picture is rather different. Among those in whom a consistent unilateral temporal seizure onset was demonstrated, interictal scalp EEG and ictal foramen ovale recordings had both correctly indicated the side of onset in only 20%, and had given false lateralization in 33%. Thus in this series 80% of the implanted patients would have been considered inoperable, or would have undergone resection on the wrong side if invasive recording had not been used. Such results obviously offer no evidence as to whether the criteria of selection for implantation were too conservative.

One author has in the past worked with two teams representing the extremes of practice. In one centre (The Maudsley Hospital, London) the majority of patients treated had mesial temporal sclerosis, which was reliably located by interictal EEG recording with confirmation if required by acute corticography (Polkey 1983). In the other (The Academic Hospital, Utrecht), mesial temporal sclerosis was rarely seen, many patients had non-temporal lesions, multiple EEG foci and a range of pathologies including penetrating injuries, sequelae of intracranial infection and hamartomata. Here ictal recordings with depth electrodes were almost always necessary (Van Veelen et al 1990). The different approaches were dictated by the patient populations, not by any theoretical position adopted by the investigators. More recently we have both changed our working practices to adapt to a changing patient population referred for treatment, and the expanding range of surgical and investigative options available (see Fig. 16.1).

Localization of normal and abnormal cerebral function. Where a decision in principle has been taken to perform surgical resection for treatment of epilepsy, it is essential to determine what neurological or psychological deficit may result. This is the more difficult as the majority of resections for epilepsy involve the temporal lobes and a patient with temporal damage may have abnormal lateralization of speech and memory. When subacute intracranial recording is performed, the opportunity may also be taken of performing leisurely mapping of cerebral function, if necessary over several days, determining location of cerebral functions by electrical stimulation and by evoked potentials (Gregorie & Goldring 1984).

For functional mapping large electrode matrices are ideal, whereas narrow flexible bundles are unsuitable because attempts at electrical stimulation generally elicit pain from the dura. Typically, electrical stimulation employs pulses of alternating polarity and about 1 ms duration applied at about 50 Hz, in trains of up to 10 seconds, between adjacent electrode pairs (bipolar stimulation) at constant currents up to 10 mA. Threshold stimulus intensities for producing cerebral damage do not appear to have been established in man; however, current densities up to $57\ \mu$ C/cm^2 per pulse are known not to produce histological change and may be regarded provisionally as the limit of safety (Gordon et al 1990).

Electrical stimulation is used both to determine the cerebral localization of normal functions and as an aid to identifying the primary focus. An attempt may also be made to evoke an attack corresponding to the patient's habitual seizure pattern from stimulation at the site of the presumed primary focus. This is not reliable as evidence of localization if an after-discharge occurs, as this may spread to involve structures at a distance from the site of stimulation (Gloor 1975). However, provided no after-discharge occurs, in patients with a single, established site of seizure onset, there is a high concordance with the locus from which the habitual aura can be obtained (Bernier et al 1990); thus, arguably, stimulation may be used to reinforce the evidence of recording spontaneous seizures.

At the primary focus the threshold for eliciting an after-discharge is usually altered with respect to the contralateral, presumably normal, side: it is most often lowered but is elevated in some 25% of subjects, presumably as a consequence of severe neuronal loss (Bernier et al 1990). How-ever, once an after-discharge has been elicited, the threshold may be markedly changed. After-discharge threshold is therefore probably not a reliable guide to localizing an epileptogenic focus (Ajmone Marsan 1973).

Neurophysiological studies—II

Acute intracranial recording. Acute electro-corticography (ECoG) has been a standard procedure in epilepsy surgery since the work of Penfield & Jasper (1954). It will usually be per-formed through a craniotomy and will therefore rarely be undertaken unless a decision has already been made concerning the site of a possible resec-tion. In patients with seizures thought to be of temporal lobe origin, this implies that a focal EEG abnormality will already have been found and the role of corticography will be limited to confirming previous findings. The chances of recording a spontaneous seizure at acute cortico-graphy are poor, and the only new evidence this procedure can usually offer is more precise locali-zation of the site and extent of the interictal EEG disturbances. Seizures may be induced by electri-cal stimulation at the site of the primary focus; although it is gratifying if these resemble the pa-tient's habitual seizure pattern, this finding does not have any value for predicting the therapeutic outcome (Engel et al 1975).

If little or no epileptiform activity occurs, this can be activated by intravenous thiopentone or methohexitone, usually up to a dose producing burst-suppression, but there is some dispute as to the utility of this procedure. Wyler et al (1987) find that small doses of methohexitone (25–100 mg) selectively activate the primary focus so that it can be more easily defined, without

producing discharges in other regions. Others report the appearance of new foci not apparently relevant to the origin of seizures, and find that activation of the ECoG before resection provides no information of value for planning the operation and that the ECoG response to methohexitone after the procedure is not predictive of prognosis (Fiol et al 1990).

In many centres, acute corticography is con-ducted whenever possible under local anaesthesia, both to permit mapping of cortical functions by electrical stimulation, and because general anaes-thetics may suppress epileptiform activity.

Both surface and depth electrodes may be used, the latter ranging in sophistication from one or two needles placed manually in such structures as the amygdala or hippocampus to stereotactic placement of several multicontact electrodes (Bancaud et al 1965, Talairach & Bancaud 1973, 1974). Surface ECoG electrodes are of two types, either fixed arrays mounted on plastic sheets or separate contacts which can be posi-tioned independently at the surgeon's discretion. Experienced teams usually choose the flexibility offered by the latter; moreover, the use of plastic sheets virtually precludes functional mapping by electrical stimulation. Separate contacts are mounted on an electrode holder bolted to the skull, supplemented by flexible leads passed under the margins of the craniotomy, and needle elec-trodes to be inserted into deep structures such as the hippocampus (Fig. 16.5).

Frequent, high amplitude discharges of spikes or spike-wave complexes may be expected in the epileptogenic zone. Sometimes it is necessary to adjust (either lighten or deepen) general anaes-thesia, if used, to demonstrate them satisfactorily. A low discharge rate such as less than one event in 4 minutes is rare, and implies a poor outcome of surgery (possibly indicating that the epileptogenic zone has not been correctly identified) (McBride et al 1991). The grapho-elements are of higher amplitude, often 500μ V to 1.5 mV, and contain more fast components than in the scalp EEG. Spikes of predominantly positive polarity are not uncommon, and discrete dipoles may be found across a single gyrus. Ongoing rhythms contain large amounts of beta activity over the frontal lobes in particular, which may be of some value in

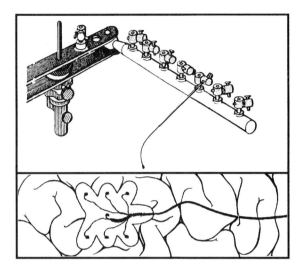

Fig. 16.5 Two types of ECoG electrode. Reprinted with permission from Binnie et al 1982.

identifying the Rolandic fissure. Delta activity is common, even with light anaesthesia and may be due in part to surgical manipulation. It is often maximal within the epileptogenic zone, but not with sufficient consistency to be of localizing value (Panet-Raymond & Gotman 1990).

The importance of acute ECoG for clinical decision making varies very much between centres. Although most centres aim to remove either the epileptogenic lesion, or the primary focus, or both, there is a French school which advocates removal of the entire epileptogenic zone and a North American tradition of resections tailored to remove only tissue from which discharges are recorded. By contrast, the British school do not regard the mapping of the epileptogenic zone during a brief acute interictal ECoG recording as very relevant, and favour so far as possible anatomically standardized procedures to remove as much tissue surrounding the focus as is compatible with the avoidance of unacceptable neurological or cognitive deficits. For temporal foci, this implies a choice between en bloc resection and amygdalo-hippocampectomy. A restricted area of interictal discharge over the middle of the midtemporal and inferior temporal convolutions, together with an anterior maximum of hippocampal discharges favours the latter (Polkey et al 1989). ECoG findings will only rarely lead to an extension of the resection, if discharges persist at

a very circumscribed area at the margin of the operative site.

Outside the temporal lobes, there are no standard resections, and the ECoG plays a more important role in determining the extent of the primary excision and possibly its subsequent extension. This will arise both in patients who have been monitored with intracranial electrodes and, more particularly, in those undergoing resection of radiologically demonstrable lesions without previous detailed electrophysiological investigation. So far as is compatible with avoidance of neurological deficit, regions of epileptiform discharge, areas with clearly reduced beta activity, radiologically demonstrable lesions, and visibly abnormal tissue will be removed. Tailored procedures may be combined with functional mapping under local anaesthesia to determine the boundaries of the region that can be excised without causing deficits. In patients with simple partial seizures with sensorimotor symptoms, suggesting a focal origin in the Rolandic area, the interictal EEG is often normal and even ictal records may fail to show a focus. Here there may often be a case for exploratory corticography at a site determined by the clinical findings. This is usually successful and, if the focal discharges occur over an area of visibly abnormal tissue, resection is likely to be followed by seizure reduction. Again, electrical stimulation can be employed. This will of course elicit sensorimotor seizures in normal subjects, but a progressive spread of the discharge and 'march' of the clinical manifestations reinforces the view that the site of origin of the patient's habitual seizure has been found.

Where multiple subpial transection (MST) is performed, it is reasonable to check how far discharges have been abolished and desynchronized, and to carry out further transection of areas showing residual synchronous discharge. It should, however, be stressed that this strategy is based on a priori considerations: evaluation studies of ECoG in MST are not yet available.

After callosotomy, ECoG, or combined EEG and ECoG recording, shows desynchronization of bilateral discharges; it appears reasonable that this should be used as a guide to determine the extent of the procedure, but the reliability of this criterion is unknown.

If acute corticography is being performed, then it is usual also to obtain a further registration following the resection. Only in exceptional circumstances will the finding of residual, or new, epileptiform activity at the margin of the resection justify removal of additional tissue, but the postresection ECoG may be of some prognostic significance. The persistence of substantial amounts of epileptiform activity is generally regarded as an unfavourable sign by the Montreal school (Jasper et al 1951, Bengzon et al 1968), but this is disputed by others (Ajmone Marsan & Baldwin 1958, Walker et al 1960). In our experience it is not the absolute amount of residual epileptiform activity, but rather the percentage reduction which is significant (McBride et al 1991); if the discharge rate after temporal lobectomy is not reduced by more than 50%, a successful outcome is unlikely. It should also be noted that the ECoG is of little relevance after amygdalo-hippocampectomy (possibly because this procedure does not necessitate removing the entire epileptogenic zone) (McBride et al 1991).

The reader may with some justification conclude from the above that, although recording of the ECoG during epilepsy surgery has been routine for many years, amazingly little attention has been directed to optimizing techniques, to developing interpretative criteria, or to determining its value.

Postoperative EEG follow-up

Assessment of EEG findings after operation is hampered by the fact that preoperative assessment is generally much more intensive than subsequent follow-up. It is unrealistic to compare short, waking postoperative records with prolonged recordings using additional electrodes and various activation techniques prior to surgery. However, Van Buren et al (1975) showed a marked reduction in epileptiform discharges in most patients postoperatively and, more importantly, a strong association between EEG improvement and seizure remission. The predictive reliability of the EEG increases in the second postoperative year. Van Buren et al (1975) found that, of those patients with epileptiform EEG discharges after 2 years, only 7% remained seizure-free; whereas

an absence of epileptiform discharges at 2 years was accompanied by clinical improvement in 87%. Taking EEG and clinical findings together, the presence of persisting EEG abnormality in a patient with early seizures confirms a poor prognosis, whereas a negative EEG carries a possibility of subsequent clinical improvement (in about 50% of patients). Even less formal study has been directed to postoperative EEG findings after the newer procedures. However, our experience of EEGs following amygdalo-hippocampectomy parallels the acute ECoG findings, in that persistent epileptiform activity is not predictive of adverse outcome.

Psychometric studies

Psychometric studies are important both to detect focal brain dysfunction and to predict the cognitive effects of surgery, especially operations on the temporal lobe. The assessment of intellectual abilities in patients is to some extent biased by the particular tests used in clinical practice. For example many tests depend upon verbal competence, or upon the ease of assessing a particular function, such as memory, which has many facets and is therefore subject to frequent and complex tests. In most centres a standard group of tests is used. These tests have been validated in normal populations and it may be necessary to use separate versions for children. This neuropsychological profile usually includes assessments of general intellectual competence such as the WAIS for full scale IQ, and subtests which evaluate verbal and non-verbal function and can be combined as estimates of verbal and non-verbal IQ. There are also tests of memory function both immediate and delayed. There are yet others which will estimate frontal lobe function and so on. Details of how such a neuropsychological profile is obtained are to be found in the review by Rausch (1987). In addition in many centres special methods will have been devised to look at particular aspects of cognitive functioning of interest to the investigators. There are also procedures which attempt to isolate the function of a particular cerebral area temporarily, in clinical practice this amounts to the carotid amytal or Wada test first described by Wada (1949). This has many variants which are described and discussed in the section on selection of patients for temporal lobe surgery.

In some schemes of assessment a minimum IQ level is quoted as a bar to surgery, but this depends upon the type of surgery which is envisaged, the clinical state of the patient and the disease process involved in the production of the severe epilepsy. One factor which can influence cognitive performance is structural damage accompanying the basic disease and its effects depend upon the site of the damage, its extent and the age of the patient at the time when it occurs. In some patients, such as one who has been the victim of severe meningitis as a child, or some metabolic or ischaemic disease, there may be an overall reduction in intellectual performance which will manifest itself as a low overall IQ score without any reduction on some subtests compared with others. In such a patient, without evidence of focal brain damage on brain imaging studies, one might infer diffuse brain damage and suspect that any epilepsy would be multifocal in origin and therefore not susceptible to resective surgery. On the other hand a patient who sustained unilateral hemisphere damage of a non-progressive nature in early childhood might also have a low IQ score and also a uniform performance on subtests but in the presence of a unilateral lesion, such as gross hemisphere atrophy, might benefit from surgery without gross further reduction in cognitive ability. However if such a patient sustained hemisphere damage later in childhood, or if it were progressive over a number of years, as we shall see when we consider selection for hemispherectomy, then the effects of surgery may be more drastic. In a similar way damage to one temporal lobe early in life can often lead to a picture of cognitive impairment with overall loss, whereas later in life there will be a greater risk of material specific deficits.

In addition however there is another mechanism which may affect intellectual performance. If there are frequent electrical discharges in one or several areas of the brain this may also affect cognitive function as has been demonstrated by Aarts et al (1984) and others. If this abnormal electrical activity is relieved by surgery then cognitive function may improve, but if it is not relieved then there may even be a deterioration.

The particular tests which are useful and the effects of surgery on cognitive function will be described in detail in relation to particular surgical procedures.

Brain imaging

The application of neuroimaging techniques to the investigation and treatment of epilepsy is dealt with elsewhere in this textbook. This section looks at the relevance of these techniques to the selection of patients for surgery. This is an appropriate point to state that the use of these investigations depends as much upon their availability as upon their suitability. For those working under financial or other constraints it may be necessary to use some of the older methods or to accept that the selection process cannot be taken beyond a certain point. For these reasons, although they will not be dealt with in detail here, plain skull radiographs, angiograms and air studies in particular should not be forgotten.

Computerized tomography of the head, hereafter CT, is now a standard technique which is widely available. Early studies show a high percentage of abnormalities in patients with epilepsy varying between 40% and 70% with a high frequency in patients with partial epilepsy as reviewed by Fish (1989). It is difficult to know what proportion of patients have undisclosed lesions since it depends to some extent upon the sophistication of the scanner used in the investigation and the scanning technique. However figures from specialist centres suggest that between 15% and 54% of patients with drug-resistant epilepsy have undisclosed focal CT lesions (Spencer et al 1984a, Rich et al 1985, Munari et al 1987). Scanning technique, especially in the temporal lobes, is important and the Oxford group first showed that altering the angle of the scanner gantry to a plane parallel to the main axis of the temporal lobes produced scans which were more informative and less susceptible to artifact (Adams et al 1987). The use of intrathecal contrast in this situation, as described from Oxford and also by Wyler & Bolender (1983), may be useful. Even with these modern techniques however it may be difficult to detect focal gliosis in the temporal lobe, such as the lesion of mesial temporal sclerosis (Schorner et al 1987), but there is no doubt that most but not all other lesions such as indolent gliomas, hamartomas, etc. will be demonstrated by CT.

Magnetic resonance imaging, hereafter MRI, is clearly superior in the demonstration of most focal pathology important to the surgeon. Thus Sperling and colleagues demonstrated seven structural lesions in 35 patients with negative CT scans using MRI. These were all small gliomas and the like, and in 18 patients who had mesial temporal sclerosis proven in the specimen resected at temporal lobectomy, they failed to demonstrate the gliosis of this lesion by MRI (Sperling et al 1986). Other groups have described similar findings, for example Schorner and colleagues who investigated 50 patients with epilepsy—CT scanning revealed 12 lesions and MRI 11 of these 12 and a further five lesions (Schorner et al 1987). It is becoming clear in our own practice that certain lesions such as those of cortical dysplasia are seen more easily and more frequently with MRI. The detection of small areas of gliosis such as those associated with mesial temporal sclerosis is more contentious. As with CT, it is dependent upon the mode of examination and the interpretation of the results. A report from Montreal suggests that in virtually all cases of 'foreign tissue' lesions they can be detected with MRI and that mesial temporal sclerosis can frequently be detected especially when the changes are severe (Kuzniecky et al 1987). Some claim that with scanning in an appropriate coronal plane parallel to the brain stem and use of the proper sequences virtually all cases of unilateral mesial temporal sclerosis can be detected. In 41 patients where the pathology in the temporal lobe had been established by subsequent operation, mesial temporal sclerosis was known to be present in 27 patients and found by MRI in 25 with two false negatives. In the 14 patients without mesial temporal sclerosis there were two false positives with MRI examination (Berkowicz, unpublished data, 1990).

Both CT and MRI in their present forms are methods of demonstrating structural abnormalities in the brain, and although MRI has the potential to reveal other aspects of brain function through MRI spectroscopy this has not yet been done and a preliminary report from Erlangen in 1990 suggests there are still considerable technical difficulties (Stefan et al 1990).

However there are other methods of brain imaging which are based on cerebral function rather than structural detail. Thus xenon-enhanced CT has been used to try to lateralize temporal lobe dysfunction by Fish and his colleagues (1987). However the main methods of investigation are proton emission tomography, hereafter PET, and single photon emission computerized tomography, hereafter SPECT. Both methods have been in use for some time and assessment of the results is bedevilled by the different ways in which they have been used by different groups, and by the fact that their spatial resolution is inferior to that of CT and MRI.

PET can measure both regional cerebral blood flow and regional cerebral metabolic rate. Both of these are useful parameters, especially in attempting to demonstrate the origin of focal epileptic seizures. Most studies have used deoxyglucose labelled with fluorine[18] and Engel and colleagues have demonstrated unilateral hypoperfusion in 70% of 50 patients studied who had partial epilepsy (Sperling et al 1987). In the same review it is noted that studies of bloodflow using oxygen[15] have also shown hypoperfusion in patients with partial seizures. These areas always seem to be greater than the area of structural abnormality. Wieser has reported the results of preoperative and postoperative PET scans in 21 patients undergoing unilateral selective amygdalo-hippocampectomy. Patients are selected for this operation on the basis of having unilateral mesial temporal onset for their seizures. Although all the patients reported by Wieser showed unilateral glucose hypometabolism prior to surgery which was appropriate to the side of operation this always involved the whole temporal lobe and in patients re-examined up to 7 years after surgery there was no restoration of normal metabolism in the lateral cortex on the operated side (Wieser personal communication). Attempts are being made around the world to enable CT, MRI, and PET or SPECT from the same patient to be accurately superimposed to allow anatomical identification of the functionally abnormal areas but no practical system yet exists. The other difficulty with

PET is that because of the technical constraints it is rarely possible to obtain ictal scans. Where such studies are available they have shown areas of hypermetabolism corresponding to the hypometabolism seen in the interictal scan, although as we shall see with SPECT it can be dependent upon the interval between the scan and the seizure.

SPECT depends almost totally on regional bloodflow, it has a much lower spatial resolution than PET, but it is also a technology which is more accessible and ictal scans can be carried out much more easily than with PET because ligands can be injected at the time of the seizure and the scan carried out at a convenient time up to 4 hours later. Early results reviewed by Sperling et al (1987) suggested that SPECT would show decreased uptake interictally in the affected temporal lobe of patients with partial epilepsy and increased uptake ictally. Typical of these kind of studies is that by Ryding et al (1988) in which they describe the result of interictal and ictal studies in 14 patients with partial epilepsy. These studies showed regional abnormalities in 93% of these patients corresponding to a known EEG focus. However, the EEG studies were with sphenoidal telemetry and as we have already seen such crude EEG assessments will not always reveal the side of origin of the seizures; in the same group of patients CT and MRI showed abnormalities in only 30%. A similar report from Duncan et al (1990) in Glasgow in which SPECT, CT and MRI were compared in 30 patients showed that abnormalities could be demonstrated in more patients using SPECT, however in these 30 patients only 17 had lateralized abnormalities on EEG which again comprised only interictal scalp and sphenoidal recordings.

In a more sophisticated study Rowe and colleagues (Rowe et al 1989) from the Austin Hospital in Australia have examined the findings in 32 patients examined with SPECT in whom detailed neurophysiological studies of seizure onset were available, including depth electrode studies in 25 patients. They were also able to decrease the time between seizure onset and injection of the ligand, (^{99m}Tc-HMPAO) to an average of 6.3 minutes. They noted that interictal scans were unreliable, indicating the correct localization compared with other methods in only 53% of patients, although in those 20 patients where lateralized hypoperfusion was seen it corresponded to the primary EEG focus in 17 (53%). When interictal and postictal scans were interpreted together the correct localization was increased to 72%. They note that the appearance of the postictal scan changes with time and that the closer the injection of ligand is to the seizure onset the more reliable are the changes seen, thus the 11 patients where injection occurred within 3 minutes of seizure onset an appropriate focal change was seen in 73%. On another occasion Berkowitz noted that in six patients with simultaneous bitemporal onset of seizures detected by depth electrodes only one showed a unilateral SPECT focus whereas it appeared to be bilateral in the other five patients. It should be recalled with respect to all lateralization techniques, that the correct side would be selected by chance in 50% of patients. The conclusion of all these studies must be that both PET and SPECT have only limited, chiefly confirmatory, value in preoperative localization.

The first requisite in assessing the results of surgery is to have a solid base of preoperative assessment. Where possible the pathology in the resected specimen should be known. Although the majority of these operations should be carried out in a few specialized centres, for reasons which will also be discussed later, nevertheless the technical details of the surgery should be such that it can be repeated by an adequately trained neurosurgeon, otherwise the procedure will die with the originator. In general it is reasonable to assert that much of the success of resective surgery depends not upon surgical technique but upon the selection of patients and the underlying pathology.

Because of the variety of operations used to treat epilepsy, and the different protocols used to select patients for those operations, detailed comparison between different centres is difficult. Certain broad principles can be adopted however in judging the results of such operations, and the following criteria would be appropriate. There should be a minimum follow-up of 5 years after surgery, since it is known that the number of patients remaining fit-free diminishes with time (Engel 1987). The follow-up data should include freedom from, or significant control of seizures, complications of surgery including intellectual changes, long-term and short-term mortality, and social and behavioural changes.

NEUROPATHOLOGY

Because the pathology in the resected specimen plays a considerable role in the result of the surgery it is appropriate, before considering the surgery in detail, to give a brief resumé of the pathology commonly found in these specimens. The following account is not a neuro-pathological text, but a brief guide to enable the reader to understand the selection procedures and results of resective surgery. Certain obvious lesions such as meningiomas, aneurysms and gliomas have been omitted, even though they may be associated with epilepsy, because they are commonly encountered and treated in general neurosurgical practice. The lesions described here, which are encountered in our resected specimens, with one or two exceptions, are universally distributed throughout the cerebral cortex and may also vary in their size. In some cases the precise nature or origin of the lesions is in dispute.

Two types of 'congenital' lesions are seen, namely cortical dysplasia and related lesions and hamartomas. As far as we know they are present in the brain from the time of its development and change little in size or distribution once formed. Both show considerable variation in their histological appearance, size and distribution. Cortical dysplasia is thought to occur in two forms, focal cortical dysplasia where there are one or several discrete areas with the characteristic histological appearance (Taylor et al 1971, Janota & Polkey 1985, Andermann et al 1987), or as diffuse, microscopic cortical dysplasia (Nordborg et al 1986) and these forms have been described by some groups in different patients and by others in the same patient. The histological picture consists of large bizarre neurones and glial cells occurring in groups with disordered connections which can be demonstrated with silver stains. Clearly these features are more easily seen in the focal aggregations than in the diffuse microscopic form. Sometimes very large areas of brain may be affected and the condition then tends to merge with the findings in patients with megalencephaly who present for surgical treatment (King et al 1985, Barkovich & Chuan 1990). In this condition there is clearly a cortical migration defect which may be restricted even to parts of one hemisphere and intermediate forms may be seen between the gross megalencephaly and cortical dysplasia as described be Marchal et al (1989) and Kuzniecky et al (1989). The relationship between these two conditions and tuberous sclerosis is also difficult to discern. In other pathological classifications they might also be seen as heterotopias.

Hamartomas are equally difficult to classify. The definition by Willis (1958) designate them as 'tumour-like, but primarily non-neoplastic malformations, or inborn errors of tissue development, characterized by an abnormal mixture of tissue indigenous to the part, with an excess of one or more of these'. On the whole they tend to be discrete and solitary.

Trauma now plays a relatively minor part, especially in practice in the UK where penetrating cerebral wounds are rare and closed head injury, which tends to cause widespread pathology, is the commonest type of cerebral trauma. In larger series the commonest area for scar resection is the frontal region.

Perinatal disease, including perinatal trauma, is rare with improvement in prenatal and obstetric care, but occasionally one still sees large areas of tissue destruction from such causes, and these may be susceptible to major resections.

Local lesions from infective causes are rare in our practice, but occasionally the late effects of pyogenic abscess may be seen. In other parts of the world tuberculosis and parasitic infections produce the same effects.

The progressive pathology known as Rasmussen's encephalitis with epilepsy, first described by Rasmussen and his colleagues in 1958 (Rasmussen et al 1958) is a distinct condition about which little is known. The clinical and other details will be described later, but it presents a pathological picture as if some kind of encephalitis was affecting parts of the brain to varying degrees. In its most severe form it may affect the whole of one cerebral hemisphere, as described in postmortem reports by Mizuno et al (1985) and Gray et al (1987). The histological picture is one of perivascular lymphocytic cuffing, and glial nodules in the areas where the brain tissue is relatively preserved and in later stages there are elements of marked microcystic degeneration and neuronal fallout with no evidence of inflammatory elements (Rasmussen 1987). Despite attempts to isolate an infective agent none has been found either in the patients or the specimens, although a recent paper by Power and colleagues suggests that cytomegalic virus is present in this material (Power et al 1990).

Vascular lesions include not only localized arteriovenous malformations and cavernous angiomas but also Sturge–Weber disease, the clinical details of which will be dealt with under hemispherectomy and major resections.

Neoplasms of various kinds are also encountered. The lesions peculiar to long-standing drug-resistant epilepsy are usually indolent and include tumours of mixed origin such as gangliogliomas. These tumours have been described as dysembryonoplastic tumours by Daumas-Duport et al (1988). In addition to this a number of low grade astrocytic tumours are found and the occasional epidermoid.

Mesial temporal sclerosis is a pathology peculiar to the temporal lobe, and was first described by Bouchet and Cazauvieilh in 1825. It is not necessary here to deal with the pathological changes in detail, there is an excellent review by Babb & Jann-Brown (1987). However certain salient facts from that review are worth noting because they may affect temporal lobe surgery and its results. It is known from numerous studies that the hippocampal damage seen after anoxic and similar episodes in humans differs in detail from the picture seen in hippocampal sclerosis associated with temporal lobe epilepsy. There is evidence from a large number of publications that mesial temporal sclerosis is nearly always asymetrical with 80% being predominantly unilateral. In nearly every series there are a few patients with dual pathology, that is mesial temporal sclerosis together with some other lesion in the temporal lobe such as a glioma or an hamartoma. It is probable that the extent of the sclerosis within the mesial temporal structures affects the results of operation. Babb et al (1984) described how local onset in the anterior hippocampus recorded through depth electrodes was associated with

neuronal loss restricted to the anterior hippocampus in the resected specimen, whereas in patients with more widespread electrical seizure onset the sclerotic changes tended to extend to the posterior limit of the resection.

RESECTIVE SURGERY

Temporal lobe resections

Introduction

Some form of temporal lobe resection is the commonest operation for drug-resistant epilepsy. This is shown in Table 16.2 which lists frequency of operations at the Montreal Neurological Institute and the Maudsley Hospital and also in an international survey (Engel 1987) where 71.9% of the reported resective operations involved the temporal lobe.

Selection details

The criteria outline above for selection for resective surgery are used to select patients for temporal lobe resections. The preoperative assessment is aimed chiefly at demonstrating a discrete pathology in the temporal lobe, or a discrete onset for the seizures in some part of the temporal lobe.

In patients where temporal lobe surgery is contemplated the previous medical history may help. It is well established that in 80% or more of patients with mesial temporal sclerosis there is

Table 16.2 Frequency of resective surgery at the Montreal Neurological Institute and the Maudsley Hospital

Resection	Montreal Neurological Institute (1929–1980)		Maudsley Hopsital (1975–1990)	
	Number	%	Number	%
Temporal	1210	56	192	69
Frontal	402	18	28	10
Central	151	7	4	2
Parietal	141	6	19	7
Occipital	30	1	4	2
Multilobe including hemispherectomy	243	11	28	10
Total	2177		279	

* From Rasmussen 1987.

a history of an atypical febrile convulsion, either unilateral or prolonged beyond 30 minutes or similar episodes in childhood (Falconer 1974). As first suggested by Ounstead (1966) if there is no history of such a convulsion, or birth trauma, and there is normal intelligence then the possibility of some other lesion should be considered. This is especially true if the epilepsy is of late onset.

The ictal history is of importance as already described. The occurrence of an aura is of localizing value and it is now well established from depth electrode studies in the mesial temporal lobe that these auras represent simple partial seizures in these structures. Falconer & Taylor (1968) suggested that an aura was more likely to be present in patients with mesial temporal sclerosis and that in those patients the aura was more likely to have a somatosensory or viscerosensory content such as a rushing cephalic or a rising epigastric aura as distinct from patients with hamartomas and the like who were likely to experience a taste or smell.

The way in which an attack begins has been held by some to be of importance, Delgado-Escueta & Walsh (1983) claimed that seizures which began with a motionless stare, especially if consistent when the attacks are video-taped, had their origin in the medial temporal structures and respond well to surgery. Later workers have shown that such a seizure onset occurs consistently in very few patients (Schmidt et al 1982, Binnie & Van der Wens 1986). The seizures themselves, in addition to the well–recognized features of mumbling, lip-smacking and so forth may also include more bizarre components such as rushing about, trying to hide etc., which are automatisms for which the patient is amnesic and are usually associated with the seizure discharge becoming bilateral. Serafetidines & Falconer (1963) found two types of speech disorders during their seizures in 100 subjects who subsequently underwent temporal lobectomy. In one type there was paroxysmal dysphasia in which the patients were unable to express themselves during a period of awareness, and this was usually found in those who were offered a left temporal lobectomy. In the second type there were speech automatisms in which the patients uttered identifiable stereotyped words and phrases for which they were subse-

quently amnesic and this was usually found in those who offered a right temporal lobectomy.

The occurrence of other kind of seizures in addition to partial seizures has not been considered a bar to operation by most authors. Falconer & Serafetidines (1963) noted that the results of temporal lobectomy in patients who suffered tonic-clonic seizures were no different from those in patients who did not, and Van Buren et al (1975) also noted 50% of their patients habitually suffered tonic-clonic attacks. However Jensen (1976) analysing the results of Vaernet's 74 operations noted that tonic-clonic seizures were a bad prognostic indicator. These authors make no distinction between those seizures which secondarily generalized after a clear partial onset and those which were apparently generalized from the start.

A significant number of the patients proposed for temporal lobe resections have personality, social and behavioural difficulties. The proportion varies from one series to another. Jensen (1975a) in a survey of the world literature on temporal lobectomy comprising over 2000 cases, noted that between 15% and 50% were described as having such difficulties. In most cases the behaviour disorder corresponded to that described by Pond (1974) consisting of irritability, unpredictable mood variation, quarrelsome behaviour and so forth. It is difficult to obtain accurate estimates for the true incidence of behaviour or personality disorder, including frank psychiatric illness, in this group of patients because few are subjected to preoperative assessment of these points with the same rigour or perseverance that is applied to other parameters such as neurophysiology or neuropsychology. Taylor, looking at Falconer's material in 1972 (Taylor 1972), estimated that only 13% were normal before operation. In their excellent account of a prospective study of children with temporal lobe epilepsy Ounstead and colleagues (Ounstead at al 1987) note that although 85% of their children had some form of psychological abnormality at initial coding in 1964, which at that time included mental subnormality, nevertheless, among the survivors into adult life some 70% were normal. A sophisticated explanation of the personality disorder seen in temporal lobe epileptics was suggested in a series of papers by Bear and Fedio (Bear & Fedio 1977,

Bear et al 1982), although recent opinion has suggested that these characteristics may well apply to any group of those with epilepsy.

The occurrence of psychosis in this group is equally interesting. The figure of 12% quoted by Falconer (1973) probably relates to the level in the epileptic population attending psychiatric hospitals and clinics (Fenton 1978), rather than the level in the general population more typically represented from the figures from Currie's study of 2% (Currie et al 1971). In the majority of these patients the psychosis is of a paranoid type, tends to supervene upon a long period of uncontrolled epilepsy and has been shown to be unaffected by operation (Serafetidines & Falconer 1962). It was originally suggested by Flor-Henry (1969) that there might be an association between left temporal lobe disease and schizophreniform illness and Taylor noted that in Falconer's material this illness was usually associated with alien tissue lesions in the left (dominant) hemisphere (Taylor 1975). We have not been able to confirm this association in our material.

In the past a full scale IQ of 70 or more was thought to be necessary for the patient to benefit from operation, but modern brain imaging reveals structural lesions in some patients which merit surgery even in the presence of a low IQ which may be produced by the functional effects of the lesion as discussed in the section on neuropsychological assessment. However, because recent memory is probably the most important function of the temporal lobes in man, it is necessary to estimate this function as exactly as possible before surgery and to try to predict accurately the effect of operation upon it. Using appropriate tests, and making assumptions about cerebral dominance in any particular patient, a disparity between verbal and spatial or performance IQ may indicate lateralized temporal dysfunction, although quite often such differences do not have a high reliability (Milner 1975). A recent study from the Maudsley Hospital has shown that there may be small non-significant trends in a group of 59 patients examined prior to temporal lobectomy with those candidates subsequently undergoing left temporal lobectomy having a better performance on non-verbal tests and the converse being true for those subsequently undergoing right temporal lobectomy. It was also shown that the age of onset of the seizures influenced both the results of preoperative testing and also the results of operation. Of equal importance are the results of memory testing and poor performance in the Wechsler Logical Memory Tests (dominant temporal lobe) or the Rey–Osterreith Memory Tests (non-dominant temporal lobe), accepted as evidence of corresponding damage.

When the psychometric findings conflict with other data there may be several explanations. One may be that the patient is of mixed cerebral dominance. Another is that if temporal lobe damage has been sustained early in life there may have been reorganization of cerebral function. Finally it may be that the patient genuinely has bitemporal damage. The only practical way to resolve this problem is by use of the carotid amytal test or one of its variants. First described by Wada in 1949 (Wada 1949) as a means of determining cerebral dominance for speech it was subsequently realized by Milner and colleagues (Milner et al 1962) that memory could also be tested in the same way. In our institution the carotid amytal test is usually carried out in the following way.

The test is carried out under EEG control, the EEG electrodes are applied, an arterial catheter is inserted into each internal carotid artery in turn, and angiography performed to confirm the location of the catheter and to determine whether or not any cross-flow occurs from one internal carotid to the contralateral cerebral-vessels. The patient is instructed in the performance of several simple neuropsychological tests, chiefly concerned with speech and verbal and non-verbal memory. The patient is then asked to elevate both hands and sodium amytal is injected into the carotid artery, at the rate of 25 mg every 5 seconds, the dose required is usually 75–150 mg. A falling away of the contralateral hand signals onset of hemiparesis and anaesthesia of the hemisphere. Test materials are presented and recognition and naming ability tested during the period of unilateral suppression of cerebral function, which usually lasts only 2–5 minutes. Recall of the material is assessed 10 minutes after full recovery. Ideally the investigation should demonstrate preservation of speech and memory function during anaesthesia of the hemisphere on which it is proposed to operate, and abolition of these functions when the contralateral hemisphere is anaesthetized. Often some function is preserved when either side is anaesthetized, suggesting incomplete lateralization.

This classical intracarotid sodium amytal test, in which each hemisphere is anaesthetized separately by injection through the appropriate internal carotid artery, presents certain theoretical difficulties, although it has proved a useful way of examining cerebral speech dominance and lateralization of memory in many units carrying out presurgical evaluation, each of which has a slightly different way of performing the classical test. The injected drug does not recessarily reach all the hippocampal structures since some of them are supplied by the posterior cerebral circulation and this may vary from one individual to the next. Furthermore the gross hemispheric dysfunction which occurs with the injection makes memory testing and its interpretation difficult on occasions. Two variants of the test are currently described which aim to restrict the effects of the sodium amytal to the hippocampal structures. In one the anterior choroidal artery is injected, or the injection is prevented from going into the remainder of the internal carotid circulation (Wieser et al 1989). In the other the posterior cerebral artery is cannulated and only the posterior choroidal artery is injected (Jack et al 1988). Both of these methods require very expert neuroradiological facilities and carry more risk than the classical internal carotid injection. None of the three methods achieve the ideal situation which would anaesthetize the whole of the hippocampus by selectively injecting the anterior and posterior choroidal arteries simultaneously. Even with the classical method of examining memory function it is clear that in patients with temporal lobe disease there may be complex arrangements. Thus in a group of 27 patients, 16 of whom subsequently underwent 'en bloc' temporal lobectomy, only 11% appeared to have substantial memory function in both hemispheres (Powell et al 1987). In 44% all the memory appeared to be in the hemisphere opposite to a known lesion, a further 7% showed only minimal memory in the lesioned hemisphere; however in 22% neither hemisphere alone was able to sustain normal memory suggest-

ing bilateral damage and in 15% most memory seemed to be in the lesioned hemisphere.

We have already noted that epileptic discharges may interfere with cognitive function. It has been shown by Aarts et al (1984) that focal epileptic discharges could cause focal cognitive impairment so that left-sided discharges tended to interfere more with verbal tasks relative to spatial tasks, and the converse for right-sided discharges. Wieser and Landis (Wieser et al 1985a) have described a patient in whom there were anomalies of verbal processing during active discharges seen from depth electrodes in the left temporal lobe which resolved after left amygdalo-hippocampectomy. Regard et al (1985) describe a patient in whom discharges were accompanied by enhanced function of the contralateral hemisphere.

The available neuroradiological tests, including functional brain imaging, have already been described. The important part played by clinical neurophysiological investigation has also been described in detail.

Surgical techniques

A diversity of operations on the temporal lobe have been described. Historically temporal lobe surgery has proceeded from superficial gyrectomies and topectomies, through more extensive removals to include the deep structures and the use of the 'en bloc' technique to preserve the pathology, and in the last few years to the use of a number of techniques which improve the results of operation by improving seizure control and minimizing morbidity.

Currently there are three options for temporal lobe resection; neocortical removal with preservation of the deep structures, removal of both neocortical and deep structures, and removal of the deep structures alone or virtually so as in selective amygdalo-hippocampectomy.

Neocortical removal only. This is currently practised by only a minority of surgeons. The earliest operations, based upon corticographic findings, were of this nature. The first case operated upon by Bailey was a success (Bailey 1954) but this was not consistent and later it was seen that seizure relief was poor (Bailey 1961). This technique was revived by Coughlan and co-workers in Dublin who used a standard block removal of temporal neocortex (Coughlan et al 1987).

Removal of neocortical and deep structures. This is the conventional temporal lobectomy. It is the most frequently reported procedure and is subject to variation and modification in various centres. In most centres the surgeon removes, in an adult, between 4.5 cm and 6.5 cm of temporal neocortex as measured from the pole. In many centres the extent of this resection may be determined by the findings at acute electrocorticography. An equivalent portion, usually 2–3 cm of hippocampus and a variable amount of the amygdala is removed either 'en bloc' (Falconer 1971) or separately. In addition the dominant and non-dominant resections are dealt with in different ways by different operators, a good description is given by Olivier (1987). It is appropriate at this point to discuss the use of the techniques of acute electrocorticography, and local anaesthesia in these resections.

The anatomical boundaries of temporal lobectomy are set in order to minimize the neurological complications of the procedure, and although sometimes the findings on electrocorticography will enable one to spare a small amount of tissue, quite often these boundaries may dictate the sparing of tissue which seems to be electrically abnormal so that it is not always possible in this region to remove the 'zone épileptogénique' completely. In our practice, where it has been customary to use corticography routinely, we have seldom found reasons for removing less temporal lobe until recently when we have performed corticography in patients where we were concerned to make a decision between lobectomy and amygdalo-hippocampectomy. Therefore, if because within the anatomical limits of the classical lobectomy there seldom seems to be any advantage in sparing tissue, then perhaps it is not essential to carry out cortical recording, although in our view it has prognostic value (McBride et al 1991). Except in the circumstance mentioned below there does not seem to be much advantage in the use of local anaesthesia in these temporal lobe resections either. Although it may be possible in the left, dominant, temporal lobe to map out speech areas under local anaesthesia, there is no reliable comparison of operations carried out under these conditions, which aim to minimize speech deficit and maximize the size of the resection, with anatomically determined operations carried out under general anaesthesia.

There are two important variations in gross temporal lobectomy. The first attempts to overcome the verbal memory deficit which may follow left temporal lobectomy. The neocortical removal is restricted to preserve the relevant verbal memory area after mapping it under local anaesthesia (Ojemann & Dodrill 1985). The deep structures are also removed. Unfortunately the effect of the restriction of the neocortical removal on the relief of epilepsy is not known.

The second variation has been introduced because with some pathologies, especially hippocampal sclerosis, the extent of hippocampal involvement may vary. Where the pathology extends to the posterior margin of the hippocampal resection the outcome of surgery may be poor (Babb & Jann-Brown 1987). In those patients where chronic depth recordings have shown spikes in the mid-posterior hippocampus the Yale group have restricted the neocortical removal to 4.5 cm from the pole. Having thus gained access to the temporal horn the hippocampal removal is extended with good results and no extra complications (Spencer et al 1984b).

Removal of deep structures alone. Niermeyer (1958) described a transventricular approach to enable removal of the deep structures alone. This selective amygdalo-hippocampectomy has been revived more recently. The indications suggested by the Zurich group are that a unilateral mediobasal electrical focus can be demonstrated by foreman ovale telemetry, or by chronic SEEG studies, or that there is a structural lesion in or adjacent to the hippocampus or amygdala (Wieser 1990). Another indication, suggested by Olivier (1987), is the presence of significant memory on the side of operation.

There are two methods of performing this operation. Yasargil (Yasargil et al 1985) describes a microsurgical approach through the insular cortex after splitting the Sylvian fissure and this is more difficult than that described by Olivier where a similar removal is made through an incision in the middle temporal gyrus about 1.5 cm from the temporal pole. Both techniques require experience in the use of the operating microscope, but at a recent international meeting on the surgical treatment of epilepsy a number of authors presented results using the latter approach, suggesting that it is becoming widely adopted. Wieser has recently suggested that in his material the efficacy of the operation may be related to the completeness of the removal of the parahippocampal gyrus.

Kelly (1987) has described an approach through the occipital region to the diseased hippocampus using a sophisticated method of stereotactic microsurgery, but this has been abandoned because of difficulties with visual field changes. However the same method of microscopic stereotactic resection can be applied through the midtemporal approach used for selective amygdalo-hippocampectomy.

Results of temporal lobe resections

As we have already observed neocortical resections alone are uncommon and the only substantial modern series is reported from Dublin. In the original report (Coughlan et al 1987), among 24 patients followed for at least 2 years after operation 54% are fit-free and 33% improved. A more recent report on 50 patients followed up between 3 and 15 years notes that the best predictors of a good outcome in this series was a clear unilateral interictal mid-anterior temporal focus, a stereotyped onset for the seizures and a greater volume of tissue removed at operation. Sixty-two percent of these patients were in Engel's groups I and II, and it was felt that the method had reasonable results in a highly selected population where limited resources were available. Morbidity and mortality were similar to those of other temporal lobe resections.

As far as conventional temporal lobectomy is concerned there is a vast literature indicating that seizure control is improved by these operations. The position up to 1973 was summarized by Jensen (1975a). Reports of 2282 cases of anterior temporal lobectomy from the literature were analysed and 885 cases had been adequately investigated and followed, the majority of these were from the Montreal Neurological Institute. Overall 43.6% of these patients were free of seizures (range 29–62%) and the unimproved

patients, those with less than a 75% reduction in their seizure frequency, averaged 33.8% (range 14–58%). Where several consecutive series were quoted from the same centre there was always an improvement in the seizure relief in the later series. Engel (1987) analysed data provided by participants in an international symposium on the surgical treatment of epilepsy. He classified 'seizure-free' as meaning having a period of at least 2 years free of seizures, with or without auras. There were 2336 lobectomies, reported from 40 centres, and 55.5% of the patients were fit-free (range 26–80%) and 16.8% (range 6–29%) were unimproved. Perhaps these results are not surprising in view of the diverse methods of selection and the periods of time over which these patients were treated. The variation could be attributed to differences in the population presented to each surgeon and in the pathology in the resected specimens. The improvements in neurophysiological assessment and brain imaging must be responsible for some of the improvement seen when compared with Jensen's figures.

The most plentiful data about the durability of resective surgery relates to temporal lobe resections. It is the common experience that the longer the patients are followed-up after operation the fewer remain absolutely fit-free. Whether this represents a total failure of the operative treatment is a matter of philosophy. Patients who obtain significant relief from operation, say a greater than 75% reduction in their seizure frequency, seldom relapse to their preoperative seizure frequency. Among 90 consecutive lobectomies at the Maudsley Hospital only one patient reverted to the preoperative seizure frequency after a substantial period of relief. Fits can recur after a seizure-free period of many years. Thirteen patients among these 90 had recurrent seizures after periods of freedom ranging from 2 years to 10 years. In 11 patients the fits were generalized seizures which in six of them were completely abolished by a restitution of one antiepileptic drug. In this group of 90 patients there were 16% who failed to benefit from the operation and this was clear by the end of the first postoperative year.

Awad recently described the experience at the Cleveland Clinic in patients undergoing all kinds of resective surgery. He noted that only 14% of recurrences of seizures occurred more than 1 year after operation and that 85% of patients having one or more seizures after surgery continued to do so as long as 6 years after operation. Half of those having one fit per month after operation continued at this rate if it persisted for 1 year. In the 23 cases who were re-investigated, there were no cases of mislateralization, prior mislocalization was suspected in six patients and proven in three. Fifteen patients were re-operated and 58% became seizure free. On the same occasion Rasmussen described the results of re-operation in 115 patients with freedom from seizures in 25%. A report from the Georgia group at the same conference described the effects of antiepileptic drug withdrawal after surgery. They described 104 patients of whom 52 were seizure-free following surgery. Drugs were withdrawn in 39 of the seizure-free patients and 77% remained seizure free at 1 year after withdrawal, 72% at 2 years and 66% at 3 years. The majority of the recurrent seizures occurred in the first year after withdrawal.

In Van Buren's series of patients undergoing temporal lobectomy, if a patient had remained seizure-free for 5 years their chance of relapsing thereafter was about 10% (Van Buren et al 1975). Similar data is available for 106 patients undergoing temporal lobectomy at UCLA (Engel 1987). They note, as we have, that in any particular year after operation, say the third year, up to 40% of patients may be fit-free but that these are not the same patients who will constitute the 40% who are fit-free the following or previous year. This has to be partly an artificial effect of grouping patients together and could perhaps be overcome by using actuarial methods of analysis, as described by Elwes and colleagues (Elwes et al 1991).

The perioperative mortality from temporal lobe resection is low. In Jensen's review (Jensen 1975a) the overall mortality was 1%, it has now fallen to 0.39% (Van Buren 1987) with no mortality in more recent series. The late mortality is another matter. Taylor & Marsh (1977) looked at the deaths in Falconer's series. There were 37 deaths in 193 patients who were followed for at least 5 years. Twenty-three of these deaths occurred in circumstances which might be related to either epilepsy or suicide. The suicides tended to occur a decade earlier than the expected peak for suicide and half the patients who died by suicide were fit-free. In the more recent series of 150 consecutive temporal lobectomies from the Maudsley hospital there have been six late deaths, two committed suicide, three died in seizures and one in a road traffic accident. Jensen found a late mortality of 4.76%, two-thirds of whom died of suicide or in an epileptic attack (Jensen 1975b). Although the death rate in these patients (47.6/1000) is in excess of that expected for a similar Danish population (2.9/1000) it is better than that quoted for a representative group of Danish patients (59.4/1000) (Brink-Hendriksen et al 1970).

The morbidity is equally low. Jensen (1975a) gives a rate of 1% for permanent hemiparesis and the more recent figures (Van Buren 1987) are about the same. It seems more likely with 'en bloc' resections. Other hazards such as a transient third nerve palsy and a complete homonymous hemianopia are equally rare. In all series the majority of patients have an upper quadrantanopia, usually not complete. Focal fits in the immediate postoperative period are also uncommon and have no influence on the eventual outcome of operation.

The intellectual sequelae of temporal lobectomy are complex and important. They depend upon the pathology in the resected temporal lobe and the age of onset of the illness. Blakemore & Falconer (1967) described an auditory learning deficit after dominant temporal lobectomy and other workers also began to describe material specific deficits. The early work on this topic has been well reviewed by Milner (1975). A study of the Maudsley series (Powell et al 1985) has shown that changes in cognitive function across the operation are small. Whereas the intellectually more able and older patients, whose epilepsy tends to be of later onset, acquire material-specific deficits; the opposite group, in whom the pathology tends to be medial temporal sclerosis, do not. This is thought to be because the insult to the brain occurs at an age when there is still some ability to reorganize cognitive function. Recently the group at the Cleveland Clinic, using a quantitative measurement of the extent of resection by MRI, has described a correlation between the extent of medial temporal removal and verbal learning on the left side, and visuo-spatial learning on the right side (Katz et al 1989). Improvement in cognitive function after operation is also related to improvement in seizure control (Novelly et al 1984). Lieb and his colleagues have shown that cognitive outcome parallels seizure control and that those factors which are predictors of poor outcome with regard to seizure control are also predictors of a poor cognitive outcome (Lieb et al 1982). Behavioural changes after temporal lobectomy are well documented and fall into two groups.

The first consists of those patients with uncontrolled partial seizures who have an aggressive behaviour disorder, the proportion varies from series to series. In Falconer's series few of the patients were of normal personality and behaviour and only 13% were normal before operation but 32% were normal afterwards (Taylor & Falconer 1968). In another review of 100 patients there were 17 who had troublesome aggressive behaviour before operation, 10 of whom improved (Falconer 1973). Jensen (1976) reports 74 patients who were socially disadvantaged prior to operation but 39% were in full-time employment afterwards. The effects of uncontrolled epilepsy on the behaviour and development of children and the beneficial results of surgery have been reviewed in a careful longitudinal study by the Oxford group (Ounstead et al 1987).

The second group consists of patients who either have a recognizable psychosis before operation or acquire one afterwards. Psychosis supervening upon chronic epilepsy, usually a schizophreniform psychosis, occurs late in the illness. Serafetidines & Falconer (1962) described 12 such patients in none of whom temporal lobectomy had any effect on the psychosis. The same findings were reported by Jensen & Larsen (1979).

Operation can also produce psychoses, both a schizophreniform psychosis usually associated with left-sided lobectomy, and a depressive psychosis usually associated with right-sided lobectomy. Jensen & Larsen (1979) report the development of psychosis in 12% of their patients and Taylor (1975) the appearance of a schizophreniform psychosis in 15% of Falconer's series. He also noted that this was more likely to be associated with 'alien tissue' pathology. Stevens (1990) has recently described the psychiatric outcome in a small sample of 14 patients followed up for between 20 years and 30 years after an anterior temporal lobectomy. Among these patients there were four in whom psychiatric problems worsened and another two who developed psychosis de novo. Two patients actually achieved an improvement in their psychiatric state and in the remaining six there was no psychiatric problem before or after operation. She notes that psychiatric problems were likely either to appear or worsen in patients where the epilepsy was of late onset, had unreality or déjà vu as auras, had pre-existing brain damage or persisting clinical or electrical seizure activity. Both Jensen & Larsen (1979) and Taylor (1975) report depressive psychoses which may be resistant to treatment and lead to suicide. In our own material we have found that schizophreniform psychoses are much rarer, there have only been six in over 150 operations. One of these was transient and one occurred 12 years after the lobectomy in a previously well patient. Finally only one followed a left-sided lobectomy, but the pathology was not 'alien tissue' and we do not have the same findings with regard to 'alien tissue' as Taylor. The discrepancy may well be due to the different population in our later series where the proportion of referrals from psychiatric sources is much lower. By contrast the occurrence of depression after right-sided lobectomy is much higher, around 35% on an informal survey, but only one suicide. All of these aspects have been reviewed in detail by Taylor (1987).

The results from selective amygdalo-hippocampectomy are equally impressive. Wieser (1986) reports 80% seizure relief. This is a reflection of the high proportion of patients with benign tumours in their series and in patients with mesial temporal sclerosis the seizure relief rate is 61%, which is similar to that achieved with 'en bloc' lobectomy. Similar results have been reported by other authors. Kruse-Larsen and colleagues report that the seizures were abolished in 65% of their group although 20% underwent re-operation which was not successful (Kruse-Larsen et al 1990). Another substantial series has been reported by Renella (1989). They report a recurrence of seizures in 16 of 41 patients operated upon, but not all operations were amygdalohippocampectomies as described by Yasargil and in 13 of these 16 patients there was evidence of further extension of the tumour in the original specimen. Awad and his colleagues have reported an analysis of the results of temporal lobe resections in 45 patients using MRI scanning and an anatomical compartmental model to measure the extent of the resection. They have shown that in mediobasal-limbic epilepsy the freedom from seizures could be related to the extent of the resection of the amygdalo-hippocampal complex (Awad et al 1989).

The Zurich series is virtually free of morbidity. As noted by Renella (1989) this relates to immaculate microsurgical technique, especially in the trans-Sylvian approach and therefore morbidity may be greater in less skilled hands, but it is to be expected that the morbidity with practice will be similar to that for formal lobectomy. These patients do not have the quadrantanopia which is inevitable with lobectomy.

The intellectual consequences of the operation seem much less than those of formal lobectomy, even in cases with more risk of amnesia. Wieser 1990, analysing in detail the effects on cognitive function in 17 patients, found only one to have deteriorated and we have had the same experience in a series of 19 patients. Wieser describes a beneficial effect on patients whose epilepsy is relieved and we have had the same experience. However he also reports patients in whom the epilepsy was not relieved and their cognitive performance deteriorated, and we have had the same experience.

The pathology in the specimens from temporal lobe resections determine the outcome, to some extent independently of the operative procedure. In both 'en bloc' resection and selective amygdalo-hippocampectomy benign lesions such as indolent tumours have an 80% seizure relief rate, MTS about 60% and nonspecific pathology about 15%.

The choice of which resective procedure to use in any particular patient with temporal lobe focus is one of the interesting challenges in modern resective surgery. It is difficult to give guidance about when each of these procedures should be employed. In some centres one is used to the exclusion of others, although most major centres have now adopted selective amygdalo-hippocampectomy by one route or another.

Our own practice is to try to use the procedure which is most likely to produce the greatest relief of seizures with minimal loss of normal function. Of course the first consideration must be the demonstrated pathology and clearly the resection must encompass this as far as is possible. The next consideration must be the intellectual performance of the involved temporal lobe. If it can be shown that it makes little or no contribution to cognitive function then either a full temporal lobectomy is performed or the decision is made on the findings at intraoperative corticography. If, on the other hand, there is evidence that cognitive function will be compromised then amygdalo-hippocampectomy may be the only choice whatever the corticographic findings. We have noted, in a small series, a particular corticographic pattern associated with mesial temporal sclerosis in patients undergoing amygdalo-hippocampectomy (Polkey et al 1989). These considerations have led to a change in the way in which patients with temporal lobe pathology are dealt with. Table

Table 16.3 Laterality and pathology in 78 temporal lobe resections over a 3-year period

Temporal lobe resection		Pathology			Total
		MTS	Other	Non-specific	
'En bloc' lobectomy	Left	12	12	2	26
	Right	3	8	9	20
	Total	15	20	11	46
Amygdalo-hippocampectomy	Left	16	1	4	21
	Right	9	1	1	11
	Total	25	2	5	32

16.3 summarizes the laterality and pathology in 78 temporal lobe resections over a 3-year period. As might be expected from the foregoing discussion it will be seen that among patients selected for amygdalo-hippocampectomy there are a higher proportion with mesial temporal sclerosis than with other pathologies and that there are more left-sided amygdalo-hippocampectomies than right-sided.

Frontal lobe resections

Cortical resection from a frontal lobe is the commonest procedure after temporal lobe resections. In many cases there is a discrete pathology within the frontal lobe and modern methods of brain imaging have made the detection of cortical dysplasia and benign tumours much easier. Although there are a number of well recognized patterns for seizures originating in the frontal lobe as described by Penfield & Jasper (1954), nevertheless the recognition of frontal lobe seizures may be difficult and they can take bizarre forms (Williamson et al 1985a). The neurophysiological investigation of these patients can be difficult. Some authors recommend the use of invasive subdural and depth electrodes in all these patients. Depth electrode studies have shown that the adversive movements of the head and eyes are a poor lateralizing feature (Robillard et al 1983). When the causative lesion lies on the medial side of the hemisphere ictal changes in the scalp EEG may be absent, bilateral or contralateral to the lesion.

The range of pathology encountered in frontal lobe resections is different from that seen in temporal lobes. Rasmussen (1975a) reporting 346 frontal resections over 45 years notes that 97 (28%) had tumours, five (1.4%) arteriovenous malformations, and 167 (48%) scarring, often caused by head trauma. In our own smaller series the distribution of pathology is somewhat different and this may reflect advances in brain imaging. When there is a clear abnormality in the frontal region the size and position of the resection can be guided by that abnormality with corticographic control. The resection may be limited by corticographic findings or by the practical size of a frontal lobe resection which should leave one gyrus anterior to the pre-central gyrus, and respect Broca's area in the dominant hemisphere.

The results of frontal resection in respect of seizure control are somewhat less satisfactory than those of temporal lobe resections. The largest series from the Montreal Neurological Institute reports 212 patients followed for 2–39 years. There were 22 patients (10%) who had been absolutely seizure-free and a total of 76 patients had suffered less than one seizure per year of follow-up (36%), with a further 42 patients experiencing a significant reduction of seizures, so that a total of 118 patients (55%) had benefited from the surgery. There has been no mortality in the last 160 operations and no morbidity. There are minor intellectual sequelae to frontal lobe resections.

Cortical resections from other areas

The number of patients submitted to surgery in the centroparietal regions is low because this is an eloquent area, and in the occipital cortex because it is rarely affected by focal epilepsy. The focal motor and focal sensory seizures which emanate from the central and parietal areas are easy to identify. Occipital seizures may begin with visual auras. Again the Montreal Neurological Institute has the only substantial series of resections from the centroparietal and occipital regions. Goldring (1987) reported cortical resections from the central areas after assessment of the seizure origin and identification of motor and sensory cortex using epidural mat electrodes. Surgery was offered to 40 of the 58 patients investigated by this means—42% were rendered seizure-free and a further 20% were improved with a mean follow-up of 5.4 years. There was no significant morbidity. In a number of these cases unsuspected indolent gliomas were found. Rasmussen (1975b) reports 68 patients undergoing central resections in 40 years. Eighteen percent were rendered absolutely fit-free, 45% were down to less than one fit per year of follow-up and overall 59% were improved significantly. In parietal resections, of which there were 132 cases, the results were almost identical. In Rasmussen's material 266 patients underwent central or parietal resections, 103 patients had tumours (38.7%) and 110 (41.3%) some other pathology leaving 45 (16.9%) with no specific pathology. Rasmussen describes 23 patients undergoing occipital resections and notes that 68% achieved a significant reduction in their epilepsy.

Resection in these areas has to be tailored, often by operation under local anaesthesia, to avoid worsening a pre-existing deficit or introducing one. In children Goldring, using his epidural mat electrodes, has managed to identify motor areas during chronic recording and by careful transfer of the position of the electrodes at subsequent operation to be aware of their position (Goldring & Gregorie 1984). In occipital operations there may be a high risk of producing a homonymous hemianopia.

Major resections

Where there is a large area of damaged or diseased brain it may still be possible to resect to one-third or half of the hemisphere, operations classified as multi-lobe resections, but the surgery and its complications are similar to those experienced with more restricted operations. However, sometimes the damage or disease process is so widespread that resection of 80% or more of the hemisphere is needed. This major procedure, known as hemispherectomy, was first described by Krynauw (1950).

The indications for hemispherectomy are varied according to the pathology involved. However certain broad indications can be stated. There must be a pathological process which can be shown on brain imaging to be confined to one hemisphere, or to be largely affecting one hemisphere, or to be known by its natural history to be usually confined to one hemisphere. The patient must have chronic drug-resistant epilepsy, which usually includes focal seizures and often epilepsia partialis continua. The patient should

have an established hemiplegia, usually of the infantile type, or because of the effect of the seizures an effective hemiplegia. In some patients with Rasmussen's disease, or hemimegalencephaly, there may not be a pre-existing homonymous hemianopia and this may be the penalty to be paid for the control of seizures. These indications are summarized in the accompanying diagram.

Applied to patients with an infantile hemiplegia and drug-resistant seizures, who often had a behaviour disorder and were dementing, it was very successful with between 70% and 80% of the patients becoming seizure-free with improvement in the behaviour. This was soon confirmed by others (Wilson 1970). Within 10 years or so it became clear from numerous reports (Falconer & Wilson 1969) that there was a serious morbidity and mortality in between one-third and one-quarter of patients from late complications associated with chronic or delayed bleeding. In Montreal it was noticed that such complications occurred in 35% of patients undergoing anatomically complete hemispherectomy but was virtually absent after lesser resections. They therefore modified their practice twice. Between 1968 and 1974 they carried out only subtotal hemispherectomies, sparing the least epileptogenic area, usually either the frontal or occipital pole. This reduced the late complications but also reduced the seizure relief so that whereas 80% of patients were virtually fit-free after complete hemispherectomy only 69% were so relieved by subtotal hemispherectomy. Since 1974 they have carried out a functionally complete hemispherectomy in which the central and temporal areas including the deep temporal structures are removed and the corpus callosum divided in the frontal and parietal regions. They have 80% of the patients seizure-free and only one late delayed complication in 14 cases followed for between 2 and 10 years (Rasmussen 1987).

Adams (1983) modified the classical hemispherectomy technique to avoid the late complications. This modification consists of preserving the septum pellucidum and blocking the foramen of Monro with a plug of muscle to separate the main CSF space from the remainder, sewing the dural flap down around the falx and tentorial hiatus to create a large extradural space, and

---

CRITERIA FOR HEMISPHERECTOMY

1. Long-standing unilateral hemispheric damage evidenced by hemiplegia, and brain imaging changes

2. Partial seizures, whether or not secondarily generalized, arising from the diseased hemisphere

Diagram 10

ensuring meticulous haemostasis to reduce the amount of blood present which might cause fibrosis and blockage of CSF pathways. Occasionally hydrocephalus of the remaining ventricle occurs, usually soon after the operation, and needs a shunt. A recent report describes 10 patients operated upon using this technique (Beardsworth & Adams 1988). There was total seizure relief in 70% of these patients with improvement of behaviour and of intellectual function in some, similar to the results reported for classical hemispherectomy (Wilson 1970).

At the present time the surgeon is presented with three different methods of hemispherectomy. There are some who still use the classical Krynauw technique, relying upon acute drainage of the cavity which remains in communication with the CSF space, often followed by a permanent shunt. Other surgeons use the current Montreal technique of a functionally complete hemispherectomy whereas others use the technique described by Adams. At present there is no way of recommending one method over the others although the classical technique is the least popular.

It should also be noted that the kind of pathology for which hemispherectomy is used is changing. In the 50 hemispherectomies performed by McKissock between 1949 and 1964 and later reported by Wilson (1970), 54% of the patients had suffered perinatal trauma or hypoxia, and a further 30% an acute febrile illness followed by hemiatrophy. However in our own series of 23 hemispherectomies performed between 1978 and 1990 there were only five patients who had cerebral atrophy secondary to an acute infection or vascular accident. The remaining 16 patients were more difficult both to assess and to operate upon. In cases of hemimegalencephaly or other cortical migrational disorders the results of operation in relation to seizure control are excellent but the complication rate in our hands has been higher. There continues to be a controversy about the treatment of Sturge–Weber disease by surgical means. Some of these patients have benefited from hemispherectomy, as described and discussed by Hoffmann and his colleagues (Hoffman et al 1979). However it was suggested by some that early excision of the lesions perhaps before they had come to involve the whole hemisphere would prevent subsequent spread of the disease.

Finally mention should be made at this point of the clinically distinct, but ill-understood disease process know as Rasmussen's disease. This has been described in a variety of papers from Montreal by Rasmussen and colleagues between 1957 and 1987 (Rasmussen et al 1958, Rasmussen 1978, 1987). Rasmussen has recently described his experience at the Cleveland Symposium and our own corresponds with theirs. He has now collected a total of 52 cases over 35 years, comprising 1–2% of the Montreal material. There were four key elements. Firstly it was essentially a disease of childhood, only one of the 51 patients had an onset of symptoms after 14 years of age. As well as the intractable epilepsy, usually involving focal motor seizures in the appropriate limbs, he noted that there was a progressive neurological deterioration comprising hemiparesis, retardation and speech difficulty, and in half the patients this picture appeared within 1 year of the onset of the epilepsy. The radiological picture was one of atrophy. Finally, as already described, the pathological picture was of 'encephalitis'.

The median age of seizure onset was 5 years, in 86% it was less than 10 years of age. In 20% there had been focal motor status, 50% had epilepsia partialis continua and in 30% the initial event was a generalized tonic-clonic seizure. The disease itself was rarely fatal, only one patient died of the disease itself, although five patients died of status epilepticus and three from postoperative haemosiderosis. Although 90% of patients were intellectually normal before onset only 15% remained so after the disease had stabilized.

It about half the patients their CSF was normal and in the other half there were non-specific changes. Rasmussen reported that in his patients the EEG was at first bilaterally abnormal but subsequently became lateralized. Atrophy could be seen in some patients as soon as 2–3 months after the onset of the disease. We have encountered a patient with a normal CT and a suggestion of swelling on an MRI. It is reported that in some cases there are areas of hypoperfusion on PET scanning.

There have been some attempts to treat the disease with steroids and immunosuppressive drugs. It is possible that the finding of material from cytomegalic virus by Power et al (1990), may result in a trial of antiviral agents in these patients. But at present the only reliable method of treatment is hemispherectomy. Rasmussen has shown consistently that lesser resections are ineffective. Among his patients 21 of the 51 had undergone hemispherectomy, 10 as the only or initial operation. Of these 21 patients 11 were seizure-free, five had less than two attacks per year and four of the remaining six obtained some improvement.

Lesional surgery

Finally it should be mentioned that there are some circumstances in which removal of the lesion alone may be sufficient. This kind of lesional surgery is becoming more widespread and tends to come into the repertoire of the general neurosurgeon because it demands few sophisticated investigations, apart from brain imaging which is becoming easily available in most neuroscience centres. In these patients the lesions are usually either hamartoma or low grade tumours, which are easy targets to resect and have a very high success rate anyway. The application of microsurgical techniques to these lesions by Kelly has been very successful (Cascino et al 1990).

FUNCTIONAL SURGERY

This is less widely practised than resective surgery. There are a number of options but they depend upon three principles which are: firstly to attempt to ablate a focus, usually by making lesions in the appropriate part of the brain using stereotactic techniques to reach the target: secondly to prevent the spread of the epileptic discharge by dividing neuronal connections; and lastly brain stimulation.

Stereotactic lesions

The application of the techniques of stereotactic neurosurgery to the treatment of epilepsy is superficially attractive. The basis of such surgery is well known from its application to the treatment of movement disorders and to a lesser extent psychiatric illness. The original method developed by Horsley & Clarke 1908, for experimental purposes,

was subsequently adapted by others for use in the human brain. In essence, if an accurate map can be made of the brain in three axes with reference to fixed points, then a needle inserted through a small drill hole in the skull can be guided under X-ray control, using coordinates from the fixed points in three planes to any particular structure known as the target. Modern brain imaging with CT and MRI, to which the stereotactic method can be adapted, has made the identification of targets easier and more certain because of the detailed way in which these methods demonstrate brain anatomy, and also allow subsequent verification of the target which was impossible with previous methods. It is therefore theoretically possible to place electrodes for SEEG recording as previously described and with the information so gained to determine sites for functional surgery.

Stereotactic lesions in subcortical structures

These procedures have a long history. Pallidal lesions to control seizures were reported by Spiegel as early as 1958 (Spiegel et al 1958). Subsequently various subcortical targets were used including the fields of Forel, thalamus and globus pallidus. These methods were used to treat the more difficult cases, usually with multiple targets and in small numbers, and tended to control rather than cure the fits. Most reviewers feel that they are of limited value (Ojemann & Ward 1975, Flanigin et al 1985, Spencer 1987). It is possible that the improvements in brain imaging will improve the efficacy of these techniques using subcortical lesions.

Stereotactic lesions in temporal lobe structures

Lesions in the temporal structures have been more rewarding possibly because the patient population is more uniform and it is also easier to compare with resective surgery. Narabayashi et al (1963) noted that in patients where he was using amygdala lesions to treat aggression if they also had resistant epilepsy then both tended to respond to the lesion. He described improvement both in children (Narabayashi & Shima 1973) and in adults (Narabayashi 1979, with improvement in both behaviour and seizure control in about half of these patients. It was noted by Mundinger that the best results were seen in patients with unilateral foci (Mundinger et al 1976). Describing 33 patients they noted that treatment of unilateral foci was twice as successful as that of bilateral foci. The Paris group noted that only 23% of 44 patients were rendered fit-free by stereotactic lesions. They felt that this method of treatment was less successful than open surgery and were anxious about the possibility of memory difficulties in patients with bilateral disease having encountered such problems in three of their patients (Talairach et al 1974). The Zurich group have reported a single unique case in which seizures were shown by SEEG to begin in one amygdala and abolished by stereotactic amygdalotomy (Hood et al 1983).

The result of 45 amygdalotomies reported by the Danish group (Vaernet 1972) is of particular interest. Both bilateral amygdalotomies, which were performed in 18 patients, and unilateral amygdalotomies, which were performed in 27 patients, rendered 18% of these patients fit-free. Eight of the 12 patients who did badly with unilateral amygdalotomies subsequently underwent unilateral temporal lobectomy with a good result. How can one summarize this work? It is clear that both the selection procedures used, and the multiplicity of lesions produced makes it difficult to compare the results of the various groups. The kind of patients treated by Vaernet are clearly very different from those treated by Narabayashi. However it seems that as the selection criteria for amygdalectomy approach those for temporal lobe resection the results of stereotactic intervention improve, but it is possible that some patients who do not fulfil the strict criteria for open surgery could benefit from these procedures.

It should be mentioned that the method of producing the stereotactic lesion does not seem to matter so long as it produces discrete, accurately delineated and reproducible tissue destruction. It has been suggested in recent years that if an epileptic focus could be accurately defined it could be destroyed by stereotactically directed radiotherapy. The advocates of this approach make no mention of the type of lesion produced by radiotherapy. There has been a recent, unconvincing, anecdotal account of one patient with a unilateral temporal focus treated by this means.

Disconnection procedures

Section of the corpus callosum

This operation was first introduced in 1940 (Van Wagenen & Herren 1940). It fell into disrepute mostly because of the undesirable neuropsychological sequelae until it was shown subsequently that these could be ameliorated if the splenium was spared (Gordon et al 1971). At the same time it was used for patients with unilateral cerebral disease (Luessenhop et al 1970). The Dartmouth group described a microsurgical technique which gave better results with fewer complications (Wilson et al 1982).

The scientific basis for callosal section is not simple. It was originally proposed as a means of preventing secondary generalization of seizures by propagation of discharges between the hemispheres. Morrell has investigated these matters with appropriate animal models over many years and summarized his findings in 1985 (Morrell 1985). He shows that although the corpus callosum is essential to secondary epileptogenesis, it is not the sole factor, and that suitably isolated slabs of cortex will not provoke secondary epileptogenesis even though their trans-callosal connections with the opposite hemisphere are intact. Furthermore he also demonstrates that axonal conduction and protein synthesis may also play an important part in secondary epileptogenesis. Other authors have also shown that in experimental animals complete division of the corpus callosum is difficult, and that even when it is virtually complete interhemispheric connections can still be demonstrated.

The current indications for the use of callosotomy are complex and empirical and are summarized in the accompanying diagram.

CRITERIA FOR CALLOSOTOMY

1. Generalized seizures, particularly atonic or tonic-clonic seizures, resulting in injury and arising in the context of partial or symptomatic generalized epilepsy.

2. This may be a preferred solution in patients with unilateral hemisphere disease, not severe enough for hemispherectomy.

3. Associated partial seizures, if any are not amenable to resective surgery.

Diagram 11

Certain points emerge, first there is some but not complete desynchronization of the EEG after callosotomy. This can be seen at acute corticography during the operation and perhaps can be used to determine when the section is sufficient (Marino 1985). A complete section is more effective than a partial section and carries perhaps less risks of complications if carried out in stages at least 2 months apart. Patients with known unilateral cerebral pathology do better than those without (Williamson 1985b). Akinetic seizures are most likely to be controlled and complex partial seizures are least affected by the operation and may be exacerbated. Precise figures are variable between the series but an overall reduction of 50% in seizure frequency occurs in 60% or more of patients (Spencer et al 1987b).

After anterior section there may be a period of mutism, incontinence and variable limb weakness lasting between a few days and weeks which generally recovers. The neuropsychological sequelae of anterior, posterior and complete section are demonstrable and well documented but are not necessarily of great practical significance. In some patients the emergence or exacerbation of lateralized deficits after callosotomy suggest that the corpus callosum may have been compensating for these deficits. This is especially so when the hemisphere of language dominance is not the hemisphere controlling handedness when the operation may leave permanent language deficits. This may be determined preoperatively by a carotid amytal test and patients of mixed dominance should have a carotid amytal test (Spencer et al 1987b). Some authors such as Rayport and colleagues (Ferguson et al 1985), note long-lasting effects of complete callosal section on everyday life in relation to hemisphere competition, language, and attention-memory sequencing, but report that on the whole, despite these effects, the operations were beneficial.

Temporal lobotomy

Brief mention is made of the operation of temporal lobotomy described by Turner (1963), in which the deep white matter of the temporal lobe is divided unilaterally or bilaterally. In a summary of his work, which is methodologically difficult to understand, it appears that 25–30% of patients were rendered fit-free, but some patients had lesions made in other parts of the brain (Turner 1982).

Multiple subpial transection

The operation of multiple subpial transection described by Morrell should be mentioned (Morrell et al 1989). It is based on the idea that epileptic discharges propagate tangentially through the cortex whereas the impulses controlling voluntary movement propagate radially. Thus if a series of vertical cuts are made in the motor cortex the epilepsy will be controlled and normal function unaffected. In 32 patients, there has been no practical neurological deficit although subtle changes could be detected on formal examination. In 20 patients followed for more than 5 years there has been complete seizure control in 55%. Seizures recurred in some patients with progressive pathology such as Rasmussen's disease but always away from the treated area. Morrell and his colleagues have also suggested the use of this procedure in Landan–Kleffner syndrome and report good results in the four patients that they had treated.

Brain stimulation

There are currently no effective methods of chronic brain stimulation for control of epilepsy. Cerebellar stimulation introduced by Cooper (1973) has been discredited in controlled trials (Wright et al 1985).

ECONOMICS

Estimates of the number of patients needing surgical treatment of their epilepsy are difficult to make and in all the published estimates there are areas of uncertainty. Most of this uncertainty arises from the paucity of data on the long-term outlook for epilepsy. Elwes and co-workers suggest that if newly diagnosed seizures have not been controlled within 2 years the probability of subsequent control falls by half (Elwes et al 1984). Dreifuss quotes Rayport as suggesting that there could be 800 000 persons in the USA with focal epilepsy of whom perhaps 360 000 (45%) will be poorly controlled (Dreifuss 1987). A *Lancet* editorial in 1988 suggests that in the UK there might be 2000 persons who would benefit from epilepsy surgery (Lancet 1988). There is reason to believe that this is a very gross underestimate based on the idea that 1% of partial epilepsy is refractory whereas Elwes and colleagues thought that up to 30% of partial epilepsy would be refractory to medical treatment comprising about 18% of all patients (Elwes et al 1984). A recent survey by Hart & Shorvon (1990) showed that in the UK only 147 surgical procedures for the relief of epilepsy were performed in 1 year. This kind of shortfall is duplicated throughout Europe and North America. Although there is currently a resurgence of interest in epilepsy surgery in these places this presents a problem of maintaining standards and training appropriate specialists in the multidisciplinary team required for this kind of work. In the USA attempts have been made to specify minimum standards for centres in which such treatment and training is carried out (National Association of Epilepsy Centers 1990).

In the current climate of health care in the UK the total effects of surgical treatment of epilepsy, and whether it is cost-effective or not, have become matters of importance to clinicians. The long-term effects of epilepsy surgery have already been referred to in detail in preceding parts of this chapter. A particularly important survey has recently been completed in Oslo by Løyning and colleagues (Guldvog et al 1991). They describe the fate of 201 patients undergoing resective surgery with that of 185 matched controls between 1949 and 1988. The overall conclusion was that there was a significant reduction in the frequency of seizures compared with the control group but that there was a penalty to be paid in the form of complications. Short-term complications occurred in 14.1% of the 68 operated patients below the age of 20 and some lasting neurological complications in 9% of this group. There was no difference in survival between the two groups.

It is difficult to know the precise cost-benefit of these procedures. If the operation is successful the financial benefits accrue to the budget of a different government department from the one that continues to support the patient if the operation is unsuccessful or followed by complications. In our own neurosurgical unit over a period of 2 years from 1987 to 1989 approximately 23% of the beds were used for the presurgical evaluation and surgical treatment of drug-resistant epilepsy. The average cost per admission was at least £2540, the cost of each therapeutic operation was £11 239, and the cost of a successful therapeutic operation, assuming 70% success, was £15 854. These are minimum figures because they have, for example, distributed expensive neurophysiological costs between all the patients treated in the Neurosurgical Unit. It is difficult to go beyond this point without using complex methods of analysis such as those proposed for the work of a regional neurosurgical unit by Pickard and colleagues (Pickard et al 1990).

REFERENCES

Aarts J H P, Binnie C D, Smit A M et al 1984 Selective cognitive impairment during focal and generalized EEG activity. Brain 107: 293–308

Adams C B T 1983 Hemispherectomy—a modification. Journal of Neurology, Neurosurgery and Psychiatry 46: 617–619

Adams C B T, Anslow P, Molyneux A et al 1987 Radiological detection of surgically treatable pathology. In: Engel J (ed) Surgical treatment of the epilepsies. Raven Press, New York, 213–233

Ajmone Marsan C 1973 Electrocorticography. In: Rémond A (ed) Handbook of electroencephalography and clinical neurophysiology, Vol 10 Part C. Elsevier, Amsterdam

Ajmone Marsan C 1980 Depth electrography and electrocorticography. In: Aminoff M J (ed) Electrodiagnosis in clinical neurology. Churchill Livingstone, New York, p 167–196

Ajmone Marsan C, Baldwin M 1958 Epileptiform activity in cortical and subcortical structures in the temporal lobe of man. In: Baldwin M, Bailey P (eds) Temporal lobe epilepsy. Thomas, Springfield, p 78–108

Ajmone Marsan C, Van Buren J M 1958 Epileptiform activity in cortical and subcortical structures in the temporal lobe of man. In: Baldwin M, Bailey P (eds) Temporal lobe epilepsy. Thomas, Springfield, p 78–108

Andermann F, Olivier A, Malanson D et al 1987 Epilepsy due to focal cortical dysplasia with macrogyria and the forme fruste of tuberous sclerosis: A study of 15 patients. In: Wolf P, Dam M, Janz D, Dreifuss F E (eds) Advances in epilepsy, vol 16. Raven Press, New York, p 35–38

Awad I A, Katz A, Hahn J F et al 1989 Extent of resection in temporal lobectomy for epilepsy. I. Interobserver analysis

and correlation with seizure outcome. Epilepsia
30: 756–762

Babb T L, Jann-Brown W 1987 Pathological findings in
epilepsy. In: Engel J (ed) Surgical treatment of the
epilepsies. Raven Press, New York p 511–540

Babb T L, Jann-Brown W, Pretorius J et al 1984 Temporal
lobe volumetric cell densities in temporal lobe epilepsy.
Epilepsia 25: 729–740

Bailey P 1954 Betrachtungen uber die chirugische
Behandlung der psychomotorische Epilepsie. Zeitblatt
Neurochirugie 14: 195–206

Bailey P 1961 Surgical treatment of psychomotor epilepsy.
Five year follow-up. Southern Medical Journal 5: 299–301

Bancaud J, Talairach J, Bonis A et al 1965 La
stéréoélectroencéphalographie dans l'épilepsie.
Informations neurophysiopathologiques apportées par
l'investigation fonctionelle stéréotaxique. Masson, Paris

Barkovich A J, Chuang S H 1990 Unilateral megalencephaly:
correlation of MR imaging and pathological characteristics.
America Journal of Neuroradiology 11: 523–531

Bear D M, Fedio P 1977 Quantative analysis of interictal
behaviour in temporal lobe epilepsy. Archives of Neurology
34: 454–467

Bear D M, Levin K, Blumer D et al 1982 Interictal behaviour
in hospitalized temporal lobe epileptics; relationship to
idiopathic psychiatric syndromes. Journal of Neurology,
Neurosurgery and Psychiatry 45: 481–488

Beardsworth E D, Adams C B T 1988 Modified
hemispherectomy for epilepsy: Early results in 10 cases.
British Journal of Neurosurgery 2: 73–84

Bengzon A R A, Rasmussen T, Gloor P et al 1968 Prognostic
factors in the surgical treatment of temporal lobe epileptics.
Neurology 18: 717–731

Bernier G, Richer F, Giard N et al 1990 Electrical
stimulation of the human brain in epilepsy. Epilepsia
31: 513–520

Bernoulli C, Siegfried J, Baumgartner C et al 1977 Danger of
accidental person-to-person transmission of Creutzfeldt–
Jakob disease by surgery. Lancet 1: 478–479

Binnie C D 1989 Depth electrodes in seizure mapping:
selection of patients. In: Chadwick D (ed) Fourth
International Symposium on Sodium Valproate and
Epilepsy, International Congress and Symposium Series.
Royal Society of Medicine, London, p 36–49

Binnie C D, Van der Wens P 1986 Diagnostic re-evaluation
by intensive monitoring of intractable absence seizures.
In: Schmidt D, Morselli P (eds) Intractable epilepsy:
experimental and clinical aspects. Raven Press, New York,
p 99–107

Binnie C D, Dekker E, Smit A et al 1982 Practical
considerations in the positioning of EEG electrodes.
Electroencephalography and Clinical Neurophysiology
53: 453–458

Binnie C D, Marston D, Polkey C E 1989 Distribution of
temporal spikes in relation to the sphenoidal electrode.
Electroencephalography and Clinical Neurophysiology
73: 403–409

Binnie C D, Polkey C E, Volans A 1990 Consistency of
lateralization in intracranial recordings of seizures of
temporal lobe origin. Acta Neurologica Scandinavica 133
(suppl): 20

Blakemore C B, Falconer M A 1967 Long-term effects of
anterior temporal lobectomy on certain cognitive functions.
Journal of Neurology, Neurosurgery and Psychiatry
30: 364–367

Bloom D, Jasper H, Rasmussen T 1959 Surgical therapy in
patients with temporal lobe seizures and bilateral EEG
abnormality. Epilepsia 1: 351–365

Bouchet and Cazauvieihl 1825 De l'épilepsie considerée dans
ses rapports avec l'aliénation mentale. Archives General
Medicine 9: 510–542

Brazier M A B 1973 Electrical seizure discharges within the
human brain. The problem of spread. In Brazier M A B
(ed) Epilepsy, its phenomena in man. Academic Press,
New York, p 151–170

Brink-Henriksen P, Juul-Jensen P, Lund M 1970 The
mortality of epileptics. In: Brackenridge R D C (ed) Life
Assurance Medicine. Proceedings of the 10th International
Congress of Life Assurance Medicine. Pitman, London,
p 139–148

Broseta J, Barcia-Salorio J L, Lopez-Comez L 1980 Burr-hole
electrocorticography. Acta Neurochirurgica 30 (suppl):
91–96

Cascino G D, Kelly P J, Hirschorn K A et al 1990
Stereotactic resection of intra-axial cerebral lesions in
partial epilepsy. Mayo Clinic Proceedings 65: 1053–1060

Christodoulou G 1967 Sphenoidal electrodes. Acta
Neurologica Scandinavica 43: 587–593

Cooper I 1973 Chronic stimulation of the paleo-cerebellum
in man. Lancet 1: 206

Coughlan A, Farrell M, Harriman O et al 1987 Appendix II.
Presurgical evaluation protocols. In: Engel J (ed) Surgical
treatment of the epilepsies. Raven Press, New York, p 689

Currie S, Heathfield K W G, Henson R A 1971 Clinical
course and prognosis of temporal lobe epilepsy. A survey of
666 patients. Brain 94: 173–190

Daumas-Duport C, Scheithauer B W, Chodkiewicz J et al
1988 Dysembryoplastic neuroepithelial tumor: A surgically
treatable tumor of young patients with intractable partial
seizures. Neurosurgery 23: 545–556

Delgado-Escueta A V, Walsh G O 1983 The selection
process for surgery of intractable complex partial seizures:
surface EEG and depth electrography. In: Ward A A, Penry
J K, Purpura D (eds) Epilepsy. Raven Press, New York,
p 295–326

Delgado-Escueta A V, Bascal F E, Treiman D M 1982
Complex partial seizures on closed-circuit television and
EEG. A study of 691 attacks in 79 patients. Annals of
Neurology 11: 292–300

Dreifuss F E 1987 Goals of surgery for epilepsy. In: Engel J
(ed) Surgical treatment of the epilepsies. Raven Press, New
York, p 31–49

Duncan R, Patterson J, Hadley D M et al 1990 CT, MR and
SPECT imaging in temporal lobe epilepsy. Journal of
Neurology, Neurosurgery and Psychiatry 53: 11–15

Elwes R D C, Johnson A L, Shorvon S D et al 1984 The
prognosis for seizure control in newly diagnosed epilepsy.
New England Journal of Medicine 311: 944–947

Elwes R D C, Dunn G, Binnie C D et al 1991 Outcome
following resective surgery for temporal lobe epilepsy: A
prospective follow-up study of 102 consecutive cases.
Journal of Neurology, Neurosurgery and Psychiatry
54: 949–952

Engel J 1987 Outcome with respect to epileptic seizures. In:
Engel J (ed) Surgical treatment of the epilepsies. Raven
Press, New York , p 553–571

Engel J, Crandall P H 1983 Falsely localizing ictal onsets with
depth EEG telemetry during anticonvulsant withdrawal.
Epilepsia 14: 344–355

Engel J, Driver M V, Falconer M A 1975 Electrophysiological

correlates of pathology and surgical results in temporal lobe epilepsy. Brain 98: 129–156

Engel J, Crandall P H, Brown W J 1980 Consistent false lateralization of seizure onset with sphenoidal and scalp telemetered ictal EEG recordings in two patients with partial complex epilepsy. Electroencephalography and Clinical Neurophysiology 50: 160

Engel J, Rausch R, Lieb J P et al 1981 correlation of criteria used for localizing epileptic foci in patients considered for surgical therapy of epilepsy. Annals of Neurology 9: 215–241

Falconer M A 1967 Brain mechanisms suggested by physiologic studies. In: Brain mechanisms underlying speech and language. Grune and Stratton, New York, p 185–203

Falconer M A 1971 Anterior temporal lobectomy for epilepsy. In: Logue V (ed) Operative surgery, vol 14 Neurosurgery. Butterworths, London, p 142–149

Falconer M A 1973 Reversibility by temporal lobe resection of the behavioural abnormalities of temporal lobe epilepsy. New England Journal of Medicine 289: 451–455

Falconer M A 1974 Mesial temporal (Ammon's Horn) sclerosis as a common cause of epilepsy. Aetiology, treatment and prevention. Lancet 2: 767–770

Falconer M A, Kennedy W A 1961 Epilepsy due to small focal temporal lesions with bilateral independent spike-discharging foci. A study of seven cases relieved by operation. Journal of Neurology, Neurosurgery and Psychiatry 24: 205–212

Falconer M A, Taylor D C 1968 Surgical treatment of drug-resistant epilepsy due to mesial temporal sclerosis. Archives of Neurology 19: 353–361

Falconer M A, Wilson P J E 1969 Complication related to delayed haemorrhage after hemispherectomy. Journal of Neurosurgery 30: 413–426

Fenton G W 1978 Epilepsy and psychosis. Journal of the Irish Medical Association 71: 315–324

Ferguson S M, Rayport M, Corrie W S 1985 Neuropsychiatric observations on behavioral consequences of corpus callosum section for seizure control. In: Reeves A G (ed) Epilepsy and the corpus callosum. Plenum Press, New York, p 501–514

Fiol M E, Torres F, Gates J R et al 1990 Methohexital (Brevital) effect on electrocorticogram may be misleading. Epilepsia 31: 524–528

Fish D R 1989 CT and PET in drug-resistant epilepsy. In: Trimble M (ed) Chronic epilepsy, its prognosis and management. J Wiley & Sons, New York, p 59–72

Fish D R, Lewis D D, Brooks D J et al 1987 Regional cerebral blood flow in patients with focal epilepsy studied using xenon enhanced CT brain scanning. Journal of Neurology, Neurosurgery and Psychiatry 50: 1584–1588

Flanigin H, King D, Gallagher B 1985 Surgical treatment of epilepsy. In: Pedley T A, Meldrum B S (eds) Recent advances in Epilepsy. Churchill Livingstone, Edinburgh, p 515–559

Flor Henry P 1969 Psychosis and TLE: A controlled investigation. Epilepsia 10: 363–395

Garretson H, Gloor P, Rasmussen T 1966 Intracarotid amobarbital and metrazol test for the study of epileptiform discharges in man: a note on its technique. Electroencephalography and Clinical Neurophysiology 21: 607–610

Gastaut H 1948 Presentation d'une électrode pharyngée bipolaire. Revue Neurologique 80: 623–624

Gloor P 1975 Contributions of electroencephalography and electrocorticography to the neurosurgical treatment of the epilepsies. In: Penry J K, Walter R D (eds) Advances in neurology, vol 8. Raven Press, New York p 59–105

Gloor P 1987 Volume conductor principles, their application to depth and surface EEG. In: Wieser H G, Elger C E (eds) Methods of presurgical evaluation of epileptic patients. Springer, Munich, p 59–68

Goldring S 1978 A method of surgical management of focal epilepsy, especially as it relates to children. Journal of Neurosurgery 49: 344–356

Goldring S 1987 Surgical management of epilepsy in children. In: Engel J (ed) Surgical treatment of the epilepsies. Raven Press, New York p 445–464

Goldring S, Gregorie E M 1984 Surgical management of epilepsy using epidural mats to localize the seizure focus. Review of 100 cases. Journal of Neurosurgery 60: 457–466

Gordon B, Lesser R P, Rance, N E et al 1990 Parameters for direct cortical electrical simulation in the human: histopathologic confirmation. Electroencephalography and Clinical Neurophysiology 75: 371–377

Gordon H W, Bogen J E, Sperry R W 1971 Absence of deconnexion syndrome in two patients with partial section of the neocommissure. Brain 94: 327–336

Gray F, Serdaru M, Baron H et al 1987 Chronic localized encephalitis (Rasmussen's) in an adult with epilepsia partialis continua. Journal of Neurology, Neurosurgery and Psychiatry 50: 747–751

Gregorie E M, Goldring S 1984 Localization of function in the excision of lesions from the sensorimotor region. Journal of Neurosurgery 61: 1047–1055

Guldvog B, Løyning Y, Hauglie-Hanssen E et al 1991 Surgical vs medical treatment for epilepsy I. A retrospective parallel cohort study. Results on outcome with regard to survival, seizures and neurologic deficit. Epilepsia 32: 375–388

Gupta P C, Dharampaul S N, Singh B 1973 Secondary epileptogenic EEG focus in temporal lobe epilepsy. Epilepsia 14: 423–426

Hart Y M, Shorvon D S 1990 Surgery for epilepsy in the United Kingdom. Acta Neurologica Scandinavica 82 (Suppl: 113)

Hoffman H J, Hendrick E B, Dennis M et al 1979 Hemispherectomy for Sturge–Weber syndrome. Child's Brain 5: 223–248

Homan R W, Jones M C, Rawat S 1988 Anterior temporal electrodes in complex partial seizures. Electroencephalography and Clinical Neurophysiology 70: 105–109

Hood T W, Siegfried J, Wieser H G 1983 The role of stereotactic amygdalotomy in the treatment of temporal lobe epilepsy associated with behavioural disorders. Applied Neurophysiology 46: 19–25

Horsley V, Clarke R W 1908 The structure and function of the cerebellum examined by a new method. Brain 31: 45–124

Hufnagel A, Elger D K, Böker D K 1990 Activation of the epileptic focus during carotid amytal test. Electrocorticographic registration with subdural electrodes. Electroencephalography and Clinical Neurophysiology 75: 435–463

Hughes J R, Schlagendorf R E 1961 Electro-clinical correlation in temporal lobe epilepsy with emphasis on inter-areal analysis of the temporal lobe.

Electroencephalography and Clinical Neurophysiology 13: 333–339

Ives J R, Gloor P 1977 New sphenoidal electrode assembly to permit long-term monitoring of the patients' ictal or interictal EEG. Electroencephalography and Clinical Neurophysiology 42: 575–580

Jack C R, Nichols D A, Sharbrough F W et al 1988 Selective posterior cerebral amytal test for evaluating memory function before surgery for temporal lobe seizure. Radiology 168: 787–793

Janota I, Polkey C E 1985 Focal dysplasia of the cerebral cortex in surgery for epilepsy. Neuropathology and Applied Biology 11: 325–326

Jasper H H 1958 Report on the committee on methods of clinical examination in electroencephalography. Electroencephalography and Clinical Neurophysiology 10: 370–375

Jasper H H, Pertuiset B, Flanigin H 1951 EEG and cortical electrograms in patients with temporal lobe seizures. Archives of Neurology and Psychiatry 65: 272–290

Jensen I 1975a Temporal lobe surgery around the world. Results, complications, mortality. Acta Neurologica Scandinavica 52: 354–373

Jensen I 1975b Temporal lobe epilepsy. Late mortality in patients treated with unilateral temporal lobe resections. Acta Neurologica Scandinavica 52: 374–380

Jensen I 1976 Temporal lobe epilepsy: Social conditions and rehabilitation after surgery. Acta Neurologica Scandinavica 54: 22–44

Jensen I, Larsen J K 1979 Mental aspects of temporal lobe epilepsy. Follow-up of 74 patients after resection of a temporal lobe. Journal of Neurology, Neurosurgery and Psychiatry 42: 256–265

Jones D P 1951 Recording of the basal EEG with sphenoidal electrodes. Electroencephalography and Clinical Neurophysiology 3: 100

Katz A, Awad I A, Kong A K et al 1989 Extent of resection in temporal lobectomy for epilepsy. II. Memory changes and neurologic complications. Epilepsia 30: 763–771

Kelly P J, Sharbrough F W, Ball K A et al 1987 Magnetic resonance imaging-based computer-assisted stereotactic resection of the hippocampus and amygdala in patients with temporal lobe epilepsy. Mayo Clinic Proceedings 62: 103–108

Kennedy W A, Hill D 1958 The surgical prognostic significance of the electroencephalographic prediction of Ammon's horn sclerosis in epileptics. Journal of Neurology, Neurosurgery and Psychiatry 21: 24–30

King M, Stephenson J B B, Ziervogel M et al 1985 A case for hemispherectomy? Neuropediatrics 16: 46–55

Kruse-Larsen C, Dam M, Smed M et al 1990 Amygdalo-hippocampectomy in partial complex epilepsy. Acta Neurologica Scandinavica 82 (Suppl): 24

Krynauw R A 1959 Infantile hemiplegia treated by removing one cerebral hemisphere. Journal of Neurology, Neurosurgery and Psychiatry 13: 243–267

Kuzniecky R, DeLaSayette D, Ethier R et al 1987 Magnetic resonance imaging in temporal lobe epilepsy: pathological correlations. Annals of Neurology 22: 341–347

Kuzniecky R, Andermann F, Tampieri D et al 1989 Bilateral central macrogyria: epilepsy, pseudobulbar palsy, and mental retardation—a recognizable neuronal migration disorder. Annals of Neurology 25: 547–554

Lancet Leading Article 1988 Surgery for temporal lobe epilepsy. 2: 1115–1116

Lange H H, Lieb J P, Engel J et al 1983 Temporospatial patterns of preictal spike activity in human temporal lobe epilepsy. Electroencephalography and Clinical Neurophysiology 56: 543–555

Laxer H 1984 Mini-sphenoidal electrodes in the investigation of seizures. Electroencephalography and Clinical Neurophysiology 58: 127–129

Lehtinen L O J, Bergstrom L 1970 Naso-ethmoidal electrode for recording the electrical activity of the inferior surface of the frontal lobe. Electroencephalography and Clinical Neurophysiology 29: 303–305

Lesser R P, Dinner D S, Luders H et al 1984 Differential diagnosis and treatment of intractable seizures. Cleveland Clinic Quarterly 51: 217–240

Lieb J P, Walsh G O, Babb T L et al 1976 A comparison of EEG seizure patterns recorded with surface and depth electrodes in patients with temporal lobe epilepsy. Epilepsia 17: 137–160

Lieb J P, Woods S C, Siccardi A et al 1978 Quantitative analysis of depth spiking in relation to seizure foci in patients with temporal lobe epilepsy. Electroencephalography and Clinical Neurophysiology 44: 641–663

Lieb J P, Engel J, Gevins A et al 1981a Surface and deep EEG correlates of surgical outcome in temporal lobe epilepsy. Epilepsia 22: 515–538

Lieb J P, Engel J, Jann-Brown W et al 1981b Neuropathological findings following temporal lobectomy related to surface and deep EEG patterns. Epilepsia 22: 539–549

Lieb J P, Rausch R, Engel J et al 1982a Changes in intelligence following temporal lobectomy: relationship to EEG activity, seizure relief, and pathology. Epilepsia 23: 1–13

Lieb J P, Rausch R, Engel J et al 1982b Psychological status related to surgical control of temporal lobe seizures. Epilepsia 23: 191–202

Lombroso C T, Erba G 1970 Primary and secondary bilateral synchrony in epilepsy. A clinical electroencephalographic study. Archives of Neurology 22: 321–334

Lüders H, Hahn J, Lesser R L et al 1982 Localization of epileptogenic spike foci; comparative study closely spaced scalp electrodes, nasopharyngeal, sphenoidal, subdural and depth electrodes. In: Akimoto H, Kazamatsuri H, Seino M, Ward A (eds) Advances in epileptology (XIIIth Epilepsy International Symposium). Raven Press, New York, p 185–189

Luessenhop A J, Dela-Cruz T C, Fairchild D M 1970 Surgical disconnection of the cerebral hemispheres for intractable seizures. Results in infancy and childhood. Journal of the American Medical Association 213: 1630–1636

Maclean P D 1949 A new nasopharyngeal lead. Electroencephalography and Clinical Neurophysiology 1: 110–112

Marchal G, Andermann F, Tampieri D et al 1989 Generalized cortical dysplasia manifested by diffusely thick cerebral cortex. Archives of Neurology 46: 430–434

Marciani M G, Gotman J, Andermann F 1985 Patterns of seizure activation after withdrawal of antiepileptic medication. Neurology 35: 1537–1543

Margerison J H, Corsellis J A N 1966 Epilepsy and the temporal lobes: a clinical, electroencephalographic and neuropathological study of the brain in epilepsy, with particular reference to the temporal lobes. Brain 89: 499–530

Margerison J H, Binnie C D, McCaul I R 1970

Electroencephalographic signs employed in the location of ruptured intracranial arterial aneurysms. Electroencephalography and Clinical Neurophysiology 28: 296–306

Marino R 1985 Surgery for epilepsy. Selective partial microsurgical callosotomy for intractable multiform seizures: Criteria for clinical selection and results. Applied Neurophysiology 48: 404–407

Mars N J J, Lopes da Silva F H 1983 Propagation of seizure activity in kindled dogs. Electroencephalography and Clinical Neurophysiology 56: 194–209

Maxwell R E, Gates J R, Flol M E et al 1983 Clinical evaluation of a depth electroencephalography electrode. Neurosurgery 12: 561–564

McBride M C, Polkey C E, Binnie C D 1991 Correlates of preoperative clinical and interictal EEG findings with outcome from resective surgery for intractable epilepsy 30: 526–532

Milner B 1975 Psychological aspects of focal epilepsy and its management. In: Purpura D P, Penry J K, Walter R D (eds) Advances in neurology, vol 8. The surgical management of the epilepsies. Raven Press, New York, p 299–314

Milner B, Branch C, Rasmussen T 1962 Study of short-term memory after intracarotid injection of sodium amytal. Transactions of the American Neurological Association 87: 224–226

Mizuno Y, Chou S M, Ester M L et al 1985 Choronic localized encephalitis (Rasmussen's) with focal cerebral seizures revisited. Journal of Neuropathology and Experimental Neurology 29: 44–351

Morrell F 1985 Callosal mechanisms in epileptogenesis. Identification of two distinct kinds of spread of epileptic activity. In: Reeves A G (ed) Epilepsy and the corpus callosum. Plenum Press, New York, p 99–130

Morrell F, Wada J, Engel J 1987 Appendix III Potential relevance of kindling and secondary epileptogenesis to the consideration of surgical treatment of epilepsy. In: Engel J (ed) Surgical treatment of the epilepsies. Raven Press, New York, p 701–707

Morrell F, Whisler W W, Bleck T P 1989 Multiple subpial transection: A new approach to the surgical treatment of focal epilepsy. Journal of Neurosurgery 70: 231–239

Morris H H, Lüders H 1985 Electrodes. In Gotman J, Ives R, Gloor P (eds) Long-term monitoring in epilepsy. Electroencephalography and Clinical Neurophysiology 37 (suppl): 3–25

Morris H H, Lüders H, Lesser R L et al 1983 Value of multiple electrodes in addition to standard 10/20 system electrodes in localizing epileptiform foci. XVth Epilepsy International Symposium, abstracts. Washington DC

Morris H H, Dinner D S, Luders H et al 1988 Supplementary motor seizures: Clinical and electroencephalographic findings. Neurology 38: 1075–1082

Munari C, Giallonardo A T, Musolino et al 1987 Specific neuroradiological examinations necessary for stereotactic procedures. In: Wieser H G, Elger C E (eds) Presurgical evaluation of epileptics. Springer-Verlag, Berlin, p 141–145

Mundinger F, Becker P, Grolkner E et al 1976 Late results of stereotactic surgery of epilepsy, predominantly temporal lobe type. Acta Neurochirurgica 23 (suppl): 177–182

Narabayashi H 1979 Long-range results of medial amygdalotomy on epileptic traits in adult patients. In:

Rasmussen T, Marino R (eds) Functional neurosurgery. Raven Press, New York p 243–252

Narabayashi H, Shima F 1973 Which is the better amygdalar target, the medial or lateral nuclei? (For behaviour problems and paroxysm in epileptics). In: Laitinen L V, Livingstone K E (eds) Surgical approaches in psychiatry. MTP, Lancaster, U K, p 129–134

Narabayashi H, Nagao T, Sato Y et al 1963 Stereotactic amygdalotomy for behaviour disorder. Archives of Neurology 9: 1–16

National Association of Epilepsy Centers 1990 Recommended guidelines for diagnosis and treatment in specialised epilepsy centres. Epilepsia 31: Suppl l

Niemeyer P 1958 The transventricular amygdalo-hippocampectomy in temporal lobe epilepsy. In: Baldwin M, Bailey P (eds) Temporal lobe epilepsy. Charles C Thomas, Springfield, Illinois, p 461–482

Nordborg C, Sourander P, Silfvenius H et al 1986 A histological study on mild cortical dysplasia in patients with intractable seizures. Abstracts of the Xth International Congress of Neuropathology, Stockholm, No 163, p 84

Novelly R A, Augustine E M, Mattson R H et al 1984 Selective memory improvement and impairment in temporal lobectomy for epilepsy. Annals of Neurology 15: 64–67

Ojemann G A, Ward A A 1975 Stereotactic and other procedures for epilepsy. In: Purpura D P, Penry J K, Walter R D (eds) Neurosurgical management of the epilepsies. Raven Press, New York, p 241–263

Ojemann G A, Dodrill C B 1985 Verbal memory deficits after left temporal lobectomy for epilepsy. Mechanism and intraoperative prediction. Journal of Neurosurgery 62: 101–107

Olivier A 1987 Commentary: cortical resections. In: Engel J (ed) Surgical treatment of the epilepsies. Raven Press, New York, p 405–416

Olivier A, Gloor P, Quesney L F 1983 The indications of and the role of depth electrode recording in epilepsy. Applied Neurophysiology 46: 33–36

Ounstead C, Lindsay J, Normal J 1966 Biological factors in temporal lobe epilepsy. Heinemann, London

Ounstead C, Lindsay J, Richards P 1987 Developmental aspects of focal epilepsies of childhood treated by neurosurgery. In: Temporal lobe epilepsy. A biographical study 1984–1986. Blackwell Scientific Publications, Oxford, p 70–86

Pampiglione G 1956 Some anatomical considerations upon electrode placement in routine EEG. Proceedings of the Electrophysiological Technologists Association 7: 20–30

Pampiglione G, Kerridge J 1956 EEG abnormalities from the temporal lobe studied with sphenoidal electrodes. Journal of Neurology, Neurosurgery and Psychiatry 19: 117–129

Panet-Raymond D, Gotman J 1990 Can slow waves in the electrocorticogram (ECoG) help localize epileptic foci? Electroencephalography and Clinical Neurophysiology 75: 464–473

Penfield W, Jasper H 1954 Epilepsy and the functional anatomy of the human brain. Churchill, London

Pickard J D, Bailey S, Sanderson H et al 1990 Steps towards cost–benefit analysis of regional neurosurgical care. British Medical Journal 301: 629–635

Polkey C E 1981 Selection of patients with chronic drug resistant epilepsy for resective surgery: 5 years' experience. Journal of the Royal Society of Medicine 74: 574–579

Polkey C E 1983 Prognostic factors in selecting patients with drug-resistant epilepsy for temporal lobectomy. In: Rose F C (ed) Research progress in epilepsy. Pitman, London, p 500–506

Polkey C E, Binnie C D, Janota I 1989 Acute hippocampal recording and pathology at temporal lobe resection and amygdalo-hippocampectomy for epilepsy. Journal of Neurology, Neurosurgery and Psychiatry 52: 1050–1057

Pond D A 1974 Epilepsy and personality disorder. In: Vinken P J, Bruyn G W (eds) Handbook of clinical neurology, vol 15. The epilepsies. North Holland Publishing, Amsterdam, p 576–592

Powell G E, Polkey C E, McMillan T M 1985 The new Maudsley series of temporal lobectomy I: Short term cognitive effects. British Journal of Clinical Psychology 24: 109–124

Powell G E, Polkey C E, Canavan A G M 1987 Lateralization of memory function in epileptic patients by use of the sodium amytal (Wada) technique. Journal of Neurology, Neurosurgery and Psychiatry 50: 665–672

Power C, Poland S D, Blume W T et al 1990 Cytomegalovirus and Rasmussen's encephalitis. Lancet 336: 1282–1284

Quesney L F, Gloor P, Andermann F 1981 Role of naso-ethmoidal electrodes in the preoperative localization of seizure activity involving the fronto temporal convexity. Epilepsia 22: 243

Rasmussen T 1975a Surgery of frontal lobe epilepsy. In: Purpura D P, Penry J K, Walter R D (eds) Advances in neurology, vol 8. Neurosurgical management of the epilepsies. Raven Press, New York p 197–205

Rasmussen T 1975b Surgery for epilepsy arising in regions other than the temporal or frontal lobes. In: Purpura D P, Penry J K, Walter R D (eds) Advances in neurology, vol 8. Neurosurgical management of the epilepsies. Raven Press, New York, p 207–226

Rasmussen T 1976 The place of surgery in the treatment of epilepsy. In: Morley T P (ed) Current controversies in neurosurgery. Saunders, Philadelphia, p 463–477

Rasmussen T 1978 Further observations on the syndrome of chronic encephalitis with epilepsy. Applied Neurophysiology 41: 1–12

Rasmussen T 1987 Cortical resection for multilobe epileptogenic lesions. In: Wieser H G, Elger C E (eds) Presurgical evaluation of epileptics. Springer-Verlag, Berlin, p 344–351

Rasmussen T, Olszewski J, Lloyd-Smith D 1958 Focal seizures due to chronic localized encephalitis. Neurology 8: 435–445

Rausch R 1987 Psychological evaluation. In: Engel J (ed) Surgical treatment of the epilepsies. Raven Press, New York, p 181–201

Regard M, Landis T, Wieser H G, Hailemariam S 1985 Functional inhibition and release: unilateral tachistoscopic performance and stereoelectroencephalographic activity in a case with left limbic status epileptic. Neuropsychologia 23: 575–581

Renella R R 1989 Outcome of surgery. In: Microsurgery of the temporal region. Springer-Verlag, Wien, p 158–164

Rich K M, Goldring S, Gado M 1985 Computed tomography in chronic seizure disorder caused by glioma. Archives of Neurology 42: 26–27

Robillard A, Saint Hilaire J M, Mercier M et al 1983 The localizing and lateralizing value of adversion in epileptic seizures. Neurology 33: 1421–1422

Rossi G F 1973 Problems of analysis and interpretation of electrocerebral signals in human epilepsy. A neurosurgeon's view. In: Brazier M A B (ed) Epilepsy, its phenomena in man. Academic Press, New York, p 259

Rovit R L, Gloor P, Henderson L R 1960 Temporal lobe epilepsy—a study using multiple basal electrodes. I. Description of method. Neurochirurgia 3: 5–18

Rowe C C, Berkovic S F, Benjamin S T et al 1989 Localization of epileptic foci with postictal single photon emission computed tomography. Annals of Neurology 26: 660–668

Ryding E, Rosen I, Elmqvist D et al 1988 SPECT measurements with ^{99}TC-HM-PAO in focal epilepsy. Journal of Cerebral Blood Flow and Metabolism 8: S95–100

Sadler R M, Blume W T 1989 Significance of bisynchronous spike-waves in patients with temporal lobe spikes. Epilepsia 30: 143–146

Schorner W, Meencke H J, Felix R 1987 Temporal lobe epilepsy: comparison of CT and MR imaging. American Journal of Neuroradiology 8: 773–781

Schmidt D, Machus B, Porter R J, Penry J K 1982 The variability of ictal signs in complex partial seizures: a videotape analysis. In Stefan H, Burr W (eds) Mobile long-term EEG monitoring: Proceedings of the MLE symposium, Bonn. G. Fischer, Stuttgart, p 149–159

Serafetinides E A, Falconer M A 1962 The effects of temporal lobectomy in epileptic patients with psychosis. Journal of Mental Science 108: 584–593

Serafetinides E A, Falconer M A 1963 Speech disturbances in temporal lobe seizures: a study in 100 epileptic patients submitted to anterior temporal lobectomy. Brain 86: 333–346

Siegal A M, Wieser W G, Wickmann W, Yasargil G M 1990 Relationship between MR-imaged total amount of tissue removed, section scores of specific mesiobasal, limbic subcompartments and clinical outcome following selective amygdalo–hippocampectomy. Epilepsy Research, Vol 6, 56–65

Silverman D 1960 The anterior temporal electrode and the 10/20 system. Electroencephalography and Clinical Neurophysiology 12: 735–737

Spencer S S 1981 Depth electroencephalograph in selection of refractory epilepsy for surgery. Annals of Neurology 9: 207–214

Spencer D D 1987 Postscript: Should there be a surgical treatment of choice and if so how should it be determined? In: Engel J (ed) Surgical treatment of the epilepsies. Raven Press, New York, p 477–484

Spencer S S, Spencer D D, Williamson P D 1981 Ictal effects of anticonvulsant medication withdrawal in epileptic patients. Epilepsia 22: 297–307

Spencer S S, Spencer D D, Williamson P D et al 1982 The localizing value of depth electroencephalography in 32 patients with refractory epilepsy. Annals of Neurology 12: 248–253

Spencer D D, Spencer S S, Mattson R H et al 1984a Intracerebral masses in patients with intractable partial epilepsy. Neurology 34: 432–436

Spencer D D, Spencer S S, Mattson R H et al 1984b Access to the posterior medial temporal lobe structures in the surgical treatment of epilepsy. Neurosurgery 15: 667–671

Spencer S S, Williamson P D, Bridgers S L et al 1985 Reliability and accuracy of localization by scalp ictal EEG. Neurology 35: 1567–1575

Spencer S S, Williamson P D, Spencer D D et al 1987a

Human hippocampal seizure spread studied by depth and subdural recording: the hippocampal commissure. Epilepsia 28: 479–489

Spencer S S, Gates J R, Reeves A R et al 1987b Corpus callosum section. In: Engel J (ed) Surgical treatment of the epilepsies. Raven Press, New York, p 425–444

Sperling M R, Wilson G, Engel J et al 1986 Magnetic resonance imaging in intractable partial epilepsy: Correlative studies. Annals of Neurology 20: 57–62

Sperling M R, Sutherling W W, Nuwer M R 1987 New techniques for evaluating patients for epilepsy surgery. In: Engel J (ed) Surgical treatment of the epilepsies. Raven Press, New York, p 235–257

Sperling M R, O'Connor M J, Tougas P 1988 Utility of depth and subdural electrodes in recording temporal lobe seizures. Epilepsia 29: 679

Spiegel E A, Wycis H T, Baird M W 1958 Long-range effects of electropallido-ansotomy in extra-pyramidal and convulsive disorders. Neurology 8: 734–740

Stefan H, Schüler P, Witting R et al 1990 First results with high-field MR spectroscopy in patients with temporal lobe epilepsy: An additional tool for focus localization? Second International Cleveland Epilepsy Symposium. Abstract 114, p 39

Stevens J R 1990 Psychiatric consequences of temporal lobectomy for intractable seizures: a 20–30 year follow-up of 14 cases. Psychological Medicine 20: 529–545

Storm van Leeuwen W 1982 Neurophysiosurgery in the Netherlands since 1971. Acta Neurochirurgica 61: 249–256

Talairach J, Bancaud 1973 Stereotactic approach to epilepsy. Progress in Neurological Surgery 5: 297–354

Talairach J, Bancaud J 1974 Stereotactic exploration and therapy in epilepsy. In: Vinken P J, Bruyn G W (eds) The epilepsies. Handbook of Clinical Neurology 15: 758–782

Talairach J, Bancaud J, Szilka G et al 1974 Approche nouvelle de la neurochirurgie de l'épilepsie. Methodologie stéréotaxique et resultats theraupeutiques. Neuro-chirurgie Suppl 2

Taylor D C 1972 Mental state and temporal lobe epilepsy. A correlative account of 100 patients treated surgically. Epilepsia 13: 727–765

Taylor D C 1975 Factors influencing the occurrence of schizophrenia-like psychosis in patients with temporal lobe epilepsy. Psychological Medicine 5: 249–254

Taylor D C 1987 Psychiatric and social issues in measuring the input and outcome of epilepsy surgery. In: Engel J (ed) Surgical treatment of the epilepsies. Raven Press, New York, 485–503

Taylor D C, Falconer M A 1968 Clinical, socio-economic and psychological changes after temporal lobectomy for epilepsy. British Journal of Psychiatry 114: 1247–1261

Taylor D C, Marsh S M 1977 Implications of long-term follow-up studies in epilepsy: With a note on the cause of death. In: Penry J K (ed) Epilepsy, the eight international symposium. Raven Press, New York, p 27–34

Taylor D C, Falconer M A, Bruton C J et al 1971 Focal dysplasia of the cerebral cortex in epilepsy. Journal of Neurology, Neurosurgery and Psychiatry 34: 369–387

Turner E A 1963 A new approach to unilateral and bilateral lobotomies for psychomotor epilepsy. Journal of Neurology, Neurosurgery and Psychiatry 26: 285–299

Turner E A 1982 Temporal lobe operations. In: Surgery of the mind. Carver Press, Birmingham, UK, p 126–169

Vaernat K 1972 Stereotactic amygdalotomy in temporal lobe epilepsy. Confinia Neurologica 34: 176–180

Van Buren J M 1987 Complications of surgical procedures in the diagnosis and treatment of epilepsy. In: Engel J (ed) Surgical treatment of the epilepsies. Raven Press, New York, p 465–475

Van Buren J M, Ajmone Marsan C, Mutsuga N et al 1975 Surgery of temporal lobe epilepsy. In: Penry J K, Walter R D (eds) Advances in Neurology, 8. Raven Press, New York, p 155–196

Van Veelen C W M, Debets R M, Van Huffelen A C et al 1990 Combined use of subdural and intracerebral electrodes in preoperative evaluation of epilepsy. Neurosurgery 26: 93–101

Van Wagenen W P, Herren R Y 1940 Surgical division of commissural pathways in the corpus callosum. Archives of Neurology and Psychiatry 44: 740–759

Wada J 1949 A new method for the determination of the side of cerebral speech dominance. A preliminary report on the intra-carotid injection of sodium amytal in man. Medicine and Biology 14: 221–222

Walker A E, Lichenstein R S, Marshall C 1960 A critical analysis of electroencephalography in temporal lobe epilepsy. Archives of Neurology 2: 172–182

Wieser H G 1983 Electroclinical features of the psychomotor seizure. Fischer, Stuttgart

Wieser H G, Hajek M, Leenders K L 1990 PET findings before and after selective amygdalo-hippocampectomy. Second International Cleveland Clinic Epilepsy Symposium, Abstracts p 41, No 121

Wieser H G 1986 'Selective amygdalo-hippocampectomy': indications, investigative technique and results. In: Symon L (ed) Advances and technical standards in neurosurgery, vol 13. Springer-Verlag, Wien, p 39–133

Wieser G H, Yasargil M G 1982 Die 'selektiv Amygdalo-Hippokampektomie' als chirurgische Behandlungsmethode der mediobasal-limbischen Epilepsie. Neurochirurgia 25: 39–50

Wieser H G, Elger C E, Stodieck S R G 1985a The 'Foramen Ovale Electrode': A new recording method for the preoperative evaluation of patients suffering from mesiobasal temporal lobe epilepsy. Electroencephalography and Clinical Neurophysiology 61: 314–322

Wieser H G, Hailemariam S, Regard M et al 1985b Unilateral limbic epileptic status activity: Stereo EEG, behavioral and cognitive data. Epilepsia 26: 19–29

Wieser H G, Valavanis A, Roos A et al 1989 'Selective' and 'superselective' temporal lobe amytal tests: I. Neuroradiological, neuroanatomical, and electrical data. In: Manelis J et al (eds) Advances in Epileptology, vol 17. Raven Press, New York, p 20–27

Wilkus R J, Thompson P M 1984 Positions of sphenoidal electrodes at the beginning and end of extended EEG monitorings. Epilepsia 15: 654

Williamson P D 1985 Corpus callosum section for intractable epilepsy: criteria for patient selection. In: Reeves A G (ed) Epilepsy and the corpus callosum. Plenum Press, New York, p 243–257

Williamson P D, Spencer D D, Spencer S S et al 1985 Complex partial seizures of frontal origin. Annals of Neurology 18: 497–504

Willis R A 1958 The borderland of embryology and pathology. Butterworths, London

Wilson D H, Reeves A G, Gazzaniga M 1982 'Central'

commissurotomy for intractable generalized epilepsy: series two. Neurology 32: 687–697

Wilson P J E 1970 Cerebral hemispherectomy for infantile hemiplegia: A report of 50 cases. Brain 93: 147–180

Wright G D S, McLellan D L, Brice J G 1985 A double-blind trial of chronic cerebellar stimulation in twelve patients with severe epilepsy. Journal of Neurology, Neurosurgery and Psychiatry 47: 769–774

Wyler A R, Bolender N F 1983 Preoperative CT diagnosis of mesial temporal sclerosis for the surgical treatment of epilepsy. Annals of Neurology 13: 59–64

Wyler A R, Ojemann G A, Lettich E et al 1984 Subdural strip electrodes for localizing epileptogenic foci. Journal of Neurosurgery 60: 1195–1200

Wyler A R, Richey E T, Atkinson R A et al 1987 Methohexital activation of epileptogenic foci during acute electrocorticography. Epilepsia 28: 490–494

Yasargil M G, Teddy P G, Roth P 1985 Selective amygdalo-hippocampectomy. Operative anatomy and surgical technique. In: Symon L (ed) Advances and technical standards in neurosurgery, vol 12. Springer-Verlag, Wien p 93–123

17. Epilepsy in developing countries: epidemiology, aetiology and health care

S. D. Shorvon   N. E. Bharucha

INTRODUCTION

Epilepsy in developing countries deserves a separate chapter in a book such as this, not because of any inherent characteristics of the condition in developing countries, nor any distinctive biological differences amongst the sufferers; indeed, it is striking to see how similar are most of the medical and scientific aspects of the condition in the most diverse of populations. Differences do occur, however, due to largely indirect factors. These will form the substance of this chapter, under three headings: 1. epidemiological differences, 2. aetiological differences, 3. differences in health care and treatment models. As scientific data concerning epilepsy from developing countries are sparse, there has been a tendency to extrapolate in many clinical areas from experience in developed countries to the developing world. However, such extrapolation needs to be interpreted with caution, as the impact of these demographic, environmental and organizational issues on the clinical practice of epilepsy may be profound, and should not be underestimated.

EPIDEMIOLOGY

Population structure in developing countries

There are over 210 countries and dependencies in the world, with a total population of over 5 000 000 000 persons. Over three-quarters of the world population live in the 'developing world'; the largest populations being that of China (1 040 600 000 persons), India (750 900 000 persons), Indonesia (163 393 000 persons), Brazil (135 564 000 persons), Bangladesh (98 657 000 persons), Pakistan (96 180 000 persons) and

Nigeria (96 198 000 persons; all 1985 figures). In 1985, of the 210 countries, only 33 (15%) had an average income of over $7000 per year (none of the above), and over 122 (57%) an average income of less than $1000. Of people in the developing world, 75% live in rural areas, although over 20 cities in the developing world have populations in excess of 5 million; and Mexico City, Sao Paulo, Shanghai and Cairo have populations over 10 million (Economist 1987).

From the point of view of epilepsy, the most important demographic distinction between developing and developed countries lies in the age structure of the populations (Table 17.1). In most developing countries, because of the high birth rate, falling infantile mortality and low life expectancy, there is a preponderance of young persons, and there are few in the elderly age groups; this contrasts greatly with the developed world where the proportion of young persons is falling, and of the elderly, particularly the very elderly, is increasing considerably. Thus, a profile of the population of the developing world will reveal it as teeming, mostly poor, mostly rural and mostly young. In this setting, medical issues are very different from those amongst the rich, urban and relatively elderly populations of the West.

Table 17.1 Population age structures (for a year or an average of years 1980–85; Economist 1987)

	Under 15 (%)	15–64 (%)	65 or over (%)
UK	19	66	15
USA	22	66	12
Europe	22	67	11
Africa	46	51	3
Asia	35	61	4
South America	35	59	6

Incidence and prevalence

The usually quoted incidence and prevalence rates for epilepsy are based largely on studies from Western populations. Incidence rates of between 30 and 100 cases per 100 000 persons in the population per year are commonly accepted (Sander & Shorvon 1987, Hauser & Hesdorffer 1990). Incidence rates might be expected to be higher in developing countries, because of the higher risks of symptomatic epilepsy and the age structure of the population, but this has been difficult to demonstrate. However in a recent study from Ecuador (see below), in which considerable attention was paid to complete case ascertainment and to precise methodological details, an annual incidence rate of 122–190 cases per 100 000 persons in the population was found (Placencia et al 1991a,b); similar rates are likely to apply in other developing countries. In the handful of studies of cumulative incidence, it has been suggested that 2–5% of persons in a population will experience a seizure at some time. Prevalence rates of epilepsy both in the first and third worlds have usually been found to lie between 4 and 10 per 1000 persons (Zielinski 1974, Sander & Shorvon 1987, Hauser & Hesdorffer 1990). Findings from published studies from developing countries are shown in Table 17.2, and as can be seen a wide variation is shown, although how much this reflects true regional difference is unknown. In surveys confined to children in developing countries, particularly high rates are found (e.g. 27.6/1000 in Chile (Chiofalo et al 1979), or 18/1000 in Mexico (Garcia-Pedroza et al 1983)). In all countries surveyed, epilepsy is a major health problem; and indeed it is the commonest serious neurological disease. Based on a standardized prevalence figure of 5/1000 (almost certainly an underestimate), in Table 17.3 are shown the estimated numbers of active patients in a range of developing countries; the global total can be similarly estimated to be in the region of 30 000 000 (of whom about 25 000 000 live in the developing world).

Table 17.2 Published prevalence figures from 12 developing countries

Country	Prevalence rate (per 1000 persons)
Brazil	13.3
China	4.4
Colombia	19.5
Ecuador	6.7–8.0
Ethiopia	5.3–8.0
India	2.5–9.0
Libya	2.3
Mexico	3.5
Nigeria	4.4–37
Pakistan	9.8
Sri Lanka	9.0
Turkey	4.6–9.0

Sources: Aziz et al 1991 (personal communication), Bharucha et al 1988a, Dada 1970, Geil 1970, Gomez et al 1978, Gutierrez et al 1980, Guvener et al 1991, Koul et al 1988, Isaac 1987, Li et al 1985, Marino et al 1987, Mathai 1971, Olivares 1972, Osuntokun et al 1987, Placencia et al 1991b, Senanayake 1987, Shridharan et al 1986.
Published figures from studies of general populations without age restrictions (crude rates given, not age, sex, race or geographically specific).
Rates for active epilepsy given where stated. The studies quoted have a variety of study methodologies, with various inclusion criteria, sample sizes, and levels of sophistication.

Table 17.3 Population and population per physician in 18 developing countries, and estimated number of cases of epilepsy

Country	Population ($\times 10^6$)[*]	Number of cases of epilepsy[†]	Population per physician[‡]
Afghanistan	17	850 000	16 700
Angola	8	40 000	15 000
Bangladesh	98	480 000	11 000
Brazil	135	675 000	1700
China	1040	5 200 000	1800
Colombia	27	135 000	1700
Ecuador	8	40 000	800
India	750	3 750 000	3700
Iran	43	215 000	6000
Iraq	14	70 000	1800
Kenya	19	95 000	7900
Libya	3	15 000	700
Liberia	2	10 000	9600
Malaysia	14	70 000	7900
Nigeria	96	480 000	12 600
Pakistan	96	480 000	3500
Peru	18	90 000	1400
Sri Lanka	16	80 000	7100

[*] Mid 1985 population figures to nearest million
[†] A very rough approximation of the number of patients with epilepsy which is based on an estimated standard point prevalence of 5/1000, and not age adjusted.
[‡] A very rough approximation, based on government statistics for physicians numbers, which may be in some instances subject to considerable error.
For the UK and US equivalent figures are respectively: Population ($\times 10^6$) 55 and 255; number of cases of epilepsy 275 000 and 1 275 000; population per physician 800 and 600).

Comparisons between findings from different studies of incidence and prevalence findings are often complicated by methodological problems which introduce potential bias (Sander & Shorvon 1987, Hauser & Hesdorffer 1990). Case ascertainment is especially problematic. In developed countries, the most common published method of case ascertainment is a review of medical records. In developing countries, where medical records are much less complete, this approach will usually underestimate grossly the number of epileptic cases and normally should not be used. A better method is to apply a screening questionnaire to a community or selected population and then examine patients giving a positive result to the screen. Such surveys depend on the sensitivity and specificity of the screening questionnaires and these need careful design and should be piloted in known populations (Placencia et al 1991c). In epilepsy studies these points are frequently neglected and some questionnaires show considerable naivety. Furthermore, the screening questionnaires are invariably administered by non-medical personnel, sometimes without training. Inadequate screening instruments or methodology may result particularly in the failure to identify patients with mild or inactive epilepsy, or partial seizures, and this may explain the high proportion of generalized seizures found in some surveys. In rural populations, it is important to understand local concepts and beliefs about epilepsy. In Indonesia, for example, the question, 'Do you suffer from convulsions?' may be answered in the negative as the term 'convulsion' also implies a hereditary incurable disease which is a disgrace for the family (Chandra 1988). For varying reasons, such concealment is common in many populations.

A second problem in field studies in developing countries concerns the criteria for the diagnosis. Epilepsy is essentially a clinical diagnosis, and in epidemiological studies one should specify the clinical criteria used in the diagnosis. Commonly, an operational definition of epilepsy as 'a specialist confirmed diagnosis' is used, but this introduces considerable subjectivity, and such a method has been rejected in the epidemiological studies of other conditions (e.g. angina or schizophrenia). A research study should also specify what constitutes 'epilepsy'. The inclusion of single seizures,

neonatal seizures, febrile seizures, seizures with an obvious precipitant, for instance alcohol, or seizures in acute illness will vary from study to study, and may influence heavily incidence and prevalence figures. A particular source of difficulty concerns inactive epilepsy. In most treated patients with epilepsy, the seizures cease but there is no general agreement as to what length of remission should occur before a patient is no longer designated 'epileptic'. Usually, a definition of epilepsy should indicate a condition in which a seizure had occurred in a defined previous period i.e. the last 5 years. As cumulative incidence figures are several-fold higher than prevalence figures, a failure to specify criteria for epilepsy may result in serious potential misinterpretation.

Age is the most important variable affecting incidence figures. In all populations studied, the incidence rates are greatest in the first year of life, remain high in the first decade and then fall to low levels in mid life. In developed countries, a second peak of cases occur in late life; for instance, in a recent population-based study of 596 patients from the UK with newly diagnosed epilepsy, 140 (25%) were aged 60 or over at the onset of seizures (Sander et al 1990). In the developing world, because of the demographic structure, this second peak is not yet noticeable.

Race and socioeconomic factors may contribute to differences in the prevalence of epilepsy in developed and developing countries. Higher rates for epilepsy have been found in blacks than in whites in three American studies and also amongst lower socioeconomic groups (Cowan et al 1989, Shamanski & Glaser 1979, Haerer et al 1986). Lower standards of perinatal care may be relevant and as an indication of this for instance, amongst blacks in America infant mortality rates are twice that of whites. In developing countries, no published study as compared racial groups or socioeconomic status, although higher prevalence rates amongst rural than urban populations in Pakistan (Aziz et al, personal communication) and Turkey (Guvener et al 1991) have been reported.

ICBERG study in Ecuador (Placencia et al 1991a,b,c,d)

ICBERG (the International Community Based

Epilepsy Research Group) carried out a number of population based studies of epilepsy between 1986 and 1990. The largest was a study in an Andean region of Ecuador, the methodology of which may act as a model for future studies, and is here outlined in some detail. The aim of the study was to identify directly, in the general population of the region, all residents with a history of non-febrile epileptic seizures, and establish their demographic and epidemiological profile. The study was carried out in a highland Andean region of Ecuador, with a population of about 75 000 persons. A total of 72 121 persons were surveyed (97% of the total population), of whom 18% lived in an urban setting (one of the three provincial towns in the region) and 82% in a rural setting. The majority are mestizo of amerindian and white descent and approximately 12% are black.

The study design was divided into a series of six steps (Placencia et al 1991a):

Step 1: A house-to-house survey was carried out using a screening instrument, which had been previously piloted and validated, with the aim of identifying all persons in the population with a possible history of non-febrile epileptic seizures. The survey was conducted by 54 screening personnel. The screening instrument had a specificity of 92.9%, a sensitivity of 79.3%, an adjusted positive predictive value of 18.3% and negative predictive value of 99.6%.

Step 2: The possible cases identified in step 1 were examined by one of a team of rural doctors trained in the use of precise operational definitions. Cases were categorized as: epileptic seizures, doubtful cases, false positives.

Step 3: Cases defined as epileptic seizures and all doubtful cases were then seen by one of a team of specialist neurologists, using the same operational definitions. All those confirmed as having afebrile epileptic seizures by the neurologist, were then given a standardized neurological interview and examination to record clinical details.

Step 4: A research case record review by an international neurological panel of all cases from step 3 was carried out, using stringent diagnostic criteria, and the cases divided into definite and probable cases.

Step 5: A random sample of 1.4% of all negatives from the original door to door screening (step 1) were interviewed by one of the rural doctor team, to ascertain the false negative rate from step 1.

Step 6: A random sample of 4.6% of the false positives from step 2 were examined by one of a team of specialist neurologists. This was to identify the false negative rate from step 2.

The screeners (step 1) were secondary school leavers who received basic training. The rural doctors (steps 2 and 5) were recently qualified doctors carrying out an obligatory 1 year pre-registration tour in rural medicine. One of a team of 12 senior neurologists from the Ecuadorian Society of Neurology carried out the final field examination (steps 3 and 6), which acted as the diagnostic gold standard for the field identification of cases. The international panel (step 4) consisted of neurologists with a special training in epilepsy from Ecuador and England. There was always a neurologist in the study area and he also participated in standardization workshops with the investigators. One epidemiologist based in Quito collaborated in the planning and the cartographic aspects. Five rural physicians were trained to co-ordinate the field work. The principal investigator lived in the study area for 2 years. Data was entered in the field into floppy diskettes using the DataEase software. Data analysis was carried out partly in England and partly in Ecuador.

Of the 72 121 persons screened, 65 791 were found to be negatives and the remaining 6330 (8.8%) were positive (step 1). Of the 6330 positives, 6155 (97%) were examined by a rural doctor, and 1235 were considered to be cases of epileptic seizures or doubtful cases (step 2). The neurologists interviewed 1199 (97%) of the 1235 cases identified by the rural doctor, and confirmed 958 as true positives, 34 as febrile convulsions only, 184 as false positives and the remaining 23 cases as doubtful. In addition the neurologist also confirmed a history of non-febrile seizures in another 71 cases, who had incomplete documentation from the previous stages. Of these 38 were positive at the screening, but were not seen by the rural doctor, and 33 were cases about whom the rural doctor had some diagnostic query. Therefore, the neurologist diagnosed 1029 cases of afebrile seizures (958 + 71) (step 3). The panel review of the 1029 research case records confirmed 881 as definite cases, and 148 as probable cases (step 4). In a random sample of 1.37% of the screened negatives, i.e. 904 of 65 791, four (0.44%) were found to be positives missed in the door to door screening. If this proportion is projected to all negative cases, a further 291 false negatives could be expected (step 5). Neurologists examined a random sample of 4.6% of the cases classified as false positive by the rural doctors (i.e. 227 of 4920) and identified four cases (1.76% of 227) as positive. If this proportion is projected to all rural doctor false positive cases, a further 87 cases could be expected (step 6).

The minimum lifetime prevalence in the population was thus calculated as 12.2/1000 (881/ 72 121), and the maximum lifetime prevalence 19.5/1000 (1407/72 121). The annual incidence rates range from a minimum estimate of 122/ 100 000 to a maximum 190/1 000 000. The prevalence of active cases ranged between 6.7/ 1000 and 8.0/1000; rates in rural areas with a high proportion of blacks were greater than in urban areas.

The study design addressed deliberately certain methodological problems of large scale epilepsy surveys. Case ascertainment was achieved by a house-to-house survey of the entire population, which did not rely on existing medical records or previous medical contact. The potential logistical difficulties which such a large scale study might raise were circumvented by the use of a cascade system for diagnostic confirmation. Cases were first screened by non-medical personnel, then examined by rural doctors, then by specialized neurologists, and finally reviewed by an international panel. This cascade system allowed the input of specialists to be focused and therefore their efficiency maximized. The screening instruments and procedure had been previously piloted and validated by application to known epilepsy cases in a clinic and then a small population in a village adjacent to the study area. Quality control exercises were undertaken at each stage of the screening process to identify false negative rates. A proportion of the general population were interviewed by the rural doctors, and a proportion of the rural doctor negative cases were interviewed by specialists to derive false negative rates. The diagnosis of epilepsy was carried out according to stringent standardized clinical algorithms, and as such was reliable and reproducible. These aspects are emphasized as they are important features of any such neuro-epidemiological investigation in rural developing country settings, where the existing medical infrastructure may be limited.

AETIOLOGY OF EPILEPSY IN DEVELOPING COUNTRIES

The causes of epilepsy in developing and developed countries are similar, but their frequency may differ considerably.

Congenital

One of the commoner causes of epilepsy in developing countries is perinatal asphyxia leading to hypoxic ischaemic encephalopathy, and intracranial haemorrhage. Metabolic disturbances in the neonate, such as low glucose, calcium or magnesium levels, and possibly a raised bilirubin level also figure prominently. Intracranial infections, whether a bacterial meningitis due to group B *Streptococci* or *E. Coli* or non-bacterial due to one of the TORCH organisms (toxoplasma, syphilis, rubella, cytomegalovirus, *Herpes simplex*) are also important. Common pathological findings either on CT or MRI scans are porencephalic cysts, hydranencephaly or multicystic encephalomalacia. A porencephalic cyst is a single unilateral cavity in a hemisphere which may not communicate with the lateral ventricle. Hydranencephaly represents massive bilateral lesions, and multicystic encephalomalacia consists of multiple, usually bilateral foci of cerebral necrosis with cavitation. These three conditions are the response of the brain to different degrees of insult by infection, trauma, haemorrhage, ischaemia or hypoxia at any time between 6 months of gestation and the early postnatal period. Three factors are responsible for this kind of reaction. The immature brain has a high water content, there are few myelinated fibres and no response by astrocytes to brain damage. Hence, fluid-containing cavities form. Patients present with spastic cerebral palsy, either hemiplegia or quadriplegia (often with mental retardation), and seizures. Occasionally a porencephalic cyst that fails to communicate with the subarachnoid space may behave as a mass lesion. In inflammatory and infectious causes of porencephaly, there may be associated hydrocephalus.

Trauma

Seizure following head injuries due to traffic accidents and falls from a height are common. The incidence of head injury due to such accidents is thought to be higher in newly industrialized societies, especially in males, although actual figures are lacking.

Infection

Infections are a particularly important cause of epilepsy in developing countries (Volpe 1981), the frequency of which may differ widely in different locations. Knowledge of these conditions is also important in developed countries, because of immigration, international air travel, and the recent advent of AIDS.

Bacterial infections

Bacterial meningitis. Bacterial meningitis is caused by *Haemophilus influenzae*, *Neisseria meningitidis*, *Streptococcus pneumoniae*, as in developed countries, and *Mycobacterium tuberculosis*. The relative frequency of these organisms in developing countries is unknown. Other organisms are less often responsible. These include Gram-negative bacillae, *Staphylococci* and *Norcardia asteroides*. Seizures occur in up to 50% of patients with meningitis, usually during the acute stage, and more commonly in children. They usually remit. Seizures occurring late in the course of the illness should suggest a focal intracranial lesion.

Focal lesions. *Brain abscess.* Brain abscess is usually due to the same organisms as in developing countries. Unusual causes in the developed countries but commoner in developing countries include tuberculosis, cysticercosis and schistosomiasis.

Cranial epidural abscess and subdural empyema. These are now rare in developed countries but still occur in developing countries because of untreated middle ear disease and sinusitis.

Intracranial thrombophlebitis. Septic intracranial thrombophlebitis is commoner for the same reason. Aseptic thrombophlebitis is still seen in developing countries and occurs in three situations:

1. In pregnancy. Four per 1000 deliveries in one study resulted in thrombophlebitis (Srinivasan and Natarajan 1974).
2. In children, due to dehydration, marasmus and untreated congenital heart disease.
3. In haemoglobinopathies such as sickle cell disease which is common in central Africa.

Seizures are a common feature of intracranial thrombophlebitis, particularly if there is cortical venous involvement.

Subacute bacterial endocarditis. This condition can present with seizures.

Other bacterial causes of chronic meningitis. These must also be borne in mind. *Treponema pallidum* is now less common than in the past. Other spirochaetes such as *Borellia recurrentis*, spread by louse bite, are endemic in Ethiopia and Sudan. *Leptospira interrogans* from contact with animal urine is the most widespread zoonosis in the world, particularly in the tropics. *Brucella* is spread by farm animals in Mediterranean countries, Latin America and Asia, and *Nocardia asteroides* is a widespread opportunistic infection.

Viral infections

Viral infections of the brain cause either aseptic meningitis or encephalitis. The viruses causing aseptic meningitis include enteroviruses, more common in developing countries because of faecal–oral transmission, mumps because of lack of vaccine in developing countries, arenaviruses such as lymphocytic choriomeningitis and Lassa fever in Africa, *Herpes simplex* type 2, *Varicella zoster* and HIV.

The main group of viruses causing epidemic encephalitis is the arbovirus group. Important arboviruses in developing countries are Japanese encephalitis found in Asia where it is endemic and dengue haemorrhagic fever in China, SE Asia, Cuba and Latin America. In Japanese encephalitis, seizures are frequent in children.

The causes of sporadic encephalitis are *Herpes simplex* type 1, mumps, adenoviruses and Epstein–

Barr virus. These are no more common in developing countries than developed countries.

The zoonotic cause of encephalitis is rabies, which is much more common in developing than developed countries. Seizures may be a part of the encephalitic phase.

The main chronic encephalitis of interest in developing countries is SSPE which is common because of the occurrence of measles at an early age and the lack of measles vaccine.

Viruses affecting the developing nervous system, include cytomegalovirus and rubella.

Para-infectious encephalomyelitis occurs after any viral infection, but most commonly after measles. Immunization has reduced its incidence. Another important cause of encephalomyelitis in developing countries is the use of rabies vaccine containing nervous tissues. In developed countries this has been replaced by other vaccines such as the human diploid cell vaccine.

Fungal infections

There are two large groups of fungi—the pathogenic fungi, restricted to certain geographic areas such as *Blastomyces dermatitidis* in parts of the Americas and Africa, and the opportunistic fungi such as *Candida albicans* which are much more widely distributed and invade debilitated or immunosuppressed hosts, or take advantage of a breach in the host defence mechanism. In addition, some widely-distributed pathogenic fungi such as *Cryptococcus neoformans* are found in Western countries in immunosuppressed people, but in developing countries are often found in otherwise normal hosts. Seizures occur in fungal infection which may present as a number of clinical pictures—meningitis, granuloma, cerebral abscess, arteritis or mycotic aneurysms. Clinically it is often hard to distinguish fungal infections from tuberculosis, because of difficulty in identifying both fungi and mycobacteria. The immunological tests useful in making these distinctions are often not available in developing countries.

Parasitic infections

Over one thousand million people throughout the world are estimated to be infected by parasites. There are no reliable figures available for frequency of infection by different parasites, nor for frequency with which the nervous system may be affected. To date, there are no vaccines available to protect humans from parasites.

Parasites are an important cause of epilepsy in tropical countries with poor sanitation and hygiene, although they also occur less frequently in non-tropical countries with good sanitation and hygiene. Parasites may be divided into two main groups, the unicellular protozoa (first animals) and multicellular worms or helminths. The major protozoan diseases which affect the nervous system are malaria, trypanosomiasis, toxoplasmosis and amoebiasis (Table 17.4). The worms are divided into round worms (nematodes), flat worms (trematodes) and segmented worms (cestodes).

Worms differ from other infectious agents in that they are unable to multiply within the definitive human host. The degree of infection is therefore determined by how many worms enter the host at one time. Cestodes usually require two hosts, a definitive host in which the adult form lives and one or more intermediate hosts in which the eggs or larvae mature (Table 17.5). Eating raw or partly-cooked hosts is an important source of infection. The occurrence of worm infestation in a particular area requires not only the correct conditions for the worm and for human infection but also for a variety of other hosts. Infection is not transmitted directly from one person to another except in rare instances, as when *Strongyloides stercoralis* spreads when there is close human contact.

Seizures may occur in several clinical settings. The acute eosinophilic meningitis of angiostrongyliasis is an example of meningitis. Cerebral malaria produces seizures in the setting of an acute encephalitic illness. Seizures occur in gambian trypanosomiasis in chronic encephalitis. Strongyloidiasis and amoebiasis produce abscesses which then act as epileptic foci. Toxoplasmosis, cysticercosis, schistosomiasis, paragonimiasis and echinococciasis produce either granulomas or cysts which can give rise to seizures, or present as space-occupying lesions.

The diagnosis of a parasitosis of the central nervous system by recovery and identification of the organism is very difficult without cerebral

Table 17.4 Protozoan diseases

Type of protozoan	Disease	Transmission	Type of reproduction	Hosts	Geographical distribution
Sporozoa *Plasmodium falciparum* *P. malariae* *P. ovale* *P. vivax*	Malaria Cerebral malaria caused by *P. falciparum*	Arthropod-borne (anopheles mosquitoes) or blood transfusion, congenital (rare)	Alternating asexual (schizogony)/sexual (sporogony) cycles occur in different hosts	Human	Tropical, developing countries. *P. falciparum*, everywhere, but most common in Africa
Sporozoa *Toxoplasma gondii*	Toxoplasmosis Congenital acquired: toxoplasma encephalitis in immunosuppressed	Ingestion of cysts from cat's faeces, blood transfusion, transplacental	Alternating sexual/asexual cycles in same host	Birds Mammals Reptiles	Worldwide
Haemoflagellate *Trypanosoma brucei* *T. gambiense* *T. rhodesiense*	Trypanosomiasis Sleeping sickness Chronic Gambian sleeping sickness Acute Rhodesian sleeping sickness	Arthropod-borne (tsetse fly)	Asexual binary fission	Humans (Gambian type) Primarily zoonosis antelope, cattle, sheep (Rhodesian type)	Gambian: western and central Africa Rhodesian: eastern Africa
T. cruzi	Chagas disease (S. American Trypanosomiasis) Acute, rare meningoencephalitis Chronic cerebral embolism secondary to cardiomyopathy	By insects, Reduviidae Transplacental and by blood transfusion less frequently	Asexual binary fission	Rodents, dogs, pigs, marsupials especially opossums	Latin America
Amoebae *Entamoeba histolytica*	Amoebiasis Brain abscess, usually metastatic from the liver	Faecal–oral person-to-person or food contamination by cysts	Asexual binary tission	Primarily humans	Worldwide, but invasive form commoner in tropics
Naeglaria	Primary amoebic meningoencephalitis	Swimming in fresh water		Free living in soil and water	
Acanthamoeba	Naeglaria acute Acanthamoeba chronic	Unknown			

biopsy. Sometimes the parasite is accessible from other sites, such as trypanosomiasis and malaria in the blood, cysticercosis in the subcutaneous tissues, or *Trichinella spiralis* in striated muscle. A variety of immunological tests are available to look for antibodies or antigens in blood or CSF (Wilson et al 1991). Sensitivity and specificity of these tests varies from one centre to another. Each centre should establish its own norms. A problem with immunological tests from an endemic area is that the serological test may be positive in a proportion of healthy controls; the CSF test will however be negative, and a positive CSF test is much more significant than a positive serological

Table 17.5 Nematodes and trematodes

Type of worm	Disease	Definitive host	Intermediate host	Transmission to humans	Geographic distribution
Nematodes					
Tissue nematodes					
Angiostrongylias (Rat lungworm)	Angiostrongyliasis Cantonensis Eosinophilic meningitis in 97% of CNS infestation Encephalomyeloradiculitis in a small proportion	Cantonensis Rat (pulmonary artery and right heart)	1st: Molluscs 2nd: Freshwater shrimps, prawns, crabs, frogs which feed on molluscs	Eating raw molluscs snails and other carriers	South-east Asia and Western Pacific islands
Gnathostoma spinigerum	Gnathostomiasis Eosinophilic meningitis with prominent radiculomyeloencephalitis, often fatal	Gastric mucosa of dogs, cats	1st: Cyclops 2nd: Freshwater fish, frogs, snails, poultry fed on 1st and 2nd	Eating raw or partly cooked fish or poultry	South-east Asia
Filariasis					
Wuchereria bancrofti *Brugia malayi*	Wucheriasis or lymphatic filariasis CNS involvement uncommon. Usually due to migration of microfilariae through brain, causes headaches, focal deficits, and seizures	Humans	Mosquitoes	Mosquito bite	Throughout the tropics
Loa loa	Loiasis As for *W. bancrofti*, but more severe	Humans	Chrysops	Bite of the chrysops	West and central Africa
Trichinosis					
Trichinella spiralis	Trichinosis Meningoencephalitis, also cerebral infarcts and hemorrhages; may also contribute to seizures	Primarily rodents also pig and other mammals	None	Eating uncooked or partly cooked meat	Worldwide, but more important in USA and Europe than the tropics
Toxocara canis *Toxocara cati*	Toxocariasis (visceral larva migrans) Granulomas lead to seizures or focal deficits	Cats and dogs	None Eggs incubate in soil	Eating soil contaminated with eggs	Worldwide
Intestinal nematodes					
Strongyloides stercoralis	Strongyloidiasis. Disseminated strongyloidiasis secondary to massive acute infection in the immunodepressed results in meningo-encephalitis, cerebral microinfarcts and Gram-negative cerebral abscesses.	Human Sometimes free living adults in soil	None Eggs hatch in intestine. Rhabditiform larvae passed out in stools. Enter soil. Become infective filariform larvae	Filariform larvae in soil penetrate skin. Sometimes autoinfection. Rhabditiform larvae mature into filariform larvae in the intestine. These invade intestinal mucosa or perianal skin	Worldwide, especially tropics and subtropics and in immunosuppresed in temperate regions

Table 17.5 Contd.

Type of worm	Disease	Definitive host	Intermediate host	Transmission to humans	Geographic distribution
Trematodes (blood flukes)					
Schistosomatidae	Schistosomiasis (bilharziasis). Brain more commonly affected by *S. japonicum*. Acute infection, 2–3% have an encephalopathy Chronic (eggs + granulomas) present as SOL with focal seizures and hemiplegia in some	Human	Snail infected by miracidia which hatch from eggs deposited in water by stools or urine	Cercariae develop in snails from miracidia. These cerceriae are free swimming and and penetrate human skin	Worldwide
S. haematobium		Adult worms inhabit vesical plexus			Africa, Near and Middle East
S. mansoni		Inhabit inferior mesenteric veins			Central & South America, Africa, Middle East
S. japonicum		Inhabit superior meenteric veins			Far East
Other flukes					
Paragonimus westermani (Oriental lung fluke)	Paragonimiasis (endemic haemoptysis) Acute: meningo-encephalitis Chronic: granulomas	Man, dog, cat, pig, rat, wild carnivores	Crabs, crayfish infected by miracidia	Eating undercooked infected meat or crabs or playing crabs	Far East
Cestodes					
Taenia sodium	Cysticercosis (encysted larval form in tissues. Cyst contains single scolex) *Parenchymal*: live cysts, dying cysts or granulomas, 'encephalitis', miliary form, disseminated calcificaton. 50% or more of these forms have seizures. Meningeal: meningitis, arachnoidcysts, intraventricular cysts, hydrocephalus Epilepsy less frequent in meningeal form	Human	Usually pig Sometimes human	Human acquires cysticercosis by eating food contaminated by human faeces containing eggs. Occasionally autoinfection by gravid segments of worm returned to stomach by reverse peristalsis. Human acquires taeniasis by eating undercooked pork containing cysticerci	
Multiceps multiceps (dog tapeworm)	Coenurosis (cysts contain multiple scolices) Cysts	Dog	Mammals, herbivorous	Faecal–oral	Africa, USA, UK.
Echinococcus granulosus	Echinococciasis (multiple d. , nter cysts each containing several scolices) Usually solitary, large cysts—SOL epilepsy, in children. May be primary or secondary	Dog	Sheep, cattle, dogs, camels	Eating food contaminated by dog faeces containing ova	Areas of sheep and cattle raising with the help of dogs, i.e. East and South Africa Middle East, Central Europe, South America, Australia and New Zealand

Table 17.5   Contd.

Type of worm	Disease	Definitive host	Intermediate host	Transmission to humans	Geographic distribution
Echinococcus multilocularis	Usually in adults, secondary or metastatic from liver	Wolves, foxes, dog, cat	Rodents, Human also for both types		
Sparganum	Sparganosis or or plerocercoid larva of diphyllobothrium related tapeworms. Genus: spirometra. Cyst or granuloma	Dogs, cat	1st: Cyclops 2nd: Frogs	Drinking water containing cyclops bearing procercoid larvae or eating or coming in contact with infected frog	South-east Asia and east central Africa

one. The new molecular biological techniques have enabled the development of DNA probes which can identify the genome of the parasite.

Parasitic infections are difficult to treat, especially in the central nervous system. Prevention remains of paramount importance, and is usually feasible. The number of drugs available is limited, they are often toxic and organisms become resistant or render themselves inaccessible by encysting or developing a cuticle. Even if the organism is susceptible to the drug, massive release of foreign antigen in the brain may set up an immunological response causing cerebral oedema with raised intracranial pressure, which may be fatal. If the organism is in the eye and the patient is given a drug lethal to that organism, blindness may result. Nowhere are treatment difficulties better exemplified than in the case of cysticercosis. If there are dying cysts or granulomas in the brain, as suggested by contrast enhancement on the CT scan or oedema around the cysts, or granulomas, it may be wiser to treat the patient symptomatically only using antiepileptic drugs and perhaps non-steroidal anti-inflammatory agents (NSAIDs). If there are cysts in the brain, as shown on CT or MRI scans, and there is no surrounding oedema or contrast enhancement, then these cysts are considered to be alive and the patient should be given definitive drug treatment with caution. Albendazole or praziquantel should be started in small doses with liberal use of NSAIDs or even steroids and cerebral dehydrating measures and, of course, antiepileptic drugs. Some patients may die, even with such cautious treatment, because of the massive immunological reaction. If there is a cyst which is surgically accessible in the eye, it is

better to operate before giving drug treatment in order to preserve vision. In patients with meningitis, NSAIDs may be used prior to starting specific treatment. Racemose cysts in the subarachnoid space or the ventricles are difficult to diagnose and to treat, and surgical removal may be necessary. These cysts often lack scolices, and like other prescolicial forms of the parasite are not significantly affected by albendazole and praziquantel. Dead cysts, seen as punctate calcification on CT scan, are treated symptomatically if necessary. Before beginning treatment of any sort, it is always wise to recall that the disease may recover without treatment.

Approach to the patient with suspected infectious cause of epilepsy

In addition to facts usually elicited when taking a history of infection such as tuberculosis, enquiries should also be made about contact with other people with infectious disease now and in the past, travel, usual country of residence, occupation (especially involving contact with animals), pets, food habits (eating unwashed, unpeeled vegetables or raw meat, or milk), history of immunization, and any medication, whether allopathic, traditional or illicit.

Skin and subcutaneous tissues, eyes, ears and paranasal sinuses, lymph nodes, liver and spleen must be looked at particularly carefully for evidence of infection, in addition to the full physical examination of all systems. Immunosuppression must be enquired about and supporting evidence sought. Laboratory investigation may be extensive and should include consideration of all body fluids (blood, urine, stools, sputum, CSF, gastric aspirate) and possibly biopsy from skin, muscle, liver, rectum, lymph nodes or even brain.

Seizures are usually secondarily generalized and occur either with or without overt evidence of CNS infection. In both situations, non-infectious causes of seizure must always be considered. In the absence of overt CNS infection, the infectious causes of seizures are those which produce cysts, granulomas or chronic abscesses in the brain, whether bacterial, fungal or parasitic. Symptoms and signs of an intracranial space-occupying lesion are often absent.

When infection of the CNS is overt, seizures occur as part of one of the following neurological syndromes: acute pyogenic meningitis, acute lymphocytic meningitis, suppurative intracranial conditions with focal signs, chronic meningitis, or encephalitis.

Cerebral mass lesions

Infections causing cysts, granulomas and chronic abscess have been considered elsewhere.

Since the advent of CT scanning, there have been a number of reports from India of young patients with seizures in whom a CT scan has been done within a month of the last seizure (Joseph et al 1990, Sethi et al 1985, Goulatia et al 1987, Wadia et al 1987, Bhatia & Tandon 1988). The scan showed a small subcortical lesion less than 1 cm in diameter of hypo- or mixed density, ring or disc enhancing and surrounded by an area of hypo-intensity suggesting oedema. When some of these patients are treated for seizures with antiepileptic drugs alone, and a repeat CT scan is done 6–8 weeks afterwards, the lesions have often disappeared. Such lesions appear much more frequently in India than elsewhere. It is not known whether these lesions are the cause or the effect of the seizures. If these are the result of seizures possibly due to altered blood–brain barrier, it is hard to explain why they are not seen in other parts of the world. If they are the cause of the seizures, why should they disappear without specific treatment? A number of possibilities have been raised, e.g. tuberculoma, cysticercus, other parasitic lesions, abscess, focal encephalitis, vascular malformation, a gliotic scar, or tumour. It is thought that the seizure may make obvious an occult focus, or that an immunological phenomenon might be occurring in an inflammatory focus.

Although the majority of these lesions disappear in 6-8 weeks, some may take longer to resolve. A sound general approach therefore to such a lesion is that if there is no other evidence for a particular aetiology, and marked peri-lesional oedema is absent, antiepileptic drugs alone should be given, and a repeat CT scan done after 2 or 3 months. If the lesion still persists, anti-tuberculous or anti-cysticercal treatment or biopsy should be considered. When all lesions persisting after 3 months observation were biopsied, a Vellore group found that 22 out of 45 patients had cysticercosis and only four of 45 had tuberculomas (Joseph et al 1990). Interestingly, this group also found that 16 of 18 patients who were taken off drugs immediately after surgery had no seizures on follow-up from 4 to 30 months.

Cerebrovascular disease

Seizures are a prominent feature of certain kinds of stroke which are seen more commonly in developing countries. These include:

1. Cerebral embolism secondary to rheumatic heart disease, subacute bacterial endocarditis and congenital heart disease. The underlying heart disease often goes unrecognized until the patient presents with seizures. There may be no history of stroke.
2. Arteritis due to a variety of infections, particularly tuberculosis.
3. Intracranial thrombophlebitis (see section on infection).
4. Haemoglobinopathies such as sickle cell disease.
5. Eclampsia

Toxic and metabolic causes

Seizures may occur due to acute toxic or metabolic conditions. Alcoholism is as big a problem in developing countries as elsewhere. Pesticides are extensively used in agriculture in developing countries, and may cause chronic or acute intoxication. Acute intoxication is usually due to improper handling and storage of the chemicals. An illustrative example is the family of patients with epilepsy from Uttar Pradesh in India (Nag et al 1977). Eight members of the family were affected. Physical signs were few, except for extensor plantar responses. Seizures were imperfectly controlled despite adequate antiepileptic treatment. Only family members who ate wheat husks had generalized tonic-clonic seizures. It was found that the wheat sacks had been stored next to the pesticide containing 10% benzahexachlorine (BHC) and BHC residues were detected in the wheat. In the same area at about the same time, other cases of epilepsy occurred in association with more chronic encephalopathic symptoms, and it was found that BHC had been used as a food preservative (Khare et al 1977).

Plant poisons, whether ingested suicidally, therapeutically, accidentally or as stimulants rarely cause seizures, unless secondary to hypoglycaemia, cardiac arrhythmias, encephalopathy or respiratory arrest. Venomous bites and stings also rarely cause seizures unless secondary to cardiorespiratory collapse or a bleeding diathesis.

Other causes

Nutritional deficiency, though common in developing countries, rarely leads to seizures. An unusual kind of reflex epilepsy has been reported from Southern India, in which simple or complex partial seizures occur when hot water is poured rapidly over the head (Satishchandra et al 1988). Some of these patients may have spontaneous seizures. In a five-centre hospital collaborative study on epilepsy, hot water precipitated seizures in 10.1% of patients in Bangalore, 5.3% of patients in Madras, 1.2% of patients in Bombay, 0.3% of patients in Delhi and none in Calcutta (Tandon 1989).

Risk factors for epilepsy

In the foregoing sections are listed a number of factors which could cause seizures. Case control studies are necessary to evaluate the relative importance of these factors in a given population. One of the first such studies in a developing country was that carried out amongst 14 010 persons in

the Parsi community of Bombay (Bharucha et al 1988b). A history of febrile seizure was found to be the only factor statistically significantly associated with epilepsy. Birth trauma, CNS infection, and head injury were not significant factors, although this may have been due partly to the low power of a study of this size. It is interesting that in a five-centre hospital-based study of epilepsy in India in the era before CT scans, febrile convulsions were found in 6.5% of patients with epilepsy, birth trauma was found in 3.1% of patients, CNS infection in 3.4%, and head injury in 4.7% of patients with epilepsy (Tandon 1989).

HEALTH CARE FOR EPILEPSY IN DEVELOPING COUNTRIES

Medical personnel and practice

A fundamental difference between the treatment of epilepsy in developed and developing countries concerns the number of doctors practising and the relative proportion of hospital-based and primary care doctors. In Table 17.3 the population and population per physician is compared in 18 developing countries and the UK and USA. These figures are based on official government sources, which in some cases may over estimate the true number of practising doctors; for instance, Osuntokun (1977) stated that the doctor:patient ratio in most African countries was less than 1:20 000, and the figures may also be influenced by the high levels of underemployment or unemployment of doctors in some countries. Moreover, in many developing countries, the medical services are concentrated in the major cities, and the supply of doctors to rural areas may be even lower. The proportion of specialists/primary care physicians is also another important factor influencing medical practice. At one extreme, in the United States there are about 1200 neurologists, about one per 25 000 persons in the population. In many developing countries, a figure of one per 5 000 000 would not be unusual.

Investigatory facilities, considered routine in developed countries, such as EEG/CT/MRI/ biochemistry/serum antiepileptic drug-level monitoring may also be scarce in the developing world. Thus in Kenya, a developing country with a good health care record, in 1988 there was no CT nor facilities for serum level monitoring and EEG only in Nairobi; in Nigeria, the African country with the largest population, CT was available in only one centre. This scarcity applies widely in the developing world. It is a further irony that the proportion of the costs of medical care provided by Government sources is considerably less in developing compared with developed countries (as indeed is the total amount of money spent). For this reason, and in the absence of widespread health insurance, the high costs of medical care are proportionally borne much more heavily by the patient in the developing than the developed world.

The model of care for epilepsy in the developed world, which is medically led, hospital-specialist based, supported by sophisticated investigations, relatively disinterested in costs, is thus very different from that which applies in the developing world; yet it has been common practice to try to transplant treatment and health care programmes, which have evolved largely from hospital practice in developed countries to rural settings in the developing world.

Treatment gap

Perhaps it is not surprising therefore that the treatment of epilepsy is often deficient. Almost the only published indication of 'outcome' of treatment in developing countries has been the work on 'treatment gap' (Shorvon & Farmer 1988,

Ellison et al 1989). The treatment gap is defined as the percentage of persons with active epilepsy who at any time are not receiving treatment. This is an indirect approximation, simply calculated from an estimated prevalence figure of epilepsy 5/1000 (a conservative estimate), the assumption that patients will be taking monotherapy with standard daily regimens (e.g. 300 mg phenytoin, 600 mg carbamazepine, 90 mg phenobarbitone), and the available drug supply figures to a country (based on imported and locally produced industrial and government figures). These calculations are a guide only, and are subject to bias in several ways; nevertheless, they give a rough approximation of the success of health care services in the provision of treatment.

In Table 17.6 are shown treatment gap figures for three developing countries; as can be seen, in these countries between 80 and 93% of all cases with active epilepsy are untreated at any one time, and very similar figures have been produced for other developing countries. A direct measurement of the number of untreated patients has been possible in two recent house-to-house surveys in developing countries. In the ICBERG survey of 72 121 persons in Ecuador, 881 persons with active epilepsy were identified of whom 85% were not taking and 71% had never taken antiepileptic drugs (Placencia et al 1991d). In a parallel ICBERG survey of 11 497 persons in Turkey, 29% of identified cases were taking antiepileptic drugs and a further 27% had been treated in the

Table 17.6   Treatment gap figures in three developing countries

Country	I: Estimated number of persons with epilepsy*	II: Number of patients receiving drug treatment[†]	III: Treatment gap[‡]
Pakistan	450 000	22 000	95%
Philippines	270 000	14 000	95%
Ecuador	55 000	11 000	80%

  * The number of persons with epilepsy is estimated on the basis of a standard prevalence rate of 5/1000 of the population (1985 figures, based on the Economist 1987); this is a crude prevalence rate, not age adjusted, and is a minimum estimate of the true prevalence of epilepsy.
  [†] The total number of persons receiving drug treatment is an estimate derived from drug supply figures, institutional consumption figures, Government production figures and local data. It is an approximation only, assuming standard dosage regimens and monotherapy.
  [‡] The treatment gap is defined as the proportion of those with active epilepsy without treatment at any one time (calculated as I–II × 100/I).
  Derived from Shorvon & Farmer 1988.

past (Guvener et al 1991). Thus, direct survey results and the indirect treatment gap calculations demonstrate that most cases of epilepsy are untreated; this can be taken as a fundamental index of the failure of medical provision.

That treatment is not reaching the majority of persons with epilepsy in developing countries is indisputable; but the reasons are complex. The large treatment gap reflects both a failure of the medical system to identify cases and also a failure to deliver treatment to identified cases. Inadequate case identification may be due to the attitudes and expectations of the patients, the practice of the medical and paramedical personnel, government health policy (which may give chronic conditions such as epilepsy a low priority), a lack of public knowledge and understanding, and poorly organized medical services and referral mechanisms. A failure to deliver treatment to identified cases may also be due to public or professional misunderstanding concerning the nature of drug treatment (e.g. the need for continuous therapy, good compliance), poorly organized medical systems, absence of medical notes or records (precluding effective follow up), inadequate or unreliable drug supply, and the attitudes and practices of patients.

Cost is an obvious factor, although treatment gap figures for the cheapest drugs are in fact worse than those for the most expensive (Shorvon & Farmer 1988), and many patients spend considerable amounts of family money on obtaining traditional cures. It is not uncommon in Africa for instance to hear of a patient travelling hundreds of miles, donating cattle or treasured items to a healer. Attitudes to treatment are also very important; a patient's experience of western medicine may be confined to the cure of infection by antibiotics, and alien to the concept that drug treatment may need to be continued on a daily basis for long periods. Traditional beliefs about the nature of epilepsy and its treatment are important, and the skilful practitioner will not try to contradict these beliefs but rather to incorporate them; indeed there is no reason why a spiritual as well as a biological reason for an illness or a treatment should not co-exist. Traditional practitioners are often held in high regard, as they are from the local people, often resident in the village, and can relate to the local culture more easily than can a medical doctor with a scientific training and different background.

A particularly important reason for treatment failure in many developing countries is inadequate drug supply. It is common for drugs to be available only irregularly in rural pharmacies, with interruptions in supply usually due to bureaucratic or logistical inefficiency. The result may be frequent cessation or switching of medication. This problem will of course interfere totally with the successful treatment of epilepsy. The concept of the 'essential drugs list' was introduced by the WHO in recognition of this issue for a variety of illnesses.

The structure of health care systems for epilepsy in the developing world

A recent report from an ICBERG workshop considered all aspects of the management of epilepsy in developing countries (Shorvon et al 1991), and a number of particular issues were emphasized. Firstly, the complementary roles of the paramedical health workers and doctors were examined. The paramedical health worker in many developing countries has a central role in epilepsy management. This is particularly so where there is a relative shortage of medical staff, and a high incidence of acute illness, especially infection, which demand more immediate medical attention than chronic conditions such as epilepsy. The paramedic, by being closely involved with and living in the community, is also often in an ideal position to identify possible cases, and encourage their attendance in a medical clinic. Because of their acceptance by local people, the paramedic may be instrumental in reducing stigma, and their understanding of local attitudes and practices may allow them to instruct about epilepsy in a way which is comprehensible and compatible with the local culture. The paramedical worker can also carry out long-term monitoring of treatment and counselling. The doctors role in the treatment of epilepsy in rural areas is complementary to that of the paramedic. He must confirm the diagnosis of cases presenting to him, classify the case, identify aetiology where appropriate, and initiate treatment. He should be available for re-referral for problems and where complications arise, but in most settings is not involved in continuous follow up at a routine level. He must organize clinics, and mobile out-reach clinics may be particularly helpful in rural areas (Watts 1989). The doctor should monitor and train paramedical workers. Both the doctor and the paramedical workers should be involved in public education and in promoting health care programmes.

Many rural health care delivery programmes fail because interventions are aimed at single issues and do not address the complexities of rural health as a whole (birth control programmes are a classic example); an integrated approach to treatment is a critically important point. For epilepsy control, a programme must be multi-pronged, addressing social and medical issues at a local level concerning the patient, the community and the medical system. In addition there should be a clear division of responsibilities of the public and private sector agencies involved. Social services, medical services, voluntary agencies, government, industry are all important players. A public health promotion campaign is also an important ingredient to a successful health care programme.

Government has a role in setting up medical systems, controlling medical manpower, training, ensuring drug availability and quality control, setting drug costs, and determining health care priorities. Government should also be encouraged to set legislation to promote rather than restrict the well being of the epileptic patient; although in many countries the law remains highly restrictive (Mani & Rangan 1990). Non-governmental organizations are also crucial in determining the quality of health care. Their advantages over government are usually less bureaucracy, more enthusiasm and motivation, efficiency, and often an absence of political interference and wide acceptance in the population. Their disadvantages are lack of continuity, often small size and limited scope, and financial uncertainty. Non-government organizations which might be involved in developing a health care programme for epilepsy include: professional medical bodies, international medical bodies, philanthropic and religious organisations and clubs, patient groups, communication media, industry and business, and educational institutions. Each may have a role in an integrated epilepsy programme.

Two examples of model epilepsy programmes have been recently reported from Africa, in which some of these principles are illustrated.

Malawi (Watts 1989)

Dr A. E. Watts, single handed in a charitable hospital in a rural area of Malawi, designed a programme which balanced efficacy with simplicity of use. The model required: adequate publicity, availability of treatment, simple treatment programme, adequate drug supply, treatment without charge, monthly clinics to review patients, review each month by the same member of staff, and out-reach clinics. Treatment was using a simple standardized regimen of phenobarbitone or phenytoin, adjusted for age, according to simple treatment protocols. An emphasis was placed on education of the patient on the first visit about the cause and treatment of epilepsy, often taking the form of: 1. epilepsy is due to a scar on the brain; 2. it takes time for this scar to heal, and so treatment must be long-lasting; 3. fits may not stop immediately, but take months, and the dose of drug may need to be adjusted, and the patient should not be discouraged during this time; 4. side effects; and 5. avoid alcohol, but otherwise there are no dietary restrictions (traditionally certain foods are prohibited).

Publicity was extensive via an action committee and other informal networks, and after a short time began to appear from long distances. The results of this simple programme were impressive. A total of 254 cases were seen in the first 18 months of this programme and 172 (68%) were still attending after 6 months. Attendance was 91–98% in each of the monthly clinics at the hospital and 71–88% in the mobile clinic. Before treatment, 88% had had seizures at least once a month. Of those followed up, 56% were seizure free at 6 months, and 40% at 12 months, and in only 15% were the seizures not improved considerably. This programme was also notable for a number of other reasons: reliance on non-governmental organizations, the success of local publicity for case identification, simple treatment regimens, attempts to counsel patients about treatment without contradicting local beliefs, reliable drug supply, and limited resources.

Kenya (ICBERG study) (Kaamugisha & Feksi 1988, Feksi et al 1991a,b)

A more ambitious project was initiated in Nakuru, a provincial hospital in Rift valley province in Kenya, by Feksi and colleagues, under the auspices of ICBERG. This consisted first of a screening process (using the key informant method, which is a highly cost-effective method of case finding in rural settings), in which 302 patients with untreated active tonic-clonic epilepsy were identified and who agreed to take part in the treatment programme. The essential features of the treatment programme were: 1. the allocation of a health worker to each patient, who visited the patient fortnightly initially and then monthly, whose role was to provide information and explanation and to monitor treatment compliance; 2. monthly hospital visits where seizure control was reviewed (by a non-specialist doctor—who for research purposes was overseen by a senior specialist); 3. simple regimens of carbamazepine or phenobarbitone, with dosages adjusted according to simple protocols; and 4. urgent recall to the clinic for side effects. Again, the results of this treatment programme were excellent; 82% completed 12 months of follow up, 53% of cases were rendered seizure free in the 6–12-month period of treatment (i.e. after dosage adjustments), and 26% markedly improved. This project is notable for several reasons: collaboration between government and non-government agencies, a large public information campaign, emphasis on health worker role, counselling and information which did not compromise local beliefs, a multidisciplinary research effort, simple treatment regimens, and reliable drug supply.

In both these programmes, treatment was highly successful in spite of the fact that the epilepsy was often long-standing, and also that the pre-treatment seizures frequency was often high (usually more than one per month). The successful outcome of these large-scale integrated health programmes in epilepsy should provide a model for other projects in other developing countries.

REFERENCES

Bharucha N E, Bharucha E P, Bharucha A E et al 1988a Prevalence of epilepsy in the Parsi community of Bombay. Epilepsia 29: 111–115

Bharucha N E, Bharucha E P, Bharucha A E, Bhise A V, Schoenberg B S 1988b Case-control study of epilepsy in the Parsi community of Bombay. A population-based study. Neurology 38: 312

Bhatia R, Tandon P N 1988 Solitary 'microlesions' in CT: A clinical study and follow-up. Neurology India 36: 139–150

Chandra B 1988 Epilepsy in Indonesia. In: Laidlaw J, Richens A, Oxley J (eds) A textbook of epilepsy. Churchill Livingstone, Edinburgh, p 511–517

Chiofalo N, Kirschbaum A, Fuentes A, Cordero M, Madsen J 1979 Prevalence of epilepsy in Melipilla, Chile. Epilepsia 20: 261–266

Cowan L D, Bodensteiner J B, Leviton A, Doherty L 1989 Prevalence of the epilepsies in children and adolescents. Epilepsia 30: 94–106

Dada T 1970 Epilepsy in Lagos, Nigeria. African Journal of Medical Science 1: 161–184

Economist 1987 The world in figures. The Economist Publications Ltd, London

Ellison R H, Placencia M, Guvener A et al 1989 A program of transcultural studies of epilepsy: outline of study objectives and design. Advances in Epileptology 17: 432–434

Feksi A T, Kaamugisha J, Gatiti S, Sander J W A S, Shorvon S D l991a A comprehensive community epilepsy programme: the Nakuru project. Epilepsy Research 8: 252–259

Feksi A T, Kaamugisha J, Sander J W A S, Gatiti S, Shorvon S D 1991 Comprehensive primary health care antiepileptic drug treatment in rural and sermi-urban Kenya. Lancet 337: 406–409

Garcia-Pedroza F, Rubio-Donnadieu F, Garcia-Ramos G, Escobedo-Rios F, Gonzales-Cortes A 1983 Prevalence of epilepsy in children: Tlalpan, Mexico City, Mexico. Neuroepidemiology 2: 16–23

Giel R 1970 The problem of epilepsy in Ethiopia. Tropical and Geographical Medicine 22: 439–442

Gomez J G, Arciniegas E, Torres J 1978 Prevalence of epilepsy in Bogota, Colombia. Neurology 28: 90–95

Goulatia R K, Verma A, Mishra N K, Ahuja G K 1987 Disappearing CT lesions in epilepsy. Epilepsia 28: 523–527

Gutierrez H, Rubio F, Escobedo F, Gonzalez A, Heron J 1980 Prevalencia de epilepsia en ninos de edad escolar de una communidad urbana de la Ciudad de Mexico. Gaceta Medica Mexicana 116: 497–501

Guvener A, Isik A, Ilbars Z et al 1991 The prevalence and phenomenology of epilepsy in a community based survey in 3 districts in central Anatolia, Turkey. Submitted for publication.

Haerer A F, Anderson D W, Schoenberg B S 1986 Prevalence and clinical features of epilepsy in a bi-racial United States population. Epilepsia 27: 66–75

Hauser W A, Hesdorffer D C 1990 Epilepsy: frequency, causes and consequences. Demos Publications, New York

Joseph T, Ghosh S, Chandy S M 1990 Study of the pathogenesis of focal epilepsy in India. Abstract No. 026 presented at the symposium on Neurosciences and Biotechnology and Meeting of the Indian Academy of

Neurosciences Society of India. New Delhi, India, Dec 12–14. 1990. Cited in Mani K S, Rangan G 1991.

Kaamugisha J, Feksi A T 1988 Determining the prevalence of epilepsy in the semi-urban population of Nakuru, Kenya, comparing two independent methods not apparently used before in epilepsy studies. Neuroepidemiology 7: 115–121

Khare S B, Rizvi A G, Shukla O P, Singh R R P, Prakash O, Mishra V D 1977 Epidemic outbreak of neuromuscular manifestations due to chronic BHC poisoining. Jounal of the Association of Physicians of India 25: 215–222

Koul R, Razdan S, Motta A 1988 Prevalence and pattern of epilepsy in rural Kashmir, India. Epilepsia 29: 116–122

Isaac M K 1987 Collaborative study on severe mental morbidity. Indian Council of Medical Research and Development of Science and Technology, New Delhi, India 1987. Cited in Mani K S, Rangan G 1991.

Li Shi-chuo, Schoemberg B S, Chung-Cheng W, Xueming-Ming C, Shu-Shun Z, Bolis C L, 1985 Epidemiology of epilepsy in urban areas of the People's Republic of China. Epilepsia 26: 391–394

Mani K S, Rangan G 1990 Asian aspects. In: Dam M, Gram L (eds) Comprehensive epileptology. Raven Press, New York, p 781–793

Marino R, Cukiert A, Pinho E 1987 Epidemiological aspects of epilepsy in Sao Paulo, Brazil. Advances in Epileptology 16: 759–764

Mathai K V 1971 Final report on investigations on methods for the rehabilitation of persons disabled by convulsive disorder. Department of Neurological Science, Christian Medical College and Hospital, Vellore, India

Nag D, Singh G C, Senon S 1977 Epilepsy epidemic due to benzahexachlorine. Tropical and Geographical Medicine 29: 229–232

Olivares L 1972 Epilepsy in Mexico. In: Milton A, Hauser A (eds) The epidemiology of epilepsy: a workshop. NINDS Monograph no 14. DHEW, Washington DC, p 53–78

Osuntokun B O, Adeuja A O G, Nottidge V A et al 1987 Prevalence of the epilepsies in Nigerian Africans: a community-based study. Epilepsia 23: 272–279

Placencia M, Suarez J, Crespo F et al 1991a A large scale study of epilepsy in Ecuador: methodological aspects. Neuroepidemiology (In press)

Placencia M, Shorvon S D, Paredes V et al 1991b Epileptic seizures in an Andean region of Ecuador: Incidence and prevalence and regional variation. Brain (In press)

Placencia M, Sander J W A S, Ellison R H, Shorvon S D, Cascante S M 1991c Validation of a screening questionnaire for the detection of epileptic seizures in epidemiological studies. Brain (In press)

Placencia M, Sander J W A S Shorvon S D, Cascante S M 1991d A prospective 12 month study of antiepileptic drug treatment with carbamazepine and phenobarbitone in a rural area of highland Ecuador. Submitted for publication

Sander J W A S, Shorvon S D 1987 Incidence and prevalence studies in epilepsy and their methodological problems: a review. Journal of Neurology, Neurosurgery and Psychiatry 50: 829–839

Sander J W A S, Hart Y M, Johnson A L, Shorvon S D 1990 The National General Practice Study of Epilepsy: newly diagnosed epileptic seizures in a general population. Lancet 336: 1267–1271

Satishchandra P, Shivaramakrishna A, Kaliaperunal V G, Schoenberg B S 1988 Hot water epilepsy: A variant of reflex epilepsy in Southern India. Epilepsia 29: 52–56

Senanayake N 1987 Epilepsy control in a developing country. Ceylon Medical Journal 32: 181–199

Sethi P K, Kumar B P, Maden V S, Mohan V 1985 Appearing and disappearing CT scan abnormalities and seizures. Journal of Neurology, Neurosurgery and Psychiatry 48: 866–869

Shamanski S L, Glaser G H 1979 Socioeconomic characteristics of childhood seizure disorders in the New Haven area. Epilepsia 20: 457–474

Shorvon S D, Farmer P J 1988 Epilepsy in developing countries: a review of epidemiological, socio-cultural and treatment aspects. Epilepsia 29: S36–S54

Shorvon S D, Hart Y M, Sander J W A S, van Andel F 1991 The management of epilepsy in developing countries: an ICBERG manual. ICSS 175, Royal Society of Medicine Publications, London

Shridharan R, Radhakrishnan K, Ashok P P, Mouse M E 1986 Epidemiological and clinical study of epilepsy in Benghazi, Libya. Epilepsia 27: 60–65

Srinivasan K, Natarajan M 1974 Cerebral venous and arterial thrombosis in pregnancy and puerperium: a study of 90 patients. Neurology India 22: 131–140

Tandon P N 1989 Epilepsy in India (Report based on a multicentric study of epidemiology of epilepsy carried out as a PL 480 funded project of the Indian Council of Medical Research). ICMR Publication, New Dehli, India

Volpe J J 1981 Non-bacterial intracranial infections In: Neurology of the new born, major problems in clinical paediatrics. Saunders, Philadelphia, vol 22, p 489–535

Wadia R S, Makhale C N, Kelkar A V, Grant K B 1987 Focal epilepsy in India with special reference to lesions showing rings and disc like enhancement on contrast computerized tomography. Journal of Neurology, Neurosurgery and Psychiatry 50: 1298–1301

Watts A E 1989 A model for managing epilepsy in a rural community in Africa. British Medical Journal 298: 805–807

Wilson J D, Braunwald E, Isselbacher K J et al 1991 Harrison's principles of internal medicine, 12th edn, McGraw–Hill, New York, p 775–778

Zielinski J J 1974 Epidemiology and medicosocial problems of epilepsy in Warsaw. Final Report on research program no. 19–P–58325–F–01. Psychoneurological Institute, Warsaw, p 50–55

18. Epilepsy and mental handicap

J. Corbett

INTRODUCTION

Epilepsy is one of the most frequent additional major handicaps in people with mental retardation, coexistence of the two impairments tending to compound the disability rather than being merely additive. Even when the symptom is well controlled, the label of epilepsy often places the person with a mental handicap at an increased social disadvantage. It is therefore important that the handicapped person has access to the same modern services for the treatment of epilepsy as his or her follows which will enable him or her to live as normal a life as possible.

No longer is epilepsy associated with the inevitability of mental deterioration. Although subtle impairments of cognitive function are seen in people receiving long-term treatment, marked and sustained deterioration, following a period of apparently normal development, is only seen in a minority. Most people with well-controlled seizures function within the normal range of intelligence.

PREVALENCE

The frequency of epilepsy in people with intellectual impairment provides a good indicator of the degree of underlying cerebral dysfunction and hence the organicity of the learning difficulties. The percentage of people having more than one seizure in the past year increases progressively with the degree of retardation. Estimates are most readily available for children of school age, where a number of studies has shown that epilepsy defined in this way occurs in between 0.4% and 0.7% (Ross & Peckham 1983, Corbett & Pond 1986).

In children with mild mental retardation (IQ 50–76) a rate between 3% and 6% (depending on whether simple or complicated seizure patterns are seen) has been reported from the National Child Development Study (Peckham 1974).

In people with learning disability who were in contact with mental handicap services, most estimates were derived from institutional studies and these were influenced by the fact that severe epilepsy was one cause of long-term hospitalization.

Recently the pattern has changed, with a move towards community care, and there are now two epidemiological studies related to epilepsy and mental retardation which provide more accurate data (Corbett et al 1975, Richardson et al 1981). These are both based on case register studies, in Camberwell in South London and Aberdeen respectively, and include long-term follow-up data extending into early adult life. Although comprising somewhat different age and IQ-related population samples, the findings from these two studies are remarkably similar and provide a clearer picture of epilepsy and mental handicap than was previously available.

In Camberwell, for children under the age of 14 functioning in the severely retarded range (IQ <50), the percentage with seizures in the year prior to the initial study was nearly 20%, with a lifelong history of seizures in 30%. In children with the most severe brain damage, functioning in the profoundly handicapped range (IQ <20), almost 50% had had a seizure sometime during life.

When this cohort of 150 children was followed up for 14 years (until 14–28 years of age) the number still suffering from epilepsy (defined as at least one seizure in the year prior to study) was similar. Although the seizures had remitted in a number, they were replaced by a similar proportion who developed seizures for the first time in adolescence (Corbett 1983).

These findings were confirmed in the Aberdeen study. The population, which comprised more mildly retarded people than in Camberwell, was followed up until a minimum of 22 years of age: 24% had a history of persistent seizures, which had occurred in 19% in the preschool years and 13% in each subsequent period of early-, late- and postschool years. Of the young people with *severe* mental retardation, that is with an IQ of less than 50, 44% had experienced one or more seizures by the age of 22 years compared with 19% of those with IQs of 50 or more who were in contact with the mental retardation services. For those with some history of seizures there was no significant association between IQ and degree of seizure impairment, but 40% had experienced seizures for more than 10 years and only 21% for less than one year; attesting to the chronicity of epilepsy in people with a mental handicap.

AETIOLOGY

Epilepsy and mental retardation are outward manifestations of a common underlying brain dysfunction and the age at which they are first seen gives a guide to both underlying pathology and prognosis. Some of the main syndromes associated with epilepsy are listed in Table 18.1.

Convulsions with onset in the first year of life associated with gross evidence of pre- or perinatal brain damage have a poor prognosis for subsequent mental development and persistence of seizures (Matsumoto et al 1983, Cavazzuti et al 1984). The same general principle applies with infantile spasms occurring between 3 and 18 months of age (Jeavons et al 1973, Lombroso 1983) and in the severe myoclonic epilepsies of early childhood, particularly the Lennox–Gastaut syndrome (onset 1 to 6 years) (O'Donohoe 1985). In each case, the progress tends to be worse if the epilepsy is symptomatic of some underlying brain pathology such as congenital malformation, perinatal brain damage, infection, biochemical disorder or progressive condition e.g. tuberous sclerosis.

The same poor prognosis may be anticipated in cases of infantile or febrile convulsion associated with status epilepticus and encephalopathy. In many of these situations it is difficult to distinguish between the effects of the underlying neuropathology on intellectual functioning and the damaging effect of subsequent seizures, particularly if these are frequent or prolonged.

The apparently beneficial effect of steroids in infantile spasms and other difficult-to-control epilepsies of early childhood (Corbett et al 1975, Snead et al 1983) suggests a specific link with biochemical changes occurring in the brain during seizures, and supports the idea that the seizures themselves may play a part in further damaging the brain. However, ACTH (adrenocorticotrophic hormone) tends to be of most benefit in 'idiopathic' infantile spasms which are likely to have a better prognosis.

PREVENTION

There is considerable scope for the prevention of mental retardation by early and energetic prophylaxis of prolonged infantile convulsions; the early diagnosis and treatment of bacterial meningitides; protection of the head from repeated injury in myoclonic astatic epilepsy in childhood; the early recognition and treatment of subconvulsive status (minor status epilepticus); and increased awareness of the iatrogenic dangers of prolonged antiepileptic medication to the developing brain. It is conceivable that if our present knowledge of the potential for prevention of childhood epilepsy was to be effectively applied in practice this would be one of the most important contributions to the medical prevention of mental retardation.

Conversely, it follows that strategies primarily directed to preventing underlying brain damage leading to mental retardation will have a significant impact on the overall prevalence of epilepsy. These will include general improvements in antenatal care and maternal screening to prevent genetic disorders; reduction in perinatal morbidity resulting from prematurity, anoxia, intracerebral haemorrhage, biochemical disorders such as hypoglycaemia and hypocalcaemia and infections. Postnatal prevention will comprise infantile screening and prevention of later onset encephalopathies resulting from dehydration, infection and head injury.

Table 18.1   Epilepsy particularly associated with specific mental retardation syndromes

	Epilepsy	West syndrome	Lennox–Gastaut syndrome	Epilepsy with onset in later childhood or adolescence
Perinatal brain injury	+		+	
Metabolic abnormalities				
Phenylketonuria	+	+	+	
Maple Syrup urine disease	+	+		
Hyperornithaemia	+	+		
Isovaleric acidaemia	+	+		
Non-ketotic hyperglycaemia	+	+		
Pyridoxine dependency	+	+		
Leucine-sensitive hypoglycaemia	+	+	+	
Tay–Sachs disease	+	+		
Lipoidosis GM 1 & GM 3	+		+	
Metachromatic leucodystrophy	+		+	+
Homocysteinuria			+	
Dysplastic conditions				
Tuberous sclerosis	+	+	+	+
Sturge–Weber syndrome	+	+	+	+
Megalencephaly	+		+	
Other cerebral malformations	+	+	+	
Aicardi syndrome	+	+		
Prenatal infections				
Cytomegalovirus	+	+		
Syphillis	+	+		
Toxoplasmosis	+	+		
Postnatal infections				
Purulent meningitis	+		+	+
Acute encephalitis	+		+	+
Subacute sclerosing panencephalitis	+		+	
Postimmunization encephalopathy	+	+		
Post-traumatic	+			+
Chromosomal abnormalities				
Down syndrome		+		
Autistic syndromes	+	+		+
Others				
Retts syndrome	+			+

DIAGNOSIS AND TREATMENT

The general principles of diagnosis and treatment in people with a mental handicap are similar to those employed in people with epilepsy who are not otherwise disabled. However, a number of general and specific points do need to be borne in mind.

In the past, health and social services for those with a mental handicap were predominantly provided separately from the mainstream services. This has led to a labelling of people as 'the mentally handicapped' in a similar fashion to the labelling of people as 'epileptics' rather than as

people first. A major consequence has been that people with a mental handicap and epilepsy have tended to be denied access to specialized services for the investigation and treatment of epilepsy. This been compounded by the tendency to base specialized services for people with mental handicap in institutions which have also been their only home.

With an increasing trend towards community care, there is both an increasing recognition of the need to improve access of people with mental handicap to generic services but it has also meant that some people with epilepsy in the community who have not needed admission to institutions have had difficulty in obtaining services for epilepsy. This situation will only be resolved by improving the education of personnel working in the primary health care, social services and specialized hospital services about both epilepsy and mental retardation.

Greatest importance will be attached to the developmental history and description of the person's skills, behaviour and additional handicaps in interview with the parents or carer of the handicapped person. It must be remembered that there are likely, by definition, to be difficulties in obtaining a clear account from the disabled persons themselves of subjective experiences associated with seizures. The account obtained from an observer will be influenced by pre-existing neurological abnormality giving rise, for example, to other forms of movement disorder such as motor stereotypes or tics. Absence attacks or brief complex partial seizures are particularly difficult to detect in people whose attention and concentration may be impaired for other reasons. Ictal events with a basis in the temporal lobe or elsewhere in the limbic system may be profoundly disturbing to the handicapped person who is unable to give an account of the subjective experience. The introduction of ambulatory monitoring has produced evidence that, while the seizure itself may be quite brief, prolonged aggressive outbursts and other disturbed restless behaviour may be seen pre- or postictally.

Because of the difficulty in obtaining subjective accounts of the seizures and carrying out EEGs it was said, in the past, that temporal lobe epilepsy did not occur in people with mental handicap. It is clear that this is not the case: with careful observation and the help of EEG technicians with particular experience of mentally handicapped people, most can be trained to wear EEG leads without the need for sedation or anaesthesia. In occasional cases, where the person is very disturbed or frightened by the investigations, light anaesthesia while the leads are being applied with recording continuing into the recovery phase may be preferable to sedation with barbiturates or epileptogenic major tranquillizers, which may only increase the disturbed behaviour. Blood may also be taken at this time for screening of the more common mental retardation syndromes and for antiepileptic drug levels.

TREATMENT

As with non-handicapped people, the mainstay of treatment of the seizure disorder is antiepileptic drug therapy, but it should be remembered that young handicapped people are particularly vulnerable to isolated seizures or even self-limiting episodes. For example, febrile convulsions may occur in early childhood in those with pre-existing brain damage, and isolated seizures in adolescence occur in up to 30% of severely handicapped people with symptoms of childhood autism. In each case a careful judgement needs to be made between the advantages of early treatment limiting the chance of recurrence, with reduction in parental or staff anxiety, and the disadvantages of committing a person who already has learning difficulties to lengthy treatment with drugs which may suppress brain activity and impair learning further.

It is always essential to consider alternative or additional strategies of management which will reduce the need to depend totally on pharmacological treatments. First and most essential is the reduction of anxiety in the child's caring network and a realization that the presence of a handicapped child in the family will have already been experienced as a partial bereavement. The occurrence of seizures, particularly of a generalized tonic-clonic variety, is likely to compound this anxiety. A parent may take a handicapped child in to their own bed for fear that they may not awake when seizures occur at night and this may lead to increased anxiety when the dependency needs cannot be met. This may engender fear in the child and contribute to an increase in seizure frequency; these anxieties have to be weighed against the fact that seizures are now the main cause of death in childhood in the severely and profoundly handicapped.

Such considerations will extend to the person's total network of dependent relationships and care staff and teachers may, understandably, be even more reluctant than parents to allow the handicapped person the dignity of risk to lead as normal a life as possible while maintaining sensible precautions.

Nowadays, swimming with staff trained in both life saving and the emergency treatment of seizures, respite care in homelike environments or with foster families who are familiar with the child's individual needs and whom parents can trust, and a range of other normative experiences should be available. These will not only enrich the quality of the disabled person's life, but by reducing anxiety help to minimize seizures.

The role of diet and behavioural strategies of management of seizures remain controversial and experimental. There is little doubt that in some brain-damaged people sensitivity to particular dietary components, such as food additives, gluten and stimulants, may provoke both episodic behaviour disturbance and precipitate seizures.

In some handicapped people with drug-resistant seizures a trial of ketogenic diet using medium triclyceride oil may be considered (De Vivo 1983 and O'Donohoe 1985). It is also well established that even quite severely handicapped people can learn strategies to avoid seizure precipitants and abort attacks. It is, however, generally true that in our present state of knowledge these techniques can only very rarely be relied upon as the sole strategy of seizure management and may be more usefully viewed as an adjuvant to drug treatment, rather than an alternative.

COMPLICATIONS

A distinction must be made between the complications of epilepsy and the treatment of secondary handicaps associated with mental retardation and the underlying neurological damage. An understanding of the interaction between these influences calls for careful detective work and assessment of the situation in an individual patient.

It is well recognized that the side-effects of antiepileptic medication, such as slowing, inattention, apparent confusion, restlessness, dysarthria, ataxia and movement disorder, may be difficult to distinguish from the signs of underlying neurological disorder (Reynolds & Travers 1974). It is likely that the damaged brain is more vulnerable to the side-effects of antiepileptic medication. Phenobarbitone can provoke hyperkinetic and irritable aggressive behaviour. Prolonged use of phenytoin may lead to a 'subacute encephalopathy' with few gross neurological signs and serum antiepileptic drug levels within the normal range (Corbett et al 1985). Diazepam derivatives may release disinhibited or aggressive behaviour and, with sustained use, tolerance develops, so that these compounds may become ineffective in the treatment of status epilepticus.

Adverse behavioural and cognitive side-effects occur in a minority of people receiving carbamazepine and sodium valproate and there are many interactions between these drugs which need to be borne in mind. There is a need for monitoring and constant re-evaluation using careful records to reduce the number of drugs to a minimum.

Finally, little is known about the side-effects of long-term antiepileptic drug treatment. People tend to be labelled as 'epileptic' long after their seizures have remitted, and judicious and careful withdrawal should be considered after a seizure-free period of 2 to 3 years, avoiding vulnerable periods of brain development such as the adolescent growth spurt.

A small minority of people with epilepsy, receiving long-term medication, show either progressive cognitive deterioration or arrest in development. Recent research suggests that this is more likely to occur in people with pre-existing brain damage and particularly complicated and drug-resistant seizure patterns. As mentioned earlier, a number of factors may be incriminated. These tend to interact so that it may be difficult to tease them out in an individual patient. This may add to the burden of handicap but severe impairment is fortunately rare and it must constantly be restated that epilepsy is not inevitably linked with mental deterioration or abnormality of personality.

CONCLUSION

It can be seen that there is a close association between seizure disorders and mental retardation. This presents a particular challenge in terms of prevention and treatment and an increased awareness and sensitivity on the part of primary health care workers, paediatricians, psychiatrists and neurologists meeting the needs of disabled people. It also necessitates a continuing dialogue with community mental handicap teams who will be concerned with linking these services.

REFERENCES

Cavuzzuti G B, Ferrari P, Lalla M 1984 Follow-up study of 482 cases with convulsive disorder in the first year of life. Developmental Medicine & Child Neurology 26: 425–437

Corbett J A 1983 Epilepsy and mental retardation—a follow-up study. In: Parsonage M, Grant R H E, Craig A G et al (eds) Advances in epileptology. XIVth Epilepsy International Symposium. Raven Press, New York, p 207–214

Corbett J A, Harris R, Robinson R 1975 Epilepsy. In: Wortis J (ed) Mental retardation and developmental disabilities vol VII. Raven Press, New York, p 79–111

Corbett J A, Trimble M R, Nicol T 1985 Behavioural and cognitive impairments in children with epilepsy; the long term effects of anticonvulsant therapy. Journal of American Academy of Child Psychiatry 24: 17–23

Corbett J A, Pond D A 1986 The management of epilepsy. In: Craft M, Bicknell J, Hollis S (eds) Mental handicap. Baillière Tindall Cox, London

De Vivo D C 1983 How to use other drugs (steroids) and the ketogenic diet. In: Maselli P L, Pippenger C E, Penry J K (eds) Antiepileptic drug therapy in paediatrics. New York, Raven Press, p 283–292

Jeavons P M, Bower B D, Dimitrakoudi M 1973 Long term prognosis of 150 cases of 'West's Syndrome'. Epilepsia 141: 153–164

Lombroso C T 1983 A prospective study of infantile spasms; clinical and therapeutic correlations. Epilepsia 24: 135–158

O'Donohoe N V 1985 Epilepsies of childhood, 2nd edn. Butterworths, London

Matsumoto A, Watanabe K, Sugiura M, Negoro, Takaesu E, Iwase K 1983 Long term prognosis of convulsive disorders in the first year of life: mental and physical development and seizure persistence. Epilepsia 24: 321–329

Peckham C S 1974 National child development study (1958 cohort) personal communication.

Reynolds E H, Travers R D 1974 Serum anticonvulsant concentrations in epileptic patients with mental symptoms. A preliminary report. British Journal of Psychiatry 124: 440–445

Richardson S A, Koller H, Katz M, McLaren J 1981 A functional classification of seizures and its distribution in a mentally retarded population. American Journal of Mental Deficiency 85: 457–446

Ross E M, Peckham C S 1983 School children with epilepsy. In: Parsonage M, Grant R H E, Craig A G et al (eds) Advances in epileptology. XIVth Epilepsy International Symposium. Raven Press, New York, p 215–220

Snead O C, Benton J N, Myers G J 1983 ACTH and prednisolone in childhood seizure disorder. Neurology 33: 966–997

19. Epilepsy in women

D. Schmidt

INTRODUCTION

About every second person with epilepsy is female and 80% of all epilepsies begin before age 25. In addition, women with epilepsy are less often discouraged from marriage and pregnancy today compared to previous decades. As a consequence, several aspects of epilepsy in women have received growing interest in recent years. These are: epilepsy and menstruation, fertility, contraception, pregnancy and birth, the newborn period and lactation and finally the risk for malformation and impaired psychomotor development in the offspring. These aspects will be briefly reviewed in this chapter.

EPILEPSY AND MENSTRUATION

The effect of menarche on the onset of epilepsy is difficult to study because of the high incidence of menarche in the age range when epilepsy normally begins both in male and female patients. No prospective studies exist on the course of epilepsy with onset during puberty either in female or male persons. One retrospective study showed no changes in antiepileptic drug concentrations during puberty (Diamantopoulos & Crumrine 1986). Given the cyclical exacerbation of epileptic seizures it is not surprising that menstruation has been invoked quite often. As ever so often, Gowers was among the first to examine this question in 1885. In 82 of his 461 cases the seizures were worse at the monthly period. Unfortunately, Gowers and most subsequent investigators did not examine male patients for comparison, except for Helmchen (1964) who promptly found similar cyclical changes in male patients with complex partial seizures. In a few women, seizures may occur only during the days immediately preceding menstruation or during menstruation itself. This was the case in 10 of 226 women with epilepsy in a recent study (Rosciszewska 1980). The term catamenial epilepsy should in a strict sense be limited to these relatively uncommon cases (Rosciszewska 1980). A number of explanations have been offered to understand the mechanism of catamenial seizures. Water retention and electrolyte imbalance have been invoked as contributing factors. Surprisingly, poor sleep in the days prior to menstruation does not seem to have been studied as a further mechanism of seizures exacerbation in women with catamenial epilepsy. A drop in phenytoin plasma concentration occurs in some patients on premenstrual days (Rosciszewska 1987). Hormonal changes are obviously most often considered, e.g. increased circulating levels of putatively proconvulsant oestrogen during days with seizures or higher levels of putatively anticonvulsant progesterone on days without seizures in women with catamenial epilepsy (Rosciszewska 1987).

A higher seizure frequency was found in the menstrual phase with its high oestrogen–progesterone ratio compared to the remainder of the cycle with a rapid fall in sex hormone concentration at the end of the luteal phase with a low oestrogen-progesterone ratio (Bäckstrom 1976, Mattson et al 1981). In addition, spike suppression was demonstrated in women with epilepsy during intravenous progesterone use (Bäckstrom et al 1984). An improvement in seizure frequency was observed when progesterone was used as on oral contraceptive or as medicine in women with catamenial seizures (Hall 1977). A moderate improvement was reported in six women when they were given medroxy-progesterone (Mattson et al 1982), in contrast to a negative report of the effect of norethisterone (Dana-Haeri & Richens, 1983). In view of the equivocal efficacy, the well documented side effects of hormonal exposure would suggest a very limited role of hormonal treatment for seizure control, if any, in women with catamenial epilepsy. Another treatment strategy is intermittent treatment for 10 days with clobazam during the expected increase of seizures (Feely & Gibson 1984).

In addition to cyclical changes in seizure frequency, menstrual disorders have been reported in women with epilepsy. Menstrual problems were found in 28 of 50 consecutive women with partial seizures of temporal lobe origin (Herzog et al 1986). Of those 28, 19 had reproductive endocrine disorders. Polycystic ovarian syndrome and hypogonadotropic hypogonadism occurred significantly more often in women with temporal lobe epilepsy than in the general population. Polycystic ovarian syndrome was associated with predominantly left-sided interictal paroxysmal electroencephalographic discharges. Hypogonatropic hypogonadism was more often found with right-sided paroxysmal discharges. Hyposexuality occurred more often in women with predominantly right-sided interictal discharges and was associated with low oestrogen hormone levels. Three major explanations have been proposed: 1. Epileptic discharges in medial temporal limbic structures lead to hypothalamic dysregulation of pituitary gonadotropin secretion. 2. Reproductive endocrine disorders with anovulatory cycles may promote the development of epileptic discharges. 3. Temporal lobe epilepsy and some associated reproductive endocrine disorders may be caused by prenatal damage common to the developing brain and the developing reproductive system.

In addition, the effect of menopause on epilepsy may be of interest. In fact there is no evidence that menopause has a consistent effect on the seizure frequency with random results ranging from no effect, a recurrence of seizures at the time of menopause and, finally, suppression of seizures during menopause (Rosciszewska 1987).

EPILEPSY AND FERTILITY

The effects of epilepsy, seizures, and antiepileptic drugs on fertility are not entirely understood. A recent report found approximately half the expected marriage rate among 100 men with epilepsy and one of 83% among 100 women with epilepsy. Marriage rates were lower in persons with an early onset epilepsy (Dansky et al 1980). In addition, the married women had only two-thirds of the number of children expected in the general population. The lower birth rate among women was partly attributable to a higher incidence of therapeutic abortions and a general increase in medical and socioeconomic problems. A similar reduction in the fertility rate to 80% and 85% was found in the Mayo Clinic records for married women and men with epilepsy, respectively (Weber et al 1986). In this report, patients with generalized epilepsy were less disadvantaged than those with partial epilepsy. In addition, a further review of the Mayo Clinic records studied the pregnancy outcome for women with epilepsy and the spouses of men with epilepsy. The proportion of spontaneous abortions was similar to that of the general population and did not differ in both groups. The conclusion was that fetal loss was not significantly associated with maternal or paternal epilepsy or with the use of antiepileptic drugs (Anneghers et al 1988).

A number of reasons may explain the lower fertility rate of women with epilepsy. These include diminished sexual interest and associated reproductive endocrine disorders (Herzog et al 1986). In addition in a recent Finnish study, mothers with epilepsy had a more severe natural history of epilepsy and a lower socioeconomic status than fathers with epilepsy (Hiilesma 1982). Prospective studies of the relationship between type of anti-epileptic drug and fertility are not available. Spermatogenesis may be influenced by antiepileptic drugs. A low sperm count and reduced semen volume and motility was found in eight of 24 patients treated with phenytoin (Stewart-Bentley et al 1976). Further studies showed that valproate did not influence semen motility (Swanson et al 1978). The presence of an antiepileptic drug in semen may cause hypersensitivity in the uterus, leading to mucosal changes and reduced fertilization or implantation. Fortunately the fertility rates have improved over recent decades (Weber et al 1986) and a recent study did not find any reduction in fertility (Bjerkedal & Egenaes 1982), perhaps reflecting better treatment of epilepsy and changing attitudes with less stigmatization for people with epilepsy.

CONTRACEPTION

As early as 1974, single case reports suggested that women with epilepsy suffered from a reduced contraceptive efficacy of oral contraceptives when taking antiepileptic drugs (Janz & Schmidt 1974). The most likely mechanism was induction of steroid biotransformation through antiepileptic drugs. Breakthrough bleeding and unwanted pregnancy were the result. In a prospective study in Berlin 8.5% of pregnant women with epilepsy reported failure of oral contraceptives (Koch et al 1983). A number of antiepileptic drugs have been implicated including phenytoin, carbamazepine, phenobarbitone primidone, and possibly ethosuximide, while valproate and benzodiazepine are not associated with an increased risk. An increase of oestrogen in the contraceptive medication or alternative protective procedures are recommended.

PREGNANCY, DELIVERY AND PUERPERIUM

With better treatment and improved social acceptance of people with epilepsy more epileptic women may choose to become pregnant. Several questions are of obvious concern. What will be the effect of pregnancy on seizures and on antiepileptic drugs? Will the epilepsy have a negative impact on pregnancy, delivery and puerperium?

Effects of pregnancy on epilepsy

The effects of pregnancy on the seizure frequency have been observed in several hundred women over the last 100 years with the reassuring result that pregnancy has a very limited influence on the natural history of epilepsy, if any (Schmidt 1982).

Several prospective studies have shown that in over half of all patients, no change occurs compared to the year preceding the pregnancy, in approximately 15% the number of seizures decrease, and in the final 35% the number of seizures increases. In patients with an increased number of seizures, poor compliance has been found to be a major variable. Poor compliance mainly out of concern about the teratogenic potential of antiepileptic drugs, loss of sleep due to emotional stress, and unjustified and ill-advised reduction of medication urged by non-specialists was associated with an increase in the number of seizures in approximately two-thirds of all women in one study (Schmidt et al 1983). Additional factors may include pregnancy-related changes in seizure propensity and drug disposition.

Deterioration is most often seen during the first trimester, the third trimester, and during lactation. The peak during the first trimester may be related to a high oestrogen–progesterone ratio during early pregnancy, with oestrogen as a potentially proconvulsant agent, and poor drug compliance. During pregnancy the plasma concentration of antiepileptic drugs decreases to a variable degree in approximately one-third to only half of the patients taking phenobarbitone, phenytoin, carbamazepine, primidone, valproate and ethosuximide. The mechanism(s) again include poor compliance and to a much lesser and more variable degree impaired absorption, increased bio-transformation, a higher volume of distribution, and reduced protein-binding (Philbert & Dam 1982).

During the third trimester and during lactation loss of sleep may occur due to inconvenience and interruption during the night for breast feeding. An increase in the number of seizures is more likely in women with a high seizure frequency before pregnancy, multiple types of seizures and a history of poor compliance (Schmidt et al 1983). The course of epilepsy cannot be reliably predicted from paroxysmal discharges in the EEG (Bardy et al 1988) during a previous pregnancy, type of epilepsy, maternal age and sex of the fetus (Knight & Rhind 1975). Women with idiopathic generalized epilepsy, who have not had tonic-clonic seizures for a year prior to pregnancy, those with only one type of seizure, and those with previous good compliance are least likely to suffer from an increase of seizures during pregnancy (Schmidt et al 1983). Status epilepticus is not more common during pregnancy, and epilepsy does not seem to begin more often during pregnancy than expected in the general population (Schmidt 1982).

From these data suggestions can be made for the management of epileptic women during pregnancy. Prior to pregnancy the number of antiepileptic drugs should be reduced as much as possible, aiming for single drug therapy, preferably without valproate, if possible. The daily dose of the antiepileptic drug should be slowly reduced to the lowest clinically effective concentration prior to pregnancy. If possible, withdrawal of antiepileptic drugs should be considered. Diagnostic re-evaluation reveals nonepileptic seizure phenomena in the occasional patient (Schmidt & Lempert 1990) or unnecessary prophylactic medication given for several years.

When pregnancy has been confirmed, it is useful to calmly reassure the patient that drug treatment should continue as before and that there is no need for reduction of daily dose or even withdrawal. Unfortunately patients may have heard otherwise from non-specialists. Confident reassurance is essential. In patients with no change in seizure frequency, the daily dose will not be changed, even in the face of lower total plasma concentrations. If there is an increase in seizures the daily dose will be increased as one would in any patient. In summary, the management of the pregnant patient with epilepsy follows the general rules with no cause for extra measures except possibly more frequent outpatient visits (Brodie 1990).

Effects of epilepsy on pregnancy

The effect of epilepsy on pregnancy is difficult to assess mainly because of regional differences in obstetric concepts and care and lack of nonepileptic controls with a similar socioeconomic background. Women with epilepsy do not seem to differ in the majority of obstetric aspects from controls in the general population (Knight & Rhind 1975, Yerby et al 1985) except for vaginal bleeding (Egenaes 1982). Without apparent association to type of antiepileptic drug treatment during pregnancy, a protracted course of delivery has been reported in single cases, possibly related to antiepileptic drug induced reduction in uterine contractibility, even though controlled trials offer no confirmation (Hiilesmaf 1982). The most serious complication is a 1.2–2-fold increase in perinatal mortality which has been carefully documented in Norway (Bjerkedal 1982) and in the US (Nelson & Ellenberg 1982). A recent study showed perinatal mortality in 2.6% of the pregnancies. The reasons for the increased perinatal mortality are not known but the increased mortality does not seem to be caused by major malformations (Nelson & Ellenberg 1982).

A further concern is the effect of individual seizures on the outcome of pregnancy. Unfortunately no data are available for absence seizures and simple or complex partial seizures. In one case, the effect of maternal generalized tonic-clonic seizures on fetal heart rate could be monitored leading to transient fetal bradycardia. It should be mentioned however that maternal diazepam exposure could be partly responsible for this effect (Teramo et al 1979). In addition, other antiepileptic drugs enter the fetal circulation and may thus exert influences on the fetus. However, no reliable data are available for individual antiepileptic drugs.

NEWBORN PERIOD AND LACTATION

Postpartal Apgar scores are lower in newborns of epileptic women (Göpfert-Geyer et al 1982) and the risk for asphyxia is increased 2–3-fold (Yerby et al 1985). In contrast, physiological icterus and hyperbilirubinaemia are less frequent in newborns of epileptic women, because increased enzyme induction leads to increased biotransformation of bilirubin. The same mechanism is held responsible for increased biotransformation of vitamin K in newborns prenatally exposed to antiepileptic drugs leading to an increased risk of bleeding in the newborn (Battino et al 1982). Administration of 1 mg/kg body weight of vitamin K is generally given prophylactically. Prenatal exposure to antiepileptic drugs is responsible for the measurable concentration of antiepileptic drugs in umbilical cord blood. For most antiepileptic drugs the concentration in umbilical cord is similar to maternal plasma except for valproate and benzodiazepines (Nau et al 1981) which are found in higher concentrations in umbilical cord plasma (Nau et al 1982). The pharmacokinetics of antiepileptic drugs in newborns show lower protein binding, decreased clearance and longer half-lives, depending on the extent of intrauterine enzyme induction. Intrauterine exposure to phenobarbitone or primidone may lead to postnatal sedation, muscular hypotonia and poor sucking. If this is the case, reduction of breast feeding is recommended. In newborns who are not breast-fed a hyperexcitability syndrome may develop for up to several weeks following withdrawal of intrauterine drug exposure with tremor and agitation. Counselling about breast feeding should include the physiological and psychological advantages of breast feeding, the wishes of the mother and the health status of the newborn. Antiepileptic drugs do enter maternal breast milk. The lower the protein binding and the higher the lipophilic properties, the more of the drug is found in the breast milk. Percentages of serum concentration of drugs found in breast milk are: valproate 3%, benzodiazepines 15%, phenytoin 10–15%, phenobarbitone 40%, carbamazepine 45%, primidone 80% and ethosuximide 90%. Recently, intrauterine exposure to valproate was partly held responsible for infantile liver failure in two sisters (Legius et al 1987).

Postnatal development of the offspring

The effect of maternal epilepsy and antiepileptic drug therapy on malformations, postnatal growth and development of the offspring is a major concern for people with epilepsy and has been investigated carefully in recent years. Malformations occur most often in the offspring of epileptic mothers exposed to antiepileptic drugs during gestation. The offspring of epileptic women have a two- to three-fold risk of major malformations compared with the general population (Speidel & Meadow 1972, Gaily 1990) but the role of maternal antiepileptic treatment is still debatable. The results of two population-based studies are controversial. A higher risk of major malformations in drug-exposed children was found in Wales

(Lowe 1973) but not in the much larger US project (Shapiro et al 1976). A higher malformation risk was also observed in children exposed to polytherapy compared to single drug therapy (Kaneko et al 1988). Only one study has shown a correlation of the malformation risk to maternal phenytoin plasma concentrations (Dansky et al 1982). In a human cohort study, no individual drug was singled out as having higher malformation risk (Bertollini et al 1987). No drug specificity for certain malformations has been clearly established, with the possible exception of valproate and neural tube defects (Lindhout & Schmidt 1986).

In a recent review of 20 case-control studies of teratogenicity of antiepileptic drugs, 2523 children were born to treated epileptic mothers and 590 children to untreated epileptic mothers (Friis 1990). In these groups the mean general malformation rate was 89.3 and 22.7/1000 live births respectively. Congenital heart defects (10.9/1000) and facial clefts (8.6/1000) were most common. A comparison of malformation rates in infants of epileptic mothers and epileptic fathers showed that malformations were 2.1- and 3.4-fold more common in the offspring of epileptic mothers (Friis 1990). The unselected material of one study which contributed 71% of the congenital heart defect cases showed, however, that congenital heart defects were as frequent in children of female and male epilepsy patients (Friis & Hauge 1985). Cohort studies of the teratogenicity of antiepileptic drugs give information on 2820 children born of epileptic mothers. The mean overall malformation rate in children of all epileptic women in 14 cohort studies was 51.1/1000 live births. The corresponding control figure is 22.7/1000 live births for children not exposed to antiepileptic drugs (Friis 1990).

Possible genetic, i.e. epilepsy-related, influences on the rate of major congenital malformations in children of epileptic patients have recently been investigated. As for facial clefts no significant association with epilepsy per se could established. The observed/expected ratios for facial clefts in the children were increased only when the mother had epilepsy: 4.7 when antiepileptic drugs were given before and during pregnancy, 2.7 in children of untreated epileptic mothers, and none in children born before the onset of maternal epilepsy. The prevalence of facial clefts in children of epileptic males and in siblings was not increased (Friis 1990). No evidence was found for a common genetic predisposition to congenital heart defects and epilepsy (Friis 1990). Another possible harmful factor to be considered in the development of malformations is seizures during pregnancy. No influence of seizures during pregnancy was found on the rate of major malformations in the offspring in one study (Shapiro et al 1976). Prospective studies of seizure type and frequency in relation to pregnancy outcome are not available.

Fetal antiepileptic drug syndromes

In addition to a number of minor physical abnormalities (Table 19.1), major syndromes of fetal antiepileptic drug syndromes include mental deficiency, growth retardation and microcephaly. Following the initial observations in five children exposed to phenytoin (Hanson & Smith 1975), similar syndromes have been reported in children exposed to other antiepileptic drugs (Dieterich et al 1980), e.g. primidone (Rating et al 1982), valproate (Di Liberti et al 1980, Jäger-Roman et al 1986), carbamazepine (Jones et al 1989) and oxazolindinediones (Zackai et al 1975). In all relevant studies, children of epileptic mothers have been observed to have more minor anomalies than children of nonepileptic mothers. In addition, exposure to antiepileptic drugs, especially more than one drug, is associated with more minor anomalies (Koch et al 1983). No single antiepileptic drug has been singled out as causing

Table 19.1 Fetal antiepileptic drug syndrome: individual minor anomalies (Koch et al 1983)

Epicanthus
Hypertelorism
Ptosis
V-shaped eyebrows
Prominent metopic ridge
Short low-bridged nose
Long philtrum
Wide mouth with full lips
Low set/ abnormal ears
Webbed neck
Hirsutism/low hairline
Distal digital hypoplasia

more minor anomalies than other antiepileptic drugs. During prospective studies hypertelorism was observed in 52% of those exposed to antiepileptic drugs in 17% of unexposed children, and in 10% of controls (Rating et al 1982). Digital hypoplasia was seen in 26% of those exposed to antiepileptic drugs but not in the two other groups. The definition of the different fetal antiepileptic drug syndromes has been carried out on a rather limited number of in-utero, antiepileptic drug exposed children and the syndromes are clearly not specific. Furthermore, few controlled studies are available and the selection criteria and methods of ascertainment are usually not fully described. Finally, no extensive family investigations have been performed.

In a recent prospective Finnish study of children at 5.5 years of age, minor anomalies were significantly more common in the children of epileptic than nonepileptic mothers. The association between prenatal phenytoin exposure and distal digital hypoplasia was confirmed. Hypertelorism also seemed to be associated with phenytoin exposure. Other features were independent of drug exposure. The results suggested a common aetiology for many of the minor anomalies of fetal antiepileptic syndromes and maternal epilepsy (Gaily 1990). Obviously there is a need for further investigation of the genetic susceptibility to develop minor anomalies.

Finally, our knowledge of the comparative risk of individual antiepileptic drugs is scarce. Clearly, oxazolindinediones should not be used in fertile women. Valproate increases the risk of neural tube defects and should be employed only after careful counselling and a provision for careful ultrasound examination and serial determination of serum alpha fetoprotein during early pregnancy. Phenytoin, carbamazepine, phenobarbitone and primidone have not been adequately compared and appear to share a similar risk for major malformations and minor anomalies. Data on ethosuximide are too scanty.

POSTNATAL GROWTH AND MENTAL DEFICIENCY

A delay in length and weight gain in the first postnatal month was observed in antiepileptic drug exposed children compared to non-exposed children of epileptic mothers and control children (Gaily 1990). The sedative drug effects (particularly of barbiturates) transmitted from the mother through the placenta and breast milk appeared to explain the delay in weight but not in length gain. Height at 5.5 years of age was not affected in a large prospective Finnish study (Gaily 1990). Reduced mean head circumference at 5.5 years without associated intellectual impairment was found in children exposed to carbamazepine monotherapy and barbiturates. The relevance of drug exposure remained uncertain. Reduced parental mean head circumference was an obvious confounding factor. In one large prospective study, the prevalence of mental deficiency in the children of epileptic mothers was found to be similar or only very slightly higher than in the general population (Gaily 1990).

General intelligence scores were lower, and the prevalence of specific cognitive dysfunction was higher in the children of epileptic mothers than in control children. No evidence was found in this study that prenatal exposure to antiepileptic drugs caused cognitive impairment. Instead, the results in this study suggested a genetic association between maternal epilepsy and cognitive dysfunction in the offspring. The reliable detection of mild cognitive and behavioural disturbances is difficult, and many confounding factors exist. An assessment of very large numbers of children with randomized drug exposure but similar maternal epilepsy is required to explore further this question.

REFERENCES

Annegers J F, Baumgartner K B, Hauser W A, Kurland L T 1988 Epilepsy, antiepileptic drugs, and the risk of spontaneous abortion. Epilepsia 29: 451–458

Bäckström T 1976 Epileptic seizures in women related to plasma estrogen and progesterone during the menstrual cycle. Acta Neurologica Scandinavica 54: 321–347

Bäckström T, Zetterlund B, Blom S, Romano M 1984 Effects of IV progesterone infusions on the epileptic discharge frequency in women with partial epilepsy. Acta Neurologica Scandinavica 69: 240–248

Bardy A H, Hiilesmaa V K, Teramo K A W 1988 Effect of pregnancy on the electroencephalogram of epileptic women. Acta Neurologica Scandinavica 78: 22–25

Battino D, Bossi L, Canger R et al 1982 Coagulation function in newborns treated in utero with antiepileptic drugs. In: Janz D, Bossi L, Dam M, Helge H, Richens A, Schmidt D (eds) Epilepsy, pregnancy and the child. Raven Press, New York, p 289–295

Bertollini R, Källen B, Mastroiacovo P, Robert E 1987 Anticonvulsant drugs in monotherapy—effect on the fetus. European Journal of Epidemiology 3: 164–171

Bjerkedal I 1982 Outcome of pregnancy in women with epilepsy. In: Janz D, Bossi L, Dam M, Helge H, Richens A, Schmidt D (eds) Epilepsy, pregnancy and the child. Raven Press, New York, p 175–178

Bjerkedal T, Egenaes J 1982 Outcome of pregnancy in women with epilepsy. In: Janz D, Bossi L, Dam M, Helge H, Richens A, Schmidt D (eds) Epilepsy, pregnancy and the child. Raven Press, New York, p 99–101

Brodie M J 1990 Management of epilepsy during pregnancy and lactation. Lancet 1: 29–30

Dana-Haeri J, Richens A 1983 Effect of norethisterone on seizures associated with menstruation. Epilepsia 24: 377–381

Dansky L, Andermann E, Andermann F 1980 Marriage and fertility in epileptic patients. Epilepsia 21: 261–271

Dansky L, Andermann E, Andermann F, Sherwin A L, Kinch R A 1982 Maternal epilepsy and congenital malformations: Correlations with maternal plasma anticonvulsant levels during pregnancy. In: Janz D, Bossi L, Dam H, Helge H, Richens A, Schmidt D (eds) Epilepsy, pregnancy and the child. Raven Press, New York, p 251–258

Diamantopoulos N, Crumrine P K 1986 The effect of puberty on the course of epilepsy. Archives of Neurology 43: 873–876

Dieterich E, Steveling A, Lukas A, Seyfeddinipur N, Spranger J 1980 Congenital anomalies in children of epileptic mothers and fathers. Neuropediatrics 11: 274–283

Di Liberti J H, Forndon P A, Dennis N R, Curry C J R 1980 The fetal valproate syndrome. American Journal of Genetics 19: 473–481

Egenaes J 1982 Outcome of pregnancy in women with epilepsy. In: Janz D, Dam M, Richens A, Bossi L, Helge H, Schmidt D (eds) Epilepsy, pregnancy and the child. Raven Press, New York, p 81–85

Feely M, Gibson J 1984 Intermittent clobazam for catamenial epilepsy. Journal of Neurology, Neurosurgery and Psychiatry 47: 1279–1282

Friis M L 1990 Malformations in children of epileptic patients. In: Comprehensive epileptology Vol 24. Raven Press, New York, p 309–316

Friis M L, Hauge M 1985 Congenital heart defects in live-born children of epileptic parents. Archives of Neurology 42: 374–376

Gaily E 1990 Development and growth in children of epileptic mothers. Academic dissertation, Helsinki

Göpfert-Geyer I, Koch S, Rating D et al 1982 Delivery, gestation, data at birth and neonatal period in children of epileptic mothers. In: Janz D, Bossi L, Dam M, Helge H, Richens A, Schmidt D (eds) Epilepsy, pregnancy and the child. Raven Press, New York, p 167–187

Gowers W G 1885 Epilepsy and other chronic convulsive diseases: their causes, symptoms, and treatment. William Wood, New York, p 255

Hall S M 1977 Treatment of menstrual epilepsy with a progesterone-only oral contraceptive. Epilepsia 18: 235–236

Hanson J W, Smith D W 1975 The fetal hydantoin syndrome. Journal of Pediatrics 87: 285–290

Helmchen H, Künkel H, Selbach H 1964 Periodische Einflüsse auf die individuale Häufigkeit cerebraler Anfälle. Archiv für Psychiatrie und Nervenkrankheiten 206: 293–297

Herzog A G, Seibel M M, Schomer D L, Vaitukaitis J L, Geschwind N 1986 Reproductive endocrine disorders in women with partial seizures of temporal lobe origin. Archives of Neurology 43: 341–346

Hiilesmaa V K 1982 A prospective study on maternal and fetal outcome in 139 women with epilepsy. Dissertation, University of Helsinki

Jäger-Roman E, Deichl A, Jakob S, et al 1986 Fetal growth, major malformations and minor anomalies in infants born to women receiving valproic acid. Journal of Pediatrics 108: 997–1004

Janz D, Schmidt D 1974 Antiepileptic drugs and failure of oral contraceptives. Lancet 1: 1113

Jones K L, Lacro R V, Johnson K A, Adams J 1989 Patterns of malformations in the children of women treated with carbamazepine during pregnancy. New England Journal of Medicine 320:1661–1666

Kaneko S, Otani K, Fukushima Y et al 1988 Teratogenicity of antiepileptic drugs: analysis of possible risk factors. Epilepsia 29: 459–467

Knight A H, Rhind E G 1975 Epilepsy and pregnancy: A study of 153 pregnancies in 59 patients. Epilepsia 16: 99–110

Koch S, Göpfert-Geyer J, Jäger-Roman E et al 1983 Antiepileptika während der Schwangerschaft. Deutsche Medizinische Wochenschrift 108: 250–257

Legius E, Jaecken J, Eggermont E 1987 Sodium valproate. Pregnancy and infantile fatal liver failure. Lancet 1: 1518–1519

Lindhout D, Schmidt D 1986 In-utero exposure to valproate and neural tube defects. Lancet 1: 1392–1393

Lowe C R 1973 Congenital malformations among infants born to epileptic women. Lancet 1: 9–10

Mattson R H, Kamer J A, Caldwaell B V, Cramer J A 1981 Seizure frequency and the menstrual cycle: A clinical study. Epilepsia 22: 242

Mattson R H, Klein P E, Caldwell B V, Cramer J A 1982 Medroxyprogesterone treatment of women with uncontrolled seizures. Epilepsia 23: 436–437

Nau H, Rating D, Koch S, Häuser I, Helge H 1981 Valproic acid and its metabolites: Placental transfer, neonatal pharmacokinetics, transfer via mothers milk and clinical status in neonates of epileptic mothers. Journal of Pharmacology and Experimental Therapeutics 219: 768–777

Nau H, Kuhnz W, Egger H J, Rating D, Helge H 1982 Anticonvulsants during pregnancy and lactation. Transplacental maternal and neonatal pharmacokinetics. Clinical Pharmacokinetics 7: 508–543

Nelson K B, Ellenberg J H 1982 Maternal seizure disorder outcome of pregnancy and neurological abnormalities in the children. Neurology 32: 1247–1254

Philbert A, Dam M 1982 Antiepileptic drug disposition during pregnancy. In: Janz D, Bossi L, Dam M, Helge H, Richens A, Schmidt D (eds) Epilepsy, pregnancy and the child. Raven Press, New York, p 101–114

Rating D, Nau H, Jäger-Roman E et al 1982 Teratogenic and pharmacokinetic studies of primidone during pregnancy and in the offspring of epileptic women. Acta Paediatrica Scandinavia 71: 301–311

Rosciszewska D 1980 Analysis of seizure distribution during menstrual cycle in women with epilepsy. In: Majkowski J (ed) A clinical and experimental research. Karger, Basel, p 280–284

Rosciszewska D 1987 Epilepsy and menstruation. Epilepsia 12: 373–378

Schmidt D 1982 The effect of pregnancy on the maternal history of epilepsy. In: Janz D, Bossi L, Dam M, Helge H, Richens A, Schmidt D (eds) Epilepsy, pregnancy and the child. Raven Press, New York, p 3–14

Schmidt D, Lempert Th 1990 Differential diagnoses in adults. In: Dam M, Gram L (eds) Comprehensive Epileptology. p 449–471

Schmidt D, Canger R, Avanzini G et al 1983 Change of seizure frequency in pregnant epileptic women. Journal of Neurology, Neurosurgery and Psychiatry 46: 751–755

Shapiro S, Hark S C, Siskind V 1976 Anticonvulsants and parental epilepsy in the development of birth defects. Lancet I: 272–275

Speidel B D, Meadow S R, 1972 Maternal epilepsy and abnormalities of the fetus and newborn. Lancet II: 839–843

Stewart-Bentley M, Virgi A, Chang S, Hiatt R, Horton R 1976 Effect of dilantin on FSH and spermatogenesis. Clinical Research 24: 101

Swanson B N, Harland R C, Dickinson R G, Gerber N 1978 Excretion of valproic acid into semen of rabbits and man. Epilepsia 19: 541–546

Teramo K, Hiilesmaa V K, Bardy A, Saarikosi S 1979 Fetal heart rate during a maternal grand mal epileptic seizure. Journal of Perinatal Medicine 7: 3–6

Weber M P, Hauser W A, Ottman R, Annegers J F 1986 Fertility in persons with epilepsy. Epilepsia 27: 746–752

Yerby M, Koepsell T, Daling J 1985 Pregnancy complications and outcomes in a cohort of women with epilepsy. Epilepsia 26: 631–635

Zackai E H, Mellman W J, Neiderer B, Hanson J W 1975 The fetal trimethadione syndrome. Journal of Pediatrics 87: 280–284

20. Epilepsy and the law

D. M. Treiman

INTRODUCTION

References to epilepsy in the law date back to Babylonian, Greek and Roman times when contracts were prepared which allowed for restitution to the buyer if a recently purchased slave turned out to have epilepsy (Temkin 1971). Until very recently epileptics were prohibited from marriage in many societies (Barrow & Fabing 1966). The last law limiting the right of persons with epilepsy to marry in the United States was repealed in 1982 (Schmidt & Wilder 1988). Currently, the major restriction of activities for individuals with epilepsy in most jurisdictions relates to the operation of motor vehicles. However, the most important aspect of epilepsy and the law at the present time is the issue of criminal liability for an act (usually a violent act) committed during an epileptic seizure.

This is not a new issue. Temkin (1971), when discussing psychomotor epilepsy in his book on the history of epilepsy, commented '. . . states of rage and acts of violence were noticed often enough in the literature from Aretaeus to the nineteenth century'. In the eighteenth and early part of the nineteenth century psychiatric complications of epilepsy were of great interest, perhaps because of the special character of many hospitals as lunatic asylums and because many of the physicians responsible for the care of patients with epilepsy were psychiatrists. *Furor epilepticus* or epileptic mania (which may well have been what we now call postictal psychosis) was particularly well studied. 'The *furor epilepticus* was dangerous; patients in this condition might even commit murder' (Portal 1827). Even as late as 1881 Gowers described epileptic mania as sudden par-

oxysmal outbursts of violence to others, usually occurring after a fit. Concomitant with the study of *furor epilepticus* there was an appreciation by some physicians of the importance of making the proper diagnosis and of circumstances where an individual should not be held liable for a committed crime: 'Dangerous epileptics had to be certified, and they had also to be diagnosed in court, lest they be punished for their criminal acts' (Temkin 1971). Foderé (cited in Temkin 1971) described what we would now call resistive violence. Delasiauve (1854) collected a number of examples of court procedures against epileptics from the first half of the nineteenth century, some of whom were acquitted because of their epilepsy. However, there was a considerable difference of opinion regarding criminal liability for crimes committed by individuals with epilepsy. Some physicians (for example, Platner 1824) held that an epileptic should not be considered guilty of a crime, whether or not there was any relation of the timing of the crime to an ictal event. Others suggested that this would lead to absurd consequences, giving epileptics a free hand to commit crimes (Temkin 1971).

These same issues persist today. This chapter will focus on this aspect of epilepsy and the law, that is, the question of epilepsy and criminal responsibility and will consider the following topics:

1. What is the nature of epilepsy and of an ictal event? Under what circumstances could violent or aggressive behaviour occur as the result of an epileptic seizure?
2. Does violent or aggressive behaviour occur more often in individuals with epilepsy?

3. Does epilepsy occur more often in violent and aggressive people?
4. Legal aspects of epilepsy and criminal liability. The insanity defence and the epilepsy defence.

NATURE OF ICTAL EVENTS

In 1873 Hughlings Jackson wrote, 'Epilepsy is the name for occasional, sudden, excessive, rapid and local discharges of gray matter'. We now know that Jackson was fundamentally correct, and that seizures are the behavioural manifestations of brief paroxysmal hypersynchronous abnormal discharges of neurons. Most seizures have a stereotyped sequence of behaviours from event to event in the same patient, although a patient may have more than one seizure pattern. Partial onset seizures begin locally in one area of the cortex and the associated behaviour is a reflection of the anatomical localization of the paroxysmal discharge. As long as the epileptic discharge remains localized consciousness is retained and the abnormal behaviour remains limited to stereotypic behaviour specific to the epileptic focus. This is what is now known as a simple partial seizure (Commission 1981). The patient is fully conscious and capable of differentiating right from wrong.

All behaviours during a simple partial seizure which require a sequence of acts are voluntary and dependent on the individual's intent to carry out the act. Myoclonic and atonic seizures, although generalized from onset, also are not associated with any alteration of contact with the environment and thus are also unlikely to be associated with involuntary directed aggressive behaviour. The focal abnormal electrical discharge of the simple partial seizure may spread to engage both hemispheres, at which time consciousness will be impaired. If the seizure activity spreads to engage the limbic system, or sometimes frontal or occipital cortex, there may be an impairment of consciousness associated with automatisms. This is what is known as a complex partial seizure (Commission 1981).

It is now recognized that there is a predictable sequence of behaviours which occur during the course of a complex partial seizure, frequently starting with a motionless stare, followed by stereotyped automatisms, and finally by reactive automatisms. Sometimes there is no stare and the initial manifestation of the seizure may be impairment of consciousness and stereotyped automatisms (Delgado-Escueta et al 1977, 1979, 1982). 'Stereotyped automatism' is a term which refers to automatic behaviour which is repetitive from seizure to seizure whereas 'reactive automatism' applies to automatic behaviour which can be modified by the environment but for which the patient is amnestic. Although absence seizures are sometimes associated with mild clonic movements and other automatisms, the nature of these automatisms is that they are simple and repetitive and are never sufficiently complex to account for directed aggression.

Either a simple partial or complex partial seizure may spread to engage diencephalic structure, at which time the patient will exhibit generalized tonic and/or clonic behaviour. Again, the sequence is predictable: initial tonic posturing, followed by clonic jerking of the face, trunk, and/or extremities which increases in amplitude and decreases in frequency, until there is an abrupt cessation of the jerking and the patient remains in a motionless, comatose state from which there is gradual or rapid recovery. During the recovery period (the postictal phase) the patient may be confused and disoriented and may experience an impairment of normal social inhibitions.

Given this description of the behavioural patterns of the seizure types recognized in the International Classification (Commission 1981), is it possible that an individual could commit a violent or aggressive act, for which he had little or no memory, as the result of a seizure? In the case of a simple partial seizure, the answer is clearly no, because consciousness is retained during the duration of the seizure. In the case of complex partial and primarily or secondarily generalized tonic and/or clonic seizures under what circumstances could ictal aggression occur? Treiman (1991) has suggested five theoretical circumstances under which ictal violence or aggression could occur, although, as will be discussed below, there is little evidence that some of these possible types of ictal aggression actually exist:

1. *Primary ictal aggression*—aggressive behaviour which is directly stimulated by the epileptic

discharge, as was suggested by some of the early human brain stimulation studies (Chapman 1958, Chatrian & Chapman 1960, Delgado et al 1952, 1968, Ervin et al 1969, Heath 1955, 1962, 1964, Heath et al 1955, Kalyanaraman 1975, King 1961, Mark & Ervin 1970, Mark et al 1969, 1975, Sem-Jacobsen 1968, Sheer 1961, Ursin 1960). For critical review of these reports see Kligman & Goldberg (1975) and Treiman (1991).

2. *Secondary ictal aggression*—aggressive behaviour which is released by disinhibition of normal social controls by a seizure discharge or which occurs in response to an epileptic discharge which produces a noxious or aversive stimulus. There is evidence that patients in spike-wave stupor (Treiman & Delgado-Escueta 1980) or in what Treiman (1990) has termed 'subtle complex partial status epilepticus' are capable of carrying out quite complex acts for a sustained period of time, for which they subsequently have little or no memory. There are no documented cases of acts of violence or aggression occurring during such prolonged attacks. However, in a recently reported case what may have been simple partial seizures were manifested by intense feelings of hate and aggression which were always directed at a 20-month-old baby for whom the patient was caring (Hindler 1989). If these feelings were ictal in origin then the violent behaviour Miss A exhibited could have been secondary ictal aggression. The very rare cases of violent automatisms during epileptic seizures, discussed below, may also be examples of secondary ictal aggression.

3. *Nonaggressive violent automatisms*—violent behaviour which occurs as a stereotyped automatism but which is not directed toward a person or object and has no aggressive intent.

4. *Resistive violence*—violent behaviour which occurs at the end of a well documented seizure while the patient is still exhibiting reactive automatisms or is in a postictal confused state.

5. Violence or aggression which occurs in the context of postictal psychosis.

ICTAL VIOLENCE—DOES IT OCCUR?

What is the evidence that ictal aggression has actually occurred under any of these circumstances listed above? Forty cases of possible ictal aggres-

sion or violence have been reported in the medical literature. Treiman & Delgado-Escueta (1983) reviewed 29 of them in detail. In their opinion, out of the 29 only three cases (two cases of Gunn & Fenton and one described by Knox) were strongly suggestive of a relationship between ictal epileptic attacks and violent automatisms. In none of the other 26 cases was sufficient detail provided in the original description to establish clearly an ictal basis for the alleged violence. In 1980 an international panel of 18 epileptologists reviewed videotapes and EEGs of 33 epileptic attacks in 19 patients who were believed to have exhibited aggressive behaviour during the recorded seizures (Delgado-Escueta et al 1981). These cases were the only examples of possible ictal violence the 18 investigators could find out of a total of 5400 seizures recorded on video-tape and EEG which were screened for presentation at the workshop. In the opinion of the panel, seven patients exhibited ictal aggression ranging from violence toward property to mild aggression directed toward a person. Of the remaining 12 patients, six only had pseudoseizures and six had minimal or no aggression.

Five of the patients in the Delgado-Escueta series have been described in greater detail elsewhere (Ashford et al 1980, Saint Hilaire et al 1980, Treiman & Delgado-Escueta 1981). These five cases and two reported subsequently by Wieser (1983) are the only patients who are known to have clear histories of assault and whose epileptic attacks have been well studied by closed circuit television and electroencephalography. The case of Patrick Sullivan, even though not documented by CCTV-EEG, seems to be a clear example of aggressive behaviour during a complex partial seizure. Thus there are only a few patients who have been reported in the medical literature who have been observed to exhibit aggressive behaviour and in whom there is reasonable evidence that their aggressive behaviour may have been related temporally to an ictal event. It is, therefore, worth reviewing these cases in some detail.

In two cases described by Gunn & Fenton (1971) violent behaviour may have been related to an ictal event. One was a 49-year-old alcoholic who had seizures since the age of 25. One evening, after having been drinking, he left the pub and had a seizure. He was recovering from the seizure when a policeman tried to remove him for being a nuisance. The patient lashed out and tried to hit the policeman. In the other case a 32-year-old man developed generalized convulsions at the age of 18. Two years later, while staying at his girlfriend's house, he had a generalized convulsion early in the morning. While still in a postictal confused state he violently attacked his girlfriend, and an elderly couple who also lived in the house. On admission to the hospital shortly thereafter he was mentally confused and amnestic for all events following the seizure. He subsequently had a generalized tonic-clonic seizure once every 1–2 years. Each seizure was followed by a period of confusion lasting 15 to 60 minutes during which the patient appeared perplexed and frightened and if restrained would become dangerously aggressive. Both of these cases are examples of 'resistive violence' in which attempts to restrain a patient while still in a postictal confused state produces violent reactive automatisms for which the patient is completely amnestic.

Knox (1968) also described six patients who exhibited resistive behaviour if an attempt was made to restrain them at the end of a seizure. One patient, a 50-year-old man, had several episodes of automatisms while under observation. During these episodes he would stagger about and if assisted would shout, 'Leave me alone'. On one occasion he grabbed an orderly by the throat, held him for several minutes and yelled, 'I'll kill you'. He kicked the doctor on another occasion. He reported that if he had a seizure at work his colleagues knew not to approach him: 'It seems I don't attack them if I'm not touched'.

Resistive violence has also been observed in other series of patients with complex partial seizures (Delgado-Escueta et al 1982, King & Ajimone Marsan 1977). In Ashford's patient (1980) and in Treiman's two patients (1981), fear apparently induced automatic destruction of property, defensive kicking and flailing. These behaviours observed on the CCTV-EEG were similar to those described in the patients' histories.

Of the 19 patients reviewed by the international panel only one (one of Saint-Hilaire's patients) exhibited ictal aggressive acts which could have resulted in serious harm to another person. This was a mentally retarded young woman of 20 who

at the age of 3 had 'a generalized infection with encephalopathy and henceforth manifested unmotivated aggressive paroxysms . . .'. Saint-Hilaire et al (1980) further described her history as follows: 'The aggressive outbursts happen suddenly, without any warning. She quickly moves toward a target and physically assaults it . . . When the targets are objects, she breaks them and/or throws them. When she directs these behaviours toward humans, she will often grab the eyeglasses and break them; if a person does not wear glasses, she will direct her attack toward the face while grabbing and/or hitting. The outbursts suddenly abate and the patient declares herself tired, she 'does not feel well' but her contact with the environment is restored to its usual level. These paroxysms happen many times a week despite heavy medication.'

During scalp EEG observations a secondarily generalized tonic-clonic seizure was recorded without evidence of aggressive behaviour.

During depth SEEG observations several 'absences' were noted during which the patient lost contact with the environment and exhibited epileptiform activity limited to the right amygdala and right temporal cortex. Stimulation of the right hippocampus only produced a local afterdischarge without behavioural change. On one occasion stimulation of the left hippocampus was followed 95 seconds later by loss of contact with the environment, irregular movements and breathing at 104 seconds after the end of the electrical stimulation, and an aggressive outburst at 117 seconds after the stimulation in which she rose suddenly from a prone position, attempted to grab the neuropsychologist's eyeglasses and verbally accused him: 'It's your fault, it's not right, you've done it' (Saint Hilaire et al 1980). Apparent epileptiform activity is seen in the right hippocampus throughout the 67 seconds of recording presented in the figure—unfortunately the entire recording from the time of the electrical stimulation throughout the entire episode is not presented, so the time the epileptiform activity began cannot be seen and is not reported in the text.

Saint Hilaire's other patient was a 30-year-old bachelor sheet metal worker who began having seizures at the age of 6, 1 year after head trauma (Saint Hilaire et al 1980). During adolescence his seizures assumed their adult pattern. They began with an aura consisting of a shiver at the level of the thorax followed by loss of consciousness. The patient then would talk or yell or insult people and spit in their faces. He remained ambulatory and was able to carry out relatively complex activities during these seizures, after which he would be amnestic.

This patient was studied with stereo electroencephalography. During a typical seizure the patient warned the staff that an aura was beginning at the time low voltage fast activity could be seen in the right amygdala and right anterior temporal leads. Seven seconds later the patient whistled and struck his right thigh with his right hand at the time when the EEG frequency in the amygdala and anterior temporal cortex slowed. Twenty seconds after onset of the initial EEG change and behavioural warning, the patient yelled vulgar insults toward a nurse in the adjacent room. Insults directed toward the nurse (even though an EEG technician was closer to him) continued when, 26 seconds after the onset of the seizure, rhythmic spike activity was seen not only from the amygdalar and anterior temporal leads but also the right parahippocampal gyrus. The seizure stopped 1 minute 15 seconds after onset and the patient was amnestic for all events.

Wieser (1983) described a boy with a socially disabling behaviour disorder and frequent rage attacks sometimes starting with fear and gastric sensations. There was left frontal temporal flattening on the EEG at the start of these episodes. Stereo EEG exploration was not performed because of the severe aggressive outbursts. However, selective left amygdalohippocampectomy stopped all seizures and the rage attacks. The boy was described as seizure free and a calm and good student over 2.5 years of follow up.

Wieser's other patient was a 16-year-old male with 'psychomotor' seizures from age 9 characterized by paroxysmal speech disturbances and fits of rage leading to brawls. During his attack he was said to abruptly raise his hand and rave or suddenly become speechless or indiscriminately attack and hit everyone around. A pneumoencephalogram showed a left temporal basal cyst communicating with the temporal horn. During stereo EEG exploration several rage attacks were observed and long-lasting 'clonic discharges' in

the left periamygdalar region were recorded which were not evident on the surface EEC. However, no data were presented regarding the exact temporal relationship between the periamygdalar discharges and the rage behaviour. The patient underwent a left temporal lobectomy. The pathological specimen demonstrated a small periamygdalar capillary hemangioma. Over 4.5 years of follow up, the patient remained seizure free and was described as a 'calm and peaceable' man.

Perhaps the best documented example of criminal aggression during an epileptic seizure is the case of Patrick Joseph Sullivan. Mr Sullivan had suffered from epilepsy since childhood. On occasion in the past he had been known to violently resist assistance during a seizure. On May 8, 1981 he was visiting a neighbour with a Mr Payne, an elderly man, age 80. Sullivan had a complex partial seizure, during which he kicked Mr Payne and caused significant damage. Afterwards Sullivan had no memory of the events. However, both the seizure and the attack were witnessed. In a case that caused extensive discussion in the British medical literature (see section on Epilepsy and the Law below), Sullivan was tried for 1. causing grievous bodily harm with intent to do grievous bodily harm and 2. inflicting grievous bodily harm.

Most of the episodes of aggression or violence which have occurred in relation to epileptic attacks are examples of resistive violence at the end of documented complex partial or generalized tonic-clonic epileptic seizures. This is true for the two cases described by Gunn & Fenton (1971), six cases described by Knox (1968), including his one case described in detail above, and in examples reported in other series of complex partial seizures described above. In those cases where violent activity occurred at (or nearly at) the beginning of behavioural seizures the behaviour consisted of random violence and not directed aggression. For example, in Treiman's two cases (1981), Ashworth's patient (1980), and perhaps in one of Wieser's patients (1983) the stereotyped automatisms consisted of random flailing movements, bicycling behaviour, or in the case of Ashford's patient, whirling movements while holding onto the draperies in the room. In each case the violent behaviour was not directed toward any individual and was stereotyped from seizure to seizure within the same patient. These are examples of non-aggressive violent automatisms.

In the two cases described by Saint-Hilaire et al (1980), in which directed aggressive behaviour appeared to be associated with ictal discharges recorded during stereo electroencephalography, the aggressive behaviour occurred after the onset of the seizure. This was true for the 20-year-old patient in whom one episode of aggressive behaviour appears to have been recorded simultaneously with the SEEG. In this patient the aggressive outburst associated with right hippocampal activity occurred 117 seconds after electrical stimulation of the left hippocampus. Furthermore the aggressive behaviour was preceded 22 seconds earlier by an alteration of contact with the environment.

In Saint-Hilaire et al's other patient (1980) the history suggests that the patient's habitual seizures always included episodes in which he yelled, insulted people, and spat in their faces. Again, the aggressive behaviour in the example reported did not occur until 20 seconds after the onset of the seizure.

In all the cases reviewed above in which violent or aggressive behaviour may have been associated with ictal activity, the exhibited behaviour either: 1. consisted of non-aggressive violent automatisms which were clearly stereotyped and repetitive from seizure to seizure within the same patient, 2. consisted of reactive automatisms manifested by directed aggression which always occurred after the onset of a clearly identifiable complex partial seizure which began with a typical initial loss of contact with the environment, or 3. consisted of resistive violence at the end of a complex partial or generalized tonic-clonic seizure when the patient was being restrained while still in a confused state. There are no documented cases of ictal aggression in which an organized directed attack toward another individual or object occurred as the initial or sole manifestation of an epileptic seizure, which could not otherwise be diagnosed on the basis of at least some concomitant features typical of complex partial or generalized tonic-clonic seizures.

INTERICTAL VIOLENCE—DOES IT OCCUR?

Although there are only a small number of case reports in the medical literature which are truly suggestive of ictal violence, there is still a prevailing belief in many medical circles that epilepsy, particularly temporal lobe epilepsy, is associated with an increased incidence of violent crimes. As recently as 1982 Kolb & Brodie, writing in *Modern Clinical Psychiatry*, stated with regard to psychomotor epilepsy, '... clinically the clouded state suggests a delirium with liberation of aggressive and occasionally self-destructive impulses. Acts of violence may be committed in the automatisms and may be of a strikingly brutal nature, the patient pursuing his crime to a most revolting extreme.' This view, which is stated as fact but for which no evidence is provided, has continued to colour the approach of many physicians to patients with complex partial epilepsy and has encouraged the frequently inappropriate use of the epilepsy defence in crimes of violence. The epilepsy defence will be discussed below. Here we need to consider what is the evidence that violent behaviour is more frequent in patients with epilepsy in general and with complex partial or temporal lobe epilepsy in particular?

Treiman (1986) reviewed in detail studies of the prevalence of violence in patients with epilepsy. A number of studies have reported an increased prevalence of violent and aggressive behaviour in patients with epilepsy. Most such studies (Ounsted 1969, James 1960, Serafetinides 1965, Taylor 1969) concentrated on selected small populations of patients with severe intractable seizure disorders frequently selected because of the presence of behavioural disorders as well as epilepsy. Rodin (1973) surveyed 700 unselected, noninstitutionalized patients with epilepsy. Thirty-four patients (4.8%) were coded as 'destructive-assaultive' during their initial evaluation. Most of these patients were young men with below-average intelligence who had more behavioural and psychiatric problems, poorer employment records, and more evidence of organic brain disease on neurological examination but no greater prevalence of temporal lobe epilepsy than a non-destructive-assaultive control group of patients matched for age, sex, and intelligence.

Surveys of large groups of unselected patients with epilepsy by Juul-Jensen (1964) and Currie (1971) found no greater predilection for violent behaviour in patients with temporal lobe epilepsy than in patients with other types of epilepsy. A number of studies of aggressive personality traits (Hermann et al 1980, Hermann & Riel 1981, Whitman et al 1982, Hermann 1982) also failed to demonstrate any relationship between seizure type and aggressive personality traits. Taken as a group these studies have failed to document an increased prevalence of violent behaviour in patients with epilepsy in general or temporal lobe epilepsy in particular. All the violent and aggressive personality traits which occur in such groups can be accounted for by other neurological and psychiatric deficits. However, it has been suggested that seizures may, under some circumstances, result in interictal personality changes which may be clinically significant (Engel et al 1986).

Griffith et al (1987) described an experimental model for limbic-epilepsy-induced disturbances in interictal defensive reactivity. Seizures are induced in cats by microinjection of kainic acid into the dorsal hippocampus. This induces an acute phase lasting 2–3 days characterized by recurrent partial onset seizures, some of which secondarily generalize. Between seizures, during this acute phase, the cats demonstrate an exaggerated defensive rage in response to mild threat or handling. Because the cats exhibit normal behaviour once the seizures stop it may be that this model is really one of postictal psychosis. There are patients whose behaviour changes markedly during seizure flurries but who, like the cats, exhibit normal behaviour between seizure flurries.

EPILEPSY IN CRIMINALS

Treiman (1986) has also reviewed the evidence that epilepsy occurs with greater prevalence in convicted criminals than in the normal population. A series of studies of epilepsy in the British prison system carried out by Gunn and his colleagues as well as by earlier workers have been detailed in a monograph (Gunn 1977). These studies demonstrated a two- to four-fold increase in the prevalence of epilepsy in prisoners compared with the non-incarcerated population. Two subsequent studies (Gunn & Bonn 1971) found that the prevalence rate for epilepsy in the prison

population (0.87% and 0.88%) was twice the 0.45% figure reported for Britain in a survey of the College of General Practitioners (1960). Several American studies (Epilepsy in North Carolina 1977, Novick et al 1977, King & Young 1978) have also investigated the prevalence of epilepsy in prison populations and observed a prevalence of 1.8% to 1.9%, more than three times the prevalence of 0.59% reported by Hauser & Kurland (1975) in the population of Rochester, Minnesota.

A number of studies have thus shown that epilepsy is two to four times more prevalent in prison populations than in the nonprison, middle class populations that form the basis of most prevalence studies in the general population. However, the prison prevalence rates are similar to those found in a number of underprivileged, lower socioeconomic communities, such as those from which most British and American prisoners come. A prevalence rate of 1.9% in black children has been reported for an inner city population in New Haven, Connecticut (Shamansky & Glaser 1979). Similar prevalence rates have been found in populations surveyed in rural Alabama counties (Hollingsworth 1978), Iceland (Gudmundsson 1966), Carlisle, England (Brewis et al 1966), Serbia (Korbar & Berkovic 1974), Bogota, Columbia (Gomez et al 1978), a rural Appalachian community (Baumann et al 1977, 1978), and Melipilla, Chile (Chiofalo et al 1979). A relationship between socioeconomic status and epilepsy would explain the higher incidence of epilepsy among criminals and prisoners. King & Young (1978) have pointed out that some aetiological factors for epilepsy are more prevalent among poor urban populations, including inadequate prenatal care and a higher incidence of head trauma. These data would thus suggest that the presence of epilepsy has no immediate relationship to violence or crimes. Rather the two- to four-fold increase in prevalence of epilepsy among incarcerated individuals most likely reflects a prevalence of epilepsy among economically deprived urban populations rather than an increased frequency of criminal activity among epileptics.

EPILEPSY AND THE LAW

The evidence cited above fails to support a clear

association between epilepsy and violent or aggressive behaviour. None-the-less, there are rare cases where violent behaviour may be the result of an epileptic seizure and there are many cases where a 'diminished legal responsibility' or 'insanity' defence has been used, even though there was no reason to believe the crime was in any way related to the occurrence of an epileptic seizure. For these reasons it is worth reviewing the way in which crimes allegedly committed as the result of an epileptic seizure have been handled in British and American courts.

There is a long standing tradition in Anglo-Saxon common law that a guilty deed requires two components: an illegal act and intent to commit the act. The principle that a person is not criminally liable for his conduct unless the prescribed state of mind is also present has been part of Anglo-Saxon criminal law since the 14th century (Golding 1985). This principle has led to the development of two forms of defence when a criminal act is committed without intent: insanity and non-insane automatism. This latter defence has been recognized in Great Britain since 1688 when Colonel Cheyney Culpeper shot a Guardsman and his horse one night while sleepwalking. Until 1800 in Great Britain all forms of defence based on lack of intent, including insanity, could lead to absolute acquittal. However, in 1800 James Hadfield, a French wars veteran who had suffered severe brain damage, unsuccessfully shot at King George III. He was acquitted on grounds of insanity. To prevent criminally insane but legally innocent people from wandering the streets again (and possibly committing another illegal act) Parliament rushed through a bill to require that people who were found not guilty by reason of insanity be detained in hospital at His Majesty's pleasure (Gunn 1991). In modified form, this same law exists in the United Kingdom today. People found not guilty by reason of insanity can be detained in hospital indefinitely. However, under the 1800 law a successful plea of 'noninsane automatism' would still result in complete acquittal.

Insanity was defined in Anglo-Saxon law by the M'Naghten trial in 1843. The M'Naghten rule, with subsequent modifications and refinements, has served as the basis for the legal consideration of insanity in both Great Britain and the United States ever since. The rule was established by the 15 chief justices of the common law courts of England after the trial of Daniel M'Naghten for the assassination of Prime Minister Robert Peel's secretary Edward Drummond (whom M'Naghten mistook for Peel). Sanity was to be presumed until the contrary was proved. The special verdict 'not guilty by reason of insanity' was only possible when it was established that 'at the time of committing the act the party accused was labouring under such a defect of reason, from disease of the mind, as not to know the nature and quality of the act he was doing, or as not to know that what he was doing was wrong' (10 Cl. & Fin. 200).

American law

In 1954, the United States Court of Appeals for the District of Columbia Circuit held in Durham v United States (214 F. 2d 862) 'that an accused is not criminally responsible if his unlawful act was a product of mental disease or mental defect'. This test, now known as the Durham 'Product' test, improved upon the M'Naghten test by taking account not only of the cognitive and volitional aspects of the defendant's mental condition, but also of the broad range of mental illness itself.

In 1962 the American Law Institute published its Model Penal Code which stated that 'a person is not responsible for criminal conduct if at the time of such conduct as a result of mental disease or defect he lacks substantial capacity either to appreciate the criminality [wrongfulness] of his conduct or to conform his conduct to the requirements of law'. Four years later, in 1966, in the case of the United States v Charles Freeman (357 F. 2d 606), the court gave this section of the Model Penal Code a strong endorsement and rejected the M'Naghten rule within its jurisdiction. As a result, this section is commonly referred to as the Freeman rule.

The problem with all of these rules for the establishment of insanity in criminal cases is that such a defence is not appropriate as a defence against a violent crime which may have occurred at the time of unconsciousness or automatic behaviour during an epileptic seizure. It is inherent (and written into the law in the United Kingdom) that those found 'not guilty by reason of insanity' as the result of the application of any of these rules are to be institutionalized for treatment which is intended to rehabilitate the insane defendant and, if possible, return him to society. However, there is no reason to believe that an epileptic patient is insane at the time of a seizure which causes an alteration in level of consciousness during which automatisms may occur. Certainly there is no reason to believe an epileptic patient is insane between seizures. Thus there can be no benefit either to society or to the individual patient if he is found not guilty by reason of insanity and incarcerated in a mental institution.

A solution to this legal dilemma has been recognized by some jurisdictions in the United States. The 'unconsciousness defence' is based on the concept that individuals cannot be legally liable for their actions if the actions were committed at the time of unconsciousness. This is known as the doctrine of *mens rea*—'Actus non facit reum nisi mens sit rea'—the deed does not make a man guilty unless his mind is guilty. This principle was clearly stated by a California court which noted in People v Freeman (61 Cal. App. 2d 110):

> No principle of criminal jurisprudence was ever more zealously guarded than that a person is guiltless if at the time of his commission of an act defined as criminal he has no knowledge of the deed.
> . . . [A]nd to hold that a man shall be held criminally responsible for an offense of the commission of which he was ignorant at the time would be intolerable tyranny.

British law

The 'unconsciousness defence' is quite similar to a defence which is known in the United Kingdom as non-insane automatism (*automatism simpliciter*). The legal definition of automatism currently accepted in the United Kingdom, given by Viscount Kilmuir, L.C. in the House of Lords appeal of Bratty v Attorney General for Northern Ireland (1961 3 All E.R. 523), is as follows:

> . . . the state of person who, though capable of action, is not conscious of what he is doing . . . It means unconscious, involuntary action and it is a defence because the mind does not go with what is being done. This is very like the words of the learned President of the Court of Appeal of New Zealand in R v Cottle

where he said: 'With respect, I would myself prefer to explain automatism simply as action without any knowledge of acting, or action with no consciousness of doing what was being done'.

In British courts two types of automatism are recognized: sane (*automatism simpliciter*) and insane (*automatism due to disease of the mind*). A successful use of the automatism defence will result in a finding of not guilty in either case. However, the consequences of the court finding that the act was caused by a non-insane automatism or by an insane automatism may be quite different. In the case of a non-insane automatism the defendant is fully acquitted and free to walk from the court. Before a change in the law, passed by Parliament in 1991, if a plea of not guilty because of an insane automatism was accepted by the court, the defendant would have been committed to a mental hospital for an indefinite period of time, until released by order of the Home Secretary. The recent legislation, an amendment to the Criminal Procedure (Insanity) Act 1964, has given the courts a much wider range of options. Defendants being found not guilty by reason of an insane automatism may still be committed to a psychiatric hospital or guardianship, or a supervision and treatment order can be applied. An absolute discharge can also be granted. The legal definition of a seizure as being a disturbance of the mind still remains, however.

Unfortunately, British courts have rejected the notion that an epileptic automatism should be considered a non-insane automatism, although this was not always so. In Regina v Charson (1955 1 All E.R. 859) epilepsy was defined as a non-insane automatism. This was a case where the defendant was accused of striking his son over the head with a hammer and then throwing him out of a window. Automatism was alleged. In his summing up, Mr Justice Barry said:

> If he struck his son with the mallet, knowing what he was doing, and by those blows caused injuries, then he is guilty . . . If he did not know what he was doing, if his actions were purely automatic and his mind had no control over the movement of his limbs, if he was in the same position as a person in an epileptic fit and no responsibility rests upon him at all, then the proper verdict is 'not guilty'. . .

However, in the same year in the case of Regina v.

Kemp (1956 3 All E.R. 249) before Mr Justice Devlin, it was held that an automatic act, allegedly associated with a lapse of consciousness due to arteriosclerosis, could be considered a disease of the mind:

The distinction between the two categories [mental disease and physical disease] is irrelevant for the purposes of the law, which is not concerned with the origin of the disease, or the cause of it, but simply with the mental condition which has brought about the act. It does not matter for the purpose of the law, whether the defect of reasoning is due to degeneration of the brain or to some other form of mental derangement. That may be a matter of importance medically, but it is of no importance to the law, which merely has to consider the state of mind in which the accused is, not how he got there. . . . a disease which is shown on the evidence to be capable of affecting the mind in such a way as to cause a defect, temporarily or permanently, of its reasoning and understanding . . . is . . . a disease of the mind within the meaning of the rule.

The legal concept that an epileptic automatism is an insane automatism was firmly established in British law in 1961 in Bratty v Attorney-General for Northern Ireland (3 All E.R. 523). Bratty was charged with killing a girl whom he had taken for a ride in his car. He took off her stocking and strangled her with it. He claimed that he could not remember anything because a 'blackness' came over him: 'I didn't know what I was doing. I didn't realize anything.' Medical testimony suggested that he might be suffering from psychomotor epilepsy, although Fenwick (1988) has suggested that careful consideration of the medical history could not possibly support this diagnosis. None-the-less, at the time of the trial the defence asked the jury to acquit the accused on a plea of automatism, to find him guilty of manslaughter, or to find him not guilty by reason of insanity. The trial judge instructed the jury to disregard the plea of automatism on the ground that there was no evidence for it. Bratty was convicted of murder and the case was appealed on the basis that the judge was incorrect in dismissing the plea of automatism. The appeal was upheld by the House of Lords. In his opinion, Lord Denning cited conflicting testimony regarding whether psychomotor epilepsy was present and went on to say:

All the doctors agreed that psychomotor epilepsy, if it exists, is a defect of reason due to disease of the mind:

and the judge accepted this view. No other cause was canvassed.

In those circumstances, I am clearly of opinion that, if the act of the appellant was an involuntary act, as the defence suggested, the evidence attributed it solely to a disease of the mind and the only defence open was the defence of insanity. There was no evidence of automatism apart from insanity.

It seems to me that any mental disorder which has manifested itself in violence and is prone to recur is a disease of the mind. At any rate it is the sort of disease for which a person should be detained in hospital rather than being given an unqualified acquittal.

Because there is real question as to whether Bratty had psychomotor epilepsy Fenwick (1988) has suggested that from a medical point of view the Bratty case was unsatisfactory as a foundation case on which to base the concept that violent act occurring during an epileptic seizure is an insane automatism. However, in the case of Regina v Sullivan there was strong evidence that a violent crime was committed during an epileptic seizure. This case has been discussed extensively in the British medical literature (Fenwick, 1987, 1988, Brahams 1983a,b,c,d, 1984, Anonymous 1983, Swan 1984, Golding 1985, Fenwick & Fenwick 1985, Gunn 1991) and has become the focus of efforts to change British law relating to the automatism defence and epilepsy. 'The law on automatism as it now stands is illogical, leads to much hardship and suffering, and so clearly needs revision' (Fenwick 1988). Fenwick summarized the Sullivan case as follows:

Sullivan, a man of previous good character, was a patient who suffered partial complex seizures with occasional secondary generalisation from the age of eight. He had had two severe head injuries which have resulted in widespread brain damage and some degree of personality change. His major attacks ceased in 1979, and only the partial complex seizures remained. These seizures spread rapidly and bilaterally into both amygdala and hippocampal structures, so that Sullivan had no memory for the seizure or events immediately after the seizure.

During a partial complex seizure Sullivan attacked and seriously injured an elderly neighbour. The seizure and the attack were witnessed, and both prosecution and defence accepted that there was no medical doubt that the assault took place during an epileptic automatism. Sullivan wished to establish the defence of the sane automatism (automatism simpliciter), and pleaded not guilty. The trial judge, His Honour Judge Lymbery, ruled that this plea was not available to the defence, and that if Mr Sullivan carried out the act during an epileptic fit, then he must plead not guilty because of automatism due to disease of the mind. If Mr Sullivan had pleaded 'insane automatism' and his plea had succeeded, as it undoubtedly would, it would have meant that the court would have had to send him to hospital, possibly a special hospital. Mr Sullivan's defence lawyers were not willing to risk this possibility, and so Mr Sullivan was persuaded to plead guilty to an act which he could not remember committing and over which he had no control.

Pamela Taylor (1985) summed up the dilemma faced by the defendant:

We told him that the judge was prepared to consider him not guilty by reason of insanity. 'But I am not insane,' said PS. We advised him, because of the consequences of this, to plead guilty. 'But I am not guilty,' said PS. Even the eloquent counsel paused, then PS spoke again: 'But you are three intelligent, educated people - I'll do whatever you say.'

The case was appealed to the Court of Appeal (1983 1 All E.R. 577) and ultimately to the House of Lords (1983 2 All E.R. 673), where the decision was also confirmed, 'thus enshrining in English law that a criminal act perpetrated during a seizure is an *insane* act and not one that is subject to the total acquittal of automatism' (Gunn 1991). Sullivan, in fact, was sentenced to 3 years' probation subject to the condition that he submit to treatment at the Maudsley Hospital under Dr Fenwick's direction.

The British legal position regarding epileptic automatism and insanity appears to be a pragmatic response to the perceived threat of a repeated episode of violent automatism from someone (e.g. Sullivan) who had already been guilty of such an act. As Gunn (1991) pointed out, 'British judges are in the business of trying to establish social order and control and they make up rules which are aimed in that direction'. In the Sullivan case Lord Justice Lawton expressed this view when he wrote (1983 1 All E.R. 577):

. . . this appeal must be dismissed. To some this may seem a harsh decision; but it should be remembered that persons who, through disease, cause injury to others and may do so again, are a potential danger to all who may come into contact with them. It is in the public interest that they should be put under medical care for as long as is reasonably necessary for the

protection of others, but no longer. The modern form of order for confinement following a special verdict gives the Secretary of State a wide discretion as to the kind of hospital to which a defendant should be sent and how long he should stay there.

. . .The acceptance . . . of a plea of guilty . . . might . . . be said to have been illogical, but merciful. However, in the particular circumstances of this case, it . . . enabled justice to be done.

Legal paradox

However, had Sullivan pleaded not guilty on grounds of insanity, which was the proper plea under British legal definitions, it is not at all clear that justice would have been done, especially if Sullivan had been detained in a mental hospital for a significant period of time, because he was not insane. That such a situation would have been bad enough in the case of Sullivan (whom all agreed committed his crime in the midst of an epileptic seizure) is clear. An even greater travesty of justice actually occurred in a New York case, in the Matter of Robert Torsney (394 N.E. 2d 262).

Robert H. Torsney was a New York City policeman. On the night of November 25, 1976 he and five fellow police officers were called to a housing project to settle a domestic dispute. As Torsney walked back toward his car he passed a group of teenage boys. One of them, 15-year-old Randolph Evans, asked, 'Did you just come from apartment 7-D?' The officers had not, but Torsney replied, 'You're damn right I did', pulled his gun and without further provocation shot Evans in the head. Torsney was indicted for second-degree murder and at his trial claimed that he had been suffering from a psychomotor seizure at the time of the shooting, even though he had no history of epilepsy before the shooting and his EEG was normal. In spite of conflicting testimony by expert witnesses regarding the possibility of epilepsy, the jury found him not guilty by reason of insanity and he was ordered into the custody of the New York State Department of Mental Hygiene. Five weeks after the verdict, an examining physician observed that 'neither before or after the offense (had Torsney) shown any signs of epilepsy'. Six months later a panel of physicians found no evidence of psychosis, a psychopathic disorder, or organic brain damage and recommended his release, which, although contested by the Brooklyn district attorney's office, he ultimately obtained.

Why does this case create a legal paradox and make a farce and mockery of the legal system? Because the sequence of events makes it clear that justice was not served. At trial the defence argued that Torsney had committed the crime as a result of psychomotor epilepsy and thus should be found not guilty by reason of insanity. The prosecution argued that Torsney did not have epilepsy and that therefore he should be found guilty of murder. Because he was found not guilty by reason of insanity he was hospitalized in a mental institution. Subsequently he argued that he was not insane and thus should be released. At this point the case required a reversal of the arguments presented by Torsney's attorney and the prosecution. Whereas the defence had, at the original trial, argued that Torsney should be found not guilty on grounds of insanity, it was now in the position of arguing that Torsney was not insane and therefore should be released. On the other hand, the prosecution, which at the original trial had argued that Torsney was not insane nor epileptic and therefore should be found guilty was, at the appeals trial, placed in the position of arguing that Torsney was indeed insane and should therefore not be released from the mental institution.

Use of the epilepsy defence

Of course, part of the problem with this case is that Torsney didn't really have epilepsy and certainly did not suffer from a complex partial seizure at the time of the shooting, so the original verdict was specious. This has been true of most American cases in which an epilepsy defence has been attempted. In 1986 Treiman reviewed the 75 crimes of violence where epilepsy was used as a defence which had been considered in the appellate literature from federal and state courts in the United States since 1889. Of these 75 cases only Torsney successfully used an epilepsy defence in the initial trial. In some cases the claim was made that the crime was committed during an epileptic seizure, whereas in others the defence had been based on a plea of diminished capacity (to know right from wrong) or insanity because

of chronic epilepsy, even though there was no evidence that the crime had occurred during an actual seizure. In none of these 75 cases was convincing evidence presented that the crime was the result of an epileptic seizure or in any way caused by epilepsy. None-the-less, the epilepsy defence in its various forms (insanity, diminished capacity, automatism, unconsciousness) continues to be a popular, if desperate, ploy by defence attorneys, at least in the United States. The evidence, however, suggests that ictal or even postictal aggression is extremely rare.

Even though attitudes toward epilepsy are improving in many parts of the world, including Great Britain and the United States, indiscriminate use of epilepsy as a defence is likely to perpetuate many myths and fallacies regarding the nature of epilepsy. Furthermore, the need for social order suggests that people should be held responsible for their actions, unless it can be shown that they had no conscious awareness of the action and no control over the loss of consciousness. For these reasons, it is essential that physicians who provide expert testimony to the courts in cases where an epilepsy defence is used in crimes of violence rigorously and critically consider the evidence for the existence of epilepsy and for the occurrence of a seizure at the time of the crime in the context of modern understanding of the nature of epileptic seizures.

Criteria for the diagnosis of peri-ictal violence

What should be the criteria for determining whether a violent crime was a result of an epileptic seizure? The 18 epileptologists who participated in the international workshop on aggression and epilepsy described above suggested five relevant criteria for consideration (Delgado-Escueta et al 1981):

1. The diagnosis of epilepsy should be established by at least one neurologist with special competence in epilepsy.
2. The presence of epileptic automatisms should be documented by the history and CCTV-EEG.
3. The presence of aggression during epileptic

automatism should be verified in a video recorded seizure in which ictal epileptiform patterns are also recorded on the electroencephalogram.

4. The aggressive or violent act should be

characteristic of the patient's habitual seizures as elicited in the history.

5. A clinical judgement should be made by the neurologist attesting to the possibility that the act was part of a seizure.

REFERENCES

American Law Institute 1962 Model penal code: proposed official draft. Philadelphia

Anonymous 1983 Insanity at law. British Medical Journal 287: 694–695

Ashford J W, Schulz S C, Walsh G O 1980 Violent automatisms in a partial complex seizure. Report of a case. Archives of Neurology 37: 120–122

Barrow R L, Fabing H D 1966 Epilepsy and the Law. A report on legal reform in the light of medical progress. Harper & Row, New York

Baumann R J, Marx B M, Leonidakis M G 1977 An estimate of the prevalence of epilepsy in a rural Appalachian population. American Journal of Epidemiology 106: 42–52

Baumann R J, Marx B M, Leonidakis M G 1978 Epilepsy in rural Kentucky: prevalence in a population of school age children. Epilepsia 19: 75–80

Brahams D 1983a Medicine and the law. Epilepsy and insanity at common law. Lancet i: 309

Brahams D 1983b Epilepsy is mental illness. Lancet ii: 116–117

Brahams D 1983c R v Sullivan: epilepsy, insanity and the common law. Medico-Legal Journal 51: 112–115

Brahams D 1983d Epilepsy and legal insanity. R v Sullivan. The Practitioner 227: 421–423

Brahams D 1984 Epilepsy and the law. Lancet i: 1481

Brewis M, Poskanzer D, Rolland C, Miller H 1966 Neurological disease in an English city. Acta Neurologica Scandinavica 42(suppl 24): 1–89

Chapman W P 1958 Studies of the periamygdaloid area in relation to human behaviour. In: Solomon H C, Cobb S, Penfield W (eds) The brain and human behavior. Association for Research in Nervous and Mental Diseases Research Publications, vol 36, p 258–277

Chatrian G E, Chapman W P 1960 Electrographic study of the amygdaloid region with implanted electrodes in patients with temporal lobe epilepsy. In: Ramey E R, O'Doherty D S (eds) Electrical studies on the unanesthetized brain. Paul B. Hoeber Inc, New York, p 351–373

Chiofalo N, Kirschbaum A, Fuentes A, Cordero M L, Madsen J 1979 Prevalence of epilepsy in children of Melipilla, Chile. Epilepsia 20: 261–266

College of General Practitioners 1960 A survey of the epileptics in general practice. British Medical Journal ii: 416–422

Commission on Classification and Terminology of the International League Against Epilepsy 1981: Proposal for revised clinical and electroencephalographic classification of epileptic seizures. Epilepsia 22: 489–501

Currie S, Heathfield K W G, Henson R A, Scott D F 1971 Clinical course and prognosis of temporal lobe epilepsy. Brain 94: 173–190

Delasiauve 1854 Traité de l' épilepsie. Quoted by Temkin O 1979 The falling sickness, 2nd edn. Johns Hopkins University Press, Baltimore

Delgado J M R, Halim H, Chapman W P 1952 Technique of intracranial electrode implacement for recording and stimulation and its possible therapeutic value in psychotic patients. Confinia Neurologica 12: 315–319

Delgado J M R, Mark V, Sweet W et al 1968 Intracerebral radio stimulation and recording in completely free patients. Journal of Nervous and Mental Diseases 147: 329–340

Delgado-Escueta A V, Kunze U, Waddell G, Boxley J, Nadel A 1977 Lapse of consciousness and automatisms in temporal lobe epilepsy: a video tape analysis. Neurology 27: 144–155

Delgado-Escueta A V, Nashold B, Freedman M et al 1979 Videotaping epileptic attacks during stereo electroencephalography Neurology 29: 473–489

Delgado-Escueta A V, Mattson R H, King L et al 1981 Special report. The nature of aggression during epileptic seizures. New England Journal of Medicine 305: 711–716

Delgado-Escueta A V, Bacsal F E, Treiman D M 1982 Complex partial seizures on closed circuit television and EEG: a study of 691 attacks in 79 patients. Annals of Neurology 11: 292–300

Engel J Jr, Caldecott-Hazard S, Bandler R 1986 Neurobiology of behavior: anatomic and physiological implications related to epilepsy. Epilepsia 27 (suppl 2): S3–S13

Epilepsy in North Carolina: resources and recommendations 1977 Chronic Disease Branch, Department of Human Resources, Raleigh, North Carolina

Ervin F R, Mark V H, Stevens J 1969 Behavioral and affective responses to brain stimulation in man. In: Zubin J, Shagass C (eds) Neurobiological aspects of psychopathology. American Psychopathological Association Proceedings, vol 58, p 54–65

Fenwick P 1987 Epilepsy and the law. In: Hopkins A (ed) Epilepsy. Chapman and Hall, London, p 553–562

Fenwick P 1988 Epilepsy and the law. In: Pedley T A, Meldrum B S (eds) Recent advances in epilepsy. Churchill Livingstone, Edinburgh, p 241–251

Fenwick P, Fenwick E (eds) 1985 Epilepsy and the law. Royal Society of Medicine International Congress and Symposium Series, no. 81. Royal Society of Medicine, London

Foderé, F-E Les lois éclairées par les sciences physiques; ou traité de médecine-légale et d'hygiéne publique, t. premier. Paris, l'an septième. Cited by Temkin O 1979 The falling sickness, 2nd edn. Johns Hopkins University Press, Baltimore

Golding A M B 1985 The law relating to epilepsy and allied disorders. Community Medicine 7: 278–282

Gomez J G, Arciniegas E, Torres J 1978 Prevalence of epilepsy in Bogota, Columbia. Neurology 28: 90–94

Gowers W R 1881 Epilepsy and other chronic convulsive diseases: their causes and symptoms. Churchill, London

Griffith N, Engel J Jr, Bandler R 1987 Ictal and enduring interictal disturbances in emotional behaviour in an animal model of temporal lobe epilepsy. Brain Research 400: 360–364

Gudmundsson G 1966 Epilepsy in Iceland, a clinical and epidemiological investigation. Acta Neurologica Scandinavica 43 (suppl 25): 1–124

Gunn J 1977 Epileptics in prison. Academic Press, London

Gunn J 1991 Legal implications of behavioral changes in epilepsy. In: Smith D, Treiman D M, Trimble M (eds) Advances in neurology, vol 55: Neurobehavioral problems in epilepsy. Raven Press, New York, p 461–471

Gunn J, Bonn J 1971 Criminality and violence in epileptic prisoners. British Journal of Psychiatry 118: 337–343

Gunn J, Fenton G 1971 Epilepsy, automatism and crime. Lancet 1: 1173–1176

Hauser W A, Kurland L T 1975 The epidemiology of epilepsy in Rochester, Minnesota, 1935 through 1967. Epilepsia 16: 1–66

Heath R G 1955 Correlations between levels of psychological awareness and physiological activity in the central nervous system. Psychosomatic Medicine 17: 383–395

Heath R G 1962 Brain centers and control of behavior—man. In: Nodine J H, Moyer J H (eds) Psychosomatic medicine: the first Hahnemann symposium. Lea & Febiger, Philadelphia, p 228–240

Heath R G 1964 Developments toward new physiologic treatments in psychiatry. Journal of Neuropsychiatry 5: 318–331

Heath R G, Monroe R R, Mickle W A 1955 Stimulation of the amygdaloid nucleus in a schizophrenic patient. American Journal of Psychiatry 111: 862–863

Hermann B P 1982 Neuropsychological functioning and psychopathology in children with epilepsy. Epilepsia 23: 545–554

Hermann B P, Riel P 1981 Interictal personality and behavioural traits in temporal lobe and primary generalized epilepsy. Cortex 17: 125–128

Hermann B P, Schwartz M S, Whitman S, Karnes W E 1980 Aggression and epilepsy: seizure type comparisons and high risk variables. Epilepsia 22: 691–698

Hindler C G 1989 Epilepsy and violence. British Journal of Psychiatry 155: 246–249

Hollingsworth J S 1978 Mental retardation, cerebral palsy and epilepsy in Alabama. University of Alabama, Tuscaloosa, Alabama

Jackson 1873 On the anatomical, physiological, and pathological investigation of epilepsies. West Riding Lunatic Asylum Medical Reports 3: 315

James I P 1960 Temporal lobectomy for psychomotor epilepsy. Journal of Mental Sciences 106: 543–558

Juul-Jensen P 1964 Epilepsy: a clinical and social analysis of 1020 adult patients with epileptic seizures. Acta Neurologica Scandinavica 40(suppl 5): S1–S148

Kalyanaraman S 1975 Some observations during stimulation of the human hypothalamus. Confinia Neurologica 37: 189–192

King H E 1961 Psychological effects of excitation in the limbic system. In: Sheer D E (ed) Electrical stimulation of the brain. Austin, University of Texas Press, p 477–486

King D W, Ajmone Marsan C 1977 Clinical features and ictal patterns in epileptic patients with EEG temporal lobe foci. Annals of Neurology 2: 138–147

King L M, Young Q D 1978 Increased prevalence of seizures disorders among prisoners. Journal of the American Medical Association 239: 2674–2675

Kligman D, Goldberg D A 1975 Temporal lobe epilepsy and

aggression. Journal of Nervous and Mental Disease 160: 324–341

Knox S J 1968 Epileptic automatism and violence. Medical Science and Law 8: 96–104

Kolb L C, Brodie H K H (eds) 1982 Modern clinical psychiatry, 10th edn. Saunders, Philadelphia

Korbar K, Berkovic K 1974 Epilepsy and delinquency. Neuropshijatirja 22: 6–75

Mark V H, Ervin F R (eds) 1970 Violence and the brain. Harper & Row, New York

Mark V H, Ervin F R, Sweet W H, Delgado J 1969 Remote telemeter stimulation and recording from implanted temporal lobe electrodes. Confinia Neurologica 31: 86–93

Mark V H, Sweet W H, Ervin F R 1975 Deep temporal lobe stimulation and destructive lesions in episodically violent temporal lobe epileptics. In: Fields W S, Sweet W H (eds) Neural bases of violence and aggression. Warren H Green, St Louis, p 379–391

Novick L F, Penna R D, Schwartz M S, Remmlinger E, Loewenstein R 1977 Health status of the New York City prison population. Medical Care 15: 205–216

Ounsted C 1969 Aggression and epilepsy rage in children with temporal lobe epilepsy. Journal of Psychosomatic Research 13: 237–242

Platner E 1824 Opuscula academica . . . post mortem auctoris edidit C. G. Neumann. Berlin. Cited by Temkin O 1979 The falling sickness, 2nd edn. Johns Hopkins University Press, Baltimore

Portal (Le Baron) 1827 Observations sur la nature et le traitement de l' épilepsie. Paris. Cited in Temkin O 1979 The falling sickness, 2nd edn. Johns Hopkins University Press, Baltimore

Rodin E A 1973 Psychomotor epilepsy and aggressive behaviour. Archives of General Psychiatry 28: 210–213

Saint-Hilaire J M, Gilbert M, Bouvier G, Barbeau A 1980 Epilepsy and aggression: two cases with depth electrode studies. In: Robb P (ed) Epilepsy updated: causes and treatment. Symposia Specialist, Miami, p 145–176

Schmidt R P, Wilder B J 1988 Epilepsy and the law: a commentary from the United States perspective. In Pedley T A, Meldrum B S (eds) Recent advances in epilepsy. Churchill Livingstone, Edinburgh, p 253–257

Sem-Jacobsen C W (ed) 1968 Depth-electrographic stimulation of the human brain and behavior. Charles C Thomas, Springfield

Serafetinides E A 1965 Aggressiveness in temporal lobe epileptics and its relation to cerebral dysfunction and environmental factors. Epilepsia 6: 33–42

Shamansky S L, Glaser G H 1979 Socioeconomic characteristics of seizure disorders in the New Haven area: an epidemiologic study. Epilepsia 20: 457–474

Sheer D E (ed) 1961 Electrostimulation of the brain. University of Texas Press, Austin

Swan M 1984 Epilepsy and insanity. Lancet ii: 756

Taylor D C 1969 Aggression and epilepsy. Journal of Psychosomatic Research 13: 229–236

Taylor P 1985 Epilepsy and insanity. In: Fenwick P, Fenwick E (eds) Epilepsy and the law. Royal Society of Medicine International Congress and Symposium Series, no. 81. Royal Society of Medicine, London

Temkin O 1971 The falling sickness, 2nd edn. Johns Hopkins University Press, Baltimore

Treiman D M 1986 Epilepsy and violence: medical and legal issues. Epilepsia 27(suppl 2): S77–S104

Treiman D M 1990 Subtle complex partial status epilepticus. Neurology 40(suppl 1): 298

Treiman D M 1991 Psychobiology of ictal aggression. In: Smith D B, Treiman D M, Trimble M R (eds) Advances in neurology, vol 55: Neurobehavioral problems in epilepsy. Raven Press, New York, p 341–356

Treiman D M, Delgado-Escueta A V 1980 Status epilepticus. In: Thompson R, Green J R (eds) Critical care of neurologic and neurosurgical emergencies. Raven Press, New York, p 53–99

Treiman D M, Delgado-Escueta A V 1981 Aggression during fear and fight in complex partial seizures: a CCTV-EEG analysis. Epilepsia 22: 243

Treiman D M, Delgado-Escueta A V 1983 Violence and epilepsy: a critical review. In: Pedley T A, Meldrum B S (eds) Recent advances in epilepsy, vol 1. Churchill Livingstone, Edinburgh, p 179–209

Ursin H 1960 The temporal lobe substrate of fear and anger. A review of recent stimulation and ablation studies in animals and humans. Acta Neurologica Scandinavica 35: 378–396

Whitman S, Hermann B P, Black R B, Chhabria S 1982 Psychopathology and seizure type in children with epilepsy. Psychological Medicine 12: 843–853

Wieser H G 1983 Depth recorded limbic seizures and psychopathology. Neuroscience and Biobehavioral Reviews 7: 427–440

CASES CITED

Bratty v Attorney-General for Northern Ireland 1961 All England Law Reports 3: 523–539

Daniel M'Naghten's Case 1843 Clark and Finnelly's Reports 10: 200–214

Durham v United States 1954 Federal Reporter 2d series 214: 862–876

In the Matter of Robert Torsney 1979 North Eastern Reporter 2d series 394: 262–278

Regina v Charlson 1955 All England Law Reports 1: 859–864

Regina v Kemp 1956 All England Law Reports 3: 249–254

Regina v Sullivan 1983 The Weekly Law Reports 3: 123–130

R v Sullivan 1983 All England Law Reports l: 577–582

R v Sullivan 1983 All England Law Reports 2: 673–679

The People v James A. Freeman 1943 California Appellate Reports 2d series 61: 110–119

United States of America v Charles Freeman 1966 Federal Reporter 2d series 357: 606–629

21. Social aspects of epilepsy

P. Thompson   J. Oxley

INTRODUCTION

In recent years there has been increasing awareness of the social dimensions of epilepsy and their importance to the medical profession (Whitman & Hermann 1986, Scambler 1987, Sonnen 1990). In this chapter we review, in turn, the following areas: education, employment, the family, the law including driving regulations, leisure, public education and mobility. Our aim is to be informative but also to offer practical solutions to some of the problems raised.

EDUCATION

Schooling will have a major impact on a child's academic, emotional and social development. This section focuses on factors which may influence a child's educational career. Emotional and social development are considered in a later section. In particular we will concentrate on ways of promoting normal educational and personal development in so far as this is possible in individual cases. Sweeping statements about children with epilepsy are less helpful than information about a particular child or young person with epilepsy and the factors which may influence development. The potential for discrimination inherent in formulating policies for school activities based on generalizations about children with epilepsy should be self-evident, and a positive, informed approach is required if discrimination is to be finally eradicated.

From segregation towards integration

In many countries the philosophy underlying educational provision for children with epilepsy has changed radically during the twentieth century. At the turn of the century, a policy of exclusion predominated. This was replaced by one of segregation. As we enter the last decade of the century, a policy of segregation has largely given way to one of integration. In the United Kingdom, government sponsored reports into services for epilepsy have endorsed the view that most children with epilepsy should be educated in mainstream schools. Special education provision should be made only after careful assessment of the child's needs [Central Health Services Council (CHSC) 1956, Central Health Services Council (CHSC) 1969, Kurtz & Morgan 1987, Department of Health and Social Security (DHSS) 1986]. Thus, the Reid Report (CHSC 1969) recommended that the decision to send a child with epilepsy to a special school should only be taken 'after a full assessment at a hospital diagnostic clinic' and that if the full range of medical, social and education facilities were available from 'the onset of the condition, even fewer than the present few number of children would require long-term placement in special schools'.

The Report of the Committee of Enquiry into the Education of Handicapped Children and Young People (Warnock Report 1978) and the 1981 Education Act which followed it, emphasized that children with special educational needs should be educated in normal schools wherever practicable. The most recent evaluation of epilepsy services believed placement in mainstream schools did not equate with integration and that if integration was to be truly successful and meet individual needs, schools required better support and services than were currently available (DHSS 1986).

Published figures for children with epilepsy of school age in Great Britain vary, but estimates generally fall between 30 000 and 70 000 (Ross et al 1980, O'Donohoe 1985) and most children with epilepsy do attend mainstream schools (Neafsey et al 1987, Thompson 1987). It is estimated that approximately one-third of children with epilepsy are at special schools but placement is largely due to the presence of additional handicaps, most notably severe learning difficulties and behavioural problems (Kurtz & Morgan 1987, Besag 1987).

Children face academic difficulties

Merely placing a child in a mainstream school, however, is no guarantee of educational success. Amongst those children with epilepsy in mainstream schools there is evidence that a significant number underachieve in certain subject areas. Problems in reading, and to a greater extent spelling and arithmetic, have been reported (Ross & West 1978, Yule 1980, Seidenberg et al 1986, Aldenkamp 1987). In addition, young people with epilepsy appear to do less well than their peer group in terms of educational and vocational qualifications (Britten et al 1986).

It is now widely accepted that academic difficulties may arise for many reasons and useful generalizations about children with epilepsy are difficult to make. Most attention has focused upon seizure-related factors with poor educational prognosis associated with early age of onset and a long seizure history, particularly where seizure control has proved problematic (O'Leary et al 1981, 1983, Dean 1983, Seidenberg et al 1989, Aldenkamp et al 1990). Seizure type also exerts an influence. For example, the site of epileptic discharges in complex partial seizures can affect the nature of the cognitive disturbance. Dominant hemisphere disturbances are more likely to affect language related processing and non-dominant disturbances spatial processing (Aarts et al 1984). Other factors which should be considered as a possible cause of lack of achievement include the occurrence of nocturnal attacks, brief epileptic discharges which can result in transient cognitive impairment, high levels of medication and polypharmacy (Stores 1987, Renier 1987, Cull &Trimble 1989).

Other psychosocial variables have been implicated. These include parental and teacher's expectations, misconceptions about epilepsy, absence from school, low self-esteem and anxiety due to stress at home. Until recently these have been overlooked. These factors have an important role with regard to educational prognosis. A recent longitudinal study concluded 'it is social rather than medical (neurological) factors which lead to lower school achievements in children with epilepsy' (Suurmeijer undated). We will return to consider some of these factors later in this section. Following a review of this area, Seidenberg (Seidenberg et al 1989) concludes 'a myriad of psychological, psychosocial and medication factors impinge upon the child with epilepsy and may affect the adequacy of the child's development and neuropsychological functioning'.

Special education

A minority of children with epilepsy, for the variety of reasons indicated above, may experience significant educational difficulties. In the United Kingdom such children are covered by the 1981 Education Act 'an act to make provision with respect to children with special educational needs'. The Act defines 'special educational needs' and together with the Education (special education needs) Regulations (1983) establishes a statutory code for those children under 19 years. Under the Act a child has a learning difficulty if:

1. he/she has a significantly greater difficulty in learning than the majority of children of his/ her age
2. he/she has a disability which either prevents or hinders him/her from making use of educational facilities of a kind generally provided for schools within the area of the local authority concerned for children of his/ her age
3. he/she is under the age of 5 years and is, or would be, if special educational provision were not made for him/her likely to fall within paragraphs (1) or (2) when over that age.

Where a child is considered to have special educational needs, then the Act requires specification of those needs, a process known as 'statementing'.

Local Education Authorities are required to conduct a multiprofessional assessment taking into account medical, educational, psychological and other factors, including the views of parents. If, following this assessment, the local education authority concludes that the child has special educational needs, it must make a written statement of such needs and the special educational provision that should be made to meet these needs. Special education provision may be made in various forms, such as in separate special schools, special units attached to primary and secondary schools, in special classes in day and boarding schools and in the child's home.

A working group convened by the Department of Health and Social Security to review services for people with epilepsy considered that only a few children with epilepsy would be expected to require statutory assessment and statementing of special educational needs (DHSS 1986). It felt that the majority would be identified under more informal procedures established by each local education authority. The Working Group believed that the relevant statutory authorities should encourage parents of children with epilepsy to fulfil their important role in the assessment procedure and help them to do so. The voluntary organizations were envisaged as having a potentially important role in providing information, help and advice to parents about the statementing procedure. The Advisory Centre for Education (ACE) publishes a wide range of information relating to education law and provision. ACE also offers free telephone advice (see Appendix C).

Where placement in a special school is considered to be advisable, this decision will often be made because of a learning difficulty or accompanying behavioural problems and not solely because of epilepsy. The DHSS Working Group (DHSS 1986) was concerned that special schools were sometimes unsupported regarding expert advice on epilepsy and that children did not always receive regular medical reviews.

Residential schools for epilepsy

There are three residential schools specializing in the treatment of epilepsy in the United Kingdom.

In addition, the Park Hospital for Children in Oxford has a short-term medical assessment facility for children with epilepsy with an attached school, such that children who remain there for several months do not miss out on their education. It is estimated that only about one in a hundred children with epilepsy have special needs requiring placement in a special school for epilepsy. These schools are well equipped to deal with frequent seizures, postictal problems and cases at risk for status epilepticus (Besag 1987). Placement at these schools is rarely a consequence of the severity of epilepsy per se. Other reasons include cognitive problems, behaviour difficulties, family and social problems and psychiatric problems (Besag 1987, Kurtz & Morgan 1987). A major disadvantage of residential education is the risk of weakening the child's links with parents and home and this has been highlighted by Kurtz & Morgan (1987). These authors, commenting on educational provision in these schools during the 1970s, noted that parents were often unaware of discussions and case conference proceedings that had taken place among the professional workers concerning their children. Awareness of such problems has led to improved communications between schools and families. St Piers Lingfield (formerly Lingfield Hospital School) works closely with families and offers the opportunity for parents with similar problems to meet together for mutual support and guidance from the multiprofessional team.

Provision outside the United Kingdom

Provision for children with special educational needs varies from country to country. Some, like the United Kingdom, have special provision for children with epilepsy (e.g. the Netherlands, Germany). In other countries, facilities for children with special needs are considered adequate to cater for children with epilepsy who have educational difficulties (e.g. Sweden—Molenaar 1987, Schwager 1987). In the USA, Public Law 94-141 and the Education for All Handicapped Children Act provides that those children whose epilepsy affects their educational performance are entitled to free public education or selected support services appropriate to their specific needs.

As in the United Kingdom, the argument is made for special needs to be met in mainstream schools wherever possible. The movement away from segregation was spearheaded by disabilities rights groups including the Epilepsy Foundation of America's affiliates (EFA 1990). The important role of parents is emphasized, including their right to challenge a school's educational decisions and to call upon evidence from experts. The complexity of educational needs including the value of investigation by a multidisciplinary team and broad cognitive assessments are endorsed. Individual children have individual educational programmes (IEPs) which include written educational goals and intervention strategies and are reviewed at least annually (Seidenberg personal communication).

Promoting educational success (Table 21.1)

Communication is essential

Inadequate communication can contribute to educational and social difficulties for the child with epilepsy. During the 1950s in the United Kingdom it was estimated that up to one-half of children with epilepsy were unknown to the school authorities (CHSC 1956). It is to be hoped this situation has now improved. However, non-disclosure by parents probably still occurs. If the school is unaware that a child has seizures, the impact of an attack during school hours is potentially devastating. A child may be mislabelled as lazy or a daydreamer due to absences. Complex partial seizures may be seen as truculent behaviour or madness. The Central Health Services Council (1969) report emphasized that 'communication will be of supreme importance and it will be essential to ensure that no conflicting advice is given to parents and teachers'.

Subsequent reports have endorsed the need for openness and a full exchange of information between primary health care services and school health services. Where good communication channels exist, they can exert a positive influence on treatment. Thus, a teacher is in a position to provide doctors with information, directly or indirectly, that may lead to beneficial changes in treatment. Sillanpaa (1983) writes 'teachers are in an excellent situation to identify seizures, particularly non-convulsive varieties; to facilitate diagnosis by describing the overt features, and evaluate the efficacy of pharmacotherapy, to report adverse drug effects and to promote the social and emotional development of epileptic children'.

Information must be accurate

Communication will be of limited value and may even be counterproductive unless the information exchanged is accurate and the knowledge base of the recipients is adequate. Parents may have inaccurate beliefs about epilepsy which they may pass on to the school. Teachers may have their own fears and misconceptions about the disorder. Faulty or conflicting parental and teacher expectations may have a negative impact on the child's school achievements and social functioning. Holdsworth & Whitmore (1974) found that a third of children with epilepsy had undue restrictions placed on their sporting activities at school.

The DHSS Working Group (DHSS 1986) considered school nurses to have a pivotal role within the school health services including 'allaying fears about epilepsy and promoting the ability of children with epilepsy'. Family doctors need to take time to discuss with parents the potential risks involved in various activities, taking into consideration the type and frequency of their child's seizures.

Information about epilepsy given during the training of teachers in the United Kingdom varies enormously but is generally considered to be quite limited, particularly outside special needs courses (Corbidge 1987). Packages are now available from epilepsy organizations providing teachers with background information about epilepsy and practical instruction, including how to manage different types of attacks (e.g. Craig et al 1985, Corbidge 1987, BEA 1991). The Epilepsy Foundation of America recommends that, as a minimum requirement, a teacher should:

— be familiar with the specific features of a
   child's seizure disorder
— know how to recognize an attack and how to
   manage it
— know what the child's medication is
— know how the medication might affect school
   performance and classroom behaviour.

For children where there is an increased likelihood of seizures occurring during the school day, classmates can benefit from teaching about epilepsy. A skilful teacher should be able to impart such knowledge in a way that does not embarrass the child with epilepsy. Teaching materials are available for classroom settings for use with even very young children (Craig et al 1985, Rogan 1987).

Children need a positive self-image

Strategies to achieve effective communication and an adequate understanding of epilepsy must include the child with epilepsy. The Central Health Services Council (1969) report noted 'the child should be told about his condition and encouraged to understand not only the limitations it may impose on his everyday life or on his future employment but also his capacity to participate in normal living'. If the child is kept in the dark, and particularly if teacher behaviour is shaped by misinformation, the child's emotional and social adjustment can be influenced adversely. This situation is made worse where teasing and taunting from classmates occurs. One parent commented: 'My son was teased a lot at his primary school. We transferred him to another school and they have been great. Kids and staff'. Low self-esteem, once developed, can lead to social withdrawal, reduced motivation and even school phobia (Kato et al 1979). Pazzaglia & Frank-Pazzaglia (1976) reported the main cause for educational difficulties in their sample was a depressive reaction which resulted from classmates fear of the epileptic seizures and the attitudes of classmates' parents.

Undue restrictions on sporting and other activities can contribute to a child's feelings of being different and inadequate. The child needs to have a wide opportunity to increase chances of success. A child with epilepsy wrote 'I missed out on every school excursion from the day of my first fit. My parents didn't want me to go and teachers were nervous about my epilepsy anyway'. Children with epilepsy need sound careers advice and the services of a specialist careers advisor may be warranted for some children.

A full education is required

For the child with epilepsy, minimizing time off school will be important. Teachers with adequate knowledge will be able to ensure a whole day's schooling is not lost because of a seizure occurring during the first lesson. Clinic appointments can be scheduled to reduce time off from school. Where hospitalization is required, professionals involved should ensure the period of inpatient treatment is limited and where a child is likely to miss several weeks from school, the possibility of providing education within the hospital setting should be explored. Even a short absence from regular classes can be sufficient to make a child fall significantly behind classmates.

Providing a full education involves considering pre-school and tertiary educational options. Where a child has problematic epilepsy, nursery placement may have considerable benefits academically, emotionally and socially. Equally, young people should not be dissuaded on the basis of their epilepsy from undertaking college and university courses. Although they are under-represented in tertiary education, the evidence suggests that young people with epilepsy go on to obtain degrees and comparable vocational qualifications (Harding & Betts 1987). For those young people considered to have special educational needs, the majority of further education and technical colleges in the United Kingdom now put on special courses, mainly designed for those with moderate or severe learning difficulties. These courses emphasize building confidence, basic skills and some vocational skills.

Monitoring progress is essential

Careful yet unobtrusive observation and monitoring of educational progress and social development of the child with epilepsy is recommended. Unfortunately, all problems may be perceived as an invariable consequence of having epilepsy. Strang (1987) writes 'unfortunately we have found that when a learning disabled child with epilepsy is "mainstreamed" into the regular classroom situation without proper identification of his learning disability, it is not uncommon for teachers to blame all of the learning, social and other problems on the presence of the epilepsy'. The earlier the difficulties are observed, the sooner these can be addressed. Good communica-

Table 21.1 Minimizing education failure and maximizing social development: the important steps in ensuring maximum education success

1. Ensure good communication between:
    — school
    — doctor and
    — family
2. Teaching about epilepsy
    — teachers
    — pupils
    — child with epilepsy
3. Positive self-image
    — increase chances of success
    — avoid unnecessary restrictions
    — provide good careers advice
4. Full education
    — avoid time off school due to appointments, hospital attendance, seizure recovery
    — explore nursery placements
    — encourage tertiary education
5. Monitoring
    — detect difficulties early
    — provide a full assessment

tion from teacher to parents may result in a medical review, possibly a medication change and an improvement in school performance may ensue. In other instances, a wider assessment may be required. The Central Health Services Council (1969) report emphasizes that 'the complexity of the problems facing parents and children makes it impossible for any one discipline to deal as a group with all of them and for this reason, more than with adults, a team approach is essential'. Parents are an important part of the team.

When a child presents with poor academic progress then a detailed neuropsychological evaluation should be sought. In order to be of any value this assessment needs to be more than the provision of an intellectual quotient and should include measures of memory, attention, speed of information processing and problem-solving capacity (Wehrli 1987, Strang 1987).

EMPLOYMENT

There are many reasons why the topic of employment is crucial to a consideration of the needs of people with epilepsy. People with epilepsy want to play a full part in the culture in which they live. Working, being an employee and earning a living, is an outward sign of integration and of acceptability by others. In the words of the Reid

report (Central Health Services Council 1969), 'Employment determines the way of life, social and financial status and the role in society and it is a source of personal satisfaction, of social companionship, of esteem, of discipline and of purpose.'

The work ethic remains predominant in many cultures as a way of structuring both society and time. And in those where it is not so all-pervasive, the need to earn money in order to simply survive may be the key motivating factor in the search for paid employment.

The relevance of employment issues to doctors and other health professionals has been succinctly summarized by Porter (1984): 'The degree of social adaptation in work, school and recreation is the final criterion for health care delivery to the patient with epilepsy.'

The fact that there is still a great deal more to be done has been shown by the result of a survey of nearly 2000 people with epilepsy living ordinary lives in the community in the UK, 72% of whom rated employment as presenting some or serious problems to them. This was the second highest problem area, only driving and transport being more of a problem (British Epilepsy Association 1990).

Cultural factors are crucial

It is unhelpful, however, just to make general statements about the employment needs of people with epilepsy without making reference to the society in which they live and want to work. In a similar way it is unhelpful to make recommendations about optimal drug treatment on purely scientific grounds without being aware of the many factors that influence the delivery of health care and thereby the likelihood of any particular drug being available to any particular patient.

The first key message in this section is that doctors who want to improve the employment prospects of people with epilepsy must be fully briefed about the prevailing social, political and economic circumstances affecting their patients. General statements by doctors that 'people with epilepsy ought to be given jobs' are useless. Furthermore, solutions to employment problems identified in western Europe and the USA, where most of the research has been carried out, may have little relevance to other societies. And even within this group of developed countries there are marked differences. Over the last 5 years in the UK, for example, there has been no improvement in the employment prospects of people with disabilities in general. This has been due to a persistently high level of unemployment which has offset advances in medical science, campaigns to persuade employers, and a demographic shift leading to a relative shortage of young people looking for work.

But these statements could lead to the conclusion that all effort to improve the employability of people with epilepsy is wasted unless the economic circumstances are favourable. Firstly, however, this is certainly not the case at an individual level, where properly targeted help can produce dramatic improvements in job related abilities. Secondly, at a macro level, campaigns to improve the employment image of any subgroup of the work force take a long time to gather momentum and to be effective. And thirdly, even when there is a plentiful supply of skilled labour, the situation can be made even better for employers in particular and society in general as more people with disabilities working means more tax payers sharing in the tax burden and more consumers wanting and able to pay for employers' products and services. And so, our second key message in this section is that efforts to change the employability image of people with epilepsy should be based on a long-term strategy which must be tuned to prevailing economic circumstances and the needs of employers. In other words, opportunities for improvement must both be seized and be created.

This review of a complex subject will concentrate on two main areas. Firstly, the size and nature of the problem and secondly, those interventions which are thought to be effective in improving employability in the key areas of legislation, non-statutory ways of changing attitudes and vocational guidance and training. The statements made are based on the published research findings, which have been reviewed by Floyd (1986) and Hauser & Hesdorffer (1990), and the experience of the authors. The authors have worked directly with people severely disabled by epilepsy at a UK centre and on a wider front both

nationally and internationally. The focus of this section will be the experience of people with epilepsy in the UK.

The size and nature of the problem

Just as the erroneous medical belief about the overall poor prognosis of epilepsy was based on studies of highly-selected populations of severely affected patients, so too have many of the studies on employment looked at similar groups. Therefore these results are similarly suspect. It is hardly surprising that very high levels of unemployment and high levels of occupational dissatisfaction have been found in patients attending tertiary referral centres. Such patients will have intractable seizures and other handicaps.

Lamentably few studies have attempted to survey less severely affected groups of patients and make valid comparisons with samples of the general population of working age. One study from the USA, quoted by Hauser & Hesdorffer (1990), looked at 127 non-retarded people with epilepsy living in Rochester, Minnesota. The study concluded that the unemployment rate amongst these people with epilepsy was about double that of the general population in that geographical area. A survey conducted by the Employment Commission of the International Bureau for Epilepsy (Fraser 1988, Fraser 1990) produced unemployment rates amongst people with epilepsy ranging from 15 to 50% in eight countries worldwide. But the validity of this information is not known.

It is hoped that large on-going community based studies, notably the UK's National General Practice Study of Epilepsy (Hart et al 1989) will provide more detailed accurate information about the impact of epilepsy on employment.

An alternative approach to finding out if people with epilepsy have problems getting and keeping jobs, is to look at people in employment and find out how many of them have epilepsy. If it is found that there is a lower percentage of employed people with epilepsy than in the general population of working age then this would suggest that epilepsy can be a barrier to getting work in that particular occupational area. Some early work in the UK (Scambler & Hopkins 1980) suggested that married women with epilepsy were particularly under-represented in the work force. Low social class and frequent seizures were other factors determining employment status in this study. A notable study by Lisle & Waldron (1986) looked at a sample of employees in the UK National Health Service, said to be the largest civilian employer in Europe. They found a prevalence rate of 1.35/1000 of employees known to have epilepsy, much lower than the 4 to 10/1000 people with epilepsy in the population as a whole (Zielinski 1988). However, a survey of 40 000 private households in the UK (Prescott-Clarke 1990) found a prevalence of approximately 2/1000 in a broadly defined economically active group. Epilepsy was found to be more common, however, in those looking for work than those in work.

Surveys of this kind are difficult to do. The sample has to be large and the findings can be criticized on the grounds that people with epilepsy are often reluctant to disclose their epilepsy (Scambler & Hopkins 1980) because of the fear that this information might lead to dismissal. This could result in fewer people with epilepsy being identified than there really are. Only in an occupation which has a comprehensive pre-employment medical assessment which is known not to discriminate against people with disabilities will this problem of non-disclosure be minimized. Such a system operates in the UK Civil Service which is responsible for employing all government staff (Espir et al 1987). Here all medical information is considered only by qualified staff and only after an applicant has been offered a job. A survey carried out on successful job applicants to the UK Civil Service showed that prevalence of people with epilepsy was 3.3/1000 (Espir personal communication).

Finding solutions to the problems

Assuming that people with epilepsy are under-represented in the workforce, being able to rectify the situation depends on the answers to a number of related further questions. Firstly, is there any need to employ more people with epilepsy? Secondly, do we understand all the factors which have led to this situation? And thirdly, are there mechanisms for taking action, which are known to be successful? The answers to these will vary from society to society but from a research point of view only the second and third of these have been studied in any systematic way.

The need to recruit more people from any group within society into employment will depend on two factors; firstly, the advantage to society of having them in the workforce and secondly, the disadvantage to society if they remain unemployed. Having epilepsy does not itself confer any particular job-related skills, although many organizations both for and of people with disabilities maintain that sufferers from a condition have particular aptitudes for helping others in a similar position. The number of people so employed will, however, be very small. People with disabilities are often said to make excellent employees, with high levels of commitment. Even if true, this is very difficult to quantify. But people with disabilities represent a body of people with energy and talent into whom considerable investment has often been made in terms of medical care and education. Retrieving that investment will depend on there being paid jobs for them to do. And in some countries, faced with demographic changes leading to fewer young people, people with disabilities are likely to be an increasingly relevant part of the country's earning capacity.

Many countries now subscribe to the concept of equal opportunities for all its citizens. Although originally applied to gender and race, the idea that someone should be disadvantaged in getting work merely because of a diagnostic label, rather than because of the direct effect that this condition has on ability to work, is now regarded as philosophically unacceptable by many societies. Their willingness to rectify obvious shortcomings in day-to-day employment practice is, however, often lacking. Nevertheless, if a country does subscribe to the concept of equal opportunities in employment then there is a clear need to ensure that people with epilepsy are included.

The disadvantages to society of people remaining needlessly unemployed are considerable. They are likely to be financially dependent either on their families or on the state and they will probably not contribute substantially to society's funds either as tax payers or as consumers. The cost of state funded employment and training services specifically for people with disabilities can also be considerable (£140.7 million in Great Britain in 1989/90). Unemployment itself is said to lead to an increase in ill health (Hayes & Nutman 1981) and thereby a greater cost in providing additional health care. These direct costs of unemployment are augmented by considerable indirect costs. Otherwise known as opportunity costs, they arise as a result of the loss of income sustained because society's funds are being diverted towards supporting some of its members to do nothing rather than in more profitable areas such as investment, overseas trade or consumerism.

Factors which affect employment prospects

The second supplementary question requiring an answer was concerned with our understanding of the many factors which may affect employment prospects amongst people with epilepsy. These have been reviewed by Zielinski & Rader (1984). Understanding these factors in some detail is important to devising strategies for overcoming them. Craig & Oxley (1986) have devised a framework for looking at the various barriers to employment which may be present. This framework is reproduced here as it allows for any employment situation to be analysed irrespective of its particular medical, economic or social components. The examples given are drawn for the UK but others can easily be substituted. The model differentiates between the intentional and unintentional barriers, those that are overt (obvious) and those that are covert (hidden). It also indicates whether the barriers are within the person with epilepsy (intrinsic) or in other people or due to external circumstances (extrinsic). This model is summarized in Table 21.2

It should not, however, be used to reinforce the view that people with epilepsy in general face overwhelming odds when looking for a job. Clearly

some do, but many do not. In attempting to assess any problem area, therefore, it is essential to be specific and consider a particular person in terms of a particular job. This model also permits a preliminary analysis of ways of overcoming employment barriers; or in other words opportunities to improve the employability of people with epilepsy.

Some of the major areas worthy of consideration under the main headings of this framework are listed in Table 21.3. The discussion which follows looks at some of these areas in more detail, highlighting those which can be changed.

Intentional barriers

The advantage of barriers that are both intentional and overt is that they can be identified, evaluated and, if found to be unreasonable, challenged. Their drawback is that they are often enshrined in legislation and effecting any change can be extremely difficult. In this section we will consider the legislation that governs employment in some occupations, eligibility for pension schemes and employers' accident liability, and the provision of sheltered employment.

Legislation The UK has no central source of information about what restrictions might apply to a particular person with epilepsy in respect of types of employment. Craig & Oxley (1986) compiled a list of statutory regulations derived from a variety of sources, acknowledging that this list might be incomplete (Table 21.4). In addition to these statutory barriers, the common law is not infrequently and quite legitimately used to avoid employing someone with epilepsy (Carter 1986). It would seem logical that there should be some central agency in each country which should firstly collate and disseminate information about statutory barriers to employment; secondly, examine their validity from time to time in the light of current employment practice and medical knowledge; and thirdly, issue guidance in general terms about the suitability for employment of those with epilepsy. Merely relying on legislation and the inevitable variation in its interpretation by different employing authorities only tends to perpetuate confusion and uncertainty to the disadvantage of the job seeker with epilepsy. More detailed individualized guidance may also be necessary and in

Table 21.2 Barriers to employment—a conceptual framework

Overt/Intentional	*Covert/Intentional*
Intrinsic	Intrinsic
Extrinsic	Extrinsic
Overt/Unintentional	*Covert/Unintentional*
Intrinsic	Intrinsic
Extrinsic	Extrinsic

Table 21.3 Barriers to employment

Overt/intentional

Intrinsic
None—this would negate the possibility of employment and the person with epilepsy would not be in the labour market

Extrinsic
1. Regulations backed by Act of Parliament, statutory instrument or a statutory body
2. Recruitment and selection policies barring those with epilepsy
3. Superannuation schemes barring people with a diagnosis of epilepsy
4. Scarcity of sheltered employment

Overt/unintentional

Intrinsic
1. Low educational achievement of job seeker
2. Lack of appropriate work skills/experience
3. Previous periods of unemployment
4. Inadequate personal knowledge/inappropriate presentation of epilepsy to potential employer
5. Intractable fits and/or drug side effects affecting performance or acceptability in the workplace
6. Presence of handicaps additional to epilepsy, e.g. mental handicap, psychiatric problems, physical disability

Extrinsic
1. Inadequate medical treatment of epilepsy prior to job search
2. Inappropriate professional guidance (medical and vocational)
3. Lack of access to counselling to identify and overcome any psychosocial problems
4. History of previous dismissal related to seizures
5. Disincentives to seeking employment, e.g. the 'poverty trap' of welfare benefits relative to low wages
6. Lack of public transport
7. Problems stemming from physical design of the workplace
8. Depressed local job market

Covert/intentional

Intrinsic
None identified

Extrinsic
1. Custom and practice not to engage people with epilepsy in certain occupations or workplaces/the effects of 'word of mouth' recruitment policies
2. Discrimination by staff responsible for recruitment and selection and/or management prejudice against disabled workers based on:
   i. inaccurate understanding of epilepsy
   ii. unjustified concerns about safety, insurance cover or trades union reactions
   iii. ignorance of productivity and attendance records of disabled employees generally
3. Use of 'quota' of 3% disabled employees as a maximum rather than a minimum
4. Unofficial 'quota' of employees with epilepsy operated by some organizations

Covert/unintentional

Intrinsic
1. Unrealistic ambitions and expectations of employment
2. Personality problems/negative attitudes about self and others
3. Restricted mobility (physical and/or psychological in origin)

Extrinsic
1. Employer ignorance of good practices in the employment of people with disabilities and of sources of help and guidance
2. Prevalence of 'myths about epileptics' held by some members of the public, and some professionals, such as:
   i. they have a high accident rate and are a danger to themselves and others
   ii. they put others in the workplace at risk if they have a fit at work
   iii. they have lower performance and productivity rates
   iv. they are often absent from work because of fits
   v. they have difficult personalities
   vi. they require higher employer insurance premiums

Great Britain this can be obtained through the Health and Safety Executive's Employment Medical Advisory Service, a service which is open to employers, employees and job applicants alike.

Pension schemes. A discussion of intentional and declared barriers to employment must include reference to occupational pension schemes and insurance cover for accidents at work. Employment law relating to all aspects of health and safety at work is well reviewed by Carter (1986). The Occupational Pensions Board (OPB 1977) concluded that the principle 'fit for the job, fit for the pension scheme' should apply to all workers with disabilities. However, some employers still justify refusing employment on the spurious grounds that the person with epilepsy is ineligible for the company's occupational pension scheme. Large company schemes are usually based on a group policy and, just as with company health insurance schemes, there is normally no requirement for individual health criteria to be met. However, the situation may not be so straightforward if a person takes out a so-called portable pension policy, payments into which can be continued

Table 21.4 Some occupations affected by statutory barriers

Occupation	Regulations	Effect
Aircraft pilot	Manual of Civil Aviation Medicine produced by International Civil Aviation Organization	Applicants shall have no established medical history or clinical diagnosis of epilepsy
Ambulance driver	Follow PSV regulations (see below)	Barrier if fit occurred since age of 5 for drivers or crew. Clerical work available to those who develop epilepsy in employment
Armed services		
Army	Army Act 1955; Manual of Military Law	Applicants are rejected on grounds of epilepsy and likely to be discharged if they develop epilepsy during employment. If they have had no fits since childhood, each case is considered individually
Navy		Medical regulations state any attacks at any age would debar from entry
RAF	Recruiting regulations in Air Force Act 1955 as amended in Army and Air Force Act 1961 and the Armed Forces Acts of 1966, 1971 and 1976	Proven epilepsy with a few exceptions is bar to recruitment. People developing epilepsy during service are given a medical employment standard which limits their employment
Coastguard	Civil Service Medical Advisory Service policy based on individual merit	Coastguards come into a category which requires special physical qualifications, therefore medical examination is arranged in all cases to determine fitness to undertake the full range of duties
Diver	Health & Safety at Work Act 1974. Diving Operations at Work Regs. 1981 (SI 1981/399)	Any history of fits (apart from febrile convulsions) will preclude granting a Certificate of Medical Fitness to Dive which must be renewed every 12 months
Fire brigade	Fire Service Act 1947: Fire Services Appointments (and Promotion) Regs. 1965	A history of epilepsy renders a man unsuitable for operational fire duties
HSV & PSV & Taxi driver	Statutory Instrument 1309 HGV (Drivers' Licences) Regs. 1977. Amendment 429, 1982, consolidated in 1984, 1925 Reg. 4 Section 22 Public Passenger Vehicle Act 1981 PSV 1985, Statutory Instrument 214 Reg. Sa	Absolute barrier if fit occurred after attaining age of 5. Immediate loss of licence to existing licence holder
Merchant Seaman	DoT Merchant Shipping (Med. Exam) Regs. 1983 Statutory Instrument 1983 No. 808, Merchant Shipping Notice M1144	Absolute barrier on applicants with history of fits since age 5. Serving seamen who develop epilepsy may be employed after 2 years free of seizures on a ship carrying a Medical Officer and provided they are not involved in the safety of ship or passengers.
Nurse & Midwife	Nurses, Midwives & Health Visitors Act 1979 S1 1983/873—midwives only	Epilepsy is not mentioned specifically. Nurses: each training authority sets own standards. Midwives: prospective trainees must provide evidence that they are not knowingly suffering from any disabilities which might preclude them from carrying out the duties of a midwife.
Police	Statutory qualifications contained in Police Regulations 1979. Regulation 14(1) (C) relates to general health criteria for entry—not specific to epilepsy.	Applicants currently having fits not recruited. Those with past history dealt with on individual basis. Also applies to traffic wardens, drivers, etc.
Prison Service	No Statutory Instrument regarding health standards for prison service.	Recent history of epilepsy debars an applicant on grounds of security for posts at Prison Officer Grade. Applicants to other grades of prison service are considered individually.

Continued overleaf

Table 21.4 *Contd.*

Occupation	Regulations	Effect
Teacher in state school	Education (Teachers) Regulations, 1982.	Applicants must be 3 years free of seizures. Teachers in post may be barred from teaching PE, Craft, Science and Home Economics.
Train driver	No statutory requirements for medical fitness	Absolute barrier if fit ever occurred (London Regional Transport) or if fit occurrred since age 5 (British Rail). Also applies to LRT guards and track operatives.

even if the employee changes jobs. These are policies for specific individuals and health criteria may be applied.

Employers' accident liability. The ineligibility of people with disabilities for employers' accident liability insurance has also been used incorrectly as a reason for refusing to employ someone with epilepsy. Under the Employer's Liability (Compulsory Insurance) Act 1969 an employer has to take out insurance against liability for injury and disease that may affect employees at work. The Act covers all employees with and without disabilities, and most insurance companies in the UK offer the same terms for disabled employees as for the rest of the workforce, provided that the employer takes the disability into account when allocating work. The employer's ability to do this will, of course, depend on having been told about the disability. Apart from possibly invalidating insurance cover, failure to disclose a relevant disability may put the employee in breach of the Health and Safety at Work etc Act (1974). The employee may then be dismissed and not be able to claim that the dismissal was unfair at an industrial tribunal.

Sheltered employment provision. Sheltered employment is a rather misleading but time-honoured term to describe a form of employment provision which is subsidized financially, usually from public funds. The term 'sponsored' or 'supported' employment might be more useful as there has lately been a move away from fixed employment provision in dedicated sheltered workshops and factories to a more integrated approach. This development is well established in the USA (Fraser 1991), where a variety of employment models have been used. The fundamental common principles are: 1. an integrated work setting in the competitive marketplace, 2. working for at least 20 hours per week, and 3. a guarantee to employer and employee that support and intervention will be available to the person with the disability for as long as is necessary to succeed in the job. The increasing use of such supported placements is likely to be the future pattern in the UK (Employment Department Group 1990). Under the sheltered placement scheme in Great Britain, people with disabilities work alongside able bodied colleagues in ordinary work environments but the employer receives financial assistance to employ them. Having a disability does, of course, not necessarily mean that productivity is below normal and sheltered employment provision is usually only made for those people with severe occupational handicaps whose output is reckoned to be between 30 and 80% of that of a non-disabled person doing the same job.

Whereas providing any form of sponsored employment is a way of helping disabled people, who might otherwise remain unemployed, to join the labour force, the decision to limit the number of available places is one taken deliberately by government. Failing to provide enough places can therefore be considered to be a barrier to employment. Nearly 21 000 severely disabled people were employed in Great Britain under the sheltered employment programme at March 31 1990. The number of unemployed people with eligible disabilities and who wish to work has been estimated as between 60 000 and 100 000 on the basis of a survey of a sample of 40 000 private households (Prescott-Clarke 1990). Surprisingly, this same research showed that between 130 000 and 270 000 people with severe disabilities are in fact in employment or self-employment, including those supported by the Sheltered Employment

Programme. This suggests that it may be more cost-effective to develop ways of facilitating people with severe disabilities to get ordinary jobs rather than creating more sheltered placements.

Sheltered employment consumes a large part of the government's total budget for providing employment services for people with disabilities. At £104.4 million in 1989/90 it accounted for 72% of the UK expenditure for specific disability programmes (£140.7 million in 1988/89) and 26% of all general and specific employment and training expenditure on people with disabilities (£391.7 million in 1988/89). It should not be argued, however, that sheltered employment is expensive. When the net costs are calculated, taking into account the extra revenue that is received in taxes and national insurance contributions from the disabled employees and the savings in social security payments, GB sheltered workshops and factories cost just over £2600 per employee and sheltered placements just over £260 per employee in the year 1986/87 (Dutton et al 1989).

Sheltered employment provision varies widely from country to country but the employment of people with epilepsy in sheltered jobs has not been studied in any systematic way. Mani has described the employment of young people with epilepsy within the extended family circle in rural areas of India as a form of true sheltered employment (Mani 1991). In the UK sheltered employment is provided and managed by a large number of different organizations. In contrast, the sheltered workshop places in Holland are provided under one scheme, employing 77 755 people with all disabilities in 1987 out of a total population of 14 million. The extent of sheltered employment provision varies considerably between member countries of the European Community, with relatively few places in Greece, Italy, Portugal, Spain and Ireland (Commission of the European Communities 1988).

Workshops specializing in the employment of people with epilepsy are few. In the UK, the government funded Remploy is the largest employer of people with disabilities with about 9% of its workforce having epilepsy. About 9% of all those employed in sheltered employment in Great Britain have epilepsy as their declared disability. The voluntary epilepsy organizations participate in sheltered employment schemes and there is a sheltered workshop specifically for people with epilepsy at the Chalfont Centre for Epilepsy.

Unintentional barriers

Some intentional barriers, of course, are not declared. Some employers still deliberately discriminate against people with epilepsy, helping to perpetuate myths about epilepsy and employment. Under UK law, such discrimination is perfectly legal (see later). If there are sound practical reasons why a person with epilepsy should not be employed in a particular job, these should be clearly stated and justified. This, at least, allows the person with epilepsy to make an informed choice whether to make a job application or whether to look elsewhere.

But perhaps the area where most progress can be made is in tackling the unintentional barriers to employment, those that commonly arise through misinformation and misunderstanding of the nature of epilepsy and the requirements of many occupations. These failures are not confined to employers, however, and the medical and other advisory professions could do a lot more to improve the situation. The role of people with epilepsy as advocates and educators is also crucial.

Perceptions of people with epilepsy. Australian work over 10 years ago (Beran & Read 1980) suggested that people with epilepsy perceive the attitudes of others in a widely varying way, but that the community in general is frequently seen as unaccepting and employers are perceived as hostile, fearful and indifferent. Undoubtedly this is only true in limited circumstances but as a generally held belief among the sample of people with epilepsy studied, it is certainly worrying. This study also showed that a high percentage of those interviewed believed that job opportunities generally were very restricted for people with epilepsy. Starting out in the job market with such perceptions invites the creation of self-fulfilling prophecies when employment is not obtained. Other experiences in this area are reviewed by Scambler (Scambler 1987). These findings also illustrate one area where appropriate counselling at an early stage could markedly improve opportunities for employment. Without such interventions, and in societies where there is a lot of unemployment, the prospects for those with such negative views must be grim.

A study of people with epilepsy in nine Northern Ireland general practices (Dowds et al 1983) asked about their experience of counselling and perceptions at work. Of a group of 182 adults, 35% claimed to have had no counselling or social support from any source, even their own family. Moreover, secrecy about epilepsy at work and in social settings was widespread. Nevertheless 76% of those available for work had jobs, although there was a commonly reported feeling amongst them that having epilepsy meant reduced opportunities for promotion and pay. Half of those in the study who were unemployed were young people under the age of 30 without educational qualifications. These figures must be interpreted in the light of the unusually high level of unemployment in that part of the UK at the time of the study. But the study is a good example of the complex interconnections of unintentional factors which can constitute powerful barriers to employment.

Vocational choice, social and vocational skills. Difficulties in employment are sometimes just a symbol of a more profound lack of psychosocial adjustment. The ability to recognize and tackle these underlying problems is often crucial to success in rehabilitation. It must also be remembered that a lack of social and work-related skills does not just occur overnight. The antecedent roots of these problems can often be found in poor adjustment within the family and at school. Failure to solve these problems at the appropriate time may be compounded by inappropriate guidance about realistic career options. School-leavers in many countries have to rely on mainstream employment programmes but the Epilepsy Foundation of America's Teen Work Project represents a coherent attempt to involve teenagers with epilepsy in their own vocational development pathway (Troxell personal communication).

The use of formal neuropsychological measures to gain a better understanding of the adjustment levels of individuals with epilepsy has made a lot of progress in some centres. For a review of this area, see Chapter 12 in this volume. Much more use should be made of these approaches in order to identify factors such as poor emotional adjustment to epilepsy, which may not be immediately apparent, before it is concluded that some people with epilepsy are simply 'failures' in the employment market (Cofield & Austin 1984). The great limitation of these strategies is their complexity and apparent expense in administration. However, there is evidence that they are more successful in getting 'difficult to place' people into jobs than generic programmes (Fraser et al 1984) and the economic benefits of these achievements will significantly offset the initial costs.

Many agencies that assist people with epilepsy get and retain jobs are now aware of the need for training in job-hunting skills, with a particular emphasis on the applicant's ability to present the epilepsy in a way that the prospective employer does not find threatening. The task is made even harder by the fact that job applicants with epilepsy cannot rely on employers having accurate information about epilepsy nor understanding its occupational relevance. A recent survey of employers' policies and practices in regard to people with disabilities in general (Morrell 1990) showed that 41% of employers interviewed considered that it is necessary for those employed in management jobs to be able to walk over a quarter of a mile and 25% thought it necessary for employees in management to be able to lift heavy weights. John & McLellan (1988) found in a survey of 52 companies in the Southampton area of England that 72% of the participating employers would not allow heavy machinery to be used by an employee with epilepsy who was allowed to hold a driving licence; 43% of the employers believed that their employer's liability insurance would not cover a person with epilepsy and 25% claimed that they had no jobs whatever for people with epilepsy. Other workers have, however, recorded positive changes in employer attitudes to epilepsy. Hicks & Hicks (1991) in San Francisco, USA have sampled employer attitudes on three occasions since 1956 using a questionnaire. In 1956 21% of respondents said that their companies knowingly hired people with epilepsy but by 1986 this figure had risen to 79%. The authors also comment that unsolicited letters accompanying the returned questionnaires 'were distinguished from all previous surveys in this series by their thoughtfulness and their reflection of apparent knowledge of the relevant issues'.

The need to work closely with employers is highlighted in one of the most highly developed special schemes for training and placing people with epilepsy in jobs. The Training and Placement Service (TAPS) National Project run by the Epilepsy Foundation of America (EFA) and its affiliates operates from 13 sites throughout the country. Its activities are based on the principles of active peer support and shared responsibility. Clients participate in vocational counselling and job seeking skills training and TAPS provides support during individual job search and once clients have started work. TAPS staff also work with employers through epilepsy education workshops and have produced excellent material written from the manager's point of view (EFA 1987) and video programmes emphasizing the employment potential of people with epilepsy. Employers also participate in local TAPS advisory committees. Details of the operation of the TAPS between 1983 and 1987 are given in a report available from the EFA. Its address is at the end of this chapter. Funding for the service is provided jointly in the first instance by the Foundation, through a grant from the Federal Department of Labor, and local sources of revenue.

Work is seen as a major part of success in rehabilitating young people with troublesome epilepsy in other countries, notably Holland (de Boer 1989, 1991a) and Germany, where Thorbecke (Thorbecke & Janz 1984) has devised a scheme for matching job suitability to an individual's seizure-related factors. Exercises of this kind will certainly lead to some people with epilepsy being excluded correctly from certain jobs but should also help to re-educate employers' beliefs about the safety aspects of employing people with epilepsy. Data have existed for a long time that people with epilepsy are no more prone to accidents at work than others (Dasgupta et al 1982, Dick 1986). Nor do they have more time off work overall due to sickness. However, to what extent these findings just reflect a recruitment policy designed to exclude people whose epilepsy is known to be uncontrolled, cannot be known for certain.

Knowing where employers' anxieties and prejudices may lie is an important asset to the job seeker with epilepsy and employees whose jobs are jeopardized by the onset of seizures. Unfortunately not all such people have access to the specialized services of the voluntary epilepsy organizations and so major efforts have been made to improve the quality of mainstream employment services for people with disabilities throughout the UK. The EFA has addressed this problem in the USA by creating a self-study manual suitable for those unable to attend one of the TAPS centres in person (EFA 1985). Contact with such clients is maintained by letter and on the telephone. With the increasingly widespread availability of modern technology including local radio, audio and videotape, satellite television, and audio and video-conferencing, the excuse of geographical remoteness for failure to provide proper rehabilitation services is no longer sustainable.

Appropriate professional advice. Before attributing all problems with employment to the attitude of employers, those who advise people with epilepsy should ask if all the other players in the employment game are fully conversant with modern thinking and information about epilepsy. There is no room for complacency in this matter. Advice given to employers and aspiring employees alike is often inconsistent. People with epilepsy themselves, one of the most potentially powerful factors for bringing about change, remain unnecessarily and damagingly ignorant.

Fortunately in the UK the official representative bodies of all sides of industry have wholly positive policies towards the employment of people with disabilities (TUC 1983, CBI 1983). However, official policy and individual practice may still be poles apart. And although the UK government's own efforts have been considerable to promote good practice (MSC 1984), recent research shows that many employers have not yet been reached (Morrell 1990). Nevertheless the Employment Department produces good written material about employment and epilepsy (Employment Service 1988), complementing that produced by all the voluntary epilepsy organizations, most of which is aimed at people with epilepsy.

An increasingly important link in the chain to improve the professional advice available to employers and employees is that provided by occupational health doctors and nurses. Based on his experience both as a general practitioner and an occupational physician to the UK National Coal Board, Brown (1986) gives practical advice on shift work and appropriate measures to be taken after an employee has a first seizure. Brown emphasizes the need for careful evaluation of risk factors by the physician at the place of work; for recommendations about placement at work to be made in writing with the agreement of the employee; and any restrictions that are considered necessary to be reviewed regularly. Brown & Hopkins (1988) point out, however, that only about a third of the working population of the UK are served by an occupational physician and small businesses are unlikely to make use of their services. This causes particular problems when it comes to the disclosure of epilepsy during recruitment. As Scambler & Hopkins (1980) have shown, a large proportion of people with epilepsy who get jobs do not disclose their epilepsy. In this 1980 survey, those who had only nocturnal attacks or whose seizures were very infrequent virtually never disclosed epilepsy. This may be, in part, because job applicants do not believe that they will be treated fairly and on their merits if this information is divulged before they have secured the job, particularly if the information is handled by non-medically trained or otherwise suitably qualified personnel.

The problems surrounding disclosure have been reviewed by Espir & Floyd (1986) who have proposed a code of practice concerning the disclosure of medical information. They recommend that:

1. all job application forms are accompanied by explanatory notes indicating the health standards required, any special physical qualification required and the medical conditions that would be a bar to certain types of job
2. no questions about health or disabilities are included on job application forms
3. job applicants are required to complete separate health declaration forms, which should be inspected only after candidates have been selected, subject to satisfactory health
4. the health declaration forms can be inspected only by occupational health physicians, or those delegated and qualified to do so

5. rejection on health grounds is possible only after a medical examination.

Their experience in operating such procedures successfully in recruiting government employees has also been reported (Espir et al 1987).

Overcoming the barriers; improving employability

The preceding sections have concentrated on barriers to employment and have highlighted some of the ways in which they are being tackled. There are two underlying strategies in the attempt to remove these barriers and enhance the employment prospects of people with epilepsy. The first is a purely voluntary approach, emphasizing that which constitutes good practice and the second is a statutory one, looking to the law to enforce certain practices and eradicate others.

The employment provisions that are available for people with disabilities in Great Britain largely spring from the Disabled Persons (Employment) Act, 1944. This was a response to the presence of a large number of war wounded who would otherwise have great difficulty in rejoining the workforce. It was also a time when skilled labour was scarce. Amongst other provisions, it placed a duty on all employers who employed 20 or more people to have at least 3% of their workforce as registered disabled people, the so-called Quota Scheme. It also requires that employers, with less than the 3% quota of registered disabled employees, obtain permission to employ someone who is not registered as disabled. Many new schemes have been introduced since 1944 but this Act remains the main legislative framework.

In 1984 the government's main agency in Great Britain for dealing with employment matters, the Manpower Services Commission, introduced the Disablement Advisory Service and launched its Code of Good Practice on the Employment of Disabled People (MSC 1984). Other initiatives have followed, notably the setting up of the Major Organizations Development Unit by the Employment Service. All of these have been aimed at encouraging employers to adopt good practice. Employers who self-identify that they conform to these standards may now use the new disability symbol (Fig. 21.1), launched in 1990.

Fig. 21.1   Disability symbol.

In its recent consultative document 'Employment and Training for People with Disabilities' the UK government sets out its thinking for the future. In the face of considerable exhortation to adopt a tougher approach by the disability lobby, it fails to support the introduction of anti-discrimination legislation on the grounds of disability, preferring instead to step up its attempts to persuade employers to do better. Those who support the government's view argue variously that attitudes will not be changed by new laws and that at a time of economic recession it is not appropriate to burden employers further. Those who argue against the government point out that the voluntary approach has not worked, that a law would be fair applying equally to all employers and that there will always be reasons to put off changing employment practice until tomorrow. Meanwhile, they say, individuals continue to suffer from inequality of opportunity merely because of the presence of a disability, irrespective of its impact on performance at work.

In the USA, on paper at least, the situation has changed dramatically. The signing of the Americans with Disabilities Act in 1990 could be a signal to other countries that giving rights to people with disabilities in terms of access to accommodation, transport, communication systems and employment is not only socially just but also makes good economic sense. In the words of the Executive Vice-President of the Epilepsy Foundation of America, which was one of the leaders in the campaign for the new Act (McLin personal communication): 'More people with disabilities in jobs means more tax payers and more consumers'.

The full impact of the new Act will not be felt for some time, the employment provisions not becoming effective until 1992. Doubts have already been raised about its likely effectiveness as monitoring its implementation will be left very largely

to local groups and individuals. There will also be a need for the voluntary organizations to mount special education campaigns to assist employers to adapt to the provisions of the new Act which in the employment sphere will require employers to make reasonable provision for otherwise qualified disabled employees or job applicants unless so doing would cause the employer unreasonable financial hardship.

Legislation is obviously a matter for individual countries and legislative provisions, if any, are likely to vary. The Employment Commission of the International Bureau for Epilepsy believes, however, that certain principles can be applied universally. Based on a wide ranging code of practice originally devised by Oxley & Craig (1989) the commission has published a set of principles aimed particularly at employers (Employment Commission of the International Bureau for Epilepsy 1989). After setting out some underlying precepts about epilepsy and its management, the principles list four main areas for attention: health care; job suitability; recruitment and selection; and assistance at work. The details, adapted from the commission's set of principles, are given in Table 21.5.

THE FAMILY

Childhood

The impact of epilepsy is hard to gauge, but in some cases it can have a significant and deleterious effect on relationships within the family and on social roles generally (Ritchie 1981, Berg 1982, Ferrari et al 1983, Ferrari 1989). Taylor (1989) points out that parents have expectations about children even before they are born: 'The child will be healthy not sick, at least as clever as they are and maintain their standards'. The diagnosis of epilepsy is equivalent to the loss of a perfect child. High levels of anxiety and resentment may remain unresolved, particularly where epilepsy is prominent and where seizures are uncontrolled. Taylor (1989) notes that 'seizures are associated with unexpected death with sufficient frequency to feed the possibility that any seizure may be the child's last'. Hoare & Kerley (1988) report the words of a father witnessing his child's first seizure: 'the most

Table 21.5 Principles for employing a person with epilepsy: good seizure control, work-related aptitudes and skills, and a positive approach to epilepsy are key factors in determining a person's employability

---

Health care

When assessing an employee or job applicant, the employer needs to understand some of the basic facts about epilepsy and its possible impact on work performance

- Seizures can take many forms and many people have only one seizure in their lives—in such cases a diagnosis of epilepsy is usually not made
- When a seizure occurs for the first time there may be a detrimental effect on self-confidence and the person may require psychological support and education about epilepsy
- In most cases, recurrent seizures can be controlled completely with appropriate therapy—this usually consists of treatment with drugs that need to be taken on a regular basis, often for several years

- If they are prescribed properly, drugs for epilepsy should not produce any side effects that have a noticeable effect on work performance
- In only a minority will seizures occur at work or will prescribed drugs impair work performance
- In such cases assessment by a physician expert in epilepsy will often improve seizure control and reduce these side effects
- Employees with epilepsy should be provided with the same health and accident insurance cover as other employees

Job suitability

The vast majority of jobs are suitable for people with epilepsy

- When medical advice is sought about the suitability of particular jobs for people with epilepsy, the guidance given should take into account the known facts about epilepsy and seizures—blanket prohibitions should be avoided
- In those jobs known to carry a high degree of physical risk to the individual worker or to others, the way the work practice is organized should be examined to reduce this risk to an acceptable level

- Only in those situations where this cannot be done are restrictions on the employment of people with epilepsy justified
- Where a person with epilepsy possesses the right qualifications and experience, job suitability should be assumed

Recruitment and selection

When personal health information is required, it should be processed separately from the job application form and evaluated by a skilled person

- Interviews should focus on the capabilities of the individual and not on his or her real or assumed limitations
- Suitability for a particular job should be decided by the employer before any implications arising from the job applicant's epilepsy are considered

- If a medical opinion is sought for an applicant's suitability for a job, the guidance given should be based on knowledge of the particular job and details of the individual's epilepsy

Assistance at work

When an employee has seizures for the first time, the employer should respond fairly by giving the employee adequate opportunity to receive proper medical treatment before making any decisions about job suitability

- If seizures are likely to occur at work, the employer should help the employee with epilepsy to disclose the epilepsy to work colleagues
- Some first aid training or other information should be provided to those who might be involved should a seizure occur

- If any special job restrictions are needed, there should be clearly stated policies about how they are to be implemented, reviewed or lifted in terms of set time periods
- If, despite proper medical attention, redeployment to another job is necessary, appropriate counselling and vocational guidance and, if necessary, rehabilitation services should be made available at an early stage

---

frightening experience we have ever been through'. Ward & Bower (1978) interviewed 81 families with children with epilepsy to assess the effect of the diagnosis on the family. They report that heightened family anxiety existed and this was fed by misconceptions about the disorder; for example, the fear that epilepsy was a correlate of severe personality or behaviour problems. In some

families with epilepsy, inappropriate parenting styles may develop.

Overprotection occurs frequently

The most frequently cited abnormal coping strategy is that of overprotection (Lerman 1977, Stores & Piran 1978, Ziegler 1981, Ferrari et al 1983).

Parents treat the child as sick. Any activity that makes parents nervous may be forbidden because 'it may cause fits'. Parents may shelter a child from failures and this will keep the child from becoming independent. It is crucial to avoid blaming everything on epilepsy. Ordinary living involves failures as well as successes and it is ordinary living that should be the objective. In some families epilepsy is never discussed and the child may come to take on a very passive role having limited involvement in family decision making and being considered less accountable for their actions (Long & Moore 1979). This can have two main disadvantages. Firstly, emotional, social and cognitive development can be adversely affected and this will have a significant impact on later interpersonal behaviour. Secondly, there is a rationalization for deviant behaviour which is not disciplined in the same way as the behaviour of siblings (Goodyear 1988). Children may rapidly learn to use their 'illness' to manipulate parents and grandparents. Even when seizures are fully controlled, family behaviour may develop as a response to earlier poorly-controlled seizures. However, parents are often in an unenviable position, having to balance the need to protect their child from injury during a seizure against the need to allow the child to lead as normal a life as possible. The accusation of overprotection is often levelled against parents of children with epilepsy when they are acting within the available information that their doctor or other professionals have provided.

Over indulgence leads to problems

This may arise in some families and it can result in 'emotional skewing', as Goodyear (1988) terms it. This refers to a preoccupation with the child with epilepsy to the detriment of the other family members. Consistent focusing by professionals on the mother and the child with epilepsy can also reinforce this skew. Relationships between siblings have been poorly studied. Not surprisingly, envy and rivalry between siblings can be discovered when siblings are given the opportunity to talk about it. Anecdotal remarks made by siblings may reveal deep-seated resentment. One sister wrote 'my parents mollycoddled her through school.

They kept her at home at the drop of a hat ... what still makes me wild is that the teachers went along with it'. Families may be very aware that neglect of siblings is occurring. The following remark comes from a mother. Her son is 15 and has intractable epilepsy and her daughter is 10. Her son has had seizures since the age of 6. 'My husband's work and my daughter's social life are completely distorted because of constant vigil over my boy full-time. Not a single hour can be spent by us without watching over our boy because any time he can get fits and get injured. I am concerned how to work with my younger daughter who is very disturbed and equally upset ... leading to a life totally alien to a child of her age. She is slowly trying to divert our attention towards her. Now I feel the time has come to also treat her psychologically'.

Seizures should not consume all of the parents' energies. The other children require parents' attention and affection and they should not be neglected.

Lowered expectations can be self-fulfilling

Many authors have commented upon the phenomenon of lowered expectations (Bagley 1972, Long & Moore 1979, Ferrari 1989). In a recent study Ferrari (1989) compared 21 children with epilepsy with their siblings. Within-family comparisons of personal, social and academic predictors for children with epilepsy and their healthy siblings revealed diminished expectations about the performance of the child with seizures. Children with epilepsy were perceived by mothers as being less likely to do well in the future. Ferrari (1989) asks whether mothers are responding to the child's epilepsy, or to what they perceive as being associated with the epilepsy, for example, learning difficulties, social difficulties, and madness?

Parental reactions to epilepsy such as those outlined above have been associated with high levels of psychosocial maladjustment in children with epilepsy and their siblings (Hoare 1984a, b, Fraser & Clemmons 1989). Disagreement between parents regarding how the child should be treated is a common cause of avoidable stress. One parent may tend to overprotect, while another goes toward denial. There is evidence that the divorce rate is higher than expected in families where a child has epilepsy. Research also indicates that when divorce has occurred, children have greater behaviour problems (Hermann et al 1989). Engel (1989) advocated that it is 'the physician's responsibility to uncover differences of parental attitude and help the parents develop a unified and effective approach'.

Adolescence

Adolescence is a time of change where issues of independence, identity and conformity occur. All of these can be complicated by epilepsy and its treatment (Pellock 1991). It is a time when external friendships become very important and more time is spent away from the family home. It is a time of establishing self-identity and sexual identity in preparation for adult life in society. Parental concerns in early and mid childhood may have led to restrictions on social activities and these will have had an influence upon social development. The nett result will become all too apparent during the adolescent years. Many young people with epilepsy adjust remarkably well but some will be socially very isolated and because of lack of opportunity and poorly developed skills may not have formed friendships (Thompson & Oxley 1989). This is a matter for concern as the ability to form and maintain friendships is very important for psychological health. Where this does not happen the individual is left without social support and is at risk of disorders such as depression and anxiety. Even parents who have had positive attitudes to their young child can find it difficult not to resort to overprotection during adolescence. It can be a time of testing limits. However, undue restrictions may lead to rebellion which may have adverse effects on the individual's health, for example, non-compliance with medication (Thornton 1987, Clement & Wallace 1990, Engel 1989).

Risk taking is necessary for all

The young person, particularly where epilepsy is severe, may remain within the parental home and never work through the natural separation from parents. This can cause significant problems when crises happen later, such as when parents become too old or ill to look after the young person with epilepsy. Support for families where the epilepsy is not under control can be particularly valuable during adolescence. Families and young people need to adopt an appropriate level of risk taking given the severity of their seizures. They must understand that normal activities are generally not harmful for the young person with epilepsy; for example, going to discotheques, social drinking and other leisure activities (see leisure section). Where epilepsy is uncontrolled, families may understandably find it very difficult to promote independence. Anxiety levels can rise significantly when the young person does not return home until the early hours of the morning. The waiting period can become agonizing as parents fear that a seizure has occurred, or an accident, or a hospital admission or worse. When the young person does return, having walked home because of missing the last bus, the parents do not become less anxious or less reluctant to endorse future social evening outings.

Achieving independence is a gradual process

At this stage in development it should become less appropriate for parents to be present at medical appointments. Indeed, much valuable information may be lost by continuing with this arrangement (Thornton 1987). 'In the therapeutic process we should look more to the patient with epilepsy than to the parents, aiming at greater responsibility and independence for the adolescent. Parents will often continue to accompany him/her at the appointments and make important decisions on their behalf even when s/he is fully capable of handling the problems' (Munthe-Kaas 1990).

Becoming more independent, in some instances, can be more easily promoted outside the family setting. Social rehabilitation programmes may be appropriate for some individuals including work with other family members. Available evidence suggests social rehabilitation programmes, particularly more didactic and practical courses, can have a significant impact on personal development and vocational prospects of young people with epilepsy. Research work by the group from the University of Washington, Seattle has shown that, at this time, parental concerns focus more on independent living and difficulties of employment than medical concerns (Fraser & Clemmons 1989). This group believes that, while not every adolescent with epilepsy requires social, psychosocial or vocational intervention, there is a subgroup where individually designed packages can have significant impact. In particular they have identified risk factors for psychosocial maladjustment including early age of onset, male sex, active and complex seizures and additional disabilities including neuropsychological impairment. They recommend early identification of individuals who might benefit from professional input. Parents may be assisted to establish reasonable expectations of their offspring, including community and social group involvement to promote patterns of independence. It is now increasingly possible for young people to achieve a high level of independence, even where epilepsy is poorly controlled. Practical solutions exist to reduce risk in the home, e.g. microwave ovens and showers (Kemp 1988)

Rehabilitation programmes may be taught within a variety of settings such as day centres, epilepsy associations, group homes and within private homes. Programmes appear better developed in the United States where epilepsy associations have taken an active role. In the Netherlands rehabilitation programmes with emphasis on work have also been reported to have considerable success (de Boer 1991). In the United Kingdom, projects are underway which show how young people with complicated epilepsy can follow individually tailored rehabilitation programmes, live independently or in small group living situations in the community (Thompson & Shorvon 1991). Moving away from the parental home has been observed to improve the quality of family relationships by giving parents time to develop their own interests and social life.

Sexuality may be poorly understood

Adolescence is also a time of sexual development and identity. Sexual problems and fears surrounding sexual performance may predominate (Strang 1987, Strauss et al 1982, Betts 1988). Young people need accurate information about sexual development and functioning, and where prob-lems arise, these should not be viewed just as a consequence of having epilepsy. It is our experience that young people with more problematic epilepsy have very poor understanding of sexual development and that the lack of education in this area constitutes another area of overprotection.

It is promising that in a recent United Kingdom survey of adolescents with epilepsy, which included some with severe seizure disorders, that a positive outcome was noted regarding social development. There were no marked differences in free time activities between the study group and controls. Both groups visited discotheques and clubs equally and all adolescents were allowed to go out shopping alone or to travel alone by bus (Clement & Wallace 1990).

Marriage

Studies have shown that people with epilepsy have a decreased likelihood of getting married when compared to the general population. This affects males particularly with an early age of onset and where epilepsy is symptomatic in origin (Dansky et al 1980, Lechtenberg 1984, Sillanpaa 1990a,b). One suggestion is that males have poor employment prospects and are not perceived by others as a good prospect for marriage as their role as a breadwinner is not secure. There is really very little research in this area but the limited evidence does suggest that for people with epilepsy marriages are more likely to end in separation and divorce than in the general population (Kurtz 1991). One suggestion is that the spouse with epilepsy, particularly when seizures are not controlled, can become overprotected and dependent. Couples can therefore become socially isolated. Epilepsy can thus put a strain on marriage and other intimate relationships. 'The non-epileptic partner often does not realize how much the anger and resentment they feel derives from being over-responsible for a person with epilepsy' (Lechtenberg 1984). There is a need for all spouses to be encouraged to allow the person with epilepsy to take charge of whatever he/she can reasonably do well and this can help to reduce tension.

Parenting

Many fears are associated with being a parent with

epilepsy, for example, that the children will develop seizures or that they will be unable to cope as parents. Couples need to make informed decisions and be given adequate information about contraception and pregnancy. In the first 2 years of life the child needs some protection against a parent's sudden loss of consciousness, particularly falling, jerking or loss of muscle power. Practical precautions and sound advice are needed which will reduce the risks of injury to the young child as a consequence of a parental seizure. Many epilepsy associations provide valuable practical advice and fact sheets on reducing risks for a parent with epilepsy. Health visitors provide an additional source of guidance.

Grandparents may attempt too readily to take on the mothering of the child and to prevent the child witnessing a seizure. The general view is that children should have epilepsy explained to them and be given practical instructions about what to do, for example, not to run away if mummy or daddy has a fit. Many children respond well to this approach (Betts 1988, Usiskin 1991). If parents offer no explanation of a parental seizure, a child may invent an explanation. The tendency is likely to be that the child will blame himself. One 4-year-old boy whose mother had epilepsy presented with disturbed nightmares and was very withdrawn. This was seen by the family as a consequence of having witnessed his mother's seizures. It emerged, however, that his emotional state had more to do with the grandparents' comment that if he did not behave himself then mummy would get very upset and have 'a turn'. Thus, when his mother did have a seizure, he blamed himself for its occurrence and understandably became very disturbed.

In some families, an older child may overprotect the parent with epilepsy. This is more likely to happen in single parent families. Some children as a consequence may have restricted social lives because they are frightened to leave the parent at home in case a seizure or injury occurs.

Later life

Epilepsy manifests more frequently for the first time in old age than was previously acknowledged (Tallis 1988, Sander et al 1990). Unfortunately, adequate information may not be given to elderly patients, but it is this age group that may have the greatest fears and misconceptions about epilepsy. The intermittent nature of the problem may make an elderly spouse housebound and place them under considerable emotional strain. One woman commented, 'Looking after my husband of 74 who is partly paralysed and fits several times a week is time consuming. I do not resent it . . . my question is why is there nowhere for him to go even for a few days each month to give me time to get out a bit and restore my energy'. The older person with epilepsy may also find they are denied their normal role in the family, for example, they may be forbidden to hold their grandchildren or be left alone with them for fear of a seizure

Promoting healthy family relationships

Professionals should provide factual information

Family members and the person with epilepsy require clear factual information. This needs to be given at the time of diagnosis, but also needs to be repeated and updated as the need arises. Lannon (1990) outlines how information about epilepsy can be adapted to be used successfully with individuals with severe learning difficulties. The family physician has a key role to play in providing this information and directing families to other resources such as the epilepsy organizations. In many countries the epilepsy organizations have developed a range of printed and video material and often provide specific written and telephone advice (see Appendix A). In Table 21.6 we set out a counselling checklist which highlights the breadth of coverage that may be needed.

Table 21.6 Counselling checklist

Seizures:	Management; Precipitating factors; Emergency action.
Other medical aspects:	Contraception and pregnancy; Inheritance; Intercurrent illness.
Treatment:	Purpose and objectives; Limitations; Side effects; Dosing schedules; Compliance.
Social aspects:	Driving; Education; Employment; Leisure activities; Family life.
Services provided by voluntary agencies.	

Emotional support is also required

It is generally accepted, however, that factual information about epilepsy is not enough (Hoare & Kerley 1988). Many families require emotional support. The adult with epilepsy may be expected to have fears and anxieties concerning ability to take on roles such as spouse and parent. Emotional support may be needed from the general practitioner, the specialist or other trained professionals. The role of voluntary groups should not be neglected. For example, the Danish Epilepsy Association runs annual family courses (Alving 1990) and the National Association of Finland runs rehabilitation courses for children and families (Sillanpaa 1990) (see Appendix A). Professionals need to acknowledge the emotional impact that seizures can have upon the whole family and assist members to develop adaptive coping strategies. There is a growing body of research evidence which demonstrates how fears and concerns about epilepsy underlie poor emotional adjustment (Goldstein et al 1990)

Lewis et al (1990) report the results of a controlled trial of a teaching package including role playing exercises to reduce anger and frustration and promote better coping skills. Children participating in the programme showed significant gains in knowledge about epilepsy and other areas including perceived social competence and confidence. The authors conclude that educational intervention that is 'family focused and tailored to teaching decision-making and communication skills is more effective than the traditional lecture/question and answer format'. Similarly, Hegelson and colleagues (1990) report how input, focusing on psychosocial topics in addition to factual information about epilepsy, can improve emotional adjustment in adults with epilepsy. Families may thus benefit from more active programmes which focus on emotional reaction and social functioning in addition to factual information about epilepsy.

Practical support is often appreciated

Much can be accomplished from a practical standpoint although these sorts of measures often have financial implications. An Australian survey (Australian Human Rights Commission 1985)

asked families what they felt would be of benefit. The following seven services were recorded as being of potential value: day care; emergency care; family support; holiday opportunities; home helps; home supervision; respite care.

Thus, many of the families are looking for services that provide a break, for and from, the epilepsy sufferer. Others have endorsed the importance of this. Engel (1989) writes, 'Parents should be encouraged to spend time with each other away from the patient in order to strengthen their relationship and thereby create a supportive family environment'. Unfortunately, provision of such services is limited and lack of understanding about epilepsy by providers may mean families may be unfavourably evaluated. Parents of a child with epilepsy stated, 'We found it difficult to go out and leave the child with babysitters . . . there is a babysitting service available for disabled children but our child's epilepsy was not considered severe enough'. People with epilepsy may be excluded from such services that are available because the disability is intermittent rather than permanent. The voluntary organizations have the potential to lobby for the provision of such services by highlighting the real need where epilepsy is intractable.

THE LAW

This section covers several areas where having epilepsy may have legal implications. The most commonly encountered are the regulations on driving and these are dealt with first. Later sections outlines the law relating to alleged criminal acts, the control of antiepileptic drugs, social security benefits, and personal insurance cover. Unless otherwise stated the discussion refers to the United Kingdom. The laws relating to education and employment are mentioned in the relevant sections elsewhere in this chapter.

Driving

Being able to drive is often a means of independence and social status. Restrictions on driving can have a significant impact on an individual's mobility and social functioning and this has led some authors to look upon driving restrictions as the 'most serious social constraint of epilepsy'

(Engel 1989). Laws regulating epilepsy and the holding of driving licences vary from country to country and even within countries. For example, there is considerable variation between the states of America and Engel (1989) considers existing legislation as 'confusing, contradictory and controversial from both legal and practical points of view'. Most American states require a 1-year seizure-free period before issuing a private driving licence. However, in twelve states there is no seizure-free period specified (e.g. North Carolina, California, Illinois, Tennessee) while a few states impose only a 6-month ban (e.g. Alaska, South Carolina and Washington). The longest seizure-free requirement is 18 months for Rhode Island and 24 months for Vermont, although special cases can be made either at the discretion of the Department of Transport (Rhode Island) or a doctor's recommendation (Vermont).

In some countries no specific guidelines or laws exist as far as fitness to drive a vehicle is concerned, for example, Greece and Guatemala. In certain countries people with epilepsy will not be issued with a driving licence under any circumstances and this includes, Cyprus, India, Pakistan and Japan. A 1-year seizure-free period is required before a driving licence will be issued in Denmark, but most other countries require individuals to be seizure free for 2 years. This includes most of the EC countries, Israel, Kenya, Mexico, Norway, South Africa and Sweden (IBE 1989).

Driving regulations in the United Kingdom

In the United Kingdom, the Driving and Vehicle Licencing Centre (DVLC) administers the driving licence regulations. It has its own medical staff and access to an expert medical advisory panel. When a person with epilepsy wishes to drive for the first time, the normal application form must be completed in full. A further form will then be sent to the applicant requesting details of the epilepsy and information will be requested from the applicant's doctor. A licence will be issued provided all normal requirements are fulfilled and the applicant has been completely free from seizures for 2 years. A licence can also be granted to an applicant who continues to have seizures, provided they only occur during sleep and provided 3 years have elapsed since the first attack. All applicants must also be able to drive without being likely to be a 'source of danger to the public' for any reason. If someone already holding a driving licence is diagnosed as having epilepsy, that person must notify the DVLC in Swansea and stop driving until further directed by the DVLC. A licence will not be reissued until a person fulfils the above requirements. Re-application may be made to the DVLC after the appropriate period, at which time further medical information will be requested. Licences issued to persons with epilepsy are usually subject to a periodic review.

The regulations relate to epilepsy and not to a single seizure. Usually an ordinary licence will be withheld for 1 year following a single attack pending a medical review at the end of that time.

Vocational and professional driving

In the United Kingdom stringent special provisions apply to vocational drivers who are required to hold a special licence: Large Goods Vehicle (LGV) or Passenger Carrying Vehicle (PCV) licence. Although covered by different legislation the same rules apply to taxi drivers. The regulations have recently been reviewed and a new vocational driver licensing system took effect from 1st April 1991. HGV and PCV licences will not be granted to an applicant who has suffered an epileptic attack since reaching the age of 5 years or has any medical condition likely to be a source of danger to the public. A single seizure occurring in a person already holding a vocational licence will result in immediate and permanent withdrawal.

Many people with epilepsy hold ordinary licences quite legally and some may be required to drive many hours each week as part of their work. The position of these professional drivers is less clear. However, since its inception in 1956 DVLC's Honorary Advisory Medical Panel on Epilepsy has recommended that a person who has experienced a seizure in adulthood should not drive professionally. Occupations likely to be effected by this recommendation are minibus and minicab drivers not requiring a special licence and commercial delivery drivers. Drivers who have their licence refused, revoked or restricted will no longer be able to apply to the DVLC to have the decision formally reconsidered. However, Medical Advisors will always be prepared to consider any fresh medical evidence produced. Drivers will, as before, have the right to appeal to a Magistrate's Court or in Scotland, to a Sheriff's Court. Doctors who wish to clarify how the regulations relate to specific patients can contact the Driver Enquiry Unit at the DVLC (see addresses).

Disclosure

In the United Kingdom, the onus of responsibility for notifying the licencing authorities lies with the licence holder. In contrast, in six states of America (California, Delaware, Nevada, New Jersey, Oregon and Pennsylvania) the doctor treating the patient with epilepsy is obliged by law to report the patient to the licensing authority. In these six states, physicians can be held liable for loss or injury if an unreported person with epilepsy has a car accident as a result of an epileptic attack but as Engel (1989) points out, there is no statistical evidence to show that states with such laws have a lower incidence of car accidents caused by people with epilepsy than states where the onus of responsibility is on the person with epilepsy.

In the United Kingdom there is overwhelming consensus amongst neurologists that doctors should not have to report a patient's epilepsy, but rather do everything necessary to encourage the individual to notify the authorities. Hopkins & Harvey (1987) comment '. . . the idea of mandatory reporting of epilepsy to legal authorities responsible for the issue of driving licences seems repugnant to many. It could be argued that patients knowing that they are likely to be reported may not seek medical help for conditions that might jeopardize their ability to drive. It has been argued that the breaking of confidentiality between doctor and patient leads to mistrust on the part of the patient to the detriment of the standard of care that he/she will receive'.

Family doctors and specialists should take time to highlight to the patient the risks to other motorists and pedestrians of a seizure occurring whilst driving. It is advisable for a record to be made in the patient's case notes of such a discussion or a copy kept of a letter to the patient regarding their legal responsibility to notify the DVLC and cease driving. Where a patient continues to drive in spite of a doctor's advice to the contrary the Medical

Defence Union emphasize that it is a matter for each individual doctor's discretion as to whether confidence should be breached. Attention should be drawn, however, to the rules of the General Medical Council which acknowledge that exceptions to the confidentiality rule may arise when disclosure of information is 'in the public interest'. If a doctor decides to make such a disclosure to the DVLC they are advised to let the patient know of the action they are going to take (James, personal communication).

Areas of misunderstanding

Confusion does arise about the regulations concerning driving. Harvey & Hopkins (1983) have shown an alarming diversity of knowledge and opinion amongst British neurologists who were asked in a postal survey to judge the applicability of the laws on epilepsy and driving in a number of clinical scenarios. There are, in fact, in the United Kingdom few exceptions to the regulations.

1. The duration of the attack does not result in exemption. Thus simple partial seizures and epileptic myoclonic jerks are regarded as seizures as far as the UK law is concerned. Their occurrence bans the persons concerned from driving.

2. The regulations are the same whether an individual is on or off medication.

3. Seizures that occur as a result of changes in treatment, even when undertaken on medical advice, are not exempt.

4. Arguments that an aura gives sufficient time to pull off the road and prevent an accident are not tenable. The length of time between an aura and the onset of a larger attack can vary between individuals and from occasion to occasion. Some auras are accompanied by impaired awareness.

5. Some people argue that they have never had an attack whilst driving. There is always a first time.

6. Arguments that hardship would be incurred, e.g. loss of job, loss of livelihood, cannot be used to over-rule the regulations.

The position is less clear cut in some other countries, most notably the United States, where the nature of the attacks can considerably influence whether a licence is issued or not. Engel

(1989) notes that patients who experience only simple partial seizures without marked motor disturbance are usually not functionally disabled during these events and may not present a hazard when driving. Prolonged auras may also result in a more favourable hearing, at least in certain states. For example, in Pennsylvania the set seizure-free period is 12 months, but this is less if the seizures are nocturnal or consist of auras alone.

Greater uncertainty exists where medical intervention may result in a change in risk of seizures. For example, if a patient underwent neurosurgery there might be a higher risk for seizures. In these cases, in the United Kingdom, the consensus is that such individuals should be encouraged to notify the licensing authority in the United Kingdom, so that the Medical Advisory Panel can look at the case on its merits. Where it is felt the risk of increase in seizures is high, then a driving licence may be revoked for a certain period of time and then the case reviewed. In the United Kingdom, a seizure occurring during antiepileptic drug withdrawal on medical advice is sufficient to bring in the 2-year ban. However, this is not the case in some countries (e.g. the United States). Engel (1989) writes, 'The fact that a seizure occurs during drug withdrawal does not necessitate restriction on driving unless requested by State law. If seizures come under control with reinstitution of medication there is usually no reason to recommend against driving'.

Accidents whilst driving

Studies of the relationship between epileptic seizures and road traffic accident rates have been largely uncontrolled and retrospective. This is for obvious ethical reasons. Taylor (1983) reported a series of accidents due to collapse at the wheel investigated by the police in which the driver survived: 38% were due to generalized seizures, 70% of these people had not declared their condition to the DVLC, and 11% were having their first seizure. This research suggests that many people with epilepsy are driving and failing to declare their condition to the licencing authority. In a Dutch study, 699 men holding a driver's licence had 5 years previously been found to have epilepsy on examination for military service. Only 19% of

these drivers had admitted having epilepsy when asked a direct question on the application form (Van der Lugt 1975). Engel (1989) cites data for the State of California from the Department of Motor Vehicles reporting accident rates for various diseases and disorders for individuals having two or more accidents over a 3-year period. This level of accidents occurred for 6% of people with diabetes, 12% of people with epilepsy, 16% of people with cardiac or cerebral vascular disorders, 19% of people with alcohol related problems and 32% of those with a history of drug abuse. Gastaut & Ziskin (1987) explored seizure types in relation to accidents. Of 400 drivers with epilepsy, 133 admitted having accidents and 97 were able to describe what happened or their seizures were witnessed. Complex partial seizures were responsible for 88% of the accidents. However, their study also demonstrates that simple partial seizures and auras do not necessarily have a protective effect. They quote a number of cases including the following two:

Case No. 1: F.G. A 34-year-old physician has complex partial seizures beginning with an aura of microteleopsa. A seizure occurred while he was driving around a curb in his own neighbourhood but seeing his surroundings retreating and growing smaller he continued straight on and collided with a building.

Case No. 2: P.A. A 51-year-old male schoolteacher has complex partial seizures heralded by an aura of déjà vu. He had a seizure while driving at the ages of 20 and 45 years. At the onset of the second of these he told his wife he was about to have an attack while braking and trying to stop at the roadside. In so doing he struck and killed a motorcyclist and has not driven since.

Reviews of the subject do suggest that people with epilepsy are at increased risk for accidents as a consequence of seizures at the wheel. A high relative percentage of these accidents are reported to be one car accidents. Studies reviewed include people who are driving legally and illegally (Spudis et al 1986, Hopkins & Harvey 1987, Taylor 1983).

The UK criminal law

Gunn (1981) has reviewed the medicolegal problems most usually encountered in relation to epilepsy. He concluded that although 'no neat generalizations can be drawn ... epilepsy does show very nicely that legal and social issues have a considerable impact upon clinical practice'. Important medical and social aspects relating to the criminal law and epilepsy which are outside the scope of this chapter are discussed by Gunn (1977, 1981), Oliver (1981), Channon (1982), Treiman (1986) and Fenwick (1987). This matter is also discussed fully in Chapter 20.

Most people with epilepsy are completely law abiding. Those few who commit crimes do so for the same reasons that motivate other people. However, a very few people with epilepsy have the misfortune to do something in the confused state after a fit which may be misunderstood as a criminal act. These events are rare and usually relatively trivial, such as picking up an object in a shop (which may lead to a prosecution for shoplifting) or undressing in a public place (which could lead to a charge of indecent exposure). Normally, if it is known that the person has had an epileptic seizure, no action will result. Difficulties can and occasionally do arise, however, if the person is not known in the locality, is unaccompanied or, very unusually, if physical injury occurs to a bystander as a result of the person behaving aggressively. Actions committed during or after a seizure are automatisms and it is generally agreed that persons in such a confused state have no control over what they do.

Deciding whether a patient is likely to have had a seizure just prior to an alleged criminal incident can either be clinically straightforward or very difficult. It is usually relatively straightforward if the patient and his seizure type are already known to the examining physician and there are detailed eye witness accounts of the incident. Without this information, a clinical diagnosis that the alleged incident was due to an epileptic seizure will be highly speculative.

The control of antiepileptic drugs

All drugs used in the UK for the control of epilepsy are classed as Prescription Only Medicine and are thus only obtainable on prescription from a registered medical practitioner. People taking medication for epilepsy are, along with those needing hormone replacement therapy, treatment for diabetes and sexually transmitted diseases, exempt from paying prescription charges for all drugs prescribed under the National Health Service, not just those for epilepsy. They should obtain a payment exemption certificate by completing Form P11. These are widely available from pharmacists, health centres and social security offices. Once completed, the form should be given to the patient's doctor to be counter-signed. Patients with epilepsy who choose to be treated privately, outside the NHS, should pay the full cost of their treatment.

Phenobarbitone is a controlled drug

In 1985 the Misuse of Drugs Act (1971) was extended to include the barbiturates and those compounds containing a barbiturate. This was done in order to control the availability of the shorter acting barbiturates which are widely abused. Phenobarbitone (Luminal) and methylphenobarbitone (Prominal) were included within the provisions of the Act but because of their use for the treatment of epilepsy, they were exempted from some of its provisions.

Unlike prescriptions for other barbiturates, it is not necessary for a doctor prescribing phenobarbitone (or compounds containing phenobarbitone) to handwrite the prescription but the prescription must be signed and hand-dated by the prescriber and not just stamped with the doctor's name. Additionally, the amount of the drug to be dispensed must be stated in letters and figures. Pharmacists are, however, permitted to dispense limited amounts of phenobarbitone in an emergency without a prescription. As, in certain circumstances, the police may wish to be satisfied that a person carrying phenobarbitone is legally entitled to it, the UK's National Society for Epilepsy recommended that everyone who takes phenobarbitone for the treatment of epilepsy should carry a written statement to that effect, signed by their doctor. In the USA, where laws on the possession of drugs vary from state to state, the Epilepsy Foundation of America (EFA) advises people to carry a precription for their medication and to carry it in an appropriately labelled container. Other guidance on legal issues in the USA is contained in a succinct EFA leaflet *Epilepsy: Legal Rights, Legal Issues* (EFA 1987b).

The use of some drugs is restricted

Many governments worldwide have sought to restrict expenditure on medicines and the UK government is no exception. In 1985, it restricted the number of drugs in certain pharmaceutical categories which could be prescribed under the NHS. The benzodiazepines were included in this 'limited list' but the majority of those used in epilepsy were still permitted. One of the benzodiazepines, clobazam (Frisium) was only permitted under the NHS for the treatment of epilepsy and prescriptions for it have to be endorsed with the code 'S3b'.

Although the limited list has not so far been extended, new measures were to be introduced in 1991 which are designed to exert a downward pressure on NHS drug costs. The hospital sector has for some time now had to control its prescribing for patients because of budgetary constraints but since April 1991 UK general practitioners (GPs) have been working with 'indicative drug amounts' which are based on their current level of prescribing costs. GPs who persistently exceed their designated level of expenditure on drugs are required to explain this under a system of peer review and can, in the last resort, be penalized financially.

Fortunately, compared to some treatments, epilepsy drugs are not expensive but undoubtedly the newer drugs are more costly than the old ones. Sabril (vigabatrin), for example, costs about 100 times more than Epanutin (phenytoin) for approximately equivalent daily doses. And so, because of these new regulations, there is a possibility that doctors might be deterred from prescribing the more modern treatments.

Doctors in many other countries, where some or all of the citizens receive state aided or insurance based medical treatment, prescribe under similar financial constraints. Often only certain antiepileptic drugs, usually the older and cheaper ones, can be prescribed at little or no cost to the patient. Although protests are often lodged by the epilepsy lobby based on purely clinical considerations, more powerful economic and politically persuasive arguments should be assembled to show that the more modern and initially expensive remedies are actually more cost effective in the longer term through their increased efficacy, lower incidence of side effects and improved quality of life.

Social security and other benefits

Having epilepsy does not bring with it the automatic right to any financial compensation. If the epilepsy results from an injury sustained at work or in a road traffic accident, then compensation can be sought from a third party through the civil court. If epilepsy results from a criminal act, such as a head injury due to an assault, then compensation may be payable by the Criminal Injuries Compensation Board.

State payments to people with epilepsy are usually based on the impact that the epilepsy has had on their ability to earn their own living. For a comprehensive account of the UK benefits system the reader is referred to a series of ten articles published in the *British Medical Journal* (Ennals 1990/1991). Further information up-dated each year is to be found in two publications produced by the Child Poverty Action Group (Lakhani & Read 1990, Rowland 1990) and in the Disability Rights Handbook, published by Disability Alliance, an organization which also provides advice on an individual basis. Its address is to be found in Appendix C.

Social security benefits are complex

Attempting to understand social security benefits is not, however, a task for the faint-hearted. As Ennals (1990) has pointed out: 'Social security benefits seem to be constantly changing . . . Each year at least one section of the claimant population seems to have to get to grips with a completely new system. All too often doctors and other primary health care professionals find themselves caught up in the web of confusion and administrative delays that beset the daily lives of an appreciable proportion of their patients'.

Benefits can, however, be broadly divided into three groups: contributory benefits, non-contributory benefits and means tested benefits. People with epilepsy are entitled, like other citizens, to claim contributory benefits, where appropriate, provided that the necessary National Insurance contributions have been made. These benefits include retirement pension, widows' benefit, unemployment benefit, sickness and invalidity benefit and maternity allowance.

If the disability due to epilepsy is severe, such that the ability to earn a living is severely prejudiced and insufficient previous contributions have been made, then a non-contributory benefit—Severe Disablement Allowance—may be claimed. If the epilepsy was caused by an industrial accident, then whether or not previous contributions have been made, Sickness or Invalidity Benefit may be claimable, as well as other benefits under the industrial injuries scheme. If the epilepsy is severe enough for the person to require frequent care from another person, then the non-contributory Attendance Allowance may be claimed. Once these benefits have been claimed successfully, they can act as a passport to others, such as income support, housing benefit and community charge benefit, all of which are means tested. A new benefit, called the disability working allowance, should help those people with epilepsy who, while unable to work full-time, could manage part-time work, but who, under the present arrangements, would be penalized financially for so doing.

In the small minority of cases in which the person with epilepsy requires day-to-day care from another person in their own home, the invalid care allowance is payable to the carer. If the disability due to epilepsy is such that care in a residential home is required then different benefit rules apply (Ennals 1990/1991). The financial responsibility for providing care is currently shared between the government's Department of Social Security and the person's own local authority. Local authorities may also be called upon to provide special facilities within the home for people who are registered with them as being disabled under the provisions of the Chronically Sick and Disabled Persons Act (1970) and the Disabled Persons (Representation) Act of 1986.

More changes are planned

Further changes to the benefits system are planned in the near future. The overall intention is, firstly, to shift the balance of responsibility onto local authorities for providing care and, secondly, to rationalize the benefits system by creating a single Disability Living Allowance which will incorporate the present attendance and mobility allowances. It is hoped that payment of this new allowance will depend more on self-assessment of need and that provided by involved lay people rather than doctors. Doctors will continue, however, to have a crucial role in the benefits system by alerting their patients to the fact that they may be eligible for benefits and assisting them to seek the right advice.

Personal insurance cover

People with epilepsy may often experience difficulty in getting full personal insurance cover through independent insurance companies, particularly if the epilepsy is still active. This may affect their ability to drive, go on holiday, obtain a mortgage to buy a house, or get life, health and personal accident insurance. Policies excluding cover for accidents or sickness due to epilepsy are usually obtainable and the voluntary organizations are often able to help. Pugh (1988) has, however, described a special personal accident insurance scheme arranged by the British Epilepsy Association and a leading UK insurance broker. The scheme includes cover for death or injury sustained as a result of seizures. The first 7 years of operating the scheme has shown that insuring people with epilepsy is a commercially viable proposition.

Cornaggia (1988) has argued that the reluctance of insurance companies to cover people with epilepsy is probably based on a general belief that having epilepsy confers a higher risk of accidents and a lack of understanding about the different types and effects of epilepsy. What little evidence exists on this would suggest that people with epilepsy are not more accident prone than others (Nelen 1988). De Boer (1988), reviewing the widely differing situation worldwide, has pointed out that insurance companies will base their decision whether or not to grant cover on the brief medical information given to them. If this information is provided by a doctor who is not expert in epilepsy, it is perhaps hardly surprising that cover is often refused. Under UK law (Access to Medical Records Act 1988), all medical information relating to applications for insurance cover must be made available to the applicant. Through this means, people with epilepsy are encouraged to check the accuracy of statements made about themselves as individuals and about epilepsy in general.

LEISURE

Doctors are often called upon to give opinions about the risk of a particular person with epilepsy engaging in a leisure activity. Although this is a common request, little systematic study has been made of these ordinary areas of daily life. This is a major area of neglect. It is, therefore, difficult for doctors to give clear cut advice which is appropriate to every situation. Individual assessment of both the person concerned and the proposed activity is highly desirable but not always possible. It is important, nevertheless, for doctors to have access to general guidance which can at least be a starting point to aid the individual concerned and the teacher or other responsible person organizing the activity. Many sports which are undertaken competitively now have their own clubs and medical advisors, both of which can be a valuable source of advice. The voluntary epilepsy associations can provide advice and guidance and the British Sports Association for the Disabled is another useful resource (see Appendix C).

Research findings

Bjorholt et al (1990) surveyed leisure time activities in terms of availability and utilization of 44 adult patients with epilepsy who had been inpatients at the National Centre for Epilepsy in Sandvika, Norway. Most of the sample lived in small scattered communities in the southern part of Norway where excellent facilities exist for various leisure time activities. However, the researchers found that most of their patients did not utilize the facilities and were mostly engaged in passive activities such as watching television, listening to the radio, and reading papers, books and magazines. Few participated in social activities and most only sought the company of their families. Patients were assessed to be only half as active

physically as the normal population. The authors also assessed individual's physical condition and found this to be relatively poor compared with the average Norwegian population of comparable age and sex. They suggested the lack of fitness was secondary to a sedentary lifestyle. The authors conclude, 'we believe that comprehensive care of patients with epilepsy should take into consideration possible inactivity-induced physical unfitness'. They suggest that many mechanisms may underlie this situation but they recommend that physicians alone may not be effective enough in dealing with these matters and it may be wise for them to join forces with physiotherapists or recreation specialists.

A further study from the same group of investigators explored the effect of physical training on seizure activity in patients with epilepsy. Twenty-one adult inpatients with uncontrolled epilepsy participated in a 4-week intensive physical training programme, exercising for at least 45 minutes three times a day, 6 days a week. The average seizure frequency during the 4-week exercise period was compared with 2 pre-exercise and 2 post exercise weeks. The authors found no significant difference in seizure frequency overall. However, they note that there was individual variation and one patient had so many seizures during physical activity that they were obviously 'exercise induced'. He himself was well aware of the negative influence of physical activity on his seizure susceptibility. For this reason they feel advice about physical training should be individualized according to the patient's experience and situation. Most encouraging observations were noted by instructors of a substantial improvement in patients' mental state with several patients becoming more sociable and to have improved self-esteem. The authors were aware that their sample was small but they feel their results are a sufficient demonstration that participating in regular physical activity does not usually lead to an increase in seizures (Nakken et al 1990).

Taking risks

Most problems where epilepsy and leisure activities are concerned stem from misinformation coupled with a general anxiety about taking risks.

An informed person will often need to ensure that these are corrected beforehand, especially if the question of the risk of an individual having a seizure during the activity (which might range from virtually nil to highly probable) is confused with estimating the danger which might result to the individual and others should the seizure happen. One-off accidents can happen to anyone whether epilepsy is present or not. Indeed Nelen reports (Nelen 1988) that accidents occurring at home and during leisure pursuits are less frequent in people with epilepsy than in the general population. These data could well reflect a more restricted lifestyle of people with epilepsy. But the study also looked at a small sub-group of people with severe epilepsy who were mentally handicapped. In this group there was a positive correlation between the number of accidents and the occurrence of secondary generalized tonic-clonic seizures. This suggests that it should be possible to identify factors which may make some people with epilepsy more prone to accidents and thereby assist with individualized assessment of risk.

If a seizure occurs during an activity, this is not an automatic signal that something tragic will follow and that future participation must be barred. Nor should it be concluded that the activity was necessarily responsible for the seizure (see section on physical exercise above). Anxiety on the part of family members and responsible professionals is, however, entirely normal and understandable, but it should not be allowed to lead to unreasonable restrictions and the psychological consequences that these will produce. A non-confrontational educational approach by informed professionals, patients and their families will go a long way to making most activities safe, emphasizing that responsibility for risk taking must be shared. Reasonable provision should also be made in case a seizure does occur. It is also quite reasonable to demand a better level of seizure control or a higher level of skilled supervision where a participant with epilepsy would be likely to die during an activity (e.g. parachuting or hanggliding) or where other participants could be endangered (e.g. rock climbing) if a seizure occurred. In high risk activities where such supervision is not available, the 2-year freedom from seizure rule, used to assess fitness to drive, is reasonable.

The following guidelines for risk assessment by parents have been adapted from Sonnen (1988a). When advising parents, doctors should:

1. point out the difference between safeguards appropriate to a short term illness (e.g. staying in bed) and those appropriate for a chronic condition
2. assign each patient to a high risk or a low risk group on the basis of the known facts about that patient
3. distinguish between restrictive measures (e.g. a ban on swimming) and non-restrictive measures (e.g. proper supervision during swimming)
4. emphasize that leisure is as important an activity to the child's development as school work
5. avoid giving dogmatic 'yes' or 'no' answers to parents' enquiries, however much this is requested
6. outline the facts and the options which will allow parents to make their own judgements

The following sections discuss briefly those activities which present most problems. Most of these involve some degree of physical activity. As risk evaluation is required in all these areas, doctors might be well advised to record if their opinion has been requested and the advice that they gave.

Contact sports

Boxing, wrestling and other contact sports where injury to the head is highly likely to occur are not advisable for people with epilepsy because of the possible exacerbation of the seizure disorder should brain damage occur. Field sports such as rugby, football and hockey involve possible head contact but for many individuals with epilepsy such team games if supervized adequately are appropriate.

Cycling

Where attacks are completely controlled there should be no increased risk. If seizures still occur, busy roads are best avoided and a companion is advisable. To our knowledge there are no laws regarding cycling and epilepsy, but riders may be financially liable if they cause an accident and another person is injured. However, doctors may be faced with patients who are still having seizures and who want to ride a bicycle. Although the possible risk to the individual is often accepted, the risk to others should the cyclist have a seizure and cause an accident is often a deterrent. In Holland, where bicycling is commonplace, the Epilepsy Centre at Heemstede operates a rule that cycling is allowed only if the seizures have been controlled for 2 months (de Boer personal communication). This seems to be a reasonable rule of thumb. The wearing of cycling helmets is becoming more widespread and it may be advisable for people with epilepsy to take this precaution.

Discotheques

These are a normal part of growing up and should not be needlessly avoided by the young person with epilepsy who seeks a full social life. Some people may find flashing or flickering lights unpleasant, but generally it is only bright, white strobe lights operating at more than five flashes per second that may, in some individuals with photosensitive epilepsy, induce seizures (see p. 314). It should be remembered that the majority of those with epilepsy are not photosensitive. Many local authorities have rules governing the use of such lights, restricting the flash frequency to under five flashes per second which makes the induction of seizures less likely. Should a person with epilepsy be exposed to such a light, however, turning away from the light source and covering one eye should be sufficient to prevent an attack. If a seizure should occur in a disco it may well be spontaneous or due to another cause.

Horse riding

Normal hard hats should be worn by all riders. Riding is a well established and rewarding activity for people with many types of disability and there are often voluntary organizations which specialize in this. In the United Kingdom, the organization Riding for the Disabled maintains local groups and facilities where the person with epilepsy wishing to ride can be catered for, especially if he or she is additionally handicapped (see Appendix C).

Physical exercise

Not all leisure activities involve physical exercise but many of them do. Many physicians will know of a patient whose seizures are always triggered by exertion but the mechanism for this is not understood and therefore ways of overcoming the problem have not been developed. The limited amount of research discussed above suggests that for most people with epilepsy, moderate exercise does not cause seizures and may well result in increase in self-esteem (Nakken et al 1990).

Social drinking

Medical opinion on drinking alcohol varies. Some physicians may recommend total avoidance of alcohol and others suggest it can be taken 'in moderation'. In the end it comes down to people with epilepsy weighing up the evidence—the risk of seizures, their confidence in keeping within the bounds of occasional drinking and their own experience. Some people with epilepsy choose not to drink alcohol at all and it is now more socially acceptable in some countries to drink no alcohol or low alcoholic beverages than in the past. If a person with epilepsy is under good medical control, there is usually no contradiction to moderate use of alcohol. Hoppener et al (1983) found social and occasional drinking had no deleterious effects on the seizure control of 52 chronically treated patients administered one to three measures of vodka per day for 16 weeks.

Precipitation of seizures by alcohol intake in patients with epilepsy is usually ascribed to the effects of alcohol withdrawal (Chan 1985, Simon 1988). Some patients are extremely sensitive to withdrawal effects of alcohol and experience seizure exacerbation and these individuals should avoid the use of alcohol altogether (Mattson 1983). When drinking becomes excessive or occurs in binges, then problems can arise. Heavy drinking is often associated with late nights, missed meals and forgotten tablets. Alcohol can also theoretically interfere with antiepileptic drug metabolism. Large amounts of liquid, e.g. beers, can trigger fits.

Swimming and water sports

Every person with epilepsy should have the benefit of learning to swim and enjoying themselves in the water with others. Not being able to swim could be very hazardous in some situations. Some voluntary organizations recommend seeking medical approval for swimming. Doctors should take into account the features of the person's epilepsy. Where seizure control is good and where auras exist, risks are reduced. Doctors need to ask about the occurrence of triggering factors which might increase the risk of seizures while swimming, e.g. cold water, stress and excitement, noise of a crowded pool and dazzling lights on the water surface. In properly managed swimming pools there should be little extra risk. Some pool managements and some schools insist that people with epilepsy wear coloured swimming caps. This may be more stigmatizing than helpful, although it is only right to inform the responsible authority at the swimming baths or for a teacher to keep a special check on a child with epilepsy in the water. The 'buddy' system is used extensively in some countries and places responsibility for safety in the water on pairs of children, one member of which has epilepsy. This may be well suited to cases where a seizure might occur. Many publicly run pools have special sessions for people with disabilities where extra supervision is available. The general subject is discussed in the United Kingdom's Sports Council's free publication 'Swimming and Epilepsy' (see Appendix C). Swimming alone in the sea, rivers or lakes, or in very cold water is not recommended.

The range of water sports is now very wide and guidance varies with the particular sport. Subaqua diving is not recommended. Sonnen (1988b) has pointed out that the use of properly fitted lifejackets which keep the head above water should allow participation in rowing, sailing and even surfing. Fishing can, however, be hazardous, particularly if undertaken in a remote location where life-saving facilities are inadequate. A review by Norman Croucher 'Water Sports and Epilepsy' is available from the Disabilities Study Unit (see addresses section).

Television and videogames

A few people with epilepsy may have a seizure while watching television (see p. 321), but in view of the amount of time some people spend watching television, the seizures are just as likely to be spontaneous events as to be due to photosensitivity. If normal television viewing is a problem, then sitting 2–3 metres away from the set at a level with the screen and not below it may help. A small illuminated lamp on top of the set may improve the situation. The susceptible person should avoid approaching the set to make adjustments or should cover one eye thus reducing the photo stimulation by half (Jeavons & Harding 1975). Remote controls should be used where available. Seizures due to television flicker are more common in Europe than in North America due to differing electricity supply cycles and higher flash rates.

Videogames can pose problems for a minority of patients. It is possible, however, to reduce the risk of a photoconvulsive response (Wilkins 1987). For instance, the frequency with which the beam of the VDU scans from the top to the bottom of the screen (the refresh rate) is important. VDUs with a refresh rate of 50/second are more likely to induce a photoconvulsive response than VDUs with a scan rate of 60/second or greater. Most commercially available VDUs now have a refresh rate of more than 60/second. Room illumination can also be relevant and dim lighting is recommended. The nature of the material displayed is as important as the display itself. The effect of intermittent light and patterns can be considerably reduced by covering one eye. A cosmetic and selective way of occluding one eye when using a VDU is to provide the patient with a pair of glasses with one lens paler (Wilkins 1987). Further guidance for patients and families is given by Wilkins & Lindsay (1987).

Travel

Special holiday schemes exist for people who have a physical or mental disability. For some people with epilepsy these holiday schemes may be appropriate. In the United Kingdom the Royal Association for Disability and Rehabilitation (RADAR) maintains lists of holidays for people with physical disabilities. MENCAP—the Royal Society for Mentally Handicapped Children and Adults—publishes a guide to holiday schemes which is available from their Holiday Officer (s.a.e. required). The Scottish Epilepsy Association organizes several holidays a year, offering a range of activities. Applications need to be made early in the year to the Association's Social Work Department (see Appendix C).

Most countries have no restrictions regarding entry with epilepsy. Restrictions regarding the carrying of antiepileptic drugs are variable and several countries including the United Kingdom, Spain, Denmark and Canada require a written statement from a doctor with details of type and dosage. The International Bureau for Epilepsy (IBE) has published a small book of guidelines for the traveller with epilepsy which includes details of any restrictions imposed by 58 countries (IBE 1989).

Difficulties may be encountered in some countries in obtaining exactly the same antiepileptic drugs used in the home country, and the proprietary names of most antiepileptic drugs differ from country to country. For example, proprietary names for phenytoin include Epinat (Norway), Epamin (Argentina), Lepobal (Spain) and Toin Unicelles (South Africa). Drugs supplied in the United Kingdom by the National Health Service can usually be prescribed for no longer than 1 month absence abroad. It is recommended that all people with epilepsy should carry accurate written information about their epilepsy and any drugs being taken. The various epilepsy associations can supply cards and forms for this purpose which can be signed by the doctor.

Health care provision varies widely between countries. The United Kingdom has reciprocal health arrangements with a number of countries including other EC countries. Persons are entitled to medical treatment on the same basis as insured nationals of that country. It must be remembered that treatment available in the EC countries is that provided under their own domestic legislation and in some instances, part payment for treatment is required. However, in order to obtain treatment and have the cost reimbursed at home, Form E111 must be obtained at least a month before travelling. The relevant United Kingdom leaflet is T1 which gives details of reciprocal arrangements. This is obtainable free from Post Offices, by post from the DHSS leaflet unit or by telephoning 0800 555 777.

Travel insurance offers cover for a variety of events such as illness, accidents, loss of baggage and possible cancellation costs. Most insurance packages require the person to sign a form indicating freedom from drugs or disability. However, many holiday firms now have policies without such exclusion clauses. Individuals are advised to read the small print of their policies carefully. The epilepsy associations can recommend companies who have favourable policies regarding epilepsy.

Most airlines do not have restrictions regarding persons with epilepsy. If seizures are likely to occur or if special arrangements are needed, the airline should be advised. Flying does not cause fits, but disrupted sleep as a consequence of altered biological rhythms on long distance flights may trigger fits. To avoid sleep deprivation individuals should try to compensate for loss of sleep on arrival. Time changes due to long distance travel may affect taking medication. Abrupt changes in routine should be avoided and alternatives necessitated by new time zones should be phased in gradually after arrival. Changes in diet may result in diarrhoea. This in turn may result in poor absorption of antiepileptic medication and loss of seizure control. It appears sodium valproate is more severely affected but no drug is exempt. The IBE (1989) recommend that when abroad the traveller with epilepsy needs to know how and where to obtain medical help and in addition know how to get in touch with epilepsy support organizations.

Yoga

The physical and psychological aspects of yoga may be entirely beneficial. The controlled deep breathing associated with the more common forms of yoga should not present any problems to the majority of people. Any of the national yoga associations can provide further guidance.

PUBLIC EDUCATION

Professionals in all countries recognize that there is still misconception about epilepsy sometimes leading to discrimination. To what extent this discrimination is hard reality and to what extent it conforms to the notion of 'perceived stigma' (Scambler & Hopkins 1980) cannot be measured easily. It probably varies widely. Nevertheless most voluntary organizations worldwide are committed to the concept of educating 'the public' in order to combat ignorance and prejudice. It is not, however, an activity that has been subjected to systematic analysis and detailed guidelines based on successful campaigns in epilepsy are singularly lacking. Jackson (1986) quoting the Institute of Public Relations defines a public education campaign as, 'the deliberate, planned and sustained effort to establish and maintain mutual understanding between an organization and its public'. Urging organizations to step back from the cause in which they are highly involved and adopt a commercial marketing approach, Jackson outlines a six-point programme as follows:

1. identify your purpose and your constituency
2. prepare your strategy and your materials
3. launch your campaign
4. monitor the response
5. evaluate the effect
6. capitalize on the experience.

Unfortunately evaluating the effect of any campaign on public attitudes is not easy, nor is distinguishing between the attitudes that people will admit to holding and the action they would take in reality. Both of these factors make it is extremely difficult to know for certain whether a campaign has had its desired effect.

Targetting the right audience

'The public' may, in any case, not be a very useful concept when considering how to bring about changes in attitudes and behaviour. Rutgers (1988) has shown from a survey in the Netherlands that many members of 'the public' who responded to advertising campaigns about epilepsy either had epilepsy themselves or had epilepsy in the family. The need to target educational campaigns is a theme stressed by Corbidge & Aspinall (1988) who list five groups other than the general public, namely, people with epilepsy; the families of people with epilepsy; the health care team and social workers; care assistants and care attendants; and teachers and educators. Each of these groups has its own educational requirements, often needing a different level of information, and different methods of receiving it.

The need to plan educational strategies carefully, using all available expertise about how people learn, can not be over-stressed. In the UK a package for school teachers (British Epilepsy Association 1991) was developed jointly with a university department of education and much more material of this kind should be learner-centred (based on an assessment of the learner's needs) rather than expert-centred (based on what experts feel that everyone else ought to know).

Despite the fact that informing the general public and influencing its attitude towards epilepsy is fraught with problems, epilepsy organizations in many countries attempt to do this through a variety of means. Many now produce a newssheet as well as a range of information material in the form of leaflets and booklets. The Epilepsy Foundation of America mounts an annual epilepsy awareness campaign by providing local radio stations with an information package with prepared audio tapes which can be played over the air. A series of very short video programmes, lasting 30 seconds or less, have also been made to broadcast standard and these are transmitted free by local television stations. There is no direct attempt to raise funds with these epilepsy 'commercials' and the messages are extremely simple. Companies which participate in the campaigns are sent a commemorative certificate.

Video is a valuable medium for education

The last few years have seen a dramatic increase in the number and quality of video programmes made about epilepsy. Video is, in one respect, an ideal medium for teaching about epilepsy as the wide spectrum of seizure types can be shown, thereby helping to dispel one of the common misconceptions that having epilepsy just means having tonic-clonic seizures. A catalogue of pro-

ductions on video and film has been compiled by
the International Bureau for Epilepsy (IBE 1985)
and programmes are available in most of the
major languages of the world. A list of key programmes has been drawn up by the Commission
on Audiovisual Education (Sonnen 1991).

All programme makers should have very clear
objectives before starting their work. The audience must be known and its state of knowledge
and attitudes assessed. It should be clearly identified how a programme is to be distributed and
how audiences will view it (Oxley 1991). These
steps can easily be overlooked in the enthusiasm
to create a new programme.

However worthwhile are the identified educational objectives, it is important not to reinforce
inadvertently prejudices that may exist within the
audience. This can happen even if it is a well-
informed, professional one, such as a medical audience. Many of the programmes produced so far
have concentrated purely on the medical aspects
of epilepsy, perhaps because the programme instigators are often doctors and because the sponsors
are often drug companies. They often contain
seizure sequences recorded in EEG laboratories,
only showing the person having a seizure, paying
little attention to their dignity as an individual.

In contrast the series of programmes produced
by the UK's National Society for Epilepsy (NSE
1991) contain seizure sequences recorded in more
natural surroundings, albeit often at a centre for
epilepsy. Although the appearance of the seizures
and those experiencing them are not always typical of epilepsy as a whole, these sequences have
attempted to show people with epilepsy doing
everyday activities as well as having seizures.
When a seizure is shown, the recovery phase is
also included.

MOBILITY

Participation in social life, recreational and voluntary activities as well as capacity to earn a living
are significantly affected by any impairment of
mobility. Aspects of family life can be severely restricted or interfered with, for example, shopping,
taking children to school and other activities, can
be disrupted without access to proper transport.
Epilepsy can threaten mobility in a number of

ways and solutions to the problems are not always
easy to find. In many countries, if the epilepsy
is active, driving is banned. Quite apart from
the physical inconvenience this brings, loss of a
driving licence may have severe economic effects
if a job is lost as a result. Loss or denial of a licence
can also have psychological effects with perceived
loss of status and in cultures where driving is
equated to masculinity, loss of potency.

Public transport may be inaccessible, other than
in large cities. In our survey of the social situation
of adults with intractable epilepsy, those residing
in London reported fewer difficulties in participating in social activities (Thompson & Oxley
1989) and one explanation for this is the better
transport network in a city. Even when transport
is accessible, travelling time can be considerable
with weekends and evenings having limited, or no,
service. Travelling on public transport, particularly alone late at night, may place any individual
at risk of assault. An alternative is the use of
taxis but fares can be prohibitive, particularly for
individuals with low incomes. Many people with
epilepsy come to find themselves dependent on
other people for lifts. One young person wrote,
'my friends help me. I tell them I am epileptic. It
is awful to always be asking for lifts and the
like'. Parents of another young person commented,
'He's at home on the farm nearly all the time. He
can't go into town, not that it's much but it would
be a break. He goes everywhere with me or my
husband . . . and we do find this restricting'. Even
if adequate transport is available, its use where the
seizures are frequent, sometimes with incontinence,
can still be embarrassing and even hazardous.

Some countries give extra financial benefits to
people with mobility problems. Unfortunately,
mobility allowance is not normally awarded to
people with epilepsy in the United Kingdom if
they only have frequent attacks unless the person
is also virtually unable to walk because of a physical impairment. Rationalization of these benefits
in the future may improve the situation for people
with epilepsy.

For individuals registered as disabled there is
sometimes a possibility of obtaining concessionary
travel rates on trains and other public transport.
Voluntary organizations can play a vital role in
lobbying for changes in availability of concession-

ary travel. Recently, after 4 years of campaigning by the British Epilepsy Association, British Rail have agreed that people with epilepsy are eligible for the British Rail Disabled Person's Railcard. This entitles the carrier to substantially reduced travel costs. Applications must be supported by a letter from a consultant neurologist, certifying that there is 'a continuing liability to seizures'. Application forms are sent with a remittance to British Rail and the consultant's letter to the Disability Unit at the Department of Transport (see Appendix C). It is possible individuals may experience difficulties and delays in gaining access to an appropriate consultant. Furthermore, the demands on consultant time at this stage remains unclear. Lobbying by local epilepsy groups in the United Kingdom has also resulted in concessionary public travel rates on buses, however, there is considerable variability in availability between areas.

ACKNOWLEDGEMENTS

All the information given in this chapter and the opinions expressed are the responsibility of the authors. However, the authors would like to acknowledge the invaluable help given to them by many people, including: Janice Bowler; Hanneke de Boer, secretary general, International Bureau for Epilepsy, Heemstede, Holland; Commission on employment of the International Bureau for Epilepsy: Hanneke de Boer, Cees Paper, Dr Maria Popovic, Rupprecht Thorbecke, Jim Troxell; Dr Andrew Craig, health promotion consultant; Roger Dennis, Department of Employment, London; Catherine Dowds, senior health education officer, National Society for Epilepsy, United Kingdom; Simon Ennals, consultant in welfare law, Essential Rights, Nottingham; Dr Michael Espir, consultant neurologist, Cromwell Hospital, London; Dr Michael Floyd, director, Rehabilitation Resources Centre, City University, London; Dr Bruce Hermann, associate professor, Epicare Center, Memphis, USA; Patricia Knight, health education advisor, United Kingdom; Susan Lannon, education and nursing co-ordinator, Oregon Comprehensive Epilepsy Programme, Portland, Oregon, USA; Cynthia Lehman, director Legal Advisory Services, Epilepsy Foundation of America; Joop Loeber, honorary executive director, International Bureau for Epilepsy, Holland; William McLin, executive vice-president, Epilepsy Foundation of America; Dr Maurice Parsonage, chairman of the Commission on Driving of the International League Against Epilepsy; Dr Michael Seidenberg, associate professor, Department of Psychology, Chicago Medical School, USA; Jim Troxell, director, Employment, Training and Youth Services, Epilepsy Foundation of America.

REFERENCES

Aarts J H P, Binnie C D, Smit A M, Wilkins A J 1984 Selective cognitive impairment during focal and generalised epileptiform EEG activity. Brain 107: 293–308

Aldenkamp A P 1987 Learning disabilities in children with epilepsy. In: Aldenkamp A P, Alpherts W C J, Meinardi H, Stores G (eds). Education and epilepsy. Swets and Zeitlinger, Lisse, p 21–37

Aldenkamp A P, Alpherts W C J, De Bruine-Seeder D, Dekker M J A 1990 Test–retest variability in children with epilepsy—a comparison of WISC-R profiles. Epilepsy Research 7: 165–172

Alving J 1990 Habilitation of children with epilepsy in Denmark. In: Sillanpaa M, Johannessen S I, Blennow G, Dam M (eds) Paediatric epilepsy. Wrightson Biomedical Publishing Ltd, Petersfield, p 327

Australian Human Rights Commission 1985 Epilepsy and human rights. Occasional Paper No. 7. Australian Government Publishing Service, Canberra

Bagley C 1972 Social prejudice and the adjustment of people with epilepsy. Epilepsia 13: 33–45

Beran R G, Read T 1980 Patient perspectives of epilepsy. Clinical and Experimental Neurology 17: 59–69

Berg B O 1982 Prognosis of childhood epilepsy—another look. New England Journal of Medicine 306: 861–862

Besag F 1987 The role of a special school for children with epilepsy. In: Oxley J. Stores G (eds) Epilepsy and education. Medical Tribune Group, London, p 65–71

Betts T 1988 People with epilepsy as parents. In: Hoare P (ed) Epilepsy and the family. C C Williams, Manchester, p 49–52

Bjorholt P G, Nakken K O, Rohmen K, Hansen H 1990 Leisure time habits and physical fitness in adults with epilepsy. Epilepsia 31: 83–87

de Boer H M 1988 The present attitude of the International Bureau for Epilepsy and its programme relevant to the problem of epilepsy and insurance. In: Canger R, Loeber J N, Castellano F (eds) Epilepsy and society: realities and prospects. Excerpta Medica (ICS 802), Amsterdam, p 221–224

de Boer H M 1989 The components of a good vocational program. In: Manelis J, Bental E, Loeber J N, Dreifuss F (eds) Advances in epileptology: XVII epilepsy international symposium. Raven Press, New York, p 479–482

de Boer H 1991 Counselling women towards independence. In: Trimble M R (ed) Women and epilepsy. John Wiley, Chichester, p 31–40

Britten N, Morgan K, Fenwick P B C, Britten H 1986 Epilepsy and handicap from birth to age thirty-six. Developmental Medicine and Child Neurology 28: 719–728

British Epilepsy Association 1991 Epilepsy: a guide for teachers. British Epilepsy Association, Leeds

British Epilepsy Association 1990 Towards a new understanding. British Epilepsy Association, Leeds.

Brown I 1986 Developing guidelines for epilepsy at work: The occupational physician's role. In: Edwards F, Espir M L E, Oxley J (eds) Epilepsy and employment—a medical symposium on current problems and best practices. ICSS no. 86. Royal Society of Medicine, London, p 53–58

Brown I, Hopkins A 1988 Epilepsy. In: Edwards F C, McCallum R I, Taylor P J (eds) Fitness for work—the medical aspects. Oxford Medical Publications, Oxford, p 210–232

Carter T 1986 Health and safety at work: Implications of current legislation. In: Edwards F, Espir M L E, Oxley J (eds) Epilepsy and employment—a medical symposium on current problems and best practices. ICSS no. 86. Royal Society of Medicine, London, p 9–17

Central Health Services Council 1956 Report of the sub-committee on the medical care of epileptics. HMSO, London

Central Health Services Council 1969 People with epilepsy: Report of a joint sub-committee of the Standing Medical Advisory Committee and the Advisory Committee on the health and welfare of handicapped persons. HMSO, London

Chan A W K 1985 Alcohol and epilepsy. Epilepsia 26: 323–333

Channon S 1982 The resettlement of epileptic offenders. In: Gunn J, Farrington D P (eds) Abnormal offenders, delinquency and the criminal justice system. John Wiley, London, p 339–373

Clement M J, Wallace S J 1990 A survey of adolescents with epilepsy. Developmental Medicine and Child Neurology 32: 849–857

Cofield R, Austin J K 1984 Psychosocial adjustment of adults with epilepsy. Patient Counselling and Health Education 6(3): 125–130

Commission of the European Communities 1988 Report from the Commission on the application of Council recommendation 86/379/EEC on the employment of disabled people in the community. COM (88) 746 final

Confederation of British Industries (CBI) 1983 Employing disabled people. CBI, London

Corbidge P 1987 Teacher training—attitudes towards epilepsy. In: Oxley J, Stores G (eds) Epilepsy and education. Medical Tribune Group, London, p 31–34

Corbidge P, Aspinall A 1988 Targeting audiences—have we hit the bullseye? In: Canger R, Loeber J N, Castellano F (eds) Epilepsy and society: realities and prospects. Excerpta Medica (ICS 802), Amsterdam, p 23–26

Cornaggia C M 1988 Epilepsy and private insurance—why a problem? In: Canger R, Loeber J N, Castellano F (eds) Epilepsy and society: realities and prospects. Excerpta Medica (ICS 802), Amsterdam, p 207–210

Craig A G, Oxley J 1986 Statutory and non-statutory barriers to the employment of people with epilepsy. In: Edwards F, Espir M L E, Oxley J (eds) Epilepsy and employment—a medical symposium on current problems and best practices. ICSS no. 86. Royal Society of Medicine,

London, p 21–32

Craig A G, Oxley J, Dowds C (eds) 1985 Children and young people with epilepsy: An educational package for teachers. National Society for Epilepsy, Chalfont St Peter

Cull C A, Trimble M R 1989 Effects of anticonvulsant medications on cognitive functioning in children with epilepsy. In: Hermann B, Seidenberg M (eds) Childhood epilepsies. Neuropsychological, psychosocial and intervention aspects. John Wiley, Chichester, p 83–103

Dansky L V, Andermann E, Andermann F 1980 Marriage and fertility in epileptic patients. Epilepsia 21: 261–271

Dasgupta A K, Saunders M, Dick D J 1982 Epilepsy in the British Steel Corporation: An evaluation of sickness, accident and work records. British Journal of Industrial Medicine 39: 146–148

Dean R S 1983 Neuropsychological correlates of total seizures with major motor epileptic children. Clinical Neuropsychology 5: 1–3

Department of Health and Social Security 1986 Report of the Working Group on services for people with epilepsy: A report to the Department of Social Security, the Department of Education and Science and the Welsh Office. HMSO, London

Dick D J 1986 Epilepsy in the British steel industry. In: Edwards F, Espir M L E, Oxley J (eds) Epilepsy and employment—a medical symposium on current problems and best practices. ICSS no. 86. Royal Society of Medicine, London, p 49–52

Dowds N, McCluggage J R, Nelson J 1983 A survey of the socio-medical aspects of epilepsy in a general practice population in Northern Ireland. Department of General Practice, Queen's University/British Epilepsy Association, Belfast

Dutton P, Mansell S, Mooney P, Edgell M, Evans E 1989. The net exchequer costs of sheltered employment. Research paper no. 69. Department of Employment, London

Education Act 1981 HMSO, London

Employment Commission of the International Bureau for Epilepsy 1989 Employing people with epilepsy: principles for good practice. Epilepsia 30: 411–412

Employment Department Group 1990 Employment and training for people with disabilities—consultative document. Employment Department, London, p 62–69

Employment Service 1988 Employing someone with epilepsy. Employment Department Group, London

Engel J 1989 Seizures and epilepsy. F. A. Davis Company, Philadelphia

Ennals S 1990/1991 Understanding benefits—a series of ten articles. British Medical Journal 301: 1321, 1386, 37, 95, 160, 228, 284, 342, 400 463

Epilepsy Foundation of America (EFA) 1985 The Workbook. EFA, Landover, Maryland, USA

Epilepsy Foundation of America (EFA) 1987a Management by common sense. EFA, Landover, Maryland, USA

Epilepsy Foundation of America (EFA) 1987b Epilepsy: Legal Rights, Legal Issues. EFA, Landover, Maryland, USA

Epilepsy Foundation of America 1990 EFA commentary. Journal of Epilepsy 3: 107–109

Espir M L E, Floyd M 1986 Epilepsy and recruitment. In: Edwards F, Espir M L E, Oxley J (eds) Epilepsy and employment—a medical symposium on current problems and best practices. ICSS no. 86. Royal Society of Medicine, London, p 39–46

Espir M L E, Semmence A, Floyd M 1987 The recruitment to the Civil Service of people with epilepsy. Journal of the Society of Occupational Medicine 37: 16–18

Fenwick P 1987 Epilepsy and the law. In: Hopkins A (ed) Epilepsy. Chapman and Hall, London, p 554–562

Ferrari M 1989 Epilepsy and its effects on the family. In: Hermann B, Seidenberg M (eds) Childhood epilepsies: neuropsychological, psychosocial and intervention aspects. John Wiley, Chichester, p 159–172

Ferrari M, Matthews W S, Barabas G 1983 The family and the child with epilepsy. Family Process 22: 53–59

Floyd M 1986 A review of published studies on epilepsy and employment. In: Edwards F, Espir M L E, Oxley J (eds) Epilepsy and employment—a medical symposium on current problems and best practices. ICSS no. 86. Royal Society of Medicine, London, p 3–8

Fraser R 1988 Employment and epilepsy: Proceedings of a seminar at the International Epilepsy Meeting, Jerusalem. International Bureau for Epilepsy, Heemstede, Netherlands, p 24–31

Fraser R T 1991 Vocational training: Epilepsy rehabilitation in the USA. In: Oxley J, de Boer H (eds) Proceedings of the employment workshop at the International Epilepsy Congress, New Delhi 1989. International Bureau for Epilepsy, Heemstede, Netherlands

Fraser R T, Clemmons D C 1989 Vocational and psycyhosocial interventions for youths with seizure disorders. In: Hermann B, Seidenberg M (eds) Childhood epilepsies: neuropsychological, psychosocial and intervention aspects. John Wiley, Chichester, p 201–219

Fraser R T, Trejo W, Blanchard W 1984 Epilepsy rehabilitation: evaluating specialised versus general agency outcome. Epilepsia 25: 332–337

Fraser R T, de Boer H M, Oxley J, Pederson B, Peper C, Thorbecke R 1989 Epilepsy and employment: An international survey. In: Manelis J, Bental E, Loeber J N, Dreifuss F (eds) Advances in epileptology: XVII epilepsy international symposium. Raven Press, New York, p 474–478

Gastaut H, Ziskin B G 1987 The risk of automobile accidents with seizures occurring while driving. Neurology 37: 1613–1616

Goldstein J, Seidenberg M, Peterson R 1990 Fear of seizures and behavioural functioning in adults with epilepsy. Journal of Epilepsy 3: 101–104

Goodyear I 1988 The influence of epilepsy on family functioning. In: Hoare P (ed) Epilepsy and the family. C C Williams, Manchester, p 11–18

Gunn J 1977 Epileptics in prison. Academic Press. London

Gunn J 1981 Medico-legal aspects of epilepsy. In: Reynolds E H, Trimble M R (eds) Epilepsy and psychiatry. Churchill Livingstone, Edinburgh, p 165–174

Harding G, Betts T 1987 Epilepsy in tertiary education. In: Oxley J, Stores G (eds) Epilepsy and Education. Medical Tribune Group, London, p 59–64

Hart Y M, Sander J W A S, Shorvon S D 1989 National general practice study of epilepsy and epileptic seizures: Objectives and study methodology of the largest reported prospective cohort study of epilepsy. Neuroepidemiology 8: 221–227

Harvey P, Hopkins A 1983 Views of British neurologists on epilepsy, driving and the law. Lancet i: 401–404

Hauser W A, Hesdorffer D C 1990 Epilepsy: Frequency, causes and consequences. Demos Publications, New York, p 273–296

Hayes J H, Nutman P 1981 Understanding the unemployed. Tavistock Publications Ltd, London

Hegelson D C, Mittan R, Siang-Yang Tan, Sirichai Chayasirisobhon 1990 Supulveda Epilepsy Education: The efficacy of a psychoeducational treatment programme in treating medical and psychosocial aspects of epilepsy. Epilepsia 31: 75–82

Hermann B P, Whitman S 1989 Psychosocial predictors of interictal depression. Journal of Epilepsy 2: 231–237

Hicks R A, Hicks M J 1991 Attitudes of major employers toward the employment of people with epilepsy: A 30-year study. Epilepsia 32(1): 86–88

Hoare P 1984a The development of psychiatric disorder among schoolchildren with epilepsy. Developmental Medicine and Child Neurology 26: 3–13

Hoare P 1984b Psychiatric disturbances in the families of epileptic children. Developmental Medicine and Child Neurology 26: 14–19

Hoare P, Kerley S 1988 The family's experience of epilepsy. In: Hoare P (ed) Epilepsy and the family. C C Williams, Manchester, p 65–72

Holdsworth L, Whitmore K 1974 A study of children with epilepsy attending ordinary schools 2. Information and attitudes held by their teachers. Developmental Medicine and Child Neurology 16: 759–765

Hopkins A, Harvey P K P 1987 Epilepsy and driving. In: Hopkins A (ed) Epilepsy. Chapman and Hall, London, p 563–571

Hoppener R J, Kuyer A, Van der Lugt P J M 1983 Epilepsy and alcohol: The influence of social intake on seizures and treatment in epilepsy. Epilepsia 24: 459–471

International Bureau for Epilepsy 1985 Epilepsy in focus. (Addenda in 1987 and 1989) Heemstede, Netherlands

International Bureau for Epilepsy 1989 A travellers handbook for persons with epilepsy. I B E, Netherlands

Jackson G A 1986 Guidelines to a successful public education campaign. In: An international approach to education campaigns about epilepsy. Proceedings of a Public Education seminar, Hamburg 1985. International Bureau for Epilepsy, Heemstede, Netherlands

Jeavons P M, Harding G F A 1975 Photosensitive epilepsy: A review of the literature and study of 460 patients. Heinemann, London

John C, McLellan D L 1988 Employers' attitude to epilepsy. British Journal of Industrial Medicine 45: 713–715

Kato H, Mori T, Moriuchi T, Kaiyak K 1979 Psychosocial aspects of schoolchildren with epilepsy; Schoolchildren who fell into school phobia. Folia Psychiatrica and Neurologica Japonica 33: 437–439

Kemp A 1988 Safety in the home. In: Dowds C, Craig A, Oxley J (eds) When epilepsy is a problem: A resources package for social services. National Society for Epilepsy, Chalfont St Peter, p 12–15

Kurtz Z 1991 Sex differences in epilepsy: Epidemiological aspects. In: Trimble M R (ed) Women and epilepsy. John Wiley, Chichester, p 47–64

Kurtz Z, Morgan J D 1987 Special services for people with epilepsy in the 1970s. HMSO, London

Lakhani B, Read J 1990 National welfare benefits handbook, 20th ed. Child Poverty Action Group, London

Lannon S 1990 Assessing seizure activity in mentally disabled adults. Journal of Neuroscience Nursing 22: 294–301

Lechtenberg R 1984 Epilepsy and the family. Harvard University Press, Cambridge

Lerman P 1977 The concept of preventative rehabilitation in childhood epilepsy. A plea against overprotection and overindulgence In: Penry J K (ed) VIIIth epilepsy international symposium. Raven Press, New York, p 265–268

Lewis M A, Salas I, de la Sota A, Chiofalo N, Leake B 1990 Randomized trial of a program to enhance the competencies of children with epilepsy. Epilepsia 31: 101–109

Lisle J, Waldron H A 1986 Employees with epilepsy in the National Health Service. British Medical Journal 292: 305–306

Long C J, Moore J R 1979 Parental expectations for their epileptic children. Journal of Child Psychology and Psychiatry 20: 299–312

Mani K S 1991 Vocational training: An Indian experience. In: Oxley J, de Boer H (eds) Proceedings of the employment workshop at the International Epilepsy Congress, New Delhi 1989. International Bureau for Epilepsy, Heemstede, Netherlands

Manpower Services Commission (MSC) 1984 Code of good practice on the employment of disabled people. MSC, Sheffield

Mattson R A 1983 Seizures associated with alcohol use and alcohol withdrawal. In: Browne T R, Feldman R G (eds) Epilepsy diagnosis and management. Little Brown and Co, Boston, p 325–332

Molenaar M 1987 Purpose, character and function of the Ad Interim Act for special education and special secondary education. In: Aldenkamp A P, Alpherts W C J, Meinardi H, Stores G (eds) Education and epilepsy. Swets and Zeitlinger, Lisse, p 61–70

Morrell J 1990 The employment of people with disabilities: Research into the policies and practices of employers. Employment Department Group Research paper no. 77. Department of Employment, London

Munthe-Kaas A W 1990 Habilitation of the child with epilepsy. In: Sillanpaa M, Johannessen S I, Bleanow G, Dam M (eds) Paediatric epilepsy. Wrightson Biomedical Publishing Ltd, Petersfield, p 317–326

Nakken K O, Bjorholt P G, Johannessen S I, Loyning T, Lind E 1990 Effect of physical training on aerobic capacity, seizure occurrence and serum level of antiepileptic drugs in adults with epilepsy. Epilepsia 31: 88–94

National Society for Epilepsy 1991 NSE publications list. National Society for Epilepsy, Chalfont St Peter

Neafsey P, Hayes J, Rogan P 1987 Integration of children with epilepsy into mainstream schools. In: Oxley J, Stores G (eds) Epilepsy and education, a medical symposium on changing attitudes to epilepsy in education. Medical Tribune Group, London, p 35–42

Nelen W 1988 Is epilepsy a dangerous condition? Investigation of accident rates in epilepsy. In: Canger R, Loeber J N, Castellano F (eds) Epilepsy and society: realities and prospects. Excerpta Medica (ICS 802), Amsterdam, p 169–174

Occupational Pensions Board 1977 Occupational pensions scheme cover for disabled people (Cmnd 6849). HMSO, London

O'Donohoe N V 1985 Epilepsies of childhood, 2nd ed. Butterworths, London

O'Leary D S, Seidenberg M, Berent S, Boll T J 1981 The effects of age of onset of tonic-clonic seizures on neuropsychological performance of children. Epilepsia 22: 197–203

O'Leary D S, Lovell M R, Saekellares J C et al 1983 Effects of age of onset of partial and generalised seizure on neuropsychological performance in children. Journal of Nervous and Mental Disease 171: 624–629

Oliver M J 1981 Epilepsy, crime and delinquency: A sociological account. Sociology 14(4): 417–440

Oxley J 1991 Marketing programmes about epilepsy. In: Oxley J, Jepson L (eds) Using audiovisuals in epilepsy. International Bureau for Epilepsy, Heemstede, Netherlands

Oxley J, Craig A G 1989 Proposals for a code of good practice for employing people with epilepsy. in: Manelis J, Bental E, Loeber J N, Dreifuss F (eds) Advances in epileptology: XVII epilepsy international symposium. Raven Press, New York, p 483–484

Pazzaglia P, Frank-Pazzaglia L 1976 Record in grade school of pupils with epilepsy: an epidemiological study. Epilepsia 17: 361–366

Pellock J 1991 The adolescent female with epilepsy. In: Trimble M R (ed) Women and epilepsy. John Wiley, Chichester, p 87–106

Porter R J 1984 Epilepsy—100 elementary principles. Saunders, Great Yarmouth

Prescott-Clarke P 1990 Employment and handicap. Social and Community Planning Research, London

Pugh R 1988 Personal accident insurance in the UK. In: Canger R, Loeber J N, Castellano F (eds) Epilepsy and society: realities and prospects. Excerpta Medica (ICS 802), Amsterdam, p 235–242

Renier W O 1987 Restrictive factors in the education of children with epilepsy from a medical point of view. In: Aldenkamp A P, Alpherts W C J, Meinardi H, Stores G (eds) Education and epilepsy. Swets and Zeitlinger, Lisse, p 3–13

Ritchie K 1981 Interactions in families of epileptic children. Journal of Child Psychology and Psychiatry 22: 65–71

Rogan P J 1987 Education and epilepsy. In: Ross E, Chadwick D, Crawford R (eds) Epilepsy in young people. John Wiley, Chichester, p 23–30

Ross E, West P B 1978 Achievements and problems of British 11 year olds with epilepsy. In: Meinardi H, Rowan A S (eds) Advances in epileptology 1977. Swets and Zeitlinger, Lisse, p 34–37

Ross E M, Peckham C S, West P B, Butler N R 1980 Epilepsy in childhood: Findings from the National Child Development Study. British Medical Journal 1: 207–210

Rowland M 1990 Rights guide to non-means tested social security benefits, 13th ed. Child Poverty Action Group, London

Rutgers M J (1988) Public education: Some experience in the Netherlands. In: Canger R, Loeber J N, Castellano F (eds) Epilepsy and society: realities and prospects. Excerpta Medica (ICS 802), Amsterdam, p 17–22

Sander J W A S, Hart Y M, Johnson A L, Shorvon S D 1990 National general practice study of epilepsy: Newly diagnosed epileptic seizures in a general population. Lancet 336: 1267–1271

Scambler G 1987 Sociological aspects of epilepsy. In: Hopkins A (ed) Epilepsy. Chapman and Hall, London, p 497–510

Scambler G, Hopkins A 1980 Social class, epileptic activity and disadvantage at work. Journal of Epidemiology and Community Health 34(2): 129–133

Schwager H J 1987 Education of children and adolescents suffering from epilepsy. In: Aldenkamp A P, Alpherts W C J, Meinardi H, Stores G (eds) Education and epilepsy.

Swets and Zeitlinger, Lisse, p 81–88

Seidenberg M, Beck N, Geisser M et al 1986 Academic achievement in children with epilepsy. Epilepsia 27: 753–759

Seidenberg M, Beck N, Geisser M et al 1989 Neuropsychological correlates of academic achievement of children with epilepsy. Journal of Epilepsy 1: 23–29

Sillanapaa M 1983 Social functioning and seizure status of young adults with onset of epilepsy in childhood. Acta Neurologica Scandinavica 68 (suppl 96): 1–81

Sillanpaa M 1990a Prognosis of children with epilepsy. In: Sillanpaa M, Johannessen S I, Blennow G, Dam M (eds) Paediatric epilepsy. Wrightson Biomedical Publishing Ltd, Petersfield, p 341–368

Sillanpaa M 1990b Habilitation of children with epilepsy in Finland. In: Sillanpaa M, Johannessen S I, Blennow G. Dam M (eds) Paediatric epilepsy. Wrightson Biomedical Publishing Ltd, Petersfield, p 329–330

Simon R P 1988 Alcohol and seizures. New England Journal of Medicine 319: 715–716

Sonnen A E H 1988a Acceptable risk in epilepsy. In: Canger R, Loeber J N, Castellano F (eds) Epilepsy and Society: realities and prospects. Excerpta Medica (ICS 802), Elsevier, Amsterdam, p 165–168

Sonnen A E H 1988b Practical guidelines for dealing with risk in patients with epilepsy. In: Canger R, Loeber J N, Castellano F (eds) Epilepsy and society: realities and prospects. Excerpta Medica (ICS 802), Amsterdam, p 185–189

Sonnen A E H 1990 How to live with epilepsy. In: Dam M, Gram L (eds) Comprehensive epileptology. Raven Press, New York, p 753–767

Sonnen A E H 1991 The work of the Commission on Audiovisual Education. In: Oxley J, Jepson L (eds) Using audiovisuals in epilepsy. International Bureau for Epilepsy, Heemstede, Netherlands

Spudis E V, Kiffin Penry J, Gibson P 1986 Driving impairment caused by episodic brain dysfunction. Restrictions for epilepsy and syncope. Archives of Neurology 43: 558–564

Stores G 1987 Medical aspects of learning problems in children with epilepsy. In: Oxley J, Stores G (eds) Epilepsy and education. Medical Tribune Group, London, p 25–30

Stores G, Piran N 1978 Dependency of different types of schoolchildren with epilepsy. Psychological Medicine 8: 441–445

Strang J 1987 Educational and related treatment considerations concerning the child with epilepsy: A developmental neuropsychological approach. In: Aldenkamp A P, Alpherts W C J, Meinardi H, Stores G (eds) Education and epilepsy. Swets and Zeitlinger, Lisse, p 118–134

Strauss E, Risser A, Jones H W 1982 Fear responses in patients with epilepsy. Archives of Neurology 39: 626–630

Suurmeijer T undated The education of children suffering from epilepsy: A follow–up study. Unpublished

Tallis R (ed) 1988 Epilepsy and the elderly. Royal Society of Medicine Services Ltd, London

Taylor J F 1983 Epilepsy and other causes of collapse at the wheel. In: Godwin-Austen R B, Espir M L E (eds) Driving and epilepsy—and other causes of impaired consciousness. Symposium Series no. 60. Royal Society of Medicine, London, p 5–7

Taylor D 1989 Psychosocial components of childhood epilepsy. In: Hermann B, Seidenberg M (eds) Childhood epilepsies: neuropsychological, psychosocial and intervention aspects. John Wiley, Chichester, p 119–142

Thompson P J 1987 Educational attainment in children and young people with epilepsy. In: Oxley J, Stores G (eds) Epilepsy and education. Medical Tribune Group, London, p 15–24

Thompson P J, Oxley J 1989 Social difficulties and severe epilepsy: Survey results and recommendation. In: Trimble M R (ed) Chronic epilepsy, its prognosis and management. John Wiley, Chichester, p 113–132

Thompson P J, Shorvon S D 1992 The epilepsies. In: Greenwood R J, Barnes M P, McMillan T M, Ward C D (eds) Neurological rehabilitation. Churchill Livingstone, Edinburgh

Thorbecke R, Janz D 1984 Guidelines for assessing the occupational possibilities of persons with epilepsy. In: Porter R J, Mattson R H, Ward A A, Dam M (eds) Advances in epileptology: XVth epilepsy international symposium. Raven Press, New York, p 571–576

Thornton L 1987 Personal relationships. In: Ross E, Chadwick D, Crawford R (eds) Epilepsy in young people. John Wiley, Chichester, p 39–46

Trades Union Congress 1983 TUC guide on the employment of disabled people. TUC, London

Treiman D M 1986 Epilepsy and violence: Medical and legal issues. Epilepsia 27(suppl 1): S77–S104

Usiskin S 1991 The woman with epilepsy. In: Trimble M R (ed) Women and epilepsy. John Wiley, Chichester, p 3–12

Van der Lugt P J M 1975 Is an application form useful to select patients with epilepsy who may drive? Epilepsia 16: 743–746

Ward F W, Bower B D 1978 A study of certain social aspects of epilepsy in childhood. Developmental Medicine and Child Neurology 20: 1–63

Warnock Report—Special Education Needs 1978 The Report of the Committee of Enquiry into the Education of Handicapped Children and Young People. HMSO, London

Wehrli A 1987 Function deficits and medical techniques. In: Aldenkamp A P, Alpherts W C J, Meinardi H, Stores G (eds) Education and epilepsy. Swets and Zeitlinger, Lisse, p 110–117

Whitman S, Hermann B P (eds) 1986 Psychopathology in epilepsy: social dimensions. New York, Oxford University Press

Wilkins A J 1987 Photosensitive epilepsy and visual display units. In: Ross E, Chadwick D, Crawford R (eds) Epilepsy in young people. John Wiley, Chichester, p 147–155

Wilkins A J, Lindsay J 1987 Questions and answers about photosensitive epilepsy: A patients guide. In: Ross E, Chadwick D, Crawford R (eds) Epilepsy in young people. John Wiley, Chichester, p 157–160

Yule W 1980 Educational achievement. In: Kulig B, Meinardi H, Stores G (eds) Epilepsy and behaviour 1979. Swets and Zeitlinger B V, Netherlands, p 162–168

Ziegler R G 1981 Impairments of control and competence in epileptic children and their families. Epilepsia 22: 339–346

Zielinski J 1988 Epidemiology. In: Laidlaw J, Richens A, Oxley J (eds) A textbook of epilepsy, 3rd edn. Churchill Livingstone, Edinburgh, p 21–48

Zielinski J J, Rader B 1984 Employability of people with epilepsy: Difficulties of assessment. In: Porter R J, Mattson R H, Ward A A, Dam M (eds) Advances in epileptology: the XVth epilepsy international symposium. Raven Press, New York, p 577–581

APPENDIX A

Epilepsy Organizations

United Kingdom

British Epilepsy Association
Anstey House
40 Hanover Square
Leeds LS3 1BE
England
Tel. 0345 089599
Northern Ireland Office
Tel. 0232 248 414

Irish Epilepsy Association
249 Crumlin Road
Dublin 12
Ireland
Tel. 001 516500

National Society for Epilepsy
Chesham Lane
Chalfont St Peter
Gerrards Cross
Bucks, SL9 0RJ
England
Tel. 02407 3991

Scottish Epilepsy Association
48 Govan Road
Glasgow G51 1JL
Scotland
Tel. 041 427 4911

European

Hilfe fur Epilepsie
A-4774 St. Marienkirchen 143
Austria

Les Amis de la Ligue Nat. Belge contre Epilepsie
135 Avenue Albert
Brussels 1060
Belgium

Danish Epilepsy Association
Korsgade 16 1
2200 Copenhagen NV
Denmark

Epilepsyaliitto
Kalevankatu 61
00180 Helsinki 18
Finland

Agir Informer et Sensibiliser le Public
Pour Ameliorer la Connaissance des
Epilepsies (AISPACE)
11 Avenue du President Kennedy
59800 Lille
France

Deutsche Epilepsie Vereiniging
Hochfeld 21b
8134 Pocking
Germany

Greek Nat. Ass. Against Epilepsy
45 Solonos Street
Athens 134
Greece

Associazone Italiana control l'Epilessia
2 via Laghetto
20122 Milan
Italy

Norsk Epilepsiforbund
Kristian Augustsgt 19 V1
Oslo 1
Norway

Liga Nacional Portuguesa Contra la Epilepsia
Rua da Boavista 713
4000 Porto
Portugal

Patronato contra las Enfermedades
Neurologicas Paroxisticas (PENEPH)
Calle Escuelas Pias n.89
08017 Barcelona
Spain

Svenska Epilepsiforbundet
P.O. Box 9514
10274 Stockholm
Sweden

Swiss League Against Epilepsy
C/O Pro Infirmis
P.O. Box 129
8032 Zurich
Switzerland

Epilepsie Vereniging Nederland
Hart. Nibbrigkade 71
fl.48 2597 XS Den Haag
The Netherlands

World Wide

Ass. de Lucha contra la Epilepsia
a/c SNA–Combate do los Pozas
59 p/1' DTO 5CP
1079 Buenos Aires
Argentina

Nat. Epilepsy Ass. of Australia
P.O. Box 554
Lilydale,
Victoria 3140
Australia

Associacao Bras. de Epilepsia
Caixa Postal 20265
04034 Sao Paulo SP
Brazil

Epilepsy Canada
Hospital Notre Dame
C.P. 1560 Succursale C
Montreal Quebec H2L 4K8
Canada

Ass. Liga contra la Epilepsia de Valparaiso
P.O. Box 150
Vina del Mar
Chile

Liga Colombiana contra la Epilepsia
Apart. Aero 604
Cartagena
Colombia

Ministerio de Salud Publica
Inst. Neurol/Neurochir. 21 YD
Vedade C Havana 4
Cuba

Epilepsy Foundation of Santa Ana El Salvador
3A Avenuda Sur no. 13
Santa Ana
El Salvador

Cagualice
Clinicas Herrera-Llerandi
Norte 6a Avenida 7–55 10
Guatemala Ciudad
Guatemala

Indian Epilepsy Association
LRT Medical Centre
176 M Karve Road
Cooperage
Bombay 400 021
India

PERPEI
Jl. Jelita Utara no 11
Rawamangun
Jakarta 13220
Indonesia

Israel Epilepsy Association
P.O. Box 1598
Jerusalem
Israel

Japanese Epilepsy Association Inc
5F Zenkokuzaidan Building 2–2–8
Nishiwaseda Shinjuku-ku
Tokyo 162
Japan

Kenya Ass.f/t Welfare of Epileptics
P.O. Box 44599
Nairobi
Kenya

Korean Epilepsy Association
Severance Hosp., C.P.O. Box 8044
Seoul 120
Korea

New Zealand Epilepsy Association Inc
Cnr. Seddon and Norton Roads
P.O. Box 1074
Hamilton
New Zealand

Epilepsy Foundation of Panama
P.O. Box 5333, zona 5
Panama

South Afr. Nat. Epilepsy League,
S.A.N.E.L.
P.O. Box 73
Observatory 7935
South Africa

Epilepsy Ass. of Sri Lanka
10 Austin Place
Colombo 8
Sri Lanka

Epilepsy Foundation of America
4351 Garden City Drive
Suite 406, Landover
Maryland 20785
United States of America

International

International Bureau for Epilepsy (IBE)
P.O. Box 21
2100 AA Heemstede
The Netherlands

APPENDIX B

Residential Schools for Epilepsy (United Kingdom)

David Lewis Centre
Alderley Edge
Mobberley
Cheshire SK9 7UD
Tel. 056 587 2613

St Piers Lingfield
Lingfield
Surrey RH7 6PN
Tel. 0342 832243

St Elizabeth's School
Much Hadham
Hertfordshire SG10 6EW
Tel. 027 984 3451

APPPENDIX C

Other Useful Addresses (United Kingdom)

Advisory Centre for Education (ACE) Ltd.
18 Victoria Park Square
London E2 9BP
Tel. 081 980 4596 (p.m. only)

The British Sports Association for the Disabled
Hayward House
Barnard Crescent
Aylesbury HP 21 9PP
Tel. 0296 27889

Child Poverty Action Group
1 Bath Street
London EC1 9PY
Tel. 071 253 3406

DHSS Leaflet Unit
P.O. Box 21
Stanmore
Middx. HA7 1AY

Disability Alliance Education and Research Association
25 Denmark Street
London WC2H 8NJ
Tel. 071 240 0806

Disability Unit
Department of Transport
Room S10/21
2 Marsham Street
London SW1P 3EB
Tel. 071 276 0800

Driver Enquiry Unit
DVLC
Swansea SA99 1TU
Tel. 0792 772151

MENCAP—The Royal Society for Mentally Handicapped Children and Adults
123 Golden Lane
London EC1Y 0RT
Tel. 071 253 9433

National Bureau for Students with Disabilities
336 Brixton Road
London SW9 7AA
Tel. 071 274 0565

Riding for the Disabled
Avenue R
National Agricultural Centre
Kenilworth
Warwickshire CV8 2LY
Tel. 0203 56107

Royal Association for Disability and Rehabilitation
25 Mortimer Street
London W1N 8AB
Tel. 071 637 5400

The Sports Council
16 Upper Woburn Place
London WC1H 0QP
Tel. 071 388 1277

22. Medical services

J. S. Duncan   Y. M. Hart

INTRODUCTION

The medical services provided for patients with any ailment are dependent on three principal factors:

1. epidemiological factors: the incidence, prevalence and severity of the condition in the population
2. the amount and source of available funding for provision of medical services
3. the priority accorded to the management of the condition, in competition with other demands.

This chapter will concentrate on the provision of medical services for people with epilepsy in the United Kingdom, with brief reference being made to the services in the United States of America, Denmark, the Netherlands, the Federal Republic of Germany, and France. The situation in developing countries is considered in Chapter 17.

Over 90% of health care in the United Kingdom is delivered by the National Health Service (NHS). The NHS is in the midst of a considerable administrative reorganization as a result of the White Paper 'Working for Patients', with the introduction of clinical budgeting for general practitioners, the creation of an internal market, and the change of status of some hospitals from being facilities administered by Regional and District Health Authorities, to being independent trusts. The management of the NHS is a very sensitive political issue, and further developments will largely depend on the policies of future governments. Key features of the NHS in 1992 are:

1. it is free at the point of service
2. funding is from central government,

distributed through Regional, District and Special Health Authorities
3. patients may be referred, by their medical attendants, anywhere in the NHS system, without bureaucratic intervention or the generation and sending of invoices and receipts
4. staff are salaried, and are not paid on a fee-for-service basis. Present funding of the NHS (£M23,062 in 1989) amounts to 4.5% of Gross National Disposable Income (£M513,247) (Central /Statistical Office 1990), considerably less than is spent in the United States or most Western European Countries.

EPIDEMIOLOGY

A detailed account of the epidemiology of epilepsy is given in Chapter 2. Recent community studies of epilepsy (Hauser & Kurland 1975, Goodridge & Shorvon 1983) have given different results from previous hospital-based investigations (Rodin 1968). In brief, the annual incidence of non-febrile single seizures is 20/100 000 and the incidence of new cases of epilepsy is 50/100 000. The cumulative lifetime incidence of a seizure, that is the overall risk of a person having a non-febrile seizure at some time in their life is about 20/1000. In contrast, the prevalence of active epilepsy in the population at any one time is about 5/1000. It is immediately apparent from the difference between the cumulative lifetime incidence of a seizure and the prevalence of active epilepsy, that about 75% of people who develop seizures at some time remit and do not have continuing active epilepsy. The estimated incidence and prevalence

Table 22.1 The epidemiology of epilepsy in a hypothetical UK population of 1 million persons

Prevalence and incidence	No. of cases
Annual incidence of febrile seizures (50/100 000)	500
Annual incidence of single seizures (20/100 000)	200
Annual incidence of new cases of epilepsy (50/100 000)	500
Prevalence of active epilepsy (500/100 000)	5000
Cumulative lifetime incidence of a seizure (2000/100 000)	20 000
Requirements for medical care	
Institutions	400
Residential care	300
Need for continuing medical attention	3300
Need for occasional medical attention	2600

data for epilepsy, for a sample population of 1 million people, are summarised in Table 22.1, which also gives approximate data on the requirements for medical care for the people with epilepsy. These data are only approximate and are derived from a variety of sources, including the US Commission for the Control of Epilepsy and its Consequences (1978) and the more recent National General Practice Study of Epilepsy (NGPSE) (Hart & Shorvon unpublished data).

RECOMMENDATIONS OF GOVERNMENT WORKING PARTIES ON MEDICAL SERVICES FOR EPILEPSY

There have been five government sponsored reports on medical and allied services for epilepsy in the UK in the last 40 years. In 1953 provision of services by local authorities was evaluated (Ministry of Health 1953). Three years later, the Cohen committee considered hospital services (Central Health Services Council 1956). In 1969 the Reid report reviewed the extent to which the recommendations of the previous reports had been implemented and made further recommendations (Central Health Services Council 1969). In the 1970s the Bennett report was commissioned to evaluate the response to the Reid report, this was forwarded to the Department of Health and Social Security (DHSS) in 1981 and was published in 1987 (Morgan & Kurtz 1987). In response to the Bennett report, the DHSS set up

a working group in 1983 to again consider the recommendations of the Reid report, in conjunction with the Bennett report. The DHSS working group reported in 1984 and published its findings in 1986 (Department of Health and Social Security 1986).

Services for adults

The Cohen and Reid reports and the DHSS working group stressed the importance of the general practitioner in managing epilepsy and its associated social issues, and the Reid report suggested that in large group practices it would be advantageous for one partner to take a special interest in epilepsy. There has been uniform agreement on the need for specialist services for diagnosis and management of difficult cases. In 1953 Cohen proposed the setting up of regional epilepsy clinics and in 1957 the Ministry of Health asked health authorities to carry out this recommendation. No additional finance was provided, however, and the proposals were not put into action. The Reid report suggested the setting up of multidisciplinary clinics at district level for all patients, and specialist regional centres for patients requiring detailed investigation. The DHSS working group concluded that not every patient required evaluation at a dedicated multidisciplinary clinic, that the majority of cases could be managed by a neurologist or other specialist, and that only a minority of patients required the services of such a clinic. The Reid, Bennett and DHSS working group reports, however, noted the inadequacies of present follow-up arrangements and the lack of continuity of care and facilities. All reports supported the concept of epilepsy clinics for patients with intractable epilepsy, run along the lines of diabetic clinics, and in close association with a neurology department.

The Reid report advocated the establishment of five or six special assessment centres for detailed medical evaluation, consideration of psychosocial aspects, rehabilitation, research and teaching, and concluded that they should be financed on a supraregional basis. Three assessment units were established in 1972: at the Chalfont Centre for Epilepsy, and Bootham Park Hospital in York for adults, and the Park Hospital in Oxford for children. The DHSS working group concluded that there should be a significant expansion of special assessment facilities, with at least 100 special assessment centre places for adults, to serve England and Wales, with further centres being established in South-West and the Midlands. It was recommended that the special assessment centres should receive supraregional funding, direct from the DHSS.

The Cohen and Reid reports argued that epilepsy 'colonies' should place less emphasis on care and containment and more on rehabilitation and return to the community. Reid opined that the need for residential care would decline as treatment became more successful and the standards of rehabilitation and provision of care in the community improved. The Bennett report noted that there was no evidence of a decline in admissions for residential care in the 1970s, but this has certainly occurred in the 1980s. Bennett and the DHSS working group concluded that there was an ongoing need for residential care for a small but definite group of patients with intractable epilepsy, often with associated disability and psychosocial problems, with the emphasis on rehabilitation and return to the community, if possible.

Services for children

All reports have stressed the need for good liaison between general practitioners, hospital and school medical services and teaching staff, and the need for education in mainstream schools, if possible, as supported by the Warnock report (Committee of enquiry into the education of handicapped children and young people 1978) and the 1981 Education Act. The DHSS working group concluded that, after initial evaluation by a specialist paediatrician or paediatric neurologist, the majority of patients would be followed up by their general practitioners, and only severe cases would require specialist follow-up. The need to involve school teachers in the care of children with epilepsy, and to educate teachers in the management of the condition was stressed, as was the need for a comprehensive assessment in the child's early teens, 2 years before leaving school. The Park Hospital was established in 1972, following the Reid report, to undertake the multidisciplinary

assessment of children with particularly difficult problems. The DHSS working group concluded that the Park Hospital should receive supraregional funding and that there should be another special assessment centre for children set up in the North of England.

Employment and education

Reid noted the high levels of unemployment in persons with epilepsy and the need for accurate, up-to-date medical information to be made available to potential employers. In some patients with epilepsy, social immaturity was identified as a problem that militated against full employment, and it was felt that social skills training was an important part of rehabilitation programmes. The DHSS working group concluded that much could be done to educate potential employers about epilepsy, and to generate a more positive attitude towards persons with the condition.

All reports agreed on the importance of education and counselling of patients with epilepsy and their families, and that this should be carried out largely by general practitioners, but also in epilepsy clinics and special assessment centres, where social workers and medical staff would have an important counselling role. It has been noted that voluntary groups and patient associations have a significant role in education. There was a similar consensus regarding the need for education of the public in general, and in particular teachers and employers, about the nature of epilepsy, in an attempt to dispel inappropriate negative perceptions. The DHSS working group concluded that epilepsy centres, clinics and voluntary agencies should target health service, social service and occupational health workers, career advisers and disablement rehabilitation officers for intensive education, from whom information would then be disseminated further.

CURRENT AVAILABILITY OF UK RESOURCES FOR EPILEPSY

The medical care of people with epilepsy involves a wide range of disciplines both in the community and in the hospital. At the centre of this system, at the primary health care level, is the GP, who is responsible for coordinating the patient's management, referring him or her to hospital where appropriate, prescribing antiepileptic drugs (AEDs), counselling, giving emergency care, and often for undertaking long-term follow-up. Hospital consultants, usually neurologists or general physicians in the case of adults, and paediatricians in the case of children, are involved in the majority of cases when referral is made at the onset of the epilepsy and may also play a part in the long-term care of those patients whose epilepsy proves difficult to control. For some patients, for example those with learning difficulties or psychiatric problems, referral to other agencies such as psychiatrists, clinical psychologists, or specialists in mental handicap may also become necessary. Nurses specifically trained in the management of people with epilepsy may play a useful role, as may appropriately trained counsellors.

Table 22.2 shows the medical personnel available in England and Wales in 1987 to provide medical care for the 30 000 people developing epilepsy each year and the 300 000 people with active epilepsy. These are average figures for the population served by each practitioner, and may vary considerably from area to area. A general practitioner in an 'average' practice might be expected to have one or two patients on his list developing epilepsy each year, and about 10 patients with active epilepsy.

Hospital referral patterns are inevitably affected by the accessibility of the various consultants. Although it is recommended that adults developing seizures be referred to a neurologist (or other specialist with a particular interest and expertise in epilepsy) (DHSS 1986), the ratio of neurologists to population is considerably lower in the UK than in the majority of other countries in the developed world. A survey carried out in 1987 on behalf of the Association of British Neurologists (Langton Hewer & Wood 1990) estimated that there was the equivalent of one whole-time neurologist for 373 000 persons (range 157 000–626 000). There were 38 health districts, serving a population of 7.1 million, with less than one weekly consultant neurological session per district. Overall, if every adult developing epilepsy were seen by a neurology consultant, each such consultant would see approximately 160 patients developing epilepsy each year. To this figure has to be added the number of children with intractable epilepsy referred on from paediatric to adult neurology clinics. In practice, many patients developing epilepsy are referred to general physicians, either because of lack of direct access to a neurologist by the GP, or because the patient gravitates naturally to the physician by virtue of being admitted to hospital acutely under the care of a medical team following the onset of seizures. It is anticipated that the number of neurologists in England and Wales will increase by about four posts each year (Department of Health, Medical Manpower and Education Division 1989): assuming no growth in the population, it would take until the year 2021 to reach the ratio of neurologists to population (1:200 000) recommended by the Association of British Neurologists. Geriatricians also play an important part in the management of epilepsy: in the UK NGPSE, a recent community-based study of over 1000 patients with newly diagnosed or suspected seizures (Sander et al 1990), 25% of those presenting with seizures were found to be aged 60 or more at the time of presentation. Many of these had additional nonneurological problems, and for these people, referral to a geriatrician, who has the facilities to oversee the patient's medical care and deal with social problems, may well be appropriate.

The situation with regard to children shows a similar shortfall in the provision of neurology

Table 22.2 Medical manpower provision in England and Wales (1987)

Personnel	Approx. mean no. of population per practitioner
General practitioner	1800
Consultant neurologist	280 000
Consultant neurologist (whole-time equivalent)	373 000
Consultant physician	39 000
Consultant paediatrician	14 000*
Paediatric neurologist	738 000*
Consultant psychiatrist (mental handicap)	293 000
Consultant psychiatrist (mental illness)	40 000
Consultant neurosurgeon	512 000
Consultant clinical neurophysiologist	966 000
Clinical neuropsychologist	837 000

* Figures apply to children under the age of 15 years.

services: although there are only about 14 000 children per consultant paediatrician, paediatric neurologists on average serve a population of 738 000 children (DHSS, Medical Manpower and Education Division 1988 Office of Population Censuses and Surveys 1990).

Some patients with intractable epilepsy may be suitable for epilepsy surgery. However, the ratio of neurosurgeons to population is also small (1:512 000) (DHSS, Medical Manpower and Education Division 1988, Office of Population Censuses and Surveys 1990), and only a small minority of these perform surgery for the relief of epilepsy (Hart & Shorvon 1990).

The United States Commission for the Control of Epilepsy and its Consequences (1978) estimated that the prevalence rate of people with mental handicap and epilepsy was about 0.07%, just over half of these patients being institutionalized (Table 22.1). Assuming similar figures pertain to the British situation, there are approximately 35 000 people in the UK with mental handicap and epilepsy. In 1987 there were 170 consultants in mental handicap to provide a service for these people, a ratio of 205 patients to each specialist.

Little information is available about the provision of the facilities necessary for the management of people with epilepsy. The survey by the Association of British Neurologists on neurology services in the UK (Langton Hewer & Wood 1990) found considerable difficulty in estimating the number of X-ray computerized tomography (CT) scanners available, but were able to identify 135 head scanners in the UK in June 1987. Overall, there was one head scanner to every 420 593 persons in the UK, but the proportion varied from one head scanner per 284 000 to one per 827 000 population. There has been a rapid increase in the provision of CT scanners in recent years, with many district general hospitals having their own facilities, and although the provision for scans remains poor in some parts of the country, lack of availability of the hardware is becoming less of a problem than previously. A more pressing problem, in many areas, is the shortage of skilled neuroradiologists to interpret the images. It is estimated that there are currently around 40 magnetic resonance imaging (MRI) scanners in routine clinical use in the UK, not including scanners dedicated to research into specific neurological diseases.

Basic electroencephalography (EEG) facilities are widely available, although in some areas of the country there is a waiting list of some months for this test, and access may be difficult, with many neurophysiology departments being situated in psychiatric hospitals. Specialized EEG facilities, such as ambulatory monitoring, EEG with sphenoidal electrodes, and EEG/video-telemetry, are much more limited, and mainly available in centres with specialist epilepsy clinics and those in which epilepsy surgery is undertaken. A study of specialized hospital services for adults with epilepsy in the North East Thames Region of the UK (Espir et al 1987), serving a population of about 3.5 million, found that EEG was available in 10 hospitals in the region, with sphenoidal EEG being available in seven departments, and ambulatory EEG in four departments. Video EEG telemetry was only available at the National Hospital for Neurology and Neurosurgery, Queen Square. The authors commented that the NE Thames region is not typical of UK health regions, with its relatively high concentration of neurological services, including the National Hospital, in addition to the five (now four) undergraduate teaching hospitals.

Serum drug concentration monitoring is widely available in district general hospital biochemistry laboratories, although analyses are often carried out on a 'batch' basis once or twice weekly, or even less frequently, thus limiting its benefits in the clinical management of epilepsy.

There are only approximately 50–60 clinical neuropsychologists in the UK, not including research workers (Thompson 1990) undertaking the whole range of clinical neuropsychology. Specialist psychological assessment of people with epilepsy, therefore, may be very difficult to obtain.

PRIMARY CARE

The general practitioner is responsible for the primary care of patients with epilepsy in the UK. He or she is often the first to see patients developing seizures, and is likely to refer the majority of them to hospital. In the case of an uncomplicated first seizure, particularly where the patient is not living alone, this will usually be to a specialist outpatient clinic, although immediate referral to hospital may be made if the seizure is prolonged or recurs, causes injury, or is associated with a history or signs suggestive of an acute underlying neurological disease, such as infection or tumour. When the first presentation is to a hospital casualty department, the general practitioner will usually be kept informed of developments and will often make the formal referral to a hospital outpatient clinic.

The hospital consultant usually confirms the diagnosis of epilepsy and informs the patient about the condition and its implications, for example for driving. The general practitioner, however, with his knowledge of the patient's background and domestic arrangements, will play a large part in the education and counselling of the patient with respect to his epilepsy, particularly since patients forget a considerable proportion of what is told them initially. Aspects of epilepsy which need to be discussed include the characteristics and causes of epilepsy, the nature of the various investigations undertaken and the results for the individual, types of treatment and their potential side-effects and limitations, inheritance, prognosis, contraception and pregnancy. Social aspects also need to be discussed, including the implications for employment, education, leisure activities, and marriage. The voluntary agencies can also play a major role in this regard, and in addition to giving telephone advice produce a number of useful leaflets dealing with various aspects of epilepsy, which may be used to supplement information given by the general practitioner.

Table 22.3 summarizes the role of the general practitioner in the management of the patient with epilepsy. The general practitioner may be responsible for initiating medication, particularly in those cases referred to hospital following a single seizure, when it is common to defer treatment until the occurrence of a further episode. He is very likely to see the patient with acute drug-related problems, and to need to adjust the medication even in the case of those patients whose care continues to be supervised by a hospital consultant. The general practitioner is also usually the first doctor to be called in the management of serial seizures and status epilepticus. For the majority of patients with 'uncomplicated' epi-

Table 22.3 The role of the general practitioner in the management of the patient with epilepsy

Initial diagnosis of epilepsy

Referral to specialist
—investigation
—confirmation of diagnosis
—initial recommendation for management

Continued follow-up of patient
—monitoring efficacy and toxicity of medication
—repeat prescriptions
—monitoring medical developments
—re-referral to specialist of complicated cases or for consideration of treatment withdrawal

Counselling
—nature and causes of epilepsy
—details and results of investigations
—treatment, including aims, limitations and side-effects
—prognosis
—inheritance
—potentially dangerous situations
—education and employment
—leisure activities
—driving
—contraception and pregnancy
—practical management of seizures

lepsy, which may be expected to respond well to antiepileptic drugs, the general practitioner oversees the continuing care of the patient after initial evaluation by a consultant. Even where patients are kept under follow-up at a hospital clinic, it is customary for the general practitioner to be responsible for issuing prescriptions. Often he will be responsible for advising when to discontinue medication, particularly when hospital follow-up no longer occurs.

Estimates of the frequency with which patients with epilepsy see their general practitioner have varied considerably between studies. In addition to its study of people with newly diagnosed seizures, the NGPSE undertook a study in 1988–89 of over 1500 patients with active epilepsy (defined as those people with a history of at least two non-febrile seizures, and either taking antiepileptic medication or with at least one seizure in the previous 2 years) in the community (Hart & Shorvon unpublished data). Only 28% of these were under continued hospital follow-up, with the general practitioner being responsible for on-going care in the remainder of the cases. Eighty-two per cent of those for whom the general practitioner was primarily responsible for their care had seen him one or more times (not necessarily for epilepsy) in the previous year, so that they had at least had the opportunity to discuss their epilepsy with him. In contrast, Lloyd-Jones (1980), auditing a group practice, found that 60% of patients being treated for epilepsy had seen neither their general practitioner nor a hospital doctor about their epilepsy in the previous year.

Other community-based agencies may also play a part in the long-term management of the patient with epilepsy. These include the school medical service, occupational health departments, the district mental handicap team, social workers and community nurses. A small number of liaison nurses (four are known to the authors), with special training in epilepsy, play a major role in the management of patients with epilepsy in certain areas of the country, in a similar manner to the more widely known liaison nurses specializing in diabetes.

SECONDARY CARE

The DHSS Working Group (1986) recommended that, 'General practitioners should normally refer all their patients with seizures to a consultant for diagnosis, initial assessment and recommendation for management', with children being seen by a consultant paediatrician or paediatric neurologist, and adults by a consultant neurologist or other consultant with a special interest in epilepsy. These consultants should involve other professional staff in the assessment where appropriate.

In practice, the proportion of patients developing seizures who are referred to hospital depends on several factors, including their age, the circumstances of the seizure, the area of the country, and the general practitioner himself. The Royal College of General Practitioners Research Committee, reporting in 1960 on a survey of people with chronic epilepsy under the care of 134 general practitioners from 67 practices in England and Wales, estimated that not more than three-quarters of all patients suffering from epilepsy had been seen by a specialist. Hopkins & Scambler (1977) identified all adults with epilepsy on the lists of 17 general practitioners in London. Of the 94 patients who had active epilepsy, were not in a long-term institution and agreed to be inter-

viewed, 95% had been referred to hospital, and in 81 cases this was to a hospital with a consultant neurologist on the staff. More recently, the NGPSE study of people developing or diagnosed as having seizures for the first time found that the likelihood of people having epileptic seizures being referred to hospital varied with age: whereas 98% of children under the age of 16, and 94% of those between the ages of 16 and 59, were seen by a specialist, only 82% of those aged 60 or over were referred (Hart, Sander & Shorvon unpublished data).

These figures suggest that the practice regarding hospital referral for people with epilepsy may have changed in the 1970s and 80s, with referral becoming the norm. Data from the NGPSE, however, indicates that referral is not always to a 'recommended' consultant. Forty per cent of the patients in this study saw a neurologist or paediatric neurologist, and 21% a paediatrician, while 20% saw a general physician, reflecting the inadequacy of the provision of adult neurological services. The remainder saw various specialists including neurosurgeons, geriatricians and psychiatrists.

Initial evaluation of the patient is undertaken with three main purposes in mind: to confirm the diagnosis of epilepsy, to determine its aetiology, and to classify the type of epilepsy and the seizure types.

For approximately 70 to 80% of people developing epilepsy, good control of seizures is possible, while for the remainder management is more difficult and the seizures may prove intractable to medical treatment (Hauser & Kurland 1975, Goodridge & Shorvon 1983, Reynolds 1987). The DHSS working group envisaged that, 'following initial assessment and recommendation for management by the consultant, patients would normally be cared for by the general practitioner'. Thus, 'mild' cases would only see the consultant again if they developed specific problems. It was suggested that patients with severe epilepsy should be referred to an epilepsy clinic for follow-up. The prevalence of epilepsy and the number of neurologists in the UK are such that, if all patients with active epilepsy remained under 6 monthly review by a neurologist, he or she would have to see 60 such patients for follow-up each week.

The proportion of patients with epilepsy remaining under hospital follow-up has varied considerably between studies. As described above, the NGPSE cross-sectional study found that 28% of people with active epilepsy were continuing to attend a hospital clinic (Hart & Shorvon unpublished data). These patients were more likely to have had recent seizures than the rest of the group; only 12% had been seizure free in the previous 2 years, compared with 34% for the group as a whole, while 29% had had at least one seizure within the previous week, compared with 16% for the whole group. Hopkins & Scambler, however, noted in their study that, 'Half of the few still attending hospital clinics have rare seizures, while those with very frequent seizures do not see even their general practitioners for months at a time'.

A number of those investigating the medical care of people with epilepsy have commented on deficiencies in the system. Goodman (1983), auditing the care of people with epilepsy in a group practice, identified a lack of continuity and supervision in the hospital care, and commented, 'Patients saw a different doctor at each attendance. Many of the changes in drug regimes were made by doctors seeing the patients for the first time. Most of the follow-up was performed by junior hospital doctors'.

INVESTIGATION OF EPILEPSY

There is no standardized regimen for the management of epilepsy, and the extent of investigation will depend on the individual circumstances of the case. The DHSS Working Group (1986) recommended that the facilities available should include routine EEG, CT, MRI, a routine X-ray service, electrocardiography (ECG), serum drug concentration monitoring, and haematology and chemical pathology services.

Investigations that may be required include routine haematology and biochemistry (including urea and electrolytes, blood sugar, calcium and liver function tests), serology, and an ECG. The major indications for performing a CT scan are: onset of seizures at the age of less than 1 year or greater than 20 years, any suggestion that the epilepsy may be partial on history, clinical examination or EEG (with the possible exception of

clinical and EEG data strongly suggestive of benign rolandic epilepsy), unexplained deterioration in seizure control, and intractable epilepsy. Patients in whom there is a particularly high yield of CT scan abnormalities include those with partial seizures, those with focal EEG changes, and patients with abnormal neurological signs. MRI may be of value in the case of patients with negative scans in whom an underlying structural lesion is strongly suspected or in patients for whom surgery is contemplated. About 30% of patients with partial seizures who have a negative CT scan can be shown to have a relevant abnormality on MRI scan (Lesser et al 1986, Theodore et al 1986, Franceschi et al 1989).

An EEG is an appropriate investigation in almost every person developing seizures. The main purpose is to assist in the classification of the seizure type and localization of any epileptogenic focus, rather than to assist in the diagnosis, although it is of particular value in the differentiation of some of the epileptic syndromes commonly developing in childhood, for example primary generalized epilepsy, and benign rolandic epilepsy. It should be remembered that in a routine (awake) interictal EEG, only 35% of patients with epilepsy always show abnormalities, 50% sometimes show abnormalities, while 15% never do (Ajmone-Marsan & Zivin 1970). Conversely, 10–15% of people who have never had a seizure may have a mildly abnormal EEG, although only about 1% the population without epilepsy have focal or generalized spike or polyspike and slow-wave abnormality in the EEG (Zivin & Ajmone-Marsan 1968). In practice, the number of patients with newly diagnosed seizures having CT scan and EEG falls short of that recommended. The NGPSE study of people with newly diagnosed seizures found that 65% of patients with definite seizures had had an EEG and 39% a CT scan. The likelihood of having an EEG or CT scan varied with age: the proportion of people over the age of 60, in whom the likelihood of finding an underlying structural lesion might be expected to be greater, was considerably smaller (33%). Eighty-three per cent of children had had an EEG and 23% a CT scan (Hart Y, Sander L, Shorvon J D unpublished data). In cases of diagnostic uncertainty, sleep-deprived EEG and ambulatory recordings may be helpful, and in a small minority of people, particularly those in whom pseudo-seizures are suspected, EEG/video-telemetry may facilitate the diagnosis.

While not routinely necessary in patients developing seizures, psychometric assessment may be of value in those people in whom seizures appear to be accompanied by a decline in intellectual function. Many patients with epilepsy also complain of problems with memory, and psychometry can help to elucidate the nature of this and act as a baseline against further measurements.

Serum antiepileptic drug concentration monitoring is helpful in certain situations, particularly when non-compliance is suspected, when it is not clear if a patient's symptoms may be drug side-effects, and for some drugs, as a guide to dosing. Monitoring of serum AED concentrations is of most value when the results are available on the same day, so that the patient can have his blood taken and be reviewed with the result in the clinic (Patsalos et al 1987). There are no firm data about the availability of serum AED concentration monitoring with same day results, but it seems unlikely that many centres apart from the major specialist epilepsy clinics have this facility.

EPILEPSY CLINICS

All government reports have recommended the establishment of epilepsy clinics, but have differed in their conclusion as to how widespread and comprehensive they should be (see above). The latest consensus was that there should be established a series of pilot clinics and, if these proved successful, that dedicated epilepsy clinics be established nationwide for patients with difficult epilepsy and attendant problems. It is envisaged that epilepsy clinics should have a similar scope and role to diabetic clinics, which have been widely acknowledged to improve the care of patients with diabetes (MacFarlane 1990). In the past, the UK medical profession has been ambivalent about the establishment of epilepsy clinics, as revealed by the replies to a 1976 enquiry of Health Authorities and Area Medical Officers (Morgan & Kurtz 1987), and firm evidence of their utility is required. A recent prospective, randomized study in Cardiff compared the care of patients with

epilepsy in a neurology clinic and in a dedicated epilepsy clinic. Patients who attended the epilepsy clinic had better control of seizures, reported less side-effects from medication, received and retained more information and were more satisfied with the service provided, than were those who attended the regular Neurology Clinic (Morrow 1990). A recent audit of an epilepsy clinic at Atkinson Morley's Hospital, London, showed 36% of referrals had a > 50% reduction in seizure frequency following attendance; 41% were being treated with monotherapy at presentation, and this increased to 59% (Crawford & Wilson 1990).

At present there is no organized system of epilepsy clinics in the UK, and the number of clinics is unclear. Any existing arrangements have been made at local level by interested clinicians, and vary enormously in their facilities and scope. At one extreme, there are a few highly developed clinics with a full range of facilities, for example, the National Hospitals for Neurology and Neurosurgery/Chalfont Centre for Epilepsy and Kings College/Maudsley Hospitals in London, and centres in Cardiff, Glasgow and Liverpool, which have patients referred on a regional and supra-regional basis. At the other extreme, a neurologist or paediatrician may see all his patients with epilepsy on a particular day of each month, with no dedicated resources, and refer to this as an epilepsy clinic. A survey of medical services for epilepsy in the North East Thames Health Region (population 3.5 million, divided into 15 Health Districts) showed there to be four dedicated epilepsy clinics, two of which were run by clinical neurophysiologists (Espir et al 1987). In the North West Thames region there are three epilepsy clinics for adults and four for children.

The Northampton and Kettering Health Districts provide a good example of what may be achieved with limited resources, at district level (Knight, personal communication). A joint paediatric epilepsy clinic is held twice a month in Northampton by a consultant neurophysiologist and a consultant paediatrician, with junior staff attending for training. Children attending this clinic have been referred from general paediatric clinics and have particular problems, several having mental handicap or pseudoseizures. There is continuity of care by the consultants. Patients are referred to

Oxford for consideration of epilepsy surgery, and may be referred back to the general paediatric clinic when treatment has been optimized. A joint clinic, by consultants in neurophysiology, paediatrics and child psychiatry is held in Kettering every 3 months, for difficult cases. Three adult epilepsy clinics are held every week, for patients with chronic epilepsy. New cases are generally evaluated by paediatricians and general physicians. There is a weekly neurology outpatient clinic in Kettering and in Northampton, staffed by a consultant and one registrar, which is used for providing second opinions. The epilepsy clinics are held in the neurophysiology department, and EEGs recorded on a patient's first attendance. Emergency EEGs and ambulatory records are available. CT scanning is available at Northampton. Serum AED concentrations are measured at Northampton, Kettering and Milton Keynes, with

Table 22.4 Epilepsy clinic — components and role

Location
—hospital outpatient department; access to a small number of inpatient beds.

Staff
—overall responsibility of a Consultant Neurologist and Consultant Paediatrician
—junior medical staff, Sub-Consultant grade specialists
—close liaison with Clinical Neurophysiologist and Psychiatrist (mental handicap and illness)
—nursing staff, nurse practitioners
—administrative staff, receptionist, secretary
—social worker

Facilities
—access to serum AED concentration monitoring, EEG, CT scanning, clinical psychology and other hospital services

Referrals
—from general practitioners and hospital doctors

Functions
—initial diagnostic evaluation and initiation of treatment
—long-term management and follow-up of severe or complicated epilepsy
—co-ordination of medical and non-medical services.

Education and counselling
—patient and family; liaison with schools, employers, social services
—wider education of community as a whole
—involvement with voluntary agencies

Teaching
—medical and paramedical staff
—non-medical staff, e.g. police, social workers, teachers

Research
—clinical research should be vigorously pursued

urgent results available in 24 hours. The clinical psychology service is under great demand and has a long waiting list. There is an urgent need for social work support to the epilepsy clinic. Despite several approaches there is no social worker who is trained in the management of epilepsy, but collaboration has developed on a personal basis.

If pilot studies confirm their value, epilepsy clinics should be established in each health district, and be available for the management of patients with difficult epilepsy and with associated problems, with referrals being made by general practitioners and hospital specialists, for initial diagnostic evaluation and long-term follow-up if necessary. The components and role of a specialized epilepsy clinic are summarized in Table 22.4. Epilepsy clinics would provide an efficient and logical concentration of resources. In addition to the medical aspects, an epilepsy clinic should have an important role in the education and counselling of patients and their families, schools and employers about epilepsy, and also act as a focus for the education of the community as a whole and interact with voluntary agencies and local patient support groups. In addition to District epilepsy clinics, there is a clear need for Regional epilepsy centres, usually situated at a Regional department of neurology and neurosurgery, at which there is a full range of diagnostic and therapeutic facilities, including MRI, clinical neuropsychology and video-EEG telemetry. It would be desirable for epilepsy clinics to operate under the auspices of a consultant neurologist and consultant paediatrician, with junior staff. Continuity of care is a major problem: with other demands on their time, it is not realistic for all clinical care to be provided by one or two consultants. Possible solutions, that have been shown to work well in diabetic clinics, include the use of long-term medical staff in a sub-consultant grade, e.g. specially trained general practitioners, and the use of nurse practitioners, who would undertake the routine monitoring of seizure control and medication, and counselling.

TERTIARY CARE

Special assessment centres

Two special assessment centres for adults with

epilepsy were designated in the UK in 1972: the Chalfont Centre for Epilepsy in Buckinghamshire and Bootham Park Hospital in York. The Park Hospital in Oxford is a designated National Assessment Centre for children with epilepsy. Other centres also fulfil an assessment role (see Appendix).

The Chalfont Centre for Epilepsy Assessment Unit comprises 33 beds. Funding is from the National Hospitals for Neurology and Neurosurgery and the unit forms an integral part of the epilepsy services of the National Hospitals and the Institute of Neurology. All medical, psychological biochemical and pharmacological staff have joint appointments between the three institutions. The medical staff consists of two senior lecturers in neurology, a senior lecturer in neurophysiology, a senior registrar, a senior house officer in neurology who rotates to the National Hospital, and research registrars. The accent of the unit is neurological rather than psychiatric, but a consultant psychiatrist makes regular visits. There is a full range of psychological investigation and intervention available. Assay of serum drug concentrations and ambulatory EEG/ECG and CCTV-EEG telemetry are available on site. Nearly all patients are seen by one of two part-time social workers. Detailed social work involvement is an invaluable part of the initial assessment, and also for counselling patients and their families, and for liaising with caring agencies in the referral district about the implementation of recommendations. CT and MRI scanning, detailed biochemical investigations, intracranial EEG recordings and other neurosurgical procedures are carried out at the National Hospital. In one recent year, 197 patients were admitted with a mean stay of 45 days. Referrals are from all parts of England, Wales and Ulster, and 77% are tertiary in nature. The principal reasons for admission include: clarification of diagnosis, optimization of medical treatment, consideration of surgical treatment, assessment of potential for independent living and employment and advice about future long-term arrangements, and education of patient, family and carers about epilepsy and its management. In addition to the inpatient facility, outpatient clinics for new referrals and follow-up are held at the Chalfont Centre and the National Hospitals. There is a separate 17-bed rehabilitation unit, which is funded by DSS and Local Authorities, to which patients who would benefit from a more prolonged period of psychosocial rehabilitation may be admitted after their medical treatment has been optimized.

The second supraregional epilepsy centre is at Bootham Park Hospital, York, and was established in 1965. A new medical director and neurophysiologist, who have links with the Regional Neurology and Neurosurgery Centre in Leeds, were appointed in 1989 and the activity of the 14-bed inpatient unit is increasing. Dedicated epilepsy clinics, and joint clinics with paediatricians are held in Leeds and York, in collaboration with the British Epilepsy Association. There are research links with the pharmacology, psychology and psychiatry departments of Leeds and York Universities.

The David Lewis Centre, in Cheshire, is a charity concerned with the residential care and rehabilitation of adults and children with chronic epilepsy. Detailed neurophysiological and psychological investigations are available on site and the centre is more geared to the assessment of patients with problematic behaviour and conduct, than are Chalfont and Bootham Park. Medical staff have joint appointments with hospitals in Manchester, where patients are referred for CT and MRI. There is a 29-bed adult assessment unit, staffed by a consultant psychiatrist and consultant clinical pharmacologist, and junior staff. Patients are admitted for short-term assessment and review of medication and then return to the community. A further eight beds are available for the assessment of children from the ages of 5 to 19. The assessment includes review of diagnosis and medical treatment, education, speech therapy, social work, neuropsychology and physiotherapy. Recommendations are made regarding further education and placement. Consultant care is provided by a psychiatrist, child psychiatrist and paediatric neurologist. At the Maudsley Hospital, there is a further inpatient epilepsy assessment unit, under the direction of a consultant psychiatrist, and with its emphasis on patients with concomitant psychological and psychiatric disturbance.

In Scotland, the Quarriers Village Epilepsy Centre, near Glasgow has a 10-bed Assessment Unit to which about 40 patients per year are admitted from all over Scotland, and also Northern Ireland and the North of England. The assessment facility is run by a consultant physician with a particular interest in epilepsy. The centre is not equipped to deal with patients with significant behaviour difficulties or profound physical or mental handicap. The average duration of admission is 8 weeks. Ambulatory EEGs and video-telemetry are available, a psychology department undertakes diagnostic work and behaviour modification therapy, and capability for work is assessed in a workshop. In addition to medical review, recommendations are made for future care and consideration given to admission to a linked Rehabilitation Unit.

The Park Hospital in Oxford was designated in 1972 as a National Assessment Centre for children with epilepsy. Despite this designation, the Park Hospital is funded through the District Mental Health Unit and, because of financial cuts, has recently had to reduce from 33 to 25 beds, of which about two-thirds are occupied by children with epilepsy. About 70 children with epilepsy are admitted each year and the average admission is for 2-3 months. Children are between the ages of 4 and 16 years, and are usually referred by a paediatrician, paediatric neurologist or child psychiatrist. The service includes medical, educational, psychiatric and social aspects of care. CCTV-EEG and detailed neuropsychology are available on site. CT and MR imaging and an epilepsy surgery programme are available in nearby hospitals. At discharge, recommendations for future care are made, in close liaison with local services.

Residential schools

The vast majority of children with epilepsy receive mainstream schooling, but there are a few, often with severe epilepsy and attendant difficulties with cognitive function and behaviour, who benefit from being educated in a special residential school. These schools are the Lingfield Hospital School in Surrey, St Elizabeth's at Much Hadham, Hertfordshire and the David Lewis Centre. In addition to an educational role, the residential schools provide close medical supervision and allow children to reach their maximum potential and develop in an equal peer group. Close links are maintained with the child's local school, and return made to mainstream education, if possible.

Residential care for adults

In the late 19th century several groups of philanthropists established refuges for people with epilepsy. The Chalfont Centre for Epilepsy, for example, was established in 1894 in a rural setting, as a 'colony' to which persons with epilepsy were admitted for long-term care. The accent was generally on an outdoor puritanical lifestyle, with the colony being largely self-sufficient. The medical care was very limited, being provided by a local general practitioner. In 1948, the National Assistance Act made local authorities responsible for finding residential care for persons who were unable to live independently, and many persons with epilepsy were referred to epilepsy 'colonies' In 1962 there were 2246 places in a total of eight homes and colonies specifically for people with epilepsy, and in 1967 there were 2067. In the 1970s public and professional opinion swung against institutional long-term care for patients with mental illness, and there was a fall-off of residential care for chronic epilepsy (Morgan & Kurtz 1987). In 1977, there were 1687 places. In the 1980s there has been a steady reduction in the numbers of patients with epilepsy in residential care, and in 1990 there were only 1022 places. Several reasons for this trend may be identified: elderly residents are dying, and with rehabilitation the more able are returning to living in the community. In addition, fewer people are being admitted to residential care as a result of improved medical management of epilepsy, better community support, financial stringency in local authorities and a disdain for 'institutionalization'. Over the last decade, the resident population of the Chalfont Centre for Epilepsy has been failing by about 10 persons per year. Not surprisingly, the average age of the resident population has increased, as has the overall level of disability—with a greater proportion of residents having troublesome epilepsy and other medical problems. In consequence, the centre's population has become less able-bodied, and has a greater need for care.

At present there are five centres providing long-term residential care for adults with epilepsy: Chalfont Centre for Epilepsy (263 beds), David Lewis Centre (239 beds), The Maghull Homes (240), Quarrier's Homes (126 beds), St Elizabeth's (94 beds) and The Meath Home (60 beds) (see Appendix). In addition to the above, it is estimated that about 30% of persons with mental handicap who are in institutional and residential care have epilepsy.

There remains a small but definite need for long-term residential care and attempts at gradual rehabilitation for some people with intractable epilepsy, commonly in association with other neurological, psychiatric or psychological handicap, and difficult social circumstances. It is our personal, admittedly controversial, view that the pendulum of opinion against residential care has swung too far and that there are people with epilepsy, in their 20s, 30s and 40s whose quality of life would be better in residential care than it would be if they continued living at home, often with ageing parents (Thompson & Oxley 1988), or in inappropriate local facilities. In addition to a patient's medical and social factors, the need for long-term care in an epilepsy centre will depend to a large extent on the availability of suitable resources, such as supervised group homes, in the patient's locality. At present, admission to a residential centre should only occur after a detailed evaluation in a special centre for epilepsy, with optimization of medical treatment and careful consideration of psychological and social issues. The emphasis of residential care is not one of care and containment, but of aiming for rehabilitation towards each patient achieving their maximum potential, in a safe and caring environment.

EPILEPSY SURGERY

It is estimated that approximately 20–30% of the 30 000 people in the UK developing epilepsy each year will have seizures which remain uncontrolled by medical treatment (Goodridge & Shorvon 1983, Reynolds 1987). Some of these may have epilepsy which is amenable to surgery. The usual criteria for considering surgical options are that the patient has seizures which are of focal origin (i.e. partial or secondarily generalized seizures)

which have proved intractable to medical treatment, and which are sufficiently frequent and severe to interfere significantly with the patient's life. Elwes & Binnie (1990) estimated that approximately 7% of patients developing epilepsy would be suitable candidates for presurgical evaluation—on this basis, around 2000 people per year in the UK may be potential candidates for epilepsy surgery. To this number may be added an estimated 'backlog' of 20 000 or more people with established intractable epilepsy.

There are two basic means by which surgery can be used in the treatment of epilepsy. One of these is to resect the area of the brain in which the epileptic discharge arises. The other method is to prevent the spread of seizure discharges by procedures to interrupt the pathways by which the discharge is spread, such as corpus callosotomy and multiple sub-pial transections. The majority of operations currently undertaken for the relief of epilepsy fall into the first category, and the outcome with regard to seizure control may be very good. Examples of such operations are temporal lobectomy, amygdalohippocampectomy, frontal lobectomy, and, for children with intractable epilepsy and infantile hemiplegia, hemispherectomy. Provided stringent selection procedures are undertaken, such surgery may be highly effective in controlling seizures: a survey of active epilepsy surgery centres undertaken to investigate the outcome of surgery with respect to epileptic seizures found that, on average, 77.3% of patients were rendered seizure-free by hemispherectomy, 55.5% by anterior temporal lobectomy, and 43.2% by extratemporal resection. Follow-up ranged from 2 to 37 years, and serious side-effects occurred in less than 10% (Engel 1987).

The potential for relief of seizures following epilepsy surgery is considerable. At present, however, facilities for such surgery in this country are limited. An investigation was undertaken in 1989 to discover the extent of surgery undertaken for epilepsy in the UK, during which all members of the Society of British Neurological Surgeons working in the UK were asked about the nature and extent of any epilepsy surgery which they performed (Hart & Shorvon 1990). Surgical procedures undertaken for the treatment of large or expanding structural lesions, for which epilepsy was not the primary indication for treatment, were excluded. One hundred and twenty neurosurgeons were approached, of whom 85 (71%) replied. Twenty-eight (32% of those replying) performed surgery specifically for epilepsy, though five had not done so in the past year. To the investigators' knowledge, replies were received from all the major centres undertaking epilepsy surgery. Only 5 surgeons had performed more than five of any particular type of operation in the previous year. A total of 147 operations for the relief of epilepsy had been carried out in this year, and of these, 86 (59%) were carried out in these five centres. The operations performed were mainly temporal lobectomies (81), amygdalohippocampectomies (26), hemispherectomies (13), and corpus callosotomies (10).

The figures quoted above suggest that there is a considerable shortfall in the availability of epilepsy surgery in the UK. It is generally agreed that the degree of expertise and the specialist facilities required for successful epilepsy surgery demand that it be carried out in a relatively small number of highly specialized centres. If it is assumed that 2000 people per year become suitable for epilepsy surgery, 20 centres each performing 100 operations per year would be needed—far more than at present. (Even if more conservative figures for those requiring epilepsy surgery are taken, 5–10 centres are probably necessary.) Guidelines for the facilities available in such centres have been recommended (National Association of Epilepsy Centres 1990). A multidisciplinary team is essential, and should include a neurosurgeon with a particular interest and expertise in epilepsy surgery, a clinical neurophysiologist, a neurologist, a neuropsychologist, and the services of a psychiatrist with experience in this field, and of a paediatric neurologist. Available facilities should include CT scanning, MRI scanning, cerebral angiography, 24-hour EEG/videotelemetry, facilities for invasive EEG monitoring, neuropsychology (including carotid amytal testing), neuropathology, and routine laboratory facilities including serum drug concentration monitoring.

VOLUNTARY AGENCIES

Government reports have all recognized the role of voluntary agencies in the care of persons with epilepsy, and the importance of close liaison between these agencies and the medical profession, particularly at epilepsy clinics. Charitable bodies run the six residential epilepsy centres in the UK and have contributed greatly to the care of people with epilepsy, in a time of decreasing state support. This work needs to be continued and adapted to current requirements, with the provision of more rehabilitation and small group units. The National Society for Epilepsy, based at the Chalfont Centre for Epilepsy, has an active health education department producing educational material for patients, relatives and professionals, holds frequent study days and assists several community-based patient support groups. The British Epilepsy Association, based in Leeds, assists many local support groups, produces educational material and employs social and voluntary workers. There are also active epilepsy societies in Wales, Scotland and in Merseyside (see Appendix).

In the past, the voluntary agencies in the UK have, in contrast to the Epilepsy Foundation of America, and with other UK agencies such as the British Diabetic Association and the Multiple Sclerosis Society, kept a low public profile. There is no doubt that there is untapped potential for effective action by UK voluntary epilepsy agencies and future roles should include:

1. a comprehensive national network of local support and counselling groups for patients and their relatives
2. formation of pressure groups, at local and national levels, to push for improved epilepsy services
3. education of medical and paramedical professionals, employers and the public at large about epilepsy
4. fund-raising and sponsoring of research.

MEDICAL SERVICES FOR EPILEPSY IN OTHER COUNTRIES

United States

Medical care in the United States is fundamentally different from the UK in several respects:

1. care is not free at the point of service for the

majority of cases and upwards of 30 million people are not covered by health insurance

2. there is no comprehensive network of general practitioners and direct or self referral to specialists is the norm

3. there is a greater tendency to early and more complete specialization by doctors.

Many adults use hospital emergency rooms for primary care and referral of cases of epilepsy to a neurology consultant is largely automatic. In the case of children, primary care is almost entirely provided by paediatricians, who will commonly refer children with epilepsy to a neurologist or paediatric neurologist. There are many more neurologists per head of population (1/32 400 in 1987) than in the UK (Menken et al 1989), reflecting the fact that US neurologists provide considerably more 'neurological primary care' than do their British counterparts. Epileptology has become recognized as a subspecialty of neurology and a number of specialized epilepsy centres have become established. Recent guidelines by the National Association of Epilepsy Centers (1990) have recommended the services, personnel, facilities and patient referrals that are appropriate to different levels of centre. This document recommends that a primary care physician may institute treatment and refer to a general neurologist (secondary level) and that referral should be made to a tertiary-level epilepsy centre if seizure control is not achieved within 9 months. It is envisaged that tertiary-level epilepsy centres will be established in many University and large Community Hospitals and should provide medical, psychological and psycho-social facilities, with 8-hour video-EEG telemetry, CT, MRI and ready referral to a neurosurgical unit. Fourth-level medical epilepsy centres are envisaged to act as regional or national referral centres, serving several million people. These centres are recommended to have a greater number of specialized staff, and the ability to perform 24-hour video-telemetry, carotid amytal testing and to have a comprehensive rehabilitation programme and close links with an epilepsy surgery programme. Fourth-level surgical epilepsy centres would have the facilities to undertake complete presurgical evaluations, including invasive EEG monitoring, and should perform at least 25 cerebral resections for epilepsy a year, to ensure that skills are kept adequately honed (Gumnit 1990).

The Epilepsy Foundation of America is a vigorous voluntary organization which lobbies national and state governments, sponsors teaching and research, and has been very active in improving public awareness of epilepsy.

Denmark

Denmark has a population of 5.5 million and about 40 000 patients with epilepsy. The vast majority receive their care from neurological and paediatric outpatient departments in county and university hospitals, with only a small minority being cared for by their general practitioners. It has been recently estimated that epilepsy accounts for 50% of the work of a neurology clinic. There is one special assessment centre, at Dianalund, of 60 beds, to which about 500 patients are admitted each year for an average period of 28 days. In addition, there are 150 long-stay beds and admission to these is very rare. Video-EEG monitoring is available at three sites, and there is one surgical treatment programme. Health care in Denmark is organized and financed by individual counties and referral for care across county boundaries requires bureaucratic approval, frequently making it difficult for patients to obtain specialist care and second opinions.

Netherlands

The Netherlands has a population of 15 million, and has 407 neurologists, or 1/37 000 people, almost 10 times the availability of neurologists in the UK. Care of epilepsy is shared between general practitioners and specialists (mainly neurologists and paediatricians). There are also specialized epileptologists, a Chair of Epileptology at Nijmegan University, three special assessment centres, with associated long-term residential beds, and a comprehensive network of epilepsy clinics.

Federal Republic Germany

These data refer to the situation in what was, until October 1990, West Germany. The provision of epilepsy services in what was East

Germany is unclear at this time. Care for patients with epilepsy is divided into five strata:

1. general practitioner or private neurologist
2. neurology or paediatric clinic
3. epilepsy clinic
4. neurology or paediatric clinic with special expertise in epilepsy
5. special centre for epilepsy.

It is unclear how many patients with epilepsy are cared for by general practitioners. There are 92 epilepsy clinics and 11 neurological and paediatric clinics with special expertise in epilepsy, which take supraregional referrals. The latter have a full range of diagnostic and both medical and psychosocial therapeutic facilities and fulfil education, information and research roles. There are two special assessment centres and five epilepsy surgery programmes.

France

In France, nearly all patients with epilepsy are under the care of a general practitioner. Over 75% of patients are referred for specialist opinion, and if the epilepsy is controlled, returned to the care of their general practitioner. Specialized epilepsy clinics exist in university hospitals and there are four special centres. At present epilepsy surgery is carried out only in Paris and Bordeaux, but it is scheduled to commence in Rennes, Grenoble and Lyon, and is planned in 10 other cities.

ACKNOWLEDGEMENTS

We are most grateful to all those colleagues, in the UK, USA and Europe, who took the time and trouble to reply to our enquiries and questionnaires.

REFERENCES

Ajmone-Marsan C, Zivin L 1970 Factors related to the occurrence of typical paroxysmal abnormalities in the EEG records of epileptic patients. Epilepsia 11: 361–381

Central Health Services Council 1956 Report of the sub-committee on the medical care of epileptics. HMSO, London

Central Health Services Council 1969 People with epilepsy: report of a joint sub-committee of the standing medical advisory committee and the advisory committee of the health and welfare of handicapped persons. HMSO, London

Central Statistical Office 1990 Key Data, UK Social and Business Statistics. HMSO, London

Commission for the control of epilepsy and its consequences 1978 Plan for nationwide action on epilepsy, vols 1–4. DHJEW publication no. (NIH) 78-279. US Department of Health Education and Welfare, Bethesda, MD

Committee of enquiry into the education of handicapped children and young people 1978 Special educational needs. HMSO, London

Crawford P, Wilson S 1990 Epilepsy clinics: do they improve epilepsy management? Acta Neurologica Scandinavica 82(Suppl 133): 32

Department of Health, Medical Manpower and Education Division 1989 Medical and dental staffing prospects in the NHS in England and Wales in 1988. Health Trends 21: 99–106

Department of Health and Social Security 1986 Report of the working group on services for people with epilepsy: a report to the Department of Health and Social Security, the Department of Education and Science and the Welsh Office. HMSO, London

Department of Health and Social Security 1987 Health and Personal Social Services Statistics for England, 1987 edition. HMSO, London

Department of Health and Social Security, Medical

Manpower and Education Division 1988 Health Trends 20: 101–109

Elwes R, Binnie C 1990 Assessing outcome following epilepsy surgery. In: Chadwick D W (ed) Quality of life and quality of care of epilepsy. Royal Society of Medicine, London, p 106–115

Engel J 1987 Outcome with respect to epileptic seizures. In: Engel J (ed) Surgical treatment of the epilepsies. Raven Press, New York, p 553–571

Espir M L E, McCarthy M, Shorvon S D 1987 Survey of specialized hospital services for adults with epilepsy in North East Thames Region of the United Kingdom. Neuroepidemiology 6: 94–100

Franceschi M, Triulzi F, Ferini-Strombi L et al 1989 Focal cerebral lesions found by magnetic resonance imaging in cryptogenic non-refractory temporal lobe epilepsy patients. Epilepsia 30: 540–546

Goodman I 1983 Auditing care of epilepsy in a group practice. The Practitioner 227: 435–436

Goodridge D M G, Shorvon S D 1983 Epileptic seizures in a population of 6000. 1: Demography, diagnosis and role of the hospital services. 2: treatment and prognosis. British Medical Journal 287: 641–647

Gumnit R 1990 Standards for epilepsy surgery centres. In: Surgery for epilepsy. NIH Consensus Development Conference. National Institutes of Health, Bethesda, MD

Hart Y M, Shorvon S D 1990 Surgery for epilepsy in the United Kingdom. Acta Neurologica Scandinavica 82 (Suppl 133): 21

Hauser W A, Kurland L T 1975 The epidemiology of epilepsy in Rochester, Minnesota 1935 through 1967. Epilepsia 16: 1–66

Hopkins A, Scambler G 1977 How doctors deal with epilepsy. Lancet i: 183–186

Langton Hewer R, Wood V A 1990 Neurology services in the United Kingdom. A report of the Association of British Neurologists, London

Lesser R P, Modie M T Weinstein M A et al 1986

Magnetic resonance imaging (1.5 Tesla) in patients with intractable focal seizures. Archives of Neurology 46: 367–371

Lloyd-Jones A 1980 Medical audit of the care of patients with epilepsy in one group practice. Journal of Royal College of General Practitioners 30: 396–400

MacFarlane I 1990 Quality of life and quality of care: The experience from diabetes. In: Chadwick D W (ed) Quality of life and quality of care in epilepsy. Royal Society of Medicine, London, p 50–58

Menken M, Hopkins A, Murray T J, Vates T S 1989 The scope of neurologic practice and care in England, Canada, and the United States. Archives of Neurology 46: 210–213

Morgan J D, Kurtz Z 1987 Special services for people with epilepsy in the 1970s. HMSO, London

Morrow J 1990 An assessment of an epilepsy clinic. In: Chadwick D W(ed). Quality of life and quality of care in epilepsy. Royal Society of Medicine, London, p 96–105

Ministry of Health 1953 National Assistance Act 1948: Welfare of handicapped persons: the special welfare needs of epileptics and of spastics. Circular 26/53. London, Ministry of Health

National Association of Epilepsy Centers 1990 Recommended guidelines for diagnosis and treatment in specialized epilepsy centers. Epilepsia 31(supplement 1): 1–12

Office of Population Censuses and Surveys 1990 Population Trends 62: 2

Patsalos P, Sander J W A S, Oxley J, Lascelles P T 1987 Immediate anticonvulsive drug monitoring in management of epilepsy. Lancet ii: 39

Research Committee of the Royal College of General Practitioners 1960 A survey of the epilepsies in general practice. British Medical Journal 2: 416–422

Reynolds E H 1987 Early treatment and prognosis of epilepsy. Epilepsia 28: 97–106

Rodin E A 1968 The prognosis of patients with epilepsy. Thomas, Springfield, IL

Sander J W A S, Hart Y M, Johnson A L, Shorvon S D 1990 National General Practice Study of Epilepsy: newly diagnosed epileptic seizures in a general population. Lancet 336: 1267–1271

Theodore W T, Forwart R, Homes R, Porter R J, DiChiro G 1986 Neuroimaging in refractory partial seizures: comparison of PET, CT, and MRI. Neurology 36: 750–759

Thompson P J, Oxley J 1988 Socioeconomic accompaniments of severe epilepsy. Epilepsia 29(Suppl 1): S9–S18

Zivin L, Ajmone-Marsan C 1968 Incidence and prognostic significance of 'epileptiform' activity in the EEG of non-epileptic subjects. Brain 91: 751-758

APPENDIX

Assessment centres for epilepsy

Bootham Park Hospital
Bootham
York, YO3 7BY
Tel: 0904 54664

Chalfont Centre for Epilepsy
Chalfont St Peter
Buckinghamshire, SL9 0RJ
Tel: 024 07 3991

David Lewis Centre★
Alderley Edge
Mobberley
Cheshire, SK9 7UD
Tel: 056 587 2613

Maudsley Hospital—Epilepsy Unit ★
Denmark Hill
London, SE5 8AZ
Tel: 071 703 6333

Park Hospital for Children
Oxford, OX3 7LQ
Tel: 0865 245651

★ Not designated special assessment centres, but provide an assessment facility for people with epilepsy.

National voluntary organizations

British Epilepsy Association
Anstey House
40 Hanover Square
Leeds, LS3 1BE.
for membership enquiries
Tel: 0532 439393
for general information
Tel: 0345 089599
Regional offices:
London Tel: 071 929 4069
Belfast Tel: 0232 248414

Epilepsy Association of Scotland (Glasgow)
48 Gowan Road
Glasgow, G511JR
Tel: 041 427 4911

Epilepsy Association for Scotland (Edinburgh)
13 Guthrie Street
Edinburgh, EH11JG
Tel: 031 226 5458

Irish Epilepsy Association
249 Crumlin Road
Dublin, W12
Tel: 01 557500

National Society for Epilepsy
Chalfont Centre for Epilepsy
Chalfont St Peter
Buckinghamshire, SL9 0RJ
Tel: 024 07 3991

Wales Epilepsy Association
Gwynedd Voluntary Services Council
Eldon Square
Dolgellau
Gwynedd
Tel: 0341 422575

International League Against Epilepsy
Dr. Simon Shorvon
Honorary Secretary
ILAE British Branch
National Hospital for Neurology and
Neurosurgery
Queen Square
London, WC1N 3BG

Special schools for children with epilepsy

David Lewis Centre
Alderley Edge
Mobberley
Cheshire, SK9 7UD
Tel: 056 587 2613

Lingfield Hospital School
Lingfield
Surrey, RH7 6PN
Tel: 0342 832243

St Elizabeth's School
Much Hadham
Hertfordshire, SG10 6EW
Tel: 027 984 3451

23. Audit in epilepsy

J. I. Morrow   G. A. Baker

DEFINITION

Medical audit is a systematic critical analysis of the quality of medical care (HMSO 1989).

THE NEED FOR AUDIT

Prior to the 1930s doctors tended to rely on 'clinical impressions'; if a form of treatment appeared to benefit some patients then it was accepted. Most physicians are now, however, prepared to concede that clinical impressions can be seriously misleading.

By the 1950s, for medicines at least, the randomized controlled trial had been established as the only reliable way to assess the efficacy of a new treatment. No pharmaceutical product can now be marketed without substantial evidence of both efficacy and safety based on well conducted clinical trials. The same methods of assessment have gradually been applied to wider forms of therapy such as medical versus surgical treatment. In the 1960s the principal of cost benefit analysis was introduced by health economists. This form of analysis attempts to demonstrate whether clinically successful treatment can also pay off in economic terms. In applying health economics to medicine it is important to be able to measure input and outcome reliably and so achieve a measure of the efficiency of the system. However, a number of medical and social changes have been taking place over the past 10 years or so which have meant that traditional measures of the success of treatment are now outmoded and this may be particularly true in the measurement of success in treating epilepsy. These changes include the changing pattern of mortality, increasing unemployment rates and changing attitudes to sickness and ill health. In simple terms, to render a patient with epilepsy seizure-free—a highly successful medical outcome—does not automatically allow that individual to return to paid employment. Thus in the 1990s, by prolonging life yet not necessarily increasing productivity, successful therapy may in many cases actually reduce the average national wealth rather than increase it. It has therefore become recognized increasingly that it is well-being, as opposed to wealth, that is improved by reducing sickness. Official thinking has therefore moved away from measuring health as merely an absence of disease but rather it now concerns the whole person and his relationship with the society in which he lives. In the present climate of cost containment in health resources, it will become increasingly important to demonstrate quantifiable improvements in well-being in order to justify the costs incurred in achieving them. In this regard it is likely that traditional methods of measuring epilepsy control, based entirely on clinical parameters, will prove inadequate. It seems probable that alternative measures, which take account of the individual nature of the condition, including its effects on psychosocial well-being, will arise. These measures will have to be combined with other more widely applicable measures of quality of life so as to allow cross comparisons with other disorders.

All clinicians strive to achieve a good quality of care but it is recognized that the management of patients may differ and, therefore, it is likely that quality of care also differs. These differences in care may ultimately effect the quality of life of our patients. Medical audit is a fairly new concept to clinicians in the United Kingdom, its purpose is a systematic and critical analysis of the methods and of the quality of medical care. The aim of audit is to improve the overall quality of care.

Medical audit may be performed by different methods with at present perhaps the most frequently used being case note review. In the future and particularly when assessing quality of life, prospective programmes of audit may take precedence. The purpose of this chapter is to present and discuss some outcome measures that may prove useful in the medical audit of epilepsy.

ACCESS TO CARE

Before considering outcome measures relating to medical care the access to that care may be examined. On a national level, the accessibility to neurologists and the physicians, who primarily deal with adults with epilepsy, may be audited by calculating neurologist numbers and distribution against the number and distribution of people with epilepsy. On a local level, the number of clinics available, the distance from patient domicile to clinics and the waiting time from referral to consultation are accessible to audit. Patients who fail to attend result in inefficiency within the system. The number and perhaps reasons for failure to attend may be examined.

THE MEDICAL MANAGEMENT OF EPILEPSY—OUTCOME MEASURES

Seizure frequency

In the assessment of epilepsy the most commonly chosen outcome measure is seizure frequency and this is often the only measure used. In assessing epilepsy and the effect of medical or surgical treatment on its control it is the reduction in seizure frequency or the proportion of patients becoming seizure-free that are the usual endpoints (Van Belle & Temkin, 1981). Seizure frequency is an attractive endpoint because it is the seizure that is the basis of epilepsy, because it can be easily monitored, and can be expressed numerically so that statistical methods can be easily applied to it. There are, however, problems in adopting this simplistic approach. The first is that the diagnosis of epilepsy is not straightforward, and the recogni-

tion of some seizure types by patient and/or relative may be difficult. The second is that seizure frequency is naturally variable. The third and perhaps most fundamental reason to question seizure frequency taken in isolation as an adequate measure of well-being in epilepsy is that any seizure frequency worse than being completely seizure-free will have effects on physical, mental and social well-being and it is not known whether, and probably unlikely that, these effects are in direct proportion to seizure frequency, for example one seizure per year has the same result as regards the ability to drive as one seizure per day.

Seizure severity

In terms of assessing psychological and social well-being, previous research has demonstrated that patients' perception of the overall severity of their seizure disorder may be more important than seizure frequency in determining the psychosocial consequences of poorly controlled epilepsy (Arnston et al 1986). For instance, it is possible that antiepileptic drugs may have an influence on seizures by inhibiting seizure spread without necessarily reducing seizure frequency (Glaser 1980). Clearly there is a need for a more comprehensive assessment of the efficacy of different treatments.

Seizure frequency alone also becomes an inadequate measure when considering the fact that even a 75% reduction in seizure frequency may not be considered a therapeutic success if the patient is still disabled by the remaining seizures. Infrequent but severe seizures may be more disabling than frequent but less severe seizures. There is limited sensitivity when using seizure frequency in double blind placebo cross-over studies.

In recent years a number of studies have attempted to develop seizure severity scales, including physician based scales (Mattson & Cramer 1985, Duncan & Sander 1990) and a patient based scale (Baker et al 1991). There is, however, some disagreement about the relative merits of a physician or observer rated scale versus a patient based scale. It is probably correct to assume that an observer rated scale is more likely to be able to differentiate reliably between seizure types. There are, however, a number of good reasons for supporting a patient based scale. There is often little agreement between doctors and patients regarding the severity of their condition, and there is a wide variability between the assessment of different doctors and other health professionals (Slevin et al 1988). It is possible that clinicians may often underestimate the impact that the illness is having on the overall quality of life of the patient (Fallowfield 1990). Patient based scales may be more sensitive in detecting changes related to treatment. Other factors including affect, may contribute to a patient's perception of seizure severity and the effect of these influences is more likely to be accounted for in scales completed by the patient. It is difficult not to agree with a recent review of health measures that proposed that it is the patient, not the doctor or nurse, that should complete the appropriate rating scale (Fallowfield 1990).

Seizure severity scales have been criticized previously as being unscientific and unreliable (Van Belle & Temkin 1981). Despite this however, it is universally recognized that there is a need for such a scale to complement the often unsatisfactory traditional outcome measures.

Antiepileptic medication

A number of aspects of the therapy of epilepsy lend themselves to audit. These would include the type of drugs chosen, the number of drugs, their adverse effects, their cost, the use of serum concentrations and the potential for alternative treatments.

The choice of antiepileptic medication may be important for some seizure types, particularly for some primary generalized seizure types found most often in childhood or adolescence. In terms of efficacy, though, for the majority of adult seizures there do not appear to be substantial differences between the various drugs. Whichever drug is chosen, monotherapy is now the preferred practice in the treatment of epilepsy and this should be achieved in the majority of patients. A small number, however, may derive increased benefit from combinations of antiepileptic drugs and a smaller number still will be candidates for surgical treatment. It is important, therefore, to review continually the effects of treatment in individual cases.

All antiepileptic drugs have potential adverse effects and some of these effects may be severe. Studies have suggested that 16-40% of patients with epilepsy may experience adverse effects from their treatment (Beghi et al 1986), and efforts should be made to reduce this figure.

The measurement of drug concentrations in the serum is a potential method of monitoring antiepileptic drug therapy but is a technique that is often used too much and it is only generally useful if its limitations are appreciated. The potential benefit of on the spot drug concentrations over the usual batch method has been previously audited in one study (Patsolos et al 1987) but further studies in this area are required.

In times of cost-containment, awareness of the cost of individual antiepileptic drugs is increasing with, in general terms, the newer drugs being the more expensive. It is likely, therefore, that the choice and continued use of an antiepileptic drug in an individual patient will depend on achieving a balance between efficacy on the one hand and adverse effects on the other, with cost being measured against benefit in the analysis of larger groups.

Follow-up and continuity of care

The recent DHSS report produced by the working group on services for people with epilepsy (1986) recommended that general practitioners should normally refer all patients developing seizures to a consultant with an interest in epilepsy for diagnosis, initial assessment and recommendations for further management. For the majority of patients care could subsequently devolve back to the general practitioner.

In a recent community based study of people newly developing seizures, the National General Practice Study of Epilepsy (Hart et al 1990) found that 92% of the study population were referred to hospital for a consultant opinion. This high figure corresponds to earlier studies (Hopkins & Scambler 1977, Lloyd Jones 1980, Taylor 1987). However, in the National General Practice Study, only 40% of patients saw a neurologist or paediatric neurologist, suggesting, therefore, that whilst a high proportion of patients are indeed referred to hospital-based services, the pattern of these referrals may not be as the working party had originally envisaged.

Regarding the follow-up care of epilepsy, the DHSS report suggested that, for most patients, the follow-up care of epilepsy would be undertaken by the general practitioner with only the more severe cases needing continuing hospital treatment. Studies in this area have revealed a variable proportion of patients under continued hospital follow-up from 11% in Hopkins & Scambler's study (1977) to 58% in a study by White & Buckley (1981). Hopkins & Scambler also made the observation that follow-up was in many cases inappropriate and not related to patient need. Surveys have also pointed out a lack of continuity of supervision in hospital care, often follow-up being by a succession of junior hospital doctors. These areas all require to be included in the audit of the care of epilepsy

Information and counselling

The diagnosis of epilepsy carries with it many serious social, occupational and psychological consequences. It is generally considered good practice to discuss these with patients. The recent working party report (1986) has, however, criticized the amount of information that patients either receive or, at least, retain.

Perhaps the factor that patients find most difficult to accept is the loss of a driving licence. The guidelines in this instance are fairly specific, and allow a model for the examination of the imparting of information to patients. However, it is not known accurately how many patients with active epilepsy continue to drive, though undoubtedly many do, nor is it known that of those that do continue to drive, whether they do so because they have not been given the correct information or whether they have chosen to ignore it. The opposite situation probably also attains in that some patients do not drive because they believe they are banned when, in fact, they may do so legally.

People with epilepsy require counselling in a number of areas where their epilepsy may affect their lifestyle. Information on these important areas should be offered routinely and discussion encouraged. In a recent survey of patients

attending hospital-based services in Cardiff (Morrow 1990), patients were given a checklist of seven important areas and asked if they had received any advice or counselling in these areas. Just prior to the patients first attendance at a routine neurology clinic patients agreed they had already received advice about a mean of one item. Over the next 12 months follow-up there was no significant increase in this response rate.

Patient satisfaction

There is an increasing awareness of the importance of involving patients in the evaluation of the quality of medical care. The recent NHS Management inquiry was highly critical of the organization's response to consumer satisfaction. Despite this, however, there still remains some scepticism about the value of the patients' views (Fitzpatrick 1990).

Little attention has been paid to applying patient satisfaction to the evaluation of epilepsy services. The recent report on the evaluation of three specialized epilepsy centres did conclude that there was a need to evaluate these clinics on the basis of patient satisfaction (DHSS 1988).

Patient satisfaction has always been difficult to define in a meaningful way. This is partly due to the fact that it is not a unitary concept but is made up of several different dimensions. Hopkins (1990) has proposed that patient satisfaction includes: accessibility of care, technical aspects of care, interpersonal relationships with nurses and doctors, continuity of care, clarity of information received and the hotel services or surroundings in an outpatient clinic.

The difficulties of measuring patient satisfaction have been well documented (Fitzpatrick 1990). The result of numerous studies have suggested that satisfaction with care is related to patients' perception of its outcome and the extent to which it meets their expectations (Stimson & Webb 1975). The consumers' unquestioning respect for the professional and their clinical skills and judgements ensures that the patient is unlikely to be able to make an independent assessment of the services he has received.

The use of questionnaires that include global questions tend to elicit high levels of expressed satisfaction with care (Jacoby 1987). High ratings of satisfaction may, however, reflect a combination of low self esteem, low expectations and ignorance of alternatives and the view that the physician is a kind and caring person.

Questionnaires are also time consuming to produce because they are required to be developed both in terms of reliability and validity. Alternative methods of assessing patient satisfaction include informal taped interviews but these are considered to be expensive in terms of time and cost.

Most researchers in the field of patient satisfaction would conclude that when developing a patient satisfaction scale it is necessary to focus attention on the particular group of patients or clinic under study as they may have satisfactions or dissatisfaction particular to their group (Hopkins 1990).

Studies of consumer satisfaction with medical services is an important component in the evaluation of outcome. There is a need to develop patient satisfaction scales for epilepsy services that are both reliable and valid, and will ultimately contribute to the overall assessment of the services provided.

Psychological aspects of epilepsy

The psychological and emotional problems encountered by patients with epilepsy have been well documented in terms of the frequency of seizures, the reaction of other people and society's attitude towards people with epilepsy (Dodrill et al 1983). The most significant factor may be the individual's concept of himself and his disorder (Masland 1988). It is often the unpredictability and the severity of the seizure and not necessarily the frequency that leads to the individual's sense of loss of control. An individual's loss of sense of control may have serious physiological and psychological consequences, including feelings of helplessness, depression, anxiety and low self-esteem (Garber & Seligman 1980, Betts 1988). Clearly self efficacy (Bandura 1989) is an important factor in the psychological functioning of people with epilepsy.

Traditionally, when assessing the control of epilepsy the seizure frequency is often the only factor taken into account by clinicians in clinical

trials (Van Belle & Temkin 1981). The success of surgical treatment for epilepsy is usually determined by the proportion of patients becoming seizure free although other variables including social adjustment (Bruton 1988) and psychological status (Rausch & Crandell 1982) have been taken into account.

A number of studies of unselected patients have demonstrated an increased incidence of psychological and psychiatric illness in patients with epilepsy. It is having epilepsy rather than a chronic disorder per se that is associated with psychopathology (Trimble 1989). Other factors including social isolation, real and perceived stigmatization also contribute to the psychological well-being of patients with epilepsy. Further, the long-term use of antiepileptic medication can be associated with affective disorders, irritability and instability of mood (Trimble 1989).

To treat epilepsy only in terms of seizure reduction is therefore inadequate and the disorder cannot be managed without reference to associated psychological disorders (Aird et al 1984). The most common of these are probably anxiety and depression (Betts 1988), often causing a degree of social disability disproportionate to seizure frequency (Gillham 1990). It is clear that existing services for patients with epilepsy have often failed to meet their psychological needs. A DHSS report (1986) recommended the establishment of specialized epilepsy clinics to meet the medical, social and psychological needs of patients through a multidisciplinary approach (Thompson & Oxley 1988). It is clear that failure to provide services to meet such needs may be detrimental to the patients overall quality of life.

Social aspects of epilepsy

The complexity of problems produced as a result of having epilepsy need to be understood in terms of the interaction of the psychological, social, and physical well-being of the patient. It is therefore clear that in the provision of clinical services a more comprehensive analysis is required in terms of social and psychological studies as well as neurological evaluation (Masland 1988).

Having epilepsy is more than coping with a medical diagnosis. It can influence many aspects of an individual's life. In recent years there has been evidence of an increasing awareness of the social dimensions of this disorder and their importance to the medical and other health professionals. Investigators have reported a wide range of social difficulties which are more frequently to be found in patients with poorly controlled seizures, multiple seizure types or associated problems. It seems reasonable to investigate these difficulties further to enable the more effective planning of services, thus helping to reduce their impact on the patient's overall quality of life. A recent review has suggested that factors such as unemployment, inability to drive and lack of social skills, pose a greater problem than the seizures themselves (Thompson & Oxley 1988). The impact of epilepsy on social functioning is, however, complex and involves the contribution of many factors ranging from the patient's coping strategies to the attitudes and behaviour of potential employers. Psychological adjustment, for example, can influence job seeking, as frequent job rejections may result in depression and low self esteem. There is also the importance of individual coping skills in meeting the demands of the employer, the attitudes of colleagues, and real or perceived stigma (Mitten 1986). Other problems lie with employers' knowledge and perceptions of epilepsy (Scambler 1990). Expectations and attitudes of the individuals and their respective employers may also need to be readjusted (Thompson & Oxley 1988).

Other areas of social functioning may also be affected, including the inability to form social relationships. It is therefore important to recognize that patients may need services other than those traditionally provided. Recent research has suggested that patients may benefit from the provision of an educational and counselling service for both patients and their families. Such counselling may help reduce the possibility of over-dependence, and encourage independence (Aird et al 1984). Patients who cannot ultimately benefit from such an intervention could alternatively be supported by locally organized Epilepsy Associations. It is apparent that there is a need to establish specialized clinics to meet the additional psychological and social needs of patients with epilepsy (Richens 1988). Opportunities need to

be created to help patients fulfil their individual potential, and thereby maximizing their overall quality of life. In terms of assessing the provision of services there is a need to understand to what degree existing services provided affect the social well-being of patients with epilepsy, if at all.

Financial considerations

The financial costs of an illness to the individual are related principally to the difficulty in obtaining paid employment commensurate with ability. In the most recent survey, a government commissioned report from the Office of Population Censuses and Surveys (1988), it was found that disabled people, below pensionable age, had lower incomes than the general population, because they were much less likely to be employed. The report stated that three-quarters of the 6.2 million disabled adults living in Britain were relying on state benefits as their main source of income. Of those reliant on benefits two-thirds said that they were only just getting by or had financial difficulties. Even when disabled people worked they earned significantly less than non-disabled people. Of those under pensionable age, 41% had incomes less than half the equivalent for the population as a whole. The average income for all disabled adults and their families excluding housing benefit, was £82.20 per week. Disabled people also had to spend more to cover their extra needs. They spent an average of £6.10 per week extra because of their disability.

Epilepsy falls into the category of disability and similar figures may be obtained from this diagnosis in isolation as for disability in general. Surveys in epilepsy have, however, been heterogeneous using different definitions of employment and different study groups. In an attempt to define unemployment rates, a survey of all patients referred to a teaching hospital in one calendar year, in whom the reason for referral was epilepsy or suspected epilepsy, was performed. In all, 279 patients were interviewed at their first outpatient attendance. Of these, 247 were in the employment years between 16 and 65 years. Ninety-three (37.7%) were available for work but were unemployed. Excluding patients with a serious physical or mental handicap (n = 25), which may have contributed to their inability to work, there remained 68 (30.6%) in whom epilepsy was the principal or sole disability, and who were unemployed. In the hospital catchment area 19 185 people were registered as unemployed (figures from Department of Employment) in a population aged 16–65 years of 172 400 (figures from the 1984 Census) giving a crude local unemployment rate of 11.1%. Thus the unemployment rate for the patients was 2–3 times that of the local population.

Accepting that community-based studies may give a more accurate reflection of true unemployment rates but given that the majority of people with epilepsy will be referred to hospital at some time (Hart et al 1990) these figures provide some evidence that those with epilepsy are seriously disadvantaged in employment and are in broad agreement with previous studies (Office of Health Economics 1971, Scambler & Hopkins 1980).

The social services will have to provide for the shortfall in earned income. The high rate of unemployment among those with epilepsy, and even for those in work the tendency to attract lower wages than the general population, means that for many income must be supplemented or provided completely by the state. Most may qualify for unemployment, supplementary and/or housing benefit. Those with severe epilepsy may receive an Attendance Allowance. In the most severe degrees of epilepsy, the Severe Disability Allowance may be payable. A carer may claim an Invalid Care Allowance and occasionally a Mobility Allowance may also be awarded, although this is rarely awarded to people with epilepsy unless there is an associated physical disability.

Epilepsy remains a common condition with a prevalence rate of about 0.5%. The medical supervision in the majority of cases is provided by the general practitioner but in some cases it will be provided through hospital based services. Medical supervision and investigation is expensive and, in the UK, borne by the state. Drugs for epilepsy require to be given on a daily basis and for a minimum of 2 years, with in many cases treatment being life-long. People with epilepsy qualify for free prescriptions and therefore once again the state will bear the cost. As an example of this cost in drug therapy alone: carbamazepine was the most frequently prescribed antiepileptic drug in 1987 with 1 220 500 prescriptions (Morrow & Routledge; 1989). Taking all these prescriptions to be for Tegretol, rather than for the generic forms, and for an average of just 600 mg daily with each prescription to cover only a 2-month period, the total annual cost for this one drug alone was approximately £10 million in 1987. If the average daily dose was larger and/or the time covered by the prescription longer then the cost will be higher, though the increasing use of generic formulations may help to reduce it.

For those with more severe degrees of epilepsy, drug monitoring, detailed investigation and the possibility of surgical treatment need to be considered, all of which are much more expensive. Most expensive of all is the provision of long-term residential care for those with chronic and intractable epilepsy. Cost comparisons have been made between different forms of care. Kriedal (1980) performed a cost benefit analysis of specialized epilepsy clinics. By calculating the efficacy of such clinics with reference to a health status index he demonstrated a clear advantage of the epilepsy clinics over existing services. In another direct comparison between an existing service and the specialist clinic, this time in a randomized controlled trial, increased benefit and patient satisfaction was demonstrated and the costs of the two methods of care were calculated and compared (Morrow 1980).

In the present financial climate accurate cost benefit analysis is likely to prove important to any medical audit. The immediate direct costs of any form of care should be relatively easy to calculate. However, because of the chronic nature of epilepsy, any savings produced by an improvement in well-being are likely to be in the longer term and may well prove more of a challenge to assess accurately.

SUMMARY

In the 1980s, it was possible to make a convincing case for the importance of auditing health and well-being. However, the methods to do so are still largely uncertain and in the 1990s we are likely to see a continuation of the philosophy with an increasing refinement of measures used in assessment. A number of aspects of the management of epilepsy from the accessibility of care to measuring clinical outcomes are probably already available. The measurement of the inter-related social and psychological aspects of the condition and the overall quality of life of our patients with epilepsy will provide the next logical step in the development of clinical audit. As experience grows, accurate auditing techniques using agreed outcome measures are likely to arise. The in-

creased provision of information technology and the increasing importance of resource management should allow for reliable cost benefit analysis. In the future, therefore, comparisons between different forms of management of epilepsy and comparisons between the management of epilepsy and the management of other conditions should ultimately improve the quality of medical services.

REFERENCES

Aird R B, Masland R L, Woodbury D M 1984 The epilepsies: A critical review. Raven Press, New York.

Arnston P, Droge D, Norton R, Murray E 1986 The perceived psychosocial consequences of having epilepsy. In: Whitman S, Hermann B (eds) Psychopathology in epilepsy: social dimensions. Oxford University Press, Oxford, p 143–161

Baker G A, Smith D F, Dewey M, Morrow J, Crawford P M, Chadwick D W 1991 The development of a seizure severity scale as an outcome measure in Epilepsy Research 8: 245–251

Bandura A 1989 Perceived self efficiency in the exercise of personal agency. The Psychologist. The Bulletin of The British Psychological Society 2(10): 411–424

Beghi E, Di Mascio R, Tognoni G 1986 Adverse effects of anticonvulsant drugs. A critical review. Adverse Drug Reactions and Acute Poisoning Review 2: 63–86

Betts T A 1988 Neuropsychiatry. In: Laidlaw J, Richens A, Oxley J (eds) A textbook of epilepsy, 3rd edn. Churchill Livingstone, Edinburgh, p 350–385

Bruton C J 1988 Conclusions: assessments of clinico-pathological results. In: Russell G, Marley E (eds) The Neuropathology of temporal lobe epilepsy. Oxford University Press, Oxford, p 82–85

Department of Health and Social Security working group (Chairman Miss P M C Witherton) 1986 Report of the working group on services for people with epilepsy: a report of the Department of Health and Social Security, the Department of Education and the Department of Science and the Welsh Office. HSMO, London

Doddrill C B, Batzel L, Queisser H R, Temkin N R 1980 An objective method for the assessment of psychological and social problems among epileptics. Epilepsia 21: 123–135

Duncan J S, Sander J W A S 1990 The Chalfont seizure severity scale, Acta Neurologica Scandinavica 82(Suppl): 31

Fallowfield F 1990 The quality of life; the missing measurement in health care. Souvenir Press, London

Fitzpatrick R 1990 Measurement of patient satisfaction. In: Hopkins A, Costain D (eds) Measuring the outcomes of medical care. Royal College of Physicians, London

Garber J, Seligman M (eds) 1980 Human helplessness: theory and applications. Academic Press, New York

Gillham R 1990 Refractory epilepsy: An evaluation of psychological methods in out-patient management. Epilepsia 31: 427–432

Glaser G H 1980 Mechanisms of antiepileptic drug action: clinical indicators. In: Glaser G H, Penry J K, Woodbury D M (eds) Antiepileptic drugs: mechanism of action. Raven Press, New York, p 11–20

HSMO 1989 Working for patients. Paper 6. HMSO, London

Hart Y, Sander J W A, Johnson A L, Shorvon S D 1990 The National General Practice Study of Epilepsy (Unpublished data).

Hopkins A, Scambler G 1977 How doctors deal with epilepsy. Lancet 1: 183–186

Jacoby A 1987 Women's preferences for and satisfaction with the current procedures in childbirth. Midwifery 3: 117–124

Kriedal T 1980 Cost-benefit analysis of epilepsy clinics. Social Science and Medicine 14C: 35–41

Lloyd Jones A 1980 Medical audit of the care of patients with epilepsy in one group practice. Journal of the Royal College of General Practitioners 30: 396–400

Masland R L 1988 Psychosocial aspects of epilepsy. In: Porter R J, Morselli P L (eds) The epilepsies. Butterworths, London, p 356–377

Mattson R H, Cramer J A 1981 A seizure frequency and severity rating system. Epilepsia 22: 241–242

Mitten R J 1986 Fear of seizures. In: Whitman S, Herman B P (eds) Psychopathology in epilepsy: social dimensions. Oxford University Press, New York, p 90–121

Morrow J I 1990 An assessment for an epilepsy clinic. Royal Society of Medicine Round Table Series 23: 96–105

Morrow J I, Routledge P A 1989 Poisoning with anticonvulsants. Adverse Drug Reactions and Acute Poisoning Review 8: 97–109

Office of Health Economics 1971 Epilepsy in society. Office of Health Economics, London.

Patsalos P N, Sander J W A, Oxley J, Lascelles P T 1987 Immediate anticonvulsant drug monitoring in management of epilepsy. Lancet 2: 39

Rausch R, Crandale P H 1982 Psychological status related to control of temporal lobe seizures. Epilepsia 23: 191–202

Report of the working group on services for people with epilepsy 1986 HMSO, London

Richens A 1988 Epilepsy clinics. A specialist service for families. In: Epilepsy and the family. Sanofi UK Ltd, Manchester, p 39–43

Scambler G, Hopkins A P 1980 Social class, epileptic activity and disadvantage at work. Journal of Epidemiology and Community Health 34: 129–133

Slevin M I, Plant H, Lynch D et al 1988 Who should measure quality of life, the doctor or patient? British Journal of Cancer 57: 109–112

Stimson G, Webb B 1975 On going to see the doctor. Routledge and Keegan Paul, London

Taylor M P 1987 Epilepsy in a Doncaster practice: audit and change over eight years. Journal of the Royal College of General Practitioners 37: 116–119

Thompson P J, Oxley J 1988 Socio-economic

accompaniments of severe epilepsy. Epilepsia 29(suppl 1): S9–S18

Trimble M R 1987 Anticonvulsant drugs: mood and cognitive function. In: Epilepsy, behaviour and cognitive function. John Wiley, Chichester

Trimble M R 1989 Chronic epilepsy, its prognosis and management. John Wiley, Chichester

Van Belle G, Temkin N 1981 Design strategies in the clinical evaluation of new antiepileptic drugs. In: Pedley T A, Meldrum B S (eds) Recent advances in epilepsy, 1. Churchill Livingstone, Edinburgh, p 93–111

White P T, Buckley E G 1981 The management of epilepsy— an audit of two practices. Health Bulletin (Edinburgh) 39: 82–83.

24. Coping with epilepsy

G. Scambler

INTRODUCTION

The question, 'How do people cope with epilepsy?', is a good deal more complex than it may appear for several reasons. Firstly, the medical concept of epilepsy subsumes a bewildering variety of symptoms and events in the lives of those individuals affected by it. One individual's epilepsy might consist only of occasional fleeting lapses of consciousness, over in seconds and generally not disruptive of relationships or milieux; while another person's epilepsy might entail regular blackouts, accompanied by thrashing limbs, frothing at the mouth and incontinence, which frequently intrude upon and curtail personal and social freedoms and opportunities. The equivalence between the two is in the diagnostic label only, important though that may be.

A second and related source of complexity is the dearth of research on coping with epilepsy using general or specific measures of quality of life. Research on quality of life in epilepsy is as yet in its infancy, although pilot work is underway and more is planned (Chadwick 1990). One of the few studies so far reported found that people's perceptions of themselves and their epilepsy were the variables most strongly related to overall well-being, while seizure frequency, time since diagnosis, a diagnosis of absence seizures, and being in full-time employment also seemed significant (Collings 1990). The relative paucity of studies on how epilepsy affects quality of life—when compared with work on some other chronic conditions, like diabetes—is perhaps understandable given the nature of epilepsy, namely, its strikingly varied and intermittent symptomatology and general unpredictability, with or without treatment.

Thirdly, the research that has been done on coping with epilepsy is largely ad hoc and specialized: it derives from discrete disciplines, or even sub-disciplines, and is only rarely genuinely multidisciplinary. Most extant studies bear the stamp either of biomedicine or of epidemiology or of psychology or of sociology. It is to be hoped that volumes like the present one, which collate material from a range of medical, behavioural and social sciences, will prompt more multidisciplinary endeavours.

The strategy in this chapter will be firstly, to establish a credible framework for considering coping in relation to epilepsy; secondly to explore coping in the context of a number of key arenas of life activity; and thirdly, to discuss the implications of the published research literature for the care afforded to people with epilepsy by health professionals.

DIMENSIONS OF COPING

The psychological literature is rich in definitions of coping and no attempt will be made to review them here. Instead, analytic distinctions will be drawn between five dimensions of coping. It is not being claimed that these distinctions define the concept of coping, merely that empirical investigations suggest they are especially pertinent when considering the circumstances of people with epilepsy. The five dimensions will be termed: accommodation, rationalization, conception of self, sociability, and fulfilment. Each will be considered briefly in turn.

Accommodation

Accommodation refers here to an individual's

reaction to the physical properties of epilepsy—most notably recurrent seizures—plus the iatrogenic effects of antiepileptic drugs or other forms of therapeutic intervention. There is evidence, for example, that many people fear seizures, not merely because they are intrinsically unpleasant to experience but because they are associated with dying. Mittan & Locke (1982) found widespread fears of seizures among a sample of American patients. Approximately 70% said they were afraid they might die during the next seizures; 46% reported living in perpetual dread of seizures; and 35% believed that death from seizures was common. Mittan (1986) has postulated a causal connection between such fears and psychopathology. Accommodation is sometimes required also to underlying pathology giving rise to epilepsy, as well as to investigative tests and to the occasionally marked side-effects of medication.

Rationalization

Rationalization denotes the process of making sense of one's epilepsy. In her general study of disability, Blaxter (1976) found that individuals made persistent efforts to see their medical history as a whole, to arrive at a coherent interpretation of what had happened to them and why. They displayed a deep need to make sense of their worlds. It is this 'strain towards rationality', as Blaxter describes it, that is here termed rationalization. Rationalization is directed at solving 'cognitive problems' (Locker 1983). There is some evidence that people with epilepsy are especially concerned to understand the cause of their seizures, and that they frequently generate their own theories if none are forthcoming from their physicians (Scambler 1989).

Conception of self

Conception of self refers to a person's sense of self-worth or self-esteem. Rejecting narrow medical views of suffering, Charmaz (1983) uses a broader concept to show how the suffering associated with chronic illnesses often leads to what she calls a 'loss of self' 'Chronically ill persons frequently experience a crumbling away of their former self-images without simultaneous develop-

ment of equally valued new ones . . . Over time, accumulated loss of formerly sustaining self-images without new ones results in a diminished self-concept'. People with epilepsy can experience such a loss of self, a loss which may be explicable in terms of the stigma still linked in many minds with epilepsy and its manifestations.

Sociability

Sociability is the term used here to represent the quality and extent of the relationships negotiated by the individual with epilepsy with significant others, from family, kin and close friends to more distant—but important—figures like employers and state and local bureaucrats. Clearly epilepsy can impede the formation of good relationships, although it need not. There is substantial evidence, in fact, that people commonly opt to conceal their epilepsy whenever possible in an attempt to pass as normal (Goffman 1968). This is a strategy which can be successful but entails a constant fear of exposure and subsequent role-strain and disadvantage.

Fulfilment

Fulfilment refers to an individual's sense of achievement, which may be expressed in relation to any of many social roles and contexts. Given the ubiquity of the work ethic in occidental societies, people with epilepsy are unexceptional in looking for fulfilment especially in the intrinsic and extrinsic rewards of employment. As the authors of the Reid Report on epilepsy stated in 1969: 'Now that gainful employment is customary for all men, for single and widowed women, and often for married women, it determines the way of life, social and financial status, and the role in society; and it is a source of personal satisfaction, of social companionship, of esteem, of discipline and of purpose' (Central Health Services Council 1969). But fulfilment can of course be sought successfully or unsuccessfully in many other ways in personal or social life. In some, epilepsy may constitute an obstacle.

It will be the object of this chapter to elaborate further on these five dimensions of coping in some of the main arenas or aspects of life activity.

Table 24.1 Dimensions of coping and arenas of life activity

Dimensions of coping	Arenas of life activity
Accommodation	Lay culture
Rationalization	Professional care
Concept of self	Personal identity
Sociability	Family and networks
Fulfilment	Employment opportunities
	Legal constraint

ARENAS OF LIFE ACTIVITY

As with dimensions of coping, an empirically-based typology of key arenas of life activity will be ventured here and used to structure discussion. The arenas are: lay culture, professional care, personal identity, family and networks, employment opportunities, and legal constraint. Table 24.1 summarizes the dimensions of coping and the arenas of life activity differentiated in this chapter.

Lay culture

Adults who develop epilepsy, or the parents of children who do so, are likely to have encountered the word epilepsy before and may well be aware of having witnessed an epileptic seizure (Scambler 1987). It is much less likely, however, that epilepsy will have had any real salience for them. It is when the diagnosis is applied to them, or to their child, that any cultural connotations the word may have for them will come to the fore and into play. It is relevant to ask, therefore, what these connotations are likely to be and what is known of their impact.

The study of epilepsy in lay culture appears to indicate a substantial de-mythologization of epilepsy in the post-war years in both Europe and the USA (Caveness & Gallup 1980, Canger & Cornaggia 1985). Typically people surveyed demonstrate an enhanced and credible understanding of what epilepsy is, and proffer a more sympathetic and accepting attitude towards sufferers than was the case a generation ago. It would be incautious and imprudent to infer on the basis of these putative trends, however, that the stigma traditionally associated with epilepsy is a thing of the past. What people say in surveys is not always a good predictor of how they will behave. Moreover, there are as yet no convincing empiri-

cal assessments either in Europe or the USA of rates of lay discrimination against those with epilepsy (Scambler 1989).

What is clear is that people are extremely sensitive and alert to the negative connotations of epilepsy when the diagnosis is applied to them or to their kin. One study reported that in only 20% of cases had the possibility of a diagnosis of epilepsy been anticipated. In the same study it was found that a few, 5%, received the news with equanimity, but this was mostly because they had not encountered the word before (Scambler 1989). For almost all those personally confronted with a diagnosis of epilepsy—in Britain and the USA at least—the label undoubtedly conjured up distressing images of fits, stigma and ostracism (Scambler & Hopkins 1986, Scambler 1989, West 1985, Schneider & Conrad 1983). Somehow, it seems, ordinary people, who display a reasonable knowledge of epileptic phenomena and empathy with sufferers when responding to questionnaire items, adopt an altogether different and grimmer outlook when physicians attach the diagnostic label to them or to their offspring.

It is important to emphasize the point that what people with epilepsy and their families hear about epilepsy out of the background noise of lay culture leads them to a profoundly negative view of what it is to be epileptic. Whatever the rate of de-mythologization of epilepsy in lay culture, it is clear that some of the stigma with which it has traditionally been imbued remains.

Professional care

A number of parents in one British study of children with epilepsy complained that the diagnosis was disclosed much later in their child's career than was reasonable (West 1979). In their study of adults with epilepsy in the USA, Schneider & Conrad (1983) reported that only 35% recalled a short gap between a first, unanticipated seizure and learning of the medical diagnosis of epilepsy. Also, in Scambler and Hopkins' (1988) study, lengthy delays were recorded: 48% said they learned of the diagnosis a year or more after the onset of seizures. It is difficult to exaggerate the significance of the moment of communication of the diagnosis by a physician, whether it be to the parent of a child with epilepsy or direct to an adult. Communication of the diagnosis of epilepsy by a physician confers the social (and legal) status of 'epileptic' on the diagnosed. It transforms a 'person' into an 'epileptic' (Scambler & Hopkins 1986).

Medical diagnoses, Schneider & Conrad (1981) point out, are realities with which people so designated must contend independently of the physiological aspects of their conditions. Further, as seen in the discussion of lay culture, the reality of a diagnosis of epilepsy conjures up predominantly negative images in the minds of sufferers and their families. The diagnosis is bad news beyond the probability of recurrent seizures. Typically, it marks the beginning of a disgruntled, protracted, sometimes life-long, process of adjustment to being epileptic.

The disgruntlement is often directed initially at the physician responsible for making and passing on the diagnosis. Indeed, some patients contest the attribution of a medical diagnosis of epilepsy because accepting it is perceived as entailing living and coming to terms with the epilepsy of lay culture (Scambler & Hopkins 1986). Thus:

I rather objected to having this label attached to my records from there on, and, it's probably dead ignorant on my part, but I objected to having this little stamp on my records labelling me as 'an epileptic' on what to me was just . . . I had fainted once, and then I fainted a year later a second time, and, as I said, I've got plenty of friends who faint occasionally but don't have this label attached to them. The general—not so much myself now, because I've found out a bit more about it—but the general public are still very ill-informed about epilepsy; I think they think there's some sort of demon going on . . . they're badly informed on epilepsy and they think you're something of a bit of a freak. I objected very much to the label originally (Scambler 1989).

If, following Shibutani (1962), reference groups are defined in terms of perspectives, then lay culture and the medical subculture provide patients with their two key reference groups for interpreting their epilepsy.

The significance of these two reference groups for patients' concepts of self will be discussed in the section on personal identity. But the physician's role is not of course limited to making and applying diagnoses. Physicians can exercise con-

siderable influence, for example, on accommodation. As the following brief accounts from people aware of their seizures testify, seizures can be disturbing, even frightening, to experience:

You get a warning, then panic sets in because you know what's going to happen . . . . It seems to take a long time, but obviously it's only a few seconds. But they're the worst seconds, when you know you're going to go and there's nothing you can do.

I used to get a peculiar taste in the mouth and a sort of ringing in the ears . . . and I used to feel weak; and then I'd fall down. I didn't shake. I didn't appear to be having a fit. I just appeared to pass out, although I never lost consciousness.

Well, I know I'm going to get one, just a few seconds before, and I sit down. I gulp, I can feel myself swallowing all the time; and the first thing I think is: 'Where am I? What day is it?' and 'What am I doing here?' And although I'm going through this funny thing, I'm aware of it. I think: 'Oh no, I've got one of these things coming on me!' and then, all of a sudden, I snap out of it and I feel tired and drowsy.

I had this numbness in my left arm and side: it was almost like a stroke—even my face was, sort of, half-dropped. It was a most peculiar thing. And I could feel this twitching, like an electric shock, in my left arm, and then I lost consciousness.

Well, all I know is, I come over a bit sweaty, then I start—it's like a cough; and then all of a sudden my hands start getting tight, but there's no feeling in them, they're numb; but I know—I can see them—they're shaking.

You know you're not able to cope with whoever's talking to you. And yet you still look normal, you know? You don't look ill, so they'll get you a drink of water; you just look the same. And if they're waiting for an answer, you know they are, and you can't think to speak. I always used to say: 'I'll try and have a line ready that I could say each time, like: "Excuse me, I don't feel well". But it never, ever happens that you do it. It's a horrible feeling, because people are looking and you and you can feel them waiting . . . I mean it must look terribly stupid to someone . . . You work yourself up to a pitch in those few seconds, trying to make your brain work. You never can but you do it automatically (Scambler, 1989).

Successful accommodation is likely to be facilitated by effective curative or, more probably, palliative medical interventions, aiming to reduce seizure frequency with minimal treatment. Pertinent too is therapy for possible psychological or psychiatric sequelae of epilepsy, or medication or psycho-social factors (Hermann & Whitman 1986).

Perhaps even more significantly, successful accommodation may also be a function of good communication between physician and patient: the widespread patient association of seizures with dying, for example, could be substantially relieved if acknowledged and discussed. Unfortunately, there is evidence that physician-patient communication is characterized too rarely by frank and open discussion as between equals. This issue is addressed in some detail below.

The physician's role in relation to rationalization, or the pursuit of cognitive order, is equally important, and even more contingent on good communication. Williams (1984) has argued that what he calls the narrative reconstruction prompted by chronic illness often focuses on causation. Scambler (1989) asked his group which questions they would most like answered by a physician, and by far the most related to aetiology. Typical comments were:

I know I've got epilepsy, but I don't know what it's all about. I don't know what causes it.

If I could understand the cause of it, then I could put everything together . . . but no one has told me what's the cause of it.

I did say to him: 'Why do I get these?' . . . and I said: 'Why is it me? Why do I have to have them?' I said this one day, and he said: 'There's so many thousands of people that have them, and there's so many different kinds'. He said: 'I just couldn't tell you'.

What's it in aid of? I've done no harm to anybody. (Scambler 1989).

Interestingly, none of those in this study who had been offered a medical theory of aetiology either challenged or complemented it with their own lay theories. In the absence of a medical theory, however, 60% ventured their own. Consistently with Tavriger's (1966) earlier study of parents of children with epilepsy, the most popular centred on protracted stress. Tavriger (1966) hypothesizes that a lay theory, or—to use her term—fantasy, may be an attempt to deny that the child has epilepsy, because the parents' fears of what this means have not been dealt with. There is a degree

of support for this hypothesis in West's (1979) study of families of children with epilepsy. What is clear is that people need to make sense of epileptic phenomena, and that this need will almost certainly be satisfied without, if not satisfied with, physicians' inputs.

Personal identity

If authoritative medical diagnosis of epilepsy conjures up negative images—present, salient and learned in lay culture—how do these images impinge on sufferers? What is the nature of the link between 'social labelling' and 'self-labelling' (Rotenberg 1974). Most, if not all, studies use the concept of stigma when analysing the patient's altered concept of self. Goffman (1968) has suggested that people who possess a particular stigma tend to have 'similar learning experiences regarding their plight, and similar changes in conception of self—a similar moral career that is both cause and effect of commitment to a similar sequence of personal adjustments'. Consistently with this suggestion, Scambler (1984) discerns a pattern in the changed self-perceptions of those with epilepsy.

Stebbins (1970) has argued that the way individuals interpret events and happenings—past, present and future—associated with a particular identity often evolves into a special view of the world. Whenever this identity becomes salient to them, their special view of the world predisposes them to a patterned response. Scambler & Hopkins (1986) argue that typically adults with epilepsy possess a special view of the world. At the core of this special view of the world is a sense of stigma.

Scambler & Hopkins (1986) distinguish between 'enacted' and 'felt stigma'. Enacted stigma refers to episodes of discrimination against people solely on the grounds of their social and cultural unacceptability. (This definition is designed to exclude instances of discrimination widely decreed to be reasonable, like driving bans, which are considered below.) Felt stigma has two referents. The first is the shame associated with being epileptic. The authors suggest that this derives less from any sense of moral culpability than from an often unarticulated feeling that epilepsy is evidence of imperfection, of a spoiled identity or being (Goffman 1968). Epilepsy, it seems, may be interpreted as an ontological deficit rather than a moral one (Scambler 1984). The second and perhaps more significant referent is, simply, a fear of meeting with enacted stigma.

Drawing on this distinction, a model, termed the 'hidden distress model' by Scambler (1989), has been constructed. This can be epitomized in three statements:

1. When a physician communicates the diagnosis of epilepsy to them, people quickly learn to see the status of 'epileptic' as a social and personal liability. This is fundamentally because they come to define epilepsy as stigmatizing; more specifically, it has its origin in a characteristic special view of the world in which a fear of enacted stigma predominates.

2. This special view of the world predisposes individuals, above all else, to conceal their condition and its medical label from others, to attempt to pass as normal. The fear of enacted stigma promotes a policy of non-disclosure, a policy which remains feasible for as long as people are discreditable rather than discredited (Goffman 1968).

3. This policy of strict concealment reduces the opportunuties for, and hence the rate of, enacted stigma, most obviously in the context of personal relationships and work. One important consequence of this is that felt stigma, and especially the fear of enacted stigma, is more disruptive of people's lives than enacted stigma.

Scambler & Hopkins (1986) leave the question 'To what extent is people's fear of enacted stigma justified?' unanswered on the grounds that the degree of risk of enacted stigma is as yet unknown.

Scambler & Hopkins do not of course claim that the hidden distress model, focusing on concealment induced by felt stigma, exhausts the coping strategies devised and employed by people with epilepsy. Rather, they purport to identify the most significant or typical mode of coping with epilepsy (Scambler 1989). West (1985) found that parents of children with epilepsy developed three principal ways of managing stigma: concealing, avoidance and avowal of normality. The strategy of concealing is closest to that highlighted in the hidden distress model. But Scambler & Hopkins' model can also be said to

incorporate the strategy of avoidance: 'Avoidance is closely related to concealing and involves in addition the continued avoidance of situations outside the family to minimize the risks of misadventure and stigmatization'. West (1990) found that two out of the 24 families he studied opted for the very different third strategy involving an avowal of normality. This combined maximum disclosure, to reduce the risk of misadventure, and maximum participation in activities outside the family circle, to accomplish normal identity. West stresses that parents who reported episodes of enacted stigma tended to be those whose advocated strategies of concealing and avoidance had failed.

In the USA Schneider & Conrad (1981) have produced a typology of modes of adaptation to epilepsy rooted in a distinction between adjusted and unadjusted adaptations. Individuals defined as adjusted are those able to neutralize successfully the actual or perceived negative impact of epilepsy on their lives. Three sub-types of adjusted adaptation are presented.

The first is the 'pragmatic' type. The pragmatist minimizes his or her epilepsy, personally and with regard to others, but does not seek invariably to cover it up. Rather a policy of selective disclosure to those who need to know is practised, embracing, for example, employers, official agencies, close friends and associates. By combining selective disclosure with a scepticism about the possibility of others' negative judgements were they to know, the pragmatist sustains a relatively normal life.

The second category is the 'secret' type. Here epilepsy is managed by sometimes elaborate procedures to control and conceal information about what is perceived as a stigmatizing, negative and bad quality of self. To the extent to which it is successful, this strategy permits cautious participation in most if not all walks of life, including driving, given a willingness to deceive the licensing authorities.

Thirdly, Schneider & Conrad refer to the 'quasi-liberated' type. Like the pragmatists, the quasi-liberated openly acknowledge their epilepsy, but, unlike the pragmatists, they go on to broadcast this information about themselves, to educate others and to release themselves from the tensions of concealment based on felt stigma. As Jobling (1977) observes in relation to psoriasis, such a policy of de-stigmatization shows deviance to be no more than difference and discredit is denied.

If adjusted adaptations to epilepsy are characterized by a sense of control, the unadjusted adaptation is marked by a sense of being overwhelmed by it. Schneider & Conrad (1981) write: 'People who speak of the condition as having a great negative impact on their lives and who seem to have developed no strategies for managing this impact we call unadjusted'. They identify one extreme sub-type, which they call the debilitated type. They suggest that this type approximates to a master status that floods one's identity and life with meanings and behaviour that 'figuratively constipate the social self'. Schneider & Conrad add the important rider that some people in their study seemed to have adopted different modes of adaptation at different stages of their lives.

Responding to Schneider & Conrad's account, Scambler (1984, 1989) has made three points. Firstly, in his study with Hopkins, non-disclosure or concealment appeared to be the first-choice strategy for the great majority of people with epilepsy across their various social roles. It was not of course the only strategy deployed, but other strategies, like Schneider & Conrad's pragmatism, tended to be viewed as back-up or second-choice strategies: individuals who voluntarily disclosed their epilepsy, for example, generally did so only when their first-choice strategy of concealment seemed likely to let them down or prove counter-productive (Scambler & Hopkins 1980). While there were some intermittent and typically reluctant pragmatists in Scambler & Hopkins' study, only 2% seemed to belong to West's category of avowers of normality or Schneider & Conrad's quasi-liberated.

Secondly, in Scambler & Hopkins' study people's epilepsy did not impinge on their minds or outlooks all the time, but only when some change of circumstances—like a significant life event—triggered off an engagement with or retreat into their special view of the world based on felt stigma. Probably the change in circumstances most likely to give epilepsy enhanced salience for an individual was a witnessed seizure which had the potential to expose him or her as an 'epileptic'. In this sense seizure frequency was important. However, it should be noted that many seizures were not witnessed by others, or were only witnessed by those already in-the-know. Most people for most of the time felt and acted just like everybody else.

Thirdly, people's epilepsy commonly had more salience for them in some roles than in others. Sometimes the socially 'deviant' status of 'epileptic' contaminated a particular role and its corresponding relationships, affecting people, for example, as husbands, fathers, employees and so on. Such contamination rarely seemed to affect the whole range of roles, but rather, at any given time, to be more apparent—and people's epilepsy therefore more salient for them—in some than in others. Thus, for example, a person might be content and well supported within her family but, because of a sudden increase in seizure frequency, suffering from severe felt stigma in connection with her discreditable position at work. Occasionally, however, a small minority of people admitted to moods of general pessimism, even hopelessness, when their epilepsy became a felt or enacted obsession and they judged themselves 'cursed'. At such times they might fairly be described as temporary candidates for Schneider & Conrad's debilitated sub-type of unadjusted adaptation.

This discussion of personal identity has concentrated on the impact of epilepsy on concept of self, or what Goffman (1968) terms 'ego identity' (see also Williams 1987). Clearly, this impact can be marked and threatening, and is typically reflected in a special view of the world—sometimes dormant sometimes active—characterized by a sense of shame and a fear of encountering rejection. The relevance of the concept of felt stigma is evident in virtually all studies of coping with epilepsy in the West. It informs many of the action strategies that people develop, and hence underlies much epilepsy-related behaviour in the family and at work.

Family and networks

For many children who develop epilepsy parents play a crucial role in relation to accommodation, rationalization and formation of concept of self; and concept of self, in turn, profoundly affects sociability and fulfilment. In the USA, Carter (1974) found that young children with epilepsy held beliefs and attitudes concerning epilepsy which were little more than derivatives of parental opinions. Moreover, early parental socialization in the family has been directly linked to negative views of self-worth, and anxiety about an unaccepting, even hostile, world outside of the family. Schneider & Conrad (1980) classify some parents of children with epilepsy as stigma coaches: 'Our data indicate that the more the parents convey a definition of epilepsy as something bad, and the less willing they are to talk about it with their children the more likely the child is to see it as something to be concealed'.

It is not unusual, then, for parents to construct a definition of epilepsy as something bad out of lay culture and, motivated by a genuine desire to protect their offspring, unwittingly to coach them to perceive and treat it in the same way. This may be accomplished by instruction or example. Some parents, for example, explicitly tell their children neither to talk about their condition nor to use the diagnostic label outside the safety of the family circle; while others say nothing but—equally eloquently—communicate the same message through their own studious avoidance of the subject or pointed avoidance of the word epilepsy.

If parents who become stigma coaches normally do so to protect their children from enacted stigma, a few have other reasons. Some worry that the stigma of epilepsy might spread to embrace themselves or other members of the family. West (1986), who studied the families of children with epilepsy, writes: 'That the disvalued status not merely attached to the child but implicated other family members was also indicated by a number of parents'. He gives the example of one parent who was unusually open about her sense of shame: 'People shy away, and they immediately think there's something wrong with the rest of the family because you've got one like that' (West 1986). West links this phenomenon of affiliational or, to use Goffman's term. 'courtesy stigma', with a view that all the parents in his study apparently held at some time or other, namely, that epilepsy runs in families. Epilepsy, then, can bring a sense of blame as well as a sense of shame.

Such alarm at the prospect of a diffusion of the stigma of epilepsy throughout the family is probably unusual. Stigma coaching normally re-

flects a straightforward wish, sensible or otherwise, to safeguard and protect. It is not the only form of protection typically offered by parents. Indeed, there is evidence that family, and especially parental, over-protection is a major source of anger and resentment in people with epilepsy (Hoare 1987). Arntson et al (1986) sent questionnaires to over 300 adults with epilepsy in the USA, and included the question: 'What advice would you give to the family and friends of a person with epilepsy?' A third counselled treating the individual with epilepsy normally (without pity) and one in 10 warned against over-protection. Parental over-protection has been documented since the 1950s, as has its potentially deleterious consequences. Behavioural and personality problems in young adults with epilepsy, for example, have been linked to over-protection.

Schneider & Conrad (1983) use the term 'disabling parental talk' to refer to statements which sounded the theme of restrictions and detailed the things a person with epilepsy could not hope or expect to do. They report a high prevalence of such statements in their research, as do Scambler & Hopkins (1988) in Britain. Reviewing the literature, Fenton (1983) concludes that 'parental over-protectiveness in the long term may encourage the development of life-long passive, dependent attitudes and impair the capacity to establish normal peer relationships'. Lerman (1977) characterizes the effects of parental over-protectiveness and over-indulgence as follows. Parents, he claims, generally react to the diagnosis of epilepsy with a mixture of apprehension, shame, anxiety, frustration and helplessness. This leads to an oppressive atmosphere of secrecy and despair which adversely affects the child. The child cannot discuss things openly and soon comes to see epilepsy as something undesirable. Enacted stigma may be encountered, at school or at play. The child becomes increasingly confined to the home and socially isolated. The intricate skills required in social relationships are never learned and he or she remains insecure, over-dependent, emotionally immature, and is inept when adulthood is reached. If such grim long-term consequences are almost certainly rarer that Lerman implies, they clearly do occur (Scambler & Hopkins 1988).

West (1986) discovered that parents who tended to over-protect also tended to favour a policy of concealment. Of the 24 families he studied, he defines six as successful concealers, six as failed concealers and the remainder as adopting a policy of selective disclosure. Scambler & Hopkins (1988) found that several parents banned use of the word epilepsy within the household, as well as outside it. Only half of those with epilepsy in their community sample who had siblings living with them when interviewed reported that the siblings were aware of the diagnosis. Only older siblings who had witnessed seizures tended to be told.

The pattern was similar for the children of parents with epilepsy, although far fewer children than siblings knew of the diagnosis: only 21% of children were said to know, compared with 50% of siblings. More remarkably perhaps, only 50% of those children who were aged 16 or more and who had actually seen a seizure were said to know of the diagnosis, compared with 86% of those siblings who were aged 16 or over and had witnessed a seizure. It seems, then, that parents were even more reluctant to disclose a diagnosis of epilepsy within the family when that diagnosis had been applied to one of them than they were when it had been applied to one of their children. Interestingly, Lechtenberg & Akner (1984) found that children who were not informed about a parent's epilepsy tended to feel unhappy and let down when they eventually found out. Efforts to conceal the problem, they concluded, breed distrust.

Given this level of secrecy and concealment within the family, it is not surprising that few are open about their epilepsy outside their families or immediate contacts. Scambler (1989) reports that nine out of 10 adults with epilepsy said they rarely disclosed the diagnosis to anybody who was not a close friend. Predictably, this general strategy of non-disclosure was motivated by felt stigma. It was a strategy frequently deployed with boy- or girl-friends, especially in casual relationships: of those who had had more than one boy- or girl-friend since learning of the diagnosis, 13% had always disclosed their epilepsy, 26% had done so at least once, and 61% had never done so (Scambler & Hopkins 1988).

Nor were Scambler & Hopkins' respondents always open with permanent or long-lasting friends. Revealingly, only 33% of the marriages that occurred after onset were preceded by a full disclosure incorporating the word epilepsy; and only a further 36% by a partial disclosure involving words like seizures, attacks, dizzy spells, and so on. No disclosure at all was made in 31% of the three dozen marriages. Disclosure was almost certainly influenced by the witnessing of seizures. There was no evidence that non-disclosure jeopardized marriages later (Scambler & Hopkins 1988).

To summarize at this juncture, the family is probably the most important filter and point of access to lay culture, especially when the onset of epilepsy is early. Not only is it usually intimately involved in accommodation and rationalization, but it often constitutes the milieu in which children and young adults with epilepsy are coached to develop a special view of the world characterized by felt stigma. While felt stigma and a first-choice strategy of non-disclosure may sometimes protect individuals with epilepsy from incidents of enacted stigma, a heavy price may be paid in terms of a diminished concept of self, reduced sociability and lack of fulfilment. This thesis is at the core of Scambler & Hopkins' hidden distress model (Scambler 1989). Other forms of over-protection, particularly parental, can of course exacerbate such problems.

Employment opportunities

This is not the place to review the literature on epilepsy and employment, but work is of course an important area for any consideration of coping. 'Work', writes Safilios-Rothschild (1970), 'is thought to play a crucial role in the formation of the core identity, in self-esteem, in overall organization of life, as well as in mental and physical health'. The work capacity of people whose epilepsy is uncomplicated by other problems has been shown to be good (Gloag 1985). When asked whether epilepsy is likely adversely to affect a person's career, however, 97% of participants in one community study replied in the affirmative (Scambler 1989). Thirty per cent of these spoke with certainty:

I mean, nobody's going to keep a person working for them if they're going to collapse every now and again.

I can't see them giving you the post if you're an epileptic, rather than John Smith who is perfectly normal.

The remaining 70% were more circumspect, making comments like the following:

It depends to a certain extent on what type of work you're doing. I mean, if you're coming in contact with the public a lot—well, some people get very nervous, don't they, if they see a person suddenly fall.

Well, I suppose a lot depends on the employer's attitude. People are still rather inclined to think—if you say fits, they rather treat you as a not-very-nice-to-know person.

Whether certain or circumspect, most people committed to the labour market in this study were sorely tempted to conceal their epilepsy from employers. Consistently with the authors' hidden distress model, many opted for secrecy. Fifty-three per cent of those who had had two or more full-time jobs after onset had never disclosed their epilepsy to an employer, and only 10% had always disclosed it. Of those in full-time work when interviewed, 55% had said nothing, 17% had referred—often obliquely—to their seizures but not to their epilepsy, and 28% had told their employers about their epilepsy. Only 5% had voluntarily disclosed their epilepsy before beginning the job, and each of these was having daily seizures (Scambler & Hopkins 1980). These findings are consistent with other studies in Britain (MacIntyre 1976) and the USA (Schneider & Conrad 1983).

For all their fearful anticipation, only 23% of those in Scambler & Hopkins' sample with post-onset work experience could recount a single occasion on which they suspected they had been victims of enacted stigma at their place of work, even casual or inconsequential teasing. However, felt stigma not only precipitated intermittently high levels of stress at work, but sometimes led to career inhibition in its own right. Some men and women who had not disclosed their epilepsy had clearly denied themselves opportunities for advancement because they thought promotion would increase the potential risk of exposure and consequent stresses. Furthermore, a number of married women chose not to enter the job market at all because of felt stigma: at the time of interview only 32% of them had full-time jobs, compared with 48% of the married women in the British population as whole. Not infrequently they were overprotected by their husbands.

Making full allowance for both the diversity and complexity of work arenas and the heterogeneity of the population of adults with epilepsy, it is reasonable to suggest some themes involving the dimensions of coping identified earlier. The argument had been made that people's concept of self is too often diminished by epilepsy, this diminution being epitomized by felt stigma. Felt stigma—sometimes triggered or reinforced by enacted stigma—can blunt ambition and, in more extreme cases, lead to withdrawal (Goffman 1968). Less directly, it can inhibit work opportunities by retarding the development of the social and psychological aptitudes and skills required for sociability and the purposeful pursuit of fulfilment. Because of the pervasiveness of the work ethic in modern first-world cultures, as well as material needs, lack of fulfilment in or at work may be especially damaging (Pasternack 1981).

Legal constraints

With the ascribed social status of epileptic come attendant legal obligations and responsibilities, the most threatening and intrusive of which tend to concern driving. In Britain people who experience day-time epileptic seizures must give up their licences; and they must be free of seizures for 2 years before lost licences can be regained (Hopkins & Harvey 1987). Despite an accident rate amongst licensed drivers with epilepsy 1.3 to 2.0 times higher than amongst age-matched controls, not all adults with epilepsy surrender their licences in the first place. Scambler (1989) reports one in five people driving illegally at the time of interview.

Consistently with the reasoning of those they interviewed, Scambler & Hopkins (1986) distinguish between enacted stigma and legitimate discrimination, the latter referring to instances of discrimination against people with epilepsy based on reason rather than on stigma. Legitimate discrimination, as exemplified in driving bans, can also diminish people's concept of self. Indeed, if banning an individual with epilepsy from driving does not constitute an episode of enacted stigma, there is no doubt that not being able to drive typically contributes to felt stigma. Epilepsy can in this sense be seen to involve a 'family of related stigmas' (Scambler, 1984). Not being able to drive may also affect sociability and fulfilment, particularly in employment.

THE PHYSICIAN'S ROLE IN COPING

The physician's role has a direct bearing on coping. This is not merely because it is the physician who formally attaches the diagnostic label and is therefore causally, if not morally, responsible for much of what follows. Schneider & Conrad (1983) make it clear that, without intending to, physicians can function as stigma coaches. West (1979) maintains that they sometimes do so not by explicitly addressing the stigma associated with epilepsy but by *not* addressing it. It is in fact physicians' reluctance to discuss the social and psychological ramifications of being epileptic, the biographical disruption (Bury 1982) it occasions, about which patients often complain.

West (1990) found that the somewhat negative accounts of encounters with hospital specialists proferred by the parents of children with epilepsy are often justified. He writes: 'There are delays in communicating a diagnosis. It is mainly implicit and is affected by the understandable though, in parents' terms, mistaken policy of playing the problem down. There is little information volunteered about medication or aetiology and almost none about the wider meaning of the problem and psychosocial consequences. Parents do have to work hard to obtain information from doctors who are all too often evasive'. West, then, offers a measure of empirical support for the multiplicity of patients' accounts of physicians' lack of time, training or motivation to elicit and address patients' own perspectives on their (or their children's) epilepsy (Scambler 1989).

Scambler (1989) has distinguished analytically between three common dimensions to patients' perspectives:

1. *Felt stigma.* In their own study almost all those seen perceived epilepsy as stigmatizing. The term felt stigma was coined to refer both to the shame many people experienced and to the fear of meeting with rejection (i.e. enacted stigma). Felt stigma was the principal constituent of people's perspectives on epilepsy.

2. *Rationalization.* People are known to be intolerant of uncertainty surrounding illness, especially if the symptoms are threatening, dramatic or intrusive. The process of filling in the gaps in physicians' explanatory accounts, of cognitive ordering, has here been called rationalization.

3. *Action strategy.* People need ways of coping with epilepsy as a potential personal or social burden. Schneider & Conrad (1981) have suggested that what might be called action strategies can vary between individuals and over time. In Scambler & Hopkins' study, however, the first-choice strategy was concealment: whenever possible people opted for secrecy in an attempt to pass as normal.

These dimensions are of course related. In Scambler & Hopkins' study, for example, felt stigma was typically an important factor in rationalization and the main determinant of action strategy (Scambler 1989).

Past evidence is that physicians tend to be interested in and concentrate on those aspects of patient rationalization that promise to facilitate diagnosis or management, but not in the process of rationalization per se. Neither felt stigma nor action strategy tend to be on the medical agenda for consultations, and are typically handled inexpertly or cursorily if raised by patients. In as far as coping also embraces accommodation, sociability and fulfilment, precisely the same judgement applies.

The substance of many documented complaints against physicians is that they are poor communicators: they are said to convey too little information to their patients. But they can also be poor listeners. Scambler (1989) argues that, as far as epilepsy is concerned, it is not enough for physicians to educate patients in the medical perspective, especially if compliance is the sole justification for doing so. It has generally been taken for granted that patient compliance is a valid measure of patient care. As Mischler (1984) points out, 'it requires a shift in perspective to recognize that the concept incorporates a medical bias'. It is revealing that although in several influential studies a high proportion of patients have reported that physicians did not fulfil their expectations, physicians have not as a consequence been described as non-compliant with patient expectations. Only patients, it appears, are non-compliant.

The psychosocial literature suggests that patients' own perspectives on their epilepsy need to be respected and explored in their own right, and that there is a measurable return on doing so. Schneider & Conrad (1983) have called for 'co-participation in care'. This would involve not only shared responsibility for management, with the patient as key decision-maker (Buchanan 1982, Conrad 1987), but also open agendas for consultations, thereby permitting patient-initiated discussion of felt stigma, rationalization and action strategy. In fact it is difficult to envisage how physicians can provide the kind of counselling now accepted as necessary and desirable (DHSS 1986, Oxley et al 1987) unless communication is improved.

Consider, for example, the individual with epilepsy who is trying to settle on an action strategy in the context of employment. The significance of employment—for concept of self and fulfilment in particular—has already been noted. If his or her physician is at all responsive, the advice is likely to be to disclose fully and hope for the best. And yet many physicians seem willing to acknowledge that this may be a recipe for disaster. In one study of attitudes towards epilepsy in general practice, 78% of those asked agreed that job opportunities for those with epilepsy are restricted. Moreover, 88% agreed that employers who claim not to discriminate against people with epilepsy in fact do; only 2% disagreed. And yet, 86% went on to agree that individuals with epilepsy should disclose their epilepsy to prospective employers, with nobody disagreeing (Davies & Scambler 1988). What price help with an action strategy here? Fortunately some attempts are currently being made to clarify medical thinking in this area (Edwards et al 1986). It is information and open discussion rather than instruction and advice packages that are needed; indeed, open discussion

reflective of co-participation in care can be therapeutic in itself.

Scambler (1990) argues that good quality care in epilepsy involves more than a competent up-to-date technical service covering the investigation, diagnosis and treatment of epilepsy at optimum cost. Attention has to be paid to health education oriented to the de-mythologization and de-stigmatization of epilepsy in the community. More pertinent to coping, he adds four suggestions for enhancing physician–patient encounters:

1. Acceptance of the principle of co-participation in care, which involves coming to terms with the concept of patient autonomy, with the patient as decision-maker
2. Acceptance also of an open agenda in physician–patient encounters
3. A holistic rather than biomedical orientation to care, with the emphasis on informing, advising and helping persons in context rather than merely managing disease
4. The development of counselling skills to complement technical skills, which presupposes both an awareness of the impact of epilepsy on quality of life and learned expertise in advising on coping.

CONCLUSION

The purpose behind this contribution has been to identify and illustrate some of the issues of coping in relation to epilepsy. This has been done through a consideration of core dimensions of coping, which have been elaborated and explored in key arenas or contexts of life activity. It is expected that this framework will be modified in the light of future research and reflection. In the final section an attempt has been made, firstly, to draw threads together to demonstrate that physicians—through their words and their behaviour—inevitably and unavoidably influence how people with epilepsy cope; and, secondly, to advance cautiously some ideas on how, by re-thinking the physician–patient consultation, physicians might be better able to facilitate patient coping. The obstacles in the way of effectively re-thinking the physician–patient consultation, most notably perhaps the lack of appropriate medical training and the contraints of time, are not under-estimated.

REFERENCES

Arntson P, Droge D, Norton R, Murray E 1986 The perceived psychosocial consequences of having epilepsy. In: Whitman S, Hermann B (eds) Psychopathology in epilepsy: social dimensions. Oxford University Press, Oxford

Blaxter M 1976 The meaning of disability: a sociological study of impairment. Heinemann, London

Buchanan N 1982 Treatment of epilepsy: whose right is it anyway? British Medical Journal 284: 173–174

Bury M 1982 Chronic illness as biographical disruption. Sociology of Health & Illness 4: 167–182

Canger R, Cornaggia J 1985 Public attitudes toward epilepsy in Italy: results of a survey and comparison with USA and West German data. Epilepsia 26: 221–226

Carter J 1974 Children's expressed attitudes toward their epilepsy. Nervous Child 6: 34–37

Caveness W, Gallup G 1980 A survey of public attitudes towards epilepsy in 1979 with an indication of trends over the past thirty years. Epilepsia 21: 509–518

Central Health Services Council 1969 Advisory Committee on the Health and Welfare of Handicapped Persons, People with Epilepsy. HMSO, London

Chadwick D (ed) 1990 Quality of life and quality of care in epilepsy. Royal Society of Medicine, London

Charmaz K 1983 Loss of self: a fundamental form of suffering in the chronically ill. Sociology of Health and Illness 5: 169–195

Collings J 1990 Epilepsy and well-being. Social Science and Medicine 31: 165–170

Conrad P 1987 The meaning of medication: another look at compliance. In: Schwartz H (ed) Dominant issues in medical sociology. Random House, New York

Davies D, Scambler G 1988 Attitudes towards epilepsy in general practice. International Journal of Social Psychiatry 34: 5–12

Department of Health and Social Security 1986 Report of the Working Group on Services for People with Epilepsy. HMSO, London

Edwards F, Espir M, Oxley J 1986 Epilepsy and employment —a medical symposium on current problems and best practices. Royal Society of Medicine Services Ltd, London

Fenton G 1983 Epilepsy. In: Lader M (ed) Handbook of psychiatry 2: mental disorder and somatic illness. Cambridge University Press, Cambridge

Gloag D 1985 Epilepsy and employment. British Medical Journal 291: 2–3

Goffman E 1968 Stigma: notes on the management of spoiled identity. Penguin, Harmondsworth

Hermann B, Whitman S 1986 Psychopathology in epilepsy: a multietiologic model. In: Whitman S, Hermann B (eds) Psychopathology in epilepsy: social dimensions. Oxford University Press, Oxford

Hoare P 1987 Children with epilepsy and their families. Journal of Child Psychology and Psychiatry 28: 651–655

Hopkins A, Harvey P 1987 Epilepsy and driving. In: Hopkins A (ed) Epilepsy. Chapman and Hall, London

Jobling R 1977 Learning to live with it: an account of a career of chronic dermatological illness and patienthood. In: Davies A, Horobin G (eds) Medical encounters: the experience of illness and treatment. Croom Helm, London

Lechtenberg R, Akner L 1984 Psychologic adaptation to epilepsy in a parent. Epilepsia 25: 40–45

Lerman P 1977 The concept of preventive rehabilitation in childhood epilepsy: a plea against overprotection and overindulgence. In: Penry J (ed) Epilepsy: the eighth international symposium. Raven Press, New York

Locker D 1983 Disability and disadvantage: the consequences of chronic illness. Tavistock, London

MacIntyre I 1976 Epilepsy and employment. Community Health 7: 195–204

Mishler E 1984 The discourse of medicine: dialectics of medical interviews. Ablex, Norwood, NJ

Mittan R 1986 Fear of seizures. In: Whitman S, Hermann B (eds) Psychopathology in epilepsy: social dimensions. Oxford University Press, Oxford

Mittan R, Locke G 1982 Fear of seizure: epilepsy's forgotten problem. Urban Health Jan/Feb: 40–41

Oxley J, Espir M, Shorvon S, Goodridge D, Richens A 1987 The framework of medical care for epilepsy. Health Trends 19: 13–17

Pasternack J 1981 An analysis of social perceptions of epilepsy: increasing rationalization as seen through the theories of Comte and Weber. Social Science and Medicine 15E: 223–229

Rotenberg M 1974 Self-labelling: a missing link in the 'societal reaction' theory of deviance. Sociological Review 22: 335–354

Safilios-Rothschild C 1970 The sociology and social psychology of disability and rehabilitation. Random House, New York

Scambler G 1984 Perceiving and coping with stigmatizing illness. In: Fitzpatrick R, Hinton J, Newman S, Scambler G, Thompson J (eds) The experience of illness. Tavistock, London.

Scambler G 1987 Sociological aspects of epilepsy. In: Hopkins A (ed) Epilepsy. Chapman and Hall, London

Scambler G 1989 Epilepsy. Tavistock, London

Scambler G 1990 Social factors and quality of life and quality of care in epilepsy. In: Chadwick D (ed) Quality of life and quality of care in epilepsy. Royal Society of Medicine, London

Scambler G, Hopkins A 1980 Social class, epileptic activity and disadvantage at work. Journal of Epidemiology and Community Health 34: 129–133

Scambler G, Hopkins A 1986 Being epileptic: coming to terms with stigma. Sociology of Health and Illness 8: 26–43

Scambler G, Hopkins A 1988 Accommodating epilepsy in families. In: Anderson R, Bury M (eds) Living with chronic illness: the experience of patients and their families. Allen and Unwin, London

Schneider J, Conrad P 1980 In the closet with illness: epilepsy, stigma potential and information control. Social Problems 28: 32–44

Schneider J, Conrad P 1981 Medical and sociological typologies: the case of epilepsy. Social Science and Medicine 15A: 211–219

Schneider J, Conrad P 1983 Having epilepsy: the experience and control of illness. Temple University Press, Philadelphia

Shibutani T 1962 Reference groups and social control. In: Rose A (ed) Human behaviour and social processes: an interactionist approach. Routledge and Kegan Paul, London

Stebbins R 1970 Career: the subjective approach. Sociological Quarterly 11: 32–49

Tavriger R 1966 Some parental theories about the causes of epilepsy. Epilepsia 7: 339–343

West P 1979 An investigation into the social construction and consequences of the label 'epilepsy'. PhD Thesis, University of Bristol

West P 1985 Becoming disabled: perspectives on the labelling approach. In: Gerhardt U, Wadsworth M (eds) Stress and stigma: explanation in the sociology of crime and illness. Macmillan, London

West P 1986 The social meaning of epilepsy: stigma as a potential explanation for the psychopathology in children. In: Whitman S, Hermann B (eds) Psychopathology in epilepsy: social dimensions. Oxford University Press, Oxford

West P 1990 The status and validity of accounts obtained at interview: a contrast between two studies of families with a disabled child. Social Science and Medicine 30: 1229–1240

Williams G 1984 The genesis of chronic illness: narrative reconstruction. Sociology of Health and Illness 6: 175

Williams S 1987 Goffman, interactionism and the management of stigma in everyday life. In: Scambler G (ed) Sociological theory and medical sociology. Tavistock, London

Epilogue

John Laidlaw   Mary V Laidlaw

In the comparatively short time since the first edition in 1976 there have been notable advances in both the knowledge and the understanding of epilepsy: advances reflected in this further expanded fourth edition in which specialists write on matters covering the whole range from the medico-scientific to the socio-medical. Undoubtedly those who learn from it will be better able to help their patients. In earlier editions we wrote of various problems such as prejudice and overprotection which the person with epilepsy had to face. Attitudes have changed to the extent that, although such problems still exist, they do not merit further emphasis in a book of this sort.

However, in this book written by professionals for professionals the patient is the *object*. In this Epilogue we seek briefly to make the patient — the person with epilepsy — the *subject*: to consider how he feels. Since this is our last contribution to the textbook which we both helped to initiate, we would like to pay tribute to the late Denis Williams, who was one of those who advised from the beginning, by quoting from the last of the three Prefaces which he wrote "... but throughout we attend to the needs of the whole person, the person with epilepsy".

How then does the person with epilepsy react to his seizures, how do they affect him? To assess the effect of a tonic-clonic convulsion on the patient, or on the friend with him, does not require much imagination and needs little elaboration: a cataclysmic event of which the patient is unaware, although he may live in fear of its occurrence and suffer from its consequences. Such a seizure in a public place cannot but be an embarrassment to the friend, but it is a happening which is clearly a major crisis, which is understandable as such: an event which calls for action from sympathetic if horrified onlookers. The patient who has continuing major fits needs great courage. Although the event is understandable and clearly a physical explosion, the occurrence at any particular time is not only unpredictable, but inexplicable.

With informed treatment many tonic-clonic convulsions can be well controlled and few patients should have to face recurrent major fits. However, complex partial seizures are common and are often more difficult to control. After the initial impact of the grotesque and obviously abnormal, it may be easier to accept and live with the generalized convulsion than the subtle, often barely perceptible deviation from the usual, which may imbue the lesser attack with an eerie unreality. To awake one morning to find one's garden trampled down by the neighbour's cows would cause horror, shock and anger. To look out to see that yesterday's yellow daffodils were blue would evoke an awesome fear, not of the daffodils, but of one's sanity. So it might be to watch someone we know well having a complex partial seizure. The patient wholly unaware of the happening of a major fit, in a state of partial consciousness may be terrified by his distorted experience of a complex partial seizure.

We conclude with three fables, which being memorable, may help to illustrate and emphasize just some of the problems with which the patient with such seizures has to contend.

The attack misunderstood

Mrs W. lived with her sister Mrs Y. in a respectable suburb of a large city. They had much in common, including their widowhood. Mrs W. suffered from epilepsy, but only occasionally did this disturb the settled regularity of their lives.

However, at first their happily adjusted relationship nearly foundered on the rocks of Mrs W's epilepsy. Mrs Y. could not understand why her usually easy-natured sister unpredictably should be so frankly unkind, even rude. Perhaps their decision to live together had been a disaster. However, money was tight and Mrs. Y. could not move out until she had time to make new plans. The delay was fortunate, since she came to realize that her sister's uncharacteristic and hurtful behaviour was related to her fits.

Mrs. Y. began to watch her sister more closely. When other people were present she seemed to fade out of the conversation. She became inaccessible, her face paled then her lips seemed to be blue and she started making chewing movements. Soon her normal colour returned but she would start to fumble clumsily with her clothes or anything else to hand. If she had been knitting, she would get into a terrible mess. These episodes would last only two or three minutes, but for at least 20 minutes she would be different: she would be irritable and abrasive. Back to her usual self, she would have no memory of what had happened.

Comment

Mrs W. had been having complex partial seizures with alteration of consciousness. She was in no way responsible for her behaviour. It must have been difficult for Mrs. Y. to understand what had been happening, but once she did appreciate the bizarre nature of her fits, the two widows lived happily ever after. The odd 20 minutes, now and again, could be ignored as just one of those things.

Psychic clothes

It may be said that we all wear psychic clothes. These clothes make it possible for us to present ourselves, not as we are, but as we would like to be: kind, intelligent, a good fellow, beautiful, fearless or sophisticated. Most of us are continuously in touch with our environment, affected by it, trying to relate to it, to manipulate or rather to control it. Our psychic clothes are an essential part of our relationships with our environment: putting them on should not be criticized and dismissed as an empty charade. What we imagine ourselves, or would like to be, is almost invariably better than what we are. It is no better or no worse to adjust the psychic dress than it is to glance in the mirror before going off to work or to shave on the morning of one's execution. As time goes on, we

come to fit these clothes better and we are the better for them.

Almost inevitably, a seizure involves a loss or significant alteration of consciousness, a break in the continuity of contact with and, therefore, control of environment: the inescapable removal of psychic clothes. The prospect of the slow involuntary undressing which may occur during a complex partial seizure is one with which it is difficult to live.

The von Z.s lived in North London perhaps just a little too far North, but not so far North that the 'von' would not be appreciated. Now both in late middle age, some ten years before they had moved imperceptibly into their modest cottage with its delightful garden. They were known to everyone and they had many good acquaintances: that is everyone knew Mrs von Z. at the Bridge Club and the Horticultural Society. Mr von Z. remained aloof. Invariably polite and courteous, he would go on regular shopping expeditions and, of course, to the library where he ordered books not usually in demand. Everyone realized that they did not have much money, but their cottage was full of treasures from the past. To the locals, they were still People of Importance. No one knew that Mr von Z. suffered from complex partial seizures; few would have known what they were. Anyway, now he was getting older, he was having few attacks. Soon he should be able to get back his driving licence and he would forget about the whole thing.

Mrs von Z. had finished the washing up. It was a lovely day and she went out into the garden. Mr von Z had gone off to the library. She stopped the motor mower to empty the grass box, and then she heard the telephone. Miss B., the librarian, was distraught and it was difficult to make out what she was saying: 'Mr von Z. has gone mad. He tried to rape me.'

By the time she reached the library the worst of the panic was over. Her husband was sitting hunched up, alone, pale and very shaken. Miss B. was also sitting alone looking pale and very shaken. At the far end of the room the local doctor was trying to explain things to the local policeman against opposition from a group of local experts. It did not take Mrs von Z. long to find out what had happened. When he handed in his books, Mr von Z. had been his usual charming self. He had smiled at the young librarian and patted her arm. She was a favourite of his. Some minutes later she was startled to feel an arm round her waist. Mr von Z. was at her side of the counter trying to kiss her. He looked flushed, his eyes were glazed and his trousers were undone. In the event she had had little difficulty in avoiding the advances. Mr von Z. had appeared to lose interest and had wandered off aimlessly to sit in a corner. Miss B. was now shamefaced that she had panicked and rushed to the telephone. The doctor had told her about the attack which Mr von Z. had had and how he would not have known what he was doing for a few minutes afterward. It was not long before a general attitude of shame-facedness spread though the neighbourhood. Everyone tried hard to be kind and was more than understanding which was the last thing that Mr Von Z. wanted. He wanted his psychic clothes back again.

Comment
Mr and Mrs von Z. moved and settled in a small village near Cambridge, as Mr and Mrs Z.

The lost half hour

Although he may be able to react purposefully, or semipurposefully, during a complex partial seizure, afterwards he is unlikely to be able to remember what happened during the attack. He may be very deeply concerned about what he may have done when he had lost control of his environment. Apart from reassuring him that the distorted appreciation of sensory input, which may have been experienced during his state of altered consciousness, is not a portent of impending insanity, it is useful to encourage him to discuss his attacks with people who have witnessed them. To surround his seizures with a well-meaning conspiracy of silence often arouses deep-seated fears that his behaviour must in fact have been unspeakable. At other times the lost half hour may result in some harmless embarrassment.

Mr R. was a 35-year-old civil servant. For 10 years he had been married. His wife worked as a ward sister at the Infirmary. They lived in Edinburgh in a third-floor flat of a high-class, if 90-year-old, tenement within easy walking distance of their work. Mrs R. was in charge of the flat and of Mr R. as well as her ward. Mr. R. did not resent this. He suffered from complex partial seizures which might last up to 10 minutes and be followed by several minutes of confusion. However, he knew when they were coming on and he was able to retire to a quiet place where his inappropriate behaviour did not embarrass his colleagues. Nevertheless, he never knew quite when they would hit him and appreciated the support to his insecurity that he got at work and from his wife.

Two years ago they decided that they had saved up enough to be able to afford to start a family, although they would have to do without Mrs R.'s salary. Timothy was three months old and a bonny baby. His feeding demands had been creating tensions which all too often became frank rows. Mr R. took to spending the early evenings with his friends in the pub and, as Mrs R. insisted all too frequently, this did not do his fits any good. Mr R. was more at home with his wife's undivided attention than with her criticism. Mrs R. was lonely, isolated, and getting more and more fed up with washing sheets and baby clothes. The one thing in the world which she wanted was a washing machine. The R.s were very fond of each other and one evening, after a particularly long and fruitless argument, they stopped quite suddenly and laughed. It was all too silly, they must start again. Mr R. promised faithfully to come straight home. They would save for the washing machine.

Mr R. kept to his resolution, Timothy became less demanding and they had enough saved for the washing machine. All went well, that is to say until a Friday afternoon when Timothy was nearly five months old. The telephone rang. It was the office: 'Is Mr R. all right? We have not seen him since lunch time'. Mrs R. became more and more worried. By the time her husband returned at 7 p.m. she was so frantic that she said all sorts of things which she should not have said. When it was clear that, although not drunk, he had been drinking, she said a lot more. Mr R. denied vehemently that he had been drinking. It is not on record what happened after that, but on Saturday morning they took a walk with Timothy and bought a washing machine.

On Monday morning two men struggled up three flights of stairs, rang the bell and, totally exhausted, delivered a washing machine. Mrs R. resuscitated them with tea and her delight. She then washed. In early afternoon she was feeding Timothy, happily, when the door bell rang. Two more men, who were totally exhausted, delivered a washing machine.

Comment
During the Friday lunch break Mr R had had quite a severe complex partial seizure and during his confused period he had left the office and gone for a walk to clear his head. On recovering full consciousness, he had acted quite normally: he fulfilled their decision to buy a washing machine; perhaps, he celebrated with a pint of beer. He had, of course, no memory of what had happened and was quite honest when he said that he had not been drinking. The memory of the pint had not registered any more than that of buying the washing machine.

It is not recorded how the second washing machine got down three flights of stairs.

Index